Cox's Clinical Applications of Nursing Diagnosis

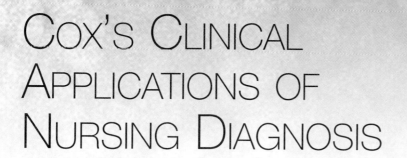

Cox's Clinical Applications of Nursing Diagnosis

Adult, Child, Women's, Mental Health, Gerontic, and Home Health Considerations

Susan A. Newfield, *PhD, RN, APRN, BC*
Associate Professor
West Virginia University
Morgantown, West Virginia

Mittie D. Hinz, *MSN, MBA, RNC*
Partner
DXT Consulting
San Antonio, Texas

Program Administrator
Hamot For Women
Hamot Medical Center
Erie, Pennsylvania

Donna Scott Tilley, *RN, PhD, CNE*
Associate Professor
Texas Christian University
Fort Worth, Texas

Kathryn L. Sridaromont, *RN, C, MSN*
Assistant Professor
Texas Tech University Health Sciences Center
Lubbock, Texas

Patricia Joy Maramba, *MSN, RN, APRN, BC*
Senior Lecturer
West Virginia University
Morgantown, West Virginia

Fifth Edition

F. A. DAVIS COMPANY • Philadelphia

F. A. Davis Company
1915 Arch Street
Philadelphia, PA 19103
www.fadavis.com

Printed in the United States of America

Last digit indicates print number: 10 9 8 7 6 5 4 3 2

Acquisitions Editor: Joanne Patzek DaCuhna, PR, MSN
Content Development Manager: Darlene D. Pedersen, RN, MSN
Senior Project Editor: Danielle J. Barsky
Art and Design Manager: Carolyn O'Brien

As new scientific information becomes available through basic and clinical research, recommended treatments and drug therapies undergo changes. The author(s) and publisher have done everything possible to make this book accurate, up to date, and in accord with accepted standards at the time of publication. The author(s), editors, and publisher are not responsible for errors or omissions or for consequences from application of the book, and make no warranty, expressed or implied, in regard to the contents of the book. Any practice described in this book should be applied by the reader in accordance with professional standards of care used in regard to the unique circumstances that may apply in each situation. The reader is advised always to check product information (package inserts) for changes and new information regarding dose and contraindications before administering any drug. Caution is especially urged when using new or infrequently ordered drugs.

Library of Congress Cataloging-in-Publication Data

Cox's clinical applications of nursing diagnosis : adult, child, women's, mental health, gerontic and home health considerations / Susan A. Newfield ... [et al.]. — 5th ed.
    p. ; cm.
  Rev. ed. of: Clinical applications of nursing diagnosis. 4th ed. c2002.
  Includes bibliographical references and index.
  ISBN-13: 978-0-8036-1655-4
  ISBN-10: 0-8036-1655-4
  1. Nursing diagnosis. 2. Nursing assessment. 3. Nursing. I. Cox, Helen C. II. Newfield, Susan A.
III. Clinical applications of nursing diagnosis. IV. Title: Clinical applications of nursing diagnosis.
  [DNLM: 1. Nursing Diagnosis. 2. Nursing Process. WY 100.4 C879 2007]
  RT48.6.C6 2007
  610.73—dc22
                                   2007009325

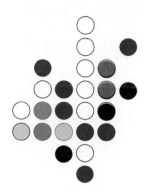

*To **Dr. Helen Cox**, colleague, mentor, and friend, on her retirement. You took ambitious, naive, young faculty members and turned us into authors and for that, we will be eternally grateful.*

*To the memory of **Dr. Mary Ann Lubno**, colleague and friend.*

PREFACE TO THE FIFTH EDITION

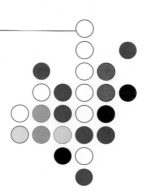

Although the fifth edition of this book has seen many author changes, our commitment and direction was clearly stated by, Dr. Helen Cox, in the preface to the fourth edition. We continue our commitment to providing a nursing focus to the process of nursing care.

The fifth edition reflects seventeen new and six revised diagnoses accepted by NANDA in 2003 and 2005 and updated information in each chapter. The chapter formats remain the same. We have revised the integration of NANDA, NIC, and NOC terminology to assist with understanding their integration. NANDA, NIC, and NOC concepts are placed in charts which identify the linkages that can be found at the beginning of each chapter. Evaluation guidance has also been revised. We provided a master evaluation flow chart in Chapter 1 rather than providing one at the end of each care plan.

Two significant trends have impacted the practice of nursing since the fourth edition; decreasing length of stay and increased emphasis on evidence based practice. The length of stay continues to decrease and this is reflected in our revision of goals, interventions, and discharge planning. As we developed care plans, current average length of stay for the setting was the litmus test for our selection of interventions. The interventions for each diagnosis reflect both current research in the area and recommended NIC interventions.

If you are new to nursing diagnosis, we encourage you to begin your journey with reading Chapter 1. Taking a few minutes to do this will provide you with an understanding of the authors' thought processes that will facilitate your use of the book.

We continue to appreciate the comments from nursing faculty, staff and students who use the book. Your thoughtful comments have inspired each edition and we urge you to continue to support us in this way. It is our sincerest wish that this book will continue to provide a map for your journey in providing excellent client care.

Susan A. Newfield, PhD, RN, APRN, BC

Preface to the Fourth Edition

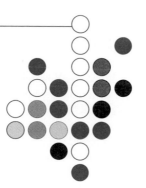

The North American Nursing Diagnosis Association (NANDA) has been identifying, classifying, and testing diagnostic nomenclature since the early 1970s. In our opinion, use of nursing diagnosis helps define the essence of nursing and give direction to care that is uniquely nursing care.

If nurses (in all instances we are referring to registered nurses) enter the medical diagnosis of, for example, acute appendicitis as the patient's problem, they have met defeat before they have begun. A nurse cannot intervene for this medical diagnosis; intervention requires a medical practitioner who can perform an appendectomy. However, if the nurse enters the nursing diagnosis "Pain," then a number of nursing interventions come to mind. Several books incorporate nursing diagnosis as a part of planning care. However, these books generally focus outcome and nursing interventions on the related factors; that is, nursing interventions deal with resolving, to the extent possible, the causative and contributing factors that result in the nursing diagnosis. We have chosen to focus nursing intervention on the nursing diagnosis. To focus on the nursing diagnosis promotes the use of concepts in nursing rather than concentrating on a multitude of specifics. For example, there are common nursing measures that can be used to relieve pain regardless of the etiologic pain factor involved. Likewise, the outcomes focus on the nursing diagnosis. The main outcome nurses want to achieve when working with the nursing diagnosis Pain is control of the patient's response to pain to the extent possible. Again, the outcome allows the use of a conceptual approach rather than a multitude-of-specifics approach. To clarify further, consider again the medical diagnosis of appendicitis. The physician's first concern is not related to whether the appendicitis is caused by a fecalith, intestinal helminths, or *Escherichia coli* run amok. The physician focuses first on intervening for the appendicitis, which usually results in an appendectomy. The physician will deal with etiologic factors following the appendectomy, but the appendectomy is the first level of intervention. Likewise, the nurse can deal with the related factors through nursing actions, but the first level of intervention is directed to resolving the patient's problem as reflected by the nursing diagnosis. With the decreasing length of stay for the majority of patients entering a hospital, we may indeed do well to complete the first level of nursing actions.

Additionally, there is continuing debate among NANDA members as to whether the current list of diagnoses that are accepted for testing are nursing diagnoses or a list of diagnostic categories or concepts. We, therefore, have chosen to focus on concepts. Using a conceptual approach allows focus on independent nursing functions and helps avoid focusing on medical intervention. This book has been designed to serve as a guide to using NANDA-accepted nursing diagnoses as the primary base for the planning of care. The expected outcomes, target dates, nursing actions, and evaluation algorithms (flowcharts) are not meant to serve as standardized plans of care but rather as guides and references in promoting the visibility of nursing's contribution to health care.

Marjory Gordon's Functional Health Patterns are used as an organizing framework for the book. The Functional Health Patterns allow categorizing of the nursing diagnoses into specific groups, which, in our opinion, promotes a conceptual approach to assessment and formulation of a nursing diagnosis.

Chapter 1 serves as the overview-introductory chapter and gives basic content related to the process of planning care and information regarding the relationship between nursing process and nursing models (theories). Titles for Chapters 2 through 12 are taken from the functional patterns. Included in each of these chapters is a list of diagnoses within the pattern, a pattern description, pattern assessment, conceptual information, and developmental information related to the pattern.

The pattern description gives a succinct summary of the pattern's content and assists in explaining how the diagnoses within the pattern are related. The list of diagnoses within the pattern is given to simplify location of the diagnoses. The pattern assessment serves to pinpoint information from the initial assessment base and was specifically written to direct the reader to the most likely diagnosis within the pattern. Each assessment factor is designed to allow an answer of "yes" or "no." If the patient's answer or signs are indicative of a diagnosis within the pattern, the reader is directed to the most likely diagnosis or diagnoses. The conceptual and developmental information is included to provide a quick, ready reference to the physiologic, psychological, sociologic, and age-related factors that could cause modification of the nursing actions in order to make them more specific for your patient. The conceptual and developmental information can be used to determine the rationale for each nursing action.

Each nursing diagnosis within the pattern is then introduced with accompanying information of definition, defining characteristics, and related factors. We have added a section titled "Related Clinical Concerns." This section serves to highlight the most common medical diagnoses or cluster of diagnoses that could involve the individual nursing diagnosis.

Immediately after the related clinical concerns section is a section titled "Have you selected the correct diagnosis?" This section was included as a validation check because we realize that several of the diagnoses appear very closely related and that it can be difficult to distinguish between them. This is, in part, related to the fact that the diagnoses have been accepted for testing, not as statements of absolute, discrete diagnoses. Thus, having this section assists the reader in learning how to pinpoint the differences between diagnoses and in feeling more comfortable in selecting a diagnosis that most clearly reflects a patient's problem area that can be helped by nursing actions.

After the diagnosis validation section is an outcome. The expected outcome serves as the end point against which progress can be measured. Different agencies may call the expected outcome an objective, a patient goal, or an outcome standard. Readers may also choose to design their own patient-specific expected outcome using the given expected outcome as a guideline.

Target dates are suggested following the expected outcome. The target dates *do not* indicate the time or day the outcome must be fully achieved; instead, the target date signifies the time or day when evaluation should be completed in order to measure the patient's progress *toward* achievement of the expected outcome. Target dates are given in reference to short-term care. For home health, particularly, the target date would be in terms of weeks and months rather than days.

Nursing actions/interventions and rationales are the next information given. In most instances, the adult health nursing actions serve as the generic nursing actions. Subsequent sets of nursing actions (child health, women's health, psychiatric health, gerontic health, and home health) show only the nursing actions that are different from the generic nursing actions. The different nursing actions make each set specific for the target population, but *must be* used in conjunction with the adult health nursing actions to be complete. Rationales have been included to assist the student in learning the reason for particular nursing actions. Although some of the rationales are scientific in nature, that is, supported by documented research, other rationales could be more appropriately termed "common sense" or "usual practice rationales." These rationales are reasons nurses have cited for particular nursing actions and result from nursing experience, but research has not been conducted to document these rationales. After the home health actions, evaluation algorithms are shown that help judge the patient's progress toward achieving the expected outcome.

Evaluation of the patient's care is based on the degree of progress the patient has made toward achieving the expected outcome. For each stated outcome, there is an evaluation flowchart (algorithm). The flowcharts provide minimum information, but demonstrate the decision-making process that must be used.

In all instances, the authors have used the definitions, defining characteristics, and related factors that have been accepted by NANDA for testing. A grant was provided to NANDA by the F. A. Davis Company for the use of these materials. All these materials may be ordered from NANDA (1211 Locust Street, Philadelphia, PA 19107). Likewise, a fee was paid to Mosby for the use of the domains and classes from McCloskey, JC, and Bulechek, GM (eds): *Nursing Interventions Classification (NIC)*, edition 3 (Mosby, St. Louis, 2000) and Johnson, M, Maas, M, and Moorhead, S (eds): *Nursing Outcomes Classification*, edition 2 (Mosby, St. Louis, 2000).

In some instances, additional information is included following a set of nursing actions. The additional information includes material that either needs to be highlighted or does not logically fall within the defined outline areas.

Throughout the nursing actions we have used the terms *patient* and *client* interchangeably. The terms refer to the system of care and include the individual as well as the family and other social support systems. The nursing actions are written very specifically. This specificity aids in communication between and among nurses and promotes consistency of care for the patient.

There has been a tremendous increase in the activity of NANDA. In 1998 alone, 16 new diagnoses were accepted, 32 diagnoses were revised, and one diagnosis was deleted. The official journal of NANDA became an international journal in 1999.

The fourth edition incorporates new and revised diagnoses from both the Thirteenth (1998) and Fourteenth (2000) NANDA Conferences. The proposed NANDA Taxonomy 2 has been inserted to replace the old Taxonomy 1, Revised. The Nursing Interventions Classification (NIC) system and the Nursing Outcomes Classification (NOC) system domains and classes have been incorporated.

Other revisions have been made to be consistent with current NANDA thought and publications. One example is the deletion of major and minor defining characteristics and their assimilation under one heading of "Defining Characteristics."

We continue to appreciate the feedback we have received from various sources and urge you to continue to assist us in this way. It is our sincerest wish that this book will continue to assist nurses and nursing students in their day-to-day use of nursing diagnosis.

Helen C. Cox, RN, C, EdD, FAAN

ACKNOWLEDGMENTS

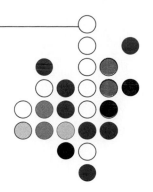

The publication of a book necessitates the involvement of many persons beyond the authors. We wish to acknowledge the support and assistance of the following persons who indeed made this book possible:

Our families and friends, who supported our taking time away from life activities.

Joanne DaCunha, Publisher, Nursing, F. A. Davis, who has provided patient direction toward our goal.

Bob Martone, Publisher, Nursing, F. A. Davis, for his continuing enthusiasm and belief in the book.

Our students and colleagues, who consistently challenge us to rethink each care plan and hold us to exacting standards.

AND

A special acknowledgment to Dr. Marjory Gordon, a most gracious lady who freely shared ideas, materials, support, and encouragement.

To each of these persons we wish to say a heartfelt "Thank you." Please accept our deepest gratitude and appreciation.

REVIEWERS

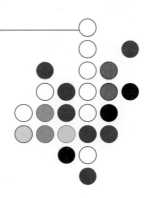

Lenora D. Follett, RN, MS
Associate Professor
Pacific Union College
Angwin, California

Mary Haase, RN, MS
Nursing Instructor
Blackhawk Technical College
Janesville, Wisconsin

Margaret Konieczny, RN, MSN
Western Nevada Community College
Carson City, Nevada

Tammie McCoy, RN, MSN, PhD
Assistant Professor
Mississippi University for Women
Columbus, Mississippi

CONTENTS

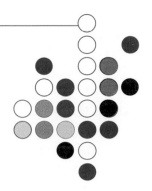

CHAPTER 9   ROLE—RELATIONSHIP PATTERN   605

CHAPTER 10   SEXUALITY—REPRODUCTIVE PATTERN   713

CHAPTER 11   COPING–STRESS TOLERANCE PATTERN   739

CHAPTER 12   VALUE–BELIEF PATTERN   799

APPENDIX A: NANDA'S AXES DEFINITIONS   829

APPENDIX B: ADMISSION ASSESSMENT FORM AND SAMPLE   831

INDEX   853

1

INTRODUCTION

WHY THIS BOOK?

When the first edition of this book was published, all the authors were faculty members at the same school of nursing. We had become frustrated with the books that were available for teaching nursing diagnosis and found that the students were also expressing some of the same frustration.

The students felt they needed to bring several books to the clinical area because the books for nursing diagnosis had limited information on pathophysiology and psychosocial or developmental factors that had an impact on individualized care planning. The students were also confused regarding the different definitions, defining characteristics, and related factors each of the authors used. They were having difficulty writing individualized nursing actions for their patients because the various authors appeared to focus on specifics related to the etiology or signs and symptoms of the nursing diagnosis rather than on the concept represented by the nursing diagnosis that had been emphasized to our students. The authors were also concerned about the number of books our students had to buy, because most books focused on just one clinical area, such as adult health or pediatrics. Thus, as the students progressed through the school, they had to buy different books for different clinical areas even though each of the books had the common theme of the use of nursing diagnosis. Another concern we, as faculty, had was the lack of information in the various books regarding the final phase of the nursing process—evaluation. This most vital phase was mentioned only briefly, and very little guidance was given on how to proceed through this phase.

The final concern that led to the writing of the book was our desire to focus on nursing actions and nursing care, not medical care and medical diagnosis. We strongly believe and support the vital role of nurses in the provision of health care for our nation, and so we have focused strictly on nursing in this book. After all, the majority of health-care providers are nurses, and statistics consistently show the general public has high respect for them.[1] In a 2004 poll conducted by *USA Today*,[2] the public considered nursing the most honest profession and trusted the information that nurses give them. This increases the importance of utilizing a standard nursing language to provide the foundation for quality nursing care and continued development of evidence-based practice.

For these reasons, we have written this book particularly geared to student use. Specifically, we wrote the first book to assist students in learning how to apply nursing diagnosis in the clinical area. By using the framework of the nursing process and the materials generated by the North American Nursing Diagnosis Association International (NANDA),[3] we believe this book makes it easier for you, the student, to learn and use nursing diagnosis in planning care for your patients. (Nursing diagnoses were developed by and used with permission of North American Nursing Diagnosis Association.[3])

Since the writing of that first book, NANDA has grown to become an international organization with nursing contributions from many countries and an alliance between NANDA International, the Nursing Interventions Classification (NIC),[4] and Nursing Outcomes Classification (NOC),[5] which resulted in the creation of the NANDA, NIC, and NOC (NNN) Taxonomy of Nursing Practice. This taxonomy was based on a modified framework of Gordon's[6] functional health patterns with "the final taxonomic structure less like Gordon's original, but with reduced misclassification errors and redundancies to near zero."[3] Taxonomy II has been recognized as an international nursing language. Designed to be multiaxial in form, it provides greater flexibility of nomenclature and allows for easy additions and modifications, thus providing a more clinically useful tool that better supports nursing practice. In spite of these revisions, some in nursing service organizations continue to view Nursing Diagnosis as an academic exercise, good for students to learn, but highly impractical in the fast-paced world of nursing operations. When service settings utilize nursing diagnosis, it is most often in electronic documentation systems. The care plans in these systems are most often standardized and demonstrate little adaptation to the individual or their health status. A review of the documentation shows that once a diagnosis is chosen the care plan is not updated during the contact with the patient. Care planning, involving telling the computer that the nurse saw the patient during that shift and looked at the care plan to determine whether it was still pertinent, simply becomes a "task" the nurse must perform. The multiaxial format of Taxonomy II can provide the clinician with the tools necessary to better format his or her clinical documentation, showing the "whole picture" of diagnosis, treatment, evaluation, re-evaluation, and nursing outcomes.

It is however, important that this tool be used correctly. "Using a multiaxial structure allows many diagnoses to be constructed that have no defining characteristics and may even be nonsense."[3] For this reason the authors of this book felt that it was important to continue to provide NANDA, NIC and NOC, and the NNN Taxonomy of nursing practice in this fifth edition. This inclusion will hopefully better clarify the work and give not only the academic setting, but also the clinical setting a guide that will provide the individual student and practitioner a resource that leads to better understanding and operational use of nursing diagnoses and, ultimately, better patient outcomes. To facilitate this integration we have provided charts in each chapter that provide basic links between the taxonomies.

THE NURSING PROCESS
PURPOSE

Gordon[7] indicates that Lydia Hall was one of the first nurses to use the term *nursing process* in the early 1950s. Since that time, the term *nursing process* has been used to describe the accepted method of delivering nursing care. Iyer, Taptich, and Bernocchi-Losey state, "The major purpose of the nursing process is to provide a framework within which the individualized needs of the client, family, and community can be met."[8] Today, the concept of the nursing process has expanded to include critical thinking processes that contribute to the decisions needed to choose the correct method of delivering nursing care.[9] The nursing process is utilized by nursing education to teach critical thinking, by professional nursing organizations to test performance (NCLEX and specialty certification exams), and by acute care institutions as a basis for care plans and critical pathways.[10]

It may be easier to think of a framework as a blueprint or outline that guides the planning of care for a patient.* As Doenges and Moorhouse write,[11] "The nursing process is central to nursing actions in any setting because it is an efficient method of organizing thought processes for clinical decision making and problem solving." Use of the nursing process framework is beneficial for both the patient and the nurse because it helps ensure that care is planned, individualized, and reviewed over the period of time that the nurse and patient have a professional relationship. It must be emphasized that patient involvement is required throughout all phases of the nursing process. If the patient is not involved in all phases, then the plan of care is not individualized.

DEFINITION

Alfaro[12] defines the nursing process as "an organized, systematic method of giving individualized nursing care that focuses on identifying and treating unique responses of individuals or groups to actual or potential alterations in health." This definition fits very nicely with the American Nurses Association (ANA) Social Policy Statement.[13] "Nursing is

---

*Throughout this book we use the terms *patient* and *client* interchangeably. In most instances these terms refer to the individual who is receiving nursing care. However, a patient can also be a community, such as in the community–home health nursing actions, or a family, such as for the nursing diagnosis Ineffective Family Coping, Compromised.

the protection, promotion, and optimization of health and abilities, prevention of illness and injury, alleviation of suffering through the diagnosis and treatment of human responses, and advocacy in the care of individuals, families, communities, and populations." Alfaro's definition is further supported by the ANA Nursing: Scope and Standards of Practice[14] (Table 1.1), practice standards written by several boards of Nursing in the United States, and the definition of nursing that is written into the majority of nurse practice acts in the United States. (The standards of Nursing Practice of the State of Texas are used as an example.[15] See Table 1.2.)

Basically, the nursing process provides each nurse a framework to utilize in working with the patient. The process begins at the time the patient needs assistance with health care, and continues until the patient no longer needs assistance to meet health-care maintenance. The nursing process utilizes the cognitive (intelligence, critical thinking, and reasoning), psychomotor (physical), and affective (emotion and values) skills and abilities a nurse needs to plan care for a patient.

ROLE IN PLANNING CARE

Perhaps the most important question is, why do we need to plan care? There are several answers to this question, ranging from consideration of a patient's individual needs to the legal aspects of nursing practice.

First, the patient has a right to expect that the nursing care received will be complete, safe, and of high quality. If planning is not done, then gaps are going to exist in the care, impacting patient outcomes. At this time, patients are being admitted to the hospital more acutely ill than in the past, and are also being discharged into their communities more seriously ill. We are now caring for patients in a general med-

---

●●●
●●● TABLE 1.1 **Standards of Care**
●●●

Standard I. Assessment: The registered nurse collects comprehensive data pertinent to the patient's health or the situation.

Standard II. Diagnosis: The registered nurse analyzes the assessment data to determine diagnoses or issues.

Standard III. Outcome Identification: The registered nurse identifies expected outcomes for a plan individualized to the patient or the situation.

Standard IV. Planning: The registered nurse develops a plan that prescribes strategies and alternatives to attain expected outcomes.

Standard V. Implementation: The registered nurse implements the identified plan.

Standard VI. Evaluation: The registered nurse evaluates progress toward attainment of outcomes.

Source: From American Nurses Association: Nursing: Scope and Standards of Practice. ANA, Silver Spring, MD, 2004, pp 21–32, with permission.

∷∷∷ TABLE 1.2 Standards of Nursing Practice

The registered nurse shall:

1. Know and conform to the Texas Nurse Practice Act and the board's rules and regulations as well as all federal, state, or local laws, rules, or regulations affecting the RN's current area of nursing practice;

2. Standards Specific to Registered Nurses. The registered nurse shall assist in the determination of health-care needs of clients and shall:

   A. Utilize a systematic approach to provide individualized, goal-directed nursing care by:

      i. performing comprehensive nursing assessments regarding the health status of the client;

      ii. making nursing diagnoses that serve as the basis for the strategy of care;

      iii. developing a plan of care based on the assessment and nursing diagnosis;

      iv. implementing nursing care; and

      v. evaluating the client's responses to nursing interventions.

Source: Adapted from Board of Nurse Examiners for the State of Texas: Standards of Nursing Practice. Texas Nurse Practice Act. Author, Austin, TX, 2004, with permission.

ical–surgical unit who would have been in a critical care unit ten years ago. We are now sending patients home in 1 to 3 days whom we previously would have kept in the hospital another 5 to 10 days. Procedures that required a 3- to 5-day hospital stay in the past are now being performed in day surgery or outpatient facilities. A variety of factors have led to this situation, including advances in technology; advent of the use of diagnosis related groups (DRGs) for patient billing; managed care insurance plans; prospective payment insurance plans, capitated payment insurance plans; movement from acute care to longer term care settings such as home health, nursing homes, and rehabilitation units; and, most importantly, the desire to contain the rapidly rising costs of health care. These problems, which together have been labeled the "quicker, sicker" phenomenon, in combination with a national shortage of registered nurses, have created a situation in which the contact time a professional nurse has with a patient is being cut to a minimum. Given this set of circumstances, if care planning is not done there is no doubt that gaps will exist in the nursing care given to a patient. Such care will be incomplete, inconsistent, unsafe, and certainly not of high quality, which will result in an increase in negative outcomes.

Second, care planning and its documentation provide a means of professional communication. This communication promotes consistency of care for the patient and provides a comfort level for the nurse. Any patient admitted to a health-care agency is going to have some level of anxiety. Imagine how this anxiety will increase when each nurse who enters the room does each procedure differently, answers questions differently, or uses different time lines for care (e.g., a surgical dressing that has been changed in the morning every day since surgery is not changed until the afternoon). Care planning provides a comfort level for the nurse because it gives the nurse a ready reference to help ensure that care is complete. In addition, when the care is planned using practices with evidence that supports their use, consistency in implementation improves efficacy resulting in improved patient outcomes. Care planning also provides a

guideline for documentation and promotes practicing within legally defined standards.

Third, care planning provides legal protection for the nurse. We are practicing in one of the most litigious societies that has ever existed. In the past, nurses were not frequently named in legal actions; however, this has changed, as a brief review of suits being filed would show. In a legal suit, nursing care is measured against the idea of what a reasonably prudent nurse would do in the same circumstances. The accepted standards of nursing practice, as published by ANA (see Table 1.1) and the individual boards of nursing (see Table 1.2), are the accepted definitions of reasonable, prudent nursing care.

Finally, accrediting and approval agencies such as the Joint Commission on Accreditation of Healthcare Organizations (JCAHO), the National League for Nursing Accrediting Commission (NLNAC), Medicare, and Medicaid have criteria that specifically require documentation of planning of care. The accreditation status of a health-care agency can depend on consistent documentation that planning of care has been done. Particularly with the third-party payers, such as Medicare, Medicaid, and insurance companies, lack of documentation regarding the planning and implementation of care results in no reimbursement for care. Ultimately, nonreimbursement for care leads to lack of new equipment, no pay raises, and, in some extreme cases, has led to hospital closures.

With the advent of electronic documentation in the acute care setting and other nursing agencies (outpatient clinics, home health care, and departments of health) it has become even more critical to possess knowledge and resources that allow practicing nurses in any setting to show the progress from nursing diagnosis to nursing interventions and finally the nursing outcomes in their documentation. Measurement of outcomes is the basis for measuring the quality, safety, and results of the care rendered to a patient or client and are today's "yardstick" on which the general public, regulatory agencies, and third-party payers base their decisions and actions.

CARE PLAN VERSUS PLANNING OF CARE

Revisions of nursing standards by JCAHO created questions regarding the necessity of nursing care plans. According to Brider,[16] Henry,[17] and Webster,[18] some authors predicted the demise of the care plan, but review of the revised nursing standards shows that the standards require not less, but more detailed care planning documentation in the patient's medical record.

The Joint Commission on Accreditation of Healthcare Organizations (JCAHO), like all health-care organizations, is experiencing change. To better serve the public and health-care organizations, JCAHO dramatically changed its accreditation process in 2005. Rather than focusing only on "nursing process," policies and procedures review, and other isolated factors within the organization, they now focus on the patients and their journey through the health-care system. This journey includes "Care, treatment, and services provided through the successful coordination and completion of a series of processes that include appropriate initial assessment of needs; development of a plan for care, treatment, and services; the provision of care, treatment, and services; ongoing assessment of whether the care, treatment, and services are meeting the patient's needs and either the successful discharge of the patient or referral or transfer of the patient for continuing care, treatment, and services."[19]

Review of the new criteria indicates that the standards require documentation related to not only the nursing process, but also the development and implementation of a plan encompassing the provision of care, treatment, and services provided the patient. Instead of defining plan, per se, the new guidelines define nursing care as: "Professional processes of assessment, diagnosis, planning, implementation, and evaluation based on the art and science of nursing to promote health, its recovery, or a peaceful and dignified death."[19]

This provision of care is still based on data gathering during patient assessment, which identifies the patient's care needs, tests the strategy for providing services to meet those needs, documents treatment goals or objectives, outlines the criteria for terminating specified interventions, and documents the individual's progress in meeting specified goals and objectives. The elements that make up the provision of care, as defined by JCAHO, are "related to each other through an integrated and cyclical process that may occur over minutes, hours, days, weeks, months, or years, depending on the setting and the needs of the patient"[19] (Fig. 1.1).

Rather than eliminating care plans, the new JCAHO requirements expand the concept and increase the importance of the coordination and documentation of the patient's journey guided by nursing assessment. This documentation must be in the medical record. The care plan is not dead; rather, it is revised to more clearly reflect the important role of nursing assessment and planning in the patient's care. No

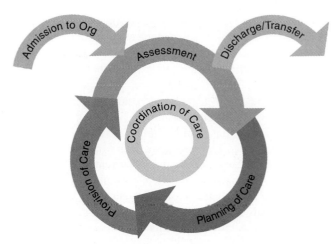

FIGURE 1.1 **Provision of care system. (*Source:* JCAHO.)**

longer a separate, often discarded, and irrelevant page, the plan of care is an integral part of the permanent record. The flow sheets developed for this book offer guidelines for computerizing information regarding nursing care.

Faculty can use the revised JCAHO guidelines[19] to assist students in developing expertise beyond writing extensive nursing care plans. This additional expertise requires the new graduate to envision the patient's journey through the health-care system and to integrate all phases of the nursing process into the permanent record. Rather than eliminating the need for care planning and nursing diagnosis, these standards have reinforced the importance of nursing care and nursing diagnosis for not only nursing, but also the entire health-care organization.

NURSING PROCESS STEPS

There are five steps, or phases, in the nursing process: assessment, diagnosis, planning, implementation, and evaluation. These steps are not distinct; rather, they overlap and build on each other. To carry out the entire nursing process, you must be sure to complete each step accurately and then build upon the information in that step to complete the next one.

ASSESSMENT

The first step, or phase, of the nursing process is assessment. During this phase, you are collecting data (factual information) from several sources. The collection and organization of these data allow you to:

1. Determine the patient's current health status.
2. Determine the patient's strengths and problem areas (both actual and potential).
3. Prepare for the second step of the process—diagnosis.

Data Sources and Types
The sources for data collection are numerous, but it is essential to remember that the patient is the primary data source. No one else can explain as accurately as the patient can the

start of the problem, the reason for seeking assistance or the exact nature of the problem, and the effect of the problem on the patient. Other sources include the patient's family or significant others; the patient's admission sheet from the admitting office; the physician's history, physical, and orders; laboratory and x-ray examination results; information from other caregivers; and current nursing literature.

Assessment data can be further classified as types of data. According to Iyer and associates,[8] the data types are subjective, objective, historical, and current.

Subjective data are the facts presented by the patient that show his or her perception, understanding, and interpretation of what is happening. An example of subjective data is the patient's statement, "The pain begins in my lower back and runs down my left leg."

Objective data are facts that are observable and measurable by the nurse. These data are gathered by the nurse through physical assessment, interviewing, and observing, and involve the use of the senses of seeing, hearing, smelling, and touching. An example of objective data is the measurement and recording of vital signs. Objective data are also gathered through such diagnostic examinations as laboratory tests, x-ray examinations, and other diagnostic procedures.

Historical data refer to health events that happened prior to this admission or health problem episode. An example of historical data is the patient statement, "The last time I was in a hospital was 1996 when I had an emergency appendectomy."

Current data are facts specifically related to this admission or health problem episode. An example of this type of data is vital signs on admission: T 99.2°F, P 78, R 18, BP 134/86. Please note, that just as there is overlapping of the nursing process steps, there is also overlapping of the data types. Both historical and current data may be either subjective or objective. Historical and current data assist in establishing time references and can give an indication of the patient's usual functioning.

Essential Skills

Assessment requires the use of the skills needed for interviewing, conducting a physical examination, and observing. As with the nursing process itself, these skills are not used one at a time. While you are interviewing the patient, you are also observing and determining physical areas that require a detailed physical assessment. While completing a physical assessment, you are asking questions (interviewing) and observing the patient's physical appearance as well as the patient's response to the physical examination.

Interviewing generally starts with gathering data for the nursing history. In this interview, you ask for general demographic information such as name, address, date of last hospitalization, age, allergies, current medications, and the reason the patient was admitted. Depending on the agency's admission form, you may then progress to other specific questions or a physical assessment. An example of an admission assessment specifically related to the Functional Health Patterns is given in Appendix B.

The physical assessment calls for four skills: inspection, palpation, percussion, and auscultation. *Inspection* means careful and systematic observation throughout the physical examination, such as observation for and recording of any skin lesions. *Palpation* is assessment by feeling and touching. Assessing the differences in temperature between a patient's upper and lower arm would be an example of palpation. Another common example of palpation is breast self-examination. *Percussion* involves touching, tapping, and listening. Percussion allows determination of the size, density, locations, and boundaries of the organs. Percussion is usually performed by placing the index or middle finger of one hand firmly on the skin and striking with the middle finger of the other hand. The resultant sound is dull if the body is solid under the fingers (such as at the location of the liver) and hollow if there is a body cavity under the finger (such as at the location of the abdominal cavity). *Auscultation* involves listening with a stethoscope and is used to help assess respiratory, circulatory, and gastrointestinal status.

The physical assessment may be performed using a head-to-toe approach, a body system approach, or a functional health pattern approach. In the *head-to-toe approach,* you begin with the patient's general appearance and vital signs. You then progress, as the name indicates, from the head to the extremities.

The *body system approach* to physical assessment focuses on the major body systems. As the nurse is conducting the nursing history interview, she or he will get a firm idea of which body systems need detailed examination. An example is a cardiovascular examination, in which the apical and radial pulses, blood pressure (BP), point of maximum intensity (PMI), heart sounds, and peripheral pulses are examined.

The *functional health pattern approach* is based on Gordon's Functional Health Patterns typology and allows the collection of all types of data according to each pattern. This is the approach used by this book and leads to three levels of assessment. First is the overall admission assessment, where each pattern is assessed through the collection of objective and subjective data. This assessment indicates patterns that need further attention, which requires implementation of the second level of pattern assessment. The second level of pattern assessment indicates which nursing diagnoses within the pattern might be pertinent to this patient, which leads to the third level of assessment, the defining characteristics for each individual nursing diagnosis. Having a three-tiered assessment might seem complicated, but each assessment is so closely related that completion of the assessment is easy. A primary advantage in using this type of assessment is the validation it gives the nurse that the resulting nursing diagnosis is the most accurate diagnosis. Another benefit to using this type of assessment is that grouping of data is already accomplished and does not have to be a separate step.

Data Grouping

Data grouping simply means organizing the information into sets or categories that will assist you in identifying the patient's strengths and problem areas. A variety of organizing frameworks is available, such as Maslow's Hierarchy of Needs, Roy's Adaptation Model, Gordon's Functional Health Patterns, and NANDA Taxonomy II.[3] Each of the nursing theorists (e.g., Roy, Levine, and Orem)[40,41] speaks to assessment within the framework of her theories. Organizing the information allows you to both identify the appropriate functional health pattern and to spot any missing data. If you cannot identify the pertinent functional health pattern, then you need to collect further data. The goal of data grouping is to arrive at a nursing diagnosis.

DIAGNOSIS

Diagnosis means reaching a definite conclusion regarding the patient's strengths and human responses. This diagnostic process is complex and utilizes aspects of intelligence, thinking, and critical thinking.[9] When planning care, one must be cognizant that "the diagnosis of human responses is a complex process involving the interpretation of human behavior related to health."[9] Therefore the patient's response and strengths facilitate their adaptation during the implementation phase. In this book, we use the diagnoses accepted by NANDA-I.

Nursing Diagnosis

The North American Nursing Diagnosis Association International (NANDA-I), formerly the National Conference Group for Classification of Nursing Diagnosis, has been meeting since 1973 to identify, develop, and classify nursing diagnoses. Setting forth a nursing diagnosis nomenclature articulates nursing language, thus promoting the identification of nursing's contribution to health, and facilitates communication among nurses. In addition, the use of nursing diagnosis provides a clear distinction between nursing diagnosis and medical diagnosis and provides clear direction for the remaining aspects of the planning of care.

NANDA accepted its first working definition of nursing diagnosis in 1990.[20] Nursing diagnosis is a clinical judgment about individual, family, or community responses to actual or potential health problems/life processes. Nursing diagnoses provide the basis for selection of nursing interventions to achieve outcomes for which the nurse is accountable.

Much debate occurred during the Ninth Conference regarding this definition, and it is anticipated this debate will continue. The debate centers on a multitude of issues related to the definition, which are beyond the scope of this book. Readers are urged to consult the official journal of NANDA-I, *Nursing Diagnosis: The International Journal of Nursing Language and Classification,* to keep up to date on this debate.

The definition of nursing diagnosis distinguishes nursing diagnosis from medical diagnosis. For example, nursing diagnosis is different from medical diagnosis in its focus. Kozier, Erb, and Olivieri[21] write that nursing diagnoses focus on patient response, whereas medical diagnoses focus on the disease process. As indicated by the definition of nursing diagnosis, nurses identify the *human responses to actual or potential* health problems while physicians place primary emphasis on identifying current health problems.

Nursing diagnosis and medical diagnosis are similar in that the same basic procedures are used to derive the diagnosis (i.e., physical assessment, interviewing, and observing). Likewise, according to Kozier and associates,[21] both types of diagnoses are designed for essentially the same reason—planning care for a patient.

A nursing diagnosis is based on the presence of defining characteristics. According to NANDA-I,[3] defining characteristics are observable cues/inferences that cluster as manifestations of an actual or wellness diagnosis. For actual nursing diagnoses (the problem is present), a majority of the defining characteristics must be present. For risk diagnoses (risk factors indicate the problem might develop), the risk factors must be present. Understanding defining characteristics improves your interpretation of human responses and assists you in making interpretations that are more accurate. This accuracy will result in implementation of interventions that have the greatest potential for the best outcomes. Your mastery of nursing diagnosis will also increase the agreement between nurses about the client's response and result in consistent, quality care.

Diagnostic Statements

According to the literature, complete nursing diagnostic statements include, at a minimum, the human response and an indication of the factors contributing to the response. The following is a rationale for the two-part statement: "Each nursing diagnosis, when correctly written, can accomplish two things. One, by identifying the unhealthy response, it tells you what should change. . . And two, by identifying the probable cause of the unhealthy response, it tells you what to do to effect change."[22]

Although there is no consensus on the phrase that should be used to link the response and etiologic factors, perusal of current literature indicates that the most commonly used phrases are *related to, secondary to,* and *due to.*

The phrase *related to* is gaining the most acceptance because it does not imply a direct cause-and-effect relationship. Kieffer[23] believes using the phrases *due to* and *secondary to* may reflect such a cause-and-effect relationship, which could be hard to prove. Thus, a complete nursing diagnostic statement would read: Pain related to surgical incision.

Gordon[6] identifies three structural components of a nursing diagnostic statement: The problem (P), the etiology (E), and signs and symptoms (S). The *problem* describes the patient's response or current state (the nursing diagnosis); the *etiology* describes the cause or causes of the response (related to); and the *symptoms* delineate the defining characteristics or observable signs and symptoms demonstrated or described by the patient. The S component can be readily connected to the P and E statements through the use of the phrase *as evidenced by.* Using this format, a complete nursing diagnostic statement would read: Pain related to surgical incision as evidenced by verbal comments and body posture.

As discussed in the preface, we recommend starting with stating the nursing diagnosis only. Therefore, the nursing diagnosis would be listed in the patient's chart in the same manner as it is given in the nomenclature: Pain. Remember that the objective and subjective data related to the patient's pain have already been recorded in the health record in the assessment section, so there is no need to repeat it.

The nursing diagnostic statement examples given previously describe the existence of an actual problem. Professional nurses are strong supporters of preventive health care—cases in which a problem does not yet exist and measures that can be taken to ensure that the problem does not arise. In such instances, the nursing diagnostic statement is prefaced by the words "Risk for." Nursing diagnoses that carry the preface "Risk for" also carry with them risk factors rather than defining characteristics.

Whereas other books include a variety of nursing diagnoses, this book uses only the actual and risk (formerly labeled "potential") diagnoses accepted by NANDA-I (30) for testing. Probable related factors (formerly "etiologic factors") are grouped, as are the defining characteristics (formerly "signs and symptoms"), under each specific nursing diagnosis. As indicated in the preface, nursing actions in this book reflect a conceptual approach rather than a specific (to related factors or defining characteristics) approach.

To illustrate this approach, let us use the diagnosis Pain. There are common nursing orders related to the incidence of pain regardless of whether the pain is caused by surgery, labor, or trauma. You can take this conceptual approach and make an individualized adaptation according to the etiologic factors affecting your patient and the reaction your patient is exhibiting to pain.

Identifying and specifying the nursing diagnoses leads to the next phase of the process— planning. Now that you know what the problems, responses, and strengths are, you can decide how to resolve the problem areas while building on the strength areas.

PLANNING

Planning involves three subsets: setting priorities, writing expected outcomes, and establishing target dates. Planning sets the stage for writing nursing actions by establishing where we are going with our plan of care. Planning further assists in the final phase of evaluation by defining the standard against which we will measure progress.

Setting Priorities

With the sicker, quicker problem discussed earlier, you are going to find yourself in the situation of having identified many more problems than can possibly be resolved in a 1-

to 3-day hospitalization (today's average length of stay). In the long-term care facilities, such as home health, rehabilitation, and nursing homes, long-range problem solving is possible, but setting priorities of care is still necessary.

Several methods of assigning priorities are available. Some nurses assign priorities based on the life threat posed by a problem. For example, Ineffective Airway Clearance would pose more of a threat to life than the diagnosis Risk for Impaired Skin Integrity. Some nurses base their prioritization on Maslow's Hierarchy of Needs. In this instance, physiologic needs would require attention before social needs. One way to establish priorities is to simply ask the patient which problem he or she would like to pay attention to first. Another way to establish priorities is to analyze the relationships between problems. For example, a patient has been admitted with a medical diagnosis of headaches and possible brain tumor. The patient exhibits the defining characteristics of both Pain and Anxiety. In this instance, we might want to implement nursing actions to reduce anxiety, knowing that if the anxiety is not reduced, pain control actions will not be successful. Once priorities have been established, you are ready to establish expected outcomes.

Expected Outcomes

Outcomes, goals, and *objectives* are terms that are frequently used interchangeably because all indicate the end point we will use to measure the effectiveness of our plan of care. Because so many published sets of standards and JCAHO talk in terms of *outcome standards* or *criteria,* we have chosen to use the term "expected outcomes" in this book.

Several authors[23–25] give guidelines for writing clinically useful expected outcomes:

1. Expected outcomes are clearly stated in terms of patient behavior or observable assessment factors.

   EXAMPLE

   POOR   Will increase fluid balance by time of discharge.

   GOOD   Will increase oral fluid intake to 1500 mL per 24 hours by 9/11.

2. Expected outcomes are realistic, achievable, safe, and acceptable from the patient's viewpoint.

   EXAMPLE

   Mrs. Braxton is a 28-year-old woman who has delayed healing of a surgical wound. She is to receive discharge instructions regarding a high-protein diet. She is a widow with three children under the age of 10. Her only source of income is Social Security.

   POOR   Will eat at least two 8-oz servings of steak daily. [unrealistic, unachievable, unacceptable, etc.]

   GOOD   Will eat at least two servings from the following list each day:

   Lean ground meat

   Eggs

Cheese
Pinto beans
Peanut butter
Fish
Chicken

3. Expected outcomes are written in specific, concrete terms depicting patient action. NOC states that outcomes among other things, should be:
Concise
Not describe nurse behaviors or interventions
Describe a state, behavior, or perception that is inherently variable and can be measured and quantified.[13]

EXAMPLE

POOR   Maintains fluid intake by 9/11.
GOOD   Will drink at least 8-oz of fluid every hour from 7 a.m. to 10 p.m. by 9/11.

4. Expected outcomes are directly observable by use of at least one of the five senses.

EXAMPLE

POOR   Understands how to self-administer insulin by 9/11.
GOOD   Accurately return-demonstrates self-administration of insulin by 9/11.

5. Expected outcomes are patient centered rather than nurse centered.

EXAMPLE

POOR   Teaches how to measure blood pressure by 9/11.
GOOD   Accurately measures own blood pressure by 9/11.

Establishing Target Dates

Writing a target date at the end of the expected outcome statement facilitates the plan of care in several ways.[19,23]

1. Assists in "pacing" the care plan. Pacing helps keep the focus on the patient's progress.
2. Serves to motivate both patients and nurses toward accomplishing the expected outcome.
3. Helps patient and nurse see accomplishments.
4. Alerts nurse when to evaluate care plan.

Target dates can be realistically established by paying attention to the usual progress and prognosis connected with the patient's medical and nursing diagnoses. Additional review of the data collected during the initial assessment helps indicate individual factors to be considered in establishing the date. For example, one of the previous expected outcomes was stated as "Accurately return-demonstrates self-administration of insulin by 9/11."

The progress or prognosis according to the patient's medical and nursing diagnosis will not be highly significant. The primary factor will be whether diabetes mellitus is a new diagnosis for the patient or is a recurring problem for a patient who has had diabetes mellitus for several years.

For the newly diagnosed patient, we would probably want our deadline day to be 5 to 7 days from the date of learning the diagnosis. For the recurring problem, we might establish the target date to be 2 to 3 days from the date of diagnosis. The difference is, of course, the patient's knowledge base.

Now look at an example related to the progress issue. Mr. Kit is a 19-year-old college student who was admitted early this morning with a medical diagnosis of acute appendicitis. He has just returned from surgery following an appendectomy. One of the nursing diagnoses for Mr. Kit would, in all probability, be Pain. The expected outcome could be "uses oral analgesic relief measures by [date]." In reviewing the general progress of a young patient with this medical and nursing diagnosis, we know that generally analgesic requirements delivered by PCA start decreasing within 48 to 72 hours. Therefore, we would want to establish our target date as 2 to 3 days following the day of surgery. This would result in the objective reading (assume date of surgery was 11/1): "Will have discontinued use of PCA and will request oral pain medication as needed for analgesia by 11/3."

To further emphasize the target date, it is suggested that the date be underlined, highlighted by using a different-colored pen, or circled to make it stand out. Pinpointing the date in such a manner emphasizes that evaluation of progress toward achievement of the expected outcome should be made on that date. Agencies which utilize electronic documentation may have automatic stop or evaluative times programmed into their system. Remember that the target date does not mean the expected outcome must be totally achieved by that time; instead, the target date signifies the evaluation date.

Once expected outcomes have been written, you are then ready to focus on the next phase—implementation.

IMPLEMENTATION

Implementation is the action phase of the nursing process. Recent literature has introduced the concept of nursing interventions, which are defined as treatments based on clinical judgment and knowledge that a nurse performs to enhance patient outcomes.[4] These interventions are the concepts that link specific nursing activities and actions. The authors of this book chose to focus on specific "nursing actions" in their plans of care rather than interventions to facilitate the student's/practitioner's development of individualized care. Two important steps are involved in implementation: The first is determining the specific nursing actions that will assist the patient to progress toward the expected outcome, and the second is documenting the care administered.

Nursing action is defined as nursing behavior that serves to help the patient achieve the expected outcome. Nursing actions include both independent and collaborative activities. *Independent activities* are those actions the nurse performs, using his or her own discretionary judgment, that require no validation or guidelines from any other health-care practitioner. An example is deciding which noninvasive technique to use for pain control or deciding when to teach the patient self-care measures. *Collaborative activities* are those actions that involve mutual decision making between two or more health-care practitioners. For example, a physician and nurse decide which narcotic to use when meperidine is ineffective in controlling the patient's pain, or a physical therapist and nurse decide on the most beneficial exercise program for a patient. Implementing a physician's order and referral to a dietitian are other common examples of collaborative actions.

Written nursing actions guide both actual patient care and proper documentation, and they must therefore be detailed and exact. Written nursing actions should be even more definite than what is generally found in physician orders. For example, a physician writes the order, "Increase ambulation as tolerated" for a patient who has been immobile for 2 weeks. The nursing actions should reflect specified increments of ambulation as well as ongoing assessment:

11/21. **a.** Prior to activity, assess BP, P, and R. After activity assess: (1) BP, P, R; (2) presence/absence of vertigo; (3) circulation; (4) presence/absence of pain.

b. Assist to dangle on bedside for 15 minutes at least 4 times a day on 11/2.

c. If BP, P, or R change significantly or vertigo is present or circulation is impaired or pain is present, return to supine position immediately. Elevate head of bed 30 degrees for 1 hour; then 45 degrees for 1 hour; then 90 degrees for 1 hour. If tolerated with no untoward signs or symptoms, initiate order 1b again.

d. Assist up to chair at bedside for 30 minutes at least 4 times a day on 11/3.

e. Assist to ambulate to bathroom and back at least 4 times a day on 11/4.

f. Supervise ambulation of one-half length of hall at least 4 times a day on 11/5 and 11/6.

g. Supervise ambulation of length of hall at least 4 times a day on 11/7.
S. J. Smith, RN

Nursing actions further differ from physician orders in that the patient's response is directly related to the implementation of the action. It is rare to see a physician order that includes alternatives if the first order has minimal, negative, or no effect on the patient. A complete written nursing action incorporates at least the following five components according to Bolander.[24]

1. Date the action was initially written.
2. A specific action verb that tells what the nurse is going to do (e.g., "assist" or "supervise").
3. A prescribed activity (e.g., ambulation).

4. Specific time units (e.g., for 15 minutes at least four times a day).
5. Signature of the nurse who writes the initial action order (i.e., accepting legal and ethical accountability).

A nursing action should not be implemented unless all five components are present. A nurse would not administer a medication if the physician order read, "Give Demerol"; neither should a nurse be expected to implement a nursing action that reads, "Increase ambulation gradually."

Additional criteria that should be remembered to ensure complete, safe, quality nursing action include:

1. Consistency between the prescribed actions, the nursing diagnosis, and expected outcome (including numbering).

EXAMPLE

Nursing Diagnosis 1
Impaired physical mobility, level 2.

Expected Outcome 1
Will ambulate length of hall by 11/8.

Nursing Action 1

11/21. **a.** Prior to activity, assess BP, P, and R. After activity assess: (1) BP, P, R; (2) presence/absence of vertigo; (3) circulation; (4) presence/absence of pain.

b. Assist to dangle on bedside for 15 minutes at least 4 times a day on 11/2.

c. If BP, P, or R changes significantly or vertigo is present or circulation is impaired or pain is present, return to supine position immediately. Elevate head of bed 30 degrees for 1 hour; then 45 degrees for 1 hour; then 90 degrees for 1 hour. If tolerated with no untoward signs or symptoms, initiate action 1b again.

d. Assist up to chair at bedside for 30 minutes at least 4 times a day on 11/3.

e. Assist to ambulate to bathroom and back at least 4 times a day on 11/4.

f. Supervise ambulation of one-half length of hall at least 4 times a day on 11/5 and 11/6.

g. Supervise ambulation of length of hall at least 4 times a day on 11/7.
S. J. Smith, RN

---

2. Consideration of both patient and facility resources. It would be senseless to make referrals to physical and occupational therapy services if these were not available. Likewise, from the patient's resource viewpoint, it would be foolish to teach a patient and his or her family how to manage care in a hospital bed if this bed would not be available to the patient at home.
3. Careful scheduling to include the patient's significant others and to incorporate usual activities of daily living (i.e., rest, meals, sleep, and recreation).
4. Incorporation of patient teaching and discharge planning from the first day of care.

5. Individualization and updating in keeping with the patient's condition and progress.

Including the key components and validating the quality of the written nursing actions help promote improved documentation. In essence, the written nursing actions can give an outline for documentation.

Properly written nursing actions demonstrate to the nurse both nursing actions and documentation to be done. Referring to the preceding example, we can see that the nurse responsible for this patient's care should chart the patient's blood pressure (BP), pulse (P), and respiration (R) rates prior to the activity, the patient's BP, P, and R rates after the activity, the presence or absence of vertigo, the presence or absence of pain, and the results of a circulatory check. Additionally, the nurse knows to chart that the patient dangled, sat up, or ambulated for a certain length of time or distance. Further, the nurse has guidelines of what to do and chart if an untoward reaction occurs in initial attempts at ambulation.

EXAMPLE

1000 BP 132/82, P 74, R 16. Up on side of bed for 5 minutes. Complained of vertigo and nausea. Returned to supine position with head of bed elevated to 30-degree angle. BP 100/68, P 80, R 24.

1100 BP 122/74, P 76, R 18. No complaints of vertigo or nausea. Head of bed elevated to 45-degree angle.

Writing nursing actions in such a manner automatically leads to reflection of the quality of care planning in the chart. Documentation of care planning in the patient's chart is essential to meet national standards of care and criteria for agency accreditation.

DOCUMENTATION

Just as development of the nursing process as a framework for practice has evolved, so documentation of that process has become an essential link between the provision of nursing care and the quality of the care provided. Several nursing documentation systems, both paper and electronic, have emerged that make it easier to document the nursing process. Four of these systems are discussed here. You will note that the narrative system is not discussed, because it tends to be fragmented and disjointed and presents problems in retrieval of pertinent information about the patient response to, and outcomes of, nursing care.

The *Problem-Oriented Record (POR)* with its format for documenting progress notes provides a system for documenting the nursing process. Additionally, POR is an interdisciplinary documentation system that can be used to coordinate care for all health-care providers working with the patient.

The POR consists of four major components:

1. The database
2. The problem list

3. The plan of care
4. The progress notes

The *database* is that information that has been collected through patient interview, observation, and physical assessment and the results of diagnostic tests. The database provides the basis for developing the problem list.

The *problem list* is an inventory of numbered, prioritized patient problems. Patient problems may be written as nursing or medical diagnoses. Problems may be actual or risk diagnoses. Because each problem is numbered, information about each problem is easily retrieved.

The *plan of care* incorporates the expected outcomes, target dates, and prescribed nursing actions as well as other interventions designed to resolve the problem. The plan of care reflects multidisciplinary care and should be agreed to by the health-care team.

The *progress note* provides information about the patient's response to or outcomes of the care provided. The full format for documenting progress is based on the acronym *SOAPIER,* which stands for *Subjective data, Objective data, Analysis/assessment, Plan, Intervention, Evaluation, and Revision.* As the plan of care is implemented for each numbered, prioritized problem, it is documented using the SOAPIER format. For example, recall the case of Mr. Kit, the 19-year-old college student who is recovering from an appendectomy. The problem list inventory would probably show Problem #1: Pain. His plan of care would state as an expected outcome: "Uses oral analgesic relief measures by [date]" and "Will have discontinued use of PCA and will request oral pain medication as needed for analgesia by 11/3."

Some of the written nursing actions would read:

1. Monitor for pain at least every 2 hours and have patient rank pain on a scale of 0–10.
2. Administer pain medications as ordered. Monitor response.
3. Spend at least 30 minutes once a shift teaching patient deep muscle relaxation. Talk patient through relaxation every 4 hours, while awake, at [list times here] once initial teaching is done.

The progress note of 11/3 would appear as follows:

Problem 1–Progress Note

S "I have had only one pain medication during the last 24 hours, and that relieved my pain." "I would rank my pain as a 1 on a scale of 0–10."

O Relaxation exercises taught, and return-demonstration completed on 11/2. No request for pain medication within past 12 hours.

A Pain relieved.

P None.

I None.

E Expected outcome met. Problem resolved. Discontinue problem.

R None.

The POR with its SOAPIER progress note emphasizes the problem-solving component within the nursing process and provides documentation of the care provided. For further information about the POR system, you are directed to the Weed[17] reference.

FOCUS charting, which is actually an offshoot of POR, is a documentation system that uses the nursing process to document care. Unlike the interdisciplinary POR, FOCUS charting is entirely oriented to nursing documentation. Like the POR system, FOCUS charting has a database, a problem list (FOCUS), a plan of care, and progress notes. However, the FOCUS (problem list) is broader than POR. In addition to nursing and medical diagnoses, the FOCUS of care may also be treatments, procedures, incidents, patient concerns, changes in condition, or other significant events. The medical record incorporates the plan of care in a three-column format (in addition to date/signature) labeled "FOCUS," "expected patient outcomes," and "nursing interventions." To illustrate, again with Mr. Kit:

DATE/SIGNATURE	FOCUS	EXPECTED PATIENT OUTCOME	NURSING INTERVENTION
11/1 *J. Jones, RN*	Pain	Will progress to 4 or more hours between requests for analgesics by 11/3.	Monitor for pain at least every 2 hours. Have pt rate pain on 0–10 scale. Administer pain med as ordered. Monitor response. *Spend at least 30 minutes once a shift teaching patient deep muscle relaxation. Talk patient through relaxation every 4 hours, while awake, at [list times here] once initial teaching is done.*

The progress notes incorporate a flow sheet for documenting daily interventions and treatments and a narrative progress note using a three-column format. The three-column format for the progress note includes a column for date, time, and signature; a FOCUS column; and a patient care note column. When the progress note is written in the patient care note column, it is organized using the acronym *DAR—Data, Action, and Response.* To illustrate, again using Mr. Kit:

DATE/TIME SIGNATURE	FOCUS	PATIENT CARE NOTE
11/1 1500 *J. Jones, RN*	Pain	D C/o pain, "My side hurts. It is a 9 on a 0–10 scale." BP 130/84, P 88, R 22.
11/1 1530 *J. Jones, RN*		A Demerol 100 mg given in rt gluteus. Turned to left side. Back rub given.
11/1 1615 *J. Jones, RN*		R States pain is better. Rates it 2 on a 0–10 scale. BP 120/80, P 82, R 18.

FOCUS charting provides a succinct system for documenting the nursing process. It reflects all the elements required by JCAHO. It is flexible, provides cues to documentation with its DAR format, and makes it easy to retrieve pertinent data. For more information on FOCUS, use the information written by Lampe.[26]

The *PIE documentation system* emphasizes the nursing process and nursing diagnosis. PIE is the acronym for *Problem, Intervention, and Evaluation.* A timesaving aspect of this system is that PIE does not require a separate plan of care. The initial database and ongoing assessments are recorded on special forms or flow sheets. Assessment data are not included in the progress note unless a change in the patient's condition occurs. If a change occurs, "A" for assessment would be recorded in the progress note. Routine interventions are recorded on a flow sheet, and the progress note is used for specific numbered problems.

When a problem is identified, it is entered into the progress note as a nursing diagnosis. Each problem is numbered consecutively during a 24-hour period, for example, P#1 and P#2. Therefore, the nurse may refer to the number rather than having to restate the problem. Interventions (I), directed to the problem are documented relative to the problem number (e.g., IP#1 or IP#2). Evaluation (E) reflects patient response to or outcomes of nursing intervention and is labeled according to the problem number (e.g., EP#1 or EP#2). To illustrate, again using Mr. Kit:

DATE	TIME	NURSE'S NOTES
11/1	1500	P#1 Pain. IP#1 BP 130/84, P 88, R 22. *J. Jones, RN*
11/1	1530	IP#1 Demerol 100 mg given IM in rt gluteus. Turned to left side. Back rub given. *J. Jones, RN*
11/1	1615	EP#1 States pain relieved. Rates pain as 2 on a 0–10 scale. BP 120/80, P 82, R 18. *J. Jones, RN*

Each problem is evaluated at least every 8 hours, and all problems are reviewed and summarized every 24 hours. Continuing problems with appropriate interventions and evaluation are renumbered and redocumented daily, thus promoting continuity of care. When a problem is resolved, it no longer is documented.

The PIE documentation system reflects the nursing process and simplifies documentation by integrating the plan of care into the progress notes. This saves time and promotes easy retrieval of pertinent data. Siegrist, Deltor, and Stocks[27] are the originators of the PIE system.

Charting by Exception was developed by nurses at Saint Luke's Hospital in Milwaukee, Wisconsin.[28] Documenting in this system differs significantly from traditional systems in that nurses chart only significant findings or exceptions to a predetermined norm.

This system centers on the development of clinical standards that describe accepted norms. The system makes extensive use of flow sheets and is becoming increasingly popular because of its streamlined format and cost-effectiveness.

A patient care plan is established based on described standards. Nursing actions are used as the base for documentation. Flow sheets are used to highlight significant findings and define assessment parameters and findings. For example, for the postpartum patient, the standard for the cardiovascular assessment is:

Cardiovascular assessment: Apical pulse, CRT, peripheral pulses, edema, calf tenderness.
Standard: Regular apical pulse, CRT <3 s, peripheral pulses palpable, no edema, no calf tenderness, nail beds and mucous membranes pink.

If the assessment findings were the same as the standard, the nurse simply makes a check mark on the flow sheet by cardiovascular assessment. If the assessment findings are different from the standard, the nurse marks an asterisk by cardiovascular assessment and explains the deviation from the standard in the narrative notes.

Charting by Exception has been shown to reduce documentation time and costs and increase attention to abnormal data. In addition, documentation is more consistent. More information about this system and examples of flow charts can be found in the publication *Charting by Exception*.[28]

To complete the nursing process cycle and, depending on its outcome, perhaps start another cycle, the final phase of the process—evaluation—must be done.

EVALUATION

Evaluation simply means assessing what progress has been made toward meeting the expected outcomes; it is the most ignored phase of the nursing process. The evaluation phase is the feedback and control part of the nursing process. Evaluation requires continuation of assessment that was begun in the initial assessment phase. In this instance, assessment is the data collection form we use to measure patient progress.

Data Collection

Initially, specific data should be collected to measure the progress made toward achieving the stated expected outcome. As an example, let us return to the outcome written for Mr. Kit, the 19-year-old college student who had an appendectomy. The expected outcome was "Will have discontinued use of PCA and will request oral pain medication as needed for analgesia by 11/3." It is now 11/3, and the nurse caring for Mr. Kit notes the date and initiates evaluation of the outcome. She first checks the chart and counts the number of complaints of pain, number and types of analgesics given, and Mr. Kit's response to the pain medication. She looks for any change in medication or a change in Mr. Kit's condition. She then interviews Mr. Kit regarding his perception of pain acuity and level of relief. At the same time, the nurse completes other assessments, such as observing the wound condition and the ease of ambulation or noting the presence of any other untoward signs or symptoms. The nurse then studies the data to see what action is necessary.

Action Following Data Collection

Action following data collection simply means making a nursing judgment of what modifications in the plan of care are needed. There are essentially only three judgments that can be made:

1. Resolved
2. Revise
3. Continue

Resolved means that the evaluative data indicate the health-care problem reflected in the nursing diagnosis and its accompanying expected outcome no longer exist; that is, the expected outcome has been met. The nurse documents the data collected and records the judgment—"Resolved." To illustrate, let us return to Mr. Kit.

First, the nurse reviews the chart. She finds that Mr. Kit requested pain medication every three to four hours for the first 18 hours after surgery. The nurses taught Mr. Kit relaxation exercises and turned him, positioned him, and gave him a back rub immediately after the administration of each analgesic. Mr. Kit has requested only one analgesic in the past 24 hours and none in the past 12 hours. He can return-demonstrate relaxation exercises and states he has only a mild "twinge" when he gets out of bed. He is looking forward to returning to school next week.

The nurse returns to the patient's chart and records the following: "11/3 Data—1 oral analgesic in past 24 hours; none in past 12 hours. Ambulates without pain; states having no pain. Resolved." She then will draw one line through the nursing diagnosis, related expected outcome(s), and nursing actions to show they have been discontinued.

Revise can indicate two actions. In one instance, the initial nursing diagnosis was not correct, so the diagnosis itself is revised. For example, the nurse may have made an initial diagnosis of Self-Esteem Disturbance. During collection of evaluation data, the patient and his family share further information that indicates that the more appropriate diagnosis is Powerlessness, Moderate. The plan of care is then modified to reflect the change in the nursing diagnosis. For evaluation purposes, the nurse again records the data and the word, "Revised." She then adds the new nursing diagnosis and marks one line through the initial nursing diagnosis.

In the second instance, while the nurse is collecting evaluation data for one nursing diagnosis and expected outcome, she finds assessment factors that show another problem has arisen. She simply records the appropriate judgment for the initial diagnosis and expected outcome (e.g., "Resolved") and revises the plan to include the new nursing diagnosis with its appropriate expected outcome and nursing actions.

Continue indicates that the expected outcome has not been met. The nurse again collects the appropriate data and, based on the data, makes the nursing judgment that the expected outcome has not been met. She records the data and adds the phrase, "Continue, reevaluate on [date]." She then modifies the plan of care by going back to the stated expected outcome, marking one line through the date, and adding a new date. Likewise, the nursing actions would be modified as necessary.

With evaluation, the nursing process cycle is completed (Fig. 1.1). Another cycle can begin with both the nurse and the patient insuring that quality care is being given and received. To assist you with the evaluation process, we have provided an evaluation flowchart template (Fig. 1.2). You can use this format to evaluate any nursing diagnosis by completing the chart with your specific information.

Building Conceptual Understandings with Care Plans

Care plans, in the format of concept maps, have emerged as an innovative teaching tool.[29,30] This format will help you, as a student, to understand the links between assessment and care, build clinical decision-making skills by increasing understanding of information relationships, and link theory to practice. Concept maps also assist with the development of critical thinking skills.[29,31-33]

The concept map care plan begins with the client's reasons for seeking health care. Branching from this are the related nursing diagnoses with the supporting data. Links that designate the relationships between the diagnoses and reasons for seeking care are developed. Links between the diagnoses show their relationships.[34] This information is then transferred to a problem or diagnosis work sheet, and the goals and interventions are developed followed by an evaluation of the client response.[29] A sample concept map for Mr. Kit is provided for you in Fig. 1.3. You can find further information on concept mapping in *Concept Mapping: A Critical-Thinking Approach to Care Planning*.[29] When you are developing a concept map you may find a program such as Inspiration® a helpful development tool. This program will assist you in developing concept boxes and linking the arrows. Some schools of nursing provide this resource for their students. You can also find this tool on the program's Web site (http://www.inspiration.com).

NURSING PROCESS AND CONCEPTUAL FRAMEWORKS

NURSING MODELS

Many nurses do not see a direct relationship between nursing models (nursing theories) and nursing process, but a direct relationship does exist. *Nursing models* present a systematic method for assessing and directing nursing practice through promoting organization and integration of what is known about human health, illness, and nursing. The *nursing process* is the action phase of a nursing model. Kataoka-Yahiro and Saylor[35] indicate that the nursing process is a method of problem solving and decision making and can be seen as a discipline specific method for critical thinking. In essence, models guide the use of the nursing process,[36] and, as previously stated, the care planning presented in this book is a result of the nursing process.

For further clarification, let us look at a few examples. If you are a supporter of Levine's Conservation Model, you would assess your patient in keeping with this model and then design your care plan to reflect prioritizing of the nursing diagnoses and nursing actions in a manner that would best promote conservation principles. Likewise, if you are a proponent of Roy's Adaptation Model, you would assess the four adaptation modes, and then prioritize your diagnoses in an order that would best promote adaptive responses. In summation, current nursing models affect care planning in terms of assessment and prioritizing of nursing diagnoses rather than requiring different diagnostic statements and different nursing actions.

PATTERNS

Several typologies have emerged as a result of the work done with nursing diagnosis. The typologies are representative of another step in theory development and are designed to facilitate the use of nursing diagnosis. The typologies provide an organizational framework that enables the nurse to focus on the pattern description and assessment rather than trying to remember all the details of individual diagnoses. The nurse can easily locate the individual diagnoses by being familiar with the patterns.

Functional Health Patterns

Gordon[7] writes that the Functional Health Patterns were identified, circa 1974, to assist in the teaching of assessment and diagnosis at Boston College School of Nursing. The Functional Health Patterns organize the individual diagnoses into categories, thus providing for the organized collection of assessment data.

The advantages offered by assessment according to the Functional Health Patterns include having a standardized

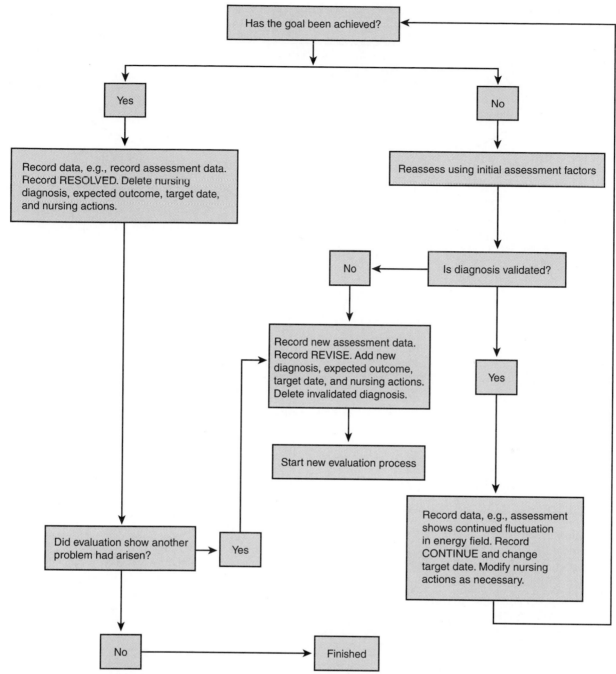

FIGURE 1.2 **Flowchart evaluation: Expected outcome. (From Cox, HC, Hinz, MD, Lubno, MA, Scott-Tilley, D, Newfield, SA, Slater, M, and Sridaromont, KL: Clinical Applications of Nursing Diagnoses: Adult, Child, Women's, Psychiatric, Gerontic, and Home Health Considerations, ed 4. FA Davis, Philadelphia, 2002.)**

method that does not have to be relearned if the setting, patient's age, or condition changes; having an assessment tool specifically designed to lead to identification of pertinent nursing diagnoses; and having an assessment method that is holistic in nature.[37]

Functional Health Patterns focus on the client's usual ways of living[37] and direct attention to all the factors that impact the individual in these ways of living. Gordon[7] defines a pattern as "a sequence of behavior across time." The Functional Health Patterns allow the nurse to assess

these behaviors by promoting the patient's describing his or her own perception as well as incorporating the nurse's observations. Both the patient's description and the nurse's observations must be included to ensure a complete assessment.

Use of the Functional Health Patterns for assessment allows identification of three major types of data:

1. **Functional patterns:** The functional patterns are client strengths that can be used to deal with either dysfunc-

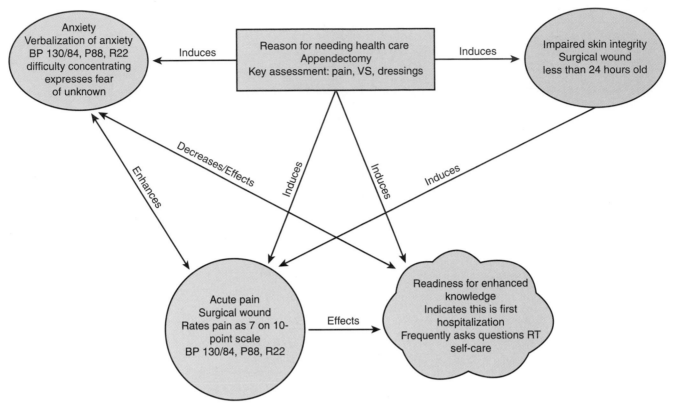

FIGURE 1.3 **Concept map.**

tional or potentially dysfunctional patterns; for example, Assessment of the Coping–Stress Tolerance Pattern shows no problem areas. The nurse can then use this functional pattern to assist the patient in learning to cope with the identified problem areas.

2. **Dysfunctional patterns:** The Dysfunctional Health Patterns identify problem areas and the nursing diagnoses related to each problem area; for example, in assessing the Elimination Pattern, the nurse identified problems with urination and specifically with Urinary Retention. Knowing that the patient has effective individual coping, the nurse then plans teaching that will utilize this strength rather than interventions that are totally nursing focused such as intermittent catheterization. The nurse could teach the patient to use Credé's maneuver, pouring warm water over the genital area, running tap water, and so on to use the client's already demonstrated strength.

3. **Potential dysfunctional patterns:** The Potential Dysfunctional Patterns are risk conditions; for example, a client who has urinary retention is at risk for the development of Excess Fluid Volume. Utilizing this knowledge, the nurse would identify areas of observation to monitor and to teach the patient to monitor.

Use of the Functional Health Patterns in assessment stresses focus on a nursing model of assessment, diagnosis, planning, intervention, and evaluation rather than a medical model. Thus, the nurse can readily differentiate between areas for independent nursing intervention and areas requiring collaboration or referral.

Table 1.3 lists the Functional Health Patterns along with a brief description of each pattern as designed by Gordon.[37] The titles of the patterns are, in essence, self-explanatory. Because the titles are self-explanatory, the Functional Health Patterns are easy to use. The chapters in this book are organized using the Functional Health Patterns and each chapter includes more detail regarding each functional health pattern as introductory information for the specific chapter.

Human Response Patterns

Patterns of Unitary Persons were first presented at the Fourth National Conference of NANDA. A group of nursing theorists met in between, as well as during, conferences to design a framework for classification of nursing diagnoses.[38,39] The NANDA Taxonomy Committee and Special Interest Group on Taxonomy[40] reviewed, clarified, and relabeled the patterns as Human Response Patterns. These revisions were presented at the Fifth and Sixth National Conferences. The patterns proposed by the theorist group describe clustering factors that represent person-environment interaction.[41] The Unitary Persons categories were not mutually exclusive; that is, one nursing diagnosis might relate to one, two, or even three of the patterns. From the Fifth through the Ninth National Conferences, refinement of the Human Response

::: TABLE 1.3 Functional Health Patterns

PATTERN	DESCRIPTION
Health Perception–Health Management	The client's perceived pattern of health and well-being and how health is managed.
Nutritional–Metabolic	Describes pattern of food and fluid consumption relative to metabolic need and pattern indicators of local nutrient supply.
Elimination	Describes pattern of excretory function (bowel, bladder, and skin). Also included are any devices used to control excretion.
Activity–Exercise	Describes pattern of exercise, activity, leisure, and recreation. Includes activities of daily living, requiring energy expenditure. Emphasis is on the activities of high importance or significance and any limitations.
Sleep–Rest	Describes patterns of sleep, rest and relaxation periods during the 24-hour day. Includes client's perception of the quantity and quality of sleep and rest.
Cognitive–Perceptual	Describes sensory-perceptual and cognitive pattern.
Self-Perception and Self-Concept	Describes self-concept pattern and perceptions of mood state.
Role–Relationship	Describes patterns of role engagement and relationships. Includes the individual's perception of the major roles and responsibilities of the current life situation.
Sexuality–Reproductive	Describes patterns of satisfaction-dissatisfaction with sexuality. Describes reproductive pattern.
Coping–Stress Tolerance	General coping pattern and the effectiveness of the pattern in terms of stress tolerance.
Value–Belief	Describes patterns of values, goals, or beliefs (including spiritual) that guide choices or decisions. Includes what is perceived as important to life, quality of life, and any perceived conflicts in values, beliefs, or expectations that are health related.

Source: From Gordon, M: Manual of Nursing Diagnosis. Tenth edition, 2002. CV Mosby, St. Louis, pp 2–5, with permission.

Patterns has continued. At the Seventh National Conference the Human Response Patterns were presented as the framework for NANDA Nursing Diagnosis Taxonomy I,[42] and the taxonomy was endorsed by NANDA members attending this conference. To assist in applying this typology, each diagnosis has information regarding its category and coding place in the Human Response Pattern.

This endorsement indicated acceptance of the Taxonomy I as a working document that would require further testing, revision, refinement, and expansion. Additional input regarding Taxonomy I Revised was solicited at the Eighth National Conference. Much of the discussion at the Eighth Conference focused on the various levels of the taxonomy with specific questions of the clinical usefulness of level I.

The first level of abstraction in Taxonomy I is the Human Response Patterns. The second level is alterations in functions. Levels II through V become increasingly concrete, with levels IV and V reflecting the diagnostic labels. Table 1.4 lists the Human Response Patterns with accompanying brief definitions. In this book we have focused on level II and include levels IV and V in the conceptual information and "Have You Selected the Correct Diagnosis?" sections.

Diagnostic Divisions: Taxonomy II

Following the Twelfth NANDA Conference, the Taxonomy Committee initiated work on Taxonomy II. NANDA members had expressed concerns regarding the ease of use of Taxonomy I Revised and the unclear classification of diagnoses into the taxonomic patterns.

After reviewing multiple taxonomic structures, the Taxonomy Committee voted to use an adaptation of Marjorie Gordon's Functional Health Patterns (FHP) as the basic taxonomic structure for Taxonomy II. The Taxonomy Committee received permission from Dr. Gordon and her publishers to adapt and use the FHP. Table 1.5 demonstrates this new structure.

At the Thirteenth Conference, the proposed Taxonomy II was presented for members' review and discussion. Additionally, members attending the conference participated in a Q-sort project. This project requested the participants to sort the individual nursing diagnoses into the proposed classes and served to validate diagnosis placement.

Subsequent to the Thirteenth Conference, the Taxonomy Committee continued to work on the refinement of Taxonomy II. At the Fourteenth Conference held in April 2000, Taxonomy II was presented to the NANDA mem-

⠿ TABLE 1.4 Human Response Patterns

PATTERN	DESCRIPTION
Exchanging	To give, relinquish, or lose something while receiving something in return; the substitution of one element for another; the reciprocal act of giving and receiving
Communicating	To converse; to impart, confer, or transmit thoughts, feelings, or information, internally or externally, verbally or nonverbally
Relating	To connect, to establish a link between, to stand in some association to another thing, person, or place; to be borne or thrust in between things
Valuing	To be concerned about, to care; the worth or worthiness; the relative status of a thing, or the estimate in which it is held, according to its real or supposed worth, usefulness, or importance; one's opinion of like for a person or thing; to equate in importance
Choosing	To select between alternatives; the action of selecting or exercising preference in regard to a matter in which one is a free agent; to determine in favor of a course; to decide in accordance with inclinations
Moving	To change the place or position of a body or any member of the body; to put and/or keep in motion; to provoke an excretion or discharge; the urge to action or to do something; leave in; to take action
Perceiving	To apprehend with the mind; to become aware of by the senses; to apprehend what is not open or present to observation; to take in fully or adequately
Knowing	To recognize or acknowledge a thing or person; to be familiar with by experience or through information or report; to be cognizant of something through observation, inquiry, or information; to be conversant with a body of facts, principles, or methods of action; to understand
Feeling	To experience a consciousness, sensation, apprehension, or sense; to be consciously or emotionally affected by a fact, event, or state

Source: From Fitzpatrick, JJ: Taxonomy II: Definitions and development. In Carroll-Johnson, RM (ed): Classification of Nursing Diagnosis: Proceedings of the Ninth Conference. Lippincott, Philadelphia, 1991, with permission.

⠿ TABLE 1.5 Taxonomy II: Domains and Classes

DOMAINS AND CLASSES	DESCRIPTION
Domain 1	**Health Promotion:** Diagnoses that refer to the awareness of well-being or normality of function and the strategies used to maintain control of and enhance that well-being or normality of function
Class 1	**Health Awareness:** Recognition of normal function and well-being
Class 2	**Health Management:** Identifying, controlling, performing, and integrating activities to maintain health and well-being
Domain 2	**Nutrition:** Diagnoses that refer to the activities of taking in, assimilating, and using nutrients for the purposes of tissue maintenance, tissue repair, and the production of energy
Class 1	**Ingestion:** Taking food or nutrients into the body
Class 2	**Digestion:** The physical and chemical activities that convert foodstuffs into substances suitable for absorption and assimilation
Class 3	**Absorption:** The act of taking up nutrients through body tissue
Class 4	**Metabolism:** The chemical and physical processes occurring in living organisms and cells for the development and use of protoplasm, production of waste and energy, with the release of energy for all vital processes
Class 5	**Hydration:** The taking in and absorption of fluids and electrolytes
Domain 3	**Elimination/Exchange:** Diagnoses that refer to secretion and excretion of waste products from the body
Class 1	**Urinary System:** The process of secretion and excretion of urine

DOMAINS AND CLASSES	DESCRIPTION
Class 2	*Gastrointestinal System:* Excretion and expulsion of waste products from the bowel
Class 3	*Integumentary System:* Process of secretions and excretion through the skin
Class 4	*Pulmonary System:* Removal of byproducts of metabolic products, secretions, and foreign material from the lung or bronchi
Domain 4	*Activity/Rest:* Diagnoses that refer to the production, conservation, expenditure, or balance of energy resources
Class 1	*Sleep/Rest:* Slumber, repose, ease, or inactivity
Class 2	*Activity/Exercise:* Moving parts of the body (mobility), doing work, or performing actions often (but not always) against resistance
Class 3	*Energy Balance:* A dynamic state of harmony between intake and expenditure of resources
Class 4	*Cardiovascular/Pulmonary Responses:* Cardiopulmonary mechanisms that support activity/rest
Class 5	*Self Care:* Ability to perform activities to care for one's body and bodily functions.
Domain 5	*Perception/Cognition:* Diagnoses that refer to the human information processing system, including attention, orientation, sensation, perception, cognition, and communication
Class 1	*Attention:* Mental readiness to notice or observe
Class 2	*Orientation:* Awareness of time, place, and person
Class 3	*Sensation/Perception:* Receiving information through the senses of touch, taste, smell, vision, hearing, and kinesthesia and the comprehension of sense data resulting in naming, associating, and/or pattern recognition
Class 4	*Cognition:* Use of memory, learning, thinking, problem solving, abstraction, judgment, insight, intellectual capacity, calculation, and language
Class 5	*Communication:* Sending and receiving verbal and nonverbal **information**
Domain 6	*Self-Perception:* Diagnoses that refer to awareness about self
Class 1	*Self-Concept:* Perception(s) about the total self
Class 2	*Self-Esteem:* Assessment of one's own worth, capability, significance, and success
Class 3	*Body Image:* A mental image of one's own body
Domain 7	*Role Relationships:* Diagnoses that refer to the positive and negative connections or associations between persons or groups of persons and the means by which those connections are demonstrated
Class 1	*Caregiving Roles:* Socially expected behavior patterns by persons providing care who are not health-care professionals
Class 2	*Family Relationships:* Associations of people who are biologically related or related by choice
Class 3	*Role Performance:* Quality of functioning in socially expected behavior patterns
Domain 8	*Sexuality:* Diagnoses that refer to sexual identity, sexual function, and reproduction
Class 1	*Sexual Identity:* The state of being a specific person in regard to sexuality and/or gender
Class 2	*Sexual Function:* The capacity or ability to participate in sexual activities
Class 3	*Reproduction:* Any process by which new individuals (people) are produced
Domain 9	*Coping/Stress Tolerance:* Diagnoses that refer to the contending with life events/life processes
Class 1	*Post-Trauma Responses:* Reactions occurring after physical or psychological trauma
Class 2	*Coping Responses:* The process of managing environmental stress
Class 3	*Neurobehavioral Stress:* Behavioral responses reflecting nerve and brain function
Domain 10	*Life Principles:* Diagnoses that refer to principles underlying conduct, thought and behavior about acts, customs, or institutions viewed as being true or having intrinsic worth
Class 1	*Values:* The identification and ranking of preferred modes of conduct or end states
Class 2	*Beliefs:* Opinions, expectations, or judgments about acts, customs, or institutions viewed as being true or having intrinsic worth
Class 3	*Value/Belief/Action Congruence:* The correspondence or balance achieved between values, beliefs, and actions

(table continued on page 20)

⣿ TABLE 1.5 Taxonomy II: Domains and Classes (continued from page 19)

DOMAINS AND CLASSES	DESCRIPTION
Domain 11	**Safety/Protection:** Diagnoses that refer to freedom from danger, physical injury or immune system damage, preservation from loss, and protection of safety and security
Class 1	**Infection:** Host responses following pathogenic invasion
Class 2	**Physical Injury:** Bodily harm or hurt
Class 3	**Violence:** The exertion of excessive force or power so as to cause injury or abuse
Class 4	**Environmental Hazards:** Sources of danger in the surroundings
Class 5	**Defensive Processes:** The processes by which the self protects itself from the nonself
Class 6	**Thermoregulation:** The physiologic process of regulating heat and energy within the body for purposes of protecting the organism
Domain 12	**Comfort:** Diagnoses that refer to the sense of mental, physical, or social well-being or ease
Class 1	**Physical Comfort:** Sense of well-being or ease
Class 2	**Environmental Comfort:** Sense of well-being or ease in/with one's environment
Class 3	**Social Comfort:** Sense of well-being or ease with one's social situations
Domain 13	**Growth/Development:** Diagnoses that refer to age-appropriate increases in physical dimensions, organ systems, and/or attainment of developmental milestones
Class 1	**Growth:** Increases in physical dimensions or maturity of organ systems
Class 2	**Development:** Attainment, lack of attainment, or loss of developmental milestones
Domain 14	**Other:** Diagnoses that are unclassifiable until new categories or classes are developed or old ones are redefined

Source: From North American Nursing Diagnosis Association: NANDA Nursing Diagnoses: Definitions and Classification 2005–2006. NANDA-I, Philadelphia, 2005, with permission.

bership for further consideration. The NANDA Board of Directors approved Taxonomy II following the Fourteenth Conference and additional revision by the Taxonomy Committee.

A unique feature of Taxonomy II is the use of axes. The use of axes simplifies wording structure of the diagnoses, allows a broader use of diagnostic terminology, is more clinically expressive, and promotes inclusion of nursing diagnoses into computerized databases. The proposed axes are illustrated in Table 1.6.

To illustrate the use of the multiaxial structure, this example is provided. A client is assessed at a clinic. The client is a 15-year-old who is 5 ft 2 in tall and weighs 190 lb. The nurse decides the applicable diagnostic concept (Axis 1) is Nutrition. She then chooses a modifier from Axis 6— "Altered" and "More than Body Requirements." The nurse does not add "Adolescent" from the Development Stage Axis (Axis 4) because further assessment documents that the client's entire family (brother, mother, and father) are also above standard weights for their age and height. Therefore, she selects "Family" from Axis 3 (Unit of Care). Because the problem is currently present, the nurse selects "Actual" from the Potentiality Axis (Axis 5). The diagnostic statement then becomes: Actual Altered Nutrition, More than Body Requirements by a Family. Stating the diagnostic statement in this fashion promotes intervention for the whole family, which, in turn, increases the probability of successful intervention for the individual patient.

Additional Taxonomy Development

With the ongoing development of language to describe the whole of nursing practice, NANDA, NIC, and NOC have developed taxonomies to organize their concepts, including human responses, nursing interventions, and nursing outcomes. Since each of these taxonomies represent stages of the nursing process, it is only logical that they be linked to assist the practitioner in the process of care plan development. To facilitate this linking, the NNN Alliance of NANDA-I, NIC, and NOC developed NNN Taxonomy of Nursing Practice. This taxonomy has blended features of each of the parent taxonomies. There are four Domains and 28 Classes[3] (see Table 1.7). In this edition, the authors of this book have provided tables that demonstrate the suggested linkages between NANDA-I,[3] NIC,[4] and NOC.[5] It is important to remember that these linkages are only suggested by NNN, and that the ultimate decisions related to diagnosis, intervention, and outcome area are those of the practitioners who are responsible for providing safe, effective, individualized care to their client systems. Our decision to present the linkages in a chart form, rather than listing the taxonomy designations, was based on the evolving nature of nursing taxonomies and a desire to provide this information to you in

TABLE 1.6 Taxonomic Axes

Axis 1	**Diagnostic Concept:** The nursing diagnosis
Axis 2	**Time:** Acute, Chronic, Intermittent, Continuous
Axis 3	**Subject of the Diagnosis:** Individual, family, community, group
Axis 4	**Age:** Fetus to elder
Axis 5	**Health Status:** Wellness, Risk, Actual
Axis 6	**Descriptor:** A Judgment that limits or specifies the meaning of a nursing diagnosis. (e.g., Ability, Anticipatory, Balance, Compromised, Decreased, Deficient, Defensive, Delayed)
Axis 7	**Topology:** Parts/regions of the body and/or their related functions-all tissues, organs, anatomical sites or structures (e.g., auditory, bowel, cardiopulmonary, gastrointestinal, intracranial, mucous membranes, olfactory, peripheral neurovascular, skin, visual)

Source: From North American Nursing Diagnosis Association: NANDA Nursing Diagnoses: Definitions and Classification 2005–2006. NANDA-I, Philadelphia, 2005, with permission.

a manner that was easily accessible to the care planning process. These tables can be found at the end of the conceptual information in each chapter.

To demonstrate the use of the various taxonomies the young man discussed above will be utilized. As you discovered previously his nursing diagnosis, according to NANDA Taxonomy II would be:

Domain 2 Nutrition
  Class 1 Ingestion
    00001 Imbalanced nutrition: More than body requirements
      The axes would then be added to increase the specificity of the diagnosis.

The NIC interventions, according to the NIC taxonomy for this NANDA diagnosis would be:

Domain I Functional Domain
  Class 2 Nutrition
    Interventions: 1100: Nutrition Management
    1260: Weight Management
    1280: Weight Reduction Assistance

The NOC outcomes measures from the NOC taxonomy would be:

Domain II Physiologic Health
  Class K Nutrition
    Level 3: 1004: Nutritional Status
      1006: Nutritional Status: Body Mass
      1008: Nutritional Status: Food & Fluid Intake
  Domain IV Health Knowledge & Behavior
    Class Q Health Behavior
      Level 3: 1612: Weight Control

Within the NNN Taxonomy for Nursing Practice the label would be:

Domain I Functional
  Class Nutrition

As demonstrated in this example, the flow of care planning across the Taxonomies can be quite cumbersome. Each of the three primary coding systems place related concepts in different categories. The Taxonomy for Nursing

TABLE 1.7 NNN Taxonomy of Nursing Practice

Domain I	**Functional:** Includes diagnoses, outcomes, and interventions to promote basic needs
Class	**Activity/Exercise:** Physical activity, including energy conservation and expenditure
Class	**Comfort:** A sense of emotional, physical, and spiritual well being and relative freedom for distress
Class	**Growth and Development:** Physical, emotional, and social growth and development milestones
Class	**Nutrition:** Processes related to taking in, assimilating, and using nutrients
Class	**Self-Care:** Ability to accomplish basic and instrumental activities of daily living
Class	**Sexuality:** Maintenance or modification of sexual identity and patterns
Class	**Sleep/Rest:** The quantity and quality of sleep, rest, and relaxation patterns
Class	**Values/Beliefs:** Ideas, goals, perceptions, spiritual and other beliefs that influence choices or decisions
Domain II	**Physiological:** Includes diagnoses, outcomes, and interventions to promote optimal biophysical health

(table continued on page 22)

●●● TABLE 1.7   NNN Taxonomy of Nursing Practice (continued from page 21)

Class	**Cardiac Function:** Cardiac mechanisms used to maintain tissue profusion
Class	**Elimination:** Processes related to secretion and excretion of body wastes
Class	**Fluid and Electrolytes:** Regulation of fluid/electrolytes and acid base balance
Class	**Neurocognition:** Mechanisms related to the nervous system and neurocognitive functioning, including memory, thinking, and judgment
Class	**Pharmacological Function:** Effects (therapeutic and adverse) of medications or drugs and other pharmacologically active products
Class	**Physical Regulation:** Body temperature, endocrine, and immune system responses to regulate cellular processes
Class	**Reproduction:** Processes related to human procreation and birth
Class	**Respiratory Function:** Ventilation adequate to maintain arterial blood gasses within normal limits
Class	**Sensation/Perception:** Intake and interpretation of information through the senses, including seeing, hearing, touching, tasting, smelling
Class	**Tissue Integrity:** Skin and mucous membrane protection to support secretion, excretion, and healing
Domain III	**Psychosocial:** Includes diagnoses, outcomes, and interventions to promote optimal mental and emotional health and social functioning
Class	**Behavior:** Actions that promote, maintain, or restore health
Class	**Communication:** Receiving, interpreting, and expressing spoken, written, and nonverbal messages
Class	**Coping:** Adjusting or adapting to stressful events
Class	**Emotional:** A mental state or feeling that may influence perceptions of the world
Class	**Knowledge:** Understanding and skill in applying information to promote, maintain, and restore health
Class	**Roles/Relationships:** Maintenance and/or modification of expected social behaviors and emotional connectedness with others
Class	**Self-Perception:** Awareness of one's body and personal identity
Domain IV	**Environmental:** Includes diagnoses, outcomes, and interventions to promote and protect the environmental health and safety of individuals, systems, and communities
Class	**Health-Care System:** Social, political, and economic structures and processes for the delivery of healthcare services
Class	**Populations:** Aggregates of individuals or communities having characteristics in common
Class	**Risk Management:** Avoidance of identifiable health threats

Source: From North American Nursing Diagnosis Association International: NANDA Nursing Diagnoses: Definitions & Classification 2005–2006. NANDA International, Philadelphia, 2005.

Practice is an attempt to resolve this issue and continues to be developed. Currently, new work of NANDA-I, NIC, and NOC continues to be placed within their unique taxonomic systems. The linking charts in each chapter will help you begin integrating these powerful languages into your nursing vocabulary and practice. To develop further expertise in these nursing languages you are encouraged to review the publications of NANDA-I,[3] NIC,[4] and NOC.[5]

VALUE PLANNING OF CARE AND CARE PLANS

The nursing process and the resultant plan for nursing care have not been given the attention or credit that they deserve. Part of the problem is that planned nursing care has not had value attached to it. All of us will make time or a place for those things that are of value to us. It is only recently that completing and evaluating the quality of care planning has begun to show up on employee evaluation forms. Likewise, it is still rare to see "complete nursing care plan" or "update care plan" on the patient assignment form.

With the changes that are occurring in health care, due to federal and state legislated mandates, completion and use of nursing care planning is going to increase in importance. Several insurance companies now audit charts, care plans, and the like in detail. No documentation of care means no reimbursement for care. Likewise, one of the first places a lawyer looks when hunting evidence for health-related court cases is the patient's chart. The basic principle in lawsuits has been "not charted, not done." Planning care as we propose in this book would furnish additional documentation that reasonably prudent care was given as well as providing a guideline for better charting.

Use of nursing diagnosis helps ensure that teaching and discharge planning are considered from the start of care. As we increase our knowledge and begin to think in terms related to nursing nomenclature, nursing actions for many of the diagnoses will relate to teaching and planning for home care.

Many of the standards supported by JCAHO, the ANA, and state boards of nursing are automatically implemented when the nursing process is completed, implemented, and documented. A review of these standards by the reader will show that the nursing process and careful planning of care can meet several standards just by writing a nursing care plan.

It is not uncommon to hear, "I don't do care plans because I don't have time to do them." It is true that there is an investment of time in completing and documenting the nursing process, but in the long-range view, such planning of care actually saves time. To illustrate, one nurse, known to the authors, works full time in nursing education but works part time at a local hospital to keep her clinical skills current. One afternoon she went to work at the hospital, received her patient assignments and a brief report, and then began to implement patient care. One nursing order read, "Change dressing as needed." Assessment of the dressing showed a change was needed. In the patient's room were all kinds of dressings, fluids, and ointments. There were no instructions for changing the dressing on the care plan or the patient's chart. The nurse then requested information from the patient who stated, "I don't like to look at it, so I don't know." The nurse then began to search for a staff member who had cared for this patient and could teach her the routine for the special dressing change. After 30 minutes, she finally found a nurse who had cared for the patient. Learning the proper dressing change took only a few minutes. The nurse then went back to the care plan, and in 3 minutes recorded the way to change the dressing under nursing orders.

Comparing the time it took to locate the information and the time it took to record the information gives a graphic example of how time can be saved by completing and documenting the nursing process. Consider the time saved if the written nursing actions are used as an outline for charting, or the time that could be saved in between shift reports if documentation of the nursing process was complete. Lastly, consider the time that could be saved by not having to go to court when questions arise over reasonable prudent care. Making time to use and document the nursing process because we can see its value to us actually saves us time in the long run.

SUMMARY

The nursing process provides a strong framework that gives direction to the practice of nursing. By completing each phase, you can reassure yourself that you are providing quality, individualized care that meets local, state, and national standards. By using the NANDA nomenclature and by providing feedback to NANDA, you can help develop this nomenclature and help ensure that nursing is recognized for the contributions it makes to our nation's health.

REFERENCES

1. Ulrich, B: A matter of trust: Public continues to regard nurses highly in honesty and ethics. Nurse Week, Dec. 17, 2001.
2. Beaumont, L: Nurses win public's trust. USA Today, January 8, 2004 www.theage.com.
3. North American Nursing Diagnosis Association International. NANDA Nursing Diagnoses: Definitions and Classification, 2005–2006, NANDA International, Philadelphia, 2005.
4. McCloskey-Dochterman, J, and Bulechek, GM: Nursing Interventions Classification. CV Mosby, St. Louis, 2004.
5. Moorhead, S, Johnson, M, and Mass, M: Nursing Outcomes Classification. CV Mosby, St. Louis, 2004.
6. Gordan, M: Nursing Diagnoses: Process and Application, ed 3. Mosby-Year Book, St. Louis, 1994.
7. Gordon, M: Manual of Nursing Diagnoses. CV Mosby, St. Louis, 2002.
8. Iyer, PW, Taptich, BJ, and Bernocchi-Losey, D: Nursing Process and Nursing Diagnosis, ed. 3. WB Saunders, Philadelphia, 1995.
9. Lunney, M: Critical Thinking and Nursing Diagnosis: Case Studies and Analyses, NANDA, Philadelphia, 2001.
10. Gardner, P: Nursing Process in Action. Thomson Delmar Learning, Clifton Park, NY, 2003.
11. Doenges, ME, and Moorhouse, MF: Nurse's Pocket Guide: Nursing Diagnosis with interventions, ed 6. FA Davis, Philadelphia, 1998.
12. Alfaro, R: Applying Nursing Diagnosis and Nursing Process: A step by step approach. Lippincott-Raven, Philadelphia, 1988.
13. American Nurses Association. Nursing's Social Policy Statement, Washington, DC: nurse books.org, 2003.
14. American Nurses Association: Nursing: Scope and Standards of Practice. American Nurses Association, Silver Spring, MD, 2004.
15. Texas Board of Nurse Examiners: Standards of Nursing Practice. Rule 217.11.2004. Texas Administrative Code Title 22 Part 11 Chapter 217, Austin, Texas, 2004.
16. Brider, P: Who killed the nursing care plan? Am J Nurs 91:35, 1991.
17. Henry, SB, Holzemer, WL, and Reilly, CA: The relationship between type of care planning system and patient outcomes in hospitalized AIDS patients. J Adv Nurs 19:691, 1994.
18. Webster, J: The effect of care planning on quality of patient care. Prof Nurse 14(2):85, 1998.
19. JCAHO: Comprehensive Accreditation Manual for Hospitals; The Official Handbook, Joint Commission Accreditation of Healthcare Organizations, Chicago, 2005.
20. Carroll-Johnson, R: Reflections on the ninth biennial conference. Nurs Diag 1:50, 1991.
21. Kozier, BB, Erb, GH, and Olivieri, R: Fundamentals of Nursing, updated ed 6. Addison-Wesley Nursing, Menlo Park, CA, 2002.
22. Tartaglia, MJ: Nursing diagnosis: Keystone of your care plan. Nursing 15:34, 1985.
23. Kieffer, JS: Nursing diagnosis can make a critical difference. Nursing Life 4:18, 1984.
24. Bolander, VB: Sorensen and Luckmann's Basic Nursing: A Psychophysiologic Approach, ed 3. WB Saunders, Philadelphia, 1994.
25. Cox, HC: Developing Nursing Care Plan Objectives: A Programmed Unit of Study. Texas Tech University Health Sciences Center School of Nursing, Continuing Education Program, Lubbock, TX, 1982.
26. Lampe, S: FOCUS Charting, ed 4. Creative Nursing Management, Minneapolis, MN, 1988.
27. Siegrist, L, Deltor, R, and Stocks, B: The PIE system: Planning and documentation of nursing care. Quality Rev Bull June, 1986
28. Burke, LJ, and Murphy, J: Charting by Exception. John Wiley & Sons, New York, 1988.
29. Schuster, P: Concept Mapping: A critical-thinking approach to care planning, FA Davis, Philadelphia, 2002
30. Schuster, P: Concept maps in clinical settings: Improved clinical performance and effective patient care. Dean's Notes 23(3):1, 2003.
31. Pehler, S, and Bodenbender, K: Concept maps as a tool for learning standardized languages. Int J Nurs Terminol Classif 14(4):39, 2003.

32. All, AC, Huycle, L, and Fisher, M: Instructional tools for nursing education: Concept maps. Nurs Educ Perspect 24(6):311, 2003.
33. Jaco, MK, Gordon, MD, and Marvin, JA: Nursing rounds link nursing diagnoses to clinical practice. Int J Nurs Terminol Classif 14(4):53, 2003.
34. Hsu, L, and Hsieh, S: Concept maps as an assessment tool in a nursing course. J Prof Nurs 21(3):141, 2005.
35. Kataoka-Yahiro, M, and Saylor C: A critical thinking model for nursing judgment. Nurs Educ 33(8):351,1994.
36. Yura, H, and Walsh, MB: The Nursing Process: Assessing, Planning, Implementing, Evaluating, ed 5. Appleton-Century-Crofts, East Norwalk, CT, 1988.
37. Gordon, M: Manual of Nursing Diagnosis: 1995–1996. McGraw-Hill, New York, 1995.
38. Roy, C, Sr: Historical perspective of the theoretical framework for the classification of nursing diagnosis. In Kim, MJ and Moritz, DA (eds): Classification of Nursing Diagnosis: Proceedings of the Third and Fourth National Conferences. McGraw-Hill, New York, 1982, p 235.
39. Roy, C, Sr: Framework for classification system development: Progress and issues. In Kim, MJ, McFarland, GK, and McLane, AM (eds): Classification of Nursing Diagnosis: Proceedings of the Fifth National Conference. McGraw-Hill, New York, 1984, p 29.
40. Kritek, PB: Report of the group who worked on taxonomies. In Kim MJ, McFarland GK and McLane AM (eds): Classification of Nursing Diagnosis: Proceedings of the Fifth National Conference. McGraw-Hill, New York, 1984, p 46.
41. Newman, MA: Looking at the whole. Am J Nurs 84:1496, 1984.
42. North American Nursing Diagnosis Association: Taxonomy I with Complete Diagnoses. Author, St. Louis, 1987.
43. Fitzpatrick, JJ: Taxonomy II: Definitions and development. In Carroll-Johnson, RM (ed): Classification of Nursing Diagnosis: Proceedings of the Ninth Conference. Lippincott, Philadelphia, 1991.

2

HEALTH PERCEPTION–HEALTH MANAGEMENT PATTERN

PATTERN DESCRIPTION

A client's perceived understanding of health and well-being and of how health is managed is a pattern description. It includes the individual's perception of health status and its relevance to current activities and future planning. Also included is the individual's health risk management and general health-care behavior, such as safety practices and adherence to mental and physical health promotion activities, medical or nursing prescriptions, and follow-up care.[1]

PATTERN ASSESSMENT

1. Review the patient's vital signs. Is the temperature within normal limits?
   a. Yes
   b. No (Risk for Infection; Ineffective Protection)
2. Review the results of the complete blood cell (CBC) count. Are the cell counts within normal limits?
   a. Yes
   b. No (Risk for Infection; Ineffective Protection)
3. Review sensory status (sight, hearing, touch, smell, and taste). Is the patient's sensory status within normal limits?
   a. Yes
   b. No (Risk for Injury)
4. Were the patient and family satisfied with the usual health status?
   a. Yes
   b. No (Health-Seeking Behavior; Ineffective Health Maintenance)
5. Did the patient, family, or community describe the usual health status as good?
   a. Yes (Readiness for Enhanced Therapeutic Regimen Management)
   b. No (Health-Seeking Behavior; Ineffective Health Maintenance)
6. Had the patient, family, or community sought any health-care assistance in the past year?
   a. Yes (Health-Seeking Behavior)
   b. No (Ineffective Health Maintenance)
7. Did the patient or family follow the routine the (doctor, nurse, dentist, etc.) prescribed?
   a. Yes (Effective Management of Therapeutic Regimen; Readiness for Enhanced Therapeutic Regimen Management)
   b. No (Noncompliance; Ineffective Management of Therapeutic Regimen; Risk for Sudden Infant Death Syndrome)
8. Did the patient or family have any accidents or injuries in the past year?
   a. Yes (Risk for Injury)
   b. No
9. Is there a disruption (change in temperature, color, field, movement, or sound) of the flow of energy surrounding the person?
   a. Yes (Disturbed Energy Field)
   b. No
10. Was the patient, family, or community able to meet therapeutic needs of all members?
    a. Yes (Effective Management of Therapeutic Regimen [Individual, Family, Community])
    b. No (Ineffective Management of Therapeutic Regimen [Individual, Family, Community])
11. Is the patient scheduled for surgery or has he or she recently undergone surgery?
    a. Yes (Risk for Perioperative-Positioning Injury)
    b. No
12. Does the patient exhibit eczema?
    a. Yes (Latex Allergy Response)
    b. No
13. Does the patient have a history of multiple surgeries or latex reactions?
    a. Yes (Risk for Latex Allergy Response)
    b. No
14. Is the patient's surgical incision healing properly?
    a. Yes
    b. No (Delayed Surgical Recovery)
15. Does the patient express a desire to manage his/her illness?
    a. Yes (Readiness for Enhanced Therapeutic Management)
    b. No

CONCEPTUAL INFORMATION

A person who practices health management techniques, such as exercising regularly, paying attention to diet, and maintaining a balance of rest and activity, has an accurate view of his or her, or his or her family's, personal health status. These individuals can also identify other ways to maintain health, and will be accurate in reporting their current health status. They also readily identify alterations or changes in health status and take active steps to correct these changes to increase their movement toward optimal health. In addition, they will initiate measures to prevent further alterations in health status. The goal of health management is to assist all patients in achieving this level of health maintenance.

Various factors influence a person's ability to achieve optimal health perception (understanding) and health management (control). Martha Rogers describes human beings as energy fields.[2] Disturbance in these fields can produce symptoms. A major factor affecting health is individual and/or family interaction with the environment.[2] Interaction with the environment increases the likelihood that environmental hazards will play a role in health management through an individual's increased exposure to problem areas. Health protection activities can reduce environmental hazards and increase optimal health management. Examples of such activities include individual and community efforts to reduce/eliminate air pollution, ensure a safe water supply, and manage sewage and hazardous waste disposal.

Another major factor affecting health promotion is an intact sensory system. Sensory organs provide information to the individual regarding the environment. An intact nervous system is required because it provides for optimum functioning of sensory, motor, and cognitive activities. An accurate cognitive–perceptual pattern and self-perception/ self-concept pattern are necessary to achieve the optimal level of health perception and management. The ability to think and understand greatly impacts basic knowledge of health and illness. Likewise, the individual's feeling of self-worth and interpretation of the meanings of health and illness to the self, influences his or her health practices. Knowledge related to health promotion and disease prevention is essential for the individual to fully maintain health management.

Cultural, societal, and familial values and beliefs influence the capacity to achieve positive health perception and health management. Values and beliefs influence what is identified as optimal health. Availability of appropriate health-care resources in a community impacts the health-care delivery system and the ability of the community to manage a therapeutic regimen. The development of nursing diagnoses for communities requires nurses to also develop interventions to influence health policy and to work with advocacy groups.[3]

The Health Belief Model[4] (Fig. 2.1) provides a framework in which to study actions taken by individuals to avoid illness. A basic assumption of the model is that the subjective state of the individual is more important in determining actions than the objective reality of the situation. The Health Belief Model states that for an individual to take action to avoid a disease, she or he needs to believe the following:

1. That she or he is personally susceptible to disease.
2. That the occurrence of the disease will have at least a moderate impact on some part of her or his life.
3. That taking action will be beneficial.
4. That such action will not involve overcoming psychological barriers such as cost, pain, or embarrassment.

These beliefs can be described as variables that define perceived benefits and barriers to taking actions under the headings "perceived susceptibility" and "severity." Because these variables do not account for the activation of the behavior, the originators of the Health Belief Model have added another class of variable called "cues to action." The individual's level of readiness provides the energy to act, and the perception of benefits provides a preferred manner of action that offers the path of least resistance. A cue to action is required to set off this appropriate action. The model suggests that by manipulating any combination of variables affecting action, the inclination to seek preventive care can be changed.

The Health Belief Model does not contain concepts related to knowledge of disease as a potential factor in determining an individual's decision to engage in preventive behavior. Several authors point out that knowledge of health consequences has only a limited relationship to the occurrence of the desired health behavior.[5-7] Yet, quite often,

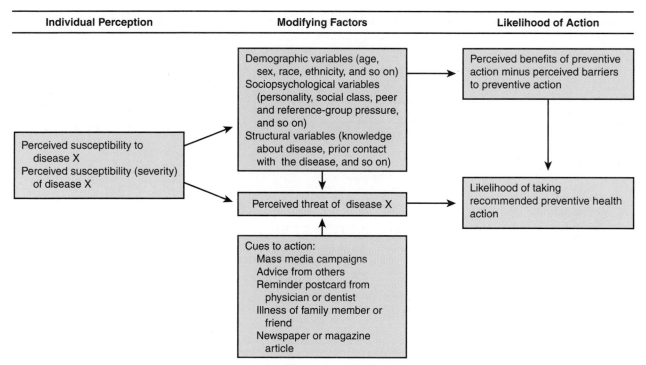

Individual Perception	Modifying Factors	Likelihood of Action

FIGURE 2.1   The Health Belief Model. (From Becker, MH, et al: Selected psychosocial models and corrrelates of individual health-related behaviors, Medical Care 15:27, 1977 [Suppl], with permission.)

imparting knowledge about diseases to the patient, in an effort to encourage future preventive behavior, is the main method used by nurses.

The Health Belief Model is disease specific. The model does not adequately explain positive health actions designed to maximize wellness, fulfillment, and self-actualization. Although the Health Belief Model is useful in predicting preventive behavior, it does not fully explain behavior motivated by health promotion.[8] More research is needed to identify the determinants of health-promoting behavior to increase our ability to assist the patient in achieving health promotion. Preventing energy field disturbances, for example, is an area of research appropriate to nursing practice.

The Health Belief Model provides the nurse with the conceptual notion that by considering the patient's perception of the situation, increasing the patient's cues to action, and decreasing the patient's barriers to action, the nurse can enhance the possibility that the patient will engage in disease prevention and early detection activities.

Pender[8] points out that health promotion and disease prevention are complementary, but very separate, concepts. Health promotion is directed toward growth and improvement in well-being, whereas disease prevention conceptually operates to maintain the status quo.[9]

The Health Promotion Model as developed by Pender[8] (Fig. 2.2) provides the framework for nursing research and practice. This model emphasizes the importance of cogni-tive–perceptual factors in behavior regulation. Cognitive–perceptual factors—for example, understanding of the importance of health, the definition of health, perceived self-competency, and perceived control of health—are primary motivational mechanisms for health-promoting behavior.

Healthy People 2010 (http://www.healthypeople. gov/)[8] describes the national health promotion and disease prevention objectives. Two major goals are addressed:

1. Increase quality and years of healthy life
2. Eliminate health disparities.

The document presents baseline epidemiologic data and projected goals for health promotion, health protection, and preventive services. Special emphasis is placed on vulnerable populations, for example, individuals who are disabled or elderly and those in lower socioeconomic status and certain ethnic groups. This document is recommended as a guide for identifying factors that influence the health perception–health management pattern. Strategies for intervention and evaluation are also included.

Whether working with individuals, families, or communities, the nurse should plan interventions appropriate for the learning needs of those being targeted. Mass media campaigns are useful when conveying general information to large groups of people, but one-to-one communication is more effective for instructing individuals in their particular circumstances. *Put Prevention into Practice* (http://www. ahcpr.gov/clinic/ppipix.htm)[11] is a comprehensive system

FIGURE 2.2 Health Promotion Model. (From Pender, NJ: Health Promotion in Nursing Practice, ed 3. Appleton-Century-Crofts, Stamford, CT, 1996, p 58, with permission.)

that was developed to assist the clinician, and the patient and his or her family, to establish a routine of preventive behaviors and services. The kit includes a clinician's handbook, preventive care timelines, office reminders, and patient-oriented materials to promote preventive behaviors.

The concepts of primary, secondary, and tertiary prevention[11] are also useful to the nurse when using the health management pattern. It is important for the nurse to recognize that a focus on the patient's strengths, not just his or her problems, is an integral part of health promotion.[12,13]

Primary prevention consists of activities that prevent a disease from occurring. A patient engaged in primary prevention activities would:

1. Maintain up-to-date immunizations.
2. Have adequate water supply and sanitation facilities.
3. Use seat belts and infant car seats, and properly store household poisons to minimize accident fatalities.
4. Eliminate tobacco products.
5. Maintain adequate nutrition, elimination, exercise, social, and personal relationships, etc.
6. Practice good oral hygiene and receive dental examinations on a regular basis.
7. Avoid excessive sun exposure and use sunscreens and protective clothing.
8. Maintain weight within normal range for age, sex, and height.
9. Maintain an environment free of chemical, biologic, and physical hazards.
10. Maintain regular sleep and rest patterns.
11. Practice healthy nutritional intake (i.e., low amounts of salt, sugar, and fat; follow food pyramid recommendations for daily servings per food group and total calories as appropriate for age, sex, and condition).
12. Maintain regular relaxation, recreation, and exercise activities.

Secondary prevention indicates activities designed to detect disease before symptoms are recognized. Screening activities are the most common type of secondary prevention activities and include:

1. Diabetes screening
2. Glaucoma screening
3. Hypertension screening
4. Hearing and vision testing
5. Pap smears
6. Breast examinations
7. Prostate and testicle examinations
8. Well-baby examinations
9. Colon and rectal examinations

Tertiary prevention refers to the treatment, care, and rehabilitation of current illness. This area indicates the patient needs to:

1. Adhere to medical and nursing treatments.
2. Make lifestyle changes necessitated by condition.

3. Seek consultation from experts in area requiring intervention, for example, individual practitioners and support groups.

DEVELOPMENTAL CONSIDERATIONS

Health-care providers can encourage the acceptance of responsibility for health-promoting activities and adherence to agreed-upon treatment plans by giving appropriate attention to the impact developmental levels have on the individual or the primary caregiver. Publications such as *Put Prevention into Practice*[11,15] can assist the nurse, patient, family, and community in establishing a routine of health-promoting behaviors and practices. The US Administration on Aging (AoA) offers many publications and programs to support the healthy aging of older Americans (http://www.aoa.gov/). One of the programs of the AoA, *You Can! Steps to Healthier Aging*, provides specific suggestions and activities for older adults to stay active and healthy (http://www.aoa.gov/youcan/youcan.asp).

INFANT AND TODDLER

Because the neonate is totally dependent on others for care, it is the primary caregiver who is entrusted with carrying out the therapeutic interventions. As the infant grows and develops, self-care abilities increase. The following information outlines developmental milestones from birth to approximately 24 months, as described by Piaget's sensorimotor stage of cognitive development.[14] During this period of development, the individual must be protected from hazards in the environment, and the primary caregiver must assume the major share of responsibility for compliance with the treatment program.

Providing a safe environment includes the following accident prevention strategies:

1. Placing infants to sleep on their back ("back to sleep")
2. Minimizing prenatal and postnatal infant smoke exposure
3. Avoiding overwrapping or overheating of infants
4. Early and regular prenatal care for expectant mothers
5. Turning pot handles away from edge of stove
6. Storing medicines, matches, alcohol, plastic bags, and house and garden chemicals in child-proofed areas
7. Using a cold-water, not a hot-water, humidifier
8. Avoiding heating formula in microwave
9. Using protection screens on heaters, fireplaces, and electrical outlets
10. Using nonflammable clothing
11. Gating stairways and windows
12. Supervising children at play, while bathing, in car, or in shopping cart
13. Controlling pets or stray animals
14. Avoiding items hung around neck
15. Providing a smoke-free environment

16. Avoiding small objects that can be inserted in mouth or nose
17. Avoiding pillows and plastic in crib
18. Removing poisonous plants from house and garden
19. Removing lead-based paint from the home

Children should be screened at birth for congenital anomalies, phenylketonuria (PKU), thyroid function, cystic fibrosis, vision impairment, and hearing deficiency. A newborn assessment should be performed, and anticipatory guidance should be provided for patients regarding growth and development, safety, health promotion, and disease prevention.

Well-baby examinations and developmental assessments are recommended at 2, 4, 6, 15, and 18 months.[11,16–18] Height and weight should be recorded on growth charts, and hemoglobin and hematocrit should be checked at least once during infancy. Parent counseling includes discussion of nutrition with attention paid to iron-rich foods; safety and accident prevention; oral, perineal and perirectal hygiene; sensory stimulation of the infant; baby-bottle tooth decay; and the effects of passive smoking. Immunizations are given during the well-baby checks according to the following schedule[19,20]:

1. Hepatitis B-1 at birth to 2 months
2. Hepatitis B-2 at 1 to 4 months
3. DTaP (diphtheria and tetanus toxoids and acellular pertussis) or DTP (diphtheria, tetanus toxoids, and pertussis), HiB (*Haemophilus influenzae* type B), pneumococcal conjugate (PCV), and polio at 2 and 4 months
4. DTaP, CPV, and HiB at 6 months
5. Hepatitis B-3 and polio at 6 to 18 months
6. HiB at 12 to 15 months[20–23]
7. MMR (measles, mumps, and rubella), varicella, PCV, and tuberculin test at 12 to 18 months
8. DTaP or DTP at 15 to 18 months
9. PCV at 2 to 5 years
10. DTaP or DTP, polio, and MMR at 4 to 6 years
11. Hepatitis B, Td (tetanus and diphtheria toxoid), MMR, and varicella at 11 to 12 years[23]

For children who have not been immunized during the first year of life, you will need to consult the latest established standards for appropriate timetables.[19,24] Hepatitis B vaccine (HBv) should be given at birth, 2 to 4 months, and 6 to 18 months.[19,24] HBv can be administered at the same time as DTP and/or *Haemophilus influenzae* type B conjugate vaccine (HibCV).[24] The Centers for Disease Control and Prevention recommends yearly administration of influenza vaccine beginning at age 6 months (2005).[25–27]

Host factors such as age and behavior affect the susceptibility to infectious disease. In general, most infectious diseases produce the greatest morbidity and mortality in the very old and the very young (http://www.cdc.gov/nip/vaccine/tdap/tdap_adult_recs.pdf).[26,28] It is also important to note that the normal newborn has a white blood cell count that is higher than that of the normal adult. The normal white blood cell count decreases gradually throughout childhood until reaching the adult norms.[27,28] It is essential that the nurse be very familiar with the blood cell count norms for this age group.

During fetal life, maternal antibodies (assuming the mother has developed them) protect the fetus from diseases such as diphtheria, tetanus, measles, and polio. This temporary immunity lasts 3 to 6 months. Colostrum contains antibodies that provide protection against enteric pathogens. Some infections can cross the placental barrier, leading to the development of congenital (present at birth) infections. Syphilis, human immunodeficiency virus (HIV), and rubella are examples of such infections. Pathogenic organisms such as herpes simplex may be acquired during passage through the birth canal. Because infants do not begin to produce immunoglobulins until 2 to 3 months after birth, they are susceptible to infections for which they have not gained passive immunity.

Infections can be of serious concern during the perinatal period, especially TORCH infections (**T**oxoplasmosis, **H**epatitis B, **R**ubella, **C**ytomegalovirus, **H**erpes). Other infections such as *Chlamydia,* group B *Streptococcus,* syphilis, HIV, and acquired immunodeficiency syndrome (AIDS) are also of great concern as all of these infections have consequences for not only the pregnancy, but also the newborn.[29] When caring for a pregnant woman or a newborn, it is important to teach techniques to prevent acquisition and transmission of these disorders and to recognize early signs and symptoms so that early interventions can be instituted. For newborns, the HBv series should be initiated at birth before discharge from the hospital.[20–24,26]

Child-care practices must include hygienic disposal of soiled diapers and cleaning of the perineum. Proper handwashing techniques are required of the care provider. Proper formula preparation and storage are also critical if the newborn is to be bottle-fed. Anatomically, the eustachian tube of the newborn and infant facilitates the passage of infection-causing organisms into the middle ear. It is important for care providers not to prop bottles, but rather to hold the newborn or infant while feeding. Passive exposure to tobacco smoke irritates the bronchial tree and increases the possibility of respiratory infection.

The infant may respond to an infection with a very high fever. Care providers should be taught how to do the following: take axillary or tympanic temperatures, provide hydration to an ill infant, give tepid baths when fever is elevated, and seek professional evaluation when an infant has a febrile illness.

TODDLER AND PRESCHOOLER

During the preoperational period, children learn how to teach themselves through trial and error, exploration, and repetition. From age 2 to 4 years, the child is egocentric, using him- or herself as a standard for others; he or she can categorize on the basis of a single characteristic. Because of the child's curiosity and exploration of the environment, it is important for the care provider to provide a safe environment. During this period the words "no," "hot," "sharp," and "hurt" should be introduced and repeatedly reinforced by the care provider. Safety rules should also be taught and reinforced repeatedly.

From ages 4 to 7 years, the child can begin to see simple relationships and is developing the ability to think in logical classes. The child can learn his or her own address and can follow directions of three steps. Rules need to be reinforced. The child can be responsible for personal hygiene with instruction and coaching.

Strategies used to provide a safe environment for the infant should also be used during childhood. Discipline, accident prevention, and the development of self-care proficiency related to eating, dressing, bathing, and dental hygiene are important areas of concern. Developmental assessments with emphasis on hearing, vision, and speech are recommended. DPT or DTaP, and OPV (oral polio vaccine) or IPV (inactivated polio vaccine) are given once between 4 and 6 years of age, at or before school entry. Consult guidelines if the child has not been immunized during the first year of life.[19–24] The Immunizations Practices Advisory Committee (ACIP) of the U.S. Public Health Service[30] recommends that a second dose of MMR be given at 4 to 5 years of age, when the child enters kindergarten.

Anticipatory guidance should be given to parents on the development of initiative and guilt, nutrition and exercise, safety and accident prevention, toothbrushing and dental care, effects of passive smoking, and skin protection from ultraviolet light.[17] In addition, the parents should be taught that, as the child begins to explore the environment and put objects and foods into his or her mouth, it will be important to ensure that contact with infectious pathogens or foreign bodies is controlled. Foreign-object-induced infection should be considered in childhood infections of the external ear, nose, and vagina.

If the preschooler has been exposed to other children, he or she most likely will have experienced several middle ear, gastrointestinal, and upper respiratory tract infections. If the child has not been around other children, he or she will likely experience such infections when entering preschool or kindergarten. Preventing injury will also assist in the prevention of infection. The adenoidal and tonsillar lymphoid tissue may normally enlarge during the early school years, partly in response to the exposure to pathogens in school.

The child will require assistance with toileting hygiene until 4 to 5 years of age. Handwashing techniques can be introduced along with toilet training and followed with consistent role modeling by the adults and older children who provide assistance to the child. Bubble baths and other scented soaps and toilet tissue may irritate the urethra in the female child and lead to urinary tract or vaginal infections. Parents, grandparents, other caregivers, and the child should be taught to avoid such items. In addition, proper dental hygiene can be taught to the child to help prevent tooth and gum infections.

SCHOOL-AGE CHILD

This period is characterized by developing logical approaches to concrete problems. The concepts of reversibility and conservation are developed, and the child can organize objects and events into classes and arrange them in order of increasing values. The child can be responsible for personal hygiene and simple household tasks. The child will need assistance when ill, but he or she can be taught self-care activities as required, such as insulin injections or taking medications on a regular basis. The child can distinguish and describe physical symptoms and report them to the appropriate caregiver, and he or she can follow instructions.

Strategies used by care providers to establish a safe environment, prevent disease, and promote health can be taught to the child. The child can perform many of these functions with supervision. Emphasis is placed on health education of the child in safety and accident prevention, nutrition, substance abuse, and anticipated changes with puberty. Anticipatory guidance for both the parents and the child should include the development of industry and avoidance of inferiority. A preadolescent immunization status check is recommended at 11 to 12 years of age.[20,21] Hepatitis B vaccine is recommended for those who did not receive the vaccine as a child. Screening of high-risk groups for tuberculosis is recommended.[11]

ADOLESCENT

True logical thought is developed and abstract concepts can be manipulated by individuals at this developmental level. A scientific approach to problem solving can be planned and implemented. The adolescent can develop, with guidance, responsibility for total self-care. With experience, the adolescent requires less guidance and can assume full decision-making responsibility and total responsibility for self-care.

Emphasis should be placed on health education of the adolescent in healthy living habits, safe driving, sex education, skin care, substance abuse, career choices, relationships, dating and marriage, breast self-examination for female adolescents, and testicular self-examination for male adolescents. Screening for pregnancy, sexually transmitted diseases, depression, high blood pressure, and substance abuse can be done. Anticipatory guidance should be given to parents and adolescents about the development of identity, role confusion, and formal operational thought.[17]

The hormonal changes of puberty may lead to acne vulgaris. If severe, proper hygiene and dermatologic evaluation will prevent serious complications. The changes in the vaginal tissue secondary to hormonal changes provide an environment conducive to yeast infections. If the adolescent is engaging in sexual activity, he or she is at risk for exposure to sexually transmitted diseases. Irritants such as soap and bubble bath may increase the possibility of urinary tract infection in female adolescents. Improper genital hygiene also predisposes the female adolescent to urinary tract infections.

Persons born after 1956 who lack evidence of immunity to measles should receive the MMR vaccine.[20,30] The MMR vaccine should not be given during pregnancy. Individuals susceptible to mumps should be vaccinated as well.[25,31] A diphtheria and tetanus vaccination (Td) should be given at 14 to 16 years of age. Hepatitis B vaccines should be given to anyone who did not receive immunizations as a child.[21] Screening of high-risk groups for tuberculosis is recommended.[11] Adolescents living in a group setting, such as a dormitory, have an increased risk of contracting a communicable disease. Good personal hygiene is important to decrease this risk.

Meningococcal vaccine is recommended for all children at their routine preadolescent visit (11 to 12 years of age). For those who have not previously received the meningitis vaccine, a dose is recommended on entry to high school. Other adolescents who want to decrease their risk of meningococcal disease can also get the vaccine. Other people at increased risk, for whom routine vaccination is recommended, are college freshmen living in dormitories.[32]

Risk-taking behavior of adolescents[32] may increase the risk of infection and accidents. Examples of these risk-taking behaviors include sexual intercourse; IV drug use; use of alcohol and tobacco; traumatic injury, tattooing or body piercing, that breaks the skin, allowing a portal of entry for pathogenic organisms; fad diets or other activities that decrease the overall health status; improper technique or equipment in water sports; motor vehicle accidents; running a vehicle or other combustion engines when not properly ventilated; substance abuse; choking on food; smoke inhalation; improper storage and handling of guns, ammunition, and knives; smoking in bed; improper use or storage of flammable items, hazardous tools, and equipment; drug ingestion; playing or working around toxic vegetation; improper preparation and storage of food; and improper precautions and use of insecticides, fertilizers, cleaning products, medications, alcohol, and other toxic substances.

ADULT

Adult thought is more refined than adolescent thought because experience and education allow the adult to differentiate among many points of view and potential outcomes in an objective and realistic manner. The adult can consider more options and can apply inductive, as well as deductive, approaches to problem solving. The adult assumes total responsibility for the care of a child. In middle adult years, the adult may also care for an elderly parent.

The adult is concerned about many of the same health promotion and disease prevention issues the adolescent worries about. Emphasis should be placed on lifestyle counseling related to family planning, parenting, stress management, career advancement, relationship enhancement, hazards at work, and development of intimacy and generativity.

Regular breast self-examination (women) and testicular self-examination (men) should be taught and encouraged. Women should have a baseline mammogram at age 35 and all women 40 and above should have a clinical breast exam and mammogram annually. Women should be advised to have Pap smears every 1 to 2 years, or more often as recommended by their primary care provider. Screening for glaucoma; high blood pressure; high blood cholesterol level; rubella antibodies; sexually transmitted diseases; and colon, endometrial, oral, or breast cancer should be done if the patient is in a risk category.

As the body develops more antibodies to pathogens, adults may find that they do not have as many colds as they used to. Some viral infections (e.g., mumps) may present serious consequences to adults (particularly men in the case of mumps). The adult female is as susceptible to genitourinary infections as the adolescent. Sexually active adults are at risk for sexually transmitted diseases.

Tetanus-diphtheria (Td) boosters should be given every 10 years. Hepatitis B vaccine should be given to people at risk for exposure. Remember, persons born after 1956 who lack evidence of immunity to measles should receive the MMR vaccine, but the MMR vaccine should not be given during pregnancy. Individuals susceptible to mumps should be vaccinated. Pneumococcal and influenza vaccines are recommended annually, especially for persons at risk for acquiring the flu, and for persons at risk for complications from infection.[25] Advanced age; conditions associated with decline in antibody levels; Native American ethnicity; and institutional settings such as military training camps, correctional facilities, and boardinghouses all are identified as risk factors[33–35] for the development of pneumonia and influenza. Tuberculosis screening of high-risk populations is recommended.[11]

OLDER ADULT

In the absence of illness affecting cognitive functioning, the older adult maintains formal operational abilities. The older adult can assume total responsibility for decision making and self-care. The older adult also often assumes responsibility for the care of others, such as a spouse, child, or grandchild. As with other developmental levels, illness or physical disability can alter the cognitive functioning and lead to self-care deficits.

Emphasis is on health education related to retirement, safety in the home, medication use, living with chronic illness, and grandparenting.[36] Anticipatory guidance is related to the development of ego integrity. The importance of regularly scheduled breast self-examinations, Pap smears, mammography (women), and testicular self-examination (men) should be taught and the practices encouraged. Glaucoma, blood pressure, cholesterol, and colon cancer screenings should also be done.[37] Podiatry care should be given as needed. Tetanus-diphtheria (Td) boosters; hepatitis B and A vaccines; and pneumonia, and varicella immunizations are given according to the same conditions discussed in the adult health section.[38,39] Older adults, who are often at risk for serious complications resulting from influenza infection, should have an annual influenza immunization.[25]

The influenza vaccine should be given annually both to people 65 and older and to younger people in high-risk groups. The pneumococcal vaccine should be given one time to people 65 years of age or older and to younger people in high-risk groups. If the older adult is at very high risk for pneumococcal infection, the vaccine may be given again 6 years after the initial immunization.[38,39] Although the worldwide incidence of tetanus is decreasing, older adults remain more susceptible to the disease. Tuberculosis cases in the United States remain disproportionately distributed in the older population and in people with acquired immunity diseases.[40]

The inability to achieve adult immunization recommendations is a serious problem in the United States. It is estimated that only 58 percent of adults age 65 and older receive the influenza vaccine, and only 35 percent receive the pneumococcal vaccine.[10] This number is markedly decreased for older Hispanic and African American adults.[10] To improve vaccination coverage of older adults, the National Guidelines Clearinghouse guidelines (http://www.guideline.gov) recommends interventions to enhance access to vaccination services, provider or system based interventions, and interventions in increase client demand for vaccination services. Interventions to enhance access to vaccination services for older adults include expanded access to vaccinations in health-care settings and reducing the client's out-of-pocket costs for vaccinations. Provider or system based interventions include provision of standing orders for clients when indicated, provider reminder systems, and provider assessment and feedback. Interventions to increase client demand for vaccination services include client reminder systems and client education.

Older adults may have a decreased ability to remove themselves from hazardous situations as a result of changes in mobility. Olfactory alterations may lead to an inability to smell smoke or gas fumes.[40] The risk for injury and increases in self-care deficits may result from sensory, motor, or perceptual difficulties.

Age-related changes in the immune system can lead to increased severity and number of infections in the older adult.[38–40] Physical aging changes in the skin, respiratory, gastrointestinal tract, and genitourinary system can lead to increases in infection. Skin breakdown due to epidermal thinning and decreased skin elasticity, less effective coughing, diminished gag reflex, decreased gastrointestinal motility, and urinary stasis can be problematic for the older adult with a less efficient immune system. Changes in the number and maturity of T-lymphocyte cells lead to decreased ability of the body to destroy infectious organisms. B-lymphocyte cells, producing immunoglobulins, are less efficient in the presence of fewer and weaker T cells.[38,41]

Older adults with chronic illnesses who are hospitalized or who are in a nursing home are at increased risk for infection. When assessing older adults for infection, it is important for the nurse to realize that the signs of infection can be altered with aging. With the aging-related changes of the immune system, and problems with temperature regulation, it is not unusual for seriously ill older adults to be afebrile while suffering from an infection. Atypical symptoms leading the nurse to suspect infection in the older adult include mental status changes, anorexia, functional decline, fatigue, falls, and new or worsened urinary incontinence.[40–43]

▪▪▪ TABLE 2.1 NNN Taxonomy Linkages

GORDON'S FUNCTIONAL HEALTH PATTERN	NANDA NURSING DIAGNOSIS	NIC PRIORITY INTERVENTIONS	NOC EVALUATIONS
Health Perception/Health Management Pattern	Energy Field Disturbed	Therapeutic Touch	Personal Health Status Personal Well-Being Spiritual Health
	Health Maintenance, Ineffective	Health System Guidance Support System Enhancement	Health Belief: Perceived Resources Health-Promoting Behavior Health-Seeking Behavior Knowledge: Health Behavior; Health Promotion; Health Resources; Treatment Regime Participation in Health-Care Decisions Personal Health Status Risk Detection Self-Care Status Student Health Status

(table continued on page 34)

TABLE 2.1 **NNN Taxonomy Linkages** (continued from page 33)

GORDON'S FUNCTIONAL HEALTH PATTERN	NANDA NURSING DIAGNOSIS	NIC PRIORITY INTERVENTIONS	NOC EVALUATIONS
	Health-Seeking Behaviors (specify)	Health Education Self-Modification Assistance	Adherence Behavior Health Beliefs Health Orientation Health-Promoting Behavior Health-Seeking Behavior Knowledge: Health Promotion Knowledge: Health Resources Personal Well-Being
	Infection, Risk for	Immunization/Vaccination Management Infection Control Infection Protection	Aspiration Prevention Community Risk Control: Communicable Disease Health Beliefs Hemodialysis Access Immobility Consequences: Physiological Immune Status Immunization Behavior Infection Severity Infection Severity: Newborn Knowledge: Infection Control; Treatment Procedure(s) Nutritional Status Risk Control Risk Control: Sexually Transmitted Diseases (STD) Risk Detection Self-Care; Hygiene Tissue Integrity: Skin and Mucous Membranes Treatment Behavior: Illness or Injury Wound Healing: Primary Intention Wound Healing: Secondary Intention
	Injury, Risk for	Electronic Fetal Monitoring: Intrapartum Fall Prevention Labor Induction Latex Precautions Malignant Hyperthermia Precautions	Abuse Protection Allergic Response: Systemic Aspiration Prevention Balance Blood Glucose Level Blood Loss Severity Coordinated Movement Fall Prevention Behavior Falls Occurrence Knowledge: Body Mechanics; Child Safety; Fall Prevention; Personal Safety Maternal Status: Postpartum Parenting: Infant/Toddler, Early/Middle Childhood Physical Safety; Psychosocial Safety Personal Safety Behavior

GORDON'S FUNCTIONAL HEALTH PATTERN	NANDA NURSING DIAGNOSIS	NIC PRIORITY INTERVENTIONS	NOC EVALUATIONS
			Physical Injury Severity
			Risk Control
			Risk Control: Hearing or Visual Impairment
			Risk Detection
			Safe Home Environment
			Seizure Control
			Self-Care Status
	Latex Allergy Response	Allergy Management Latex Precautions	Allergic Response: Localized
			Immune Hypersensitivity Response
			Tissue Integrity: Skin and Mucous Membranes
	Therapeutic Regimen Management, Effective	Anticipatory Guidance Health System Guidance	Adherence Behavior
			Compliance Behavior
			Family Participation in Professional Care
			Knowledge: Treatment Regime
			Participation in Health-Care Decisions
			Risk Control
			Symptom Control
			Treatment Behavior: Illness or Injury
	Therapeutic Regimen Management, Ineffective	Behavior Modification Self-Modification Assistance	Compliance Behavior
			Knowledge: Diet; Treatment Regimen
			Participation in Health Care Decisions
			Symptom Control
			Treatment Behavior: Illness or Injury
	Therapeutic Regimen Management, Readiness for Enhanced	* still in development	Adherence Behavior
			Compliance Behavior
			Family Participation in Professional Care
			Knowledge: Treatment Regimen
			Participation in Health-Care Decisions
			Risk Control
			Symptom Control
			Treatment Behavior: Illness or Injury
	Perioperative Positioning, Injury, Risk for	Positioning: Intraoperative Skin Surveillance	Allergic Response: Systemic
			Aspiration Prevention
			Blood Coagulation
			Blood Loss Severity
			Circulation Status
			Cognition
			Cognitive Orientation
			Fluid Overload Severity
			Immune Status
			Medication Response
			Neurologic Status: Spinal Sensory/ Motor Function
			Respiratory Status: Gas Exchange; Ventilation
			Risk Control
			Risk Detection
			Thermoregulation

(table continued on page 36)

::: TABLE 2.1 NNN Taxonomy Linkages (continued from page 35)

GORDON'S FUNCTIONAL HEALTH PATTERN	NANDA NURSING DIAGNOSIS	NIC PRIORITY INTERVENTIONS	NOC EVALUATIONS
	Protection, Ineffective	Electronic Fetal Monitoring: Intrapartum Environmental Management: Violence Prevention Infection Control Infection Protection Post-Anesthesia Care Surgical Precautions Surveillance: Safety	Tissue Integrity: Skin and Mucous Membranes Tissue Perfusion: Peripheral Abuse Protection Community Violence Level Health Beliefs: Perceived Ability to Perform Health-Promoting Behavior Immune Status Immunization Behavior Knowledge: Personal Safety Personal Autonomy
	Sudden Infant Death Syndrome, Risk for	*still in development	Knowledge: Infant Care; Parenting Parenting: Infant/Toddler Physical Safety Parenting Performance Prenatal Health Behavior Preterm Infant Organization Risk Control Risk Control: Tobacco Use Risk Detection Thermoregulation: Newborn
	Surgical Recovery, Delayed	Incision Site Care Nutrition Management Pain Management Self-Care Assistance	Ambulation Blood Loss Severity Endurance Fluid Overload Severity Hydration Immobility Consequences: Physiological Infection Severity Nausea and Vomiting Severity Pain Level Post Procedure Recovery Status Self-Care: ADL Wound Healing: Primary Intention

*Linkages to these concepts are not present in current NANDA, NIC, and/or NOC literature.

 APPLICABLE NURSING DIAGNOSES

ENERGY FIELD, DISTURBED

DEFINITION[44]

A disruption of the flow of energy surrounding a person's being that results in disharmony of the body, mind, and/or spirit.

DEFINING CHARACTERISTICS[44]

Perceptions of changes in patterns of energy flow such as:

1. Movement (wave, spike, tingling, dense, flowing)
2. Sounds (tone, words)
3. Temperature change (warmth, coolness)
4. Visual changes (image, color)
5. Disruption of the field (deficit, hole, spike, bulge, obstruction, congestion, diminished flow in energy field)

RELATED FACTORS[44]

Slowing or blocking of energy flows secondary to:

1. Pathophysiologic factors (illness, pregnancy, injury)
2. Situational factors: personal or environmental (pain, fear, anxiety, grieving)
3. Treatment related factors (immobility, labor and delivery, perioperative experience, chemotherapy)

4. Maturational factors (age related developmental difficulties or crisis—specify)

RELATED CLINICAL CONCERNS

1. Chronic or catastrophic illness
2. Trauma
3. Autoimmune deficiency syndrome
4. Insomnia
5. Chronic fatigue syndrome
6. Cancer or chemotherapy
7. Recent surgery
8. Sensory or perceptual disorders
9. Pain
10. Birthing process (labor and delivery)

 Have You Selected the Correct Diagnosis?

Fatigue
For this diagnosis, the client will report exhaustion and lack of energy. Assessment will document an overall reduction of energy, not a disruption of energy.

Activity Intolerance
The client will relate, via interview, specific activities that cannot be accomplished. Specific physical findings, such as abnormal pulse and respiration rates, will be present during activity.

Ineffective Thermoregulation
This diagnosis relates to temperature fluctuations only. Energy field disruption demonstrates other defining characteristics in addition to temperature change.

Disturbed Sleep Pattern
A problem in the sleep–rest pattern could result in alterations in the energy field. Interviewing the person regarding sleep habits will assist in clarifying whether the primary diagnosis is Disturbed Sleep Pattern or Disturbed Energy Field.

Disturbed Sensory Perception
Determining the person's orientation to time and place; his or her ability to discern objects in the environment via vision, touch, sound, or smell; and his or her problem-solving abilities will assist in distinguishing Disturbed Energy Field from Disturbed Sensory Perception.

Pain
Observing for signs and symptoms of pain (facial mask, guarding behavior, moaning, or crying) will distinguish Pain from Disturbed Energy Field.

EXPECTED OUTCOME

Assessment will demonstrate a consistent energy field by [date].

Client verbalizes an improvement in their sense of well-being by [date].

NURSING ACTIONS/INTERVENTIONS WITH RATIONALES

Adult Health

ACTIONS/INTERVENTIONS	RATIONALES
Establish trusting relationship with the patient.	Promotes accurate assessment.
Allow the patient to talk about condition.	Promotes nurse–patient relationship.
Assess energy field.	Alterations, variations, and/or asymmetry in the energy field are detected through assessment.[45]
Center self:	Promotes accurate assessment.
• Imagine self as open system with energy flow content in, through, and out of the system.	
• Consciously quiet your mind; put aside or detach from inward and outward distractions.	
• Focus full attention and *intention* on *helping* patient.	
Assess for heat or tingling over specific body areas:	
• Glide hands, palm down, and slowly move over body, head to toe, 2 to 4 inches above body.	
Be sensitive to any images that come to mind: words, symbols, pictures, colors, sound, mood, emotion, etc.[46]	There may be a loss of energy, disruption or blockage in the flow of energy, or an accumulation of energy in a part of the body.[47]
Attempt to get a sense of the dynamics of the energy field. Synthesize assessment data into an understandable format.	

(care plan continued on page 38)

NURSING ACTIONS/INTERVENTIONS WITH RATIONALES (continued from page 37)

Adult Health

ACTIONS/INTERVENTIONS	RATIONALES
Redirect areas of accumulated energy, reestablish the energy flow, and direct energy to depleted areas. Repattern or rebalance patient's energy field.	Energy transfer or transformation can occur without direct physical contact between two systems.[45] Hands are focal points for the direction and modulation of energy.[45]
Do therapeutic touch for no longer than 10 minutes.	Could disrupt the energy field of the therapist.
Assess the patient's subjective reaction to therapeutic touch. Patient should feel more relaxed, less anxious, and less pain (if there were complaints of pain prior to therapeutic touch).	Nurse acts as a conduit through which the environmental or universal energy passes to the patient.[45,46]
Teach the patient relaxation exercises using some of the same techniques as therapeutic touch: • Assist the patient to center self. • Teach the patient to imagine a peaceful place. Help the patient to visualize place through all the senses and to allow the energy of the imagined place to bring about a state of calmness. • Teach the patient to scan his or her body to self-assess areas of body or muscle tension. • Assist the patient to consciously relax that tense area of the body. • Practice relaxation at least 10 to 20 minutes a day.	Relaxation requires the patient to stop trying and to step outside of self and adopt a nontrying attitude. This allows the person to release and use the inherent energy of self.[46] Rebalances energy flow through the body.[46]

Child Health

ACTIONS/INTERVENTIONS	RATIONALES
Monitor for reciprocity of maternal–infant dyad.	Provides assessment for causative factors and the mutuality or responsiveness between infant and caregiver. *Consider potential effects of medications as antiseizure meds.
Identify developmentally appropriate parameters to determine the most conducive and therapeutic method for monitoring the child's energy field.[47,48]	Disturbed energy fields may be related to numerous other altered patterns due to the infant or child's basic coping repertoire, especially altered thermoregulation–altered neurologic status. Approaching the infant or child according to cues for behavior potential yields greater likelihood of stress reduction.
Monitor energy field with a focus on maintaining self-comforting activities for the child. May begin with soft music and/or soothing voice.[47,48]	Will enhance assessment of energy field.
Begin with gentle but firm pressure of hands on one another.	Warms hands.
Assess energy field from head to toe. Focus on determining sites where differences are present. Refer to Adult Health-Care Plan for additional details.	Routine assessment.
Attempt to redirect areas of lesser flow or greater flow within an overall free-flowing energy field, allowing $\frac{1}{2}$ to 1 inches between nurse's hands and the child.	Restores balance. The infant or child has a small energy field.

ACTIONS/INTERVENTIONS	RATIONALES
Monitor the client's responses to therapeutic touch. Focus on identifying stimulus response.	Permits evaluation of success of therapy.
Teach the client (or family, depending on client's age) to note physical and mental cues that alter energy field, especially stressors.[49,50]	Promotes early intervention.
Offer age-appropriate relaxation techniques (e.g., imaginary floating like a feather to suggest lightness for a school-ager vs. gentle rocking to rhythmic music for an infant).[51,52]	Pays attention to developmental level.
Be mindful of contributing factors of self. Offer ways to assist the caregiver in learning techniques for maintenance of energy field balance.	Provides long-term assistance.
As appropriate, assist family to develop ways to reduce sensitivity to external triggering cues.	Provides long-term balance.

Women's Health

Same as Adult Health except for the following:

ACTIONS/INTERVENTIONS	RATIONALES
Instruct in use of therapeutic touch, relaxation, imagery and visualization, paced breathing, music, acupressure, and hypnosis as a means of coping with labor pain.[53]	Provides a natural source of dealing with the discomfort of labor.[53–60] Allows the woman and her newborn to experience a drug-free labor and delivery.
Instruct women in the use of NAC for relaxation and self-care during times of illness and stress throughout their life span. Some of these therapies include such practices as acupressure and acupuncture, artistic expression, biofeedback, deep breathing, healing touch hypnosis, imagery, music, prayer, relaxation, therapeutic touch and other practices which support women's psychosocial and spiritual components, as well as their physical domain.[58–60]	NAC (Natural, alternative, complementary health-care practices) have a limited research base at the present time; but women throughout the ages have used these techniques to become tuned into the energy surrounding a person's being and the harmony of body, mind and spirit. "Women have always been healers. Cultural myths from around the world describe a time when only women knew the secrets of life and death, and therefore they alone could practice the magical art of healing."[60]

Mental Health

ACTIONS/INTERVENTIONS	RATIONALES
Explain intervention to the client in terms that facilitate reality orientation and do not exacerbate thought disorders. • Use examples that elicit the client's past experiences with personal energy fields that do not reinforce delusional beliefs (e.g., EEG and EKG measure electrical energy that flows from the body; walking across the floor and then touching something releases the buildup of energy that can be seen or felt as a mild shock). Rubbing a balloon over the hair and watching it stand up when the balloon is moved away is another example.	Prevents reinforcement of delusional system and facilitates the development of a trusting relationship.[61]

(care plan continued on page 40)

NURSING ACTIONS/INTERVENTIONS WITH RATIONALES (continued from page 39)

Mental Health

ACTIONS/INTERVENTIONS	RATIONALES
• Instruct the client that these techniques facilitate his or her own healing potential and are used in conjunction with other treatments.	
Discuss with the client his or her perceptions or concerns about their alterations.	Understanding the client's cognitive map facilitates the development of interventions that facilitate client change.[61,64]
Discuss with the client interventions that can assist with energy balance. In consultation with the client select one of the following methods for altering energy fields based on the assessment: • Therapeutic touch • Foot or hand reflexology • Visual imagery • Visualization with relaxation techniques • Acupressure • Transcutaneous electrical nerve stimulation (TENS) • Biofeedback	All these techniques have been demonstrated to have effects on the body's energy fields.[45,46,53,57,62–64] Application of these interventions by the nurse is related to having appropriate training in the technique. If the nurse is unskilled in the techniques, efforts should be made for appropriate referrals at this point. Additional information on these techniques can be found in the references.
Note referral information here with date and time of appointment with practitioner.	
If the nurse is prepared to implement the intervention, prepare the client and environment for the application of the intervention: • Provide private, quiet environment. • Teach the client about the intervention.	Increases the client's level of comfort.[55,64]
• Obtain the client's permission to utilize the intervention.	Builds trust and promotes the client's sense of control.[55,64]
• Provide appropriate music that increases the client's feelings of comfort.	Sound that is loud and irritating can have a negative impact on psychological and physiologic well-being.[44]
• Provide essential oils or other scents that enhance the client's sense of well-being.	Odors have impact on the limbic system and impact affect.
Focus own attention on the intent of the interaction.	The nurse's intention provides a crucial basis for these interventions.[45,48,58]
Inform the client that he or she should tell the practitioner if there are any differences in the way he or she feels during the application of the technique. This could include feelings of relaxation, warmth, or change in breathing patterns.	Changes that occur with alterations in the energy fields may be perceived by the client before the practitioner notices a difference. The goal of these interventions is to promote balance, so the treatment should stop when these differences are observed by the client or practitioner.[45,46,65] Also promotes the client's sense of control.[45,46]
Assist the client into a comfort position that will facilitate treatment.	It is important that the client is well supported because the techniques do promote the relaxation response.
Utilize selected technique [number] times a day for [number] minutes. Observe the client for signs that indicate that the desired effect has occurred. This could include: • Sigh • Relaxation in muscles • Slower, deeper breathing	The ability of the client to maintain balance is based on general levels of wellness, lifestyle, and stressors.[65]

ACTIONS/INTERVENTIONS	RATIONALES
• Drop in voice volume • Peripheral flush on the face and neck • Client's report of feeling different • Reassessment indicates balance has occurred	
Assist the client into a comfortable, relaxed position after treatment.	
Teach the client techniques that can maintain balance between treatments and that do not require the assistance of a practitioner, including: • Relaxation • Cross crawl exercises • Stress reduction • Cognitive reframing • Visualization • Improved nutrition • Decreasing use of tobacco and alcohol	Maintenance of energy field balance involves a holistic approach to care and has been demonstrated to have effects on human energy fields.[45–53,62,65–68]
Note teaching schedule and content here.	

Gerontic Health

ACTIONS/INTERVENTIONS	RATIONALES
Obtain medication profile (prescription and over-the-counter) to determine whether drug actions or reactions contribute to the disturbance.	Medications may contribute to disturbed energy fields.
Ensure adequate padding and proper position for any sessions.	Proper positioning prevents pain, pressure, and thus disturbances in concentration.
Adjust massage efforts and pressure to compensate for changes in an older patient's tactile sensation.	Older adults, with aging changes in the nervous system, may have a decreased perception of being touched.
Use teaching materials, as needed, that are appropriate for the patient (such as printed information of a size that is easily read, or quality audiotapes that are not distorted or high pitched).	Uncompensated sensory changes of aging can affect the ability to use audio–visual sources if the information is not adjusted to meet the older adult's needs.
Discuss with the client use of complementary or alternative therapies prior to initiating therapies.	Older adults may experience psychological or spiritual distress if therapies used cause a conflict with their belief system. (Some adults may react negatively to therapeutic touch, perceiving it as "laying on of hands" in a religious manner.)[70]
Teach clients or caregivers relaxation strategies, use of guided imagery, massage, or music therapies to promote stress reduction.	The therapies listed are recommended for older adults who would benefit from the reduced sympathetic response to stress. The physical and psychological changes associated with aging can increase stress and impede body/mind healing.[63,71]
Ensure that therapeutic touch sessions, if used, are of brief duration and gently done.	Caution is recommended when using therapeutic touch with infants, very debilitated patients, and the elderly.[59]

(care plan continued on page 42)

NURSING ACTIONS/INTERVENTIONS WITH RATIONALES (continued from page 41)

Gerontic Health

ACTIONS/INTERVENTIONS	RATIONALES
Document older adult's use of any complementary or alternative therapies, to include preferred treatment, frequency of treatments, and effects experienced.	Many adults are reluctant to discuss use of alternative therapies. Nondisclosure may lead to adverse reactions from drug, food, or herb interactions.[69,70]
Discuss with clients potential effects from complementary or alternative therapies, such as dizziness or weakness after acupuncture, risk for fractures with chiropractic, and drug or herb interactions.	Little research is currently available on the effects of complementary or alternative therapies on older adults. Cautioning clients on potential effects may reduce the risk for injury or adverse reactions.[70]

Home Health

ACTIONS/INTERVENTIONS	RATIONALES
Assist the client and family to identify disturbances in energy field.	Early identification assists in providing early intervention.
Teach the client and family techniques to prevent and/or treat disturbed energy field, such as: • Therapeutic touch • Foot or hand reflexology • Visual imagery • Visualization with relaxation techniques • TENS • Biofeedback	Involvement improves motivation and improves the outcome. Self-care is enhanced.
Assist the client and family in providing a private, quiet environment.	Client comfort is increased, and response to intervention is enhanced.[61,67]
Assist the client and family in identifying resources in the community, such as: • Massage therapist • Reflexologists • Stress reduction classes	Use of existing community services is efficient use of resources.

HEALTH MAINTENANCE, INEFFECTIVE

DEFINITION[44]

Inability to identify, manage, and/or seek out help to maintain health.

DEFINING CHARACTERISTICS[44]

1. History of lack of health-seeking behavior
2. Reported or observed lack of equipment, financial, and/or other resources
3. Reported or observed impairment of personal support systems
4. Expressed interest in improving health behaviors
5. Demonstrated lack of knowledge regarding basic health practices
6. Demonstrated lack of adaptive behaviors to internal or external environmental changes
7. Reported or observed inability to take responsibility for meeting basic health practices in any or all functional pattern areas

RELATED FACTORS[43]

1. Lack of, or significant alteration in, communication skills (written, verbal, and/or gestural)
2. Lack of ability to make deliberate and thoughtful judgments
3. Perceptual or cognitive impairment (complete or partial lack of gross and/or fine motor skills)
4. Ineffective individual coping
5. Dysfunctional grieving
6. Unachieved developmental tasks

7. Ineffective family coping
8. Disabling spiritual distress
9. Lack of material resources

RELATED CLINICAL CONCERNS

1. Dementias such as Alzheimer's disease and multi-infarct
2. Mental retardation
3. Any condition causing an alteration in level of consciousness, for example, a closed head injury, carbon monoxide poisoning, or cerebrovascular accident
4. Any condition affecting the person's mobility level, for example, hemiplegia, paraplegia, fractures, or muscular dystrophy
5. Chronic diseases, for example, rheumatoid arthritis, cancer, chronic pain, or multiple sclerosis

 Have You Selected the Correct Diagnosis?

Spiritual Distress
A problem in the Value-Belief Pattern could result in variance in health maintenance. If the therapeutic regimen causes conflict with cultural or religious beliefs or with the individual's value system, then it is likely some alteration in health maintenance will occur. Interviewing the patient regarding individual values, goals, or beliefs that guide personal decision making will assist in clarifying whether the primary diagnosis is Ineffective Health Maintenance or a problem in the Value-Belief Pattern.

Ineffective Coping
Either Ineffective Individual Coping or Compromised or Disabled Family Coping could be suspected if there are major differences between the patient and family reports of health status, health perception, and health-care behavior. Ineffective Community Coping may be present if there are inadequate resources for problem solving or deficits in social support services for community members. Verbalizations by the patient or family member regarding inability to cope also indicate ineffective coping. Community members may express dissatisfaction with meeting community needs.

Interrupted Family Process
Through observing family interactions and communication, the nurse may assess that Interrupted Family Process exists. Rigidity of family functions and roles, poorly communicated messages, and failure to accomplish expected family developmental tasks are a few observations to alert the nurse to this possible diagnosis.

Activity Intolerance or Self-Care Deficit
The nursing diagnosis of Activity Intolerance or Self-Care Deficit should be considered if the nurse observes or validates reports of inability to complete the required tasks because of insufficient energy or because of the patient's inability to feed, bathe, toilet, dress, and groom him- or herself.

Powerlessness
The nursing diagnosis of Powerlessness is considered if the patient reports or demonstrates having little control over situations, expresses doubt about ability to perform, or is reluctant to express his or her feelings to health-care providers.

Deficient Knowledge
Deficient Knowledge may exist if the patient or family verbalizes less than adequate understanding of health management or recalls inaccurate health information.

Impaired Home Maintenance
This diagnosis is demonstrated by the inability of the patient or family to provide a safe living environment.

EXPECTED OUTCOME

Will describe at least [number] contributing factors that lead to health maintenance alteration and at least one measure to alter each factor by [date].

TARGET DATES

Assisting patients to adapt their health maintenance requires a significant investment of time and also requires close collaboration with home health caregivers. For these reasons, it is recommended the target date be no less than 7 days from the date of admission.

NURSING ACTIONS/INTERVENTIONS WITH RATIONALES

Adult Health

ACTIONS/INTERVENTIONS	RATIONALES
Assist the patient to identify factors contributing to health maintenance change through one-to-one interviewing and value clarification strategies. Factors may include:	Healthy living habits reduce risk. Assistance is often required to develop long-term change. Identification of the factors significant to the patient will provide the foundation for teaching positive health maintenance.

(care plan continued on page 44)

NURSING ACTIONS/INTERVENTIONS WITH RATIONALES (continued from page 43)

Adult Health

ACTIONS/INTERVENTIONS	RATIONALES
• Stopping smoking[53,71–74] • Ceasing drug and alcohol use • Establishing exercise patterns[75] • Following good nutritional habits • Using stress management techniques • Using family and community support systems • Using over-the-counter medications • Using herb, vitamins, food supplements, or cleansing programs[76]	
Develop with the patient a list of assets and deficits as he or she perceives them. From this list, assist the patient in deciding what lifestyle adjustments will be necessary.	Increases the patient's sense of control and keeps the idea of multiple changes from being overwhelming.
Identify, with the patient, possible solutions, modifications, etc., to cope with each adjustment.	The more the patient is involved with decisions, the higher the probability that the patient will incorporate the changes.
Develop a plan with the patient that shows both short-term and long-term goals. For each goal, specify the time the goal is to be reached.	Avoids overwhelming the patient by indicating that not all goals have to be accomplished at the same time.
Have the patient identify at least two support persons. Arrange for these persons to come to the unit and participate in designing the health maintenance plan.	Provides additional support for patient in maintaining plan.
Assist the patient and significant others in developing a list of *potential* strategies that will assist in the development of the lifestyle changes necessary for health maintenance. (This list should be a brainstorming process and include both solutions that appear to be very unrealistic as well as those that appear most realistic.) After the list is developed, review each item with the patient, combining and eliminating strategies when appropriate.	People most often approach change with "more of the same" solutions. If the individual does not think that the strategy will have to be implemented, he or she will be more inclined to develop creative strategies for change.[76]
Develop with the patient a list of the benefits and disadvantages of behavior changes. Discuss each item with the patient as to the strength of motivation that each item has.	Placing items in priority according to the patient's motivation increases probability of success.
Develop a behavior change contract with the patient, allowing the patient to identify appropriate rewards and consequences. Remember to establish modest goals and short-term rewards. [Note reward schedule here.]	Positive reinforcement enhances self-esteem and supports continuation of desired behaviors. This also promotes patient control, which in turn increases motivation to implement the plan.[55]
Teach the patient appropriate information to improve health maintenance (e.g., hygiene, diet, medication administration, relaxation techniques, and coping strategies).	Provides the patient with the basic knowledge needed to enact the needed changes.
Review activities of daily living (ADLs) with the patient and support person. Incorporate these activities into the design for a health maintenance plan.	Incorporation of usual activities personalizes the plan.

● N O T E : *May have to either increase or decrease ADLs.*

ACTIONS/INTERVENTIONS	RATIONALES
Assist the patient and support person to design a monthly calendar that reflects the daily activities needed to succeed in health maintenance.	Provides a visual reminder.
Have the patient and support person return/demonstrate health maintenance procedures at least once a day for at least 3 days before discharge. Times and types of skills should be noted here.	Permits practice in a nonthreatening environment where immediate feedback can be given.
Set a time to reassess with the patient and support person progress toward the established goals. This should be on a frequent schedule initially and can then gradually decrease as the patient demonstrates mastery. [Note evaluation times here.]	Provides an opportunity to evaluate and to give the patient positive feedback and support for achievements.
Provide the patient with appropriate positive feedback on goal achievement. Remember to keep this behaviorally oriented and specific.	
Communicate the established plan to the collaborative members of the health-care team.	Provides continuity and consistency in care.
Refer the patient to appropriate community health agencies for follow-up care. Be sure referral is made at least 3 to 5 days before discharge.	Ensures the service can complete their assessment and initiate operations before the patient is discharged from the hospital. Use of the network of existing community services provides for effective utilization of resources.
Schedule appropriate follow-up appointments for patient before discharge. Notify transportation service and support persons of these appointments. Write appointment on brightly colored cards for attention. Include date, time, appropriate name (physician, physical therapist, nurse practitioner, etc.), address, telephone number, and name and telephone number of person who will provide transportation.	Facilitates patient's keeping of appointments and reinforces importance of health maintenance.

Child Health

● N O T E : *Developmental consideration should always guide the health maintenance planned for the child patient. Also, identification of primary defects is stressed to reduce the likelihood of secondary and tertiary delays.*

ACTIONS/INTERVENTIONS	RATIONALES
Determine who is the patient's primary caregiver.	Fosters the likelihood for continuity of care and who is accountable for care of child.
Teach the patient and family essential information to establish and maintain health according to age, development, and status. Well checks are suggested at time of immunization with access to a health-care provider for annual checks or in time of illness after 1 year in the absence of a chronic health-care need.	An individualized plan of care more definitively reflects specific health maintenance needs and increases the value of the plan to the patient and his or her family.
Assist the patient and family in designing a calendar to monitor progress in meeting goals. Offer developmentally appropriate methods (e.g., toddlers enjoy stickers of favorite cartoon or book characters).	Reinforcement in a more tangible mode facilitates compliance with the plan of health maintenance, especially with long-term situations.

(care plan continued on page 46)

NURSING ACTIONS/INTERVENTIONS WITH RATIONALES (continued from page 45)

Child Health

ACTIONS/INTERVENTIONS	RATIONALES
Identify risk factors that will impact health-care maintenance (e.g., prematurity, congenital defects, altered neurosensory functioning, errors of metabolism, or altered parenting).	Identification of risk factors allows for more appropriate anticipatory planning of health care, assists in minimizing crises and escalation of simple needs, and serves to reduce anxiety.
Begin to prepare for health maintenance on initial meeting with child and family.	A holistic plan of care realistically includes futuristic goals, not merely immediate health needs.
Provide appropriate telephone numbers for health team members and clinics to the child and parents to assist in follow-up.	Anticipatory planning for potential need for communication allows the patient or family realistic methods for assuming health care while enjoying the back-up of resources.

Women's Health

ACTIONS/INTERVENTIONS	RATIONALES
Assist the patient to describe her perception and understanding of essential information related to her individual lifestyle and the adjustment necessary to establish and maintain health in each cycle of reproductive life.	Allows assessment of the patient's basic level of knowledge so that a plan can begin at the patient's current level of understanding.
Develop with the patient a list of stress-related problems at work and at home as she perceives them. From this list, assist the patient in deciding what lifestyle adjustments will be necessary to establish and maintain health.	Provides essential information to assist patient in planning a healthy lifestyle.
Cigarette smoking is not only detrimental to the health of women, but it is also the causing factor involved with morbidity and mortality. One in four women smoke and more than 3.1 million adolescents in America are cigarette smokers.[78]	Experts recommend following PHS (US Public Health Service: Treating Tobacco Use and Dependence Practice Guidelines)[79] guidelines, which recommend three types of effective counseling and therapy[79,80]: • Skill training • Intra-treatment-clinician support • Extra-treatment-social support Consider psychosocial elements of women's lifestyle when offering interventions to stop smoking. Augment strategies with specific information related to each life cycle. (Adolescence, reproductive, mid-life, elder)[78]
Identify, with the patient, possible solutions and modification to facilitate coping with adjustments. Develop a plan that includes short-term and long-term goals. For each goal, specify the time frame for reaching the goal.	Provides sequential steps to alternate health maintenance within a defined time period. Keeps the patient from being overwhelmed by all the changes that might be necessary.
Provide factual information to the patient about menstrual cycle patterns throughout the life span. Include prepubertal, menarcheal, menstrual, premenopausal, menopausal, and postmenopausal phases.[81]	Provides basic information and knowledge that is needed throughout life span.
Teach the patient how to record accurate menstrual cycle, obstetric, and sexual history. Assist the patient in recognizing lifestyle changes that occur as a part of normal development.	Provides the patient with the information necessary to cope with changes throughout the reproductive cycle.

ACTIONS/INTERVENTIONS	RATIONALES
Discuss pregnancy and the changes that occur during pregnancy and childbearing. Stress the importance of a physical examination *before* becoming pregnant to include a Pap smear, rubella titer, AIDS profile, and genetic workup (if indicated by family history).	Provides patient with the information needed to plan for a healthy pregnancy.
Describe to and assist the patient in planning routines that will maintain well-being for the mother and fetus during pregnancy (e.g., reducing fatigue, eating a nutritionally adequate diet, exercising properly, obtaining early prenatal care, and attending classes to obtain information about infant nutrition, infant care, and the birthing experience).	Provides the expectant family with information to enable them to make informed choices about pregnancy, childbirth, and beginning parenting.
Provide information and support during postpartum period to assist the new mother in establishing and maintaining good infant nutrition, whether breastfeeding or formula feeding.	
Refer the patient to appropriate groups for support and encouragement after birth of baby (e.g., La Leche League and parenting groups).	
Teach terminology and factual information related to spontaneous abortion or the interruption of pregnancy. Encourage expression of feelings by the patient and her family. Provide referrals to appropriate support groups within the community.	Allows the patient to grieve and reduces fear regarding subsequent pregnancies.
Provide contraceptive information to the patient, including describing different methods of contraception and their advantages and disadvantages.	Allows the patient to plan appropriate contraceptive measures according to personal values and beliefs.
Emphasize the importance of lifestyle changes necessary to cope with postmenopausal changes in the body, such as estrogen replacement therapy, calcium supplements, balanced diet, exercise, and routine sleep patterns.	Provides the patient with basic information that will assist in planning a healthy lifestyle during and following menopause. Discuss use of alternative therapies for hormone replacement therapy.[60,80–83]
Teach the patient the importance of routine physical assessment throughout the reproductive life cycle, including breast self-examination, Pap smears, and routine examinations by the health-care provider of her choice (e.g., nurse midwife, nurse practitioner, or physician).	Provides knowledge that allows the patient to plan a healthy lifestyle.

Mental Health

ACTIONS/INTERVENTIONS	RATIONALES
Spend 30 minutes once a day discussing client's perception of current situation and life/personal goals before the changes occurred: • Use open-ended questions and reflective listening. • Let the client be the expert. • Do not provide advice.	Behavior change that is developed with the client using the client's identified needs and co-evolved solutions improves outcomes.[84-86]
Provide positive verbal reinforcement for the client's strengths and previous successes.	Positive reinforcement increases behavior.[87]

(care plan continued on page 48)

NURSING ACTIONS/INTERVENTIONS WITH RATIONALES (continued from page 47)

Mental Health

ACTIONS/INTERVENTIONS	RATIONALES
Discuss client's understanding of the options to facilitate the identified changes. Reflect to client nurse's understandings of the client's solutions and goals. Summarize the solutions and goals that the client identified. Develop a schedule for positive reinforcement when goals are attained. [Note the reinforcers and schedule of reinforcement here.]	Positive reinforcement increases behavior.[87]

Discuss with client sources of social support:
• Schedule meeting with client and social support system. Note the date and time of that meeting here.
• Spend 1 hour one time per week meeting with client and social support system to focus on:
  • With client's permission educate support system about client's health-care needs
  • Model communication and assist support system in developing positive communication skills
	Social support improves health outcomes.[88]

Include the client in group therapy to provide positive role models and peer support and to permit assessment of goals and exposure to differing problem solutions.	Group provides opportunities to relate and react to others while exploring behavior with each other.[87]

Gerontic Health

● N O T E: *Interventions provided in the adult health section are applicable to older adults. The major emphasis here is on client education. Ageism may present barriers to teaching older clients. The older adult is capable of learning new information.[89] Teaching strategies are available to enhance the learning experience for older adults.[90]*

ACTIONS/INTERVENTIONS	RATIONALES
Ensure privacy, comfort, and rapport prior to teaching sessions.	Reduces anxiety and promotes a non-distracting environment to enhance learning.
Avoid presenting large amounts of information at one time.	This encourages increased opportunity to process and store new information.
Monitor energy level as teaching session progresses.	Reduces possibility of fatigue which can impair learning.
Present small units of information, with repetition, and encourage patient to use cues that enhance ability to recall information.	Compensates for delayed reaction time associated with aging. Promotes retention of information by connecting information to previously mastered skills.[90]
Use multisensory approach to learning sessions whenever possible.	Hearing, vision, touch, and smell used in conjunction can stimulate multiple areas in the cerebral cortex to promote retention.[91]

Home Health

ACTIONS/INTERVENTIONS	RATIONALES
Assist the client and family to identify home and workplace factors that can be modified to promote health maintenance (e.g., ramps instead of steps, elimination of throw rugs, use of safety rails in showers, and maintenance of a nonsmoking environment).[92,93]	This action enhances safety and assists in preventing accidents. Promoting a nonsmoking environment helps reduce the damaging effects of passive smoke.

ACTIONS/INTERVENTIONS	RATIONALES
Involve the client and family in planning, implementing, and promoting a health maintenance pattern through: • Establish family conferences to discuss strategies for meeting client health maintenance needs. • Engage in mutual goal setting with client and family. Plan strategies with the client/family to establish goals for their involvement in managing the therapeutic regimen. • Assist family members in acquiring family or community based assistance for specified tasks as appropriate (e.g., cooking, cleaning, transportation, companionship, or support person for exercise program).	Involvement improves motivation and outcomes.
Teach the family and caregivers about disease management for existing illness: • Symptom management • Medication effects, side effects, and interactions with over-the-counter medications • Reporting the use of over-the-counter remedies, herbal supplements and medicines to the health-care provider • Wound care as appropriate. Prevention of skin breakdown for clients with illnesses contributing to immobility.	Provides a sense of autonomy and prevents premature progression of illness.
Teach the client and family health promotion and disease prevention activities: • Relaxation techniques • Nutritional habits to maintain optimal weight and physical strength • Techniques for developing and strengthening support networks (e.g., communication techniques or mutual goal setting) • Physical exercise to increase flexibility, cardiovascular conditioning, and physical strength and endurance[94] • Evaluation of occupational conditions[94] • Control of harmful habits (e.g., control of substance abuse) • Therapeutic value of pets[95]	These activities promote a healthy lifestyle.

HEALTH-SEEKING BEHAVIORS (SPECIFY)

DEFINITION[44]

A state in which an individual in stable health is actively seeking ways to alter personal health habits and/or the environment in order to move toward a higher level of health.

DEFINING CHARACTERISTICS[44]

1. Expressed or observed desire to seek a higher level of wellness
2. Demonstrated or observed lack of knowledge of health promotion behaviors
3. Stated (or observed) unfamiliarity with wellness community resources
4. Expression of concern about impact of current environmental conditions on health status
5. Expressed or observed desire for increased control of health practice

RELATED FACTORS[44]

To be developed.

RELATED CLINICAL CONCERNS

Because this diagnosis, as indicated by the definition, relates to individuals in stable health, there are no related medical diagnoses.

Have You Selected the Correct Diagnosis?

Impaired Home Maintenance
This diagnosis may be involved if the individual or family is unable to independently maintain a safe, growth-promoting immediate environment.

Powerlessness
If the client expresses the perception of lack of control or influence over the situation and potential outcomes or does not participate in care or decision making when opportunities are provided, the diagnosis of Powerlessness should be investigated. Community powerlessness may be an indicator of Ineffective Community Coping.

EXPECTED OUTCOME

Will [increase/decrease] [habit] by [amount] by [date].

EXAMPLES

Will decrease smoking by 75 percent by [date].
Will increase exercise by walking 2 miles three times per week by [date].

TARGET DATES

Changing a habit involves a significant investment of time and energy regardless of whether the change involves starting a new habit or stopping an old one. Therefore, the target dates should be expressed in terms of weeks and months.

NURSING ACTIONS/INTERVENTIONS WITH RATIONALES

Adult Health

ACTIONS/INTERVENTIONS	RATIONALES
Two hours after admission, identify post-discharge resources (e.g., classes, support groups) to reinforce positive health habits.	Allows adequate time to complete discharge planning and teaching required for home care.
Note potential risk factors that should be dealt with regarding actual health status (e.g., financial status, coping strategies, or resources).	Provides basic knowledge that will contribute to individualized discharge planning.
Teach the patient about activities for promotion of health and prevention of illness (e.g., well-balanced diet, including restricted sodium and cholesterol intake, need for adequate rest and exercise, effects of air pollutants including smoking, and stress management techniques).	Provides the patient and family with the essential knowledge needed to modify behavior.
Review the patient's problem-solving abilities, and assist the patient to identify various alternatives, especially in terms of altering his or her environment.	Promotes shared decision making and enhances patient's feeling of self-control.
Provide appropriate teaching to assist the patient and family in becoming confident in self-seeking health-care behavior (e.g., teach assertiveness techniques to the patient and family).	Increases sense of self-control and reduces feelings of powerlessness.
Assist the patient and family to list benefits of high-level wellness and health-seeking behavior.	Makes visible the reasons these activities will help the family.
Help the patient and family develop a basic written plan for achieving individual high-level wellness. Provide time for questions before dismissal to solidify plans for follow-up care. At a minimum, 30 minutes per day for 2 days prior to discharge should be allowed for this question-and-answer period. Note times here.	Demonstrates importance of follow-up care.
Give and review pamphlets about wellness community resources.	Reinforces teaching and provides ready reference for patient and family after discharge from agency.
Support the patient in his or her health-seeking behavior. Advocate when necessary.	Provides supportive environment and underlines the importance of health-seeking activities.
Refer to appropriate health-care providers and various community groups as appropriate for assistance needed by the patient and his or her family.	Provides professional support systems that can assist in health-seeking behavior.

Child Health

ACTIONS/INTERVENTIONS	RATIONALES
Monitor the child and family for perceived value of health. Incorporate into any plan personal and family needs identified through this monitoring.	Values are formulated in the first 6 years of life and will serve as primary factors in how health is perceived and enjoyed by the individual and family. If values are in question, there is greater likelihood that how health to be maintained will be subject to this values conflict. Until health-seeking behavior is identified as a value, follow-up care will not be deemed to be beneficial.
Assist the child and family to identify appropriate health maintenance needs and resources (e.g., immunizations, nutrition, daily hygiene, basic safety, how to obtain medical services when needed [including health education], how to take temperature of an infant, basic skills and care for health problems, health insurance, Medicaid, and related state resources).	Knowing available resources and incorporating these resources into the plan for health care facilitate long-term attention to health.

Women's Health

ACTIONS/INTERVENTIONS	RATIONALES
Teach the patient the importance of seeking information and support during the reproductive life cycle. Include information about prepubertal, menarcheal, menstrual, childbearing, parenting, menopausal, and post-menopausal periods of the life cycle.	Provides the basic information needed to support health-seeking behaviors.
Provide woman with information about health tests and screenings at various life stages. These tests include: • Blood glucose • Blood pressure • Bone density test (osteoporosis) • Breast cancer screenings • Cardiovascular disease risk assessment • Cholesterol • Colorectal exam • Dental checkup • Eye exam • Hearing test • Pap test and pelvic exam • Routine physical • Thyroid screening	Most chronic diseases that affect women can be prevented. Knowing the risk factors and the modifying behaviors can greatly reduce the number of women facing chronic illness and even death. Cardiac disease is the number one killer of women in this country. Research has shown that most morbidity and mortality of women can be greatly decreased by routing screening, diagnosis, counseling and behavior modification.[96]

Mental Health

ACTIONS/INTERVENTIONS	RATIONALES
Assign the client a primary care nurse.	Provides increased individuation and continuity of care, facilitating the development of a therapeutic relationship. The nursing process requires that a trusting and functional relationship exist between nurse and client.[61]

(care plan continued on page 52)

NURSING ACTIONS/INTERVENTIONS WITH RATIONALES (continued from page 51)

Mental Health

ACTIONS/INTERVENTIONS	RATIONALES
Primary care nurse will spend 30 minutes twice a day with client [note times here]. The focus of these interactions will conform to the following schedule:	Promotes the client's trust in the nurse and perception of control.[85–87]
• *Interaction 1:* Have the client identify specific areas of concern. List the identified concerns on the care plan. Also identify the primary source of this concern (i.e., client, family member, member of the health-care team, or other members of the client's social system).	Promotes the client's perception of control.
• *Interaction 2:* List *specific* goals for each concern the client has identified. These goals should be achievable within a 2- to 3-day period. (One way of setting realistic, achievable goals is to divide the goal described by the client by 50 percent.)	Promotes the client's self-esteem when goals can be accomplished.[87]
• *Interaction 3:* Have the client identify steps that have been previously taken to address the concern.	Promotes the client's self-esteem and provides motivation for continued efforts.
• *Interaction 4:* Determine the client's perceptions of abilities to meet established goals and areas where assistance may be needed. (If the client indicates a perception of inability to pursue goals without a great deal of assistance, the alternative nursing diagnoses of Powerlessness and Knowledge Deficit may need to be considered.)	
Assist client in developing strategies to achieve the established goals, developing action plans, evaluating the outcome of these plans, and then revising future actions in future interactions. [Note schedule of these interactions here.]	
Provide positive verbal reinforcement for client's achievements of goals. This reinforcement should be specific to the client's goals. [Note those things that are rewarding to the client here and the kind of behavior to be rewarded.]	

Gerontic Health

In addition to interventions for Adult Health, the following may be used with the older client:

ACTIONS/INTERVENTIONS	RATIONALES
Encourage the client to participate in health-screening and health-promotion programs such as Senior Wellness Programs. These programs are often offered by hospitals, clinics, and senior citizens centers.	Provides a cost-effective, easily accessible, long-term support mechanism for the patient.
Ensure privacy, comfort, and rapport prior to teaching sessions.	Reduces anxiety and promotes a nondistracting environment to enhance learning.
Avoid presenting large amounts of information at one time.	This encourages increased opportunity to process and store new information.
Monitor energy level as teaching session progresses.	Reduces possibility of fatigue which can impair learning.
Present small units of information, with repetition, and encourage patient to use cues that enhance ability to recall information.	Compensates for delayed reaction time associated with aging. Promotes retention of information by connecting information to previously mastered skills.[90]

ACTIONS/INTERVENTIONS	RATIONALES
Use multisensory approach to learning sessions whenever possible.	Hearing, vision, touch, and smell used in conjunction can stimulate multiple areas in the cerebral cortex to promote retention.[91]

Home Health

ACTIONS/INTERVENTIONS	RATIONALES
Help the client identify his or her personal definition of health, perceived personal control, perceived self-efficacy, and perceived health status.	Awareness of definition of health, locus of control, perceived efficiency, and health status identifies potential facilitators and barriers to action.
Assist the client in identifying required lifestyle changes. Assist the client to develop potential strategies that would assist in the lifestyle changes required.	Lifestyle changes require change in behavior. Self-evaluation and support facilitate these changes.
Assist the client and family to identify home and workplace factors that can be modified to promote health maintenance (e.g., ramps instead of steps, elimination of throw rugs, use of safety rails in showers, and maintenance of a nonsmoking environment).[74,89,90]	This action enhances safety and assists in preventing accidents. Promoting a nonsmoking environment helps reduce the damaging effects of passive smoke.
Involve the client and family in planning, implementing, and promoting a health maintenance pattern through: • Helping to establish family conferences to discuss strategies for meeting client health maintenance needs. • Engaging in mutual goal setting with client and family. Encourage the client/family to establish goals for their own involvement in managing the therapeutic regimen. • Assisting family members in acquiring family or community-based assistance for specified tasks as appropriate (e.g., cooking, cleaning, transportation, companionship, or support person for exercise program)	Involvement improves motivation and outcomes.
Teach the family and caregivers about disease management for existing illness: • Symptom management • Medication effects, side effects, and interactions with over-the-counter medications • Reporting the use of over-the-counter remedies, herbal supplements and medicines to the health-care provider • Wound care as appropriate. Prevention of skin breakdown for clients with illnesses contributing to immobility.	Provides a sense of autonomy and prevents premature progression of illness.
Teach the client and family health promotion and disease prevention activities: • Relaxation techniques • Nutritional habits to maintain optimal weight and physical strength • Techniques for developing and strengthening support networks (e.g., communication techniques or mutual goal setting) • Physical exercise to increase flexibility, cardiovascular conditioning, and physical strength and endurance • Evaluation of occupational conditions • Control of harmful habits (e.g., control of substance abuse) • Therapeutic value of pets[95]	These activities promote a healthy lifestyle.

INFECTION, RISK FOR

DEFINITION[44]

The state in which an individual is at increased risk for being invaded by pathogenic organisms.

DEFINING CHARACTERISTICS (RISK FACTORS)[44]

1. Invasive procedures
2. Insufficient knowledge to avoid exposure to pathogens
3. Trauma
4. Tissue destruction and increased environmental exposure
5. Rupture of amniotic membranes
6. Pharmaceutical agents
7. Malnutrition
8. Immunosuppression
9. Inadequate secondary defenses (e.g., decreased hemoglobin, leukopenia, suppressed inflammatory response)
10. Inadequate acquired immunity
11. Inadequate primary defenses (broken skin, traumatized tissue, decrease in ciliary action, stasis of body fluids, change in pH secretions, altered peristalsis)
12. Chronic disease

 Have You Selected the Correct Diagnosis?

Self-Care Deficit
Self-Care Deficit, especially in the areas of toileting, feeding, and bathing-hygiene, may need to be considered if improper handwashing, personal hygiene, toileting practice, or food preparation and storage have increased the risk of infection.

Impaired Skin Integrity; Impaired Tissue Integrity; Imbalanced Nutrition, Less Than Body Requirements; Impaired Oral Mucous Membrane
These diagnoses may predispose the client to infection.

Impaired Physical Mobility
This diagnosis should be considered if skin breakdown is secondary to lack of movement. Skin breakdown always predisposes the patient to Risk for Infection.

Imbalanced Body Temperature; Hyperthermia
These diagnoses should be considered when the body temperature increases above normal, which is common in infectious processes.

Ineffective Management of Therapeutic Regimen (Noncompliance)
This diagnosis may be occurring in cases of inappropriate antibiotic usage or inadequate treatment of wounds or chronic diseases.

RELATED FACTORS[44]

The risk factors serve also as the related factors.

RELATED CLINICAL CONCERNS

1. AIDS
2. Burns
3. Chronic obstructive pulmonary disease (COPD)
4. Diabetes mellitus
5. Any surgery and any condition where steroids are used as a part of the treatment regimen
6. Substance abuse or dependence
7. Premature rupture of membranes

EXPECTED OUTCOME

Will return/demonstrate measures to decrease the risk for infection by [date].

TARGET DATES

An appropriate target date would be within 3 days from the date of diagnosis.

NURSING ACTIONS/INTERVENTIONS WITH RATIONALES

Adult Health

ACTIONS/INTERVENTIONS	RATIONALES
Monitor vital signs every 4 hours around the clock. [State times here.]	Provides a baseline that allows quick recognition of deviations in subsequent measurements.
Use standard precautions and teach the patient and family the purpose and techniques of standard precautions.[98]	Protects the patient and family from infection.
Teach the patient and family about the infectious process, routes, pathogens, environmental and host factors, and aspects of prevention.	Provides basic knowledge for self-help and self-protection.

ACTIONS/INTERVENTIONS	RATIONALES
Maintain adequate nutrition and fluid and electrolyte balance. Provide a well-balanced diet with increased amounts of vitamin C, sufficient iron, and 2400 to 2600 mL of fluid daily.	Helps prevent disability that would predispose infection.
Collaborate with the physician regarding screening specimens for culture and sensitivity (e.g., blood, urine, sputum, and spinal fluid).	Allows accurate determination of the causative organism and identification of the antibiotic that will be most effective against the organism.
Monitor the administration of antibiotics for maintenance of blood levels and for side effects (e.g., diarrhea or toxicity).	Antibiotics have to be maintained at a consistent blood level, usually 7–10 days, to kill causative organisms. Antibiotics may destroy normal bowel flora, predisposing the patient to the development of diarrhea and increasing the chance of infection in the lower gastrointestinal tract.
Maintain a neutral thermal environment.	Avoids overheating or overcooling of room that would contribute to complications for the patient.
Assist the patient with a thorough shower at least once daily (dependent on age) or total bed bath daily.	Reduces microorganisms on the skin.
Provide good genital hygiene, and teach the patient how to care for the genital area.	Also enhances feeling of well being, and prevents spread of opportunistic infections.[97,99]
Wash your hands thoroughly between each treatment. Teach the patient the value of frequent handwashing.	Prevents cross-contamination and nosocomial infections.
Use sterile technique when changing dressings or performing invasive procedures.	Protects the patient from exposure to pathogens.[100]
Turn every 2 hours on [odd/even] hour	Promotes tissue perfusion.
Perform passive exercises or have the patient perform active range of motion (ROM) exercises every 2 hours on [odd/even] hour. Remember that the patient may have decreased tolerance of activity.	
Cough and deep-breathe every 2 hours on [odd/even] hour.	Mobilizes static pulmonary secretions, thereby improving gas exchange.
Consult with appropriate assistive resources as indicated.	Appropriate use of existing community service is efficient use of resources.

Child Health

ACTIONS/INTERVENTIONS	RATIONALES
Assess for all contributing factors to include pharmacologic agents, recent exposures, and deviations in immune status.	Widest consideration will likely identify how the threat of infection will be met.
Monitor axillary temperature every 2 hours on [odd/even] hour. (May be assessed per rectal or tympanic according to health-care provider's preference.)	Most appropriate route for frequent measurements for the very young child. Oral temperature measurements would not be accurate.
Institute aseptic precautions.	Provides basis for decreased likelihood of reinfection.
Provide instructions to child at developmentally appropriate level and to parents while instituting infectious precautions as applicable.	Allows for meeting child's needs for understanding as questions are answered. This helps to insure appropriate precautions are upheld to prevent spread to others including family members.
If neutropenic precautions are necessary, monitor CBC and absolute neutrophil count.	Provides essential basis for diagnosis and treatment.
Obtain specimens as required, esp. blood, urine, and stool. (May require lumbar puncture for septic work-up.)	Ensures baseline and follow-up monitoring for adequacy of treatment/status.

(care plan continued on page 56)

NURSING ACTIONS/INTERVENTIONS WITH RATIONALES (continued from page 55)

Child Health

ACTIONS/INTERVENTIONS	RATIONALES
Administer medications as scheduled with attention to appropriate dosage for weight/indication, peak and trough results, and potential for allergenic response.	Abides by safe practice of administration of medications within desired blood levels. Monitoring for side effects yields likelihood of early detection to lessen severity of possible anaphylaxis.
Encourage the child and parents to verbalize fears, concerns, or feelings related to infection by scheduling at least 30 minutes per shift to counsel with family. Note times here.	Provides support, decreases anxiety and fears, and provides teaching opportunity.

Women's Health

ACTIONS/INTERVENTIONS	RATIONALES
During prenatal period, inform the mother about and how to prevent perinatal infections: • Encourage the mother to avoid frequent changing of partners and other high-risk sexual behaviors while pregnant. Teach the mother good preventive health-care behaviors such as:	Infections acquired during pregnancy can cause significant morbidity and even mortality for both mother and/or infant.[29] Pregnancy is considered an immunosuppressed state. Responses of the immune system during pregnancy may decrease the mother's ability to fight infection.

• Maintaining good nutrition
  • Teach strategies that allow women to gain and utilize maximum energy by eating nutritiously, including identifying supplements that can augment energy levels.
  • Perform a dietary assessment and provide a nutritional education to the breastfeeding woman.
• Getting correct amount of sleep
• Exercise
• Reducing stress levels
	Researchers agree that strong links exist between good nutrition and the prevention of diseases such as osteoporosis, cardiac disease, and certain female cancers. In fact, nutrition is one of the biggest factors in women's health throughout all the stages of her life.[101,102]
	The recommended energy intake during the first 6 months of lactation can be reached by having one extra meal per day (approximately 500 kcal).[103]

Test the mother for presence of TORCH infections.	This is a group of organisms that cross the placenta and interfere with the development of the fetus and health of the newborn infant. **T**oxoplasmosis, **H**epatitis B, **R**ubella, **C**ytomegalovirus, **H**erpes. Other infections such as Chlamydia, Group B Streptococcus, Syphilis, HIV and AIDS are also of great concern as all of these infections have consequences for not only the pregnancy but also the newborn.[29]
In the presence of ruptured amniotic membranes, monitor for signs of infection at least every 4 hours at [state times here] (e.g., elevated temperature or vaginal discharge odor).	Provides clinical data needed to quickly recognize the presence of infection.
Use aseptic technique when performing vaginal examinations, and limit the number of vaginal examinations during labor.	Reduces the opportunities to introduce infection.

ACTIONS/INTERVENTIONS	RATIONALES
Teach the mother to take only showers (no tub baths) and to monitor and record temperature. Have her take temperature at least every 4 hours on a set schedule.	Teaches the patient basic information to recognize and prevent infection.
Keep linens and underpads clean and changed as necessary during labor.	Reduces the likelihood of nosocomial infections.
Monitor incisions (cesarean section or episiotomy) at least every 4 hours at [state times here] for redness, drainage, oozing, hematoma, or loss of approximation.	Provides clinical data needed to quickly recognize the presence of infection.
During postpartum period, monitor fundal height at least every 4 hours at [state times here] around the clock for 48 hours.	Provides database necessary to screen for infection.
During postpartum period, monitor the patient at least every 4 hours at [state times here] for any signs of foul smelling lochia, uterine tenderness, or increased temperature.	Provides clinical data needed to quickly recognize the presence of infection.
In instances of abortion, obtain a complete obstetric history.	
Monitor abdomen at least every 4 hours at [state times here] for any swelling, tenderness, or foul-smelling vaginal discharge following an abortion.	
If meconium is present in amniotic fluid, immediately clear airway of the infant by suctioning (preferably done by physician immediately on delivery of the infant's head).	Helps prevent aspiration pneumonia in the infant.
Suction gastric contents immediately. Observe for sternal retractions, grunting, trembling, jitters, or pallor. If any of these signs are present, notify the physician at once.	Indicates development of respiratory complications secondary to meconium.
Wash hands each time before and after you handle the baby.	Prevents development of nosocomial infections.
Avoid wearing sharp jewelry that could scratch the baby.	
Keep umbilical cord clean and dry by cleansing at each diaper change or at least every 2 hours on [odd/even] hour.	
Monitor circumcision site for swelling, odor, or bleeding each diaper change or at least every 2 hours on [odd/even] hour.	Gives parents basic information regarding prevention of infection and monitoring for the development of infection.
Demonstrate and have parent return/demonstrate: • How to take the baby's temperature measurement • How to properly care for umbilical cord and circumcision	

Mental Health

ACTIONS/INTERVENTIONS	RATIONALES
Monitor the temperature of clients receiving antipsychotic medications twice a day, and report any elevations to physician. [Note times for temperature measurement here.]	These clients are at risk for developing agranulocytosis. The greatest risk is 3 to 8 weeks after therapy has begun. Can occur any time during the first 12 weeks of treatment.[104]

(care plan continued on page 58)

NURSING ACTIONS/INTERVENTIONS WITH RATIONALES (continued from page 57)

Mental Health

ACTIONS/INTERVENTIONS	RATIONALES
Monitor the client for the presence of a sore throat in the absence of a cold or other flu-like symptoms, mouth sores, skin ulcerations, and peripheral edema at least daily. Report any occurrence. Note schedule for this assessment here.	These could be symptoms of agranulocytosis.[104]
Teach the client to report any signs of infection (lethargy, weakness, fever, sore throat, temperature elevations) symptoms to their health-care team.	
During the first 12 weeks of treatment with an antipsychotic, report any signs of infection in the client to the physician for assessment of white cell count.	
Review the client's CBC or WBC before antipsychotics are started, and report any abnormalities on this and any subsequent CBCs to the physician.	Provides a baseline for comparison after the client has begun antipsychotic therapy.
Teach client and support systems about special WBC monitoring programs (i.e., Clozapine requires a monthly WBC monitoring during the first 6 months and after 6 months every other week).	
Teach the client and family handwashing techniques, nutrition, appropriate antibiotic use, hazards of substance abuse, and universal precautions.	These measures can help prevent or decrease the risk of infection.

Gerontic Health

In addition to the interventions for Adult Health, the following may be utilized:

ACTIONS/INTERVENTIONS	RATIONALES
Encourage clients to maintain immunization status, especially annual influenza, tetanus and diphtheria every 10 years, and annual pneumonia vaccine.	Older adults, with aging changes to the immune system, are at increased risk for infection.
Teach importance of avoiding crowds in the presence of flu or cold outbreaks.	Decreases potential for contact with infectious processes at high-risk times.
Teach the client and caregiver atypical signs and symptoms that may indicate infection in an older adult.	Older adults may not have fever, localized pain, or other classic signs in the presence of infection.
Assist the client in maintaining adequate hydration of 2000 cc daily.	Adequate hydration status has a preventive effect.
Assist the client in maintaining adequate vitamin intake, particularly vitamins A, C, and E; zinc; and selenium.	These nutrients are known to assist in infection prevention.

Home Health

ACTIONS/INTERVENTIONS	RATIONALES
Teach the client and family measures to prevent transmission of infectious disease to others. Assist the patient and family with lifestyle changes that may be required: • Handwashing • Isolation as appropriate	Many infectious diseases can be prevented by appropriate measures. The client and family members require this information and the opportunity to practice these skills.

ACTIONS/INTERVENTIONS	RATIONALES
• Proper disposal of infectious waste (e.g., bagging)	
• Proper treatment of linens soiled with infectious matter.	Hot water provides an effective means of destroying
• Proper use of disinfectants	microorganisms, and a temperature of at least 160° F
• Appropriate medical intervention (e.g., antibiotics or antipyretics)	for a minimum of 25 minutes is commonly recommended for hot-water washing. Chlorine bleach provides an extra margin of safety. A total available
• Immunization as recommended by CDC	chlorine residual of 50 to 150 ppm is usually achieved
• Signs and symptoms of infection	during the bleach cycle.[98,105–107]
• Treatment for lice and removal of nits	
• Asepsis for wound care	

● NOTE: *Items can be sterilized at home by immersing in boiling water for 10 minutes. The water needs to be boiling for the entire 10 minutes. Equipment, such as bedside commodes, bedpans, and other items exposed to blood and body fluids can also be cleaned with a 1:10 bleach and water solution.*

Participate in tuberculosis screening and prevention program.[108–110]	This action serves as the database to identify the need for interventions to prevent infections.
Monitor for factors contributing to the risk for infection.	
Involve the client and family in planning, implementing, and promoting reduction in the risk for infection:	Family involvement is important to ensure success. Communication and mutual goals improve the
• Family conference	outcome.
• Mutual goal setting	
• Communication	
Teach the client and family measures to prevent or decrease potential for infection:	These measures reduce the risk of infection.
• Handwashing techniques, including the use of alcohol-based antimicrobial gels.	
• Universal precautions for blood and body fluids	
• Personal hygiene and health habits	
• Nutrition	
• Immunization schedule	
• Proper food storage and preparation	
• Elimination of environmental hazards such as rodents or insects	
• Proper sewage control and trash collection	
• Appropriate antibiotic use to include instruction to take the entire prescribed dose, to refrain from using partially used prescriptions or prescriptions written for other persons.	
• Hazards of substance abuse	
• Preparation and precautions when traveling to areas in which infectious diseases are endemic	
• Signs and symptoms of infectious diseases for which the client and family are at risk	
• Preparation for disaster (water storage, canned or dried food, and emergency waste disposal)	

INJURY, RISK FOR

DEFINITIONS[44]

Risk for Injury A state in which the individual is at risk of injury as a result of environmental conditions interacting with the individual's adaptive and defensive resources.

Risk for Suffocation Accentuated risk of accidental suffocation (inadequate air available for inhalation).

Risk for Poisoning Accentuated risk of accidental exposure to or ingestion of drugs or dangerous products in doses sufficient to cause poisoning.

Risk for Trauma Accentuated risk of accidental tissue injury, for example, wound, burn, or fracture.

DEFINING CHARACTERISTICS (RISK FACTORS)[44]

A. Risk for Injury

1. External
   a. Mode of transport or transportation
   b. People or provider: Nosocomial agents; staffing patterns; cognitive, affective, and psychomotor factors
   c. Physical: Design, structure, and arrangement of community, building, and/or equipment
   d. Nutrients: Vitamins, food types
   e. Biologic: Immunization level of community, microorganism
   f. Chemical: Pollutants, poisons, drugs, pharmaceutical agents, alcohol, caffeine, nicotine, preservatives, cosmetics, and dyes

2. Internal
   a. Psychological: Affective, orientation
   b. Malnutrition
   c. Abnormal blood profile: Leukocytosis–leukopenia, altered clotting factors, thrombocytopenia, sickle cell, thalassemia, decreased hemoglobin
   d. Immuno–autoimmune dysfunction
   e. Biochemical, regulatory function: Sensory dysfunction, integrative dysfunction, effector dysfunction, tissue hypoxia
   f. Developmental age: Physiologic, psychosocial
   g. Physical: Broken skin, altered mobility

B. Risk for Suffocation

1. External (environmental)
   a. Vehicle warming in closed garage
   b. Use of fuel-burning heater not vented to outside
   c. Smoking in bed
   d. Children playing with plastic bags or inserting small objects into their mouth or nose
   e. Propped bottle placed in an infant's crib
   f. Pillow placed in an infant's crib
   g. Eating large mouthfuls of food
   h. Discarded or unused refrigerators or freezers without removed doors
   i. Children left unattended in bathtubs or pools
   j. Household gas leaks
   k. Low-strung clothesline
   l. Pacifier hung around infant's head

2. Internal (individual)
   a. Reduced olfactory sensation
   b. Reduced motor abilities
   c. Cognitive or emotional difficulties
   d. Disease or injury process
   e. Lack of safety education
   f. Lack of safety precautions

C. Risk for Poisoning

1. External (environmental)
   a. Unprotected contact with heavy metals or chemicals
   b. Medicines stored in unlocked cabinet accessible to children or confused persons
   c. Presence of poisonous vegetation
   d. Presence of atmospheric pollutants
   e. Paint, lacquer, etc. in poorly ventilated areas or without effective protection
   f. Flaking, peeling paint or plaster in presence of young children
   g. Chemical contamination of food and water
   h. Availability of illicit drugs potentially contaminated by poisonous additives
   i. Large supplies of drugs in house
   j. Dangerous products placed or stored within the reach of children or confused persons

2. Internal (individual)
   a. Verbalization of occupational setting without adequate safeguards
   b. Reduced vision
   c. Lack of safety or drug education
   d. Lack of proper precaution
   e. Insufficient finances
   f. Cognitive or emotional difficulties

D. Risk for Trauma

1. External (environmental)
   a. Slippery floors (e.g., wet or highly waxed)
   b. Snow or ice collected on stairs, walkways
   c. Unanchored rugs
   d. Bathtub without handgrip or antislip equipment
   e. Use of unsteady ladders or chairs
   f. Entering unlighted rooms
   g. Unsteady or absent stair rails
   h. Unanchored electric wires
   i. Litter or liquid spills on floors or stairways
   j. High beds
   k. Children playing without a gate at the top of the stairs
   l. Obstructed passageways
   m. Unsafe window protection in homes with young children
   n. Inappropriate call-for-aid mechanisms for bed-resting patient
   o. Pot handles facing toward front of stove
   p. Bathing in very hot water (e.g., unsupervised bathing of young children).
   q. Potential igniting gas leaks
   r. Delayed lighting of gas burner or oven
   s. Experimenting with chemical or gasoline
   t. Unscreened fires or heaters
   u. Wearing plastic apron or flowing clothes around open flame
   v. Children playing with matches, candles, cigarettes
   w. Inadequately stored combustibles or corrosives (e.g., matches, oily rags, lye)
   x. Highly flammable children's toys or clothing
   y. Overloaded fuse boxes

z. Contact with rapidly moving machinery, industrial belts, or pulleys

aa. Sliding on coarse bed linen or struggling within bed restraints

bb. Faulty electrical plugs, frayed wires, or defective appliances

cc. Contact with acids or alkalis

dd. Playing with fireworks or gunpowder

ee. Contact with intense cold

ff. Overexposure to sun, sunlamps, or radiotherapy

gg. Use of cracked dinnerware or glasses

hh. Knives stored uncovered

ii. Guns or ammunition stored unlocked

jj. Large icicles hanging from roof

kk. Exposure to dangerous machinery

ll. Children playing with sharp-edged toys

mm. High-crime neighborhood and vulnerable clients

nn. Driving a mechanically unsafe vehicle

oo. Driving after partaking of alcoholic beverages or drugs

pp. Driving at excessive speed

qq. Driving when tired

rr. Driving without necessary visual aid

ss. Children riding in the front seat in car

tt. Smoking in bed or near oxygen

uu. Overloaded electrical outlet

vv. Grease waste collected on stoves

ww. Use of thin or worn potholders

xx. Misuse of necessary headgear for motorized cyclists or young children carried on adult bicycles

yy. Unsafe road or road-crossing conditions

zz. Play or work near vehicle pathways (e.g., driveways, laneways, or railroad tracks)

aaa. Nonuse or misuse of seat restraints

2. Internal (individual)

a. Lack of safety education

b. Insufficient finances to purchase safety equipment or effect repairs

c. History of previous trauma

d. Lack of safety precautions

e. Poor vision

f. Reduced temperature or tactile sensation

g. Balancing difficulties

h. Cognitive or emotional difficulties

i. Reduced large or small muscle coordination

j. Weakness

k. Reduced hand–eye coordination

RELATED FACTORS[44]

The risk factors serve as the related factors for risk diagnoses.

RELATED CLINICAL CONCERNS

1. AIDS
2. Dementias such as Alzheimer's disease or multi-infarct
3. Diseases of the eye such as cataracts or glaucoma
4. Medications, for example, hallucinogens, barbiturates, opioids, or benzodiazepines
5. Epilepsy
6. Substance abuse or dependence

 Have You Selected the Correct Diagnosis?

Activity Intolerance
This diagnosis should be considered if the nurse observes or validates reports of the patient's inability to complete required tasks because of insufficient energy. Insufficient energy could lead to accidents through, for example, falling or dropping of items.

Impaired Physical Mobility
This diagnosis is appropriate if the patient has difficulty with coordination, range of motion, muscle strength and control, or activity restrictions related to treatment. This could be manifested by the frequent occurrence of accidents or injury.

Deficient Knowledge
This diagnosis may exist if the client or family verbalizes less-than-adequate understanding of injury prevention.

Impaired Home Maintenance
This diagnosis is demonstrated by the inability of the patient or the family to provide a safe living environment.

Disturbed Thought Process
This diagnosis should be considered if the patient exhibits impaired attention span; impaired ability to recall information; impaired perception, judgment, and decision making; or impaired conceptual reasoning abilities. This diagnosis could certainly be reflected in increased accidents or injuries.

Risk for Violence
This diagnosis exists if the accidents or injuries can be related to the risk factors for self-inflicted or other-directed physical trauma (e.g., self-destructive behavior, substance abuse, rage, and hostile verbalizations).

EXPECTED OUTCOME

Will identify hazards [list] contributing to risk for injury and at least one corrective measure [list] for each hazard by [date].

TARGET DATES

Although preventing injury may be a lifelong activity, establishing a mindset to avoid injury can be begun rapidly. An appropriate target date would be within 3 days of admission.

NURSING ACTIONS/INTERVENTIONS WITH RATIONALES

Adult Health

ACTIONS/INTERVENTIONS	RATIONALES
Keep bed wheels locked and bed in low position. Keep head of bed elevated at least 30 degrees at all times. Utilize siderails as necessary	Siderails should be used judiciously. Use alternative methods in patients to whom side rails pose more of a danger (e.g., confused).
Assess patient safety status at least hourly. If risk for injury exists, do not leave patient unattended. Schedule sitters around the clock. Provide appropriate signage or communication if the patient has been identified as being at risk for injury (e.g., falls).	Primary preventive measures to ensure patient safety. Green dot serves to alert other health-care personnel of patient's status.
Check respiratory rates and depth and chest sounds at least every 4 hours at [Note times here].	Ongoing monitoring of risk factors.
Continuously assess airway patency. Know location of emergency airway equipment.	
Do not leave medications or solutions in the room.	Basic safety measures to prevent poisoning.
Make sure handrails are in place in the bathroom and that safety strips are in tub and shower. Do not leave patient unattended in bathtub or shower.	Basic safety measures to prevent injury.
Keep the patient's room free of clutter.	Basic safety measures to prevent injury.
Orient the patient to time, person, place, and environment at least once a shift and as necessary.	Keeps patient aware of environment.
Provide night light.	Safety measure to prevent falling at night.
Assist in correcting, to the extent possible, any sensory–perceptual problems through appropriate referrals.	Correction of sensory–perceptual problems (vision, for example) will assist in accident prevention.
Assist the patient with all transfer and ambulation. If the patient requires multiple pillows for rest or positioning, tape the bottom layer of pillows to prevent dislodging.	Assists in preventing suffocation or tripping on pillows.
Teach the patient and family safety measures for use at home:	
• Use nonskid rugs or tack down throw rug.	
• Use handrails.	
• Install ramps.	
• Use color contrast for steps, door knobs, electrical outlets, and light switches.	
• Avoid surface glare (e.g., floors or table tops). Maintain clean, nonskid floors and keep rooms and halls free of clutter.	
• Change physical position slowly.	
• Use covers for electrical outlets.	
• Position pans with handles toward back of stove.	
• Have family post poison control number for ready reference.	
• Provide extra lighting in room and night light.	
Teach the patient and significant other:	Basic safety measures.
• Alterations in lifestyle that may be necessary (e.g., stopping smoking, stopping alcohol ingestion, decreasing or ceasing drug ingestion, or ceasing driving)	
• Use of assistive devices (e.g., walkers, canes, crutches, or wheelchairs)	

ACTIONS/INTERVENTIONS	RATIONALES
• Heimlich maneuver • Cardiopulmonary resuscitation (CPR) • Recognition of signs and symptoms of choking and carbon monoxide poisoning • Necessity of chewing food thoroughly and cutting food into small bites	
Refer to appropriate agency for safety check of home. Make referral at least 3 days prior to discharge.	Allows time for checking and correction of problem areas.

Child Health

ACTIONS/INTERVENTIONS	RATIONALES
Maintain appropriate supervision of the infant at all times. Allow respite time for the parents. Do not leave the infant unattended. Have bulb syringe available in case of need to suction oropharynx. If regular equipment for suctioning is required, validate by checking label that all safety checks have been completed on equipment. Be aware of potential for young children to answer to any name. Validate identification for procedures in all young children.	Will prevent medication or treatment errors. Anticipatory safety is an ongoing requisite for care of children.
Keep siderails of crib up, and monitor safety of all attachments for crib or infant's bassinet.	Infants and small children are prone to putting small pieces in mouth, nose, or ears. Basic safety measures.
Check temperature of water before bathing and formula or food before feeding. Do not microwave formula.	Helps prevent scalding or chilling of the infant.
Maintain contact at all times during bathing. Infants unable to sit must be held constantly. Older children should be monitored as well, with special attention given to mental or physical needs for a handicapped child.	
Place the infant on back with pacifier, for sleeping. Recommendations include infant to sleep in same room as caregivers. Special instructions may be required with preterm infants and/or those with special conditions, for example, gastroesophageal reflux.	Helps maintain airway. New updates regarding sudden infant death syndrome (SIDS) now provide this mandate from the American Academy of Pediatrics. (See section on High Risk for SIDS.)
Investigate any signs and symptoms that warrant potential child protective service referral.	Provides assistance for the child and family in instances of child abuse and is mandated by law.
Teach family basic safety measures: • Store plastic bags in cabinet out of child's reach. • Do not cover mattress or pillows of the infant or child with plastic. • Make certain crib design follows federal regulations and that mattress has appropriate fit with crib frame. • Discourage co-sleeping in bed with the infant. • Avoid use of homemade pacifiers (use only those of one-piece construction with loop handle). • Do not tie pacifier around the infant's neck. • Untie bibs, bonnets, or other garments with snug fit around neck of the infant before sleep. • Inspect toys for removable parts and check for safety approval.	Ensures environmental safety for the infant or child. Prevents possible suffocation. Adheres to new guidelines to prevent suffocation/reduces SIDS risk. Same as above. Danger of infant being rolled on. Danger of aspiration. Danger of strangulation. Danger of strangulation. Danger of aspiration.

(care plan continued on page 64)

NURSING ACTIONS/INTERVENTIONS WITH RATIONALES (continued from page 63)

Child Health

ACTIONS/INTERVENTIONS	RATIONALES
• Do not feed the infant foods that do not readily dissolve, such as grapes, nuts, and popcorn.	Danger of aspiration.
• Keep doors of large appliances, especially refrigerators, closed at all times.	Danger of child being trapped inside refrigerator.
• Maintain fence and constant supervision around swimming pool.	Prevents possible drowning.
• Exercise caution while cleaning, with attention to pails of water and cleaning solutions.	Prevents possible drowning/aspiration.
• As the infant or child is able, encourage swimming lessons with supervision and foster water safety.	Offers primary prevention to foster long-term water safety.
• Use caution in exposure to sun for periods of longer than 10 minutes. Use SPF sunblock for children, avoid direct sunlight esp. from 11 A.M. to 4 P.M.	Offers protective safety measure.
• Use appropriate seat belts and car seats according to weight and development.	
• Keep matches and pointed objects, such as knives, in a safe place out of the child's reach.	
• Use lead-free paint on the child's furniture and environment.	
• Keep toxic substances locked in cabinet and out of the child's reach.	
• Hang plants and avoid placement on floor and tables.	
• Discard used poisonous substances.	
• Do not store toxic substances in food or beverage containers.	
• Administer medication as a drug, not as candy.	
• Use childproof medication containers.	
• Keep syrup of ipecac on hand in case of accidental poisoning.	
• As applicable, use any special monitoring equipment as recommended for the child.	
• Monitor mealtimes to prevent aspiration with giggling.	

Women's Health

ACTIONS/INTERVENTIONS	RATIONALES
Teach the patient and family the risk for injury to the fetus and patient when the pregnant woman smokes, is exposed to secondhand smoke, or engages in substance abuse (e.g., alcohol and drugs [legal or illegal]).	Provides initial safety information regarding the well-being of the fetus.
Ask all patients about the existence of violence in their homes. Report child and elder abuse to proper authorities and any suspicion of family violence. Some states require reporting of violence against women. (See Chapters 9 and 11 for more detailed nursing actions.)	A legal requirement in some states.
Provide atmosphere that allows the patient considering abortion to relate her concerns and experiences and to obtain detailed information about the method of abortion that is being considered.	Allows the patient to receive nonjudgmental information about the pros and cons of all choices available.

ACTIONS/INTERVENTIONS	RATIONALES
Encourage questions and verbalization of the patient's life expectations.	
Provide information on options available to the patient. This is especially important in cases of domestic violence.	Some states require that information about local women's shelters be provided when domestic violence is suspected.
Assist the patient in identifying lifestyle adjustments that the decision could entail.	
Involve significant others, if so desired by the patient, in discussion and problem-solving activities regarding lifestyle adjustments.	
In instances where the patient has performed a self-induced abortion, obtain detailed information regarding the method used. Provide atmosphere that allows the patient to relate her experience.	In self-induced abortion, there is high probability of injury and subsequent infection. This information provides the health team with basic data to begin assessing the degree of injury.
Ascertain whether abortifacients (castor oil, turpentine, lye, ammonia, etc.) or mechanical means (coat hanger, knitting needles, broken bottle, or knife) were used.	
Regardless of the type of abortion, obtain a history from the patient that includes: • Date of last menstrual period • Method of contraception, if any • Previous obstetric history • Known allergies to anesthetics, analgesics, antibiotics, or other drugs • Current drug usage • Past medical history • Note the patient's mental state (e.g., anxious, frightened, or ambivalent).	Provides basic database to initiate planning of care.
Perform physical assessment with special notice of: • Amount and character of vaginal discharge • Temperature elevation • Pain • Bleeding: consistency, amount, and color	
Teach the patient the importance of proper storage of birth control pills, spermicides, and medications.	To keep out of reach of children or others who should not use these medications.
Assist the patient in identifying drugs that are teratogenic to the fetus.	Provides information that allows the patient to plan for safety during pregnancy.
Assist the patient in becoming aware of environmental hazards when pregnant, such as x-rays, people with infections, cats (litter boxes), and hazards on the job (surgical gases, industrial hazards).	

Mental Health

In addition to the following interventions, refer to the applicable interventions provided in the Adult Health and Home Health sections of this diagnosis.

ACTIONS/INTERVENTIONS	RATIONALES
Orient the client to person, place, and time on each interaction.	Disorientation can increase the client's risk for injury if the environment is perceived as dangerous.
Provide appropriate assistance to the client as he or she moves about the environment.	Prevents falls and possible injury.

(care plan continued on page 66)

NURSING ACTIONS/INTERVENTIONS WITH RATIONALES (continued from page 65)

Mental Health

ACTIONS/INTERVENTIONS	RATIONALES
Monitor level of consciousness every 15 minutes when the client is acutely disoriented following special treatments or when consciousness is affected by drugs or alcohol. If level of consciousness is impaired, place the client on side to prevent aspiration of vomitus, and withhold solid food until level of consciousness improves. Place the client in bed with siderails, and keep siderails raised.	Patient safety is of primary importance. Provides information about the client's current status so interventions can be adapted appropriately. Prevents aspiration by facilitating drainage of fluids away from airway and prevents falls and possible injury.
Do not allow the client to smoke without supervision when disoriented or when consciousness is clouded.	
Provide supervision for clients using new tools that could precipitate injury in special activities such as occupational therapy.	
Teach the client and members of support system:	
• Risks associated with excessive use of drugs and alcohol.	
• Appropriate methods for compensating for sensory–perceptual deficits (e.g., use of pictures or colors to distinguish environmental cues when ability to read is lost).	
Remove all environmental hazards (e.g., personal grooming items that could produce a hazard, cleaning agents, foods that produce a hazard when taken with certain medicines, plastic bags, clothes hangers, belt and ties, or shoestrings). Remove unnecessary pillows and blankets from the bed.	Prevents the client from acting impulsively to injure self with items easily found in environment. This allows staff time to offer alternative coping strategies when clients are experiencing difficulty with coping.
Maintain close supervision of the client. (If the client is suicidal, refer to nursing actions for Risk for Violence, Chapter 9, for specific interventions.)	Prevents the client from acting impulsively.
Check the client's mouth carefully after oral medicines are given for any amounts that might be held in the mouth to be used at a later date.	Basic safety precaution.
If the client is at risk for holding pills in the mouth to be used later, collaborate with physician to have doses changed to liquids or injections.	
Keep lavage setup and airway and oxygen equipment on standby.	
Talk with the client and members of support system about situations that increase the risk for poisoning, and develop a list of these situations.	
Label all medicines and poisonous substances appropriately.	
If client is in physical restraints:	Safety of client, other clients, and staff are of primary importance.[87,104]
• Ensure that all least restrictive measures have been attempted before restraints were initiated and orders for restraint meet JCAHO and institutional policy.	
• Provide one-to-one monitoring at all times	

ACTIONS/INTERVENTIONS	RATIONALES
• Monitor client's vital signs every 15 minutes • Offer food, water and toileting every 15 minutes • Inform client of conditions for restraint release • Release restraints, one limb at a time, on a scheduled basis and assess circulation and sensation in affected body part. Note schedule here. • Release client from restraint when client's behavior is under control and no longer poses a risk to themselves or others.	

Gerontic Health

In addition to the following interventions, refer to the applicable interventions provided in the Adult Health and Home Health sections of this diagnosis.

ACTIONS/INTERVENTIONS	RATIONALES
Refer the independent elder to home health for home safety assessment at least 3 days prior to discharge from hospital.	Provides timely home care planning, and allows implementation of safety measures before patient is discharged.
Minimize the use of or refrain from the use of physical and chemical restraints.	Use of chemical and physical restraints in elders is associated with risk of injury.
Utilize restraint alternatives: • Environmental changes • Bed safety • Seating and position support • Toileting and continence programs • Increased supervision and staffing for high-risk clients • Alarms	These alternatives can prevent falls without using potentially dangerous restraints.
Conduct a fall evaluation including an assessment of history of falls, medications, vision, gait and balance, lower limb joints, and neurologic and cardiovascular function.	Assists in determining modifiable risk factors for falls.

Utilize the "Get Up and Go" test to determine risk for falls.[112]
  I. Technique: Direct patient to do the following
    A. Rise from sitting position.
    B. Walk 10 feet.
    C. Turn around.
    D. Return to chair and sit down.
  II. Interpretation
    A. Patient takes <20 seconds to complete test.
      1. Adequate for independent transfers and mobility.
    B. Patient requires >30 seconds to complete test.
      1. Suggests higher dependence and risk of falls.
	Assists in objectifying the client's risk for falls.

Ensure that any sensory adaptations are made prior to activities. (Client has clean glasses and/or functional hearing aid available, as needed, adequate lighting to safely move about, and clear pathway for ambulation.)	The client may experience increased risks for injury if sensory losses are not addressed.[111,112]
Initiate fall precautions, as indicated, on admission to care facility, or on an as-needed basis.	Use of fall prevention strategies reduces the risk for falls in older adults and potential loss of function associated with falls and injuries.[112,114]

(care plan continued on page 68)

NURSING ACTIONS/INTERVENTIONS WITH RATIONALES (continued from page 67)

Gerontic Health

ACTIONS/INTERVENTIONS	RATIONALES
Teach at-risk older adults fall prevention strategies: • Clients using mobility aids • Clients on medications that increase the potential for vertigo, weakness, or orthostatic changes • Clients with motor or sensory deficits	Falls at home or in health-care settings are one of the main causes of morbidity and mortality in older adults.[111–115]
Instruct the patient on safe administration of medication. Monitor for knowledge of drug dosage, reason for medication, expected effect, and possible side effects. Reinforce teaching on a daily basis.	Basic medication safety measures.
If the patient suffers from dementia, teach the caregiver the following safety adaptations[116]: • Place in a locked closet articles, such as power tools, medications, or appliances, that the individual may misuse and injure self or others. • Ensure that water temperature is low enough to prevent scalding. • Remove knobs from stove if cooking is a fire hazard. • Install gates at the top of stairs to prevent falls. • Tape door latches or remove tumblers from locks to prevent the patient from accidentally locking himself or herself in rooms. • Place two locks on entry and exit doors if the individual is prone to wandering. • Ensure that furnishings do not have sharp edges or large areas of glass that could cause injury during a fall.	Older adults with the diagnosis of dementia often display signs of poor judgment. The listed teaching factors decrease the risk for injury in the home setting.

Home Health

ACTIONS/INTERVENTIONS	RATIONALES
Assist the client and family in obtaining a referral for gait training and training for appropriate use of assistive devices. These can usually be obtained through a physical therapy department.	Prevention activities reduce the risk of injury.
Review medications with the client and family. Determine if medications may increase the client's risk for falls; clients taking more than four medications, psychotropic medications and antihypertensives. Collaborate with physician or health-care practitioner to modify medications as indicated.	These medications may increase risk of falls.
Assist the client and family in locating and accessing an exercise program with balance training as one of the components that is appropriate for the client's health status. These can usually be recommended by a physical therapy department.	Prevention activities reduce the risk of injury.
Assess the client for postural hypotension. Collaborate with a physician as indicated for treatment of postural hypotension.	Postural hypotension is a modifiable risk factor for falls.

ACTIONS/INTERVENTIONS	RATIONALES
Assist the client and family in adhering to the therapeutic regimen for cardiovascular disorders and cardiac arrhythmias.	Cardiovascular disorders and cardiac arrhythmias are modifiable risk factors for falls.
Involve the client and family in planning, implementing, and promoting reduction in the risk for injury:	Involvement of the client and family enhances motivation and increases the possibility of positive outcomes and the long-term lifestyle changes required.
• Arrange family conferences to clarify risk factors for injury and preventive measures the family can implement.	
• Assist the family to define mutual goals for prevention of injury.	
• Promote communication.	
• Assist family members with specific tasks as appropriate to reduce the risk for injury.	
● N O T E : *Restraining the client may increase, not decrease, the risk for injury.[117]*	
It is important to arrange the environment so that the client can avoid injury (e.g., use bedside commode or raised toilet seat; remove unnecessary furniture; remove throw rugs, repair or remove loose or damaged flooring, pick up objects that may be blocking pathways[118–120]; remove unsafe or improperly stored chemicals, weapons, cooking utensils, and appliances; use and store toxic substances safely; obtain certification in first aid and CPR; properly store food; obtain knowledge of poisonous plants; learn to swim; remove fire hazards from environment; design and practice an emergency plan for action if fire occurs; and properly use machines powered by petroleum products).	
• Teach the client and family injury prevention activities as appropriate:	Prevention activities reduce the risk of injury. Many people either do not know these prevention strategies or need to have them reinforced.
• Avoid the use of restraints for all clients, particularly confused clients.	Restraints have not been demonstrated to prevent falls and may increase risk for other types of injuries. (National Guideline Clearinghouse, http://www.guideline.gov.)
• Proper lifting techniques	
• Assist family in securing patient lift equipment for immobilized clients to prevent family/caregiver injury.	
• Removal of hazardous environmental conditions, such as improper storage of hazardous substances, improper use of electrical appliances, smoking in bed or near supplemental oxygen, open heaters and flames, and congested walkways	
• Proper ventilation when using toxic substances	
• First aid for poisoning	
• Proper labeling, storage, and disposal of toxic materials such as household cleaning products, lawn and garden chemicals, and medications	
• Proper food preparation and storage	
• Proper skin, lung, and eye protection when using toxic substances	
• Toxic substances out of reach of infants and young children	
• Recognition of toxic plants and removal from environment as indicated	
• Plan of action if accidental poisoning occurs	

(care plan continued on page 70)

NURSING ACTIONS/INTERVENTIONS WITH RATIONALES (continued from page 69)	

Home Health

ACTIONS/INTERVENTIONS	RATIONALES
Assist the client and family in lifestyle adjustments that may be required.	For long-term change, lifestyle adjustments are often required. Many people require assistance with these changes.
Refer to appropriate assistive community resources as indicated	Use of existing community services is an efficient use of resources.
Participate in early-return-to-work programs.[121]	Such programs lead to better client outcomes.
Participate in local, state, and national immunization initiatives.[122]	Community participation in immunization initiatives improves the rate of appropriate immunization and reduces the risk of outbreak of the diseases for which vaccines are available.

LATEX ALLERGY RESPONSE, RISK FOR AND ACTUAL

DEFINITION[44]

At risk for or demonstrates an allergic reaction to natural latex rubber products.

DEFINING CHARACTERISTICS[44]

A. Risk for Latex Allergy Response
1. Multiple surgical procedures, especially from infancy (e.g., spina bifida)
2. Allergies to bananas, avocados, tropical fruits, kiwi, or chestnuts
3. Professions with daily exposure to latex (e.g., medicine, nursing, or dentistry)
4. Conditions needing continuous or intermittent catheterization
5. History of reaction to latex (e.g., balloons, condoms, or gloves)
6. Allergies to poinsettia plants
7. History of allergies and asthma

B. Latex Allergy Response
1. Type I reactions: Immediate
2. Type IV reactions
   a. Eczema
   b. Irritation
   c. Reaction to additives causes discomfort (e.g., thiurams, carbamates)
   d. Redness
   e. Delayed onset (hours)
3. Irritant reactions
   a. Erythema
   b. Chapped or cracked skin
   c. Blisters

RELATED FACTORS[44]

No immune mechanism response.

RELATED CLINICAL CONCERNS

1. Any immune suppressed condition
2. History of multiple surgeries
3. History of multiple allergies
4. Asthma
5. Urinary bladder dysfunctions

☑ Have You Selected the Correct Diagnosis?

Impaired Tissue Integrity
In this instance, the client has actual tissue damage secondary to mechanical injury, radiation, etc. There will be actual breaks in the tissue, not just erythema or blisters.

Ineffective Protection
The patient with this diagnosis will have a decrease in the ability to guard against internal or external threats. The related factors for this diagnosis are much broader than just one response to an identified allergen.

EXPECTED OUTCOME

Will describe at least [number] different measures to use to avoid Latex Allergy Response by [date].

TARGET DATES

With appropriate therapy, the signs and symptoms of Latex Allergy Response begin to abate within 48 to 72 hours; thus, an appropriate target date would be 2 to 3 days.

NURSING ACTIONS/INTERVENTIONS WITH RATIONALES

Adult Health

ACTIONS/INTERVENTIONS	RATIONALES

Type I reaction:
• Remove all latex products possible.
• Stop treatment or procedure.
• Support airway; administer 100 percent oxygen.
• Start IV with volume expander.
• Give the following drugs according to physician order:
  • epinephrine
  • antihistamines
  • steroids
	Anaphylactic emergency.

Clearly identify patients who have a latex allergy with signs both at the bedside and on the chart and armbands.[115–118]	Alert all health-care workers that latex precautions must be taken in case emergency services are ever needed.
Isolate the patient if possible.	
Encourage patients to purchase and wear a MedicAlert® ID bracelet or necklace.[123–126]	
Report latex allergy to the Food and Drug Administration's MedWatch program at (800) FDA-1088.[123–126]	Establishes accurate data on latex allergies.
Identify routinely used supplies that contain latex.[123–126]	Ensures a latex-safe environment.
Identify latex-safe alternatives for these frequently used supplies.[123–126]	
Remove all latex-containing materials from the patient's bedside.[123–126]	
Replace latex-containing items with latex-safe alternatives.[115–118]	
Notify other departments as needed:	Ensures adequate communication among departments and coordination of care to provide a latex-safe environment.
• Pharmacy	So that medications can be prepared in a latex-free environment using nonlatex products.
• Dietary (avoid bananas, avocados, and chestnuts)	So that latex gloves worn by the personnel preparing food can be substituted with a vinyl alternative.
• Physical Therapy and Occupational Therapy, if appropriate	Ensure that all therapy equipment is latex-free.
• Surgical Services • Respiratory Therapy • Radiology • Laboratory • Material Management • Environmental Services	
Pad blood pressure cuff before taking blood pressure.	
Use nonpowdered latex gloves that have low protein content or vinyl gloves or nitrile gloves made of synthetic material with latex-like characteristics. When you must wear powdered latex gloves, never snap them on or off.	Aerosolized latex protein from the latex glove powder is one of the biggest contributing factors in triggering a latex reaction.
Use latex-free equipment and keep carts filled with these products. It is particularly critical that latex-free life-support equipment is included in the carts.	If a patient has an emergency event, it should not be compounded by having equipment that could worsen the event.

(care plan continued on page 72)

NURSING ACTIONS/INTERVENTIONS WITH RATIONALES (continued from page 71)

Adult Health

ACTIONS/INTERVENTIONS	RATIONALES
Do not inject through intravenous tubing injection ports. Use stopcock as needed. Use only latex-safe syringes.	
Do not aspirate medications through rubber stopper of multidose vials; remove stopper and aspirate contents directly.	
Check the manufacturer's product label for latex content.	Ensures a latex-safe environment.
Prohibit latex balloons in the patient's room. Mylar balloons are a latex-safe alternative.	
Include allergy information in all reports given to other departments.	
Document the use of latex-free products during care. Monitor for any adverse reactions.	Documentation is vitally important in patient care.
If a reaction does occur, document the presence of the reaction, and the steps that were taken to treat it. Document the patient's response to treatment.	
Notify the physician immediately if the patient does have an allergic reaction to latex.	
Assess the patient's and family's need for education related to latex allergy and provide that which is needed.	
Common sources of latex at home and at work:	

Common sources of latex at home and at work:
- Art supplies
- Bandages
- Balloons
- Balls
- Carpet backing
- Cleaning gloves
- Condoms or diaphragms
- Diapers
- Douche bulbs
- Elastic in clothing
- Elastic in hair accessories
- Erasers
- Eye drop bulbs
- Feeding nipples
- Food handled with latex gloves
- Handles (rubber) on tools, racquets, and bicycles
- Hot water bottles
- Infant toothbrush massager
- Koosh balls
- Pacifiers
- Paints
- Rubber clothing (e.g., raincoats)
- Rubber toys
- Shoes
- Tires
- Wheelchair cushions

Document the patient's and family's response to the teaching.

Child Health

ACTIONS/INTERVENTIONS	RATIONALES
Risk for	
Assess for signs and symptoms suggestive of latex allergy, including sneezing, coughing, rash, hives, or wheezing in the presence of balloons, Koosh balls, catheters, or other rubber items.[127,128]	Identification of at-risk populations aids in diagnosis of latex allergy.
Determine the history for the infant or child to note any allergic reactions, including triggering event or substance, actual symptoms, treatment required, and exacerbations.	Knowledge of individual's status assists in identification of at-risk or actual latex allergy and treatment as reference in event of recurrence and for preventive suggestions.
Determine whether the infant or child has undergone allergy testing, has received results, and has undergone a treatment regimen.	Documentation of known status is essential to consider possible change from potential to actual allergenic status.
Ask whether the infant or child has been diagnosed with a condition that requires contact with catheters or other hospital products, such as gloves or monitoring equipment.	Identification of risk factors assists in prevention of latex allergy development for all populations.
Ask whether the infant or child has ever experienced an allergic reaction during surgery.	Surgery imposes a risk for latex allergy development.
List any known foods, drugs, or allergenic substances for the infant or child.	Evidence of absence is essential; presence of history will be needed for risk reduction for exacerbation.
Provide appropriate identification alerts for records and identification bands as the child is cared for to signify allergenic status to latex.[127,128]	Proper identification serves to lessen the likelihood of repeated exposure and precipitation of latex allergic response.
Ask the parents how they would identify an allergic reaction in their child.	Individualized assessment provides validation of knowledge and values the importance of each possible manifestation of allergic response.
Find out whether the parents are aware of emergency equipment and treatment that may be required in the event of latex allergenic response.	Assessment for treatment is vital to management of possible allergic response to expedite intervention and minimize delay in event of emergency.
As dismissal planning is done, ensure the availability of emergency medical services (EMS), how to summon EMS, appropriate use of equipment, and how to maintain a plan in event of need.	Anticipatory planning assists in empowerment of parents to act in event of emergency, thereby ensuring best chance for treatment without delay.
Carry out health interview with focus on components to determine positive history or likelihood of latex allergy* medical diagnosis of spina bifida (myelomeningocele is a high risk).	Determination of a latex allergic client alerts all to need for precautionary measures.
Note most recent allergy testing, known allergies, current treatment, and plan for how best to prepare for elective surgery or treatments within hospital or clinic.	Exposure to latex early in life with repeated exposures in first years of life increases likelihood for latex allergy. Documentation of status provides appropriate basis for precautionary treatment of client.
Note history of allergenic responses to latex with attention to ongoing risk indices such as implants or need for special medical equipment such as catheters.[127,128]	Identification of risk indices alerts caregivers to likelihood of precautions to be implemented.
Identify appropriate treatment for known latex allergies to include need for special airway and oxygen delivery equipment, medications such as epinephrine, and specialists who will be available to assist in event of acute allergenic response.	Anticipatory planning will best provide for possible emergency without delay.

(care plan continued on page 74)

NURSING ACTIONS/INTERVENTIONS WITH RATIONALES (continued from page 73)

Child Health

ACTIONS/INTERVENTIONS	RATIONALES
Provide identification bracelet and appropriate designation of latex allergy status for the infant or child per medical record and ensure its appropriate sharing with all who will provide care for client (including daycare providers, teachers, or sitters).	Anticipatory planning and valuing of risk for acute allergenic response is best met with dissemination to significant caregivers for provision of greater freedom from risk and prevention of latex allergic recurrence.
Assess parental knowledge of current plan of care with a focus on potential allergenic triggers prior to dismissal and for ongoing care.	Anticipatory planning for the individual places value on the preventive component.
Assess for stressors related to the infant or child's latex allergy status.	Valuing feelings and perceptions of the client and family fosters open communication and provides cues for related nursing needs.

Women's Health

● N O T E : *The nursing actions for a woman with the nursing diagnosis of latex allergy are the same as those for Adult Health. Be aware that infants born to mothers with latex allergies could themselves be allergic to latex, and all the precautions taken with the mother should be followed with infants. This includes padding the crib well to keep the infant away from the crib mattress covers, which usually have latex in them.*

Research studies have shown that glove powder binds to latex proteins and is therefore a major hazard and contributor to the amount of latex found in the air in operating rooms and patient rooms where gloves are routinely used. It has been shown that patients and health-care workers are exposed on a continuous basis when working in rooms in which there is a high usage of gloves with powder, as bound proteins are aerosolized when gloves are dispensed, put on, used, and/or removed from the hands. Health-care personnel and patients in labor and delivery are particularly vulnerable and at risk for latex allergy because of the high use of gloves during vaginal examinations of the patient in labor and during cesarean sections. Likewise, the health-care worker needs to be aware of the presence of latex in nipples on infant bottles.

ACTIONS/INTERVENTIONS	RATIONALES
Replace all examination gloves and sterile gloves in obstetric units with vinyl or low-allergen, powder-free latex gloves.	A major reason for the increase in sensitization rates in health-care workers and patients is the use of products containing high levels of extractable proteins, such as powdered, high-allergen gloves.[124,125]
When using vinyl gloves during pelvic examinations, in surgery, or when dealing in any situation requiring standard precautions, always double glove.	Because of the high failure rate of vinyl gloves, it is recommended to use low-allergen, powder-free latex gloves during high-risk situations involving standard precautions; however, if there is a need for the use of no latex products (such as with the latex-sensitive patient or health-care worker), then the health-care worker using vinyl gloves should double glove for his or her own protection.
Carefully interview the pregnant client and screen for risk for latex allergy. Question about past pregnancy outcomes, particularly if they have had any infants with neural tube defects (e.g., spina bifida).	Because of the frequent use of gloves, catheters, etc. in the care of these babies, both the baby and the caretaker may have developed a sensitivity to latex. (Approximately 72 percent of patients with spina bifida are allergic to latex.)[127,128]

ACTIONS/INTERVENTIONS	RATIONALES
Pregnant mothers who have been involved with the care of a previous child that could have involved exposure to latex products, and/or their newborn infant, should be treated with latex avoidance regardless of their allergy status.	This mother and her newborn are at risk for a potential reaction to latex.[126,127]
Carefully monitor the mother and her newborn for symptoms of an allergic reaction, including a systemic reaction.	
Teach the mother and her family the essentials of latex precautions: • Review of routes of exposure • Use of infant and toddler supplies and toys	

Mental Health

Nursing interventions and rationales for this diagnosis are the same as those for Adult Health.

Gerontic Health

Use information provided in Adult Health section for this diagnosis. Currently there is no evidence available to suggest specific interventions for this diagnosis based on age of the client.

Home Health

ACTIONS/INTERVENTIONS	RATIONALES
Inquire about sensitivity to latex or other related factors at onset of care.	Allows early identification of potential for allergic reactions.
Assist the client in acquiring a MedicAlert bracelet when latex allergy is present.	Prevents further exposure to latex products.
Assist the client in securing latex-free supplies for home use.	Prevents further exposure to latex products.
Educate the client, family members, and potential caregivers about latex-containing devices and equipment, as well as the signs of acute allergic reactions.	Encourages family participation in client care and reduces potential for accidental exposure.
Educate the client, family members, and potential caregivers how to access emergency medical care should an accidental exposure precipitate an acute reaction.	Prevents further morbidity.
Assist the client and family in obtaining an epineprhrine pen for use in case of anaphylactic reaction to latex.	Prevents further morbidity.

MANAGEMENT OF THERAPEUTIC REGIMEN, EFFECTIVE

DEFINITION[44]

A pattern of regulating and integrating into daily living a program for treatment of illness and its sequelae that is satisfactory for meeting specific health goals.

DEFINING CHARACTERISTICS[44]

1. Appropriate choices of daily activities for meeting the goals of a treatment or prevention program
2. Illness symptoms are within a normal range of expectation
3. Verbalized desire to manage the treatment of illness and prevention of sequelae

4. Verbalized intent to reduce risk factors for progression of illness and sequelae

RELATED FACTORS[44]

To be developed.

RELATED CLINICAL CONCERNS

Any condition requiring long-term management; for example, cardiovascular diseases and diabetes mellitus.

 Have You Selected the Correct Diagnosis?

There are currently no other diagnoses this diagnosis could be compared with, or that are close to, the concept of this diagnosis. This diagnosis could be classified as a wellness diagnosis; that is, the patient with this diagnosis is progressing toward wellness and appropriate health maintenance.

EXPECTED OUTCOME

Subsequent assessments document continued progress toward health by [date].

TARGET DATES

Effective management of a therapeutic regimen requires a lifelong commitment by the client. Therefore, target dates will vary from weeks to years. It would be appropriate to set the first target date for 1 month after the patient's discharge.

NURSING ACTIONS/INTERVENTIONS WITH RATIONALES

Adult Health

ACTIONS/INTERVENTIONS	RATIONALES
Allow time for the patient to discuss his or her feelings about the therapeutic regimen.	
Support the patient in choices made to effectively manage therapeutic regimen.	Encourages the patient's sense of control and strengthens support systems.
Review availability and use of resources and support groups.	
Answer questions about disease process and therapeutic regimen. Provide teaching for any new components of therapeutic regimen.	
Assist the patient to solve problems as they arise.	Encourages the patient's sense of self-control.
Allow and monitor self-care while in the hospital.	Promotes independence.
Have the patient return/demonstrate activities associated with therapeutic regimen (e.g., dressing changes; glucose testing; blood pressure checks; counting calories, fat grams, carbohydrates, and sodium intake; self-administering medications). Supervise performance, critique, and reteach as necessary.	Provides feedback for skills; reaffirms motivation.
Review self-reported plan of activities with the patient, and continue to encourage its use and the sharing of the plan with the patient's employer and physician.	Provides visual record of plan that is integrated into patient's lifestyle.
Review accomplishment of goals of therapeutic regimen, and praise the patient for even small accomplishments.	Improves motivation and gives the patient a sense of achievement.
Allow at least 30 minutes a day for the patient to verbalize possible conflicts with therapeutic regimen. Role-play possible scenarios.	Provides an opportunity for patient to verbalize and act out alternate coping strategies in a nonthreatening environment.
Have the patient make follow-up appointments with appropriate resources or health-care providers prior to discharge.	Facilitates continuity and consistency of plan.
Continue to coordinate care with other health-care providers or community resources.	Promotes patient advocacy.

Child Health

ACTIONS/INTERVENTIONS	RATIONALES
Utilize appropriate age and developmental communication.	Assists in developing a trusting relationship with the client and primary caregiver.
Determine the client's and primary caregiver's perception of condition.	Provides a starting point for discussing and teaching therapeutic regimen.
Assist the family to determine when and where follow-up care will be utilized.[49,50]	Promotes long-term management.
Offer verbal and emotional reinforcement for appropriate attendance to mutually agreed-to criteria. State criteria here (e.g., maintain immunizations).	Provides positive reinforcement.
Acknowledge need for the caregiver to be relieved (at regular intervals) of total responsibilities of dependent infant or child. Encourage the caregiver to express feelings regarding responsibility. Delineate community resources that can augment care.[49,50]	Assists in preventing caregiver role strain. Promotes effective management.
Identify subsequent factors that are likely to resurface over time (e.g., developmental concerns).	Anticipatory guidance is central to nursing.

Women's Health

ACTIONS/INTERVENTIONS	RATIONALES
Utilize Prenatal Risk Indicator Tools to identify women who are high risk for pregnancy and birth. Assess and counsel those mothers identified as high risk. Assist the patient to plan changes necessary in her lifestyle to maintain pregnancy and health of mother and fetus until birth.[29]	Provides the patient with the information needed to make informed choices and necessary lifestyle changes in order to maximize health for herself and her fetus.
Provide the new mother with information about various support groups and health-care programs when early postpartum discharge occurs. Provide teaching and support on an ongoing basis from time of conception until end of postpartum period for the new mother, her family, and her baby. Provide new parents with written handouts, help-line telephone numbers, follow-up appointments with advanced practice nurse, pediatrician, and obstetrician following postpartum discharge.	Provides the patient with the information needed to make informed choices and necessary lifestyle changes in order to maximize health for herself and her fetus.

Mental Health

ACTIONS/INTERVENTIONS	RATIONALES
Sit with the client [number] minutes [number] times a day to discuss: • His or her understanding of the current situation • Strategies that assist the client in this management • Support systems • Stressors [Note important data from these discussions here.]	Promotes the development of a trusting relationship by communicating respect for the client.[69] Provides assessment data that will assist in the development of a plan to support client's current behaviors. Support systems promote healthy behaviors.[88]
Discuss with the client signs and symptoms that would indicate that assistance is needed with management.	Promotes the client's sense of control.[97]

(care plan continued on page 78)

NURSING ACTIONS/INTERVENTIONS WITH RATIONALES (continued from page 77)

Mental Health

ACTIONS/INTERVENTIONS	RATIONALES
Develop with the client a plan for obtaining the necessary assistance when needed.	
Provide positive social reinforcement and other behavioral rewards for demonstration of adaptive management. (Those things that the client finds rewarding should be listed here with a schedule for use. The kinds of behaviors that are to be rewarded should also be listed.)	Positive reinforcement encourages adaptive behavior and enhances self-esteem.[87]
Discuss with the client the impact of stress on physiologic and psychological well-being. Develop with the client a plan for learning relaxation techniques, and have client practice technique for 30 minutes 2 times a day at [times] while hospitalized. Remain with the client during practice session to provide verbal cues and encouragement as necessary. These techniques can include: • Meditation • Progressive deep muscle relaxation • Visualization techniques that require the client to visualize scenes that enhance the relaxation response • Biofeedback • Prayer • Autogenic training	Anxiety decreases coping abilities and physiologic well-being. Repeated rehearsal of a behavior internalizes and personalizes it.[87]
Develop with the client a plan for integrating relaxation techniques into daily schedule at home.	Having a concrete plan increases the probability that the behavior will be implemented in the new environment.
Develop with the client a plan to include play into daily activities. Note the plan and specific activities here.	Play provides a sense of joy and rejuvenates inner vitality, enhancing coping abilities.[69]
Establish a time to meet with the client and those members of his or her support system identified as most important. Note time here. Utilize this time to discuss: • Support system's understanding of the client's situation • Support system's perceptions of their involvement with the management of the illness • Support system's perceptions of their needs at this time	Interactions between members of the support system and the individual can impact individual health and coping.[87,88] Provides an opportunity to assess support system's perspective to assist in developing interventions and further their acceptance of the intervention.[69,88]
Develop with the members of the support system a plan to meet the perceived needs. [Note this plan here.]	Increases support system's sense of control while enhancing self-esteem. Provides opportunities for increasing support system coping by recognizing that the illness has an impact on this system.[69,88]
Identify, with the client, community support groups that can be utilized when he or she returns home. Note those groups identified here with a plan for contacting them before the client leaves the hospital.	Groups can provide hope, information, and role models for coping and support.[88]

Gerontic Health

ACTIONS/INTERVENTIONS	RATIONALES
Monitor at each subsequent contact for continued ability to effectively manage regimen.	Physiologic aging or exacerbation of chronic illness may, over time, diminish continued ability to implement regimen.

ACTIONS/INTERVENTIONS	RATIONALES
Refer to community resources as indicated.	The older patient may have concerns related to availability of support systems, costs of medication, and availability of transportation. Use of already available community resources provides a long-term, cost-effective support system.
Establish communication link with primary caregiver and family.	Family members may not be geographically available.
Advise family members of availability of managed care resources in the community where older client resides.	Provides care options for family to consider.
Provide follow-up support via home visits and telephone contacts.	Presents opportunities for continued problem solving and increasing trust.
Assist caregivers in establishing and meeting their needs.	Enables continuation of care while decreasing the potential for burnout.
Review with the client and family the therapeutic regimen.	Helps determine possible areas of difficulty for client or caregiver.
Provide multisensory teaching materials (tapes, websites, literature) on therapeutic regimen to assist client and caregiver in adhering to regimen.	Provides quick access to information for the caregiver or client.
Incorporate a variety of local, regional, or state social services to ensure that needed information about the regimen is available to older patients.	Information flow may be impeded because of temporary relocation or social isolation.
Identify older community leaders, via age-related groups or associations, who can identify strengths or weaknesses of the community (such as senior citizen center members, church groups, and support groups focused on problems common to older adults).	Peer or cohort influences may assist in identifying and promoting problem solving.

Home Health

ACTIONS/INTERVENTIONS	RATIONALES
Assess the client/family understanding of the current disease process and therapeutic regimen.	Identifies knowledge deficits or misunderstanding to prevent problems.
Assess client/family strategies for managing the therapeutic regimen and assist in the provision of community resources that might support continued use of these strategies.	Supports the continued use of effective strategies.
Discuss the therapeutic regimen and strategies for managing the regimen with client and family regularly (as determined to be appropriate by the nurse) to ensure continued accurate understanding and effective use of strategies.	Clients/families may not be able to maintain sustained management, this will allow for early identification of problems.
Provide education as the client's condition or regimen changes.	Ensures that the client/family can maintain their current therapeutic management of the regimen.
Involve the client, family, and community in planning, implementing, and promoting the treatment plan through[129,135,137]: • Assisting with family conferences. • Coordinating mutual goal setting. • Promoting increased communication.	Involvement increases motivation and improves the probability of success.

(care plan continued on page 80)

NURSING ACTIONS/INTERVENTIONS WITH RATIONALES (continued from page 79)

Home Health

ACTIONS/INTERVENTIONS	RATIONALES
• Assigning family members specific tasks as appropriate to assist in maintaining the therapeutic regimen plan (e.g., support person for patient, transportation, or companionship in meeting mutual goals). • Utilizing population surveillance to detect changes in illness patterns for the community. • Support the client, family, or community in eliminating barriers to implementing the regimen by: • Providing for privacy. • Referring to community services (e.g., church, home health volunteer, transportation service, or financial assistance). • Providing for interpreters and for community-based language classes for English speakers to learn other languages as well as for non-English speakers to learn English. • Serving as social activist to encourage necessary participants to complete their tasks. This may include fund-raising, testifying before governing bodies, or coordinating efforts of several groups and organizations.	Many barriers are institutional and can be eliminated or reduced.
Assign one health-care provider or social service worker, as much as possible, to provide continuity in care provision.	Continuity of care provides a means for effective problem solving and early identification of problems.
Make timely telephone calls to clients to discuss care (e.g., 1 day after being seen in clinic for minor acute infection, or weekly or monthly on a routine schedule for chronically ill person).[140]	Follow-up with clients reinforces positive behaviors and may aid in early identification of problems. Follow-up also implies support of health-care professionals.
Reteach the client and family appropriate therapeutic activities as the need arises.	Reinforcement of information and continued assistance may be required to improve implementation of the therapeutic regimen.[137]

MANAGEMENT OF THERAPEUTIC REGIMEN (INDIVIDUAL, FAMILY, COMMUNITY), INEFFECTIVE

● **N O T E :** *This diagnosis was proposed at the Tenth NANDA Conference with the result that a proposal to delete Noncompliance was expected to be presented at the next conference. However, this has not occurred to date. As discussed in the conceptual section of this chapter, and in additional information later in this section, there are many people who object to the diagnosis of Noncompliance. For this reason, we will not provide nursing actions for Noncompliance but will provide the definition, defining characteristics, and related factors for this diagnosis until it is officially deleted. In 1994, the categories of Family and Community were added.*

DEFINITIONS[44]

Ineffective Management of Therapeutic Regimen (Individual) A pattern of regulating and integrating into daily living a program for treatment of illness and the sequelae of illness that is unsatisfactory for meeting specific health goals.

Noncompliance (Specify) The extent to which a person's and/or caregiver's behavior coincides or fails to coincide with a health-promoting or therapeutic plan agreed upon by the person (and/or family and/or community) and health-care professional. In the presence of an agreed upon, health-promoting or therapeutic plan, person's or caregiver's behavior is fully or partially nonadherent and may lead to clinically effective, partially effective, or ineffective outcomes.

Ineffective Management of Therapeutic Regimen (Family)   A pattern of regulating and integrating into family processes a program for treatment of illness and the sequelae of illness that is unsatisfactory for meeting specific health goals.

Ineffective Management of Therapeutic Regimen (Community)   A pattern of regulating and integrating into community processes programs for treatment of illness and the sequelae of illness that is unsatisfactory for meeting health-related goals.

DEFINING CHARACTERISTICS[44]

A. **Ineffective Management of Therapeutic Regimen (Individual)**
  1. Choices of daily living ineffective for meeting the goals of a treatment or prevention program
  2. Verbalized desire to manage the treatment of illness and prevention of sequelae
  3. Verbalized that he or she did not take action to reduce risk factors for progression of illness and sequelae
  4. Verbalized difficulty with regulation and/or integration of one or more prescribed regimens for treatment of illness and its effects or prevention of complications
  5. Acceleration (expected or unexpected) of illness symptoms
  6. Verbalized that he or she did not take action to include treatment regimens in daily routines
B. **Noncompliance**
  1. Behavior indicative of failure to adhere (by direct observation or by statements of patient or significant others)
  2. Evidence of development of complications
  3. Evidence of exacerbation of symptoms
  4. Failure to keep appointments
  5. Failure to progress
  6. Objective tests (physiologic measures or detection of markers)
C. **Ineffective Management of Therapeutic Regimen (Family)**
  1. Inappropriate family activities for meeting the goals of a treatment or prevention program
  2. Acceleration (expected or unexpected) of illness symptoms of a family member
  3. Lack of attention to illness and its sequelae
  4. Verbalized desire to manage the treatment of illness and prevention of the sequelae
  5. Verbalized difficulty with regulation and/or integration of one or more effects or prevention of complication
  6. Verbalized that family did not take action to reduce risk factors for progression of illness and sequelae
D. **Ineffective Management of Therapeutic Regimen (Community)**
  1. Illness symptoms above the norm expected for the number and type of population

  2. Unexpected acceleration of illness(es)
  3. Number of health-care resources is insufficient for the incidence or prevalence of illness(es)
  4. Deficits in people and programs to be accountable for illness care of aggregates
  5. Deficits in community activities for secondary and tertiary prevention
  6. Deficits in advocates for aggregates
  7. Unavailable health-care resources for illness care

✔ Have You Selected the Correct Diagnosis?

Deficient Knowledge
This is the most appropriate diagnosis if the patient or family verbalizes less than adequate understanding of health management or recalls inaccurate health information.

Ineffective Individual Coping or Compromised or Disabled Family Coping
These diagnoses are suspected if there are major differences between the patient and family reports of health status, health perception, and health-care behavior. Verbalizations by the patient or family regarding inability to cope also indicate this differential nursing diagnosis.

Dysfunctional Family Processes
Through observing family interactions and communication, the nurse may assess that Altered Family Processes is a consideration. Poorly communicated messages, rigidity of family functions and roles, and failure to accomplish expected family developmental tasks are a few observations that alert the nurse to this possible diagnosis.

Activity Intolerance or Self-Care Deficit
These diagnoses should be considered if the nurse observes or validates reports of inability to complete the tasks required because of insufficient energy or because of inability to feed, bathe, toilet, dress, and groom self.

Disturbed Thought Processes
The nursing diagnosis of Disturbed Thought Processes should be considered if the patient exhibits impaired attention span; impaired ability to recall information; impaired perception, judgment, and decision making; or impaired conceptual and reasoning abilities.

Impaired Home Maintenance
This diagnosis is demonstrated by the inability of the patient or family to provide a safe home living environment.

RELATED FACTORS[44]

A. **Ineffective Management of Therapeutic Regimen (Individual)**
  1. Perceived barriers
  2. Social support deficits

3. Powerlessness
4. Perceived susceptibility
5. Perceived benefits
6. Mistrust of regimen and/or health-care personnel
7. Knowledge deficits
8. Family patterns of health care
9. Excessive demands made on individual or family
10. Economic difficulties
11. Decisional conflicts
12. Complexity of therapeutic regimen
13. Complexity of health-care system
14. Perceived seriousness
15. Inadequate number and types of cues to action

B. Noncompliance
1. Health-care plan
   a. Duration
   b. Significant others
   c. Cost
   d. Intensity
   e. Complexity
2. Individual factors
   a. Personal and developmental abilities
   b. Health beliefs
   c. Cultural influences
   d. Spiritual values
   e. Individual's value system
   f. Knowledge and skill relevant to the regimen behavior
   g. Motivational forces
3. Health system
   a. Satisfaction with care
   b. Credibility of provider
   c. Access and convenience of care
   d. Financial flexibility of plan
   e. Client–provider relationship
   f. Provider reimbursement of teaching and follow-up
   g. Provider continuity and regular follow-up
   h. Individual health coverage
4. Network
   a. Involvement of members in health plan
   b. Social value regarding plan
   c. Perceived beliefs of significant others

C. Ineffective Management of Therapeutic Regimen (Family)
1. Complexity of health-care system
2. Complexity of therapeutic regimen
3. Decisional conflict
4. Economic difficulties
5. Excessive demands made on individual or family
6. Family conflict

D. Ineffective Management of Therapeutic Regimen (Community)
1. Perceived barriers
2. Social support deficit
3. Powerlessness
4. Perceived susceptibility

5. Perceived benefits
6. Mistrust of regimen and/or health-care personnel
7. Knowledge deficit
8. Family patterns of health care
9. Family conflict
10. Excessive demands made on individual or family
11. Economic difficulties
12. Decisional conflicts
13. Complexity of health-care regimen
14. Complexity of health-care system
15. Perceived seriousness
16. Inadequate number and types of cues to action

RELATED CLINICAL CONCERNS

1. Any diagnosis new to the patient; that is, patient does not have education or experience in dealing with this disorder.
2. Any diagnosis of a chronic nature, for example, pain, migraine headaches, rheumatoid arthritis, or a terminal diagnosis.
3. Any diagnosis that has required a change in health-care providers, for example, referred from long-time family physician to cardiologist.

ADDITIONAL INFORMATION

Some nursing authors object to the term "Noncompliance."[135–137,140–142] Compliance can become the basis for a power-oriented relationship in which one is judged and labeled compliant or noncompliant based on the hierarchical position of the professional in relation to the patient. The diagnosis of Noncompliance is to be used for those patients who wish to comply with the therapeutic recommendations but are prevented from doing so by the presence of certain factors. The nurse can in such situations strive to lessen or eliminate the factors that preclude the willing patient from complying with recommendations.

The principles of informed consent and autonomy[143] are critical to the appropriate use of this diagnosis. A person may freely choose not to follow a treatment plan. The nursing diagnosis Noncompliance does not mean that a patient is not willing to obey, but rather that a patient has attempted a prescribed plan and has found it difficult to follow through with it. The area of noncompliance must be specified. A patient may follow many aspects of a treatment program very well and find only a small part of the plan difficult to manage. Such a patient is noncompliant only in the area of difficulty.

Several nursing authors have recognized the interdependent nature of illness and healing.[138–143] This interdependence is especially pronounced in chronic illness. As a patient and his or her family adapts to a chronic condition, noncompliance with prescribed treatment regimens may actually be constructive and therapeutic, not detrimental.[140] The nurse who learns to listen to the patient and plan treatments in collaboration with the patient will benefit from the wisdom of people experiencing illness.[130,134]

EXPECTED OUTCOME

Will return-demonstrate appropriate technique or procedures [list] for self-care by [date].

TARGET DATES

The specific target dates for these objectives will be directly related to the barriers identified, the patient's entering level of knowledge, and the comfort the patient feels in expressing satisfaction or dissatisfaction. The target date could range from 1 to 5 days following the date of admission.

NURSING ACTIONS/INTERVENTIONS WITH RATIONALES

Adult Health

ACTIONS/INTERVENTIONS	RATIONALES
Help the patient and/or family identify potential areas of conflict (e.g., values, religious beliefs, cultural mores, or cost).	Assesses motivation and decreases risk of ineffective management of therapeutic regimen.
Make a list of these potential areas of conflict and help the patient and/or family problem solve each area one at a time. Note the list here with plan for problem solving.	
From time of admission, utilize each patient encounter to provide instructions for self-care. Teach the patient and significant others knowledge and skills needed to implement the therapeutic regimen (e.g., measuring blood pressure, counting calories, administering medications, or weighing self). [Note teaching topics and schedule here.]	Provides time to incorporate changes into lifestyle and to practice as necessary before day of discharge from hospital.
Assist the patient and/or family in identifying factors that actually or potentially may impede the desired therapeutic regimen plan:	Assesses motivation and decreases risk of diagnosis development.
• Sense of control	
• Language barriers (provide translators, assign nursing personnel to care for patient who speak the patient's language)	
• Cultural concerns (cultural mores, religious beliefs, etc.; design a plan that will allow incorporation of the therapeutic regimen within the cultural norms of the patient)	
• Financial constraints	
• Knowledge deficits	
• Time constraints	
• Level of knowledge and skill related to treatment plan	
• Resources available to meet treatment plan objectives	
• Complexity of treatment plan	
• Current response to treatment plan	
• Use of nonprescribed interventions	
• Entry to health-care system	
Allow opportunities for the patient and family to express feelings and to verbalize fears related to therapeutic regimen (e.g., body image, cost, side effects, pain, or dependency) by devoting at least 30 minutes per day to this activity. [List times here.]	Increases the patient's sense of control. Facilitates continuity and consistency of plan.

(care plan continued on page 84)

NURSING ACTIONS/INTERVENTIONS WITH RATIONALES (continued from page 83)

Adult Health

ACTIONS/INTERVENTIONS	RATIONALES
Design a chart to assist the patient to visually see the effectiveness of therapeutic regimen (e.g., weight loss chart, days without smoking, blood pressure measurements). Begin the chart in hospital within 1 day of admission. Follow up 1 week after discharge.	Visualization of actual progress promotes implementation of prescribed regimen.
Assist in the development of a schedule that will allow the patient to keep appointments and not miss work. Forward plan to employer and physician.	Demonstrates importance of schedule to patient, employer, and physician. Coordinated effort encourages adherence to regimen.
Assist the patient in developing time-management skills to incorporate time for relaxation and exercise. Have patient develop a typical 1 week schedule, then work with patient to adapt schedule as needed.	Individualizes schedule and highlights need for relaxation and exercise.
Contract, in writing, with the patient and/or significant others for specifics regarding regimen. Have patient and family establish mutual goal setting sessions. Assign specific family members specific tasks. Follow up 1 week after discharge; recheck 6 weeks following discharge.	Demonstrates, in writing, the importance of the plan, and by listing definitive follow-up times, enhances the probability of regimen implementation. Involvement increases motivation and improves the probability of success.
Design techniques that encourage the patient's or family's implementation of the regimen, such as setting single, easy-to-accomplish, short-term goals first and progressing to long-term goals as the short-term goals are met. If the idea of stopping smoking is too overwhelming, help the patient design a personal adaptive program. For example, change to a lower tar/nicotine cigarette, implement timed smoking (e.g., only one cigarette every 30 or 60 minutes), stabilize, then make further reductions.	Prevents multiple changes from overwhelming patient, thus avoiding one major contributor to ineffective management of therapeutic regimen.
Teach the patient and significant others assertive techniques that can be used to deal with dissatisfaction with caregivers.	Long waiting periods in offices, unanswered questions, being rushed, etc. increase the likelihood of abandoning the regimen. Assertiveness helps the patient and family overcome the feelings of powerlessness and increases the sense of control.
Assist in correction of sensory, motor, and other deficits to the extent possible through referrals to appropriate consultants (e.g., occupational therapist, physical therapist, ophthalmologist, audiologist).	
Have the patient and/or family design a home care plan. Assist the patient to modify the plan as necessary. Forward the plan to home health service, social service, physician, etc.	
Relate any information regarding dissatisfaction to the appropriate caregiver (e.g., to physician, problems with the time spent in waiting room, cultural needs, privacy needs, costs, need for generic prescriptions).	
Make follow-up appointments prior to the patient's leaving the hospital. Do it from the patient's room, and put appropriate information regarding appointment on brightly colored card (i.e., name, address, time, date, and telephone number).	Demonstrates exactly how to make appointments for patient.

ACTIONS/INTERVENTIONS	RATIONALES
Refer the patient and/or family to appropriate follow-up personnel (e.g., nurse practitioner, visiting nurse service, social service, or transportation service). Make referral at least 3 days prior to discharge.	Allows time for home care assessment and initiation of service.
Request follow-up personnel to remind the patient of appointments via card or telephone.	Shares the responsibility for implementing the regimen, and demonstrates the importance attached to follow-up care by those providers.
When discharge is imminent, transfer responsibility of self-care to patient. Supervise performance, critique, and reteach as necessary.	Allows sufficient practice time that provides immediate feedback on skills, etc.
Have the patient and significant others restate principles at least three interactions prior to discharge.	

● N O T E : *For Ineffective Management of Therapeutic Regimen (Community), see Home Health.*

Child Health

● N O T E : *Because of the dependency of the infant or child, ineffective management will always include both the individual and the family.*

ACTIONS/INTERVENTIONS	RATIONALES
Assist in developing health values of regimen adherence before the infant's birth through emphasis of these aspects in childbirth education classes.	Initiates idea of individual health management for child's health before birth. Allows sufficient time for parents to incorporate these ideas.
Allow for the infant or child's schedule in appointment scheduling (e.g., respect for naps, mealtimes). Involve the family in planning care for the infant or child.	Facilitates comfort for the child, parents, and health-care provider. Demonstrates individuality and increases likelihood of regimen implementation.
Provide appropriate criteria for monitoring follow-up of the infant or child's status, especially in instance of chronic condition, to also demarcate when to call doctor or case manager.	Anticipatory specific planning and knowledge of condition enhances self-management behaviors, thereby valuing self-esteem and likelihood of continued appropriate follow-up.
Reward progress in the appropriate manner for age and development.	Reinforcement increases valuing for desired behaviors.
Depending on needs of the infant or child, may, when services cannot be procured, require a change in location with the goal of seeking effective therapeutic regimen services. This may depend on state and/or local funding with referral on regional basis. Language or educational needs must also be addressed.	The weakest component of many communities relates to care of the young, thus making consideration of the child a critical component.

Women's Health

ACTIONS/INTERVENTIONS	RATIONALES
Develop a sensitivity for cultural differences of women's roles and the impact on their implementation of a therapeutic regimen.[144]	Demonstration of understanding of the patient's culture and inclusion of these differences in planning increase the probability of effective management of the therapeutic regimen.
Encourage the family to share views of childbirth with health-care personnel through classes and interviews.[144]	The health-care worker needs to be aware of how cultural beliefs can impact the care of the new mother and her newborn. Understanding the cultural beliefs of the patient will help the health-care provider to plan care

(care plan continued on page 86)

NURSING ACTIONS/INTERVENTIONS WITH RATIONALES (continued from page 85)

Women's Health

ACTIONS/INTERVENTIONS	RATIONALES
	in a manner that will insure the safety of both mother and infant, as well as gain compliance from the family.[144]
Discuss with the family their traditions and taboos for mother and baby during transitional period after childbirth. For example, in some Far Eastern cultures, the mother does not touch the infant for several days after birth. The grandmother or aunts become the primary caregivers for the infant.[145,146]	Increases patient satisfaction and compliance, as well as allowing the childbirth instructor and nursing personnel to plan with the patient and family appropriate care during childbearing.

Family

ACTIONS/INTERVENTIONS	RATIONALES
Assess the pregnant woman's and her family's perception of the tasks of pregnancy complicated by high-risk factors, such as premature rupture of membranes, premature labor, maternal or fetal illness, and socioeconomic hardships.[145,146]	Provides basis for plan of care and allows the family to make informed choices about care needs during and after pregnancy.
Encourage the family to share concerns of the changes and restrictions on family lifestyle as a result of the high-risk pregnancy. (Example: Restrictions on pregnant woman involving changes in homemaking, child-rearing, sexuality, social and recreational activities, disruptions in career, and financial commitments.) Help the family identify community agencies and resources that can assist them to better follow the treatment regimen.	Allows caregivers to determine importance of compliance with treatment regimen to the family and to refer them to the proper resources.

Community

ACTIONS/INTERVENTIONS	RATIONALES
Inform appropriate agencies when new mothers (parents) exhibit signs and symptoms of nonattachment to their newborn, substance abuse, homelessness, and dysfunctional family dynamics that could result in violence or neglect.[147–149]	Allows for appropriate support and follow-up for the new mother and her newborn infant.
Refer clients to appropriate community agencies (home visiting nurses, public health nurses, child protective agencies, etc.) to provide new mothers and their infants transitional care during postpartum period (particularly after early discharge).	Ensures smooth, safe transition for new mother and her family into parenting roles. Ensures physical and psychological stability for the new mother and her infant. Provides continuity of care from the hospital to the home to the primary caregiver (physician, advanced practice nurse, etc.).

Mental Health

● N O T E: *It is important to remember that the mental health client is influenced by a larger social system and that this social system plays a crucial role in the client's ongoing participation with the health-care team. The conceptualization that may be most useful in intervention and assessment of the client who does not follow the recommendations of the health-care team in this area may be system persistence. Hoffman[148] uses this concept to communicate the idea that the system is signaling that it desires to continue in its present manner of organization. This could present a situation in which the individual client indicates to the health-care team that he or she desires change, and yet change is not demonstrated because of the constraints placed on the individual by the larger social system (i.e., the family). This places the responsibility on the nurse to initiate a comprehensive assessment of the client system when the diagnosis of Ineffective Management of Therapeutic Regimen or Noncompliance is considered.*

ACTIONS/INTERVENTIONS	RATIONALES
Involve the client system in discussions on the treatment plan. This should include: • Family • Individuals the client identifies as important in making decisions related to health (e.g., cultural healers, social institutions such as probation officers, public welfare workers, officials in the school system, etc.)	Promotes the client's perceived control and increases potential for the client's involvement in the treatment plan.[69,88,143]
Discuss with the family their perception of the current situation. This should include each family member, and each should be given an opportunity to present his or her perspective. Questions to ask the family include: • What do you think is the difficulty here? • Who is most affected by the current situation? • Who is least affected? • What have you done that has helped the most? • The least? • What happened when you tried to work on the situation? • What has changed in the family since the beginning of the current situation? • What is the best advice you have received about this situation? • What is the worst? For further guidance in this process, refer to Wright and Leahey.[69]	Communicates respect of the family and their experience of the situation, which promotes the development of a trusting relationship. Provides information about the family's strengths, and provides the nurse with an opportunity to support these strengths in a manner that will facilitate the development of treatment program that the family will implement.[69,88,143]
Discuss with the identified system those factors that inhibit system reorganization: • Knowledge and skills related to necessary change • Resources available • Ability to use these resources • Belief system about treatment plan • Cultural values related to the treatment plan	Recognition of those factors that inhibit change can facilitate the development of a plan that eliminates these problems.
Discuss with the system involvement of other systems such as social services, school systems, and health-care providers in the family situation.	Larger systems often impose "rules" on families that maintain the larger system by sacrificing the families' coping abilities or becoming overinvolved to the degree that families feel in a one-down position. The primary "rule" blames the family for problems.[69]
Assist the system in making the appropriate adjustments in system organization. Note the specific type of assistance the system requests here with the nursing actions needed identified.	Affirms and promotes client's strengths.[61]
Enhance, with positive reinforcement, current patterns that facilitate system reorganization. Note the type of positive reinforcers to be utilized and behaviors to be reinforced here.	
Role model effective communication by:	Models for the family effective communication that can enhance their problem-solving abilities.[69]

(care plan continued on page 88)

NURSING ACTIONS/INTERVENTIONS WITH RATIONALES (continued from page 87)

Mental Health

ACTIONS/INTERVENTIONS	RATIONALES
• Seeking clarification • Demonstrating respect for individual, family members, and the family system • Listening to expression of thoughts and feelings • Setting clear limits • Being consistent • Communicating with the individual being addressed in a clear manner • Encouraging sharing of information among appropriate system subgroups	
Demonstrate an understanding of the complexity of family problems by: • Not taking sides in family problem solving • Providing alternative explanations of behavior patterns that recognize the contributions of all persons involved in the situation, including health-care providers, if appropriate.	Promotes the development of a trusting relationship while developing a positive orientation.[61,69]
Make small changes in those patterns that inhibit system changes. For example, ask the client to talk with the family in the group room instead of in an open public area on the unit, or ask the client who washes his or her hands frequently to use a special soap and towel and then gradually introduce more changes in the patterns.	Promotes the client's control and provides realistic, achievable goals for the client, thus preserving self-esteem when change can be accomplished.[61]
Advise the client to make changes slowly. It is important not to expect too much too soon.	Increases self-esteem and increases desire to continue those behaviors that elicit this response.[69,139]
Provide the appropriate positive verbal feedback to all parts of the system involved in assisting with the changes. It is important not to focus on the demonstration of old patterns of behavior at this time. The smallest change should be recognized.	
Develop goals with the family that are based on the data obtained in the assessment. These goals should be specific and behavioral in nature.	Promotes the family's sense of control and the development of a trusting relationship by communicating respect for the client system. Accomplishment of goals provides positive reinforcement, which motivates continued behavior and enhances self-esteem.[61,69]
Provide positive reinforcement to families for the strengths observed during the assessment and subsequent interviews.	Positive reinforcement motivates continued behavior and enhances self-esteem.[69]
Encourage communication between family members by: • Having family members discuss alternative solutions and goal setting. • Having each family member indicate how he or she might contribute to resolution of the concerns. • Having family members identify strengths of one another and how these can contribute to the resolution of the situation.	Assists the family in developing problem-solving skills that will serve in future situations, and promotes healthy family functioning.[69]

ACTIONS/INTERVENTIONS	RATIONALES
Develop teaching plan to provide the family with information that will enhance their problem solving. Note the content and schedule for this plan here.	Lack of information about the situation can interfere with problem solving.[69]
Provide opportunities for the expression of a range of affect; this can mean having the family discuss situations that promote laughing and crying together. Express to the family that their emotional experiences are normal.	Validates family members' emotions and helps identify appropriateness of their affective responses. Persistent, intense emotions can inhibit problem solving.[69] Normalizing decreases sense of isolation and assists in making connections between family members.[69]
Contract with the family for specific behavioral homework assignments that will be implemented before the next meeting. These should be concrete and involve only minor changes in the family's normal patterns. For example, have them start with calling a resource for the information they may need to do something different. If it is difficult for the family to accomplish these tasks, the family system may be having unusual problems with the change process and should be referred to an advanced practitioner for further care.	Suggesting specific tasks can provide the family with new ways to interact that can improve problem solving.[69]
If the task is not completed, do not chastise the family. Indicate that the nurse misjudged the complexity of the task, and assess what made it difficult for the family to complete the task. Develop a new, less complex task based on this information. If the nurse and family continue to have difficulty developing a plan of cooperation, a referral may need to be made to a nurse with advanced training in family systems work. Promotes positive orientation and recognizes that the development of change strategies is an interactive process between the family and the health-care system.[61,69]	
Communicate the plan to all members of the health-care team.	Promotes continuity of care and builds trust.
Refer the family to community resources for continued support. Assist family in making these contacts by developing a specific plan. [Note the specific plan here with the types of support needed.]	Community resources can provide ongoing support. A specific plan increases opportunities for success.[61,69]
Develop with the family opportunities for them to have time together and in various subgroupings (parents, parents with children, children) that involve activities other than those directly related to the current problem. This could include respite activities, family play time, relaxation, and other stress reduction activities. Note this plan here.	Provides families with positive experiences with one another and opportunities to rebuild resources for coping. Also assists them in developing a broader identity of the family. They are more than the problem or illness.[61,69]
Before termination, praise the family's accomplishments. Give the family credit for the change.	Reinforces family's strengths and promotes self-esteem. Reminds family of the new skills they have acquired.[61,69]

● N O T E : *Refer to Home Health for primary interventions for Ineffective Management of Therapeutic Regimen (Community). The primary agencies that are available to assist with community mental health resources are the Mental Health Association and National Alliance for the Mentally Ill (NAMI). NAMI publishes a journal titled Innovations & Research. Both these associations open their membership to professionals, consumers, families of consumers, and members of the community interested in mental health issues. The purpose of these organizations is to provide community resources and support for mental health consumers and their families and advocate for mental health consumers.*

(care plan continued on page 90)

NURSING ACTIONS/INTERVENTIONS WITH RATIONALES (continued from page 89)

Gerontic Health

Refer to the Adult Health section for list of potential/actual factors present that may impede use of therapeutic regimen plan.

ACTIONS/INTERVENTIONS	RATIONALES
Refer to mental health specialist to rule out depression.	Depression in the elderly is frequently underdiagnosed and undertreated.
Refer to community resources.	The older patient may have concerns related to availability of support systems, costs of medication, and availability of transportation. Use of already available community resources provides a long-term, cost-effective support system.
Establish communication link with primary caregiver and family.	Family members may not be geographically available.
Advise family members of availability of managed care resources in the community where older client resides.	Provides care options for family to consider.
Provide follow-up support via home visits and telephone contacts.	Presents opportunities for continued problem solving and increasing trust.
Assist caregivers in establishing and meeting their needs.	Enables continuation of care while decreasing the potential for burnout.
Review with the client and family the therapeutic regimen.	Helps determine possible areas of difficulty for client or caregiver.
Provide multisensory (written, computer, audio) information on therapeutic regimen to assist client and caregiver in adhering to regimen.	Provides quick access to information for the caregiver or client.
Incorporate a variety of local, regional, or state social services to ensure that needed information about the regimen is available to older patients.	Information flow may be impeded because of temporary relocation or social isolation.
Identify older community leaders, via age-related groups or associations, who can identify strengths or weaknesses of the community (such as senior citizen center members, church groups, and support groups focused on problems common to older adults).	Peer or cohort influences may assist in identifying and promoting problem solving.

Home Health

ACTIONS/INTERVENTIONS	RATIONALES
Assist the client, family, or community to delineate factors contributing to ineffective therapeutic regimen management by helping them to assess: • Level of knowledge and skill related to treatment plan • Resources available to meet treatment plan objectives • Appropriate use of resources to meet treatment plan objectives • Complexity of treatment plan • Current response to treatment plan • Use of nonprescribed interventions • Barriers to adherence to prescribed plan or medication	Barriers and facilitators to ineffective management can be altered to improve outcomes.
Involve the client, family, and community in planning, implementing, and promoting the treatment plan.[147,148]	Involvement increases motivation and improves the probability of success.

ACTIONS/INTERVENTIONS	RATIONALES
• Assisting with family conferences. • Coordinating mutual goal setting. • Promoting increased communication. • Assigning family members specific tasks as appropriate to assist in maintaining the therapeutic regimen plan (e.g., support person for patient, transportation, or companionship in meeting mutual goals). • Identifying deficits in community resources. • Identifying appropriate community resources. • Utilizing population surveillance to detect changes in illness patterns for the community.	
Support the client, family, or community in eliminating barriers to implementing the regimen by: • Providing for privacy. • Referring to community services (e.g., church, home health volunteer, transportation service, or financial assistance). • Alerting other health-care providers and social service personnel of the problem that long waiting periods create. • Providing for interpreters and for community-based language classes for English speakers to learn other languages as well as for non-English speakers to learn English. • Identifying community leaders to develop coalitions to address the problems identified. • Serving as social activist to encourage necessary participants to complete their tasks. This may include fundraising, testifying before governing bodies, or coordinating efforts of several groups and organizations.	Many barriers are institutional and can be eliminated or reduced.
Assign one health-care provider or social service worker, as much as possible, to provide continuity in care provision.	Continuity of care provides a means for effective problem solving and early identification of problems.
Assist health-care providers and social service workers to understand the destructive nature of noncompliance in chronic illness.[148]	Provides motivation for health-care providers to take appropriate action when noncompliance is a problem.
Make timely telephone calls to clients to discuss care (e.g., 1 day after being seen in clinic for minor acute infection, or weekly or monthly on a routine schedule for chronically ill person).[148]	Follow-up with clients reinforces positive behaviors and may aid in early identification of problems. Follow-up also implies support of health-care professionals.
Collaborate with other health-care professionals and social service workers to reduce the number and variety of medications and treatments for chronically ill clients.[149–151]	Complex medication and treatment regimens may be difficult for some clients to adhere to.
Reteach the client and family appropriate therapeutic activities as the need arises.	Reinforcement of information and continued assistance may be required to improve implementation of the therapeutic regimen.[150]
Identify unmet needs of the community.	Accurate community needs assessment provides data to set community goals.
Involve community leaders and representative sampling of the community population in focus groups to identify issues and to develop action plan to meet the unmet needs.	Collaboration among community leaders and citizens provides support for long-term change

(care plan continued on page 92)

NURSING ACTIONS/INTERVENTIONS WITH RATIONALES (continued from page 91)

Home Health

ACTIONS/INTERVENTIONS	RATIONALES
Identify resources available and those needed to implement action plan.	Appropriate use of existing resources. Provides direction for development of needed resources.
Create marketing plan to disseminate information and generate interest in plan.	Communication of the plan is necessary to sustain interest and increase participation.
Foster community partnerships to ensure the continuation of the plan.	Long-term maintenance of the plan will require commitment and collaboration among many groups.

MANAGEMENT, READINESS FOR ENHANCED THERAPEUTIC REGIMEN

DEFINITION[44]

A pattern of regulating and integrating into daily living a program(s) for treatment of illness and its sequelae that is both sufficient for meeting health-related goals and that can also be strengthened.

DEFINING CHARACTERISTICS[44]

1. Expresses desire to manage the treatment of illness and prevention of sequelae.
2. Choices of daily living are appropriate for meeting the goals of treatment or prevention.
3. Expresses little to no difficulty with regulation/ integration of one or more prescribed regimens

for the treatment of illness or prevention of complications.
4. Describes reduction of risk factors for progression of illness and sequelae.
5. No unexpected acceleration of illness symptoms.

EXPECTED OUTCOME

The client will demonstrate enhanced management of their therapeutic regimen by [date].

TARGET DATES[44]

Client education and support are key interventions for Readiness for Enhanced Therapeutic Regimen. Since the client is already demonstrating positive behaviors, it is recommended that target dates be no further than 3 days from the date of initial diagnosis.

NURSING ACTIONS/INTERVENTIONS WITH RATIONALES

Adult Health

ACTIONS/INTERVENTIONS	RATIONALES
Initially, spend 30 minutes talking with client about their understanding of their current health situation, prescribed regimen, and perceived responsibility regarding management. Use language the client can understand	Allows the nurse to tailor teaching according to the patient's capacity to understand health-care information.[152]
Provide a quiet environment for instruction. Ensure that the patient is well rested, pain free, and not under the influence of medications that alter cognition. Postpone teaching when patient's condition, or the environment, does not promote focus on the content.	Information will be better retained when the patient is able to adequately focus on instruction.
Identify key decision maker in client's system based on cultural norms.	
Spend [number] minutes 2 times a day discussing with client their goals and methods they perceive would assist with goal achievement.	

ACTIONS/INTERVENTIONS	RATIONALES
Have patient identify the rewards for goal achievement.	
Have patient identify their preferred and most effective way of learning (e.g., visual, auditory, or participatory)	Appropriate teaching methods enhance transfer of information.
Spend 15 minutes one time per day reviewing the plan with the client and providing an opportunity for questions. Discuss with client rationale for various components of plan.	Imparts relevancy to the goal.
Have patient verbalize plan and ensure that patient's understanding is congruent achieving therapeutic goal	
Identify and secure adequate post-discharge support system. This could include community agencies, family and friends.[88,153]	

Child Health

ACTIONS/INTERVENTIONS	RATIONALES
Assess for all possible contributing factors related to infant or child such as new or ongoing health/safety needs that comprise the therapeutic regimen.	Provides the most realistic basis for care.
Assess for caregiver's (or child's as appropriate) current knowledge for therapeutic regimen.	Serves as a basis for validation and clarification of current knowledge and best plan for how to begin to assist in plan.
Assess the caregiver's and/or child's priorities in learning.	Provides mutual planning basis with respect for client input.
Provide environmental privacy and freedom from interruption with pediatric-appropriate setting if child is also included.	Offers a therapeutic milieu for learning.
Utilize basic knowledge/developmental level language for child in teaching.	Honors the caregiver/child's ability to best understand plan.
Offer time for question/answer with examples to generate validation of knowledge.	Reinforcement of learning in a timely manner creates likelihood for retention.
Provide appropriate resource materials and creative developmentally appropriate teaching aids (e.g., puppets).	Provides greater likelihood of learning.
Assist in development of plan for care calendar and file for maintaining important resources.	Offers reinforcement and ability to remember access to health-care providers and follow-up.

Women's Health

ACTIONS/INTERVENTIONS	RATIONALES
Women's health follows the patterns, interventions and rationales of the Adult Health section. The following comments are specifically related to diseases that occur in women and/or diseases with a high incidence among the female population.	
Discuss with women the effect of environmentally acquired diseases and how to reduce exposure to environmental toxins. Provide them with information about hazardous substances, perform risk assessment, and collaborate with community agencies. Work with legislators to pass and enforce environmentally related legislation.[154]	Usually women of poor economic and minority classes are those exposed to environmental toxins. Substandard housing, exposure to "dump sites" or exposure to environmental disaster sites (such as New Orleans' Ninth Ward after hurricane Katrina).[154]

(care plan continued on page 94)

NURSING ACTIONS/INTERVENTIONS WITH RATIONALES (continued from page 93)

Women's Health

ACTIONS/INTERVENTIONS	RATIONALES
	Agricultural pesticides have been directly linked with birth defects and some causal effects upon pregnancy, such as an increased incidence of PIH in agricultural areas of the country.[154]
Discuss the dangers of smoking and the effects of second hand smoke on those about them (families, children, co-workers, etc). Guide them to programs for smoking cessation not only during pregnancy, but for all life cycles.	Smoking has been identified as the most hazardous exposure that women today face. Even if the individual does not smoke, exposure to second hand smoke can lead to menstrual cycle irregularities, osteoporosis, decreased fertility and lung cancer.[155]
Discuss alternatives to reducing symptoms of premenstrual syndrome. Lifestyle changes to include exercise and good nutrition. Refer to classes to help decrease stress and provide emotional support.	Ninety-seven percent of women are affected by premenstrual syndrome at some point in their life.[155–157]

Mental Health

ACTIONS/INTERVENTIONS	RATIONALES
Spend 30 minutes once a day discussing client's perception of current situation and life/personal goals. • Use open-ended questions and reflective listening • Let the client be the expert • Do not provide advice Discuss client's needs and resources necessary to support ongoing care Reflect to client nurse's understandings of the client's solutions and goals Summarize the solutions and goals that the client identified	Behavior change that is developed with the client using the client's identified needs and co-evolved solutions improves outcomes.[84–86]
Develop a schedule for positive reinforcement when goals are attained. Note the reinforcers and schedule of reinforcement here.	Positive reinforcement increases behavior.[87]
Discuss with client sources of social support. • Schedule meeting with client and social support system. [Note the date and time of that meeting here.] • Spend 1 hour one time per week meeting with client and social support system to focus on: • With client's permission educate support system about client's health-care needs Model communication and assist support system in developing positive communication skills	Social support improves health outcomes.[88,153]
Include the client in group therapy to provide positive role models and peer support and to permit assessment of goals and exposure to differing problem solutions.	Group provides opportunities to relate and react to others while exploring behavior with each other.[87]
Provide client with information that will facilitate contact with health-care team. Schedule regular contact with the client to provide positive reinforcement for their efforts and refer to community support systems before discharge.	Ongoing support from the health-care team facilitates adherence to therapeutic regimens.[69,84,158]

ACTIONS/INTERVENTIONS	RATIONALES
• Schedule time for the client to talk with community support systems before discharge.	
Discuss with client potential problems that might arise and develop plans to adjust self-care as necessary.	Prevents client burnout and enhances self-esteem. Planned relapse becomes no relapse.[69]
Normalize times when client's adherence to the therapeutic regimen is not perfect and schedule "safe holidays" from perfect adherence.	
Provide client with educational materials.	Provides self–care information that is readily accessible to the client.[84]
Provide materials that address client's best learning mode (auditory/visual) and at client's level of understanding (proper reading level). [Note client's reading level here.]	

Gerontic Health

ACTIONS/INTERVENTIONS	RATIONALES
Determine the client's existing knowledge regarding the therapeutic regimen.	This allows the nurse to focus on strengths and existing knowledge and also assists in determining knowledge deficits or misunderstandings.
Determine the client's priorities for learning.	Client involvement in the learning process facilitates success.
Ensure privacy, comfort, and rapport prior to teaching sessions.	Reduces anxiety and promotes a nondistracting environment to enhance learning.
Avoid presenting large amounts of information at one time.	This encourages increased opportunity to process and store new information.
Monitor energy level as teaching session progresses.	Reduces possibility of fatigue which can impair learning.
Present small units of information, with repetition, and encourage the patient to use cues that enhance ability to recall information.	Compensates for delayed reaction time associated with aging. Promotes retention of information by connecting information to previously mastered skills.[90]
Use multisensory approach to learning sessions whenever possible.	Hearing, vision, touch, and smell used in conjunction can stimulate multiple areas in the cerebral cortex to promote retention.[91]

Home Health

ACTIONS/INTERVENTIONS	RATIONALES
Assess the client and family's understanding of the current therapeutic regimen.	Identifies potential misunderstanding or knowledge deficit.
Assist the client/family in the development of a therapeutic network to include informal relationships with informal structures in the nuclear family to select laypersons and professionals.[174]	Enhances the support and educational resources of the family/client.
Educate the client/family about risk factors and prevention for progression of their illness and sequelae.	Involvement improves motivation and improves the outcome. Self-care is enhanced.
Assist the client and family to identify home and workplace factors that can be modified to promote health maintenance (e.g., ramps instead of steps, elimination of throw rugs, use of safety rails in showers, and maintenance of a nonsmoking environment).[92,93]	This action enhances safety and assists in preventing accidents. Promoting a nonsmoking environment helps reduce the damaging effects of passive smoke.

(care plan continued on page 96)

NURSING ACTIONS/INTERVENTIONS WITH RATIONALES (continued from page 95)

Home Health

ACTIONS/INTERVENTIONS	RATIONALES
Involve the client and family in planning, implementing, and promoting a health maintenance pattern through: • Helping to establish family conferences to discuss strategies for meeting client health maintenance needs. • Engaging in mutual goal setting with client and family. Encourage the client/family to establish goals for their own involvement in managing the therapeutic regimen. • Assisting family members in acquiring family or community-based assistance for specified tasks as appropriate (e.g., cooking, cleaning, transportation, companionship, or support person for exercise program). • Teach the family and caregivers about disease management for existing illness: • Symptom management • Medication effects, side effects, and interactions with over-the-counter medications. • Reporting the use of over-the-counter remedies, herbal supplements and medicines to the health-care provider. • Wound care as appropriate. Prevention of skin breakdown for clients with illnesses contributing to immobility.	Involvement improves motivation and outcomes. Provides a sense of autonomy and prevents premature progression of illness.
Teach the client and family health promotion and disease prevention activities: • Relaxation techniques • Nutritional habits to maintain optimal weight and physical strength. • Techniques for developing and strengthening support networks (e.g., communication techniques or mutual goal setting). • Physical exercise to increase flexibility, cardiovascular conditioning, and physical strength and endurance.[94] • Evaluation of occupational conditions[92] • Control of harmful habit, such as substance abuse • Therapeutic value of pets[95]	These activities promote a healthy lifestyle.

PERIOPERATIVE-POSITIONING INJURY, RISK FOR

DEFINITION[44]

A state in which the client is at risk for injury as a result of the environmental conditions found in the perioperative setting.

DEFINING CHARACTERISTICS (RISK FACTORS)[44]

1. Disorientation
2. Edema
3. Emaciation
4. Immobilization
5. Muscle weakness
6. Obesity
7. Sensory or perceptual disturbances due to anesthesia

RELATED FACTORS[44]

The risk factors also serve as the related factors.

RELATED CLINICAL CONCERNS

1. Any condition requiring surgical intervention
2. Peripheral vascular disease
3. Diabetes mellitus
4. Malnutrition

Have You Selected the Correct Diagnosis?

Risk for Injury
This diagnosis is broader based than Risk for Perioperative-Positioning Injury. The latter would be used only when surgery is involved.

Risk for Peripheral Neurovascular Dysfunction
This diagnosis is broader based than Risk for Perioperative-Positioning Injury. A comparison of risk factors documents a wider variety of risk factors for peripheral neurovascular dysfunction.

5. Arthritis deformans
6. Dementias, such as Alzheimer's disease or multi-infarct

EXPECTED OUTCOME

Will remain free from any signs or symptoms of perioperative-positioning injury by [date].

TARGET DATES

Because of the emergency nature of this diagnosis, target dates should be set in terms of hours for the first 2 days postoperatively.

NURSING ACTIONS/INTERVENTIONS WITH RATIONALES

Adult Health

ACTIONS/INTERVENTIONS	RATIONALES
General Principles (Generally Applies to All Positions, Including Supine)	
Keep siderails up on stretcher.	Basic safety measures.
The patient should be in a comfortable position whether awake or asleep; ensure that operating room (OR) bed is dry and free from wrinkles.	Prevents softening of the skin and indentations of the skin.
Length of operative procedure should *always* be considered in positioning and supporting patient during the operation.	Certain complications can arise with extended length of operation (e.g., low back pain for patient in supine position, or pressure on heels and/or toes from drapes).
Provide adequate exposure of the operative site.	
Maintain good anatomic alignment. Pad bony prominences and pressure points.	Prevents impaired circulation, awkward position, or undue pressure.
Ensure good respiration with no restrictions.	Avoids respiratory complications and assists in providing good oxygenation.
Nerves should be protected—arms, hands, legs, ankles, and feet; use a footboard.	Maintains alignment; relieves pressure.
The elderly, very thin, or obese patients should have special consideration; assess nutritional status, level of hydration, vascular disease, etc.	Reduces the risk of complication.
Check mobility and range of motion prior to positioning. Note any physical abnormalities and/or injuries and how they may affect the proposed position.	Avoids unnecessary strain on already compromised joints, etc.
Move the patient only when anesthetist indicates patient can be moved.	Avoids startling semiconscious patient and provides basic safety.
Have a sufficient number of people available to move the patient safely or utilize appropriate transfer devices.	Ensures patient safety and prevents shearing forces on skin
Ensure that no metal is touching the patient.	Reduces pressure risk and risk of injury if cautery is used.
The dispersion pad should be on a fatty area (e.g., mid to upper thigh, depending on operative site). Recheck dispersion pad if patient has to be repositioned.	Basic safety measures.

(care plan continued on page 98)

NURSING ACTIONS/INTERVENTIONS WITH RATIONALES (continued from page 97)

Adult Health

ACTIONS/INTERVENTIONS	RATIONALES
Place arms at right angles to the patient. Do not hyperextend the arms. Secure the arms with a restraint around the wrist.	Avoids strain on arms.
Place the safety belt above the patient's knees (depending on operative site).	Avoids compromising circulation in popliteal area.
Ensure that all supports are padded.	Basic safety measures.

Specific Positions

Lithotomy

Raise or lower legs at the same time.	Reduces strain on hip joints.
Lower legs, slowly at the same time.	
Adjust height of stirrups to fit the patient's legs.	
Be sure that no part of the legs touch metal.	Prevents electrical burns.
Cover stirrups with linen or place long leg booties on the patient's legs (up to mid thigh).	Protects nerves and circulation.
Pad popliteal space.	
Ensure that the patient's buttocks are over lower break in table.	

Nephro or Thoracic Surgery

Move the patient slowly and carefully, as a unit; have sufficient assistance.	Basic safety measure.
The patient will be on side over the middle break of the table.	
Position lower arm at a 90-degree angle away from body.	
Place upper arm parallel to lower arm on a separate and high armboard or straight above the head. Restrain as needed. Protect nerves and muscles.	Facilitates respiration; maintains circulation.
Support the patient's sides with padded kidney rests.	Provides support for side and back.
Bend bottom leg 45 to 90 degrees. Top leg should be straight.	Stabilizes the patient.
Place pillow(s) between knees and legs and feet	Protects pressure points.

Jacksonian (Modified Knee–Chest)

●NOTE: *Patient will probably be put to sleep on the stretcher and then rolled onto the OR table.*

Have sufficient assistance to move the patient.	Basic safety measure.
Extend arms on armboards above the head.	Facilitates respiration; maintains circulation.
Place pillow under ankles.	Protects pressure points.
Support chest.	Stabilizes patient's position.
Turn head to side; ensure an adequate airway.	Allows good expansion of chest and promotes gas exchange.

Prone (Upper and Lower Back Surgery)

●NOTE: *Patient will probably be put to sleep on the stretcher and then rolled onto a back frame. This allows the back to be hyperextended and supports the chest for good respiration. Actions are the same as for Jacksonian position except:*

ACTIONS/INTERVENTIONS	RATIONALES
Place pillows under upper chest, thighs, legs, ankles, and feet.	Avoids pressure and strains. Provides good anatomic alignment.
Trendelenburg	
Support shoulders with padded shoulder rests.	Provides stabilization of the patient's position.

Child Health

● **N O T E :** *Any procedure requiring prolonged stabilization in a fixed position places neonates and children at risk for this diagnosis (e.g., ECMO [extracorporeal membranous oxygenation] with cannulation of major vessels requires fixed positioning for several days to 1 week).*

Safeguard the child with nursing actions relevant from Adult Health for positioning plus the following:

ACTIONS/INTERVENTIONS	RATIONALES
Monitor skin integrity from head to toes with specific attention to head, ears, elbows, back, and heels, or other body parts in direct contact with surface of mattress or lines from monitoring equipment.[49]	Decreases likelihood of impact of shearing forces or burns and demonstrates appropriate caution to diminish possible injury.
*Recognize the need for ongoing monitoring for infants, young children, or any client under the influence of anesthesia regarding loss of sensation or cues of verbal nature to warn of pain/injury.	Offers anticipatory planning for prevention and early detection of injury related to potential positional factors.
	Infants and children with spina bifida (myelomeningocele) may have diminished neuro-sensation in legs and feet depending on the level of involvement.

Women's Health

Same as for Adult Health except for the following:

ACTIONS/INTERVENTIONS	RATIONALES
Determine proper alignment and positioning of mother during the cesarean section and any other procedure in which mother must lie on back. Place a wedge cushion under the left buttock when positioning mother on surgical table.	Enhances circulation and oxygen supply to the placenta and the fetus.[159]
Assist the mother's chosen partner (support person) to prepare for the cesarean section by describing the events that will take place, explaining his role and where he will sit (a stool or chair next to the mother's head) during the surgery, and identifying who will assist him.	Reassures and supports the partner (support person) during surgery, allowing him to be supportive to the pregnant woman.

Mental Health

Nursing interventions and rationales for this diagnosis are the same as for Adult Health. Mental health clients who are most commonly at risk for this diagnosis are those receiving electroconvulsive therapy (ECT) treatments.

(care plan continued on page 100)

NURSING ACTIONS/INTERVENTIONS WITH RATIONALES (continued from page 99)

Gerontic Health

In addition to the interventions for Adult Health, the following may be applied to the older client:

ACTIONS/INTERVENTIONS	RATIONALES
Monitor closely for signs of hypothermia, especially in frail elders.	Frail elders are at high risk for hypothermia as a result of changes associated with aging. Elimination of an anesthetic agent may be reduced because of hypothermia. Older adults may have increased oxygen demand secondary to shivering if hypothermia is not treated.[151,160,161]
Provide head and neck support that prevents head rotation or hyperextension.	Hyperextension or rotation may cause vertebral circulatory compromise in older patients.
Ensure adequate padding over pressure-prone areas.	Decreases potential for circulatory compromise as well as nervous system or skin injury in older patients at risk for these problems.
Observe, especially intraoperatively, for external pressure caused by leaning on patient.	Compromised circulation or increased skin pressure can result in patient injury.
Position extremities with caution.	Older patients are at an increased risk for osteoporosis and, consequently, fractures.

Home Health

ACTIONS/INTERVENTIONS	RATIONALES
Begin preoperative teaching to the client and family as soon as possible prior to surgery. Include the need for early ambulation, deep-breathing exercises, and adequate pain control. Reinforce teaching as needed postoperatively.	Involvement of the client and family increases motivation. Correct knowledge supports the behavior and assists in preventing complications.
Instruct patient and family/caregivers about situations that require immediate intervention from their health-care provider: • abrupt increase in temperature • changes in skin integrity • alterations in the patient's level of consciousness	Early intervention prevents exacerbation of complications.
Involve the home caregiver in developing plan of care to decrease risk of complications.	Involvement in the planning increases motivation and success of the intervention.

PROTECTION, INEFFECTIVE

DEFINITION[44]

The state in which an individual experiences a decrease in the ability to guard the self from internal or external threats such as illness or injury.

DEFINING CHARACTERISTICS[44]

1. Maladaptive stress response
2. Neurosensory alterations
3. Impaired healing
4. Deficient immunity
5. Altered clotting
6. Dyspnea
7. Insomnia
8. Weakness
9. Restlessness
10. Pressure sore
11. Perspiring
12. Itching
13. Immobility
14. Chilling
15. Cough

16. Fatigue
17. Anorexia
18. Disorientation

RELATED FACTORS[44]

1. Abnormal blood profiles (leukopenia, thrombocytopenia, anemia, coagulation)
2. Inadequate nutrition
3. Extremes of age
4. Drug therapies (antineoplastic, corticosteroid, immune, anticoagulant, thrombolytic)
5. Alcohol abuse
6. Treatments (surgery, radiation)
7. Disease such as cancer and immune disorders

RELATED CLINICAL CONCERNS

1. AIDS
2. Diabetes mellitus
3. Anorexia nervosa
4. Cancer
5. Clotting disorders (e.g., disseminated intravascular coagulation, thrombophlebitis, anticoagulant medications)

☑ **Have You Selected the Correct Diagnosis?**

Risk for Infection
This diagnosis would most likely be a companion diagnosis. Risk means the individual is not presenting the actual defining characteristics of the diagnosis, but there are indications the diagnosis could develop. Ineffective Protection is an actual diagnosis.

---

6. Substance abuse or dependence
7. Any disorder requiring use of steroids

EXPECTED OUTCOME

Will return/demonstrate measures to increase self protection by [date].

TARGET DATES[44]

Ineffective Protection is a long-lasting diagnosis. Therefore, a date to totally meet the expected outcome could be weeks and months. However, since the target date signals the time to check progress, a date 3 days from the date of the original diagnosis would be appropriate.

NURSING ACTIONS/INTERVENTIONS WITH RATIONALES

Adult Health

ACTIONS/INTERVENTIONS	RATIONALES
Protect the patient from injury and infection. (See appropriate nursing actions and rationales under the diagnoses Risk for Injury and Risk for Infection.)	Protects the patient from infection or spread of infection.
Use standard precautions in caring for the patient.	
Place the patient in protective isolation, but **do not** promote an isolated feeling for the patient. Encourage frequent telephone calls and visits from significant others.	Lessens sense of isolation and maintains therapeutic relationship.
Check the patient at least every 30 minutes while awake. Spend 30 minutes with client every 2 hours on [odd/even] hour while awake to answer questions and provide emotional support while in reverse isolation. Note times for these interactions here.	
Monitor: • Vital signs, mucous membranes, skin integrity, and response to medications at least once per shift. • Unexplained blood in the urine. • Prolonged bleeding after blood has been drawn or from injection sites.	Allows comparison to baseline at admission and evaluation of effectiveness of therapy.

(care plan continued on page 102)

NURSING ACTIONS/INTERVENTIONS WITH RATIONALES (continued from page 101)

Adult Health

ACTIONS/INTERVENTIONS	RATIONALES
• Side effects of blood and blood products: Monitor for possibility of blood reaction. Take vital signs every 15 minutes, hour times an hour, then every 30 minutes until transfusion is completed. In the event of transfusion reaction, stop the transfusion immediately, maintain IV line with saline, and notify physician while monitoring patient for further anaphylactic signs and symptoms.	
• Effects and side effects of steroids: Improved general status, decreased inflammatory signs and symptoms versus untoward effects including bleeding, sodium (Na) or potassium (K) imbalance. Calculate and record intake and output at least once per shift.	
• Effects and side effects of antineoplastics, such as nausea, cardiac arrhythmias, extrapyramidal signs and symptoms. These side effects vary according to the specific agents used. Take vital signs every 5 to 10 minutes during actual administration and use a cardiac monitor.	
• Signs and symptoms of infection such as lymphoid interstitial pneumonia or recurrent oral candidiasis	
Apply pressure after each injection and after removal of IV needle.	Assists in stopping of bleeding.
Provide oral hygiene or assist the patient with oral hygiene at least 3 times per day, taking appropriate precautions for vulnerable mucous membranes.	Prevents opportunistic infection.
Provide body hygiene or assist the patient with body hygiene at least once daily at time of the patient's choosing.	
Measure and record intake and output at end of each shift.	Monitors effectiveness of bowel and bladder function.
Provide the patient with food choices and portions that will facilitate their eating nutritious meals. Collaborate with diet therapist regarding the patient's likes, dislikes, and planning for dietary needs after hospital discharge.	Ensures balanced intake of necessary vitamins, minerals, etc., to assist in tissue repair. Assists in lessening impact of infections.
Collaborate with appropriate members of the health-care team regarding therapeutic regimen	Gives guidelines for future therapeutic regimen as well as assessing effectiveness of current regimen.
Teach the patient and significant others: • Medication administration • Signs and symptoms to be reported • Special laboratory or other procedures to be done at home • Anticipatory safety needs • Routine daily care • Appropriate clean and sterile technique • Isolation or reverse-isolation technique • Common antigens and/or allergens and seasonal variations	Provides basic knowledge needed for the patient and family to make modifications necessitated by alteration in protective mechanisms.

ACTIONS/INTERVENTIONS	RATIONALES
• How to avoid or reduce exposure to antigens and/or allergens (alteration of environment) • Type and use of protective equipment • Standard precautions • Rationale for compliance with prescribed regimen • Resources available for assistance with health care, legal questions, or ethical questions	
Identify community resources for patient and family. Make referrals at least 3 days before discharge from hospital.	Allows time for agencies to initiate service. Use of existing community services is effective use of resources.

Child Health

● N O T E : *Infants at risk for this diagnosis are premature infants, infants with family history of hemophilia or sickle cell anemia, infants whose mothers have a history of drug abuse or HIV, and children who have histories of medication reaction. In infants especially, incubation for HIV depends on acquisition time. The infant may be exposed any time during pregnancy, but sero-con/retroversion to a negative HIV status may occur, with a later positive HIV status again. The more symptomatic the mother, the greater the effect on the infant due to constant reinfection (in the infant). For infants whose mothers are HIV positive, 26 percent are HIV positive in the first 5 months of life, an additional 24 percent are HIV positive by 12 months of life, and the remaining 50 percent are HIV positive by 2 years of age. Key symptoms are intercurrent infection and weight loss. Other conditions noted include failure to thrive, hepatomegaly, cardiomegaly, lymphoid interstitial pneumonia, chronic diarrhea, cardiomyopathy, encephalopathy, and opportunistic infections. Even tuberculosis may be seen in these infants, with a tendency to progress from primary to miliary phase. In these infants there may be disseminated bacille Calmette-Guérin (BCG) infection. It is important to be aware of laboratory studies requiring large amounts of blood to study the course of sero HIV status. This blood drawing is problematic in the already depressed immune and reticuloendothelial systems of these infants. It is imperative that these infants not be given live polio vaccine because of their HIV-positive status.*

ACTIONS/INTERVENTIONS	RATIONALES
Maintain monitoring for: • Observable lesions of ecchymotic nature or evidence of tendency toward bruising • Decreased absorption of nutrients (especially the premature infant because of the possibility of necrotizing enterocolitis)	Essential monitoring to avoid overwhelming of child's system by infection, etc.
Provide at least one 30 to 60 minute opportunity per day for the family to ventilate feelings about the specific illness of their child.	Reduces anxiety, fear, and anger, and provides an opportunity for teaching.
Teach the child and family essential care.	Basics of home care for child with diagnosis of Ineffective Protection.
As applicable, exercise caution for any medications or blood products to be administered.	
Provide diversionary therapy according to child's status, developmental level, and interests.	Prevents boredom and restlessness and fosters continued development of child in spite of illness.
Be aware of current frustration with use of DDC (dideoxycytidine) and AZT (zidovudine) in children. At this time, protocols dictate doses.	Avoid unrealistic hope. Ideally, toxicity is balanced against the need to reach therapeutic central nervous system (CNS) dosage levels.

(care plan continued on page 104)

NURSING ACTIONS/INTERVENTIONS WITH RATIONALES (continued from page 103)

Child Health

ACTIONS/INTERVENTIONS	RATIONALES
Remind the family that current treatment for AIDS is only palliative. Be sensitive to the unique nature of this health concern for all involved. Promote attention to the need for: • Spiritual and emotional support • Nutritional support • Treatment of HIV-related infections • Administration of IV immune globulin • Treatment of tumors and end organ failure • Chronic pain	Avoids unrealistic hope while providing knowledge and support necessary to deal with a fatal illness.
Acknowledge potential loss of mother for the infant with HIV, and plan appropriately for foster care status as indicated.	Anticipatory planning will assist in health maintenance in best interest of infant in event of need for separation from the mother.

Women's Health

ACTIONS/INTERVENTIONS	RATIONALES
HELLP syndrome (a severe form of pregnancy-induced hypertension): Monitor laboratory results for low platelets (less than 100,000/cc), elevated liver enzymes, elevated SGOT/SGPT, intravascular hemolysis, schistocytes or burr cells on peripheral smear, low hematocrit (Hct) (without evidence of significant blood loss), and hypertension.[29,159]	Understanding the laboratory values for a preeclamptic mother progressing toward HELLP syndrome allows the health-care provider to prevent and/or begin early treatment of this dangerous variant of severe preeclampsia. H = hemolysis EL = elevated liver enzymes LP = low platelets[159]
Other high-risk history in the mother such as history of preterm labor, chronic hypertension, sickle cell anemia, and other blood disorders.	Allows nursing staff time and information to plan individual care for the mother and her newborn infant.
Signs and symptoms of infection.	
Mother's history of drug abuse, alcohol abuse, HIV, or domestic violence.	Safety of the mother and the infant is of utmost importance. Provides opportunity for assessment of home environment and provision of assistance.

Mental Health

● N O T E : *Clients receiving antipsychotic neuroleptic drugs are at risk for development of agranulocytosis. This can be a life-threatening side effect and usually occurs in the first 8 weeks of treatment. Any rapid onset of sore throat and fever should be immediately reported and actively treated. Tricyclic antidepressants can cause blood dyscrasias with long-term therapy. Initial symptoms of these dyscrasias include fever, sore throat, and aching.*

ACTIONS/INTERVENTIONS	RATIONALES
Immediately report the client's complaint of sore throat or development of temperature elevation to physician. Institute nursing actions for hyperthermia. (See Chapter 3.)	Alterations could be symptoms of agranulocytosis or blood dyscrasias, which would place the client at risk for infection. Prompt recognition and intervention prevent progression and improve client outcome.[104]

ACTIONS/INTERVENTIONS	RATIONALES
Teach the client who has had this type of response to antipsychotic neuroleptics or tricyclic antidepressants that he or she should not take this drug again.	
If the client is experiencing severe alterations in thought processes, provide one-to-one observation until mental status improves or until the client can again participate in unit activities.	Client safety is of primary importance. Provides opportunity for ongoing assessment of the quality of the content of the client's thought and provides ongoing reality orientation.
Refer to the nursing care plans for Sensory Perception: Distributed and Thought Processes: Disturbed for more detailed plans of care.	

Gerontic Health

● N O T E : *The older adult is subject to impaired protection due to age related changes in the immune system which include decreased resistance to bacterial, fungal, and viral infections; increased risk of reactivating latent infections; absence of the classic signs of infection; changes in hypersensitivity responses; diminished response to vaccines; concurrent chronic diseases and debilitation; institutionalization; increased incidence of autoimmune disorders.*

ACTIONS/INTERVENTIONS	RATIONALES
Monitor sensory status at each encounter. Ensure, if necessary, that sensory-enhancing aids (glasses, contacts, hearing aids) are clean and functioning.	Uncorrected sensory impairments may negatively impact the communication process.
Monitor for subtle signs of infection, such as new onset of falls, incontinence, confusion, or decreased level of function.	Changes in immune system with aging can cause increased potential for infection. Infection may present in an atypical manner in older adults.[42]
Teach the client to avoid soaps that may cause dry skin.	Dry skin predisposes to potential skin breakdown and loss of protective barrier against pathogens.[162]
Initiate measures to maintain skin integrity such as: • Using pressure-relieving devices for use in chairs or in bed • Ensuring frequent weight shifting to reduce pressure on vulnerable areas (bony prominences) • Monitoring and documenting skin status with each contact according to care setting and client condition • Avoiding shearing forces that may cause epidermal damage • Prompting client and caregiver to change position frequently to avoid skin integrity problems	Intact skin acts as a protective barrier against infection.[162]
Teach clients and/or caregivers need for AIDS testing as appropriate.	AIDS is often undetected in older adults in the early stages because of lack of knowledge about risk for the disease and false assumptions that AIDS is not a disease present in older adults.[164,165]
Monitor renal and hepatic function in older adults who receive antiretroviral therapy.	Antiretroviral therapy can further compromise kidney and liver function.
Assist the client in maintaining adequate hydration of 2000 cc daily.	Adequate hydration status has a preventive effect.
Assist the client in maintaining adequate vitamin intake, particularly vitamins A, C and E, zinc, and selenium.	These nutrients are known to assist in infection prevention.

(care plan continued on page 106)

NURSING ACTIONS/INTERVENTIONS WITH RATIONALES (continued from page 105)

Home Health

ACTIONS/INTERVENTIONS	RATIONALES
Develop, with the client, family, and caregiver, plans for dealing with emergency situations, such as: • Decision making regarding calling ambulance • Decision tree for calling nurse or physician	Advance planning improves the response and outcomes in crisis situations.
Assist the client and family to identify learning needs such as: • Universal precautions • How to disinfect surfaces contaminated with blood or body fluids (use 1:10 solution of bleach) • Protective isolation • Proper handwashing • Use of separate razors, toothbrushes, eating utensils, etc. • Proper cooking of food • Avoidance of pet excrement • Avoidance of others with infection • Skin care, oral hygiene, and wound care • Use of protective equipment • Signs and symptoms of infection, fluid and electrolyte imbalance, malnutrition, pathologic changes in behavior, and underlying disease process • CPR and first aid • Hazardous waste disposal (e.g., soiled dressings, needles, or chemotherapy vials) • Advanced directive (e.g., living wills and durable power of attorney for health care) • Financial and/or estate planning • Symptom management and pain control • Administration of required medications • Nutrition • Care of catheters, IVs, respiratory therapy equipment, etc. • Proper treatment of linens soiled with infectious matter • Environmental cleanliness	This action describes knowledge required to protect the client and the family. Hot water provides an effective means of destroying microorganisms, and a temperature of at least 160°F for a minimum of 25 minutes is commonly recommended for hot-water washing. Chlorine bleach provides an extra margin of safety. A total available chlorine residual of 50 to 150 ppm is usually achieved during the bleach cycle.[98]
Assist the client and the family to identify resources to meet identified learning needs.	Involvement of the client and family improves their ability to identify resources and to function more independently.
Involve the client and family in planning and implementing environmental, social, and family adaptations to protect the client.	Involvement of the client and family improves motivation and outcomes.
Plan with the family and client for safe as well as meaningful activities according to the client's level of functioning and interests.	Provides for activity while protecting the client and family.
Assist the client and family in lifestyle adjustments that may be required.	Lifestyle changes often require support.

SURGICAL RECOVERY, DELAYED

DEFINITION[44]

An extension of the number of postoperative days required for individuals to initiate and perform on their own behalf activities that maintain life, health, and well-being.

DEFINING CHARACTERISTICS[44]

1. Evidence of interrupted healing of surgical area (e.g., red, indurated, draining, immobile)
2. Loss of appetite with or without nausea
3. Difficulty in moving about
4. Requires help to complete self-care
5. Fatigue
6. Report of pain or discomfort
7. Postpones resumption of work or employment activities
8. Perception that more time is needed to recover

RELATED FACTORS[44]

To be developed.

RELATED CLINICAL CONCERNS

1. Any recent major surgeries
2. Recent trauma requiring surgical intervention

 Have You Selected the Correct Diagnosis?

Risk for Infection
Risk for infection could be a companion diagnosis and would increase the probability of Delayed Surgical Recovery developing.

Ineffective Tissue Perfusion
This diagnosis could be the primary diagnosis, because any alteration in tissue perfusion to the operative site could result in delayed healing.

Impaired Physical Mobility
This diagnosis could also be a companion diagnosis or could be a contributing factor to the development of Delayed Surgical Recovery. This diagnosis would interfere with the necessary postoperative ambulation.

EXPECTED OUTCOME

Surgical incision will show no signs or symptoms of delayed healing by [date].

TARGET DATES

Because of multiple factors such as age, presence of chronic conditions, or a compromised immune system, the target date for this diagnosis could range from days to weeks. An appropriate initial target date, to measure progress, would be 3 days.

NURSING ACTIONS/INTERVENTIONS WITH RATIONALES

Adult Health

ACTIONS/INTERVENTIONS	RATIONALES
Assist patient in identifying perceived obstacles to delayed recovery.	
Incorporate patient into plan of care and display goals prominently in patient room.	Gives visual substantiation toward goal attainment (IHI Web site).
Reduce obstacles to learning. Provide a stress free environment, provide ample pain control measures without impeding mentation. [Note those actions needed by the nurse to facilitate client's learning here.]	Stress, pain, etc. reduce receptivity to instruction.[167]
Protect the patient from injury and infection. Use standard precautions.	Protects patient from infection or spread of infection.
Collaborate with diet therapist for in-depth dietary assessment and planning. Monitor the patient's food and fluid intake daily.	Adequate, balanced nutrition assists in healing and reducing fatigue.
Carefully plan activities of daily living and daily exercise schedules with detailed input from the patient. Determine how to best foster future patterns that will maintain optimal sleep–rest patterns without fatigue through planning ADLs with the patient and family.	Realistic schedules based on the patient's input promote participation in activities and a sense of success.
Assist the patient with self-care as needed. Plan gradual increase in activities over several days.	Allows the patient to gradually increase strength and tolerance for activities.

(care plan continued on page 108)

NURSING ACTIONS/INTERVENTIONS WITH RATIONALES (continued from page 107)

Adult Health

ACTIONS/INTERVENTIONS	RATIONALES
Promote rest at night. Note those things that assists client's rest here.	Increases quantity and quality of rest and sleep.
Avoid sensory overload or sensory deprivation. Provide diversional activities.	Sensory aspects can deplete energy stores. Diversional activities help prevent overload or deprivation by focusing patient's concentration on an activity he or she personally enjoys.
Address unresolved stressors by instructing the patient in stress reduction techniques. Note those techniques to be taught here.	Mental and physical stress greatly contributes to sense of inability to resume ADLs and stimulates undesirable effects from stress response.
• Have patient return—demonstrate at least once a day through day of discharge.	
Assist the patient to develop coping skills:	
• Review past coping behaviors and success or lack of success.	Determines what has helped in the past, and determines if the measures are still useful.
• Help identify and practice new coping strategies.	Allows the patient to practice and become comfortable with skills in a supportive environment.
• Challenge unrealistic assumptions or goals.	Assists the patient to avoid placing extra stress on self.
Turn, cough, and deep breathe every 2 hours on [odd/even] hour.	Mobilizes static pulmonary secretions.
Incorporate passive or active ROM exercises as appropriate every 2 hours on [odd/even] hour.	Promotes tissue perfusion and can benefit pulmonary system.[168]
Initiate early mobilization strategies	Has been shown to improve oxygen saturation and decrease length of stay.[151]
Protect with a sterile dressing for 24 to 48 hours. Wash hands before and after dressing changes or any contact with the surgical site, or when an incision dressing must be changed. Use sterile technique, and educate the patient and family regarding proper:	
• Incision care, symptoms of SSI, and the need to report such symptoms.	
• Monitor for hyperglycemia	Hyperglycemia lends to decreased wound healing.
• Assess cultural and religious norms.	Cultural and religious norms influence the perception of "the sick role."
• Collaborate with psychiatric nurse practitioner, ostomy or wound care management specialist as appropriate regarding care.	Collaboration helps to provide holistic care. Specialist may help discover underlying events for delayed surgical recovery and assist in designing an alternate plan of care.

Child Health

ACTIONS/INTERVENTIONS	RATIONALES
Monitor for all contributing factors, such as diet, altered organic or pathophysiologic functions, medications, environmental issues, psychological components, and circumstantial issues.	Thorough assessment will best offer ways to address factors that are impeding healing.
Determine appropriate treatment with attention to unique status per client's situation, with specific attention to medications, formula or diet, and surgical procedure/expected recovery.	Anticipatory planning provides holistic avenues to consider for recovery.

ACTIONS/INTERVENTIONS	RATIONALES
Note specific treatment protocols to satisfy unique healing or surgically related needs for client.	Unique protocols will best offer appropriate healing likelihood when implemented per intended plan.
Reassess every 8 hours for progress in healing (wound color, tissue status, drainage, and all related parameters).	Frequent ongoing assessment provides feedback to assist in determination of success of plan versus need for consideration of alternate modalities.
Reassess for potential additional delays of recovery as initial delays are identified.	Primary delays in surgical recovery may contribute to likelihood of delays to be noted later, with multiple delays made more likely to be noted before greater complications arise.
Assess for other nursing problems that may be identified as critical to resolution in relation to current surgical delay.	Multifactorial problems in recovery are best managed by separation and identification according to known etiology and treatment.

Women's Health

This nursing diagnosis pertains to women the same as to any other adult, with exception of the following:

ACTIONS/INTERVENTIONS	RATIONALES
After a Cesarean Section	
Monitor abdomen at least every 4 hours (state times here) for any distention, redness or swelling at incision site, tenderness, foul-smelling lochia, or vaginal discharge.	Monitor the patient for signs and symptoms of incisional and/or puerperal infection.
Wash hands each time before and after you or family members handle the baby.	Prevents development of nosocomial infection in the infant.
Maternal delay in recovering can involve a longer separation from the infant:	
• Act as a liaison between the family, nursery, and the mother.	
• Keep the mother informed and reassured about her baby.	
If the mother is unable to care for the infant, develop a schedule in which the infant is brought to the mother's room for frequent visiting.	
Let significant other or chosen family member care for the infant in the mother's room.	
If unable to transport the infant to the mother, obtain pictures of infant and set them up where the mother can view them.	
Involve other family members in the care of the infant.	
• Prepare the family to take the infant home without the mother.	
• Teach the family, and have them return—demonstrate, care and feeding of the infant.	
• If the mother desires to breast-feed:	
• Collaborate with physician regarding advisability of breast-feeding.	
• Involve lactation consultant to assist mother in pumping and	
• dumping milk if unable to use for infant, or	
• storing milk, if able to use, and sending home with the family.	

(care plan continued on page 110)

NURSING ACTIONS/INTERVENTIONS WITH RATIONALES (continued from page 109)

Mental Health

Nursing interventions and rationales for this diagnosis are the same as those for Adult Health.

Gerontic Health

● N O T E : *The older adult undergoing surgical treatment, either elective or emergency, is at great risk for problems with delayed recovery. Age-related changes in numerous systems and protective mechanisms increase the potential for complications pre-, intra-, and postoperatively. It is not uncommon for older adults to have a preexisting medical disease, atypical signs and symptoms of infection, cardiac or respiratory problems, and less ability to deal with stressors such as hypoxia, volume depletion, or volume overload. Gerontologic nursing groups are actively designing research-based protocols to ensure "best practices" in caring for older adults. The reader is referred to the work of NICHE (Nurses Improving the Care of the Hospitalized Elderly) at the Hartford Institute for Geriatric Nursing and the University of Iowa Research-Based Protocols developed by the University of Iowa Gerontological Nursing Interventions Research Center (http://www.hartfordign.org/programs/niche/)*[129,130]

ACTIONS/INTERVENTIONS	RATIONALES
Determine the client's mental status upon admission, and monitor the client for signs of acute confusion (delirium). Document results of mental status determinations in the client's record. The Mini-Mental State Exam by Folstein and/or the NEECHAM Confusion Scale are tools commonly used or recommended to determine mental status.	Older adults are at risk for developing acute confusion because of the multiple risk factors they experience (relocation, pain, physiologic changes associated with surgical procedures).
Initiate protocol (if available in your facility) for interventions addressing care of the acutely confused client if mental status changes warrant such action.	Delays in determining the presence of acute confusion may lead to extended hospital stays, decreases in functional status, and nursing home placement for older adults.
Manage postoperative acute pain aggressively to assist clients in recovery from the effects of surgery. Teach clients and family or significant others the benefits of adequate pain control in the recuperative process. Pain management can promote early ambulation, facilitate effective coughing and deep breathing, and decrease postoperative complications.	Older adults and some health-care providers may have concerns regarding use of pain medication. Some older adults may have fears of becoming addicted to medications. Health-care providers may be reluctant to medicate older adults because of concerns about overdosing or oversedating older clients.[153,154]
Plan caregiving activities that avoid stressing the client due to prolonged duration or intensity.	Physiologic reserves are decreased with aging. Too many demands can lead to increased fatigue and decreased ability to tolerate mobility efforts and postoperative activities to improve respiratory and cardiovascular status.
Monitor for evidence of poor wound healing.	Medications, poor nutritional status, systemic disease, and a history of smoking can have a negative effect on the normal wound repair response.[155]
Arrange for a nutrition consult if the client shows evidence of altered nutritional status.	Alterations in nutrition, such as protein–calorie malnutrition or nutrient deficiencies, can affect wound healing.
Refer older adults for evaluation of possible depression, especially if declining functional ability is noted.	Older adults who have depressive symptoms have negative postoperative outcomes.[156,157]

Home Health

ACTIONS/INTERVENTIONS	RATIONALES
Educate the client, family members, and potential caregivers how to care for the wound appropriately and have them demonstrate proper wound care.	Allows the family to participate in care and prevents infection or exacerbation of existing infection.
Assist the client and caregivers in obtaining necessary supplies for appropriate wound care.	Maximizes the client and caregiver's ability to provide appropriate wound care.
Instruct the client and caregivers in signs and symptoms of infection, hemorrhage, and dehiscence, as well as how and when to seek medical care.	Prevents further morbidity.
Educate the client, family members, and potential caregivers of the importance of taking all antibiotics as prescribed until the regimen is complete.	Treats existing infection and prevents possible super-infection.
Encourage the client to eat small frequent meals that are high in calories and protein.	Allows maximum nutrition without discomfort from large meals.
Weigh the client twice weekly.	Early identification of excessive weight loss can help identify complications such as dehydration.
Encourage the client to identify times of day when fatigue is worse, and space activities around the times when they are less fatigued.	Allows the client some control of activities.
Assist the client in obtaining durable medical equipment for the home (e.g., bedside commodes and shower chairs) until the fatigue improves.	Makes self-care activities less tiring.
Encourage the client to rest before scheduled activities.	May help avoid exacerbation of the fatigue.
Encourage the client to participate in walking activity as tolerated.	Fatigue seems to show improvement with walking programs
Encourage the client and caregivers to adhere to a round-the-clock analgesic regimen rather than using medications on a prn basis until pain is controlled.	Keeps pain at a tolerable level and avoids highs and lows in pain intensity.
Actively listen to the client and family members' concerns about delayed recovery and provide honest answers about the client's progress.	Allows verbalization of frustration and aids in realistic planning for the future.
Assist the client in obtaining letters and/or documentation as needed for employers regarding extended recovery time.	Helps eliminate a source of anxiety.

SUDDEN INFANT DEATH SYNDROME, RISK FOR

DEFINITION[44]

Presence of risk factors for sudden death of an infant under 1 year of age.

RISK FACTORS[44]

Modifiable

1. Infants placed to sleep in the prone or side lying position
2. Prenatal and/or postnatal infant smoke exposure
3. Infant overheating/overwrapping
4. Soft underlayment/loose articles in the sleep environment
5. Delayed or nonattendance of prenatal care

Potentially Modifiable

1. Low birthweight
2. Prematurity
3. Young maternal age

Nonmodifiable

1. Male gender
2. Ethnicity (i.e., African American or Native American race of mother)

3. Seasonality of SIDS deaths (higher in winter and fall months)
4. SIDS mortality peaks between infant age of 2 to 4 months

RELATED CLINICAL CONCERNS

1. Prematurity
2. Low birthweight
3. Young maternal age
4. Late or absence of prenatal care
5. Prenatal history of maternal smoking
6. High-risk status of the neonate, esp. males

EXPECTED OUTCOME

Will identify risk factors [list] and at least one corrective measure for each risk by [date].

    *The priority risk factor is assumed to be the need for putting infants to sleep on their back on non-soft bedding, free of pillows.

ADDITIONAL INFORMATION

For many years, apnea was thought to be the predecessor of SIDS, and home apnea monitors were considered effective as a means of preventing SIDS. Although the American Academy of Pediatrics acknowledges that home apnea monitors are being used widely, they do not recommend their use as a strategy to prevent SIDS. Monitors may be helpful to allow rapid recognition of apnea, airway obstruction, respiratory failure, interruption of supplemental oxygen supply, or failure of mechanical respiratory support in those infants

 Have You Selected the Correct Diagnosis?

Risk for Sudden Infant Death Syndrome is the most appropriate diagnosis if the parents or infant caregivers verbalize less-than-adequate understanding of infant care or if potentially modifiable or nonmodifiable risk factors are present.

who have experienced an apparent life threatening event (ALTE) according to the Sudden Infant Death Syndrome Task Force of the American Academy of Pediatrics.[173]

    The predominant hypothesis regarding the etiology of SIDS remains that certain infants, for reasons yet to be determined, may have a maldevelopment or delay in maturation of the brainstem neural network that accounts for arousal and influences the physiologic responses to life-threatening challenges during sleep. The Task Force on SIDS recommends cautious consideration for modifying those risks which can be modified while recognizing there may be additional factors to be considered by the pediatrician and healthcare team in allowing for the best practice.[173]

TARGET DATES

A long-term goal of maintaining infant safety can be met by establishing short-term goals of parent/caregiver education. Short-term goals for parents/caregivers to verbalize or demonstrate proper infant care should be established in terms of days or hours, ideally prior to discharge of the infant.

NURSING ACTIONS/INTERVENTIONS WITH RATIONALES

Adult Health

The interventions for Child/Women's Health apply to this population.

Child Health

ACTIONS/INTERVENTIONS	RATIONALES
Assess caregiver(s) readiness for learning to prevent SIDS.	Readiness offers cues for likelihood of effective learning as prevention education increases likelihood for reduction of risk for SIDS to extent possible.[173]
Provide educational materials to primary caregiver(s) to include the following as applicable. (Confirm those aspects that may be inappropriate with pediatrician or primary care provider.): • Universal precautions • Place infant on back with pacifier from birth to 6 months of age.	Adheres to standards currently endorsed by the SIDS Task Force of the American Academy of Pediatrics.[173] Assists in maintenance of airway.

ACTIONS/INTERVENTIONS	RATIONALES
• Use of firm sleep mattress with basic sheet covering. Avoid placing soft materials such as pillows, quilts, comforters, or sheepskins under a sleeping infant.	Lessens likelihood of infant airway being obstructed secondary to blanket or other surface bedding obstructing airway.
• Avoid soft objects (such as stuffed animals) and loose bedding (no pillow-like bumper pads, instead use thin, fixed to crib bumper pads). Tuck blankets from chest level down or utilize sleep sacks designed to keep infant warm but not constricted or head covering.	Lessens likelihood of objects or blankets covering infant's face or obstructing the infant's airway.
• Have infant's crib in same room as caregiver(s) but no co-sleeping.	Risk of SIDS reduced and allows for close contact for feeding and potential need for intervention.
• Refrain from smoking; do not expose the infant to second-hand smoke.	Lessens irritants to reduce SIDS and numerous other respiratory conditions.
• Consider offering a pacifier at nap time and bedtime.	Mechanism is unknown, but evidence is compelling for reducing risk of SIDS.
• Do not reinsert pacifier once infant falls asleep.	Same as above.
• If infant refuses pacifier, do not force infant to take it.	Same as above.
• Pacifiers are to be free of any sweet solution.	Lessens likelihood of infection with such organisms as botulism as found in honey.
• Pacifiers are to be cleaned often and replaced regularly every 3 to 4 weeks.	Lessens likelihood of infection or likelihood of broken pieces being aspirated by infant.
• For breast-fed infants, delay pacifier introduction until 1 month of age	Lessens likelihood of nipple confusion as breastfeeding is established.
• Avoid overheating: infant to be lightly clothed for sleep with room temperature maintained for adult with light clothing-infant should not feel hot to the touch.	Overheating is shown to be a risk factor for SIDS.
• Avoid commercial devices marketed to reduce the risk of SIDS including positional devices or rebreathing devices.	Efficacy or safety is not yet sufficiently upheld in studies done thus far.
• Do not use home monitors as a strategy for reducing the risk of SIDS. Electronic respiratory and cardiac monitors are suited to detect cardiorespiratory arrest and may be of value for home monitoring of those infants deemed to be at risk for instability from a cardiorespiratory standpoint.	Does not decrease the threat of SIDS.
• If concurrent risk exists for apnea of infancy or prematurity, caregiver(s) are taught basic CPR.	Offers caregiver(s) sense of confidence for ability to intervene in instance of actual cardiorespiratory arrest.
*May vary per institution or preference of pediatrician or neonatologist.	
• Avoid possible development of positional plagiocephaly (malshapen flatness of the occiput).	Recommendations for alternative positioning and movement during waking time is likely to prevent the malshaping of the infant's head while also fostering appropriate motor development and time for interaction with primary caregiver(s).
• Encourage tummy time while infant is awake and in close observation.	
• Avoid excessive time in carriers, car-seat carriers, or bouncers in which the occiput is pressured.	
• Alternate position of head turning week by week and alternate crib position to provide alternate views to rest of room.	
*Special attention should be addressed to these components if neurologic injury or developmental delay of the infant is suspected.	
Early referral for plagiocephaly is encouraged to help avoid the need for surgery. In some instances, orthotics may help avoid surgical intervention.	

(care plan continued on page 114)

NURSING ACTIONS/INTERVENTIONS WITH RATIONALES (continued from page 113)

Child Health

ACTIONS/INTERVENTIONS	RATIONALES
Monitor primary caregiver for support need(s).	Provides backup to help value and support caregiver(s), esp. in instance of young age or those for whom support is vital.
Teach caregiver(s) to maintain close observation of infant at all times.	Maintains safe environment.
Monitor caregiver's ability to provide this care.	
Teach caregiver(s) to utilize national and local resources for additional support for education and support in dealing with the risk for SIDS. National SIDS Resource Center: http://www.sidscenter.org, American Sudden Infant Death Syndrome (SIDS) Institute. (http://www.sids.org)	Provides support to strengthen knowledge and sense of ability to cope with reinforcement of basic risk reducing principles for SIDS with shared sense of valuing.
Monitor for concurrent risk factors that place the maternal–infant dyad at increased likelihood for stressors that suggest other nursing needs, especially role strain and primary caregiving needs.	Assists in secondary prevention of related problems.
Monitor caregiver(s) compliance with plan for reduction of SIDS risk.	Values the importance of compliance with SIDS risk reduction and offers confirmation of caregiver(s) ability to demonstrate accuracy of techniques.
• Provide positive verbal reinforcement for progress/identification of unmet preventive goals.	
Remind caregiver(s) of need for other caregivers to comply with essential SIDS risk reduction measures, especially day care and babysitters.	Ensures uniform risk reduction for SIDS to degree possible.

Women's Health

ACTIONS/INTERVENTIONS	RATIONALES
The education and advice recorded in the child health section apply to women's health, as women are the major caretakers of children. However all caregivers, whether grandparents, or other family members should be aware how to comply with the essential SIDS risk reduction measures.	
Care of self during the prenatal period can contribute to the reduction of the incidence of SIDS. Good nutrition, proper exercise, no smoking, no exposure to second-hand smoke, and no drug or alcohol use during pregnancy.	The risk of SIDS is five to ten times greater in infants of mothers who abused drugs during pregnancy. This is particularly true of the infant who goes through withdrawal after birth.[29]

Mental Health

The interventions for Child/Women's Health apply to this population.

Gerontic Health

This diagnosis does not apply to the aging population unless the infant caregiver is elderly. In such cases, the interventions for Child/Women's Health would apply.

Home Health

The interventions for Child/Women's Health would be applied in the home setting.

REFERENCES

1. Gordon, M: Manual of Nursing Diagnosis. CV Mosby, St. Louis, 2002.
2. Rogers, ME: An Introduction to the Theoretical Basis for Nursing. FA Davis, Philadelphia, 1970.
3. Kneeshaw, M, and Lunney, M: Nursing diagnosis: Not for individuals only. Geriatr Nurs 37:246, 1989.
4. Rosenstock, I: Historical origins of the health belief model. In Becker, M (ed): The Health Belief Model and Personal Behavior. Charles B. Slack, Thorofare, NJ, 1974.
5. Ridenour, N: Health beliefs, preventive behavioral intentions and knowledge of gonorrhea: Predictors of recidivism? In Monograph 1983, Proceedings of 2nd Annual Sigma Theta Tau Conference, The World of Work: Research in Nursing Practice. Sigma Theta Tau, Indianapolis, IN, 1983.
6. Fleury, J: The application of motivational theory to cardiovascular risk reduction. Image J Nursing Scholar 24:229, 1992.
7. Janz, NK: The health belief model in understanding cardiovascular risk factor reduction behaviors. Cardiovasc Nurs 24:39, 1988.
8. Pender, NJ: Health Promotion in Nursing Practice, ed 3. Appleton-Century-Crofts, Stamford, CT, 1996.
9. Brubaker, B: Health promotion: A linguistic analysis. Adv Nurs Sci 5:1, 1983.
10. U.S. Department of Health and Human Services: Healthy People 2010 (Conference Edition in Two Volumes). U.S. Government Printing Office, Washington, DC, 2000.
11. Health and Human Services: Put Prevention Into Practice. American Nurses Association, Waldorf, MD, 1994.
12. Shortridge, L, and Valanis, B: The epidemiological model applied in community health nursing. In Stanhope, M, and Lancaster, J (eds): Community Health Nursing: Process and Practice for Promoting Health, ed 3. CV Mosby, St. Louis, 1992.
13. Gleit, C, and Tatro, S: Nursing diagnosis for healthy individuals. Nurs Health Care 32:151, 1981.
14. Hockenberry, M, Wilson, D, Winkelstein, M, and Klein, N: Wong's Nursing Care of Infants and Children, ed 7. CV Mosby, St. Louis, 2003.
15. Popkess-Vawter, S: Wellness nursing diagnoses: To be or not to be? Nursing Diagnosis 2:19, 1991.
16. Knollmueller, RN: Prevention Across the Life Span: Healthy People for the 21st Century. American Nurses Publishing, Washington, DC, 1993.
17. Schuster, CS, and Ashburn, SS: The Process of Human Development: A Holistic Life-Span Approach, ed 3. JB Lippincott, New York, 1992.
18. Preventive Services Task Force: Guide to Clinical Preventive Services, ed 2. Williams & Wilkins, Baltimore, 1996.
19. American Academy of Pediatrics, Committee on Infectious Diseases: Red Book: Report of the Committee on Infectious Diseases, ed 24. Author, Elk Grove Village, IL, 1997.
20. Centers for Disease Control: Recommended childhood immunization schedule—United States, 1995. MMWR 44:RR-5, 1, 1995.
21. Centers for Disease Control: Progress toward elimination of Haemophilus influenzae type b disease among infants and children—United States, 1987–1993. MMWR 43:8, 1994.
22. Centers for Disease Control: Haemophilus b conjugate vaccines for prevention of Haemophilus influenzae type b disease among infants and children two months of age and older. Recommendation of the immunization practices advisory committee (ACIP). MMWR 40:RR-1, 1991.
23. AAFP updates childhood immunizations schedule. Am Fam Physician 51:2031, 1995.
24. Centers for Disease Control: General recommendations on immunization: Recommendations of the Advisory Committee on Immunization Practices (ACIP). MMWR 43:RR-1, 1, 1994.
25. Centers for Disease Control (CDC): Prevention and Recommended Adult Immunization Schedule—United States, October 2005–September 2006. MMWR 54:Q1–Q4, 2005.
26. Centers for Disease Control: Hepatitis B virus: A comprehensive strategy for eliminating transmission in the United States through universal childhood vaccination. MMWR 40:RR-13, 1991.
27. Baron, M, and Tafuro, P: The extremes of age: The newborn and the elderly. Nurs Clin North Am 20:181, 1985.
28. Schuster, CS: Normal physiological parameters through the life cycle. Nurse Pract 2:25, 1997.
29. Lowdermilk, DL, and Perry, S: Maternity & Women's Health Care, ed 8. CV Mosby, St. Louis, 2004.
30. Immunizations Practices Advisory Committee: Measles prevention: Recommendations of the Immunizations Practices Advisory Committee. MMWR 38:1, 1989.
31. American College of Physicians: Guide for Adult Immunization, ed 3. Author, Philadelphia, 1994.
32. Centers for Disease Control: Youth risk behavior surveillance—United States, 1993. MMWR 44:SS-1, 1995.
33. Centers for Disease Control: Update on adult immunization. MMWR 40:RR-12, 1991.
34. Immunizations Practices Advisory Committee: Pneumococcal polysaccharide vaccine. MMWR 38:64, 1989.
35. Shapiro, E, et al: The protective efficacy of polyvalent pneumococcal-polysaccharide vaccine. N Engl J Med 325:1453, 1991.
36. Slaninka, SC, and Galbraith, AM: Healthy endings: A collaborative health promotion project for the elderly. J Gerontol Nurs 24:35, 1998.
37. Rubenstein, LZ, and Nahas, R: Primary and secondary prevention strategies in the older adult. Geriatr Nurs 18:11, 1998.
38. Plichta, AM: Immunization: Protecting older patients from infectious disease. Geriatrics 51:47, 1996.
39. American Academy of Family Practitioners: Immunization policies for older patients. http://www.aafp.prg/policy/camp/aap-d_c.html, August, 1999.
40. Tyson, SP: Gerontological Nursing Care. WB Saunders, Philadelphia, 1999.
41. Staab, AS, and Hodges, AC: Essentials of Gerontological Nursing: Adaptation to the Aging Process. JB Lippincott, Philadelphia, 1996.
42. Emmett, KR: Nonspecific and atypical presentation of disease in the older patient. Geriatrics 53:50, 1998.
43. Fraser, D: Assessing the elderly for infections. J Gerontol Nurs 23:5, 1997.
44. North American Nursing Diagnosis Association: Nursing Diagnosis: Definitions and Classification, 2000–2001. Author, Philadelphia, 2000.
45. Wright, SM: Validity of the human energy assessment form. West J Nurs Res 13:635, 1991.
46. Krieger, D: The Therapeutic Touch: How to Use Your Hands to Help or Heal. Prentice-Hall, Englewood Cliffs, NJ, 1979.

47. Krieger, D: Living the Therapeutic Touch: Healing as a Lifestyle. Prentice-Hall, Englewood Cliffs, NJ, 1987.

48. Dossey, BM, Keegan, L, and Guzzetta, CE: Holistic Nursing: A Handbook for Practice, ed 3. Aspen, Gaithersburg, MD, 2000.

49. Whitis, G, and Iyer, P: Patient Outcomes in Pediatric Nursing. Springhouse Corporation, Springhouse, 1995.

50. McCoy, PA, and Votroubek, W: Pediatric Home Care: A Comprehensive Approach. Aspen Publishers, Gaithersburg, MD, 1990.

51. Miller, L: Psychotherapy of epilepsy: Seizure control and psychosocial adjustment. J Cognit Rehab 12:14, 1994.

52. Gatts, EJ, et al: Reducing crying and irritability in neonates using a continuously controlled early environment. J Perinatol 15:215, 1995.

53. Alexander, C, and Steefel, L: Biofeedback: Listen to the body. RN 51, August, 1995.

54. Nichols, F, and Gennaro, S: The childbirth experience. In Nichols, F and Humenick, S (eds): Childbirth Education, Research and Theory, ed 2. WB Saunders, Philadelphia, 2000.

55. Talton, CW: Touch—of all kinds—is therapeutic. RN 61, February, 1995.

56. Morrelli, I: Interview with author on use of therapeutic touch during labor. 1995.

57. Marks, G: Alternative therapies. in Nichols, F and Humenick, S (eds): Childbirth Education, Research and Theory, ed 2. WB Saunders, Philadelphia, 2000.

58. McKinney, JB: The Online Journal of Knowledge, Synthesis for Nursing (Therapeutic Touch, Human Energy Field Nursing, Holistic Care Practice, Research): October 1995, Document 11.

59. Meehan, TC: Therapeutic touch as a nursing intervention. J Adv Nursing 28(1), 1998.

60. Huebscher, R: Natural, alternative and complementary health care in tests. In Breslin ET, and Lucas, VA (eds): Women's Health Nursing: Toward Evidence-Based Practice. Elsevier, Philadelphia, 2003.

61. Erickson, HC, Tomlin, EM, and Swain, MP: Modeling and Role-Modeling: A Theory and Paradigm for Nursing. Prentice-Hall, Englewood Cliffs, NJ, 1983.

62. Becker, R, and Selden, G: The Body Electric. William Morrow, New York, 1985.

63. Dossey, BM: Complementary and alternative therapies for our aging society. J Gerontol Nurs 23:45, 1997.

64. Moore, T: Best practice guidelines: An invitation to reflect on therapeutic touch practice. J Nursing Care Quality 20:90, 2005.

65. Thie, J: Touch for Health. Devorss & Company, Marina del Rey, CA, 1979.

66. Quinn, J, and Strelkauskas, A: Psychoimmunologic effects of therapeutic touch on practitioners and recently bereaved recipients: A pilot study. Adv Nurs Sci 15:13, 1993.

67. Snyder, M: Independent Nursing Interventions, ed 2. Delmar Publishers, Albany, NY, 1992.

68. Kunz, L, and Kunz, B: The Practitioner's Guide to Reflexology. Prentice-Hall, Englewood Cliffs, NJ, 1985.

69. Wright, L, and Leahey, M: Nurses and Families, ed 3. FA Davis, Philadelphia, 2000.

70. Eliopoulos, C: Using complementary and alternative therapies wisely. Geriatr Nurs 20:139, 1999.

71. Lorenzi, EA: Complementary/alternative therapies: So many choices. Geriatr Nurs 20:125, 1999.

72. Anderson, R, and Anderson, K: Success and failure attributions in smoking cessations among men and women. Am Assoc Occup Health Nurs J 38:180, 1990.

73. Wewers, M, and Gonyon, D: Cigarette craving during the immediate post cessation period. Appl Nurs Res 2:46, 1989.

74. Frost, C: Implications of smoking bans in the workplace. Am Assoc Occup Health Nurs J 39:270, 1991.

75. Daughton, DM, et al: Total indoor smoking ban and smoker behavior. Prevent Med 21:670, 1992.

76. Volden, C, et al: The relationship of age, gender and exercise practices to measures of health, life-style, and self-esteem. Appl Nurs Res 3:20, 1990.

77. Brown, J, and March, S: Use of botanicals for health purposes by members of a prepaid health plan. Res Nurs Health 14:330, 1991.

78. Ibrecht, SA: Achieving Success: Nursing care for pregnant women who smoke, AWHONN Lifelines 8(3):190, 2004.

79. Hershberger, P: Smoking and Pregnant Teens. AWHONN Lifelines 2(4):26, 1998.

80. Murray, E, and Wewers, ME: Nurses can play a significant role in reducing tobacco use in the U S. AWHONN Lifelines 8(3):200, 2004.

81. Patrick, T: Female Physical Development. In Breslin, ET, and Lucas, VA (eds): Women's Health Nursing: Toward Evidence-Based Practice. WB Saunders, Philadelphia, 2003.

82. Lindsay, SH: Menopause naturally: Exploring alternatives to traditional HRT, AWHONN Lifelines 3(5):32, 1999.

83. Learn, CD, and Higgins, PG: Harmonizing herbs: Managing menopause with help from Mother Earth. AWHONN Lifelines 3(5):39, 1999.

84. McCloskey-Dochterman, J, and Bulecheck, G: Nursing Interventions Classification. CV Mosby, St. Louis, 2004.

85. Ossman, SS: Nephrology Nursing Journal 31:346, 2004.

86. Parsons, JT, Rosof, E, Punzalan, JC, and Di Maria, L: Integration of motivational interviewing and cognitive behavioral therapy to improve HIV medication adherence and reduce substance use among HIV-positive men and women. AIDS Patient Care & STDs 19:31, 2005.

87. Kneisl, C, Wilson, H, and Trigoboff, E: Comtemporary Psychiatric-Mental Health Nursing. Pearson Education, Upper Saddle River, NJ, 2004.

88. Greenx, J: Historical view of social support. J Nurs Scholar 37:300, 2005.

89. Papalia, DE, and Olds, SW: Human Development, ed 7. McGraw-Hill, Burr Ridge, IL, 1998.

90. Rice, R: Teaching strategies for special patient groups encountered in home care. Geriatr Nurs 20:220, 1999.

91. Katz, LC, and Rubin, M: Keep Your Brain Alive. Workman Publishing, New York, 1999.

92. Briasco, M: Indoor air pollution: Are employees sick from their work? Am Assoc Occup Health Nurs J 38:375, 1990.

93. Kipen, HM, et al: Measuring chemical sensitivity prevalence: A questionnaire for population studies. Am J Pub Health 85:574, 1985.

94. Bonheur, B, and Young, S: Exercise as a health-promoting lifestyle choice. Appl Nursing Res 4:2, 1991.

95. Rosenkoetter, M: Health promotion: The influence of pets on life patterns in the home. Holistic Nurs Pract 5:42, 1991.

96. Burns, M: Screening and diagnostic tests. In Breslin, ET, and Lucas, VA (eds). Women's Health Nursing: Toward Evidence-Based Practice. WB Saunders, Philadelphia, 2003.

97. Eirckson, H, Tomlin, E, and Swain, M: Modeling and Role-Modeling: A Theory and Paradigm for Nursing. Prentice-Hall, Englewood Cliffs, NJ, 1983.

98. Garner, J S: Guideline for isolation precautions in hospitals, Part I. Evolution of isolation practices, Hospital Infection Control Practices Advisory Committee: Am J Infect Control 24(1):24–31, 1996.

99. Kozier, B: Fundamentals of Nursing: Concepts, Process, and Practice, ed 7, Prentice Hall Health, Upper Saddle River NJ, 2004.

100. St. Clair, K, and Larrabee, JH: Clean versus sterile gloves: which to use for postoperative dressing changes. Outcomes Management 6(1):17, 2002.

101. Sellers, JB: Health care for older women. In Breslin, ET, and Lucas, VA (eds): Women's Health Nursing: Toward Evidence-Based Practice. WB Saunders, Philadelphia, 2003.

102. DelAngelo, D: Energize your life (unpublished speech, October 2005, Erie, PA).

103. Wilson, PR, and Pugh, LC: Promoting nutrition in breast feeding women. JOGNN 120, 2005.

104. Maxmen, J, and Ward, N: Psychotropic Drugs Fast Facts. WW Norton, New York, 2002.

105. Centers for Disease Control: Recommendations for the prevention of HIV transmission in health-care setting. MMWR 36:1, 1987.

106. Centers for Disease Control: Update: Universal precautions for prevention of transmission of human immunodeficiency virus, hepatitis B virus, and other bloodborne pathogens in health-care settings. MMWR 37:377, 1988.

107. Centers for Disease Control: Recommendations for preventing transmission of human immunodeficiency virus and hepatitis B virus to patients during exposure-prone invasive procedures. MMWR 40:1, 1991.

108. Benenson, A: Control of Communicable Diseases Manual, ed 16. American Public Health Association, Washington, DC, 1995.

109. Dooley, S, et al: Guidelines for preventing the transmission of tuberculosis in health-care settings, with special focus on HIV-related issues. MMWR 39:RR-17, 1990.

110. Centers for Disease Control: Tuberculosis control laws—United States, 1993. Recommendations of the Advisory Council for the Elimination of Tuberculosis (ACET). MMWR 42:RR-15, 1993.

111. Burke, MM, and Walsh, MB: Gerontologic Nursing: Wholistic Care of the Older Adult. CV Mosby, St. Louis, 1997.

112. Galindo-Cioca, DJ: Fall prevention. J Gerontol Nurs 21:11, 1995.

113. McCloskey, JC, and Bulechek, GM: Nursing Intervention Classification, ed 2. CV Mosby, St. Louis, 1997.

114. Commodore, D: Falls in the elderly population: A look at incidence, risks, healthcare cost, and preventive strategies. Rehabil Nurs 20:84, 1995.

115. Tyson, SR: Gerontological Nursing Care. WB Saunders, Philadelphia, 1999.

116. Mace, N, and Rabin, P: The 36-Hour Day: A Family Guide. Johns Hopkins University Press, Baltimore, 1991.

117. Evans, L, and Strumpf, N: Myths about elder restraint. Image 22:124, 1990.

118. Kilpack, V, et al: Using research-based interventions to decrease patient falls. Appl Nurs Res 4:68, 1991.

119. Hogue, CC: Managing falls: The current basis for practice. In Funk, SG, et al (eds): Key Aspects of Elder Care. Springer, New York, 1992.

120. Jech, AO: Preventing falls in the elderly. Geriatr Nurs 13:43, 1992.

121. Williams, J: Employee experiences with early return to work programs. Am Assoc Occup Health Nurs 39:64, 1991.

122. National Immunization Campaign: Community Leader's Guide for the National Immunization Campaign. Author, Washington, DC, 1991.

123. Brown, M, and Hess, R: Managing latex allergy in the cardiac surgical patient. Crit Care Nurs Q 21:8, 1998.

124. Baumann, NH: Latex allergy. Orthop Nurs 18:15, 1999.

125. Carroll, P: Latex allergy: What you need to know. RN 62:40, 1999.

126. Harrau, BO: Managing latex allergy patients. Nurs Manage 29:48, 1998.

127. Romanczuk, A: Latex use with infants and children: It can cause problems. MCN 18:208, 1993.

128. Wong, DL: Wong and Whaley's Clinical Manual of Pediatric Nursing, ed 5. CV Mosby, St. Louis, 2000.

129. Breunig, K, et al: Noncompliance as a nursing diagnosis: Current use in clinical practice. In Hurley, M (ed): Classification of Nursing Diagnosis: Proceedings of the Sixth Conference. CV Mosby, St. Louis, 1986.

130. Benner, PE, and Wrubel, J: The Primacy of Caring: Stress and Coping in Health and Illness. Addison-Wesley, Menlo Park, CA, 1989.

131. Gabbe, SG, Niebyl, JR, and Simpson, JL: Normal and Problem Pregnancies. Churchill-Livingstone, New York, 1996.

132. Mandeville, LK, and Troiano, NH: High-Risk and Critical Care Intrapartum Nursing. JB Lippincott, Philadelphia, 1999.

133. Stainton, MC: Supporting family functioning during a high-risk pregnancy. MCN Am J Matern Child Nurs 19:24, 1994.

134. Gadow, S: Covenant without cure: Letting go and holding on in chronic illness. In Watson, J, and Ray, M (eds): The Ethics of Care and the Ethics of Cure: Synthesis in Chronicity. National League for Nursing, New York, 1988.

135. Hagey, R, and McDonough, P: The problem of professional labeling. Nursing Outlook 32:151, 1984.

136. Edel, M: Noncompliance: An appropriate nursing diagnosis? Nursing Outlook 33:183, 1985.

137. Keeling, A, et al: Noncompliance revisited: A disciplinary perspective of a nursing diagnosis. Nursing Diagnosis 4:91, 1993.

138. Beauchamp, TL, and Childress, JF: Principles of Biomedical Ethics, ed 4. Oxford University Press, New York, 1994.

139. Graham, J: Motivational interviewing: A hammer looking for a nail? J Psychiatr Mental Health Nurs 11:494, 2004.

140. Thorne, S: Constructive noncompliance in chronic illness. Holist Nurs Pract 5:62, 1990.

141. Cooper, M: Chronic illness and nursing's ethical challenge. Holist Nurs Pract 5:10, 1990.

142. Jones, S, Jones, P, and Katz, J: A nursing intervention to increase compliance in otitis media patients. Appl Nurs Res 4:68, 1989.

143. Lange, N, and Tigges, BB: Influence positive change with motivational interviewing. Nurse Practitioner 30:44, 2005.

144. Upvall, MJ: Women and Culture. In Breslin, ET, and Lucas, VA (eds). Women's Health Nursing: Toward Evidence-Based Practice. Elsevier, Philadelphia, 2003.

145. Watson, J: Nursing, Human Science and Human Care: A Theory of Nursing. National League for Nursing, New York, 1991.

146. Nichols, FC, and Zwelling, E: Maternal-Newborn Nursing: Theory and Practice. WB Saunders, Philadelphia, 1997.

147. Kontz, M: Compliance redefined and implications for home care. Holist Nurs Pract 3:54, 1989.

148. Hoffman, L: A co-evolutionary framework for systemic family therapy? In Hansen, JC, and Keeney, BP (eds): Diagnosis and Assessment in Family Therapy. Aspen Systems, Rockville, MD, 1983.

149. Smith, F, and Knice-Ambinder, M: Promoting medication compliance in clients with chronic mental illness. Holist Nurs Pract 4:70, 1989.

150. Gravely, E, and Oseasohn, C: Multiple drug regimens: Medication compliance among veterans 65 years and older. Res Nurs Health 14:51, 1991.

151. Ebersole, P, and Hess, P: Toward Healthy Aging, ed 5. CV Mosby, St. Louis, 1998.

152. Nielsen-Bohlman, L, Panzer, AM, and King, DA (eds): Committee on Health Literacy. 2004.

153. Lipman, EL, and Boyle, MH: Social support and education groups for single mothers: A randomized controlled trial of a community-based program. Can Med Assoc J 173:1451, 2005.

154. Amaya, MA: Women's environmental health. In Breslin, ET, and Lucas, VA (eds): Women's Health Nursing: Toward Evidence-Based Practice. Elsevier, Philadelphia, 2003.

155. Kanusky, C: Health concerns of women in midlife. In: Breslin ET, and Lucas, VA (eds): Women's Health Nursing: Toward Evidence-Based Practice. Elsevier, Philadelphia, 2003.

156. Skillman-Hull, L: Adolescent women's health care. In Breslin, ET, and Lucas, VA (eds): Women's Health Nursing: Toward Evidence-Based Practice. Elsevier, Philadelphia, 2003.

157. Teschendorf, M: Women during the reproductive years. In Breslin, ET, and Lucas, VA (eds): Women's Health Nursing: Toward Evidence-Based Practice. Elsevier, Philadelphia, 2003.

158. Haynes, R, Yao, X, Degani, A, Kripalani, S, Garg, A, and McDonald, H: Interventions for enhancing medication adherence. The Cochrane Library, 2006.

159. Martin, EJ: Intrapartum Management Modules, ed 3. Williams & Wilkins, Baltimore, 2002.

160. Kelly, M: Surgery, anesthesia, and the geriatric patient. Geriatr Nurs 16:213, 1996.

161. Worfolk, J: Keep frail elders warm. Geriatr Nurs 18:7, 1997.

162. Skewes, SM: Skin care rituals that do more harm than good. Am J Nurs 96:33, 1996.

163. Taylor, C: Fundamentals of Nursing: The Art and Science of Nursing Care. JB Lippincott, Philadelphia, 1997.

164. Letvak, S, and Schoder, D: Sexually transmitted diseases in the elderly: What you need to know. Geriatr Nurs 17:156, 1997.

165. Szirony, TA: Infection with HIV in the elderly population. J Gerontol Nurs 25:25, 1999.

166. Pasero, CL, and McCaffery, M: Managing postoperative pain in the elderly. Am J Nurs 96:38, 1996.

167. Csokasy, J: Assessment of acute confusion: Use of the NEECHAM confusion scale. Appl Nurs Res 12:51, 1999.

168. Fanning, MF: Reducing postoperative pulmonary complications in cardiac surgery patients with the use of best evidence. J Nurs Care Quality 19:2, 9, 2004.

169. Palmer, RM, and Bolla, L: When your patient is hospitalized: Tips for primary care physicians. Geriatrics 52:36, 1997.

170. Weksler, ME: Wound repair in older patients: Preventing problems and managing the healing. Geriatrics 53:88, 1998.

171. Kurlowicz, LH: Perceived self-efficacy, functional ability, and depressive symptoms in older elective surgery patients. Nurs Res 47:219, 1998.

172. Kurlowicz, LH, and Streim, JE: Measuring depression in hospitalized, medically ill, older adults. Arch Psychiatr Nurs XII:209, 1998.

173. Task Force on Sudden Infant Death Syndrome: Pediatrics 116:1245, 2005.

174. Anderson, E, and McFarlane, J: Community as Partner: Theory and Practice in Nursing, ed 4. Lippincott, Williams & Wilkins, Philadelphia, 2004.

3

NUTRITIONAL–
METABOLIC PATTERN

PATTERN DESCRIPTION

The nutritional–metabolic pattern focuses on food and fluid intake, the body's use of this intake (metabolism), and problems that might influence intake. Problems in this pattern may have a physiologic, psychological, or sociologic base. Physiologic problems may be primary in nature, for example, vitamin deficiency, or they may arise secondary to another pathophysiologic state, such as a peptic ulcer. Psychological factors, such as stress, may result in an alteration, such as overeating or anorexia nervosa, in the nutritional–metabolic pattern. Sociologic factors, for example, low income, inadequate or unsafe storage, social isolation, and cultural food preferences, may result in an altered nutritional–metabolic state.

According to the popular truism "You are what you eat," what we eat is converted to our cellular structure and affects its functioning. The nutritional–metabolic pattern allows us to look at the whole of this relationship.

PATTERN ASSESSMENT

1. Weigh the patient. Is the patient's weight beyond the recommended range for his or her height, age, and sex?
   a. Yes (Imbalanced Nutrition, More Than Body Requirements, Risk for or Actual; Fluid Volume Excess; Imbalanced Body Temperature, Risk for; Imbalanced Fluid Volume, Risk for)
   b. No (Nutrition, Readiness for Enhanced)
2. Does the patient weigh less than the recommended range for his or her height, age, and sex?
   a. Yes (Imbalanced Nutrition, Less Than Body Requirements; Deficient Fluid Volume, Risk for or Actual; Imbalanced Body Temperature, Risk for; Adult Failure to Thrive; Impaired Dentition)
   b. No (Nutrition, Readiness for Enhanced)
3. Have the patient describe a typical day's intake of both food and fluid, including snacks and the pattern of eating. Is the patient's food intake above the average for his or her age, sex, height, weight, and activity level?
   a. Yes (Imbalanced Nutrition, More Than Body Requirements, Risk for or Actual)
   b. No (Nutrition, Readiness for Enhanced)
4. Is the patient's food intake below the average for his or her age, sex, height, weight, and activity level?
   a. Yes (Imbalanced Nutrition, Less Than Body Requirements; Adult Failure to Thrive; Impaired Dentition)
   b. No (Nutrition, Readiness for Enhanced)
5. Is the patient's fluid intake sufficient for his or her age, sex, height, weight, activity level, and fluid output?
   a. Yes (Fluid Balance, Readiness for Enhanced)
   b. No (Deficient Fluid Volume, Risk for or Actual; Imbalanced Body Temperature, Risk for; Imbalanced Fluid Volume, Risk for)

6. Does the patient show evidence of edema?
   a. Yes (Fluid Volume Excess; Imbalanced Fluid Volume, Risk for)
   b. No
7. Is the patient's gag reflex present?
   a. Yes
   b. No (Impaired Swallowing; Risk for Aspiration)
8. Does the patient cough or choke during eating?
   a. Yes (Impaired Swallowing; Risk for Aspiration)
   b. No
9. Assess the patient's mouth, eyes, and skin. Are these assessments within normal limits (e.g., no lesions, soreness, or inflamed areas)?
   a. Yes
   b. No (Impaired Tissue Integrity; Impaired Oral Mucous Membrane)
10. Assess the patient's teeth. Are teeth within normal limits?
    a. Yes
    b. No (Impaired Dentition)
11. Are intake and output, skin turgor, and weight vacillating?
    a. Yes (Imbalanced Fluid Volume, Risk for)
    b. No (Fluid Balance, Readiness for Enhanced)
12. Is the patient able to move freely in bed? Ambulates easily?
    a. Yes
    b. No (Impaired Tissue Integrity; Impaired Skin Integrity, Risk for or Actual)
13. Review the patient's temperature measurement. Is the temperature within normal limits?
    a. Yes
    b. No (Ineffective Thermoregulation; Hyperthermia; Hypothermia)
14. Is the patient's temperature above normal?
    a. Yes (Ineffective Thermoregulation; Hyperthermia)
    b. No
15. Is the patient's temperature below normal?
    a. Yes (Ineffective Thermoregulation; Hypothermia)
    b. No
16. Is the patient exhibiting signs or symptoms of infection? Vasoconstriction? Vasodilation? Dehydration?
    a. Yes (Imbalanced Body Temperature, Risk for)
    b. No
17. Ask the patient: "Do you have any problems swallowing food? Fluids?"
    a. Yes (Impaired Swallowing; Risk for Aspiration)
    b. No
18. Does the patient report chronic health problems?
    a. Yes (Adult Failure to Thrive)
    b. No
19. Does the patient complain of being nauseated?
    a. Yes (Nausea)
    b. No

● N O T E : *The next questions pertain only to a mother who is breastfeeding.*

20. Weigh the infant. Is his or her weight within normal limits for his or her age?
    a. Yes (Effective Breastfeeding)
    b. No (Ineffective Breastfeeding)
21. Ask the patient: "Do you have any problems or concerns about breastfeeding?"
    a. Yes (Ineffective Breastfeeding)
    b. No (Effective Breastfeeding)

CONCEPTUAL INFORMATION

The nutritional–metabolic pattern requires looking at four separate but closely aligned aspects: nutrition, fluid balance, tissue integrity, and thermoregulation. All four functionally interrelate to maintain the integrity of the overall nutritional–metabolic functioning of the body.

Food and fluid intake provides carbohydrates, proteins, fats, vitamins, and minerals, which are metabolized by the body to meet energy needs, maintain intracellular and extracellular fluid balances, prevent deficiency syndromes, and act as catalysts for the body's biochemical reactions.[1]

NUTRITION

Nutrition refers to the intake, assimilation, and use of food for energy, maintenance, and growth of the body.[2] Assisting the patient in maintaining a good nutritional–metabolic status facilitates health promotion and illness prevention, and provides dietary support in illness.[1]

Swallowing is associated with the intake of food or fluids. *Swallowing* is a complex activity that integrates sensory, muscular, and neurologic functions that generally occur in four phases: (1) *oral preparatory phase,* during which the food is chewed, mixed with saliva, and prepared for digestion; (2) *oral phase,* during which food is moved backward past the hard palate and downward to the pharynx; (3) *pharyngeal phase,* when the larynx closes and the food enters the esophagus; and (4) *esophageal phase,* during which the food passes through the esophagus, in peristaltic movement, to the stomach. The first two phases are voluntarily controlled, and the last two phases are involuntarily controlled.

Many factors affect a person's nutritional status, such as food availability and food cost; the meaning food has for an individual; cultural, social, and religious mores; and physiologic states that might alter a person's ability to eat.[3] In essence, we are initially concerned with the adequacy or inadequacy of the patient's nutritional state. If the diet is adequate, there is no major reason for concern, but we must be sure that all are defining "adequacy" in a similar manner. Most people are likely to define an adequate diet as one that prevents hunger; however, professionals look at an adequate diet as being one in which nutrient intake balances with body needs.

The familiar Food Pyramid was recently revised to reflect an evolving philosophy/outlook regarding the state of nutrition in the U.S. Dietary Guidelines. The guidelines moved away from using servings as the benchmark for nutrient intake to daily amounts expressed in cups or ounces. The current recommendations (based on a 2000-calorie diet) include a daily intake of:

- 6 ounces of grains, at least half of which should be whole grains
- $2^1/_2$ cups of vegetables
- 2 cups of fruits
- 3 cups of milk (or dairy products)*
- $5^1/_2$ ounces of lean meats and beans

The recommendation to limit fats and oils has remained unchanged. The new guidelines also encourage more individualization of diet plans. Individuals can tailor their diet according to age, activity, and body mass index. More information can be obtained at http://www.mypyramid.gov.

● **N O T E :** *Many adults may be lactose intolerant. Lactase enzymes are now available over-the-counter as a digestive aid for lactose intolerance.**

An inadequate nutritional state may be reflective of intake (calories), use of the intake (metabolism), or a change in activity level. Underweight and overweight are the most commonly seen conditions that reflect alteration in nutrition.[4]

Underweight can be caused by inadequate intake of calories. In some instances, the intake is within RDA, but there is malabsorption of the intake. The malabsorption or inadequate intake can be due to physiologic causes (pathophysiology), psychological causes (anorexia or bulimia), or cultural factors (lack of resources or religious proscriptions).[4]

Special notice needs to be given to maternal nutritional needs during the postpartum period. New mothers need optimal nutrition to promote healing of the tissues traumatized during labor and delivery, to restore balance in fluid and electrolytes created by all the rapid changes in the body, and, if the mother is breastfeeding, to produce adequate amounts of milk containing fluid and nutrients for the infant.[5] Infants have very little room for fluctuation in fluid balance, especially in the immediate postpartum period. Some researchers believe the infant is behind on fluid intake immediately after birth due to inadequate maternal hydration during labor and birth. Human milk has large amounts of fat content to provide the infant with the adequate amount of calories for growth, digestion, physical activity, and maintenance of organ metabolic function.[5] Breastfeeding demands energy and the mother will experience a gradual weight loss while breastfeeding, as fat deposits stored during pregnancy are used. However, mothers should not diet during breastfeeding, as fat-soluble environmental contaminants to which she has been exposed are stored in her body's fat reserves. Quick, large amounts of weight loss will release these contaminants into her breastmilk.[5]

The breastfeeding woman can generally meet her nutritional needs and those of her infant through adequate dietary intake of food and fluids; however, because the energy demand is greater during lactation, RDA standards recommend an additional 200 to 500 extra calories per day be added to the diet to provide adequate nutrients for both mother and infant, without catabolism of lean tissue of the mother.[5]

An overweight condition is rarely due to a physiologic disturbance, although a genetic predisposition may exist. Overweight is most commonly due to an imbalance between food and activity habits (i.e., increased intake and decreased activity).[4] However, research indicates there is a metabolic set point, and, in actuality, overweight people may be eating less than normal-weight people.

Either underweight or overweight may be a sign of malnutrition (inadequate nutrition), with the result that the patient exhibits signs and symptoms of less than or more than body requirements. In either instance, the nurse must assess the patient carefully for his or her overall concept of malnutrition.

FLUID VOLUME

Fluid volume incorporates the aspects of actual fluid amount, electrolytes, and metabolic acid-base balance. Regardless of how much or how little a patient's intake, or how much or how little a patient's output, the fluid, electrolyte, and metabolic acid-base balances are maintained within a relatively narrow margin. This margin is essential for normal functioning in all body systems, and so it must receive close attention in providing care.

Approximately 60 percent of an adult's weight is body fluid (liquid plus electrolytes plus minerals plus cells), and approximately 75 percent of an infant's weight is body fluid. These various parts of body fluid are taken in daily through food and drink and are formed through the metabolic activities of the body.[1,3] The body fluid distribution includes *intracellular* (within the cells), *interstitial* (around the cells), and *intravascular* (in blood cells) fluids. The combination of interstitial and intravascular is known as *extracellular* (outside the cells) *fluid*. Distribution of body fluid is influenced by both the fluid volume and the concentration of electrolytes. Body fluid movement, between the compartments, is constant and occurs through the mechanisms of osmosis, diffusion, active transport, and osmotic and hydrostatic pressure.[1,3]

Body fluid balance is regulated by intake (food and fluid), output (kidney, gastrointestinal [GI] tract, skin, and lungs), and hormones (antidiuretic hormones, glucocorticoids, and aldosterone). The largest amount of fluid is located in the intracellular compartment, with the volume of each compartment being regulated predominantly by the solute (mainly the electrolytes).

Electrolytes are either positively or negatively charged particles (ions). The major positively charged electrolytes (cations) are sodium (the main extracellular electrolyte), potassium (the most common intracellular electrolyte), calcium, and magnesium. The major negatively charged electrolytes (anions) are chloride, bicarbonate, and phosphate. The electrolyte compositions of the two extracellular compartments (interstitial and intravascular) are nearly identical. The intracellular fluid contains the same number of electrolytes as the extracellular fluid does, but the intracellular electrolytes carry opposite electrical charges from the electrolytes in the extracellular fluid. This difference between extracellular and intracellular electrolytes is necessary for the electrical activity of nerve and muscle cells.[1,3] Therefore, electrolytes help regulate cell functioning as well as the fluid volume in each compartment.

Usually the body governs intake through thirst and output through increasing or decreasing body fluid excretion via the kidneys, GI tract, and respiration. Because of the way the body governs intake and output, in addition to the effects of pathophysiologic conditions such as shock, hemorrhage, diabetes, and vomiting on intake and output, the patient may enter a state of metabolic acidosis or alkalosis.

Acid–base balance reflects the acidity or alkalinity of body fluids and is expressed as the pH. In essence, the pH is a function of the carbonic acid:bicarbonate ratio.[3] Acid–base balance is regulated by chemical, biologic, and physiologic mechanisms. Chemical regulation involves buffers in the extracellular fluid, whereas biologic regulation involves ion exchange across cell membranes. Physiologic regulation is governed in the lungs by carbon dioxide excretion, and in the kidneys through metabolism of bicarbonate, acid, and ammonia.[1]

Metabolic acidosis is caused by situations in which the cellular production of acid is excessive (e.g., diabetic ketoacidosis), high doses of drugs (e.g., aspirin) have to be metabolized, or excretion of the produced acid is impaired (e.g., renal failure).[3] Weight reduction practices (fad diets or diuretics) can contribute to the development of acidosis, as can chemical substance abuse.[1]

Fluid volume is affected by regulatory mechanisms, body fluid loss, or increased fluid intake. Because fluid volume is so readily affected by such a variety of factors, continuous assessment for alterations in fluid volume must be made.

TISSUE INTEGRITY

Nutrition and fluid are vitally important to tissue maintenance and repair. Underlying tissues are protected from external damage by the skin and mucous membranes. Thus, the integrity of the skin is extremely important in the promotion of health, because the skin and mucous membranes are the body's first line of defense. The skin also plays a role in temperature regulation and in excretion.

The skin and mucous membranes act as protection through their abundant supply of nerve receptors that alert the body to the external environment (i.e., temperature, pressure, or pain). The skin and mucous membranes also act as barriers to pathogens, thus protecting the internal tissues from these organisms.[3]

The skin's superficial blood vessels and sweat glands (eccrine and apocrine) assist in thermoregulation. As the body temperature rises, the superficial blood vessels dilate and the sweat glands increase secretion. These two actions result in increased perspiration, which, through evaporation, cools the body. During instances of excessive perspiration, water, sodium chloride, and nonprotein nitrogen are excreted through the skin; this affects fluid volume and osmotic balance. As the body temperature drops, the opposite reactions occur; there is vessel constriction and decreased sweat gland secretion so that body heat is retained internally.

To fulfill their protective function of the underlying tissues, the skin and mucous membranes must be intact. Any change in skin or mucous membrane integrity can allow pathogen invasion, and will also allow fluid and electrolyte loss. Skin and mucous membrane integrity relies on adequate nutrition and removal of metabolic wastes (internally and externally), cleanliness, and proper positioning. In emergency surgical settings or in cases of patients in poor health (e.g., very elderly and medically indigent), age and serum albumin levels might also be predictive of increased risk for skin breakdown.[6] Any factor that compromises nutrition, fluid, or electrolyte balance can result in impairment of skin or mucous membrane integrity or, at least, a high risk for impairment of skin integrity or mucous membrane integrity.

THERMOREGULATION

Thermoregulation refers to the body's ability to adjust its internal core temperature within a narrow range. The core temperature must remain fairly constant for metabolic activities and cellular metabolism to function for the maintenance of life. The core temperature rarely varies as much as 2°F. In fact, the range of temperature that is compatible with life ranges only from approximately 90 to 104°F.

Both the hypothalamus and the thyroid gland are involved in thermoregulation. The hypothalamus regulates temperature by responding to changes in electrolyte balances. Both extracellular cations—sodium and calcium—affect the action potential and depolarization of cells. When there is an imbalance of sodium and calcium within the hypothalamus, hypothermia or hyperthermia can result. The thyroid glands regulate core body temperature by increasing or decreasing metabolic activities and cellular metabolism, thus altering heat production.

Many factors influence thermoregulation. The skin has previously been mentioned as a thermoregulatory organ. Heat is gained or lost to the environment by evaporation, conduction, convection, and radiation. *Evaporation* occurs when body heat transforms the liquid on a person's skin to vapor. *Conduction* is the loss of heat to a colder object through direct contact. When heat is lost to the surrounding cool air, it is called *convection*. *Radiation* occurs when heat is given off to the environment, helping to warm it.

A person generally loses approximately 70 percent of all heat from radiation, convection, and conduction. Another 25 percent is lost through insensible mechanisms of the lungs and evaporation from the skin and about 5 percent is lost in urine and feces. When the body is able to produce and dissipate heat within a normal range, the body is in heat balance.[7]

SUMMARY

The interrelationship of nutrition, fluid balance, thermoregulation, and tissue integrity explains the nursing diagnoses that have been accepted in the nutritional–metabolic pattern. Indeed, if there is an alteration in any one of these four factors, it would be wise for the nurse to assess the other three factors to ensure a complete assessment.

DEVELOPMENTAL CONSIDERATIONS
INFANT

Swallowing is a reflex present before birth, because during intrauterine life the fetus swallows amniotic fluid. Following the transition to extrauterine life, the infant learns very rapidly (within 12 to 24 hours) to coordinate sucking and swallowing. There are really no developmental considerations of the act of swallowing, because it is a reflex.

The normal process for swallowing involves both the epiglottis and the true vocal cords. These two structures move together to close off the trachea, and to allow saliva or solid and liquid foods to pass into the esophagus. The respiratory system is thus protected from foreign bodies.

Salivation is adequate at birth to maintain sufficient moisture in the mouth. However, maturation of many salivary glands does not occur until the third month, and corresponds with the baby's learning to swallow at other than a reflex level.[8] Tooth eruption begins at about 6 months of age and stimulates saliva flow and chewing. The infant has a small amount of the enzyme ptyalin, which breaks down starches.

Water constitutes the greatest proportion of the infant's body weight. Approximately 75 to 78 percent of an infant's body weight is water, with about 45 percent of this water found in the extracellular fluid. The newborn infant loses significant water through insensible methods (approximately 35 to 45 percent) because of the relatively greater ratio of body surface area to body weight. The respiratory rate of an infant is approximately two times that of the adult; therefore, the infant is also losing water through insensible loss from the lungs. The newborn also loses water through direct excretion in the urine (50 to 60 percent) and through fairly rapid peristalsis as a result of the immaturity of the GI tract.

The newborn is unable to concentrate urine well, so is more sensitive to inadequate fluid intake or uncompensated water loss.[9] The body fluid reserve of the infant is less than that of the adult, and because the infant excretes a greater volume per kilogram of body weight than the adult, infants are very susceptible to deficient fluid volume. The infant needs to consume fluids equal to 10 to 15 percent of body weight. Fluid and electrolyte requirements for the newborn are 70 to 100 mL/kg per 24 hours, 2 mEq of sodium and potassium per kilogram per 24 hours, and 2 to 4 mEq of chloride per kilogram per 24 hours.

The kidney function of the infant does not reach adult levels until 6 months to 1 year of age.[9] The functional capacity of the kidneys is limited, especially during stress. In addition, the glomerular filtration rate is low, tubular reabsorption or secretory capacity is limited, sodium reabsorption is decreased, and the metabolic rate is higher. Therefore, there is a greater amount of metabolic wastes to be excreted. An infant's kidney is less able to excrete large loads of solute-free water than a more mature kidney.[10]

Feeding behavior is important not only for fluid, but also for food. The caloric need of the infant for the first 3 months is 110 kcal/kg per day, from 3 to 6 months 100 kcal/kg per day, and from 6 to 9 months 95 kcal/kg per day.[5] Breast milk contains adequate nutrients and vitamins for 6 months of life. The American Academy of Pediatrics recommends breastfeeding exclusively for the first 6 months of life, and continued breastfeeding with inclusion of other foods for at least 12 months.[5] Some bottle formulas are overly high in carbohydrates and fat (especially cholesterol), which may lead to an increase in fat cells.

Solid foods should not be introduced until the infant is 6 months of age. Studies have indicated that there is a relationship between the early introduction of solid food (younger than 4 months of age) and overfeeding of either milk or food, leading to infant and adult obesity.[5] The infant should be made to feel secure, loved, and unhurried at feeding time, regardless of whether the mother is breastfeeding or bottle feeding. Skin contact is very important for the infant for brain development and other physiologic and psychological reasons.

The skin of an infant is functionally immature, and thus the baby is more prone to skin disorders. Both the dermis and the epidermis are loosely connected, and both are relatively thin, which easily leads to chafing and rub burns.[8] Epidermal layers are permeable, resulting in greater fluid loss. Sebaceous glands, which produce sebum, are very active in late fetal life and early infancy, causing milia and "cradle cap," which goes away at about 6 months of age. Dry, intact skin is the greatest deterrent to bacterial invasion. Sweat glands (eccrine or apocrine) are not functional in response to heat and emotional stimuli until a few months after birth, and their function remains minimal through childhood. The inability of the skin to contract and shiver in response to heat loss causes ineffective thermal regulation.[4] Also, the infant has no melanocytes to protect against the rays of the sun. This is true of dark-skinned infants as well as light-skinned infants.

The infant's core body temperature ranges from 97 to 100°F. Temperature in the infant fluctuates considerably, because the regulatory mechanisms in the hypothalamus are not fully developed. (It is not considered abnormal for the newborn infant to lose 1 to 2°F immediately after birth.) The infant is not able to shiver to produce heat, nor does the infant have much subcutaneous fat to insulate the body. However, the infant does have several protective mechanisms by which he or she is able to conserve heat to keep the body temperature fairly stable. These mechanisms include vasoconstriction so that heat is maintained in the inner body core, an increased metabolic rate that increases heat production, a closed body position (the so-called fetal position) that reduces the amount of exposed skin, and the metabolism of adipose tissue. This particular adipose tissue is called "brown fat" because of the rich supply of blood and nerves. Brown fat comprises 2 to 6 percent of body weight of the infant. Brown fat aids in adaptation of the thermoregulation mechanisms.[8] The ability of the body to regulate temperature at the adult level matures at approximately 3 to 6 months of age.

TODDLER AND PRESCHOOLER

By the end of the second year, the child's salivary glands are adult size and have reached functional maturity.[8] The toddler is capable of chewing food, so it stays longer in his or her mouth, and the salivary enzymes have an opportunity to begin breaking down the food. The saliva also covers the teeth with a protective film that helps prevent decay. Drooling no longer occurs because the toddler easily swallows saliva.

Dental caries occur infrequently in children younger than 3 years; but rampant tooth decay in very young children is almost always related to prolonged bottle feeding at nap time and bedtime (bottle mouth syndrome). The toddler should be weaned from the bottle, or at least not allowed to fall asleep with the bottle in her or his mouth.[11] Parents should be taught that the adverse effects of bedtime feeding are greater than thumb sucking or the use of pacifiers.

Affected teeth remain susceptible to decay after nursing stops. If deciduous teeth decay and disintegrate early, spacing of the permanent teeth is affected, and immature speech patterns develop. Discomfort is felt and emotional problems may result.[11]

The first dental examination should occur between the ages of 18 and 24 months. Dental hygiene should be started when the first tooth erupts by cleansing the teeth with gauze or cotton moistened with hydrogen peroxide and flavored with a few drops of mouthwash. After 18 months, the child's teeth may be brushed with a soft or medium toothbrush.[11] Fluoride supplements are believed to prevent cavities.

In the toddler, the transition to the appropriate proportion of body water to body weight (62 percent water) begins.[12] The extracellular fluid is about 26 percent, whereas the adult has about 19 percent extracellular fluid. Toddlers have less reserve of body fluid than adults and lose more body water daily, both from sensible and insensible loss. This age group is highly predisposed to fluid imbalances.[13] These imbalances relate to the fact that the kidney still is immature, so water conservation is poor, and the toddler still has an increased metabolic rate and therefore greater insensible water loss than the adult. However, GI motility slows, so this age group is better able to tolerate fluid loss through diarrhea. The 2- to 3-year-old needs 1100 to 1200 mL (four to five 8-ounce glasses) of fluid every 24 hours, whereas the preschooler needs 1300 to 1400 mL of fluids every 24 hours.

The caloric need in the toddler is 1000 calories/day or 100 calories/kg at 1 year and 1300 to 1500 calories/day at 3 years. A child should not be forced to "clean the plate" at mealtime, and food should not be viewed as a reward or punishment. Instead, caloric intake should be related to the growing body and energy expenditures.

The caloric need of the preschooler is 85 calories/kg. Eating assumes increasing social significance, and continues to be an emotional, as well as a physiologic, experience.[4] Frustrating or unsettled mealtimes can influence caloric intake, as can manipulative behavior on the part of the child or parent. The child may also be eating foods with empty calories between meals.

In the toddler, functional maturity of skin creates a more effective barrier against fluid loss; the skin is not as soft as the infant's, and there is more protection against outside bacterial invasion. The skin remains dry because sebum secretion is limited. Eccrine sweat gland function remains limited, eczema improves, and the frequency of rashes declines.

Skin, as a perceptual organ, experiences significant development during this period. Children like to "feel" different objects and textures and like to be hugged. Melanin is formed during these years, and thus the toddler, preschooler, and school-age child are more protected against sun rays.[8] In addition, small capillaries in the periphery become more capable of constriction and thus thermoregulation. Also, the child is able to sense and interpret that he or she is hot or cold, and can voluntarily do something about it.

SCHOOL-AGE CHILD

At this age, the child begins losing baby teeth as permanent teeth erupt. The child should not be evaluated for braces until after all 6-year molars have erupted. The permanent teeth are larger than the baby teeth and appear too large for the small face, causing some embarrassment. Good oral hygiene is important.

For the school-age child, the percentage of total body water to total body weight continues to decrease until about 12 years of age, when it approaches adult norms.[13] Extracellular fluid changes from 22 percent of body weight at 6 years to 17.5 percent at age 12 as a result of the proportion of body surface area to mass, increasing muscle mass and connective tissue, and increasing percentage of body fat.

Water is needed for excretion of the solute load. Balance is maintained through mature kidneys, leading to mature urine concentration and acidifying capacities. Fluid requirements can be calculated in terms of height, weight,

surface area, and metabolic activity. The school-age child needs approximately 1.5 to 3 quarts of fluid a day. In addition, the child needs a slightly positive water balance. The electrolyte values are similar to those for the adult except for phosphorus and calcium (because of bone growth).[13]

The caloric need of the school-age child is greater than that of an adult (approximately 80 calories/kg or 1600 to 2200 calories/day). The ages of 10 to 12 reflect the peak ages of caloric and protein needs of the school-age child (50 to 60 calories/kg per day), because of accelerated growth, muscle development, and bone mineralization. "The school age child reflects the nutritional experiences of early childhood and the potential for adulthood."[4]

ADOLESCENT

By age 21, all 32 permanent teeth have erupted. The adolescent needs frequent dental visits because of cavities, and also for orthodontic work that may be in progress. There is a growth spurt and sexual development changes. A total increase in height of 25 percent and a doubling of weight are normally attained.[14] Muscle mass increases and total body water declines with increasing sexual development.[15] The adolescent needs 34 to 45 calories/kg per day and tends to have eating patterns based on external environmental cues rather than hunger. Eating becomes more of a social event. There is a high probability of eating disorders such as anorexia and bulimia arising during this age period.

The basal metabolic rate increases, lung size increases, and maximal breathing capacity and forced expiratory volume increase, leading to increased insensible loss of fluid through the lungs. Total body water decreases from 61 percent at age 12 to 54 percent by age 18 as a result of an increase in fat cells. Fat cells do not have as much water as tissue cells.[15] The water intake need of the adolescent is about 2200 to 2700 mL per 24 hours.

Sebaceous glands become extremely active during adolescence and increase in size. Eccrine sweat glands are fully developed and are especially responsive to emotional stimuli (and are more active in males); apocrine sweat glands also begin to secrete in response to emotional stimuli.[16] Stopped-up sebaceous glands lead to acne, and the adolescent's skin is usually moist.

YOUNG ADULT

The amount of ptyalin in the saliva decreases after 20 years of age; otherwise the digestive system remains fully functioning. The appearance of "wisdom teeth," or third molars, occurs at 20 to 21 years. There are normally four third molars, although some individuals may not fully develop all four. Third molars can create problems for the individual. Eruptions are unpredictable in time and presentation, and molars may come in sideways or facing any direction. This can force other teeth out of alignment, which makes chewing difficult and painful. Often these molars need to be removed to prevent irreparable damage to proper occlusion of the jaws. Even normally erupting third molars may be painful. The young adult must see a dentist regularly.

Total body water in the young adult is about 50 to 60 percent. There is a difference between males and females because of the difference in the number of fat cells. Most water in the young adult is intracellular, with only about 20 percent of fluid being extracellular. Growth is essentially finished by this developmental age.

ADULT

Ptyalin has sharply decreased by age 60 as well as other digestive enzymes. Total body water is now about 47 to 54.7 percent. Diet and activity indirectly influence the amount of body water by directly altering the amount of adipose tissue. The basal metabolic rate gradually decreases along with a reduced demand for calories. Caloric intake should be adjusted for age and activity level.

Tissues of the integumentary system maintain a healthy, intact, glowing appearance until age 50 to 55 if the individual is receiving adequate vitamins, minerals, other nutrients, and fluids and maintains good personal hygiene. Wrinkles do become more noticeable, however, and body water (from integumentary tissues) decreases, leading to thinner, drier skin that bruises much more easily. Fat increases, leading to skin that is not as elastic and will not recede with weight loss, so bags develop readily under the eyes.[8] Also, skin wounds heal more slowly because of decreased cell regeneration.

OLDER ADULT

The nutritional status of the older adult is receiving increased scrutiny by health-care professionals because of the impact poor nutrition has on health status and quality of life.[17,18] Since the early 1990s, many states and organizations working with older adults have begun nutritional screening to identify those at high risk for poor nutrition. The Nutrition Screening Initiative (NSI) program encourages use of a 10-item checklist entitled "DETERMINE" to identify at-risk elders. The checklist is easily administered and results in a score ranging from 0 (lowest risk) to 21 (highest risk).[19] Scores of 4 or more on the checklist usually indicate that the older adult should undergo further nutritional evaluation. Many older adults experience aging changes that can affect nutritional status. Older adults also experience risk factors, such as polypharmacy, social isolation, low income, altered functional status, loneliness, and chronic and acute diseases, that impact nutritional status.[20]

Older adults may experience changes in the mouth that can affect nutrition. Tooth decay, tooth loss, degeneration of the jaw bone, progressive gum regression, and increased reabsorption of the dental arch can make chewing and eating a difficult task for the older adult if good dental health has not been maintained.[21] Reduced chewing ability, problems associated with poorly fitting dentures, and a decrease in salivation, secondary to disease or medication,

effects compound nutritional problems for older adults.[22] Aging causes atrophy of the olfactory organs and with diminished smell often comes decreased enjoyment of foods and decreased consumption.[23] Research continues to evolve concerning taste discrimination in older adults. More recent studies support limited changes in taste associated with aging when healthy, nonmedicated adults are sampled. The impact of medications, poor oral hygiene, or cigarette smoking may cause older adults to complain of an unpleasant taste in their mouth called *dysgeusia*.[24]

Changes in olfaction and decreased salivation secondary to disease or medications can influence the taste of food. When compounded by gum disease, poor teeth, or dentures, problems with food intake can occur. The number of older adults who are *edentulous* (without teeth) is gradually declining and is estimated to be approximately 37 percent of adults 70 years of age or older.[21] Caries, especially occurring on the crowns of the tooth, occur in more than 95 percent of the elderly population.[21] Older adults are especially vulnerable to oral carcinomas.[25]

Total body water of the older adult is about 45 to 50 percent. Older adults have problems tolerating extremes of temperature. Aging results in skin changes such as dryness and wrinkling. Skin assessment for alterations in fluid volume must be carefully interpreted. Skin turgor assessment should be done on the abdomen, sternum, or the forehead. Skin turgor is not a reliable indicator of hydration status in older adults. Assessment should focus on tongue dryness, furrows in the tongue, confusion, dry mucous membranes, "sunken" appearance of the eyes, or difficulty with speech.[26] Older adults also have a diminished thirst sensation secondary to changes in brain osmoreceptors; thus thirst is not readily triggered in older adults.[25] Changes in blood volume are minimal. Serum protein (albumin) production is decreased, but globulin is increased.

Aging changes do bring about changes in nephrotic tubular function, which affects removal of water, urine concentration, and dilution. This leads to a decrease in specific gravity and urine osmolarity. There is a decrease in bladder capacity, often leading to nocturia. With the change in bladder capacity, older adults may limit fluid in the evenings to offset nocturia, but limiting fluids may lead to nocturnal dehydration. Sodium and chloride levels remain constant, but potassium decreases.

Many changes occur in the GI tract, such as decreased enzyme secretion, gastric irritation, decreased nutrient and drug absorption, decreased hydrochloric acid secretion, decreased peristalsis and elimination, and decreased sphincter muscle tone, making nutrition a primary concern. Older adults need decreased and nutrient-dense calories. Adequate intake of vitamins and trace elements along with adequate protein, fat, carbohydrates, bulk, and electrolytes is important. The decreased intake of milk and fresh fruits, commonly found in older populations, is a source of concern because of the continuing need for calcium, fiber, and vitamin intake.[27]

Integumentary changes result in skin that is drier and thinner, and skin lesions or discolorations, and scaliness (keratosis) may appear. Wrinkling occurs in areas commonly exposed to the sun, such as the face and hands. Fatty layers lost in the trunk, face, and extremities leads to the appearance of increased joint size throughout the body. The skin becomes less elastic with aging and may lose water to the air in low-humidity situations, leading to skin chapping.

The older adult has difficulty tolerating temperature extremes. Body temperature may increase because of a decrease in the size, number, and function of the sweat glands. Decreased fat cells and changes in peripheral blood flow make older adults more sensitive to cooler conditions. Older adults may wear sweaters or additional layers of clothing when the external temperature feels comfortable or warm to younger individuals. Melanocyte decreases lead to pale skin color and gray hair. Hair loss is common. Older women, with imbalances in androgen–estrogen hormones, may have noticeable increases in facial and chin hairs. Aging changes to the skin can result in tactile changes, and therefore, the ability to perceive temperature, touch, pain, and pressure is diminished.[23] Decreased tactile ability may lead to thermal, chemical, and mechanical injury that is not readily detected by the older adult.

TABLE 3.1 NANDA, NIC, and NOC Taxonomy Linkages

GORDON'S FUNCTIONAL HEALTH PATTERN	NANDA NURSING DIAGNOSIS	NIC PRIORITY INTERVENTIONS	NOC EVALUATIONS
Nutritional– Metabolic Pattern	Failure to Thrive, Adult	Hope Instillation Mood Management Self-Care Assistance	Appetite Cognition Endurance Nutritional Status Nutritional Status: Food & Fluid Intake Physical Aging Self-Care: ADL Weight: Body Mass Will to Live
	Aspiration, Risk for	Aspiration Precautions Teaching: Infant Safety Vomiting Management	Aspiration Prevention Body Positioning: Self-Initiated Cognition Cognitive Orientation Immobility Consequences: Physiological Knowledge: Treatment Procedure(s) Mechanical Ventilation Response: Adult Nausea & Vomiting Severity Neurological Status Post Procedure Recovery Status Respiratory Status: Airway Patency; Ventilation Risk Control Risk Detection Seizure Control Self-Care: Non-Parenteral Medication Swallowing Status
	Body Temperature, Risk for Imbalanced	Temperature Regulation: Intraoperative Vital Signs Monitoring	Hydration Immune Status Infection Severity Infection Severity: Newborn Medication Response Neglect Recovery

(table continued on page 128)

TABLE 3.1 NANDA, NIC, and NOC Taxonomy Linkages *(continued from page 127)*

GORDON'S FUNCTIONAL HEALTH PATTERN	NANDA NURSING DIAGNOSIS	NIC PRIORITY INTERVENTIONS	NOC EVALUATIONS
			Neurological Status: Autonomic Risk Control Risk Detection Thermoregulation Thermoregulation: Newborn
	Breastfeeding, Effective	Lactation Counseling	Breastfeeding Establishment: Infant; Maternal Breastfeeding Maintenance Breastfeeding Weaning
	Breastfeeding, Ineffective	Breastfeeding Assistance Lactation Counseling	Breastfeeding Establishment: Infant; Maternal Breastfeeding Maintenance Breastfeeding Weaning Knowledge: Breastfeeding
	Breastfeeding, Interrupted	Bottle Feeding Emotional Support Lactation Counseling	Breastfeeding Maintenance Breastfeeding Weaning Knowledge: Breastfeeding Parent-Infant Attachment
	Dentition, Impaired	Oral Health Maintenance Oral Health Restoration	Oral Hygiene Self-Care: Oral Hygiene
	Fluid Balance, Readiness for Enhanced	*Still in development*	Fluid Balance Fluid Overload Severity Hydration Kidney Function
	Fluid Volume, Deficient, Risk for and Actual	Electrolyte Monitoring Fluid Management Fluid Monitoring Hypovolumia Management Intravenous IV Therapy Shock Management: Volume	**Actual** Electrolyte & Acid/Base Balance Fluid Balance Hydration Nutritional status: Fluid and Food Intake **Risk for** Appetite Blood Loss Severity Bowel Elimination Breastfeeding Maintenance Electrolyte & Acid/Base Balance Fluid Balance Hydration Knowledge: Disease Process; Health Behaviors; Medication; Treatment Regimen Nausea & Vomiting Severity Food Intake Risk Control Risk Detection Self-Care Status Swallowing Status Thermoregulation Thermoregulation: Neonate Urinary Elimination

GORDON'S FUNCTIONAL HEALTH PATTERN	NANDA NURSING DIAGNOSIS	NIC PRIORITY INTERVENTIONS	NOC EVALUATIONS
	Fluid Volume, Excess	Electrolyte Monitoring Fluid Management Fluid Monitoring Hypervolemia Management	Electrolyte & Acid–Base Balance Fluid Balance Fluid Overload Severity Kidney Function
	Fluid Volume, Risk for Imbalanced	Electrolyte Monitoring Fluid Management Fluid Monitoring IV Therapy	Appetite Blood Loss Severity Bowel Elimination Breastfeeding Establishment: Infant Breastfeeding Maintenance Cardiac Pump Effectiveness Electrolyte & Acid–Base Balance Fluid Balance Fluid Overload Severity Hydration Kidney Function Knowledge: Disease Process; Health Behavior; Medication; Treatment Regimen Nausea & Vomiting Severity Nutritional status: Food & Fluid Intake Physical Aging Post Procedure Recovery Status Risk Control Risk Detection Thermoregulation Thermoregulation: Newborn Urinary Elimination Vital Signs Wound Healing: Secondary Intention
	Hyperthermia	Fever Treatment Malignant Hyperthermia Precautions Temperature Regulation Vital Signs Monitoring	Thermoregulation Thermoregulation: Newborn Vital Signs
	Hypothermia	Hypothermia Treatment Temperature Regulation Temperature Regulation: Intraoperative Vital Signs Monitoring	Thermoregulation Thermoregulation: Newborn Vital Signs
	Infant Feeding Pattern, Ineffective	Enteral Tube Feeding Lactation Counseling Nonnutritive Sucking Tube Care: Umbilical Line	Aspiration Prevention Breastfeeding Establishment: Infant Breastfeeding: Maintenance Hydration Nutritional Status: Food & Fluid Intake Swallowing status
	Nausea	Medication Management Nausea Management	Appetite Comfort level Hydration Nausea & Vomiting Control Nausea & Vomiting: Disruptive Effects Nausea & Vomiting Severity Nutritional Status: Food & Fluid Intake

(table continued on page 130)

TABLE 3.1 NANDA, NIC, and NOC Taxonomy Linkages *(continued from page 129)*

GORDON'S FUNCTIONAL HEALTH PATTERN	NANDA NURSING DIAGNOSIS	NIC PRIORITY INTERVENTIONS	NOC EVALUATIONS
	Nutrition: Readiness for Enhanced	*Currently in development	Knowledge: Diet Nutritional Status Nutritional Status: Food & Fluid Intake Nutritional Status: Nutrient Intake
	Nutrition: Imbalanced, Less than Body Requirements	Eating Disorders Management Nutrition Management Weight Gain Assistance	Appetite Breastfeeding Establishment: Infant Nutritional Status Nutritional Status: Food & Fluid Intake; Nutrient Intake Self-Care: Eating Weight: Body Mass
	Nutrition: Imbalanced, More than Body Requirements, Risk for and Actual	Eating Disorders Management Nutrition Management Weight Reduction Assistance	**Actual** Nutritional Status Nutritional Status: Food & Fluid Intake; Nutrient Intake Weight: Body Mass Weight Control **Risk for** Knowledge: Diet Nutritional Status Nutritional Status: Food & Fluid Intake; Nutrient Intake Risk Control Risk Detection Stress Level Weight: Body Mass Weight Control
	Swallowing, Impaired	Aspiration Precautions Swallowing Therapy	Aspiration Prevention Swallowing Status Swallowing Status: Esophageal Phase, Oral Phase, Pharyngeal Phase
	Thermoregulation, Ineffective	Temperature Regulation Temperature Regulation: Intraoperative	Thermoregulation Thermoregulation: Newborn
	Tissue Integrity Impaired	Wound Care	**Tissue Integrity, Impaired** Allergic Response: Localized Ostomy Self-Care Tissue Integrity: Skin & Mucous Membranes Wound Healing: Primary Intention; Secondary Intention
	A. Skin Integrity, Impaired Risk for and Actual	**Actual** Incision Site Care Pressure Ulcer Care Skin Surveillance Wound Care	**Actual** Allergic Response: Localized Hemodialysis Access Tissue Integrity: Skin & Mucous Membranes Wound Healing: Primary Intention; Secondary Intention

GORDON'S FUNCTIONAL HEALTH PATTERN	NANDA NURSING DIAGNOSIS	NIC PRIORITY INTERVENTIONS	NOC EVALUATIONS
		Risk for Pressure Management Pressure Ulcer Prevention Skin Surveillance	
			Risk for Allergic Response: Localized Child Development: Adolescence Fluid Overload Severity Hemodialysis Access Immobility Consequences: Physiological Infection Severity Infection Severity: Newborn Nutritional Status Nutritional Status: Biochemical Measures
	B. Oral Mucous Membrane, Impaired	Oral health restoration	Ostomy Self-Care Physical Aging Risk Control Risk Detection Self-Mutilation Restraint Tissue Integrity: Skin & Mucous Membranes Tissue Perfusion: Peripheral Wound Healing: Primary Intention; Secondary Intention Oral Hygiene Tissue Integrity: Skin & Mucous Membrane

 APPLICABLE NURSING DIAGNOSES

ADULT FAILURE TO THRIVE

DEFINITION[28]

A progressive functional deterioration of a physical and cognitive nature; the individual's ability to live with multisystem diseases, cope with ensuing problems, and manage his or her care is remarkably diminished.[30]

DEFINING CHARACTERISTICS[28]

1. Anorexia—does not eat meals when offered
2. States does not have an appetite, not hungry, or "I don't want to eat"
3. Inadequate nutritional intake—eating less than body requirements
4. Consumes minimal to no food at most meals (i.e., consumes less than 75 percent of normal requirements at each or most meals)
5. Weight loss (decreased body mass from baseline weight—5 percent unintentional weight loss in 1 month, 10 percent unintentional weight loss in 6 months)
6. Physical decline (decline in body function)
7. Evidence of fatigue, dehydration, and incontinence of bowel and bladder
8. Frequent exacerbations of chronic health problems such as pneumonia or urinary tract infections
9. Cognitive decline (decline in mental processing) as evidenced by problems with responding appropriately to environmental stimuli, demonstrates difficulty in reasoning, decision making, judgment, memory, and concentration, and decreased perception
10. Decreased social skills or social withdrawal—noticeable decrease from usual past behavior in attempts to form or participate in cooperative and independent relationships (e.g., decreased verbal communication with staff, family, and friends)
11. Decreased participation in activities of daily living that the older person once enjoyed

12. Self-care deficit—no longer looks after, or takes charge of, physical cleanliness or appearance
13. Difficulty performing simple self-care tasks
14. Neglects home environment and/or financial responsibilities
15. Apathy as evidenced by lack of observable feeling or emotion in terms of normal activities of daily living and environment
16. Altered mood state—expresses feelings of sadness or being low in spirit
17. Expresses loss of interest in pleasurable outlets such as food, sex, work, friends, family, hobbies, or entertainment
18. Verbalizes desire for death

RELATED FACTORS[28]

1. Depression
2. Apathy
3. Fatigue

RELATED CLINICAL CONCERNS

1. Any terminal diagnosis (e.g., cancer, AIDS, or multiple sclerosis)
2. Chronic clinical depression
3. Any chronic disease
4. Cerebrovascular accident or paralytic conditions

 Have You Selected the Correct Diagnosis?

Imbalanced Nutrition, Less Than Body Requirements
This diagnosis could be a companion diagnosis because Imbalanced Nutrition, Less Than Body Requirements would be a defining characteristic in Adult Failure to Thrive. Adult Failure to Thrive appears in chronic conditions, and involves much more than just altered nutrition.

Impaired Swallowing
This diagnosis relates only to the swallowing process and is not inclusive enough to cover all the problem areas of Adult Failure to Thrive.

EXPECTED OUTCOME

Will gain [number] pounds of weight by [date].
    Makes [number] of decisions related to care by [date].

TARGET DATES

Adult Failure to Thrive will require long-term intervention. Target dates should initially be stated in terms of weeks. After improvement is shown, target dates can be expressed in terms of months.

NURSING ACTIONS/INTERVENTIONS WITH RATIONALES

Adult Health

● N O T E : *A study[29] demonstrated a relationship between Adult Failure to Thrive and Helicobacter pylori infection. The clinical presentation of the infection was characterized by the lack of symptoms typically associated with gastric diseases, such as nausea, vomiting, dyspepsia, and abdominal pain. Instead, the patient exhibited signs of aversion to food, decline in mental functions, and the inability to perform activities of daily living (ADLs).*

ACTIONS/INTERVENTIONS	RATIONALES
Refer to Nutrition, Imbalanced, Less Than Body Requirements for basic nursing actions or interventions.	Basic methods and procedures that improve nutrition and appetite.
Administer nutritional liquids via gastric enteral tube as ordered. (See Additional Information for Imbalanced Nutrition, Less Than Body Requirements.)	
Monitor for: • Swallowing deficit • Occult blood in stools • Dehydration; replace with IV fluids as ordered. • Electrolytes • Document intake and output.	Allows early detection of complications and assists in monitoring effectiveness of therapy.
Offer soft, regular diet with nutritional liquid supplement.	Easily chewed and digested food.

ACTIONS/INTERVENTIONS	RATIONALES
Schedule periods of rest and activity.	
Develop contract with patient to assume increasing responsibility ADLs. [Note patient's contract here.]	
Do not force feed.	Risk for aspiration pneumonia.
Collaborate with:	Provides basic resources and information needed; promotes holistic approach to treatment.
• Psychiatric nurse clinician	To address underlying emotional and cognitive problems.
• Nutritionist/dietician	Formulate appropriate nutrient intake to support health restoration.
• Physical/occupational therapist	To preserve and improve physical abilities to assume responsibility of ADLs.

Child Health

This diagnosis would not be used with infants or children.

Women's Health

Nursing actions for this diagnosis are the same as those for Adult Health, Mental Health, and Gerontic Health.

Mental Health

● N O T E : *For clients with severe or life-threatening compromised physiologic status, refer to Adult Health for interventions. When the client is psychologically unstable, refer to the following plan of care. The adult and psychiatric interventions can be combined based on client need. Monitor client for suicidal ideation. If this is determined to be an issue, appropriate interventions should be implemented utilizing the Risk for Suicide diagnosis. Also utilize plans for Ineffective Individual Coping and Disturbed Thought Process as appropriate.*

ACTIONS/INTERVENTIONS	RATIONALES
Spend [number of] minutes with the client [number of] times per shift to establish relationship with the client.	
Discuss with the client and client's support system the client's food/fluid preferences. [Note here special foods and adaptations needed.]	
Provide the client with opportunity to make food/fluid choices. Initially these should be limited so the client will not be overwhelmed with decisions. [Note client choices here.]	Opportunities to increase personal control improve self-esteem and have a positive impact on mood.[30–32]
Provide the client with necessary sensory and eating aids. [Note here those needed for this client. This could include eyeglasses, dentures, and special utensils.]	
Provide quiet, calm milieu at mealtimes.	Clients with mood disorders may have difficulty with concentration.[33]
Provide the client with adequate time to eat.	Clients with mood disorders may experience psychomotor retardation that can expand the time it takes them to eat.[33]

(care plan continued on page 134)

NURSING ACTIONS/INTERVENTIONS WITH RATIONALES (continued from page 133)

Mental Health

ACTIONS/INTERVENTIONS	RATIONALES
Provide foods that meet the client's preferences, are of high nutritional value, and require little energy to eat. [Note client's preferences here.]	Meeting basic health needs improves stamina.[33]
Sit with the client during meals and provide positive verbal reinforcement. [Note here client-specific reinforcers.]	Fatigue may limit the client's physical energy.[33]
When the client's mental status improves, spend [number of] minutes each shift with the client discussing issues and concerns. [Note here those issues important for the client to discuss.]	This demonstrates acceptance of the client and facilitates problem solving.[31]
Provide prescribed medications and monitor for effects.	
When the client's mental status improves, engage the client in [number of] therapeutic groups per day. [Note here the groups the client will attend.]	Decreases sense of loneliness and isolation, increases self-understanding, increases social support, and facilitates the development of relationship and coping skills.[31,32]

Gerontic Health

ACTIONS/INTERVENTIONS	RATIONALES
Review the older adult's medication list for possible medication-induced failure to thrive.	Adverse reactions to medications such as antidepressants, beta-blockers, neuroleptics, anticholinergics, benzodiazepines, potent diuretic combination drugs, and anticonvulsants and polypharmacy (more than four to six prescription drugs) can lead to cognition changes, anorexia, dehydration, or electrolyte problems and result in failure to thrive.[34]
Monitor weight loss pattern according to care setting policy or client contact opportunities. Maintain weight information in an easily retrievable place to allow quick access and ease in comparison of weights.	In older adults, a percentage weight loss over a 6- to 12-month time period is associated with increased risk of disease, disability, and mortality.[35]
Review nutritional pattern with the client and/or caregiver to determine whether adequate nutritional support is present.	Poor nutrition can lead to adverse clinical outcomes for older adults.[35]
Arrange for psychological supports for the older client, such as validation therapy, reminiscing, life review, or cognitive therapy.	The therapies listed promote self-worth, decrease stress, focus on the client's strengths, and provide the opportunity for resolution of prior unfinished conflicts.[36]
Refer the older client for evaluation of depression.	Depression is frequently underdiagnosed in the older adult and is often associated with unintentional weight loss in the older population.[35]
Review the social support system available to the client.	Social isolation is considered a significant feature in depression, malnutrition, and decreased function in older adults.[37]
Encourage the client to participate in a regular program of exercise.	Exercise can prevent further loss of muscle mass often found with failure to thrive and improve strength and energy.[25]

Home Health/Community Health	
ACTIONS/INTERVENTIONS	RATIONALES
Monitor the client's ability to provide basic self-care; provide referrals for community agencies to augment deficits in self-care. Many agencies offer assistance with personal hygiene, transportation, meal preparation, and light housework in the home.	Difficulty in performing self-care and ADLs are defining characteristics of Adult Failure to Thrive.
Provide with information and resources to facilitate the client keeping a food diary to track intake. Monitor the adequacy of the diet in terms of calories and nutrients. Secure a dietary consult as appropriate.	Poor nutrition can lead to adverse clinical outcomes.
Weigh the client on each home visit.	Weight loss is a defining characteristic of Adult Failure to Thrive. Significant weight loss may lead to increased risk of disease and exacerbation of the condition.
Facilitate the delivery of meals for home bound clients. Refer the client to services available in his or her area. [Note support needed from nursing here to sustain this support.]	Increases the availability of well rounded, nutrient-dense meals.
Refer the client to age- and condition-specific community exercise programs available in his or her area. Develop, with the client, a reward system that would reinforce his or her involvement in the program. [Note the client's plan here.]	Physical decline is a defining characteristic of Adult Failure to Thrive.
Spend [number] minutes each visit talking with the client and family about their social support system. Make referrals as needed to community agencies that provide needed services. Many agencies provide services such as counseling and volunteer visitors. [Note the support needed from nursing to facilitate and sustain these interactions.]	Social isolation is a defining characteristic of Adult Failure to Thrive.

ASPIRATION, RISK FOR

DEFINITION[28]

The state in which an individual is at risk for entry of GI secretions, oropharyngeal secretions, or solids or fluids into tracheobronchial passages.[28]

DEFINING CHARACTERISTICS (RISK FACTORS)[28]

1. Increased intragastric pressure
2. Tube feedings
3. Situations hindering elevation of upper body
4. Reduced level of consciousness
5. Presence of tracheostomy or endotracheal tube
6. Medication administration
7. Wired jaws
8. Increased gastric residual
9. Incompetent lower esophageal sphincter
10. Impaired swallowing
11. GI tubes
12. Facial, oral, or neck surgery or trauma
13. Depressed cough and gag reflexes
14. Decreased GI motility
15. Delayed gastric emptying

RELATED FACTORS[28]

The risk factors also serve as the related factors for this nursing diagnosis.

RELATED CLINICAL CONCERNS

1. Closed head injury
2. Any diagnosis with presenting symptoms of nausea and vomiting
3. Bulimia
4. Any diagnosis requiring use of a nasogastric tube
5. Spinal cord injury

Have You Selected the Correct Diagnosis?

Impaired Swallowing

Swallowing means that when food or fluids are present in the mouth, the brain signals both the epiglottis and the true vocal cords to move together to close off the trachea so that the food and fluids can pass into the esophagus and thus into the stomach. Impaired Swallowing implies that there is a mechanical or physiologic obstruction between the oropharynx and the esophagus that prevents food or fluids from passing into the esophagus. In Risk for Aspiration there may or may not be an obstruction between the oropharynx and the esophagus. The major pathophysiologic dysfunction that occurs in Risk for Aspiration is the inability of the epiglottis and true vocal cords to move to close off the trachea. This inability to close off the trachea may occur because of pathophysiologic changes in the structures themselves, or because messages to the brain are absent, decreased, or impaired.

Ineffective Airway Clearance

In Ineffective Airway Clearance, the patient is unable to effectively clear secretions from the respiratory tract because of some of the same related factors as are found with Risk for Aspiration. However, in Ineffective Airway Clearance, the defining characteristics (abnormal breath sounds, cough, change in rate or depth of respirations, etc.) are associated directly with respiratory function, whereas the defining characteristics of Risk for Aspiration are directly or indirectly related to the oropharyngeal mechanisms that protect the tracheobronchial passages from the entrance of foreign substances.

EXPECTED OUTCOME

Will describe [number] of strategies to decrease risk for aspiration by [date].

TARGET DATES

Aspiration is life threatening. Initial target dates should be stated in hours. After the number of risk factors has been reduced, the target dates can be moved to 2- to 4-day intervals.

NURSING ACTIONS/INTERVENTIONS WITH RATIONALES

Adult Health

ACTIONS/INTERVENTIONS	RATIONALES
Considerations for the naso/orogastric intubated patients:	
Confirm placement at least once every shift when the patient is receiving continuous feeds, prior to bolus feeds, or prior to medication administration.	To assure correct placement of feeding tubes.
Monitor residual of feeding tube at least once every shift when the patient is receiving continuous feeds and prior to bolus feeds.	Monitors patient tolerance of tube feeding regimen.
Considerations for endotrach intubation:	
• Maintain head of bed 30 to 45 degrees unless contraindicated.	
• Provide mouth care at least every four hours. [Note times here.]	Secretions in the oropharyngeal cavity are a source of microaspiration.
• Ensure that balloon cuff is appropriately inflated.	Underinflated balloon cuffs allow passage of oral secretions into the trachea.
• Extubate at the earliest opportunity.	Extubation will allow the normal capacities of swallowing with which endotracheal intubation interferes.
• Suction above and below the balloon cuff prior to extubation.	To eliminate oral secretions that can be aspirated.
Considerations for the patient with noninvasive positive pressure ventilation (e.g., bi-PAP).	
• Implement gastric decompression via naso/orogastric intubation.	Gastric distention can occur with positive pressure masks, increasing the potential for aspiration.
• Devise alternative oxygenation strategies during oral intake.	Food and fluids become projectiles under the influence of positive pressure masks.

ACTIONS/INTERVENTIONS	RATIONALES
In preparation for discharge: • Teach the patient to eat when calm and in a relaxed, nonstimulating atmosphere. • Teach the patient and family the Heimlich maneuver and have them return-demonstrate at least daily for 3 days before discharge. • Teach the patient and family suctioning technique as needed, including appropriate ordering of supplies.	Would assist in episodes of choking, and allow the patient and family to feel comfortable with level of expertise before going home.

Child Health

ACTIONS/INTERVENTIONS	RATIONALES
Determine best position for the patient as determined by underlying risk factors (e.g., head of bed elevated 30 degrees with the infant propped on right side after feeding). • Confirm need for special positioning with pediatrician or primary health-care provider as this constitutes a deviation from the BACK TO SLEEP protocol to prevent risk for SIDS, especially in infants from birth to 6 months of age.	Natural upper airway patency is facilitated by upright position. Turning to right side decreases likelihood of drainage into trachea rather than esophagus in the event of choking.
Check bilateral breath sounds every 30 minutes or with any change in respiratory status.	In the event of aspiration, increased gurgling and rales with correlated respiratory difficulty (from mild to severe) will be noted.
Measure amount of residual, immediately before feeding, in nasogastric tube and report any excess beyond 10 to 20 percent of volume or as specified.	Monitors the speed of digestion and indicates the patient's ability to tolerate the feeding.
Note and record the presence of any facial trauma or surgery of face, head, or neck with associated drainage.	Monitoring for these risk factors assists in preventing unexpected or undetected aspiration.
Monitor for risk factors that would promote aspiration (e.g., increased intracranial pressure, Reye's syndrome, nausea associated with medications, cerebral palsy, or neurologic damage).	An increased stimulation or sensitivity to the gag reflex increases the likelihood of choking and possible aspiration.
Assist the patient and family to identify factors that help prevent aspiration (e.g., avoiding self-stimulation of gag reflex, avoiding deep oral or pharyngeal suctioning, and chewing food thoroughly).	
Provide opportunities for the patient and family to ask questions or ventilate regarding risk for aspiration by scheduling at least 30 minutes twice a day at [times] for discussing concerns.	Allows an opportunity to decrease anxiety, provides time for teaching, and allows individualized home care planning.
Teach the family and patient (if old enough) age-appropriate cardiopulmonary resuscitation (CPR), first aid, and Heimlich maneuver.	Basic safety measures for dangers of aspiration.

(care plan continued on page 138)

NURSING ACTIONS/INTERVENTIONS WITH RATIONALES (continued from page 137)

Women's Health

● **N O T E :** *The following actions pertain to the newborn infant if meconium is present in amniotic fluid.*

ACTIONS/INTERVENTIONS	RATIONALES
Alert obstetrician and pediatrician of the presence of meconium in amniotic fluid.	Presence of meconium alerts health-care providers to possible complications.
Assemble equipment and be prepared for resuscitation of the newborn at the time of delivery.	Basic emergency preparedness.
Be prepared to suction the infant's nasopharynx and oropharynx while head of the infant is still on the perineum.	
Immediately evaluate and record the respiratory status of the newborn infant.	
Assist pediatrician in viewing the vocal cords of the infant (have various sizes of pediatric laryngoscopes available). If meconium is present, be prepared to insert endotracheal tube for further suctioning.	
Continue to evaluate and record the infant's respiratory status.	There is no designated time frame for observation; however, the nurse needs to continue to evaluate the infant for at least 12 to 24 hours for respiratory distress and the complications of pulmonary interstitial emphysema, pneumomediastinum, pneumothorax, persistent pulmonary hypertension, central nervous system (CNS) dysfunction, and renal failure. These infants should be placed in a level 2 or 3 nursery.
Reassure the parents by keeping them informed of actions.	Reduces anxiety.
Allow opportunities for the parents to verbalize fears and ask questions.	Reduces anxiety and provides teaching opportunity.

Mental Health

● **N O T E :** *Clients receiving electroconvulsive therapy (ECT) are at risk for this diagnosis.*

ACTIONS/INTERVENTIONS	RATIONALES
Remain with the client who has had ECT until gag reflex and swallowing have returned to normal. Monitor gag reflex and swallowing every [number] minutes until return to normal.	Basic safety measures until the client can demonstrate control.
Place the client who has had ECT on right side until reactive.	Lessens the probability of aspiration through the influence of gravity on stomach contents.
Clients in four-point restraint should be placed on right side or stomach. Elevate the client's head to eat, and remove restraints one at a time to facilitate eating. Request that oral medications be changed to liquid forms.	Lessens probability of aspiration due to difficulty in swallowing tablets or pills that might cause gagging.
Observe clients receiving antipsychotic agents for possible suppression of cough reflex.	One side effect of these medications is suppression of the cough reflex. Loss of this reflex promotes the likelihood of aspiration.[38]

Gerontic Health

ACTIONS/INTERVENTIONS	RATIONALES
Older adults may develop a decreased gag reflex. To reduce the risk of aspiration: • Monitor gag reflex before any procedures involving anesthesia such as bronchoscopy, esophagogastroduodenoscopy (EGD), or general surgery.	Establishes baseline data to use for comparison after the procedure is completed.
Monitor gag reflex post procedure before giving fluids or solids.	Ensuring return of gag reflex decreases risk of aspiration once oral intake is resumed.

Home Health/Community Health

ACTIONS/INTERVENTIONS	RATIONALES
Secure proper equipment for patient's home to prevent aspiration, including a bed with adjustable head and suction machine. Ensure that caregivers are thoroughly familiar with equipment and its proper use.	Proper supplies are required in the home for prevention of aspiration and emergency relief of aspiration.
Teach caregivers and patient how to thicken drinks to the proper consistency as ordered.	Ensures patient safety and family comfort in the home setting.
Teach patient and caregivers about the importance of maintaining head elevation during and after enteral feedings.	Basic safety measure.
Assess the caregiver's ability to provide CPR and Heimlich maneuver. Provide re-teaching as needed to ensure competence.	Ensures patient safety and family comfort in the home setting.
Educate caregivers of signs that patient has aspirated.	To allow early detection and facilitate appropriate caregiver response.
Educate caregivers of patient symptoms of complications of aspiration that indicate the need to seek immediate medical attention.	To allow early detection and facilitate appropriate caregiver response.

BODY TEMPERATURE, IMBALANCED, RISK FOR

DEFINITION[28]

The state in which the individual is at risk for failure to maintain body temperature within the normal range.[30]

DEFINING CHARACTERISTICS (RISK FACTORS)[28]

1. Altered metabolic rate
2. Illness or trauma affecting temperature regulation
3. Medications causing vasoconstriction or vasodilation
4. Inappropriate clothing for environmental temperature
5. Inactivity or vigorous activity
6. Extremes of weight
7. Extremes of age
8. Dehydration
9. Sedation
10. Exposure to cold or cool or warm or hot environments

RELATED FACTORS[28]

The risk factors also serve as the related factors for this nursing diagnosis.

RELATED CLINICAL CONCERNS

1. Any infectious process
2. Hyperthyroidism/hypothyroidism
3. Any surgical procedure
4. Head injuries

Have You Selected the Correct Diagnosis?

Risk for Imbalanced Body Temperature
Risk for imbalanced body temperature needs to be differentiated from Hypothermia, Hyperthermia, and Ineffective Thermoregulation.

Hypothermia
Hypothermia is the condition in which a person maintains a temperature lower than normal for him or her. This means that the body is probably dissipating heat normally but is unable to produce heat normally. In Risk for Imbalanced Body Temperature both heat production and heat dissipation are potentially nonfunctional. In Hypothermia, a lower than normal body temperature can be measured. In Risk for Imbalanced Body Temperature, temperature measurement may not show an abnormality until the condition has changed to Hyperthermia or Hypothermia.

Hyperthermia
Hyperthermia is the condition in which a person maintains a temperature higher than normal. This means that the body is probably producing heat normally but is unable to dissipate the heat normally. Both heat production and heat dissipation are potentially nonfunctional in Risk for Imbalanced Body Temperature. As with Hypothermia, a temperature measurement shows an abnormal measurement.

Ineffective Thermoregulation
Ineffective Thermoregulation means that a person's temperature fluctuates between being too high and too low. There is nothing wrong, generally, with heat production or heat dissipation; however, the thermoregulatory systems in the hypothalamus or the thyroid are dysfunctional. Again, a temperature measurement shows an abnormality.

EXPECTED OUTCOME

Will have no alteration in body temperature by [date].

TARGET DATES

Initial target dates would be stated in hours. After stabilization, target dates could be extended to 2 to 3 days.

NURSING ACTIONS/INTERVENTIONS WITH RATIONALES

Adult Health

ACTIONS/INTERVENTIONS	RATIONALES
Monitor for factors contributing to Risk for Imbalanced Body Temperature at least every 2 hours on [odd/even] hour. (Refer to Risk Factors.)	Detects overproduction or underproduction of heat.
Monitor temperature for at least every 2 hours on [odd/even] hour.	
Note pattern of temperature for last 48 hours.	Assists in ascertaining any trends. Typical viral–bacterial differentiation may be possible to detect on temperature curves.
Monitor skin and mucous membrane integrity every 2 hours on [odd/even] hour.	Can provide early clues for fluid imbalance. Adequate hydration assists in maintaining normal body core temperature.
Monitor intake and output every hour.	To maintain fluid balance.
If temperature is above or below parameters defined by health-care provider, take appropriate measures to bring temperature back to normal range. Refer to nursing actions for Hypothermia and Hyperthermia.	
Collaborate with health-care team in identifying causative organisms.	Identification of organism allows determination of most appropriate antibiotic therapy.
Maintain consistent room temperature.	Prevents overheating or overcooling due to environment.
Teach the patient to wear appropriate clothing and modify routines to prevent alterations in body temperature:	Regulates constant metabolism and provides warmth.
• Teach the patient how to manage activity with regard to environmental conditions that can influence temperature imbalance (e.g., not engaging in outdoor activities in extreme temperatures).	

ACTIONS/INTERVENTIONS	RATIONALES
Avoid sedatives and tranquilizers that depress cerebral function and circulation.	Risk factors for this diagnosis.
Assist the patient to learn to assess biorhythms.	Generally, early morning is the period of lowest body metabolic activity. Add extra clothes until food and physical movement stimulate increased cellular metabolism and circulation. Helps determine peak and trough of temperature variations.
Teach patient to balance physical and sedentary activity.	Assists in maintaining consistency in metabolic functioning.
Refer to nursing diagnoses Hypothermia or Hyperthermia for interventions related to these situations once the alteration has occurred.	

Child Health

ACTIONS/INTERVENTIONS	RATIONALES
Monitor temperature at least every hour.	The young infant and child may lack mature thermoregulatory capacity. Temperatures that are either too high (102°F or above) or too low (below 97°F) may bring about spiraling metabolic disruption of acid–base status. Seizures and shock may follow.
If temperature is less than 97°F rectally (or parameters defined by physician), take appropriate measures for maintaining temperature:	Young infants and children may not be able to initiate compensatory regulation of temperature, especially in premature and altered CNS/immune conditions. These basic measures must be taken to safeguard a return to the homeostatic condition.
• Infants: Radiant warmer or isolette	Best method of warming newborn infant is to place infant on mother's chest skin to skin and cover both with warm blanket. Sometimes infants placed under warmers or in isolettes can become dehydrated if not monitored adequately.
• Older child: Thermoblanket • Administer medications as ordered.	
Be cautious to not overdose in a 24-hour period. Abide by recommended dosage schedule every 8 hours or pediatric medication recommendations.	Using caution in dosage calculation and abiding by appropriate guidelines minimize inadvertent overdosing and subsequent untoward effects of medication.
If temperature is above 101°F, take appropriate measures to bring temperature back to normal range (or at least 98 to 100°F):	Young infants and children may have febrile seizures due to immature thermoregulatory mechanisms and must be appropriately safeguarded against further sequelae.
• Administer Tylenol, antibiotics, or other medications as ordered.	
• Monitor and document related symptoms with specific regard for potential febrile seizures.	
• Monitor for the development of febrile seizures, and check for history of febrile seizures.	
• If the infant or child has reduced threshold for seizures during times of fever, be prepared to treat seizures with anticonvulsants, maintain airway, and provide for safety from injury.	Anticipatory planning promotes optimal resuscitation efforts.
• Provide appropriate teaching to the child and parents related to hyperthermia and hypothermia (e.g., temper-	Self-care empowers and fosters long-term confidence as well as reduces anxiety.

(care plan continued on page 142)

Child Health

ACTIONS/INTERVENTIONS	RATIONALES
ature measurement, wearing of proper clothing, use of Tylenol instead of aspirin, consuming adequate amounts of food and fluid, and use of tepid baths).	
• Be cautious and do not overtax the infant or child with congestive heart failure or pulmonary problems by allowing a temperature elevation to develop.	Increased metabolic demands in the presence of an already taxed cardiopulmonary status can become severe, resulting in life-threatening conditions if left untreated.
• Avoid use of aspirin and aspirin products.	Standards of care per the American Academy of Pediatrics to decrease the potential for Reye's syndrome.
• Avoid use of tympanic membranous thermometer in infants age 6 months or younger.	Studies indicate that tympanic thermometers are inaccurate in infants, especially those younger than 3 months of age.

Women's Health

ACTIONS/INTERVENTIONS	RATIONALES
Assist the patient in identifying lifestyle adjustments necessary to maintain body temperature within normal range during various life phases (e.g., perimenopause or menopause).	So-called hot flashes related to changes in the body's core temperature can be somewhat controlled in women via estrogen replacement therapy; however, as hormone levels fluctuate with the aging process, some hot flashes will occur. These can be helped by adjusting the environment (e.g., room temperature, amount of clothing, or temperature of fluids consumed).
Maintain house at a consistent temperature level of 70 to 72°F.	
Keep bedroom cooler at night and layer blankets or covers that can be discarded or added as necessary.	
Have the patient drink cool fluids (e.g., iced tea or cold soda).	
Have the patient wear clothing that is layered so that jackets, etc., can be discarded or added as necessary.	
In collaboration with physician, assist the patient in understanding role of estrogen and the amount of estrogen replacement necessary during perimenopause and menopause.	Individuals have unique, different requirements as to the amount of estrogen necessary to maintain appropriate hormone levels. It is of prime importance that each patient can recognize what her body's needs are and communicate this information to the health-care provider.[39]

Mental Health

ACTIONS/INTERVENTIONS	RATIONALES
Observe clients receiving neuroleptic drugs for signs and symptoms of hyperthermia. Teach clients these symptoms and caution them to decrease their activities in the warmest part of the day and to maintain adequate hydration, especially if they are receiving lithium carbonate with these drugs.	Neuroleptic drugs may decrease the ability to sweat, and therefore make it difficult for the client to reduce body temperature.[38,40]

ACTIONS/INTERVENTIONS	RATIONALES
Observe clients receiving antipsychotics and antidepressants for loss of thermoregulation. Elderly client, especially, should be monitored for this side effect. Provide the client with extra clothing and blankets to maintain comfort. Protect this client from contact with uncontrolled hot objects such as space heaters and radiators. Heating pads and electric blankets can be used with supervision.	Antipsychotics and antidepressants can cause a loss of thermoregulation. The client's learned avoidance behavior can be altered and consciousness can be clouded as a result of medications. Hypothermia is more common that hyperthermia.[38,40]
Do not provide electric heating devices to the client who is on suicide precautions or who has alterations in thought processes.	Basic safety measure.
Notify physician if the client receiving antipsychotic agents has an elevation in temperature or flu-like symptoms.	Antipsychotics, especially chlorpromazine and thioridazine, can cause agranulocytosis. This risk is greatest 3 to 8 weeks after therapy has begun.[38,40] Clients who have experienced this side effect in the past should not receive the drug again because a repeat episode is highly possible.
Review the client's complete blood count (CBC) before drug is started, and report any abnormalities on subsequent CBCs to the physician.	Basic monitoring for agranulocytosis.
Clients receiving phenothiazines should be monitored for hot, dry skin, CNS depression, and rectal temperature elevations (can be as high as 108°F). Monitor the client's temperature three times a day while awake at [times]. Notify physician of alterations.	These medications can produce hyperthermia, which can be fatal. This hyperthermia is due to a peripheral autonomic effect.[38,40]
Monitor clients receiving tricyclic antidepressants (TCAs) and the monoamine oxidase inhibitors (MAOIs) for alterations in temperature three times a day while awake. [Note times here.] Notify physician of any alterations.	The side effect of a hyperpyretic crisis can be produced in clients receiving these medications.[38,40]

Gerontic Health

● **N O T E :** *Normal changes of aging can contribute to altered thermoregulation. Age-related changes that may be associated with altered thermoregulation are a decrease in febrile response, inefficient vasoconstriction, decreased cardiac output, decreased subcutaneous tissue, diminished shivering, diminished temperature sensory perception, and diminished thirst perception. Thus, older clients are at high risk for alterations in thermoregulation, both hyperthermia and hypothermia.*

In addition to the interventions for Adult Health the following can be utilized with the older adult client.

ACTIONS/INTERVENTIONS	RATIONALES
Check on older adults often who are at risk: • During heat alerts • During cold weather • In homes without air conditioning or heating • During electrical outages or electrical service interruptions	Primary preventive measure.
Instruct/assist client to select proper clothing: • Layers during cold weather and lighter garments during warmer weather	Primary preventive measure

(care plan continued on page 144)

NURSING ACTIONS/INTERVENTIONS WITH RATIONALES (continued from page 143)

Gerontic Health

ACTIONS/INTERVENTIONS	RATIONALES
Monitor and record the temperature of older clients often and regularly during high-risk times: • Intra- and postoperative period • When infection is present • When fluid imbalance is present	Tracks client norms and provides a mechanism for early identification of changes.
Use warmed IV solutions in older clients in the intra-/postoperative period unless hyperthermia is present.	Prevent episodes of hypothermia.

Home Health/Community Health

ACTIONS/INTERVENTIONS	RATIONALES
Teach measures to decrease or eliminate Risk for Imbalanced Body Temperature: • Wearing appropriate clothing • Taking appropriate care of underlying disease • Avoiding exposure to extremes of environmental temperature • Maintaining temperature within norms for age, sex, and height • Ensuring appropriate use of medications • Ensuring proper hydration • Ensuring appropriate shelter	Appropriate environmental temperature regulation provides support for physiologic thermoregulation.
Assist the client and family to identify lifestyle changes that may be required: • Learn safety and thermal injury prevention measures if client works or plays outdoors. • Measure temperature in a manner appropriate for the developmental age of the person. • Maintain ideal weight. • Avoid substance abuse.	Support is often helpful when individuals and families are considering lifestyle alterations.
Involve the client and family in planning, implementing, and promoting reduction or elimination of the Risk for Imbalanced Body Temperature by establishing family conferences to set mutual goals and to improve communication.	Involvement of the client and family provides opportunity to increase motivation and enhance self-care.
Monitor the patient's need for assistive resources and provide referrals as needed.	Utilization of existing resources can prevent injury or illness.
Pay particular attention to the client's ability to pay for heat and cooling in the home. Many communities have financial assistance programs for vulnerable persons who cannot afford appropriate heating and cooling.	

BREASTFEEDING, EFFECTIVE

DEFINITION[28]

The state in which a mother–infant dyad–family exhibits adequate proficiency and satisfaction with the breastfeeding process.

DEFINING CHARACTERISTICS[28]

1. Mother–infant communication patterns (infant cues, maternal interpretation, and response) are effective.
2. Regular and sustained suckling and swallowing at the breast.

3. Appropriate infant weight patterns for age.
4. Infant is content after feeding.
5. Mother able to position infant at breast to promote a successful latch-on response.
6. Signs and/or symptoms of oxytocin release (let-down or milk ejection reflex).
7. Adequate infant elimination patterns for age.
8. Eagerness of infant to nurse.
9. Maternal verbalization of satisfaction with the breast-feeding process.

RELATED FACTORS[28]

1. Infant gestational age more than 34 weeks
2. Support sources
3. Normal infant oral structure
4. Maternal confidence
5. Basic breastfeeding knowledge
6. Normal breast structure

RELATED CLINICAL CONCERNS

Because this is a wellness diagnosis, there are no related clinical concerns.

 Have You Selected the Correct Diagnosis?

Effective Breastfeeding
Effective Breastfeeding is a wellness diagnosis. It signifies a successful experience for both the mother and the baby. If there is a problem with breastfeeding, then the appropriate diagnosis is Ineffective Breastfeeding. These two diagnoses could be considered to be at opposite ends of a continuum.

Impaired Parenting
Effective Breastfeeding focuses on the nutrition and growth of the infant, rather than on the degree of attachment with the infant. Although Effective Breastfeeding contributes to the attachment of the infant to the mother and the mother to the infant, the supplying of the infant with nutrition by breastfeeding or by formula feeding should be differentiated from attachment processes, which are addressed in Impaired Parenting, Risk for or Actual, and Parental Role Conflict.

EXPECTED OUTCOME

The infant will have all of the following:

1. Adequate weight gain and return to birth weight by 3 weeks of age
2. Six or more wet diapers in 24 hours, after 2 days
3. At least two stools every 24 hours, after 2-3 days

TARGET DATES

Although it usually takes 2 to 3 weeks for the mother and infant to establish a synchronized pattern of feeding, an initial target date of 4 days should be set to ensure an effective beginning to the breastfeeding process.

NURSING ACTIONS/INTERVENTIONS WITH RATIONALES

Adult Health

For this diagnosis, Women's Health nursing actions serve as the generic actions. This diagnosis would probably not arise on an adult health unit.

Child Health

While the infant and mother typically have established effective breastfeeding within the first week or so of life there are instances when a need for intervention does occur on the child health-care unit. Obviously the reason for hospitalization is considered in the plan for effective breastfeeding, especially when surgical intervention is a part of the plan of care. In such instances mothers are encouraged to pump during times when the infant is NPO or unable to breastfeed, and freeze the expressed milk in individual bottles labeled for future use. Please see nursing actions under Women's Health for additional interventions.

Women's Health

● N O T E : *If the diagnosis of Effective Breastfeeding has been made, the most appropriate nursing action is continued support for the diagnosis. Successful lactation can be established in any woman who does not have structural anomalies of the milk ducts and who exhibits a desire to breastfeed. Adoptive mothers can breastfeed as well as birth-mothers. The following actions serve to facilitate the development of Effective Breastfeeding.*

(care plan continued on page 146)

NURSING ACTIONS/INTERVENTIONS WITH RATIONALES (continued from page 145)

Women's Health

ACTIONS/INTERVENTIONS	RATIONALES
Review the mother's knowledge base regarding breast-feeding prior to the initial breastfeeding of the infant. Information on benefits of breastfeeding must be given to the patient's extended family as well as the patient. The nutritional merit of breastfeeding must be embraced by the extended family. Social, emotional, and spiritual aspects of breastfeeding must be addressed. Education must be tailored culturally and to each community's beliefs.	Success or failure to breastfeed is strongly influenced by family and community, their values and beliefs. Sisters, aunts, mothers, and grandmothers play a large role in breastfeeding success. Determining the basis for assistance and teaching is essential to avoid nonessential repetition and confusion for the mother.[41–43]
	Confidence is gained through knowledge. Research has shown that providing pregnant women with accurate breastfeeding information increases breastfeeding initiation rates.[44]
The baby is kept with the mother immediately after birth so that breastfeeding can be initiated at the time the newborn is most receptive (within the first hour after birth).	Research has shown that not separating the mother and baby after birth leads to higher success rates with breastfeeding.[41–49]
Demonstrate and assist the mother and significant other with correct breastfeeding techniques (e.g., positioning and latch-on).	Successful lactation depends on understanding the basic how-to's and correct techniques for the actual feeding act. Women who attend prenatal breastfeeding skills education and a breastfeeding class before discharge increased breastfeeding knowledge. These women had a significantly higher rate of breastfeeding at 6 months postpartum.[44,49]
Teach the mother and significant other basic information related to successful breastfeeding (e.g., milk supply, diet, rest, breast care, breast engorgement, infant hunger cues, and parameters of a healthy infant).	Informing the family about how they can support and help the new mother increases the success rate of breastfeeding after return home. Small things such as fixing a cup of tea (hydration for the mother), running a bath, minding the older siblings, or making a quick trip to the grocery store, gives the new mother time to breastfeed.[5,41]
Assess the mother's breasts for graspable nipples, surgical scars, skin integrity, and abnormalities prior to the initial breastfeeding of the infant.	Provides the assessment base for diagnosing of potential problems as well as the base for developing strategies for success.
Assess the infant for ability to breastfeed prior to breastfeeding (e.g., state of awareness or physical abnormalities).	
Place the infant to breast within the first hour after birth.	It is important to work with the infant's sleep–wake cycle in establishing breastfeeding. If the infant can successfully suckle immediately after birth, a successful and encouraging pattern is usually established for both the mother and the infant.
To initiate or maintain lactation when the mother is unable to breastfeed the infant, encourage the mother to express breast milk either manually or by using a breast pump at least every 3 hours.	This assists in establishing and maintaining the milk supply. The hospital-grade electric pump with a double collecting kit is essential equipment in helping mothers maintain milk supply when the infant cannot suckle at a breast. This is an important part of the success of this mother to provide nutrition and emotional support as well as nutritional support to the infant who cannot breastfeed because of prematurity or illness.[50,51]

● N O T E : *Always use a hospital-grade electric pump with a double collecting kit when assisting mothers of babies in neonatal units to pump.*

ACTIONS/INTERVENTIONS	RATIONALES
Observe the infant at breast, noting behavior, position, latch-on, and sucking technique with the initial breastfeeding and then as necessary. Document these observations in the mother's and infant's charts.	Using a written scale is an excellent method of measuring the self-efficacy of mothers who are breastfeeding, as well as identifying high-risk mothers, build confidence in breastfeeding mothers, assess breastfeeding behaviors, and evaluate the effectiveness of interventions.[52]
Encourage the mother and significant other to identify support systems to assist her with meeting her physical and psychosocial needs at home.	The majority of women who are successfully breastfeeding when leaving the hospital quit as soon as they are home for 2 weeks. Support systems are a critical component in the maintenance of successful lactation.[41–43,52]
Encourage the mother to drink at least 2000 mL of fluids a day, or 8 ounces of fluids every hour.	
To provide sufficient amounts of calcium, proteins, and calories, encourage the mother to eat a wide variety of foods from the Food Pyramid.[5]	Breastfeeding mothers should increase their caloric intake to 2000 to 2500 calories/day in order to maintain successful lactation.[5]
Encourage the mother to breastfeed at least every 2 to 3 hours to establish milk supply, then regulate feeding according to infant's demands (feed effectively at least 8 times per day).	Newborns need frequent feeding to satisfy their hunger and to establish their feeding patterns. It is important that the mother understand that the infant's suckling will determine the supply and demand of breast milk.
Monitor the infant's output for number of wet diapers. Document the number of diapers and the color of urine. A well hydrated infant will have six to eight wet diapers and at least three bowel movements every 24 hours after day 4.[5]	Helps determine intake, hydration, and nutritional status of infant.
Weigh the infant at least every third day and record.	
Assist the mother in planning a day's activities when breastfeeding to ensure that the mother gets sufficient rest.	Helps the new mother establish a schedule that is beneficial for both the mother and infant.[41]
Encourage advanced planning for the working mother if she intends to continue to breastfeed after returning to work.	
Involve the father or significant other in breastfeeding by encouraging the "provider–protector" role.	The breastfeeding mother requires a great deal of support and encouragement. Fathers can supply this by providing her with time for rest and assistance with infant care. For example, the father can bring the infant to the mother at night rather than the mother having to get up each time for the feeding. Fathers can intervene with family and friends to provide nursing mothers with privacy and a quiet environment.

Mental Health

This diagnosis will not be applicable in a mental health setting.

Gerontic Health

This diagnosis is not applicable in gerontic health.

Home Health

The Home Health nursing actions for this diagnosis are the same as those for Women's Health.

BREASTFEEDING, INEFFECTIVE

DEFINITION[28]

The state in which a mother, infant, or child experiences dissatisfaction or difficulty with the breastfeeding process.

DEFINING CHARACTERISTICS[28]

1. Unsatisfactory breastfeeding process
2. Nonsustained sucking at the breast
3. Resisting latching on
4. Unresponsiveness to other comfort measures
5. Persistence of sore nipples beyond the first week of breastfeeding
6. Observable signs of inadequate infant intake
7. Insufficient emptying of each breast per feeding
8. Inability of infant to attach onto maternal breast correctly
9. Infant arching and crying at the breast
10. Infant exhibiting fussiness and crying within the first hour after breastfeeding
11. Actual or perceived inadequate milk supply
12. No observable signs of oxytocin release
13. Insufficient opportunity for sucking at the breast

RELATED FACTORS[28]

1. Nonsupportive partner or family
2. Previous breast surgery
3. Infant receiving supplemental feedings with artificial nipple
4. Prematurity
5. Previous history of breastfeeding failure
6. Poor infant sucking reflex
7. Maternal breast anomaly
8. Maternal anxiety or ambivalence
9. Interruption in breastfeeding
10. Infant anomaly
11. Knowledge deficit

RELATED CLINICAL CONCERNS

1. Any diseases of the breast
2. Cleft lip; cleft palate
3. Failure to thrive
4. Prematurity
5. Child abuse

 Have You Selected the Correct Diagnosis?

Ineffective Breastfeeding
Ineffective Breastfeeding should be differentiated from the patient's concern over whether she wants to breastfeed or not. Although a mother who does not want to breastfeed will more than likely be ineffective in her breastfeeding attempts, ineffective breastfeeding can be related to problems other than just unwillingness to breastfeed. Other diagnoses that need to be differentiated include:

Anxiety
Anxiety is defined as a vague, uneasy feeling, the source of which is often nonspecific or unknown to the individual. If an expression of perceived threat to self-concept, health status, socioeconomic status, role functioning, or interaction patterns is made, this would constitute the diagnosis of Anxiety.

Impaired Parenting
Impaired Parenting is defined as the inability of the nurturing figures to create an environment that promotes optimum growth and development of another human being. Adjustment to parenting, in general, is a normal maturation process following the birth of a child.

Delayed Growth and Development: Self-Care Skills
This diagnosis is defined according to a demonstrated deviation from age group norms for self-care. Inadequate caretaking would be defined according to specific behavior and attitudes of the individual mother or infant.

Ineffective Individual Coping
This diagnosis is defined as the inability of the individual to deal with situations that require coping or adaptation to meet life's demands and roles. All the changes secondary to the birth of a new baby could result in this diagnosis.

EXPECTED OUTCOME

Infant will require no supplemental feedings by [date].

TARGET DATES

Because Ineffective Breastfeeding can be physically detrimental to the infant as well as emotionally detrimental to the mother, an initial target date of 3 days is best.

NURSING ACTIONS/INTERVENTIONS WITH RATIONALES

Adult Health

For this nursing diagnosis, the Women's Health nursing actions serve as the generic nursing actions.

Child Health

ACTIONS/INTERVENTIONS	RATIONALES
Monitor for factors contributing to the infant's ability to suck: • Structural abnormalities (e.g., cleft lip or palate) • Altered level of consciousness, seizures, or CNS damage • Mechanical barriers to sucking (e.g., endotracheal tube or ventilator) • Pain or underlying altered comfort or medication • Prematurity with diminished sucking ability	Assessment of the infant's ability to suck assists in meeting goals for effective breastfeeding.
Determine the effect the altered or impaired breastfeeding has on the mother and infant by providing at least one 30-minute period per day for talking with the mother. Monitor maternal feelings expressed, maternal–infant behaviors observed, and excessive crying or unrelenting fussiness in the infant.	The maternal–infant responses provide the essential database in determining how serious the breastfeeding issues are. This information dictates how to approach the problem and promote realistic follow-up.
To the degree possible, provide emotional support for the infant in instances of temporary inability to breastfeed (e.g., gavage feedings with appropriate cuddling). Include the parents in care. Allow the infant to suck on pacifier if possible.	Before attempting any formula feedings try various artificial feeding techniques using the mother's own milk for the infant.[51] Provides temporary substitutions for breastfeeding that promote trust and sense of security for the infant. Also, bonding with the mother is still possible.[50,51,53,54]
Coordinate the parents' visitation with the infant to best facilitate successful breastfeeding in such areas as rest, natural hunger cycles, and comfort of all involved.	
Assist with plan to manage impaired breastfeeding to best provide support to all involved (e.g., breast-pumping for period of time with support for this effort until normal breastfeeding can be resumed). Breast milk may be frozen or even given in gavage feeding. Support the mother's choice for whatever alternatives are chosen.	Maintain the mother's confidence in breastfeeding. Supporting her choice for alternative feeding demonstrates valuing of her beliefs.[50,51,53,54]
Provide appropriate resources that may include local lactation specialist or in house assistance, plus those available via the Internet, library, and book stores.	

Women's Health

ACTIONS/INTERVENTIONS	RATIONALES
Ascertain the mother's desire to breastfeed the infant through careful interviewing and reviewing of the mother's knowledge of breastfeeding.	Provides intervention base for nursing actions. Allows planning of support, teaching, and evaluation of motives and desires to breastfeed.
List the advantages and disadvantages of breastfeeding for the mother.	Assists the mother to make an informed decision about breastfeeding.[5,44,52]
Obtain a breastfeeding and bottle-feeding history from the mother (e.g., did she breastfeed before, and if so, was it successful or unsuccessful)?	
Allow for uninterrupted breastfeeding periods.	Providing the mother and infant with uninterrupted breastfeeding times allows them to become acquainted with each other and allows time for learning different breastfeeding techniques.

(care plan continued on page 150)

NURSING ACTIONS/INTERVENTIONS WITH RATIONALES (continued from page 149)

Women's Health

ACTIONS/INTERVENTIONS	RATIONALES
Collaborate with physician, lactation consultant, perinatal clinical nurse specialist, etc. to determine ways to make abnormal breast structure amenable for breast-feeding.	Assists the mother who has strong desire to breastfeed to be successful.
Observe the mother with the infant during breastfeeding. Explain and demonstrate methods to increase infant sucking reflex. Demonstrate to the mother various positions for breastfeeding and how to alternate positions with each feeding to prevent nipple soreness (e.g., sitting up, lying down, using football hold, holding the baby "tummy to tummy," using pillows for the mother's comfort, or using pillows for supporting the baby).	Provides basic information and visible support to assist with successful breastfeeding.
Ascertain the mother's need for privacy during breast-feeding.	Promotes the mother's comfort with the physical act of breastfeeding.
Monitor for poor or dysfunctional sucking by checking: • Position the mother is using to hold the baby • Baby's mouth position on areola and nipple • Position of the baby's head (e.g., inappropriate hyper-extension)	Proper positioning facilitates satisfaction with breastfeeding for both the mother and baby.
Ascertain the mother's support for breastfeeding from others (e.g., husband or significant other, patient's female family members, obstetrician, pediatrician, and nurses on postpartum unit).	Support from others is essential for attaining successful breastfeeding. Success or failure to breastfeed is strongly influenced by family and community, their values and beliefs. Sisters, aunts, mothers, and grandmothers play a large role in breastfeeding success. To determine the basis for assistance and teaching is essential in order to avoid nonessential repetition and confusion for the mother.[41–43]
Discuss the infant's needs and frequency of feedings.	Provides basic information and visible support to assist with successful breastfeeding.
Assist the mother in planning a day's activities when breastfeeding, ensuring that the mother gets plenty of rest.	Provides information necessary for the mother to plan the basics of her self-care.
Teach the patient: • The proper diet for the breastfeeding mother, listing important food groups and necessary calories to adequately maintain milk production. • The idea of advanced planning for the working mother who plans to breastfeed • That it takes time to establish breastfeeding (usually a month) • The use of various hand pumps, battery-operated pumps, and electric pumps • How to hand-express breast milk • How to store expressed breast milk properly	The breastfeeding woman can generally meet her nutritional needs and those of her infant through adequate dietary intake of food and fluids; however, because the energy demand is greater during lactation, RDA standards recommend an additional 200 to 500 extra calories per day to be added to the diet to provide adequate nutrients for both mother and infant without catabolism of the mother's lean tissue.[5]
Schedule specific times for consultation and support for the mother. Plan at least 30 minutes per shift (while awake) for talking with the mother.	

ACTIONS/INTERVENTIONS	RATIONALES
If the baby is separated from the mother, such as in neonatal intensive care unit (NICU), involve the baby's nurses in planning with the mother routines and times for breastfeeding the infant.[50,51]	
Refer the mother to breastfeeding support groups.	Provides basic information and visible support to assist with successful breastfeeding.
For the mother who has had a cesarean section, place a pillow over the abdomen before putting the infant to the breast.	Assists in keeping pressure off the incision line while breastfeeding.
Breastfeeding after breast surgery: • Prenatal nipple and breast assessment along with history and description of breast surgery • Teach appropriate interventions for mother's use. • Supplemental methods of feeding (using a supplemental nursing system) • Ensure that mothers know how to assess for infant dehydration. • Sunken anterior fontanel • Weak, high-pitched cry and insufficient and infrequent wet diapers (early days—one or two wet diapers per day; after days 3 and 4—six to eight wet diapers per day) • Availability of galactogogues (increase milk supply). ***Should be taken only when a low milk supply is documented by the mother.***[55]	Research has shown that breast surgery may not have an impact on a women's ability to breastfeed as much as the support around her.[41,55]
Assist the mother of a premature baby to pump breast routinely to initiate milk production.	See effective breastfeeding diagnosis for correct pump setup for these mothers.
Demonstrate proper storage and transportation of breast milk for the premature baby.	Basic teaching to ensure safe nutrition for infant.
Assist the mother who has to wean a premature baby from tube feedings to breastfeeding by: • Teaching the mother to place the infant at the breast several times a day and during tube feeding • Encouraging the mother to hold, cuddle, and interact with the infant during tube feedings • Allowing the mother and infant privacy to begin interaction with breastfeeding • Being available to assist with the infant during breastfeeding interaction • Reassuring the mother that it might take several attempts before the baby begins to breastfeed	Provides needed support during this process.
Give breastfeeding mothers copies of educational materials.	Provides a readily available information source.
If breastfeeding is not possible because of an infant physical deformity, teach the mother how to pump breasts and how to feed the infant breast milk in bottles with special nipples.	Allows the mother the option of breastfeeding in the event that the deformity can be surgically corrected.
Encourage maternal attachment behavior by not separating mother and baby after birth.	Assists the mother in adjustment to parenting and effective caretaking of the infant.

Mental Health

Refer to Women's Health nursing actions for interventions related to this diagnosis.

(care plan continued on page 152)

NURSING ACTIONS/INTERVENTIONS WITH RATIONALES (continued from page 151)

Gerontic Health

This diagnosis is not appropriate for gerontic health.

Home Health/Community Health

ACTIONS/INTERVENTIONS	RATIONALES
Assist the client and family in identifying risk factors pertinent to the situation: • Premature infant • Infant anomaly • Maternal breast dysfunction • Infection • Previous breast surgery • Supplemental bottle feedings • Nonsupportive family • Lack of knowledge • Anxiety	Identification of and early interventions in high-risk situations provide the opportunity to prevent problems.
Consult with, or refer to, appropriate community resources as indicated (e.g., WIC).	Appropriate and cost-effective use of available resources.

BREASTFEEDING, INTERRUPTED

DEFINITION[28]

A break in the continuity of the breastfeeding process as a result of inability or inadvisability to put the baby to the breast for feeding.[30]

DEFINING CHARACTERISTICS[28]

1. Infant not receiving nourishment at the breast for some or all feedings
2. Lack of knowledge regarding expression and storage of breast milk
3. Maternal desire to maintain lactation and provide (or eventually provide) her breast milk for her infant's nutritional needs
4. Separation of the mother and infant

RELATED FACTORS[28]

1. Contraindications to breastfeeding (e.g., drugs or true breast milk jaundice)
2. Maternal employment
3. Maternal or infant illness
4. Need to abruptly wean infant
5. Prematurity

RELATED CLINICAL CONCERNS

1. Any condition requiring emergency admission of the mother to hospital
2. Any condition requiring emergency admission of the infant to hospital

3. Prematurity
4. Postpartum depression

 Have You Selected the Correct Diagnosis?

Ineffective Breastfeeding
Ineffective Breastfeeding is expressed dissatisfaction or problems with breastfeeding. With Interrupted Breastfeeding, there is no expressed dissatisfaction or major problems; however, Breastfeeding has temporarily ceased as a result of factors beyond the mother's control.

Ineffective Infant Feeding Pattern
In this diagnosis, there is a defined problem with the infant's ability to suck, swallow, and breathe. Breastfeeding for this infant has not ever been successful. With Interrupted Breastfeeding, the infant has no problems with sucking or swallowing, and the stoppage of breastfeeding can be overcome by storing breast milk and feeding the infant via a bottle.

EXPECTED OUTCOME

Infant will demonstrate no weight loss secondary to adaptations for Interrupted Breastfeeding by [date].

TARGET DATES

Because this interruption might occur as a result of an emergency, initial evaluation should occur within 24 hours after the initial diagnosis. Thereafter, target dates can be moved to every 3 days.

NURSING ACTIONS/INTERVENTIONS WITH RATIONALES

Adult Health

Refer to Women's Health for appropriate interventions.

Child Health

ACTIONS/INTERVENTIONS	RATIONALES
Monitor for infant's ability to suck. Encourage sucking on a regular basis, especially if gavage feedings are a part of the therapeutic regimen.	Provides basic data critical to success. In times of non-breastfeeding, it is beneficial to encourage sucking to reinforce the feeding time as pleasurable and to enhance digestion, unless contraindicated by a surgical or medical condition (e.g., cleft repair of lip or palate, prolonged NPO [nothing by mouth] status with concerns for air swallowing).
Provide support for the mother–infant dyad to facilitate breastfeeding satisfaction.	Feedback may provide essential valuing during times of stress.
Monitor infant cues suggesting satisfaction: • Weight gain appropriate for status • Ability to sleep at intervals	The fact that the infant's satisfaction and input are valued provides a critical component in the entire process of breastfeeding.

Women's Health

ACTIONS/INTERVENTIONS	RATIONALES
Provide appropriate information on why breastfeeding needs to be interrupted. Be specific about length of time (i.e., days, weeks, or months), and offer options for maintaining breast milk until able to resume breast-feeding.[49-51,53]	Assists breastfeeding families in establishing and maintaining breastfeeding capabilities when it is inadvisable or impossible to put the baby to the breast for feeding.
Describe routine for pumping, expressing, and storing of breast milk during emergency period.	
Contact lactation consultant and/or perinatal nurse who can assist with plan of nursing care and with maintenance of breast milk during mother's illness (e.g., emergency surgery, medical regimen [medications] that contradict breastfeeding, or injury requiring hospitalization of mother).[45,46]	
Provide the mother with appropriate information about breast pumps and how to obtain one (rent or buy) to aid in expression of breast milk (i.e., semiautomatic breast pump, automatic breast pump, battery-operated breast pump, or manual breast pump).	
Demonstrate and have the mother return-demonstrate proper assembly and use of breast pump.	
Assist the mother in learning manual expression of breast milk.[46] • Good handwashing technique before expressing milk • Correct positioning of hand and fingers so as not to damage breast tissue	

(care plan continued on page 154)

NURSING ACTIONS/INTERVENTIONS WITH RATIONALES (continued from page 153)

Women's Health

ACTIONS/INTERVENTIONS	RATIONALES
• Sterile wide-mouth funnel and bottle for storage of breast milk	
Discuss options for maintaining breastfeeding with the mother who is returning to work. Provide assistance to help the mother establish feeding schedule with work schedule (e.g., breastfeed a.m. and p.m., pumping at noon, etc.)[45,46,56]	
Provide resources (e.g., printed materials or consultant) to assist the mother when negotiating with her employer for time and place to pump or breastfeed during working hours.[46]	
Assist the mother and family to arrange schedule to bring the infant to her during working hours.	
Encourage the mother and significant other to verbalize their frustrations and concerns about establishing and maintaining lactation when the infant is ill or premature.[47,50,51,53]	
Refer to lactation consultant/clinical nurse specialist who can support the parents and assist the nurse in developing a program of breastfeeding or supplementing of the infant with the mother's breast milk.[53–55]	Provides basic information that assists in promoting effective breastfeeding.

Mental Health

● N O T E : *This diagnosis will not, in all likelihood, be applicable in a mental health setting. Should a mother be admitted with a mental health–related diagnosis, the physician would probably suggest changing the infant to bottle-feedings. Should the physician agree that breastfeeding could continue, the Women's Health actions would be applicable for the mental health client.*

Gerontic Health

This diagnosis is not appropriate for gerontic health.

Home Health/Community Health

● N O T E : *If home care is needed because of either mother or infant illness or disability, the nurse will need to address the underlying problem in order to promote Effective Breastfeeding. It is not likely that home health care would be initiated if the only diagnosis was Ineffective Breastfeeding; however, there are lactation consultants whose entire practice is home health. This practice has been specifically designed to assist with maintenance of successful lactation.*

ACTIONS/INTERVENTIONS	RATIONALES
Support the mother, infant, and family dynamics for successful breastfeeding.	Encouragement and support increase the potential for positive outcomes.

ACTIONS/INTERVENTIONS	RATIONALES
Recognize cultural variations in feeding practices when assessing effectiveness of breastfeeding.	Feeding patterns vary according to cultural norms.
Provide additional education or referrals as requested or as the situation changes.	Community-based support is ongoing; early intervention as the situation changes increases the potential for continued effectiveness. Support from others is essential in attaining successful breastfeeding. Success or failure to breastfeed is strongly influenced by family and community, their values and beliefs. Sisters, aunts, mothers, and grandmothers play a large role in breastfeeding success. Determining the basis for assistance and teaching is essential in order to avoid nonessential repetition and confusion for the mother.[41–43]

DENTITION, IMPAIRED

DEFINITION[28]

Disruption in tooth development, eruption patterns, or structural integrity of individual teeth.[30]

DEFINING CHARACTERISTICS[28]

1. Excessive plaque
2. Crown or root caries
3. Halitosis
4. Tooth enamel discoloration
5. Toothache
6. Loose teeth
7. Excessive calculus
8. Incomplete eruption for age (may be primary or permanent teeth)
9. Malocclusion or tooth misalignment
10. Premature loss of primary teeth
11. Worn down or abraded teeth
12. Tooth fractures
13. Missing teeth or incomplete absence
14. Erosion of enamel
15. Asymmetric facial expression

RELATED FACTORS[28]

1. Ineffective oral hygiene
2. Sensitivity to heat or cold
3. Barriers to self-care
4. Access or economic barriers to professional care
5. Nutritional deficits
6. Dietary habits
7. Genetic predisposition
8. Selected prescription medications
9. Premature loss of primary teeth
10. Excessive intake of fluoride
11. Chronic vomiting

12. Chronic use of tobacco, coffee, tea, or red wine
13. Lack of knowledge regarding dental health
14. Excessive use of abrasive cleaning agents
15. Bruxism

RELATED CLINICAL CONCERNS

1. Dental surgery
2. Elderly wearing dentures
3. Facial trauma
4. Anorexia or bulimia
5. Malnutrition

 Have You Selected the Correct Diagnosis?

Imbalanced Nutrition, Less Than Body Requirements
Impaired Dentition might be a primary factor in the development of Imbalanced Nutrition, Less Than Body Requirements. Impaired Dentition is a very specific diagnosis related only to the teeth and would require intervention before working on the broader diagnosis of Imbalanced Nutrition, Less Than Body Requirements.

Adult Failure to Thrive
Again, Impaired Dentition might contribute to the development of Adult Failure to Thrive. This means Impaired Dentition would need to be resolved before the broader definition of Adult Failure to Thrive.

EXPECTED OUTCOME

Will return-demonstrate complete oral hygiene by [date].

TARGET DATES

One week would be an appropriate time period to check initial progress toward resolving this problem area.

NURSING ACTIONS/INTERVENTIONS WITH RATIONALES

Adult Health

ACTIONS/INTERVENTIONS	RATIONALES
Educate and provide patient with well-balanced diet including fiber.	Provides essential nutrition.
Assist the patient with oral hygiene at least after meals and at bedtime.	Cleans and lubricates the mouth.
If Impaired Dentition predisposes to Imbalanced Nutrition, Less Than Body Requirements, refer to that nursing diagnosis.	
If Impaired Dentition predisposes to Imbalanced Nutrition, More Than Body Requirements, refer to that nursing diagnosis.	
If Impaired Dentition is related to chronic vomiting, refer to the nursing diagnosis for Nausea or Disturbed Body Image and/or Alteration in Nutrition, Less than Body Requirements Psychiatric Care Plan.	Impaired Dentition related to chronic vomiting can be a symptom of an eating disorder and the client needs to be assessed for this.
If Impaired Dentition is related to chronic use of tobacco, coffee, tea, or red wine, educate the patient in methods to stop this usage. [Note education plan here.]	Encourages health promotion and decreases factors related to Impaired Dentition.
Consult with dietitian to provide soft, nonmechanical diet.	Makes food easier to chew, thereby encouraging essential nutrition.
Consult with social worker to help the patient find affordable access to professional dental care.	
Teach the patient about dental health.	Assists in preventive maintenance and good oral health.
Refer to a dentist.	
Consult oral surgeon if extraction is deemed necessary.	

Child Health

ACTIONS/INTERVENTIONS	RATIONALES
Monitor for all possible contributing factors to include, but not limited to, organic, genetic, familial, medical, prenatal, or neonatal factors; prematurity; jaundice; significant injuries or exposures; and nutritional possibilities.	Consideration of all possible etiologies best helps identify treatment modalities.
Determine whether there are coexistent congenital anomalies or risk factors. • Risk for caries increased by the infant or toddler being given fruit juices or high corn syrup/fructose content beverages, especially in a bottle.	Primary deficits may exist in isolation or in combination with other deficits.
Identify current dental hygiene for the client (expectations according to age norms; e.g., 6 months—gentle cleansing of gums with soft cotton cloth). • Teach the child and significant others practices that increase the risk of caries.	Preventive maintenance knowledge offers a baseline for hygiene routines and reduction of risk factors for age.
Monitor the mouth fully for status of gums and teeth, if present, type and location, condition of enamel, and alignment or malocclusion.	Actual observation assists in accuracy of diagnosis and treatment.

ACTIONS/INTERVENTIONS	RATIONALES
Determine pattern of tooth appearance and correlation to norms for primary and secondary teeth.	Expected norms assist in identification of deviations.
Determine patterns of tooth loss according to norms for primary and secondary teeth.	Expected norms assist in identification of deviations.
Make appropriate recommendations for maintenance, prophylactic, and restorative care of the client's teeth and gums.	Appropriate referral to specialists offers maximum potential for long-term maintenance of dentition health.
Offer appropriate education for safeguarding permanent teeth for the client and family, to include indications for mouth guards during contact sports, ways to minimize risk of injury, and importance of seeking immediate attention of dentist in event of accidental loss of tooth.	Anticipatory planning assists in dentition health maintenance.
Ascertain client and parental knowledge regarding medications, dietary factors, special orthodontia, or other related maintenance issues.	Validation of actual knowledge or care issues affords optimum likelihood of adherence to regimen for the individual client.
Provide information for local support groups when applicable (e.g., Dental Association).	Support groups foster shared experience with validation of peer input.
Determine resources for continued maintenance, including financial, as determined on an individual basis.	Resources help provide appropriate care as situation permits.
• Refer to community resources to facilitate continued maintenance of dental health.	

Women's Health

Nursing interventions for Women's Health are the same as those for Adult Health.

● N O T E : *It is important to practice good dental health during pregnancy. A pregnant woman needs approximately 1.2 g of calcium and phosphorus daily during pregnancy to help maintain bony stores.*

Mental Health

The nursing actions for this diagnosis in the mental health client are the same as those for Adult Health.

Gerontic Health

ACTIONS/INTERVENTIONS	RATIONALES
Determine the client and/or caregiver's ability to perform oral hygiene measures.	Physical aging changes associated with chronic disease such as arthritis may limit the ability to perform oral care.[56]
Review and/or teach the client strategies for good oral hygiene as necessary (i.e., daily flossing, brushing after meals, and using correct equipment [soft-bristled tooth brush]).[54]	Many older adults have not been taught how to adequately clean their teeth by brushing and flossing.[56]
Refer the client to an occupational therapist, if needed, for assistive equipment and techniques to enhance oral hygiene practices.[57]	Older adults may experience problems with gripping toothbrushes or using dental floss, and thus adequate oral care is inhibited.[57]
Advocate for clients to ensure access to dental services.	Many older adults are reluctant to use dental services because of cost concerns.[58]

(care plan continued on page 158)

NURSING ACTIONS/INTERVENTIONS WITH RATIONALES (continued from page 157)

Gerontic Health

ACTIONS/INTERVENTIONS	RATIONALES
If dentures are present, monitor for appropriate fit, bedtime removal of dentures, and presence of food trapping under dentures after meals.	There is continuous resorption of ridges beneath dentures over time, causing a slow change in how well dentures fit. Failure to remove dentures at bedtime may result in oral trauma or breathing problems if the dentures are loose. Food trapping can lead to mucosal inflammation from organisms trapped under dentures.[56]

Home Health/Community Health

ACTIONS/INTERVENTIONS	RATIONALES
Assist the client in obtaining dentures when appropriate.	Assists the client to increase nutritional intake and improve appearance.
Assist the client in replacing poorly fitting dentures when necessary. Older clients will require correction of denture fit every few years.	Decreases multiple problems created by poorly fitting dentures.
Teach the client proper oral care: • Brushing teeth after each meal • Vigorous mouth rinsing • Flossing at least once daily	Prevents exacerbation of existing conditions.
Teach the client appropriate dietary modifications: • Reducing refined carbohydrates • Reducing between-meal snacks	
Assist the client in obtaining oral care products as necessary.	Encourages proper oral hygiene.
Educate clients about signs and symptoms of tooth decay and periodontal disease and when to seek medical or dental care.	Encourages self-care and prevention.

FLUID BALANCE, READINESS FOR ENHANCED

DEFINITION[28]

A state in which an individual's pattern of equilibrium between fluid volume and chemical compositions of body fluids is sufficient for meeting physical needs and can be strengthened.

DEFINING CHARACTERISTICS[28]

1. Expresses willingness to enhance fluid balance
2. Stable weight
3. Moist mucous membranes
4. Food and fluid intake adequate for daily needs
5. Straw-colored urine with specific gravity within normal limits
6. Good tissue turgor
7. No excessive thirst
8. Urine output appropriate for intake
9. No evidence of edema or dehydration

RELATED FACTORS

None listed.

RELATED CLINICAL CONCERNS

Illness that has potential of impacting fluid balance

Have You Selected the Correct Diagnosis?

Risk for Imbalanced Fluid Volume
Indicates a potential for fluid shifts.

Readiness for Enhanced Fluid Balance
Readiness for Enhanced Fluid Balance is the more appropriate diagnosis for patients who are starting to exhibit behaviors that demonstrate the ability to maintain adequate fluid balance.

EXPECTED OUTCOME

The client will demonstrate enhanced fluid balance by [date].

Demonstrates balance in 24-hour intake and output.

Verbalizes [number] of lifestyle adaptations that will enhance fluid balance by [date].

TARGET DATES

Client education and support are key interventions for Readiness for Enhanced Fluid Balance. Since the client is already demonstrating positive behaviors, it is recommended that target dates be no further than 3 days from the date of initial diagnosis.

NURSING ACTIONS/INTERVENTIONS WITH RATIONALES	

Adult Health

ACTIONS/INTERVENTIONS	RATIONALES
Assist the patient in documenting plan for adequate fluid intake including types and amounts of fluids.	Assures that devised plan has food choices based on dietary guidelines.
Educate patient to obtain necessary information from food labels.	Assists patient in making appropriate fluid intake choices based on content.
Have patient verbalize appropriate choices for fluid intake.	Demonstrates patient understanding of appropriate fluids for consumption.
Educate patient in regard to adjusting fluid intake relative to physical activity, disease processes, and medications.	Gives patient fundamental basis for decision making.
Educate patient regarding signs and symptoms of fluid imbalances: dependent edema, shortness of breath, concentrated urine, dry mucous membranes, decreased skin turgor, urinary tract infections.	
Have patient document weight on a daily basis.	Assists in trending progress.
Follow-up with patient 3 days after initial diagnosis.	Allows to monitor progress and adjust plan as necessary.
Educate patient regarding signs and symptoms of fluid imbalances: dependent edema, concentrated urine, dry mucous membranes, decreased skin turgor, urinary tract infections.	
Have patient to document weight on a daily basis to assist in trending.	
Follow-up with patient 3 days after initial diagnosis.	Allows to monitor progress and adjust plan as necessary.

Child Health

Oral rehydration offers a realistic treatment option for mild and moderate dehydration and often is suited to home as opposed to hospital management.[58]

ACTIONS/INTERVENTIONS	RATIONALES
Monitor for all contributory patterns to provide a basis for fluid and electrolyte needs, especially prior 24-hour intake and output, losses per stool, surgical losses, and post-op drainage.	Provides fullest database for considering plan for success.
Offer fluids according to plan-see that fluids and electrolytes are offered according to hydration needs* (based on metabolic requisites for size by surface area calculations). Clarify with pediatrician, nurse practitioner, or primary care physician. May also consult	Appropriate fluid amount and composition will best satisfy rehydration needs according to dehydration risk.*

(care plan continued on page 160)

Child Health

ACTIONS/INTERVENTIONS	RATIONALES
Harriet Lane handbook with a desired urinary output of 2 mL/kg minimally.[59] [Note those fluids preferred by the child here.]	
Teach the family to have appropriate fluid and electrolyte solutions including Pedialyte, Infalyte, Resol, Lytren, Nutrilyte, and others, on hand.	Provides guidance for future situations.
Avoid simple sugars, such as soft drinks or Kool-Aid.	Osmotic effects may worsen diarrhea.
Monitor for tolerance of fluid and avoid overfeeding—small feedings regularly are better tolerated.	Lessens likelihood of increased intolerance during initial rehydration phase.
Reassess for hydration status with a focus on urinary output of 2 mL/kg, minimally, level of consciousness, skin turgor, and anterior fontanel status for infants.	
Maintain strict intake and output for the duration of the rehydration experience.	Offers a record for evaluation of effectiveness of plan.
Reassess the caregiver's knowledge for need for rehydration. [Note teaching needs and plan here.]	Provides anticipatory guidance.[59]

Women's Health

The nursing actions for the women's health client with this diagnosis are the same as those for the adult health clients and gerontic health clients. For breastfeeding women, see Effective Breastfeeding diagnosis.

Mental Health

The nursing actions for the mental health client with this diagnosis are the same as those for the Adult Health client.

Gerontic Health

● NOTE: *Dehydration has been reported to be the most common fluid and electrolyte imbalance in older people. Hospitalized elders with dehydration have mortality rates as high as 46 percent. Elders are particularly susceptible to dehydration because of age-related changes such as decreased renal perfusion and sensitivity to antidiuretic hormone (ADH), decreased sense of thirst, decreased mobility, and confusion. In addition, some pathological conditions; such as hypertension and heart and renal disease, make elders highly susceptible to fluid and electrolyte imbalances.[60]*

In addition to the interventions for Adult Health, the following may be utilized for the aging client:

ACTIONS/INTERVENTIONS	RATIONALES
Facilitate client receiving at least 1500 cc/day of oral intake.	Less than this can lead to rapid dehydration.
Regularly and frequently monitor dependent and semidependent clients for adequate fluid intake. These clients should be considered for a restorative fluid program.	Preventive practice.
Utilize a fluid intake sheet to monitor daily fluid intake.	Tracks oral intake and allows for early identification of less than optimal intake.

ACTIONS/INTERVENTIONS	RATIONALES
Regularly and frequently present fluids to bedridden clients. [Note the client's preferred fluids here.]	Facilitates maintenance of adequate hydration status.
Utilize medication time to encourage increased fluid intake.	Medication time can be an important source of fluids.[60]

Home Health/Community Health

In addition to the interventions for Adult Health, the following may be utilized in the community setting:

ACTIONS/INTERVENTIONS	RATIONALES
Monitor the patient's ability to access and pay for adequate beverages. Refer to community resources as appropriate.	Adequate resources facilitate adherence to plan of care. Promotes self-care.
Monitor the patient's ability to obtain adequate beverages. When travel or mobility issues are present, refer to community resources.	Adequate resources facilitate adherence to plan of care. Promotes self-care.
Teach the caregiver and client to maintain oral fluid intake of at least 1500 cc/day.	Minimal amount of fluid required to maintain adequate hydration status.

FLUID VOLUME, DEFICIENT, RISK FOR AND ACTUAL

DEFINITIONS[28]

Risk for Deficient Fluid Volume
The state in which an individual is at risk of experiencing vascular, cellular, or intracellular dehydration.

Deficient Fluid Volume
The state in which an individual experiences decreased intravascular, interstitial, and/or intracellular fluid. This refers to dehydration, water loss alone without change in sodium.

DEFINING CHARACTERISTICS[28]

A. Risk for Deficient Fluid Volume
1. Factors influencing fluid needs (e.g., hypermetabolic state)
2. Medications, for example, diuretics
3. Loss of fluid through abnormal routes (e.g., indwelling tubes)
4. Knowledge deficiency related to fluid volume
5. Extremes of age
6. Deviations affecting access to or intake or absorption of fluids (e.g., physical immobility)
7. Extremes of weight
8. Excessive losses through normal routes, for example, diarrhea
B. Deficient Fluid Volume
1. Weakness
2. Thirst
3. Decreased skin/tongue turgor
4. Dry skin/mucous membranes

5. Increased pulse rate, decreased blood pressure, decreased pulse volume/pressure
6. Decreased venous filling
7. Change in mental state
8. Decreased urine output
9. Increased urine concentration
10. Increased body temperature
11. Elevated hematocrit
12. Sudden weight loss (except in third spacing)

RELATED FACTORS[28]

A. Risk for Deficient Fluid Volume
   The risk factors also serve as the related factors for this diagnosis.
B. Deficient Fluid Volume
   1. Active fluid volume loss
   2. Failure of regulatory mechanisms

RELATED CLINICAL CONCERNS

1. Addison's disease (adrenal insufficiency or crisis)
2. Hemorrhage
3. Burns
4. AIDS
5. Crohn's disease
6. Vomiting and diarrhea
7. Ulcerative colitis

 Have You Selected the Correct Diagnosis?

Impaired Oral Mucous Membrane and Imbalanced Nutrition, Less than Body Requirements
The client may not be able to ingest food or fluid because of primary problems in the mouth, or the

(box continued on page 162)

Have You Selected the Correct Diagnosis? *(box continued from page 161)*

client just may not be ingesting enough food from which the body can absorb fluids.

Bowel Incontinence, Diarrhea, or Urinary Incontinence
These diagnoses may be causing an extreme loss of fluid before it can be absorbed and used by the body.

Impaired Skin Integrity
This diagnosis could be the primary problem. For example, the patient who has been burned has grossly impaired skin integrity. The skin is supposed to regulate the amount of fluid lost from it. If there is relatively little intact skin, the skin is unable to perform its regulatory function and there is significant loss of fluid and electrolytes.

Self-Care Deficit or Impaired Parenting
In the infant or young child, the problem may primarily be a Self-Care Deficit or Impaired Parenting. The infant or young child is not able to obtain the fluid he or she wants and must depend on others. If the parents are unable to recognize or meet these needs, then the infant or young child may have a Risk for or Actual Deficient Fluid Volume. Even in an adult, the primary nursing diagnosis may be Self-Care Deficit. Again, if the adult is unable to obtain the fluid he or she requires because of some pathophysiologic problem, then he or she may have a Risk for or Actual Deficient Fluid Volume.

EXPECTED OUTCOME

Intake and output will balance within 200 mL by [date].

TARGET DATES

Normally, intake and output will approximately balance only every 72 hours; thus, an appropriate target date would be 3 days.

NURSING ACTIONS/INTERVENTIONS WITH RATIONALES

Adult Health

ACTIONS/INTERVENTIONS	RATIONALES
Take vital signs every 2 hours on [odd/even] hour and include apical pulse.	Essential to monitoring of cardiovascular response to illness state and replacement therapy.
Carefully observe any surgical sites for signs of bleeding, hematomas, etc.	
• Observe for signs and symptoms of shock at least every 1 hour at [state times here] (e.g., weakness, diaphoresis, hypotension, tachycardia, or tachypnea).	
Measure and record total intake and output every shift: • Check intake and output hourly. • Document amount and quality of all urine, stools, and vomitus. • Check urine specific gravity every 4 hours at [state times here].	Determines extent of fluid loss, need for replacement, or progress of replacement therapy.
Monitor intravenous fluids in conjunction with I & O. (See Additional Information for Imbalanced Nutrition, Less Than Body Requirements.)	Monitoring of fluid replacement and prevention of fluid overload.
Monitor: • Mental status and behavior at least every 2 hours on the [odd/even] hour	
Weigh daily at [state time here]. Teach the patient to weigh at the same time each day in same-weight clothing.	Monitoring for fluid replacement. Allows consistent comparison of weight.
• Skin turgor at least every 4 hours at [state times here] while awake	
• Electrolytes, blood urea nitrogen, albumin hematocrit, and hemoglobin (Collaborate with health-care provider regarding frequency of laboratory tests.) • Central venous pressure every hour, if appropriate	Essential to determining potential contributing factors to fluid imbalance.

ACTIONS/INTERVENTIONS	RATIONALES
Force fluids to a minimum of 2000 mL daily: Offer small amount of fluid (4 to 5 ounces) at least every hour while awake and at every awakening during night. [Note client's fluid preferences here.] • Interspace fluids with high-fluid-content foods (e.g., popsicles, gelatin, pudding, ice cream, or watermelon). Avoid beverages with diuretic effects. Collaborate with health-care team to determine medications that address source of fluid loss (e.g., antidiarrheals or antiemetics). Assist the patient to eat and drink as necessary. Provide positive verbal support for the patient's consuming fluid.	Prevents dehydration and easily replaces fluid loss without resorting to IVs. Frequent fluids improve hydration; variation in fluids is helpful to encourage the patient to increase intake.
Monitor and address insensible fluid losses. Monitor gastric tubes to suction for large amounts of gastric drainage. Initiate replacements if necessary. Teach the patient, prior to discharge, to increase fluid intake at home during: • Elevated temperature episodes • Periods when infection and elevated temperatures are present • Periods of exercise • Hot weather	
Measures to ensure adequate hydration: • Need to drink fluids before feeling of thirst is experienced • Recognizing signs and symptoms of dehydration such as dry skin, dry lips, excessive sweating, dry tongue, and decreased skin turgor • How to measure, record, and evaluate intake and output	Support the patient's self-care by pointing out measures he or she can use to control fluid imbalance. Adequate intake and early intervention will prevent undesirable outcomes.
Refer to other health-care professionals as necessary.	Provides support and fosters collaboration through use of readily available resources.

Child Health

ACTIONS/INTERVENTIONS	RATIONALES
Measure and record total intake every shift and note 24-hour totals: • Check intake and output hourly (may require weighing diapers or insertion of a Foley catheter [infants may require use of a 5 or 8 feeding tube if size 10 Foley is too large]).	A 24-hour fluid assessment is meaningful for diagnosing deficits and also provides a basis for replacement needs.
• Check urine specific gravity every 2 hours on [odd/even] hour or every voiding or as otherwise ordered.	Specific gravity is a good indicator of degree of hydration.
Force fluids to a minimum appropriate for size (will be closely related to electrolyte needs and cardiac, respiratory, and renal status). [Note fluids preferred by child here.] • Infants: 70 to 100 mL/kg in 24 hours • Toddler: 55 to 70 mL/kg in 24 hours • School-age child: 20 to 50 mL/kg in 24 hours	Prompt replacement and maintenance of appropriate fluids prevents further circulatory or systemic problems. Specific attention is also required with respect to sodium, potassium, and caloric intake. Infants are subject to fluid volume depletion because of their relatively greater surface area, higher metabolic rate, and immature renal function.[61]

(care plan continued on page 164)

NURSING ACTIONS/INTERVENTIONS WITH RATIONALES (continued from page 163)

Child Health

ACTIONS/INTERVENTIONS	RATIONALES
Weigh the patient daily at the same time of day, on the same scale, and in the same clothing (weigh infants without diaper).	Accuracy of weight cannot be overstressed. The weight often serves as a major indicator of the effectiveness of the treatment regimen. Iatrogenic problems are more likely to occur with inaccuracies.
Assist in individualizing oral intake to best suit the patient's needs and preferences. Include parents in designing this plan.	When options exist, honoring them facilitates better compliance with goals and helps the patient and family to feel valued.

Women's Health

ACTIONS/INTERVENTIONS	RATIONALES
Assist the patient to identify lifestyle factors that could be contributing to symptoms of nausea and vomiting during early pregnancy. • Eat small, frequent meals. • Eat dry toast or crackers before arising. • Avoid foods with bothersome smells. • Avoid rich, fatty foods, spicy foods, and greasy foods. • Drink fluids separately from meals. • Drink herbal teas (raspberry leaf or peppermint). • Suck on a cinnamon stick. Identify the patient's support system. Monitor the patient's feelings (positive or negative) about pregnancy. Evaluate social, economic, and cultural conditions. Involve significant others in discussion and problem-solving activities regarding physiologic changes of pregnancy that are affecting work habits and interpersonal relationships (e.g., nausea and vomiting). Teach the patient measures that can help alleviate pathophysiologic changes of pregnancy. In collaboration with the dietitian: • Obtain dietary history. • Assist the patient in planning diet that will provide adequate nutrition for her and her fetus's needs.	Provides basis for treatment of symptoms and basis for teaching and support strategies. There are homeopathy methods of controlling nausea and vomiting of pregnancy including yoga, acupuncture, and rearranging eating patterns during the first 3 to 4 months of pregnancy.[5,62,63]
Teach methods of coping with gastric upset, nausea, and vomiting: • Eat bland, low-fat foods (no fried foods or spicy foods). • Increase carbohydrate intake. • Eat small amounts of food every 2 hours (avoid empty stomach). • Eat dry crackers or toast before getting up in the morning. • Take vitamins and iron with night meal before going to bed (vitamin B, 50 mg, can be taken twice a day but never on an empty stomach).	Provides information, education, and support for self-care during pregnancy. There are homeopathy methods of controlling nausea and vomiting of pregnancy including yoga, acupuncture, and rearranging eating patterns during the first 3 to 4 months of pregnancy.[5,62,63]

ACTIONS/INTERVENTIONS	RATIONALES
• Drink high-protein liquids (e.g., soups or eggnog).[5,62,63] • Avoid foods with bothersome smells. • Avoid rich, fatty foods, spicy foods, and greasy foods. • Drink fluids separately from meals • Drink herbal teas (raspberry leaf or peppermint). • Suck on a cinnamon stick.[5,62,63]	
Monitor the patient for: • Variances in appetite • Vomiting between 12 and 16 weeks of pregnancy • Weight loss • Intractable nausea and vomiting	Provides basis for therapeutic intervention if necessary as well as support of that patient, which can decrease fear and feelings of helplessness.
Collaborate with physician regarding monitoring for: Dehydration • Electrolyte imbalance: hemoconcentration, ketosis with ketonuria, hyponatremia, hypokalemia	Provides support and information to increase self-awareness and self-care.
● NOTE: *"During pregnancy, gastric acid secretion normally is reduced because of increased estrogen stimulation. This places the women at risk for alkalosis, rather than the acidosis that usually occurs in an advanced stage of dehydration."*[64]	
• Hydration (approximately 3000 milliliters/24 hours) and providing vitamin supplements • Restriction of oral intake and providing parental administration of fluids and vitamins.	
● NOTE: *"Vitamin B$_6$ has been found effective and safe for use in nausea and vomiting of pregnancy."*[5]	
Allow expression of feelings and encourage verbalization of fears and questions by scheduling at least 30 minutes with the patient at least once per shift.	
Provide the patient and family with diet information for the breastfeeding mother to prevent dehydration: • Increase daily fluid intake. • Drink at least 2000 mL of fluid daily. • Extra fluid can be taken just before each breastfeeding (e.g., water, fruit juices, decaffeinated tea, or milk). • Eat well-balanced meals to include the basic food groups.	Provides information that allows for successful lactation and healthy recovery from childbirth.
Teach the parents fluid intake needs of the newborn.	Feeding behavior is important not only for fluid but also for food. The caloric need of the infant for the first 3 months is 110 kcal/kg per day, from 3 to 6 months 100 kcal/kg per day, and from 6 to 9 months 95 kcal/kg per day.[5] Breast milk contains adequate nutrients and vitamins for 6 months of life. The American Academy of Pediatrics recommends breastfeeding exclusively for the first 6 months of life and continue breastfeeding with other food induction for at least 12 months.[5]
Monitor the newborn for fluid deficit, and teach the parents to monitor via the following factors: • "Fussy baby," especially immediately after feeding • Constipation (remember, breastfed babies have fewer stools than formula-fed babies) • Weight loss or slow weight gain	Provides information and support for healthy growth and development of the newborn.
Evaluate the baby, mother, and nursing routine: • Is the baby getting empty calories (e.g., a lot of water between feedings)?	

(care plan continued on page 166)

Women's Health

ACTIONS/INTERVENTIONS	RATIONALES
• Monitor the baby for nipple confusion from switching the baby from breast to bottle and vice versa many times. • Count the number of diapers per day (should have six to eight very wet diapers per day). • Monitor the infant for intolerance to the mother's milk or bottle formula. Monitor the baby for illness or lactose intolerances. Monitor how often the mother is nursing the infant (infrequent nursing can cause dehydration and slow weight gain).	

Mental Health

ACTIONS/INTERVENTIONS	RATIONALES
If the client is confused or is unable to interpret signs of thirst, place on intake and output measurement, and record this information every shift.	Medications and/or clouded consciousness may affect the client's ability to recognize need for fluids.
Evaluate potential for fluid deficit resulting from medication or medication interaction (e.g., lithium and diuretics). If this presents a risk, place the client on intake and output measurement every shift.	Estimated daily requirement for adults is 1500 to 3000 mL/day.[65]
Evaluate mental status every shift at [times]. If the client's values and beliefs influence intake: • Alter environment as necessary to facilitate fluid intake, and note alterations here (e.g., if the client thinks fluids from cafeteria are poisonous, have the client assist in making drink on unit). • Provide positive attention to the client at additional times to avoid not drinking as a way of obtaining negative attention.	Basic monitoring to determine the client's ability to independently take fluids.

Gerontic Health

In addition to the interventions for Adult Health, the following may be utilized for the aging client.

ACTIONS/INTERVENTIONS	RATIONALES
Encourage the patient to drink at least 8 ounces of fluid every hour while awake.	Older adults may not experience thirst sensation in response to fluid deprivation. Older clients may not feel thirst or dry mouth, even when dehydrated. When given free access to fluids, older adults tend to drink less than their younger counterparts. Older clients, unprompted, may fail to drink enough fluids to stay adequately hydrated. Thus, frequent offering of fluids to the older adult is essential.
Be sure fluids are within reach of the patient confined to bed.	For those confined to bed or with restricted movement, this action is a simple, basic measure to promote fluid intake.

Home Health/Community Health

ACTIONS/INTERVENTIONS	RATIONALES
Assist the client and family in identifying risk factors pertinent to the situation: • Diabetes • Protein malnourishment • Extremes of age • Excessive vomiting or diarrhea • Medication for fluid retention or high blood pressure • Confusion or lethargy • Fever • Excessive blood loss • Wound drainage • Inability to obtain adequate fluids because of pain, immobility, or difficulty in swallowing	Early intervention in risk situations can prevent dehydration.
Assist the client and family in identifying lifestyle changes that may be required: • Avoiding excessive use of caffeine, alcohol, laxatives, diuretics, antihistamines, fasting, and high-protein diets • Using salt tablets • Exercising without electrolyte replacement	Avoidance of dehydrating activities will prevent excessive fluid loss.

FLUID VOLUME, EXCESS

DEFINITION[28]

The state in which an individual experiences increased fluid retention and edema.[30]

DEFINING CHARACTERISTICS[28]

1. Jugular vein distention
2. Decreased hemoglobin and hematocrit
3. Weight gain over short period
4. Dyspnea
5. Intake exceeds output
6. Pleural effusion
7. Orthopnea
8. S_3 heart sounds
9. Pulmonary congestion
10. Change in respiratory pattern
11. Change in mental status
12. Blood pressure changes
13. Pulmonary artery pressure changes
14. Oliguria
15. Specific gravity changes
16. Azotemia
17. Altered electrolytes
18. Restlessness
19. Anxiety
20. Anasarca
21. Abnormal breath sounds, rales (crackles)
22. Edema
23. Increased central venous pressure
24. Positive hepatojugular reflex

RELATED FACTORS[28]

1. Compromised regulatory mechanisms
2. Excess fluid intake
3. Excess sodium intake

RELATED CLINICAL CONCERNS

1. Congestive heart failure
2. Renal failure
3. Cirrhosis of the liver
4. Cancer
5. Toxemia

☑ Have You Selected the Correct Diagnosis?

Decreased Cardiac Output and Impaired Gas Exchange
The body depends on both appropriate gas exchange and adequate cardiac output to oxygenate tissues and circulate nutrients and fluid for use and disposal. If either of these is compromised, then the body will suffer in some way. One of the major ways the body suffers is in the circulation of body fluid. Fluid will be left in tissue and not absorbed into the general circulation to be redistributed or eliminated.

Imbalanced Nutrition, More Than Body Requirements
This diagnosis could be the primary problem. The person ingests more food and fluid than the body can metabolize and eliminate. The result is excess fluid volume in addition to the other changes in the body's physiology.

(box continued on page 168)

Have You Selected the Correct Diagnosis? *(box continued from page 167)*

Urinary Retention
One way the body compensates fluid balance is through urinary elimination. If the body cannot properly eliminate fluids, then the system "backs up" so to speak, and excess fluid remains in the tissues.

Impaired Physical Mobility
Besides appropriate gas exchange and adequate cardiac output, the body also needs movement of muscles to assist in transporting food and fluids to and from the tissue. Impaired Physical Mobility might lead to an alteration in movement of food and fluids. Waste products of metabolism and excess fluid are allowed to remain in tissues, creating a fluid volume excess.

ADDITIONAL INFORMATION

Excess fluid volume can occur as a result of water excess, sodium excess, or water and sodium excess.[58] Careful assessment and monitoring is needed to recognize the difference in precipitating causes.

Edema: Mild or 1+ means that the skin can be depressed 0 to $1/4$ inch; moderate or 2+ means that the skin can be depressed $1/4$ to $1/2$ inch; severe or 3+ means that the skin can be depressed $1/2$ to 1 inch; and deep pitting edema or 4+ means that the skin can be depressed more than 1 inch and it takes longer than 30 seconds to rebound.

EXPECTED OUTCOME

Intake and output will balance within 200 mL by [date].

● N O T E : *May want difference to be only 50 mL for a child.*

TARGET DATES

In a healthy person, intake and output reach an approximate balance over a span of 72 hours. An acceptable target date would then logically be the third day after admission.

NURSING ACTIONS/INTERVENTIONS WITH RATIONALES

Adult Health

ACTIONS/INTERVENTIONS	RATIONALES
Take vital signs every 2 hours at [state times here], and include apical pulse.	Permits monitoring of cardiovascular response to illness state and therapy.
Check lung, heart, and breath sounds every 2 hours on [odd/even] hour.	Essential monitoring for fluid collection in lungs and cardiac overload due to edema.
Elevate head of bed 30 degrees if not contraindicated.	Facilitates respiration.
Check intake and output hourly (urinary output not less than 30 milliliters/hour).	
Measure and record total intake and output every shift.	Determines extent of fluid balance, need for diuresis, or progress of therapy.
Observe and document quantity and character of urine, vomitus, and stools.	
Check urine specific gravity at least every 2 hours on [odd/even] hour.	
Monitor: • Skin turgor at least every 4 hours while awake. [Note times here.] • Electrolytes, hemoglobin, and hematocrit. Collaborate with health-care team regarding frequency of laboratory tests. • Mental status and behavior at least every 2 hours on [odd/even] hour.	Essential monitoring for fluid and electrolyte imbalance.
Weigh daily at [state times here]. Weigh at same time each day and in same-weight clothing.	Monitoring for fluid replacement. Allows consistent comparison of weight.
Administer medication (e.g., diuretics) as prescribed. Monitor medication effects.	
Collaborate with health-care provider to develop fluid restriction regimen clearly indicating amount per shift.	Restricting fluids prevents cardiovascular system overload and potential pulmonary effects.

ACTIONS/INTERVENTIONS	RATIONALES
Teach the patient to monitor his or her own intake and output at home.	Supports the patient's self-care by pointing out measures he or she can use to control fluid imbalance. Adequate intake and early intervention will prevent undesirable outcomes.
In collaboration with dietitian: • Obtain nutritional history. Refer to other health-care professionals, as appropriate.	Cost-effective use of readily available resources. Promotes interdisciplinary care and thus better care for the patient.

Child Health

ACTIONS/INTERVENTIONS	RATIONALES
Measure and record total intake, output, blood pressure, and pulse every shift: • Check intake and output hourly, and weigh diapers. • Monitor specific gravity at least every 2 hours or as specified.	A strict assessment of intake and output serves to guide treatment for indication of hydration status. The specific gravity assists in determining cardiac, renal, and respiratory function and electrolyte status.
Reposition as tolerated every half-hour.	Prevents stasis of fluids in any one part of body. Assists in circulation of fluid and in preventing skin integrity problems.
Weigh daily at the same time under the same conditions of dress (infants without clothes, children in underwear).	Accuracy of weight is critical; it serves as a major indicator for treatment effectiveness, and is an ongoing parameter for treatment.
Administer medications as ordered with attention to appropriate dosage and potential effect on electrolytes.	Potassium and sodium alterations may be present and must be addressed to prevent further fluid or electrolyte imbalance.
Anticipate potential for respiratory distress and monitor appropriately by cautious checking of breath sounds, respiratory effort, and level of consciousness.	Fluid overload and fluid and electrolyte deviations may lead to respiratory and/or cardiac arrest if undetected or untreated.
Administer fluids per IV with appropriate equipment; i.e., when using Buretrol clamp off main supply of fluids even while on IV pump. Place enough fluid for 2 hours at a time in the Buretrol, and use medium infusion pumps for medications. In young infants, 1 hour of fluid may be used.	Likelihood of iatrogenic fluid overdose is lessened with appropriate safeguards.

Women's Health

● N O T E : *Pregnancy-induced hypertension (PIH), often called the "disease of theories," has been documented for the last 200 years. Numerous causes have been proposed but never substantiated; however, data collected during this time do support the following:*

1. Chorionic villi must be present in the uterus for a diagnosis of PIH to be made.
2. Women exposed for the first time to chorionic villi are at increased risk for developing PIH.
3. Women exposed to an increased amount of chorionic villi (e.g., multiple gestation or hydatidiform mole) are at greater risk for developing PIH.
4. Women with a history of PIH in a previous pregnancy are at increased risk for developing PIH.
5. Women who change partners are more likely to develop PIH in a subsequent pregnancy.
6. There is a genetic predisposition for the development of PIH, which may be a single gene or multifactorial.
7. Vascular disease places the patient at greater risk for developing superimposed PIH.[64]

(care plan continued on page 170)

NURSING ACTIONS/INTERVENTIONS WITH RATIONALES (continued from page 169)

Women's Health

ACTIONS/INTERVENTIONS	RATIONALES
Review the client's history for factors associated with pregnancy-induced hypertension (PIH): • Family and personal history such as diabetes or multiple gestation • Rh incompatibility or hypertensive disorder • Chronic blood pressure 140/90 mm Hg or greater prior to pregnancy, or in the absence of a hydatidiform mole, that persists for 42 days postpartum	Basic database required to assess for potential of PIH.
During current pregnancy, observe for the following characteristics of PIH: • Nulliparous women younger than 20 or older than 35 years of age • Multipara with multiple gestation or renal or vascular disease • Presence of hydatidiform mole	Increased knowledge for the patient will assist the patient with earlier help-seeking behaviors.
Monitor the patient for chronic hypertension[65]: • Increase in systolic blood pressure of 30 mm Hg or diastolic blood pressure of at least 15 mm Hg above baseline on two occasions at least 2 hours apart • Development of proteinuria	
Monitor and teach the patient to immediately report the following signs of PIH: • Increase of 30 mm Hg in blood pressure or 140/90 blood pressure and above • Edema: Weight gain of 5 pounds or greater in 1 week • Proteinuria: 1 g/L or greater of protein in a 24-hour urine collection (2+ by dipstick) • Visual disturbances: blurring of vision or headaches • Epigastric pain	Increased knowledge for the patient will assist the patient with earlier help-seeking behaviors.
Observe closely for signs of severe preeclampsia in any patient who presents with[64]: • Blood pressure greater than or equal to 160 mm Hg systolic, or greater than or equal to 110 mm Hg diastolic, on at least two occasions 6 hours apart with the patient on bedrest • Proteinuria greater than or equal to 5 g in 24 hours or 3+ to 4+ on qualitative assessment • Oliguria: less than 400 mL in 24 hours • Cerebral or visual disturbances • Epigastric pain • Pulmonary edema or cyanosis • Impaired liver function of unclear etiology • Thrombocytopenia	Knowledge of the complexity and multisystem nature of the disease assists with early detection and treatment.
Monitor, at least once per shift, for edema. Teach the patient to: • Monitor swelling of hands, face, legs, or feet. (**Caution:** May need to remove rings.) • Be aware of a possible need to wear loose shoes or a bigger shoe size.	Basic safety measures.

ACTIONS/INTERVENTIONS	RATIONALES
• Schedule rest breaks during day and to elevate feet. • When lying down, to lie on left side to promote placental perfusion and prevent compression of vena cava. In collaboration with the dietitian: • Obtain nutritional history. • Place the patient on high-protein diet (80 to 100 g of protein). • Place the patient on reduced sodium intake (not more than 6 g daily or less than 2.5 g daily). Monitor: • Intake and output: urinary output not less than 30 mL/h or 120 mL/4 h • Effect of magnesium sulfate ($MgSO_4$) and hydralazine hydrochloride (Apresoline) therapy (have antidote for $MgSO_4$ [calcium gluconate] available at all times during $MgSO_4$ therapy) • Deep tendon reflexes (DTR) at least every 4 hours [state times here] • Respiratory rate, pulse, and blood pressure at least every 2 hours on the [odd/even] hour • Fetal heart rate and well-being at least every 2 hours on the [odd/even] hour Institute seizure precautions.	
Ensure bedrest and reduction of noise level in the patient's environment.	Decreases sensory stimuli that might increase the likelihood of a seizure.

Mental Health

ACTIONS/INTERVENTIONS	RATIONALES
Observe chronic psychiatric clients and clients with preexisting alcoholism[66] for signs and symptoms of polydipsia and/or water intoxication. The observations include[66-68]: • Frequent trips to sources of fluid and excessive consumption of fluids • Client stating, "I feel as if I have to drink water all of the time," or a similar statement • Fluid-seeking behavior • Dramatic or rapid fluctuations in weight • Polyuria • Incontinence • Carrying large cups • Urine specific gravity of 1.008 or less[66] • Decreases in serum sodium	A pattern of extreme polydipsia and polyuria can develop in clients with psychiatric disorders. This may be related to dopamine central nervous system activity and dysfunction in antidiuretic hormone activity in combination with psychosocial factors. The sense of thirst can also be increased by certain medications.[67,68]
Discuss the client's explanations for excessive drinking to determine causes of excessive fluid intake. If it is determined that drinking is a diversionary activity or an attempt to avoid interaction, implement nursing actions for Social Isolation and/or Deficient Diversional Activity, as appropriate. If it is determined that fluid intake is related to testing concern of staff or testing limits, refer to nursing actions for Powerlessness or Self-Esteem disturbances.	Determining exact reason for polydipsia allows for more effective intervention.

(care plan continued on page 172)

NURSING ACTIONS/INTERVENTIONS WITH RATIONALES (continued from page 171)

Mental Health

ACTIONS/INTERVENTIONS	RATIONALES
If it is determined that the client is at risk for water intoxication, implement the following actions: • Monitor and document fluid intake and output and weight fluctuations on a daily basis. • Restrict fluids as ordered by physician.	Water intoxication can be life-threatening.[66]
Provide small medicine cup (30 mL) for the client to obtain fluids.	
Provide fluids such as chipped ice on a schedule. [Note schedule here.]	
Instruct the client in need for reducing nicotine consumption. If the client cannot do this, it may be necessary to initiate a "rationing" plan. If so, note plan here.	Nicotine increases release of antidiuretic hormone (ADH), a water-conserving hormone.[66]
Provide the client with sugarless gum and/or hard candy to decrease dry mouth. [Note the client's preference.]	
Identify with the client those activities that would be most helpful in diverting attention from fluid restriction. [Note specific activities here with schedule for use.]	
Refer to occupational and recreational therapists.	
If the client continues to have difficulty restricting fluids, provide increased supervision by limiting the client to day area or other group activity rooms where he or she can be observed. Note restrictions here. If necessary, place the client on one-to-one observation.	
Talk with the client about feelings engendered by restrictions for 15 minutes per shift. [Note times here.]	
Discuss the client's restriction in a community meeting if: • Restrictions are impacting others on the unit. • Support from peers would facilitate client's maintaining restrictions.	
Provide positive verbal support for the client's maintaining restriction(s).	Promotes the client's self-esteem and provides motivation for continued efforts.
Identify with the client appropriate rewards for maintaining restrictions and reaching goals. Describe rewards and behaviors necessary to obtain rewards here.	Promotes the client's self-esteem and sense of control and provides motivation for continuing his or her efforts.

Gerontic Health

Nursing actions for the gerontic health patient with this nursing diagnosis are the same as those for Adult Health and Home Health.

Home Health/Community Health

ACTIONS/INTERVENTIONS	RATIONALES
Teach methods to protect edematous tissue:	Tissue is at risk for injury. The client and family can be taught to minimize risks and damage.

ACTIONS/INTERVENTIONS	RATIONALES
• Practice proper body alignment. • Use pillows, pads, etc. to relieve pressure on dependent parts. • Avoid shearing force when moving in bed or chair. • Alter position at least every 2 hours.	
Assist the client and family to set criteria to help them determine when a physician or other intervention is required.	Planned decision making to prepare for potential crisis.
Assist the client and family in identifying risk factors pertinent to the situation (e.g., heart disease, kidney disease, diabetes mellitus, diabetes insipidus, liver disease, pregnancy, or immobility).	Identification of risk factors and understanding of relationship to fluid excess provide for intervention to reduce or prevent negative outcomes.
Teach signs and symptoms of fluid excess: • Peripheral and dependent edema • Shortness of breath • Taut and shiny skin	Early recognition of signs and symptoms provides data for early intervention.
Assist the client and family in identifying lifestyle changes that may be required: • Avoid standing or sitting for long periods of time; elevate edematous limbs. • Avoid crossing legs. • Avoid constrictive clothing (girdles, garters, knee-high stockings, rubber bands to hold up stocking, etc.). • Consider wearing antiembolism stockings. • Avoid excess salt. Teach the patient and family to read labels for sodium content. Avoid canned and fast foods. • Use spices other than salt in cooking. • Avoid lying in one position for longer than 2 hours. • Raise head of bed or sit in chair if having difficulty breathing. • Restriction of fluid intake as necessary (e.g., usual in kidney and liver disease). • Weigh at the same time every day wearing the same clothes and using the same scale.	Knowledge and support provide motivation for change and increase potential for positive outcome.
Teach purposes and side effects of medication (e.g., diuretics or cardiac medications).	Appropriate use of medication and reduction of side effects.

FLUID VOLUME, IMBALANCED, RISK FOR

DEFINITION[28]

A risk of a decrease, increase, or rapid shift from one to the other of intravascular, interstitial, and/or intracellular fluid. This refers to the loss or excess or both of body fluids or replacement fluids.

DEFINING CHARACTERISTICS[28]

None given.

RISK FACTORS[28]

1. Scheduled for major invasive procedures
2. Other risk factors to be determined

RELATED CLINICAL CONCERNS

1. Any major surgical procedure
2. Any kidney or adrenal gland disease
3. Hemorrhage
4. Burns
5. Any disease impacting the intestines

 Have You Selected the Correct Diagnosis?

Risk for Deficient Fluid Volume
This diagnosis refers to the danger of fluid loss, whereas Risk for Imbalanced Fluid Volume can be either a deficit or an excess. Risk for Fluid Volume Imbalance should be used until the nurse can definitively evaluate in which direction the fluid shift is going.

(box continued on page 174)

Have You Selected the Correct Diagnosis? *(box continued from page 173)*

Excess Fluid Volume
This is an actual diagnosis and signifies a fluid overload.

EXPECTED OUTCOME

Will not exhibit any signs or symptoms of deficient fluid volume or excess fluid volume by [date].

Will have a 24-hour balance in intake and output of fluids by [date].

TARGET DATES

In a healthy person, intake and output reach an approximate balance over a span of 72 hours. An acceptable target date would then logically be the third day after admission.

NURSING ACTIONS/INTERVENTIONS WITH RATIONALES

Adult Health

ACTIONS/INTERVENTIONS	RATIONALES
Measure and record total intake and output every shift.	Determines fluid loss or fluid retention and need for replacement or restriction of fluids.
Check intake and output hourly.	
Check urine specific gravity every 4 hours at [state times here].	
Observe and document color and character of all urine, stools, and vomitus.	
Take vital signs every 2 hours on [odd/even] hour and include apical pulse.	Permits monitoring of cardiovascular response to illness state and therapy.
Check lung, heart, and breath sounds every 2 hours on [odd/even] hour.	
Elevate head of bed as needed.	Facilitates respiration.
Monitor:	Essential monitoring for fluid and electrolyte balance.
• Weight: Weigh daily at [state time here]. Teach the patient to weigh at same time each day in same-weight clothing.	Monitoring for fluid replacement. Allows consistent comparison of weight.
• Skin turgor at least every 4 hours at [state times here] while awake	
• Electrolytes, blood urea nitrogen, hematocrit, and hemoglobin (Collaborate with physician regarding frequency of laboratory tests.)	
• Central venous pressure every hour (if appropriate)	Essential monitoring for intravascular fluid volume balance.
• Mental status and behavior at least every 2 hours on [odd/even] hour	
• For signs and symptoms of shock at least once per hour (e.g., weakness, diaphoresis, hypotension, tachycardia or tachypnea)	
If evidence suggests a fluid volume deficit, see actions for Fluid Volume Deficit, Actual.	
If evidence suggests a fluid volume excess, see actions for Fluid Volume Excess, Actual.	Restricting fluids prevents cardiovascular system overload and reduces workload.

Child Health

ACTIONS/INTERVENTIONS	RATIONALES
Monitor at-risk populations, especially those infants and children scheduled for surgery or procedures in which NPO status is necessary for fluid inbalances.	Greater likelihood exists for fluid volume imbalances with infants or children who undergo surgery during which fluids may be lost or gained in a short period of time.
Determine preoperatively or prior to onset of procedures the ongoing fluid plan for the client with specifications for: • Type of fluid and status of oral feedings • Rate of administration of IV fluid • Electrolyte status and additives to be administered • Accurate weight • Accurate 24-hour intake and output • Recent essential preoperative laboratory tests with abnormal results addressed • Allowance for special drainage or physiologic demands • Past 24-hour specific gravity record	Anticipatory planning provides appropriate focus on risk for deficit or overload for vulnerable infants and children in advance of actual occurrence.
Identify appropriate parameters to be addressed by all members of the health-care team during and after surgery or procedure to include cardiac, renal, neurologic, metabolic, and related physiologic alterations.	Pre-identification of coordination of multidisciplinary specialists assists in appropriate fluid maintenance.
Maintain the patient's temperature during and after surgery or procedure.	Metabolic demands are lessened in the absence of cold stress or hyperthermia.

Women's Health

● N O T E : *Bleeding can occur rapidly during pregnancy, delivery, and postpartum. There is potential for maternal exsanguination within 8 to 10 minutes because of the large amount of blood flowing to the uterus and placenta during pregnancy.*

ACTIONS/INTERVENTIONS	RATIONALES
Monitor the patients presenting to labor and delivery for signs and symptoms of: • Severe abruptio-persistent uterine contractions • Shock out of proportion to blood loss • Rigid, tender, localized uterine pain, and tetanic contractions • Bright red bleeding without pain	Abruptio placentae accounts for approximately 15 percent of all perinatal deaths.
	Placenta previa occurs in 0.005 percent of pregnancies but has a reoccurrence rate of 4 to 8 percent.
Carefully monitor for uterine involution and signs and symptoms of bleeding during delivery and postpartum.	Subinvolution, retained products of conception, uterine atony, and lacerations of the birth canal are the leading causes of postpartum hemorrhage.

Mental Health

The nursing actions for this diagnosis in the mental health client are the same as those for Adult Health.

(care plan continued on page 176)

NURSING ACTIONS/INTERVENTIONS WITH RATIONALES (continued from page 175)

Gerontic Health

● N O T E : *See interventions for Adult Health. Older adults are at risk for this diagnosis as a result of aging changes that affect the ability to respond to volume changes. Renal system changes make responses to volume overload or depletion difficult. Older adults experience a delayed response to a decrease in sodium and are at higher risk for volume depletion. A delay in the ability to excrete salt and water leads to an increased risk for fluid overload and hyponatremia. Postoperatively, the older adult may have excessive or prolonged aldosterone/ADH responses, causing difficulty eliminating excess fluids.*

Home Health/Community Health

ACTIONS/INTERVENTIONS	RATIONALES
Monitor the client for the presence of ascites (e.g., abdominal distention with weight gain) or edema, and report to physician.	Prevents complications of fluid shifts.
Monitor for signs of dehydration: • Dry tongue and skin • Sunken eyeballs • Muscle weakness • Decreased urinary output	Dehydration may accompany fluid shifts such as ascites or edema.
Educate the client and caregivers about the importance of adhering to a sodium-restricted diet (e.g., 250 to 500 mg per day).	Promotes normal fluid balance.
Educate the client and caregivers about medications prescribed to control the fluid volume imbalance (e.g., potassium-sparing diuretics) and possible side effects.	Promotes compliance with prescribed medications.
Assist the client in obtaining supplies necessary to measure intake and output, and teach the client and caregivers how to measure and record intake and output.	Basic monitoring for imbalances.
Monitor balance each nursing visit.	Allows for early identification of progressing fluid imbalances.

HYPERTHERMIA

DEFINITION[28]

A state in which an individual's body temperature is elevated above his or her normal range.

DEFINING CHARACTERISTICS[28]

1. Increase in body temperature above normal range
2. Seizures or convulsion
3. Flushed skin
4. Increased respiratory rate
5. Tachycardia
6. Warm to touch

RELATED FACTORS[28]

1. Illness or trauma
2. Increased metabolic rate
3. Vigorous activity
4. Medications or anesthesia
5. Inability or decreased ability to perspire
6. Exposure to hot environment
7. Dehydration
8. Inappropriate clothing

RELATED CLINICAL CONCERNS

1. Any infectious process
2. Septicemia

3. Hyperthyroidism
4. Any disease leading to dehydration (e.g., diarrhea, vomiting, hemorrhage)
5. Any condition causing pressure on the brainstem
6. Heat stroke

 Have You Selected the Correct Diagnosis?

Risk for Imbalanced Body Temperature
This diagnosis indicates that the person is potentially unable to regulate heat production and dissipation within a normal range. In Hyperthermia, the patient's ability to produce heat is not impaired. Heat dissipation is impaired to the degree that Hyperthermia results.

Ineffective Thermoregulation
Ineffective Thermoregulation indicates that the patient's body temperature is fluctuating between being elevated and being subnormal. In Hyperthermia, the temperature does not fluctuate; it remains elevated until the underlying cause of the elevation is negated

or until administration of medications such as Tylenol and aspirin show a definitive effect on the elevation.

Hypothermia
Hypothermia means the patient's body temperature is subnormal. This indicates the exact opposite measurement from Hyperthermia.

EXPECTED OUTCOME

Will return to normal body temperature (range between 97.3 and 98.8°F) by [date].

TARGET DATES

Because hyperthermia can be life-threatening, initial target dates should be in terms of hours. After the patient has demonstrated some stability toward a normal range, the target date can be increased to 2 to 4 days.

NURSING ACTIONS/INTERVENTIONS WITH RATIONALES

Adult Health

ACTIONS/INTERVENTIONS	RATIONALES
Monitor temperature every [odd/even] hour while the patient is awake and temperature remains elevated. Measure temperature every 2 hours during night. [Note times here.] After temperature begins to decrease, lengthen time between temperature measurements.	Hyperthermia is incompatible with cellular life.
Implement strategies to decrease temperature including sponging the patient with cool water, applying continuous cold packs, providing a tepid bath, or use of a cooling blanket until temperature is lowered to at least 102°F. Dry the patient well, and keep dry and clean.	Basic measures to assist in temperature reduction via heat dissipation. Overchilling could cause shivering, which increases heat production.
Use a fan to cool environment to no less than 70°F.	Promotes cooling via heat dissipation.
Give antipyretic drugs as prescribed. Closely monitor effects, and document effects within 30 minutes after medications given.	Antipyretics assist in temperature reduction. Allows the health-care team to assess the effectiveness of the antipyretic. Ineffectiveness would require repeating medication or changing to a different antipyretic.
Maintain seizure precautions until temperature stabilizes.	Hyperthermia can lead to febrile seizures as a result of overstimulation of the nervous system.
Monitor intake and output, and daily weights.	To avoid fluid volume deficits.
Give skin, mouth, and nasal care at least every 4 hours while awake. [Note times here.]	Hyperthermia promotes mouth breathing in an effort to dissipate heat. Mouth breathing dries the oral mucous membrane.
Change bed linens and pajamas as often as necessary.	Keeping bed linens and pajamas dry helps avoid shivering.
Do not give stimulants.	Stimulants cause vasoconstriction, which could increase hyperthermia.
Gather data relevant to underlying contributing factors at least once per shift.	Control of underlying factors helps prevent occurrence of hyperthermia.

(care plan continued on page 178)

NURSING ACTIONS/INTERVENTIONS WITH RATIONALES (continued from page 177)

Adult Health

ACTIONS/INTERVENTIONS	RATIONALES
Provide health-care teaching, beginning on admission, regarding: • Need for frequent temperature checks • Related medical or nursing care • Safety needs when using ice packs or electric cooling blanket • How family can assist in care • Importance of hydration • Possible fear or altered comfort of patient with fever because of discomfort, fast heart rate, dizziness, and general feeling of illness • Possible seizure activity	Relieves anxiety and allows the patient and family to participate in care. Initiates home care planning.
Carry out appropriate infection control process, in the event or potential event of infectious disease, according to actual or suspected organisms.	Prevents spread of infection.
Assist in obtaining specimens for culture.	Assists in identifying potential causative source.
Assist in promoting a quiet environment.	Allows for essential sleep and rest. Hyperthermia causes increased metabolic rate.

Child Health

ACTIONS/INTERVENTIONS	RATIONALES
Monitor temperature every 30 minutes until temperature stabilizes. • In malignant hyperthermia secondary to response to anesthetic agent such as halothane, prevention includes pre-operative assessment for family history, but risk is still present with each successive surgery.	Frequent assessment per tympanic (aural) thermometer or as specified provides cues to evaluate efficacy of treatment and monitors underlying pathology.
Administer antipyretic, antiseizure, or antibiotic medications as ordered with precaution for: • In diagnosed malignant hyperthermia, dantrolene or similar agent will be given. • Maintenance of IV line • Drug safe range for the child's age and weight • Potential untoward response • IV compatibility • The infant's or child's renal, hepatic, GI status and risk for cardiac arrhythmias secondary to tachycardia	Unique components for each individual patient must be considered within usual treatment modalities to help bring safe and timely return of temperature while avoiding iatrogenic complications.
Provide padding to siderails of crib or bed to prevent injury in event of possible seizures.	Protection from injury in likelihood of uncontrolled sudden bodily movement serves to protect the patient from further problems. Uses universal seizure precautions.
Ensure that airway maintenance is addressed by appropriate suctioning and airway equipment according to age.	As a part of seizure activity, there is always the potential of loss of consciousness with respiratory involvement.
During acute phase of treatment, as applicable, recognizing need for cooling blanket, gastric lavage, and possible cardiopulmonary bypass, assist in explaining procedures to family and provide updates on child's status on a regular basis.	Regular and timely informative updates alleviate fears and assist family in coping.

Women's Health

● N O T E : *Women's Health will have the same nursing actions and rationales as Adult Health, Geronic Health, and Psychiatric Health, except for the following: (Newborn is included with Women's Health because newborn care is administered by nurses in mother-baby units.)*

ACTIONS/INTERVENTIONS	RATIONALES
When under heat source or bililights, monitor the infant every hour for increased redness and sweating. Check heat source at least every 30 minutes (overhead, isolettes, or bililights).	Provides safe environment for the infant.
Monitor the infant's temperature, skin turgor, and fontanels (bulging or sunken) for signs and symptoms of dehydration every 30 minutes while under heat source. First temperature measurement should be rectal; thereafter can be axillary.	Provides essential information as to the infant's current status and promotes a safe environment for the infant.
Check for urination; the infant should wet at least six diapers every 24 hours.	Basic monitoring of the infant's physiologic functioning.
Replace lost fluids by offering the infant breast, water, or formula at least every 2 hours on [odd/even] hour.	Decreases insensible fluid loss and maintains body temperature within normal range. This action decreases the infant's needs for IV glucose.
Pregnancy: • Teach the patient to avoid use of hot tubs or saunas. • During first trimester: Concerns about possible CNS defects in fetus and failure of neural tube closure.[69] • During second and third trimesters: Concerns about cardiac load for mother.[69] • Provide cooling fans for mothers during labor and for patients on $MgSO_4$ therapy. • Keep the labor room cool for the mother's comfort.	Provides safe environment for the mother and prevents injury to the fetus.

Mental Health

Adult Health plan of care provides the foundation care of the mental health client with the following considerations:

ACTIONS/INTERVENTIONS	RATIONALES
Monitor clients receiving neuroleptic drugs for decreased ability to sweat by observing for decreased perspiration and an increase in body temperature with activity, especially in warm weather. Monitor these clients for hyperpyrexia (up to 107°F). Notify physician of alterations in temperature. Note alteration in the client's plan of care and initiate the following actions: • The client should not go outside in the warmest part of the day during warm weather. • Maintain the client's fluid intake up to 3000 mL every 24 hours by (this is especially important for clients who are also receiving lithium carbonate; lithium levels should be carefully evaluated): • Having client's favorite fluids on the unit. • Having the client drink 240 mL (8-ounce) glass of fluids every hour while awake, and 240 mL with each meal. If necessary, the nurse will sit with the client while the fluid is consumed.	Clients who are receiving neuroleptic medications are at risk for developing neuroleptic malignant syndrome, which can be life-threatening.[65]

(care plan continued on page 180)

NURSING ACTIONS/INTERVENTIONS WITH RATIONALES (continued from page 179)

Mental Health

ACTIONS/INTERVENTIONS	RATIONALES
• Maintaining record of the client's intake and output. • Dress the client in light, loose clothing. • If the client is disoriented or confused, provide one-to-one observation. Decrease the client's activity level by: • Decreasing stimuli • Sitting with the client and talking quietly, or involving the client in a table game or activity that requires little large muscle movement. [Note activities that that client enjoys here.] • Assigning room near nurse's station and dayroom areas Monitor the client's mental status every hour. **Do not** provide clients with alteration in mental status with small electrical cooling devices unless they receive constant supervision. Give the client as much information as possible about his or her condition and measures that are implemented to decrease temperature. Teach the client and family measures to decrease or eliminate risk for hyperthermia. (See Home Health for teaching information.) Consult with appropriate assistive resources as indicated.	High fevers can alter mental status and thus decrease the client's ability to make proper judgments. Increased physical activity increases body temperature, and the decreased ability to sweat, secondary to medications, inhibits the body's normal adaptive response.[65]

Gerontic Health

● N O T E : *Normal changes of aging may alter the older client's experience of hyperthermia. Older clients may exhibit diminished sweating and a diminished sensory perception of heat. Thus, careful assessment is essential in older clients.*

In addition to the interventions for Adult Health, the following may be utilized for the aging client.

ACTIONS/INTERVENTIONS	RATIONALES
Facilitate the client's maintenance of adequate hydration, especially during periods of infection, activity, or heat.	Primary prevention.
Teach the client symptoms of heat cramps: • Painful musculoskeletal cramps and spasms • Tender muscles • Moist skin • Normal or slightly elevated body temperature	Allows for early recognition and prevents complications.
For clients with heat cramps, provide oral saline solution, and rest in a cool place.	Prevents complications.
Teach the client symptoms of heat syncope: • Sudden episode of unconsciousness • Weak pulse • Cool and moist skin	Allows for early recognition and prevents complications.
For clients with heat syncope, place the client in a recumbent position, provide oral or IV fluids, and allow for rest in a cool place.	Prevents complications.

ACTIONS/INTERVENTIONS	RATIONALES
Teach clients symptoms of heat exhaustion: • Thirst • Fatigue • Nausea • Reduced urine output • Giddiness or delirium	Allows for early recognition and prevents complications.
For clients with heat exhaustion, allow for rest in a cool environment, and replace fluids with saline solution (oral or IV).	Prevents complications.
Teach clients/caregivers signs of heat stroke: • Absence of sweating • Loss of consciousness	Signifies the need for emergency interventions.
For clients with heat stroke, access emergency services immediately, remove excess clothing, and cool the client rapidly (cold water immersion, ice packs, tepid water spray, fans) without inducing shivering.	Prevents further complications.

Home Health/Community Health

ACTIONS/INTERVENTIONS	RATIONALES
Monitor for factors contributing to hyperthermia. (See Defining Characteristics.)	Identification of risk factors provides for intervention to reduce or prevent negative outcomes.
Teach the client and family signs and symptoms of hyperthermia: • Flushed skin • Increased respiratory rate • Increased heart rate • Increase in body temperature • Seizure precautions and care	Provides data for early intervention.
Teach measures to decrease or eliminate the risk of hyperthermia: • Wearing appropriate clothing • Taking appropriate care of underlying disease • Avoiding exposure to hot environments • Preventing dehydration • Using antipyretics • Performing early intervention with gradual cooling	Provides basic knowledge that increases the probability of successful self-care.
Involve the client and family in planning, implementing, and promoting reduction or elimination of the risk for hyperthermia.	Involvement provides opportunity for increased motivation and ability to appropriately intervene.
Assist the client and family to identify lifestyle changes that may be required: • Measure temperature using appropriate method for developmental age of person. • Learn survival techniques if the client works or plays outdoors. • Ensure proper hydration. • Transport to health-care facility. • Use emergency transport system.	Knowledge and support provide motivation for change and increase potential for a positive outcome.

HYPOTHERMIA

DEFINITION[28]

The state in which an individual's body temperature is reduced below normal range.[28]

DEFINING CHARACTERISTICS[28]

1. Pallor (moderate)
2. Reduction in body temperature below normal range
3. Shivering (mild)
4. Cool skin
5. Cyanotic nail beds
6. Hypertension
7. Piloerection
8. Slow capillary refill
9. Tachycardia

RELATED FACTORS[28]

1. Exposure to cool or cold environment
2. Medications causing vasodilation
3. Malnutrition
4. Inadequate clothing
5. Illness or trauma
6. Evaporation from skin in cool environment
7. Decreased metabolic rate
8. Damage to hypothalamus
9. Consumption of alcohol
10. Aging
11. Inability or decreased ability to shiver
12. Inactivity

RELATED CLINICAL CONCERNS

1. Hypothyroidism
2. Anorexia nervosa
3. Any injury to the brainstem

 Have You Selected the Correct Diagnosis?

Risk for Imbalanced Body Temperature
This diagnosis indicates that the person is potentially unable to regulate heat production and heat dissipation within a normal range. In Hypothermia, the patient's ability to dissipate heat is not impaired. Heat production is impaired to the degree that Hypothermia results.

Ineffective Thermoregulation
The body temperature fluctuates between being too high and too low. In Hypothermia, the temperature does not fluctuate; it remains low.

Hyperthermia
The patient's temperature is above normal, not below normal.

EXPECTED OUTCOME

Will identify at least [number] measures to use in correcting hypothermia by [date]

Body temperature and vital signs will be within normal limits by [date].

TARGET DATES

Hypothermia can be life-threatening; therefore, initial target dates should be in terms of hours. After the patient has demonstrated some stability toward a normal range, target dates can be increased to 2 to 4 days.

NURSING ACTIONS/INTERVENTIONS WITH RATIONALES

Adult Health

ACTIONS/INTERVENTIONS	RATIONALES
Monitor temperature measurement every hour until temperature returns to normal levels and stabilizes.	Assesses effectiveness of therapy.
Warm the patient quickly. Increase room temperature. Use warming blankets and warmed IV fluids; close doors to room.	Basic measures that assist in increasing core temperature and prevent excess heat dissipation. Heat lamps and hot-water bottles warm only a limited area and increase the likelihood of local tissue damage.
Prevent injury. Gently massage body; however, do not rub a body part if frostbite is evident.	Massage helps stimulate circulation; however, massage of a frostbitten area promotes tissue death and gangrene. In frostbite, circulation has to be gradually reestablished through warming.

ACTIONS/INTERVENTIONS	RATIONALES
Address skin protective needs by frequent monitoring for breakdown or altered circulation.	Hypothermia causes peripheral vasoconstriction, which leads to a risk for impaired skin integrity.
Monitor respiratory rate, depth, and breath sounds every hour. Provide for airway suctioning and positioning as needed.	Hypothermia and its related factors promote the development of respiratory complications.
Bathe with appropriate protection and covering.	Prevents heat loss.
Devote appropriate attention to prevention of major complications such as shock, cardiac failure, tissue necrosis, infection, fluid and electrolyte imbalance, convulsions or loss of consciousness, respiratory failure, and renal failure.	Awareness of the complications of hypothermia will help prevent the complication.
Administer medications as prescribed.	
Monitor effects of medication, and record within 30 minutes after administration.	Assists in monitoring effectiveness of therapy.
Obtain a detailed history regarding: • Onset • Related trauma and causative factors • Duration of hypothermia	
Provide opportunities for the patient and family to ask questions and relay concerns by including 30 minutes for this every shift. [Note times here.]	Decreases anxiety and facilitates home care teaching.
Allow for appropriate attention to resolution of psychological trauma, especially in instances of severe exposure to cold at least once per shift. [Note times here.]	Helps in reducing patient's anxiety, and facilitates patient's resolving lingering effects of trauma.
Teach the patient and family measures to decrease or eliminate the risk for hypothermia, to include: • Wearing appropriate clothing when outdoors • Maintaining room temperature at minimum of 65°F • Wearing clothing in layers • Covering the head, hands, and feet when outdoors (especially the head) • Removing wet clothing	Permits the patient to participate in self-care, and promotes compliance to prevent future episodes.
Teach the patient about the kinds of behavior that increase the risk for hypothermia: • Drug and alcohol abuse • Working, living, or playing outdoors • Poor nutrition, especially when body fat is reduced below normal levels as in anorexia nervosa	
Teach the patient and family signs and symptoms of early hypothermia: • Confusion, disorientation • Slurred speech • Low blood pressure • Difficulty in awakening • Weak pulse • Cold stomach • Impaired coordination	
Make appropriate arrangements for follow-up after discharge from hospital. Identify support groups in the community for the patient and family.	Fosters resources for long-term management in terms of adequate housing, financial resources, and social habits.
Consult with appropriate assistive resources as indicated:	Promotes effective long-term management and prevention of future episode.

(care plan continued on page 184)

NURSING ACTIONS/INTERVENTIONS WITH RATIONALES (continued from page 183)

Adult Health

ACTIONS/INTERVENTIONS	RATIONALES
• Obtain an energy audit by public service company to identify possible sources of heat loss. • Refer the patient to social services to provide information on emergency shelters, clothing, and food banks. • Recommend financial counseling if heating the home is financially difficult.	

Child Health

ACTIONS/INTERVENTIONS	RATIONALES
Monitor for level of involvement according to history and contributing factors, and address client's initial stabilization as appropriate. • During the immediate treatment phase, the infant or child may require intensive care to include assisted ventilation and cardiac and renal monitoring as stabilization is achieved.	Treatment is determined by level of involvement with anticipatory planning to restore normal homeostasis.
Provide for maintenance of body temperature by hat (stockinette for infant) and using open radiant warmer, isolette, or heating blanket.	Heat loss is greatest via the head in young infants, as well as by convection and evaporation. Suitable maintenance of temperature by appropriate equipment helps maintain neutral body core temperature.
Incorporate other health-care team members to address collaborative needs.	Provision of support for long-term follow-up places value on the need for care and the importance of compliance. Assists in reducing anxiety.
Monitor for knowledge needs and provide teaching to address unknown and necessary information for the child and family in developmentally appropriate terms (e.g., temperature measurement).	Serves to establish foundation of trust, and provides essential basis for follow-up care.
Anticipate safety needs according to the patient's age and development status. [Note adaptations necessary to meet safety needs here.]	Each opportunity for reinforcing the importance of safety as a part of well-child follow-up should not be overlooked. Emphasize caution with rectal thermometer to prevent trauma to anal sphincter and tissue, and caution the family regarding the use of mercury-glass thermometer and breakage. If electronic equipment is used, emphasize the importance of protection to skin, constant surveillance, and unique safety needs per manufacturer.
Teach caregiver(s) preventive measures to decrease likelihood of recurrence, especially related to minimizing cold exposure with use of clothing appropriate to the season such as suitable bunting and snowsuits in cold climates.	Assists in ensuring careful consideration of dangers of cold exposure for infants and children.

Women's Health

Newborn

● N O T E : *This nursing diagnosis pertains to the woman the same as to any other man. The reader is referred to the other sections for specific nursing actions pertaining to women and hypothermia. Infants control their body temperature with nonshivering thermogenesis; this process is accompanied by an increase in oxygen and calorie consumption. Therefore, use of a radiant warmer or prewarmed mattress for initial care provides environmental heat giving rather than heat losing. However, it is important to note that hypothermia and cold stress in the neonate are related to the amount of oxygen needed by the infant to control apnea and acid–base balance. It is estimated that to replace a heat loss during a temperature drop of 6.3°F, the infant requires a 100 percent increase in oxygen consumption for more than 1½ hours. Metabolic acidosis can occur quickly if the infant becomes hypothermic.[5]*

ACTIONS/INTERVENTIONS	RATIONALES
To prevent hypothermia in the newborn: • Dry the new infant thoroughly. • Cover with blanket. • Lay next to the mother (cover the mother and the infant by placing the blanket over them). • Place the infant under a radiant heat source. • Keep the infant and mother out of drafts. Observe the infant for hypothermia. Check temperature every hour until stable, then every 4 hours times 4, then once a shift in the hospital. Do not use rectal thermometers; take newborn temperatures by axilla or skin probe (continuous probe).	Prevention of heat loss in the infant reduces oxygen and calorie consumption and prevents metabolic acidosis. Skin-to-skin contact with the mother is absolutely the best method of producing and maintaining the infant's thermal balance.

Mental Health

ACTIONS/INTERVENTIONS	RATIONALES
Monitor the client's mental status every 2 hours [note times here]; report alterations to the physician.	Antipsychotic and antidepressant medications can alter thermoregulation, which results in hypothermia.[65]
If the client is receiving antipsychotics or antidepressants, report this to the physician when the alteration is first noted.	
Protect the client from contact with uncontrolled hot objects such as space heaters and radiators by teaching clients and family to remove these from the environment.	
Allow the client to use heating pads and electric blankets only with supervision.	Basic safety measures.
Teach the client the potential for medication to affect body temperature regulation, especially in the elderly.	

Gerontic Health

● N O T E : *Aging clients may experience a diminished sensory perception of temperatures. Other normal changes of aging such as inefficient vasoconstriction, decreased cardiac output, decreased subcutaneous tissue, and decreased shivering may contribute to the development of hypothermia in the aging client.*

(care plan continued on page 186)

Gerontic Health

In addition to the interventions for Adult Health, the following may be utilized for the aging client:

ACTIONS/INTERVENTIONS	RATIONALES
Teach caregivers to recognize the stages of hypothermia: **Early**—no feeling of cold, temperature lower than usual baseline **Mid**—impaired mental functioning, slurred speech, slowed or irregular pulse, diminished tendon reflexes, slow and shallow respirations **Late**—rapid progression of hypothermia, muscular rigidity, diminished urinary output, stupor, coma, cool and pink skin	Older clients may not verbalize typical symptoms of hypothermia owing to a decreased sensory perception of temperatures. Regular and frequent assessment of client status during high-risk times is essential.
Monitor temperature frequently and regularly.	Establishes a baseline and allows for early identification of changes.
Use warming blankets with caution.	Warming blankets may be effective but should be monitored closely, as clients may not verbalize or experience possible hyperthermia that may result.
Utilize warmed IV solutions as appropriate.	Prevention of complications or further hypothermia.
Utilize cardiac monitoring in high-risk clients.	Older clients may experience dysrythmias secondary to hypothermia.
For late-stage hypothermia, consider core rewarming techniques such as cardiac bypass.	Prevention of further complications.

Home Health/Community Health

ACTIONS/INTERVENTIONS	RATIONALES
Involve the client and family in planning, implementing, and promoting reduction or elimination of the risk for hypothermia.	Involvement provides likelihood of increased motivation and ability to intervene appropriately.
Assist the client and family to identify lifestyle changes that may be required: • Avoiding drug and alcohol abuse • Learning survival techniques if the client works or plays outdoors (e.g., camping, hiking, or skiing) • Keeping the person dry • Transporting to health-care facility • Using emergency transport system	Knowledge and support provide motivation for change and increase the potential for a positive outcome.

INFANT FEEDING PATTERN, INEFFECTIVE

DEFINITION[28]

A state in which an infant demonstrates an impaired ability to suck or coordinate the suck-swallow response.

DEFINING CHARACTERISTICS[28]

1. Inability to coordinate sucking, swallowing, and breathing
2. Inability to initiate or sustain an effective suck

RELATED FACTORS[28]

1. Prolonged NPO status
2. Anatomic abnormality
3. Neurologic impairment or delay
4. Oral hypersensitivity
5. Prematurity

RELATED CLINICAL CONCERNS

1. Prematurity
2. Cerebral palsy

3. Thrush
4. Hydrocephalus
5. Any condition that would require major surgery immediately after birth

---

 Have You Selected the Correct Diagnosis?

Ineffective Breastfeeding
With this diagnosis, the infant is able to suckle and swallow, but there is dissatisfaction or difficulty with the breastfeeding process. The key difference would be based on the defining characteristics of Ineffective Breastfeeding versus Ineffective Infant Feeding Pattern. If the infant demonstrates problems with initiating, sustaining, or coordinating sucking, swallowing, and breathing, then Ineffective Infant Feeding Pattern is the most appropriate diagnosis.

Imbalanced Nutrition, Less Than Body Requirements
Certainly this diagnosis could be the result of Ineffective Infant Feeding Pattern if the feeding problem is not remedied. However, correction of the primary problems would prevent the development of this diagnosis.

EXPECTED OUTCOME

Will demonstrate normal ability to suck-swallow by [date].

TARGET DATES

This diagnosis would be life-threatening; therefore, progress should initially be evaluated every few hours. After the infant has begun to exhibit at least some sucking-swallowing, then the target date can be moved to every 2 days, as improvement is made.

NURSING ACTIONS/INTERVENTIONS WITH RATIONALES

Adult Health

For this diagnosis, Child Health and Women's Health (Newborn) serve as the generic actions. This diagnosis would not be used in Adult Health.

Child Health

ACTIONS/INTERVENTIONS	RATIONALES
Monitor for all possible contributory factors: • Actual physiologic sucking potential • Other objective concerns (e.g., swallowing or respiratory) • Objective history data (e.g., prematurity or congenital anomalies) • Maternal or infant reciprocity and degree to which the mother tunes in to infant's cues for readiness for feeding • Subjective data from the caregivers or parents	A thorough assessment and monitoring serves as the critical basis for appropriately individualizing and prioritizing a plan of health care.
Provide anticipatory support to the infant for respiratory difficulties that could increase the probability of aspiration.	Airway maintenance is a basic safety precaution for this infant. Airway and suctioning equipment are standard. (See nursing actions for Risk for Aspiration.)
Ascertain the most appropriate feeding protocol for the infant with attention to:	A realistic yet holistic approach provides a foundation for multidisciplinary management with best likelihood for success.
• Nutritional needs according to desired weight gain • Actual feeding mode (i.e., modified nipple, larger hole nipple, syringe adapted for feeding, position for feeding, or gastric tube)	Specific criteria provide measurable progress parameters.

(care plan continued on page 188)

NURSING ACTIONS/INTERVENTIONS WITH RATIONALES (continued from page 187)

Child Health

ACTIONS/INTERVENTIONS	RATIONALES
• Health status and prognosis • Compliance factors • Socioeconomic factors • Maternal–infant concerns	
Explore the feelings the caregivers or parents have related to the Ineffective Feeding Pattern.	Often the expression of feelings reduces anxiety and may allow further potential alterations to be minimized by early intervention.
Strictly monitor and calculate intake, output, and caloric count on each shift, and total each 24 hours.	Caloric intake and hydration status are indirectly and directly used to monitor the infant's progress in tolerance of feeding and feeding efficacy.
Weigh the infant daily or more often as indicated.	Weight gain would serve as a major indicator of effective feeding and assist in assessment of hydration.
Collaborate with other health-care professionals to better meet the infant's needs.	A multidisciplinary approach is most effective in level and cost of care.
Allow for appropriate time to prepare the infant for feeding, and provide a calm, soothing milieu.	A nonhurried, nonstressful milieu promotes the infant's relaxation and allows the infant to perceive feeding as a pleasant experience.
Facilitate family to participation in feeding and plans for feeding.	Inclusion of the family empowers the family and augments their self-confidence and coping.
Provide teaching based on an assessment of parental knowledge needs and/or deficits. [Note teaching plan here.]	Knowledge provides a means of decreasing anxiety. When based on assessed needs, it will reflect the individualized needs and more likely meet the parents' learning needs.
Allow for time to clarify feeding protocols, questions, and discharge planning. Schedule follow-up with lactation specialist as needed.	Appropriate attention to questions and concerns the parents may have assists in reducing anxiety, thereby allowing for learning and a greater likelihood of adherence to the therapeutic regimen.

Women's Health

ACTIONS/INTERVENTIONS	RATIONALES
Provide support and information to the mother and significant other. Explain the infant's inability to suck, and provide suggestions and options (based on etiology of sucking problem) to correct or reduce the problem.[50,53,70–73]	The basic rationale for all the nursing actions in this diagnosis is to provide nutrition to the infant in the most appropriate, cost-effective, and successful manner.
Describe the anatomy and physiology of sucking to the mother.	Assists in decreasing anxiety, provides a base for teaching, and permits long-range planning.
Explain importance of positioning for both bottle- and breastfeeding.[71–73]	Encourages proper suckling by the infant.
Provide support and supervision to assist the mother in encouraging the infant to suck properly.	

ACTIONS/INTERVENTIONS	RATIONALES
Assist the mother and family to assess appropriate intake by observing the infant for at least six to eight wet diapers in 24 hours (after milk has come in).	Ensures that the infant is getting enough nutrition and is not becoming dehydrated.[50,53,71]
If necessary, provide supplemental nutrition system while teaching the infant to suck (e.g., dropper, syringe, spoon, cup, or supplementation device).[74,75]	Pays attention to basic nutrition while also attending to problem with sucking.
Refer the mother to lactation consultant or clinical nurse specialist for assistance and support in teaching the infant to suck.	
Assist the mother and significant others to choose feeding system for the infant (breast, bottle, cup, or tube) that will supply best nutrition.	Provides basic support to encourage essential nutrition.

Mental Health

This diagnosis would not be used in Mental Health.

Gerontic Health

This diagnosis is not appropriate for the aging patient.

Home Health/Community Health

The nursing actions for Home Health would be the same as for Women's Health.

NAUSEA

DEFINITION[28]

An unpleasant, wave-like sensation in the back of the throat, epigastrium, or throughout the abdomen, that may or may not lead to vomiting.

DEFINING CHARACTERISTICS[28]

1. Reports nausea or "sick to stomach"
2. Increased salivation
3. Aversion toward food
4. Gagging sensation
5. Sour taste in mouth
6. Increased swallowing

RELATED FACTORS[28]

1. Treatment related:
   a. Gastric irritation—pharmaceuticals (e.g., aspirin, non-steroidal anti-inflammatory drugs, steroids, antibiotics, alcohol, iron, and blood)
   b. Gastric distention—delayed gastric emptying caused by pharmacological interventions (e.g., narcotics administration, anesthesia agents)
   c. Pharmaceuticals (e.g., analgesics, antivirals for HIV, aspirin, opioids, chemotherapeutic agents)
   d. Toxins (e.g., radiotherapy)
2. Biophysical
   a. Biochemical disorders (e.g., uremia, diabetic ketoacidosis, pregnancy)
   b. Cardiac pain
   c. Cancer of stomach of intra-abdominal tumors (e.g., pelvic or colorectal cancers)
   d. Esophageal or pancreatic disease
   e. Gastric distention due to delayed gastric emptying, pyloric intestinal obstruction, genitourinary and biliary distention, upper bowel stasis, external compression of the stomach, liver, spleen or other organ enlargement that slows the stomach functioning (squashed stomach syndrome), excess food intake
   f. Gastric irritation due to pharyngeal and/or peritoneal inflammation
   g. Liver or splenetic capsule stretch
   h. Local tumors (e.g., acoustic neuroma, primary or secondary brain tumors, bone metastases at the base of the skull)
   i. Motion sickness, Ménière's disease, or labyrinthitis

j. Physical factors (e.g., increased intracranial pressure, meningitis)
k. Toxins (e.g., tumor produced peptides, abnormal metabolites due to cancer)
3. Situational
Psychological factors (e.g., pain, fear, anxiety, noxious odors, taste, unpleasant visual stimulation)

RELATED CLINICAL CONCERNS

1. Any surgical procedure
2. Cancer
3. Any gastrointestinal disease
4. Viruses
5. Pregnancy

 Have You Selected the Correct Diagnosis?

There really are no other diagnoses that could be confused with this diagnosis.

EXPECTED OUTCOME

Will self-report no nausea by [date].

TARGET DATES

Because uncontrolled nausea and vomiting can quickly lead to fluid and electrolyte imbalance, target dates should be at 24-hour intervals until the nausea is controlled.

NURSING ACTIONS/INTERVENTIONS WITH RATIONALES

Adult Health

ACTIONS/INTERVENTIONS	RATIONALES
Avoid food smells or unpleasant odors.	Olfactory sense is important in the total dining experience.
Avoid greasy, fatty meals.	Greasy foods promote nausea.
Collaborate with the patient and dietitian about food likes and dislikes. [List foods here.]	Helps patient feel a part of his or her health-care regimen.
Try small, frequent feedings. Drink fluids between meals rather than with meals.	Reduces the amount of food in the stomach and avoids the feeling of fullness.
Elevate the head of bed or position on right side for 30 minutes after eating if not contraindicated.	Promotes digestion by gravity.
Teach diversion, guided imagery, and relaxation.[76]	Reduces stress and takes the mind off the nausea.
Place a cold washcloth over eyes and cheeks.	Cools the face and diverts blood and attention away from the stomach.
Collaborate with the health-care provider regarding alternative treatments.[77]	
Consider alternative therapies such as ginger, peppermint, or cinnamon. [Note use for client here.]	Alternative treatments to calm the stomach.
Administer antiemetic medications as prescribed. Monitor for effects.[78–83]	

Child Health

ACTIONS/INTERVENTIONS	RATIONALES
Monitor for all possible contributory factors including: • Actual physiologic components (electrolyte imbalances, history of cancer, altered metabolic status, bilirubin elevations, increased intracranial pressure, gastrointestinal irritation/deviations, etc.) • Potential pharmacologic agents (chemotherapy agents, medications, or allergens) • Emotional concerns of the client and family or significant others • Subjective data from all who have influence in the care of the client	A thorough assessment provides the most appropriate base of data for individualized care.

ACTIONS/INTERVENTIONS	RATIONALES
Identify the pattern of nausea, including known precedent auras or sensations, triggering stimuli, correlation of stimuli to perception of nausea or suggestion of nausea, physical signs and symptoms noted, length of duration of symptoms, factors noted to ameliorate perceived nausea, and ongoing effects nausea exerts.	A thorough assessment of the pattern assists in individualization of care with the intent of remaining open to ongoing priorities, as well as the identification of other nursing problems.
Develop a plan for dealing with nausea with an element of ongoing monitoring every 1 hour, or more often as needed, for goal of lessening of perceptions or suggested nausea if the client is unable to express sensations.	An individualized plan of care with specific needs addressed will best afford successful management of nausea.
• Note signs and symptoms suggestive of nausea.	
• Correlate signs and symptoms with other sensations, stimuli, or events.	
• Identify measures to alleviate perceived sensation of nausea, such as cold cloth on forehead, administration of antiemetics, or other specific antinausea medications.	
• Provide a therapeutic milieu to promote rest. Eliminate noxious stimuli of noise, odors, and light. Maintain room temperature at a comfortable and steady level.	
• Determine the need for presence of the parent or significant other to provide a sense of security for the infant or child. [Note client-specific management plan here.]	
Collaborate with other health professionals as needed to best address needs for the client and family.	A multidisciplinary approach offers the most inclusive and cost-effective approach for care.
Offer developmentally appropriate coping mechanisms to enhance the child's sense of self-worth and likelihood of cooperation.	Appropriate developmental approach is critical to success in creating the best effort for self-worth of the infant or child and the parent.

Women's Health

The nursing actions for this diagnosis are the same as for Adult Health.

Mental Health

The nursing actions for this diagnosis in the mental health client are the same as those in Adult Health.

Gerontic Health

In addition to the interventions for Adult Health, the following may be utilized for the aging client:

ACTIONS/INTERVENTIONS	RATIONALES
Carefully assess fluid and volume status frequently and regularly.	Nausea, even in the absence of vomiting, may lead to fluid and electrolyte imbalances as the client may avoid any oral intake when nauseated. Older clients are at increased risk for fluid and volume status imbalances.
Consider dietary modifications as appropriate to include: • Small frequent meals • Reduced fat content • Avoidance of indigestible or partially indigestible materials • Avoiding carbonated beverages	Reduces exposure to factors that may contribute to nausea.

(care plan continued on page 192)

NURSING ACTIONS/INTERVENTIONS WITH RATIONALES (continued from page 191)

Gerontic Health

ACTIONS/INTERVENTIONS	RATIONALES
Consider antiemetic agents or prokinetic agents as appropriate.	Pharmacologic therapy, when given as prescribed, can alleviate existing nausea and prevent further episodes.
Review the older adult's medications to determine whether GI problems are noted as a side effect.[23]	Many drugs taken by older adults, such as opioids, antidepressants, and anticholinergics, have nausea as a side effect.[84]
Determine whether the older adult is using herbs (aloe, senna, cascara) to alleviate problems with constipation.	Using large amounts of herbal laxatives may cause nausea.[85]
Discuss with the client, if noted, stress effects on the GI system, and assist the client with relaxation strategies as needed to reduce stress.	Stress can lead to reductions in peristalsis and digestive enzymes and cause nausea, anorexia, abdominal distention, or vomiting.[57]
Monitor the infusion rate of tube feeding, if present, to prevent rapid feeding.	Rapid feeding rates can produce nausea.[86]

Home Health/Community Health

ACTIONS/INTERVENTIONS	RATIONALES
Educate the client and caregivers on how to deal with nausea: • Avoid sudden changes in position. • Keep the environment clean and free of noxious odors. • Keep the environment well ventilated; a fan or open window is often helpful. • Use relaxation or diversion. • Apply cool washcloths to the face and neck. • Avoid hot baths or a hot environment.	Increases the ability to manage situations quickly and independently. Prevents episodes of nausea from external factors.
Help the client identify foods that may precipitate episodes of nausea.	Prevents future episodes.
Educate the client and caregivers in the administration of prescribed antiemetics. Help the client to clearly identify accompanying symptoms to assist the physician in prescribing the correct type of antiemetics.	Promotes a sense of independence by the client, and facilitates obtaining appropriate prescriptions.
Help the client to identify prescription medications, particularly antibiotics and opioids, that may be causing the nausea.	Facilitates changing prescriptions as necessary.
When the client believes that foods can be tolerated, encourage him or her to start with clear liquids at moderate temperatures and progress to soft bland foods in small amounts.	Rapidly reintroducing solid food may stimulate nausea and vomiting.

NUTRITION, READINESS FOR ENHANCED

DEFINITION[28]

A state in which an individual's pattern of nutrient intake is sufficient for meeting metabolic needs and can be strengthened.

DEFINING CHARACTERISTICS[28]

1. Expresses willingness to enhance nutrition
2. Eats regularly
3. Consumes adequate food and fluid
4. Expresses knowledge of healthy food and fluid choices
5. Follows an appropriate standard for intake (e.g., the food pyramid or American Diabetic Association guidelines)

6. Safe preparation and storage for food and fluids
7. Attitude toward eating and drinking is congruent with health goals

RELATED FACTORS[28]

1. Mechanical (pressure, shear, and friction)
2. Radiation (including therapeutic radiation)
3. Nutritional deficit or excess
4. Thermal (temperature extremes)
5. Knowledge deficit
6. Irritants
7. Chemical (including body excretions, secretions, and medications)
8. Impaired physical mobility
9. Altered circulation
10. Fluid deficit or excess

RELATED CLINICAL CONCERNS

1. New diagnoses that would necessitate nutritional alterations, such as Diabetes.
2. Treatments that require alterations in nutrition
3. Developmental change in nutritional needs.

 Have You Selected the Correct Diagnosis?

Risk for Imbalanced Nutrition: More Than Body Requirements.
If the patient's nutrient intake exceeds his or her metabolic needs, then the most correct diagnosis is Risk for Imbalanced Nutrition: More than Body Requirements. Readiness for enhanced nutrition would be the most appropriate diagnosis if the patient has behaviors demonstrating a tendency toward nutrient intake that is appropriate for metabolic needs.

EXPECTED OUTCOME

The client will verbalize plan to enhance nutrition by [date].
The client will identify [number] of alterations in current nutritional patterns that will enhance nutrition by [date].

TARGET DATES

Client education and support are key interventions for Readiness for Enhanced Nutrition. Since the client is already demonstrating positive behaviors, it is recommended that target dates be no further than 3 days from the date of initial diagnosis.

NURSING ACTIONS/INTERVENTIONS WITH RATIONALES

Adult Health

ACTIONS/INTERVENTIONS	RATIONALES
Assist the patient in devising a dietary plan that meets recommended dietary allowances.	Ensures that the devised plan has food choices based on dietary guidelines.
Educate the patient regarding supplements if he or she is unable to meet nutrient intake needs through dietary intake.	
Assist patient in devising schedule that facilitates regular meals.	
Have the patient verbalize appropriate food choices.	Demonstrates patient understanding of appropriate food choices.
Review with the patient appropriate food handling strategies including refrigeration, heating, handling, etc.	Integral to safety.
Educate the patient in regard to adjusting caloric intake in accordance with physical activity.	Helps balance caloric intake with expenditures.
Educate the patient to obtain necessary information from food labels.	Assists the patient in making appropriate food choices when considering content.
Consult with a nutritionist as necessary.	
Follow-up with the patient 3 days after initial diagnosis [list date here].	Monitors patient progress and need for modification of plan.

(care plan continued on page 194)

NURSING ACTIONS/INTERVENTIONS WITH RATIONALES (continued from page 193)

Child Health

ACTIONS/INTERVENTIONS	RATIONALES
Assess for all contributory factors, especially reasons for disruption in usual nutrition pattern, such as surgery, illness, or other.	Offers the fullest database for consideration of a plan that is individualized.
Determine the ability of the caregiver to provide feedings as determined by schedule and type, especially if formula is difficult to obtain or costly.	Offers anticipatory guidance for prevention of inability to follow regimen.
Refer to community resources for nutritional assistance, i.e., WIC. [Note referral information here.]	Provides resources for the essential plan.
Teach the caregiver when and how to weigh infant or young child, and when to notify primary care physician or pediatrician.	Provides anticipatory support to boost the confidence of the caregiver.
Teach the caregiver about the importance of a calm environment during feedings and about providing adequate rest periods.	Assists in creation of a stress-free environment to facilitate normal digestive processes.

Women's Health

Nursing actions for this diagnosis are the same as those for Adult Health.

Mental Health

Nursing actions for this diagnosis are the same as those for Adult Health.

Gerontic Health

Nursing actions for this diagnosis are essentially the same as those for Adult Health and Home Health.

Home Health/Community Health

Nursing actions for this diagnosis in the home patient are essentially the same as those for Adult Health and Home Health with the following additions:

ACTION/INTERVENTIONS	RATIONALES
Monitor the patient's ability to pay for adequate quality and quantity of foods. Refer to community resources as appropriate.	Adequate resources facilitate adherence to plan of care. Promotes self-care.
Monitor the patient's ability to obtain adequate quality and quantity of foods. When travel or mobility issues are present, refer to community resources.	Adequate resources facilitate adherence to plan of care. Promotes self-care.

NUTRITION, IMBALANCED, LESS THAN BODY REQUIREMENTS

DEFINITION[28]

The state in which an individual experiences an intake of nutrients insufficient to meet metabolic needs.

DEFINING CHARACTERISTICS[28]

1. Pale conjunctival and mucous membranes
2. Weakness of muscles required for swallowing or mastication
3. Sore, inflamed buccal cavity

4. Satiety immediately after ingesting food
5. Reported or evidence of lack of food
6. Reported inadequate food intake less than RDA (recommended daily allowance)
7. Reported altered taste sensation
8. Perceived inability to ingest food
9. Misconception
10. Loss of weight with adequate food intake
11. Aversion to eating
12. Abdominal cramping
13. Poor muscle tone
14. Abdominal pain with or without pathology
15. Lack of interest in food
16. Body weight 20 percent or more below ideal
17. Capillary fragility
18. Diarrhea and/or steatorrhea
19. Excessive loss of hair
20. Hyperactive bowel sounds
21. Lack of information; misinformation

RELATED FACTORS[28]

Inability to ingest or digest food or absorb nutrients as a result of biologic, psychological, or economic factors.

RELATED CLINICAL CONCERNS

1. Anorexia nervosa or bulimia
2. Cancer
3. AIDS
4. Alzheimer's disease
5. Anemia
6. Ostomies
7. Schizophrenia, paranoid

 Have You Selected the Correct Diagnosis?

Impaired Oral Mucous Membrane
If the oral mucous membranes are severely inflamed or damaged, food intake could be so painful that the person ceases intake to avoid the pain. Although the end result might be Imbalanced Nutrition, Less Than Body Requirements, initial intervention needs to be aimed at handling the oral mucosal problem.

Diarrhea
In this instance, the body cannot absorb the necessary nutrients because the food passes through the gastrointestinal tract too rapidly.

Ineffective Tissue Perfusion
Once the food has been ingested, digested, and absorbed, its components must get to the cells. If there is Altered Tissue Perfusion, the nutrients may not be able to get to the cells in sufficient quantities to do any good.

Self-Care Deficit, Feeding, or Disturbed Sensory Perception: Visual, Olfactory, and/or Gustatory, or Ineffective Health Maintenance
One of these diagnoses may be the primary problem. If the person does not sense hunger through the usual means—seeing, smelling, or tasting—or if the person thinks he or she has already eaten, then the desire to eat may not exist. Even if the person senses hunger, the inability to feed oneself, to shop for food, or to prepare food could result in less than adequate nutrition.

Pain
If the preparation or actual eating of food increases pain level, then the patient might elect to avoid eating to assist in pain control.

Fear, Dysfunctional Grieving, Social Isolation, Disturbed Body Image, Alteration in Self-Esteem, and Spiritual Distress
These diagnoses are psychosocial problems that can impact nutrition. Each of these may create a decreased desire to eat, or even if food is eaten, the person may vomit because the stomach will not accept the food. In addition, if the person eats, he or she may only pick at the food and not ingest enough to maintain the body's need for nutrients.

Deficient Knowledge
The person may not really know how much or what kind of food is more beneficial to his or her body.

EXPECTED OUTCOME

Will gain [number] pounds by [date].

TARGET DATES

This diagnosis reflects a long-term care problem; therefore, a target date of 5 days or more from the date of admission would be acceptable.

NURSING ACTIONS/INTERVENTIONS WITH RATIONALES

Adult Health

ACTIONS/INTERVENTIONS	RATIONALES
Include patient in collaboration efforts with dietitian/ nutritionist menu to achieve desired nutritional intake.	

(care plan continued on page 196)

Adult Health

ACTIONS/INTERVENTIONS	RATIONALES
• Administer appropriate medications 30 minutes before meals (e.g., analgesics or antiemetics); record effects of medications within 30 minutes of administration.	
Provide a rest period of at least 30 minutes prior to meal.	Conserves energy for feeding self and digestion.
Provide an environment that entices the patient to eat and facilitates the patient's eating: • Reduce noxious stimuli. • Open all food containers and release odors outside the patient's room. • Raise the head of bed. • Open carton and packages. • Cut food into small, bite-size pieces. • Provide assistive devices (e.g., large-handled spoon or fork, all-in-one utensil, or plate guard).	
Offer small, frequent feedings every 2 to 3 hours rather than just three meals per day. Allow the patient to assist with food choices and feeding schedules.	Three large meals a day give a sense of fullness, and the size of servings may be overwhelming to the patient. Smaller meals facilitate gastric emptying, thus promoting a larger food intake overall.
Offer between-meal supplements. Focus on high-protein diet and liquids.	Provides additional caloric intake. Providing high-protein foods and fluids helps prevent muscle-tissue loss.
Encourage significant others to bring special food from home.	Familiar food promotes appetite and empowers the patient and family in regard to the diet. Allows an opportunity for teaching diet.
Maintain calorie count with every meal. Review daily intake.	Monitors goal attainment or identifies areas for improvement.
As goal weight is achieved, allow patient to increase physical activity. Coordinate with physical/occupational therapy.	Stimulates appetite.
Monitor: • Vital signs every 4 hours while awake at [state times here] and as required based on measurement results • Airway, sensorium, chest sounds, bowel sounds, skin turgor, mucous membranes, bowel function, urine specific gravity, and glucose level at least once per shift • Laboratory values (e.g., electrolyte levels, hematocrit, hemoglobin, blood glucose, serum albumin, and total protein)	Allows early detection of complications, and assists in monitoring effectiveness of therapy.
Make sure intake and output is balancing at least every 72 hours.	Ensures that weight gain is not due to fluid retention.
Weigh daily at [state time] and in same-weight clothing. Have the patient empty bladder before weighing. Teach the patient this routine for continued weighing at home.	Assesses effectiveness of therapy and interventions. Promotes the patient's control of weight after discharge.
Provide frequent positive reinforcement for: • Weight gain • Increased intake • Using consistent approach	

ACTIONS/INTERVENTIONS	RATIONALES
Teach the patient and significant others: • Balanced diet based on the dietary recommendations • Role of diet in health (e.g., healing, energy, and normal body functioning) • How to keep food diary with calorie count • Adding spices to food to improve taste and aroma • Use of exchange lists • Relaxation techniques	Provides essential information needed to prevent future episodes.
Teach patient strategies that lend to success of goal: • Encourage the patient to eat slowly. • Avoid gas-producing foods and carbonated beverages. • Allow rest periods of at least 30 minutes after feeding.	Facilitates the digestion process. Gas-producing foods promote nausea and a feeling of fullness. Facilitates digestion and reduces stress.
Educate the patient on consuming nutrient-dense foods.	
Refer, as necessary, to other health-care providers.	Provides ongoing support for long-term care.

ADDITIONAL INFORMATION

There will be situations in which the patient's nutritional condition has progressed or clinical situation warrants that tube feedings or total parenteral nutrition will become necessary. In addition to the nursing actions for the overall nursing diagnosis of Imbalanced Nutrition, Less Than Body Requirements, the following actions should be added:

NURSING ACTIONS/INTERVENTIONS WITH RATIONALES

Tube Feedings

ACTIONS/INTERVENTIONS	RATIONALES
Check placement and patency prior to each feeding. Initial placement should be checked using radiographic verification because auscultatory methods are not always accurate. Check gastric aspiration for acidic pH.[87,88]	Prevents aspiration.
Aspirate the tube prior to each feeding. If 150 mL or more, delay feeding and notify appropriate health-care provider.	Assesses for patient tolerance of enteral feeds.
Check the temperature of the feeding before administering. The temperature should be slightly below room temperature.	Prevents abdominal cramping and reflux.
Measure the amount of feeding exactly. Monitor infusion rate at least every 4 hours around the clock at [times].	Assures consistency with prescribed feeding regimen.
Keep the patient in a semi-Fowler's position or on right side for at least 30 minutes following feeding if not contraindicated.	Prevents reflux and aspiration of feeding.
If feeding is to be administered by gravity method (preferred), make sure all air is out of tubing and use caution to not feed too quickly.	Air in stomach creates a feeling of fullness and gas.
Collaborate with the health-care team regarding initiation of protein supplements.	
Monitor respiratory rate, effort, and lung sounds at least every 4 hours around the clock at [times].	Allows monitoring for possible aspiration.
Monitor for side effects including diarrhea.	Diarrhea can exacerbate nutritional imbalance.

(care plan continued on page 198)

NURSING ACTIONS/INTERVENTIONS WITH RATIONALES (continued from page 197)

Total Parenteral Nutrition

ACTIONS/INTERVENTIONS	RATIONALES
Check insertion site for warmth, redness, swelling, leakage, and pain at least every 4 hours at [state times here].	Basic monitoring for infiltration and venous irritation.
Verify order for appropriate formula.	
Check flow rate once every hour.	Prevents fluid overload.
Implement institution appropriate standards for administration, including tubing and dressing changes, and use of filters. [Note schedule here.]	
Do not administer without pump.	The pump allows for accurate flow rate.
Check for signs and symptoms of circulatory overload at least every 2 hours [state times here] (e.g., headache, neck vein distention, tachycardia, increased blood pressure, or respiratory changes).	

Child Health

● N O T E : *This diagnosis represents a long-term care issue. Therefore, a series of subgoals of smaller amounts of weight to be gained in a lesser period of time may be necessary. Long-term goals are still to be formulated and revised as the patient's status demands. Also, there will undoubtedly be instances in which overlap may exist for other nursing diagnoses. Specifically, as an example, in the instance of an alteration in nutrition related to actual failure to thrive, one must refer to appropriate role performance on the part of the mother with consideration for holistic nursing management. It would be most critical to include a few specific nursing process components to reflect the critical needs for the mother–infant dyad.*

Adult health interventions can be utilized as indicated with the following considerations:

ACTIONS/INTERVENTIONS	RATIONALES
Determine all contributory factors, especially underlying malabsorptive conditions secondary to congenital anomalies.	Variable degrees of involvement will demand appropriate follow-up to consider the fullest needs for nursing intervention.
*Short bowel syndrome may constitute a long term need for treatment with in-depth teaching needs.	
Feed the infant on a regular schedule that offers nutrients appropriate to metabolic needs. For example, an infant of less than 5 pounds will eat more often, but in lesser amounts (2 to 3 ounces every 2 to 3 hours) than an infant of 15 pounds (4 to 5 ounces every 3 to 4 hours).	The stomach capacity and digestive concerns for each patient must be considered to realistically plan for weight gain over a slow, steady, incremental time frame.
Assist or feed the patient:	Appropriate attention to aesthetic, physical, and emotional details related to feeding helps provide the optimal potential for pleasant, long-lasting eating patterns. The limitation of psychological and emotional duress cannot be overemphasized, and must be considered in each parent–child unit.
• Elevate the head of bed, or place the infant in infant seat, and older infant or toddler in high chair with safety belt in place. If necessary, hold the infant. (This will be dictated in part by the patient's status and presence of various tubes and equipment.)	Facilitates digestion and provides interactive times for caregiver(s) and infant or young child.

ACTIONS/INTERVENTIONS	RATIONALES
• Help the patient wash hands. For infants and toddlers, administer diaper change as needed.	Prevents risk of infection.
• Warm foods and formula as needed, and test on wrist before feeding the infant or child.	Safety for potential hyperthermic injury.
• Provide aids appropriate for age and physical capacity as needed, such as two-handed cups for toddlers, favorite spoon, or Velcro strap for utensils for child with cerebral palsy.	Favors self-care according to developmental capacity.
• Offer small, age-appropriate feedings with input from family members regarding the child's preferences.	Offers the family input to best meet the child's need and likelihood for adequate nutrition.
• Encourage the patient to eat slowly and to chew food thoroughly. For infant, bubble before, during, and after feeding.	Assists in tolerance of feeding.
Role-model for parents, in a nonthreatening, nonjudgmental manner, feeding an infant or child.	Nonthreatening role-modeling and personal encouragement foster compliance and lessen anxiety.
Weigh the patient on same scale and at same time [state time here] daily. Weigh infants without clothes, older children in underwear.	Weight gain serves as a critical indicator of efficacy of treatment. Maintaining consistency in weighing lessens the number of potential intervening variables that would result in an inaccurate weight.
Teach the patient and family: • Balanced diet appropriate for age using basic food groups • Role of diet in health (e.g., healing, energy, and normal body functioning). If the infant is medically diagnosed as Failure to Thrive, offer appropriate emotional support and allow at least 30 minutes three times a day [state times here] for exploring dyad relationships • How to use spices and child-oriented approach in encouraging the child to eat (e.g., peach fruit salad, with peach as a face, garnished with cherries and raisins for eyes and nose, half of a pineapple round for mouth) • Monitoring for possible food allergies, especially in toddlers with history of allergies • How to weigh self appropriately, if applicable, or for parents to weigh the child	
Provide positive reinforcement as often as appropriate for the parents and child, demonstrating critical behavior.	Reinforcement of desired behaviors fosters long-term compliance, thereby empowering the family with satisfaction and confidence for ultimate self-care management with minimal intervention by others.

Women's Health

● NOTE: *Poverty and substance abuse are often associated with nutritional deficits. Remember that underweight women who are pregnant will exhibit a different pattern of weight gain than normal-weight women. This difference exhibits a rapid weight gain at the beginning of the first trimester of about 1 pound per week by 20 weeks. In the underweight woman, weight gain can be as much as 18 to 20 pounds. Remember to teach the parents signs and symptoms of weight loss in the neonate.[49]*

ACTIONS/INTERVENTIONS	RATIONALES
Collaborate with the dietitian in planning and teaching diet:	Gives baseline from which to plan better nutrition.

(care plan continued on page 200)

NURSING ACTIONS/INTERVENTIONS WITH RATIONALES (continued from page 199)

Women's Health

ACTIONS/INTERVENTIONS	RATIONALES
• Emphasize high-quality calories (cottage cheese, lean meats, fish, tofu, whole grains, fruits, and vegetables). • Avoid excess intake of fats and sugar. • Assist the patient in identifying methods to keep caloric intake within the recommended limit. Verify pre-pregnant weight. Determine whether weight loss during first trimester is due to nausea and vomiting. Check activity level against daily dietary intake. Check for food intolerances. Check environmental influences: • Hot weather • Cultural practices • Pica eating • Economic situation • Ascertain economic status and ability to buy food • Monitor woman's emotional response to the pregnancy and to additional weight gain	Assist in planning realistic diet changes within the patient's means and according to the patient's particular needs and habits.

● **N O T E**: *Dieting is never recommended during pregnancy because it deprives the mother and fetus of nutrients needed for tissue growth, and because weight loss is accompanied by maternal ketosis, a direct threat to fetal well-being.*[5,62]

ACTIONS/INTERVENTIONS	RATIONALES

Identify additional caloric needs and sources of those calories for the nursing mother.[89,90]
• An additional 500 calories/day above normal dietary intake is needed to produce adequate milk (depending on the individual, a total of 2500 to 3000 calories/day).
• Additional fluids are necessary to produce adequate milk.
 	
Collaborate with nutritionist to provide a health dietary pattern for the lactating mother.
 	
Monitor the mother's energy levels and health maintenance:
• Does she complain of fatigue?
• Does she have sufficient energy to complete her daily activities?
• Does the dietary assessment show irregular dietary intake?
• Is she more than 10 percent below the ideal weight for her body stature?
For breastfeeding the newborn or neonate during the first 6 months, teach the mother:
• The major source of nourishment is human milk.
• Vitamin supplements can be used as recommended by physician:
  • Vitamin D
  • Fluoride
  • If indicated, iron
	Provides basis for ensuring good nutrition, and assists in successful breastfeeding.

ACTIONS/INTERVENTIONS	RATIONALES
The infant should be taking in approximately 420 mL daily soon after birth and building to 1200 mL daily at the end of 3 months.	Provides for good nutritional status of the newborn.
Monitor for fluid deficit at least daily: • "Fussy baby," especially if immediately after feeding • Constipation (remember breastfed babies have fewer stools than formula-fed babies)	Allows early intervention for this problem.
Weight loss or slow weight gain: Closely monitor the baby, the mother, and nursing routine: • Is the baby getting empty calories (e.g., a lot of water between feedings)? • Avoid nipple confusion, which results from switching the baby from breast to bottle and vice versa many times. • Instruct the mother in "cup feeding" of nursing infant to ensure adequate fluid intake and avoid nipple confusion.[50,54,59] • Count the number of diapers per day (should have six to eight very wet diapers per day). • Is there intolerance to mother's milk or bottle formula? • Is there illness or lactose intolerance? • Infrequent nursing can cause slow weight gain.	Provides the infant with nutrition, while supporting the breastfeeding mother.[63]

Mental Health

● N O T E : *Because of long-term care requirements for these clients, target dates should be determined in weeks or months, not hours or days.*

ACTIONS/INTERVENTIONS	RATIONALES
Do not attempt teaching or long-term goal setting with the client until concentration has improved (symptom of starvation).	Starvation can affect cognitive functioning.[91]
Establish contract with the client to remain on prescribed diet and not to perform maladaptive behavior (e.g., vomiting or use of laxatives). State specific behavior and rewards for the client here. • Plan gradual refeeding with incremental progression Provide vitamin and mineral supplements as prescribed.	Provides the client with a sense of control, and clearly establishes the consequences and rewards for behavior. Weight gain of 2 to 3 pounds/week for inpatient care and 0.5 to 1 pound/week is reasonable.[92]
Place the client on 24-hour constant observation (this will be discontinued when the client ends maladaptive behavior, or at specific times that nursing staff assess are low risk).	Provides consistency and structure during the stressful early period of treatment.
Place the client on constant observation during meals and at high-risk times for maladaptive behavior (such as 1 hour after meals or while using the bathroom). This action will take effect when the preceding one is discontinued.	Provides support for the client during stressful period.
Do not allow the client to discuss weight or calories. Excessive discussion of food is also discouraged.	Decreases the client's abnormal focus on food and promotes normal eating patterns. This behavior is more indicative of starvation than an eating disorder.[91]
Require the client to eat prescribed diet (all food on tray each meal except for those three or four foods the client was allowed to omit in the admission contract). List the client's omitted food here.	Promotes the client's sense of control and participation in decision-making within appropriate limits.

(care plan continued on page 202)

NURSING ACTIONS/INTERVENTIONS WITH RATIONALES (continued from page 201)

Mental Health

ACTIONS/INTERVENTIONS	RATIONALES
Sit with the client during meals, and provide positive support and encouragement for the feelings and concerns the client may have.	Provides a positive, supportive context for the client.[91]
Do not threaten the client with punishment (tube feeding or IVs).	
Report all maladaptive behavior to the client's primary nurse or physician for confrontation in individual therapy sessions.	
Spend [number] minutes with the client every [number] minutes to establish relationship.	
Respond to queries related to fears of being required to gain too much weight with reassurance that the goal of treatment is to return the client to health, and that he or she will not be allowed to become overweight. Also reinforce the risks of eating disorder.	
Provide the client with information on bingeing and purging and the impact they have on dieting and the body.	Provides the client with increased information about his or her behaviors. Does not impact calorie loss and destroys the tissue of the upper GI tract.[93]
If the client vomits, have him or her assist with the cleanup, and require him or her to drink an equal amount of a nutritional replacement drink.	Provides natural consequences for behavior.
Schedule the client for group therapy (specific encouraging behavior should be listed here, such as assisting the client to complete morning care on time or other interventions that are useful for this client).	Provides support from peers and a source of honest feedback.[91]
Encourage the client's family by [list specific encouraging behaviors for this family] to attend family therapy sessions.	Provides support for the family and an opportunity for the family to work through their concerns together.[91]
Assist the client with clothing selection. Clothes should not be too loose, hiding weight loss, or too tight, assisting the client to feel overweight even though appropriate weight is achieved.	Altered body image makes it difficult for clients to make appropriate choices; honest feedback and support from the nursing staff makes the transition to "healthy" choices easier.
Have the client develop a daily food diary that records time of day, amount and type of food, and binge or purge behavior with feelings and thoughts.	Assists clients in linking thoughts with behaviors.[93]
When maintenance weight is achieved, assist the client with selection of appropriate foods from hospital menu.	As symptoms of starvation are resolved, the client is better able to make appropriate choices, and gradual returning of control prepares the client to accept responsibility at discharge.[91]
When maintenance weight is achieved, refer to the dietitian for teaching about balanced diet and home maintenance.	
When maintenance weight is achieved, refer to occupational therapist for practice with menu planning, trips to grocery stores to purchase food, and meal preparation.	
When maintenance weight is achieved, plan passes with the client for trips to restaurants for meals.	Provides further information to the client to assist in maintaining desired weight. Provides visible reward for weight maintenance.

ACTIONS/INTERVENTIONS	RATIONALES
Allow the client to exercise [number] minutes [number] times per day while supervised (this will be altered as the client reaches maintenance weight).	
Allow the client to do the following exercises during the exercise period. (These are graded to the client's physical condition. Consultation with the occupational therapist is useful.)	
Allow the client [number] of [number] minute walks on hospital grounds with a staff member each day.	Assists the client in developing realistic goals for exercise according to age and ability.
Meet with family/significant others [number] minutes [number] times per week to discuss positive family interactions and support for client. In this meeting model appropriate communication and develop plan for responding to the client's eating patterns. Refer to nursing actions for Family Processes, Interrupted for more in depth plan to address family interaction issues.	Family support, education, and therapy improve outcomes of eating disorder treatment.[92]
• Facilitate the development of a specific plan for ongoing care and support after discharge. [Note that plan here with the names of contact persons.]	

Gerontic Health

In addition to the interventions for Adult Health, the following may be utilized with the aging client.

● N O T E : *National Clinical Guidelines recommend in cases of clients with weight loss problems, that the client or their proxy have a full discussion of their health-care wishes with a health-care professional. A discussion of the treatment goals and the resident's ongoing quality of life, should be initiated. The decision they make should be documented. Certain causes of malnutrition may be irreversible.[94]*

ACTIONS/INTERVENTIONS	RATIONALES
Monitor and record client's weight each week.	Establishes a baseline and allows for early identification of changes.
Monitor and record client's hydration status regularly. Elders should ingest between 1500 and 2000 mL per day.[94]	Establishes a baseline and allows for early identification of changes.
Ensure environmental conditions at mealtime are conducive to adequate intake: • Palatable, minimally restrictive diet • Pleasant, well lit, unhurried mealtimes • Social environment at mealtime[94]	
For clients with dependency in eating, establish and adhere to restorative feeding program.[94]	Recognition of feeding problems and proper feeding techniques may improve weight loss in nursing homes.[94]
Involve family with visits or assistance with feeding at mealtimes.[94]	
Use calorie-dense foods whenever possible.[94]	
Initiate or maintain an exercise program when appropriate.[94]	Exercise may increase dietary intake.[94]
Offer nutritional supplements between meals and not to substitute for calorie intake at meals.[94]	To increase dietary intake.[94]
Evaluate the client for possible depression and treat accordingly.[94]	Depression may be a reversible cause of decreased dietary intake.[94]

(care plan continued on page 204)

NURSING ACTIONS/INTERVENTIONS WITH RATIONALES (continued from page 203)

Gerontic Health

ACTIONS/INTERVENTIONS	RATIONALES
Consult with a pharmacist to determine drugs that might be producing anorexia.[94]	Drugs have been found to be a cause of weight loss in long term care residents.[94]

Home Health/Community Health

The long-term nature of this diagnosis requires long-term goals that are measured in weeks or months. Short-term goals can be established to assess patient understanding of interventions.

ACTIONS/INTERVENTIONS	RATIONALES
Monitor the client's ability to pay for adequate quantity and quality of food. Refer client to community resources for assistance as appropriate.	Financial factors and availability of food should be addressed prior to other factors.
Reduce associated factors, for example: • Minimize noxious odors by using foods that require minimal cooking; or if someone else is cooking for the client, arrange for the client to be away from the cooking area. • Provide social atmosphere desired by the client. • Plan medications to decrease pain and nausea around mealtime. • Plan meals away from area where treatments are performed. • Maintain oral hygiene before and after meals. Instruct the client and family in proper brushing, flossing, and use of water pick. • Facilitate client's request for or preparation of favorite foods. • Avoid foods that contribute to noxious symptoms such as gas, nausea, or GI distress. • Discourage fasting. Teach stress-reduction exercises. • Maintain exercise program as tolerated.	Provides positive environment to promote nutritional intake.
Teach to add high-calorie, high-protein, and high-fat items to meal preparation activities (e.g., use milk in soups; add cheese to food, and use butter or margarine in soups and vegetables).	Promotes weight gain and prevents loss of muscle mass.
Teach or provide assistance to rest before meals. If the client is doing the meal preparation, teach to cook large quantities and freeze several meals at a time and to seek assistance in meal preparation when fatigued.	Provides optimal conditions to avoid excess fatigue.

NUTRITION, IMBALANCED, MORE THAN BODY REQUIREMENTS, RISK FOR AND ACTUAL

DEFINITIONS[28]

Risk for Imbalanced Nutrition: More Than Body Requirements The state in which an individual is at risk of experiencing an intake of nutrients that exceeds metabolic needs.

Imbalanced Nutrition: More Than Body Requirements The state in which an individual is experiencing an intake of nutrients that exceeds metabolic needs.

DEFINING CHARACTERISTICS[28]

A. Risk for (presence of risk factors such as):
  1. Reported use of solid food as major food source before 5 months of age
  2. Concentrating food intake at end of day

3. Reported or observed obesity in one or both parents
4. Reported or observed higher baseline weight at beginning of each pregnancy
5. Rapid transition across growth percentiles in infants or children
6. Pairing food with other activities
7. Observed use of food as reward or comfort measure
8. Eating in response to internal cues other than hunger, such as anxiety
9. Eating in response to external cues such as time of day or social situation
10. Dysfunctional eating patterns

B. **More Than Body Requirements**
1. Triceps skin fold greater than 15 mm in men, or 25 mm in women
2. Weight 20 percent more than ideal for height and frame
3. Eating in response to external cues such as time of day or social situation
4. Eating in response to internal cues other than hunger (e.g., anxiety)
5. Reported or observed dysfunctional eating pattern (e.g., pairing food with other activities)
6. Sedentary activity level
7. Concentrating food intake at end of day

RELATED FACTORS[28]

1. Risk for: The risk factors also serve as the related factors.
2. More Than Body Requirements: Excessive intake in relation to metabolic needs.

RELATED CLINICAL CONCERNS

1. Alzheimer's disease
2. Morbid obesity
3. Hypothyroidism
4. Disorders requiring medicating with corticosteroids

5. Any disorder resulting in prolonged immobility
6. Metabolic syndrome

 Have You Selected the Correct Diagnosis?

Deficient Knowledge
The patient, because of his or her cultural background, may not know the appropriate food groups and the nutritional value of the foods. In addition, the cultural beliefs held by a patient may not value thinness. Therefore, the people of a particular culture may actually promote obesity.

Ineffective Health Maintenance
Because of other problems, the patient may not be able or willing to modify nutritional intake even though he or she has information about good nutritional patterns.

Other Possible Diagnoses
Several diagnoses from the psychosocial realm may be the underlying problem that has resulted in Risk for or More Than Body Requirements. Powerlessness, Self-Esteem Disturbance, Social Isolation, Disturbed Body Image, or Ineffective Individual Coping may also need to be dealt with in the patient who is at risk for or actually has Imbalanced Nutrition, More Than Body Requirements.

EXPECTED OUTCOME

Will lose [number] pounds by [date].
　　Will verbalize plan for healthy weight loss by [date].
　　Will identify [number] behaviors that facilitate weight loss by [date].

TARGET DATES

Because this diagnosis reflects long-term care in terms of both cause and correction, a target date of 5 days or more would not be unreasonable.

NURSING ACTIONS/INTERVENTIONS WITH RATIONALES

Adult Health

ACTIONS/INTERVENTIONS	RATIONALES
Assist the patient to identify dysfunctional eating habits, during first day of hospitalization, by: • Associating times of eating and types of food with corresponding events (e.g., in response to internal cues or in response to external cues) • Review the patient's dietary and activity patterns	Provides basic information needed to plan changes in dysfunctional habits to begin weight-loss program.
Discuss with the patient potential or real motivation for desiring to lose weight at this time.	Assists in understanding the patient's rewards for goals, and assists in establishment of goals and rewards.

(care plan continued on page 206)

NURSING ACTIONS/INTERVENTIONS WITH RATIONALES (continued from page 205)

Adult Health

ACTIONS/INTERVENTIONS	RATIONALES
Discuss with the patient past attempts at weight loss and factors that contributed to their success or failure.	Provides increased individualization and continuity of care, which facilitates the development of a therapeutic relationship.[95]
Weigh the patient daily at [state time]. Teach the patient to weigh self at the same time each morning in same clothing. Help the patient to establish a graphic to allow visualization of progress (e.g., bar chart, chart with gold star for each weight-loss day).	Provides a visible means of ascertaining weight-loss progress.
Limit the patient's intake to number of calories recommended by the physician and/or nutritionist.	Reduces calories to promote weight loss yet maintain body's nutritional status.
Have the patient design own weight-loss plan at least 3 days prior to discharge to allow practice and revision as necessary: • Maintain accurate calorie count every shift. Review every 24 hours.	Allows the patient to assume control for long-term therapy. The more the patient is involved in planning care, the higher the probability for compliance. Monitors progress toward goals. Gives tangible feedback to patient.
Collaborate with physical therapist in establishing an exercise program. Assist the patient in selecting an exercise program by providing the patient with a broad range of options, and have the client select one he or she will enjoy. [Note client's plan for exercise here.]	Exercise burns calories and tones muscles. Assists in narrowing the range between calories consumed and calories burned. Facilitates development of adaptive coping behaviors.
Assist the patient to establish a food diary, during first day of hospitalization, which should be maintained until weight has stabilized to desired goal. The diary should include specific details of eating habits including the foods, where consumed, when consumed, and specific factors surrounding consumption and physical activity.	Helps the patient to identify real intake and to identify behavioral and emotional antecedents to dysfunctional eating behavior.[32,33,96]
Teach the patient the principles of a balanced diet, or refer to dietitian for instructions, at least 3 days before discharge.	Provides basic knowledge needed to control weight at home. Promotes self-care. Promotes the patient's perception of control.
Review pros and cons of alternate weight-loss options with the patient: • Fad diets • Enrollment in weight loss programs • Surgery	Promotes safety in weight-loss plan. Avoids serious complications such as heart failure due to questionable weight-loss ideas.
Demonstrate adaptations in eating that could promote weight loss: • Smaller plate • One-half of usual serving • No second servings	Assists in behavior modification needed to lose weight.
Suggest that the patient contract with a significant other or home health nurse prior to discharge. Consult with the family and visitors regarding importance of the patient's adhering to diet. Caution against bringing food, etc., from home.	Provides added reinforcement and support for continued weight loss. Involves others in supporting the patient in weight-loss effort.

ACTIONS/INTERVENTIONS	RATIONALES
Refer to community resources at least 3 days before discharge from hospital. Refer the patient and family to psychiatric nurse practitioner for appropriate techniques to use at home, as well as assistance with guilt, anxiety, etc. over being obese.	Provides long-range support for continued success with weight loss.

Child Health

Orders are the same as for the adult. Make actions specific to the child according to the child's developmental level.

Women's Health

ACTIONS/INTERVENTIONS	RATIONALES
Verify the pre-pregnancy weight.	Provides basis for planning diet with the patient.
Obtain a 24-hour diet history. Ask the patient to select a typical day.	
Calculate the woman's calorie and protein intake.	
Rule out excessive edema and hypertension. Measure ankles and abdominal girth and record. Remeasure each day. Measure blood pressure every 4 hours while the patient is awake at [state times here].	
Encourage the client to increase her activity by: Joining exercise groups for pregnancy (usually found in childbirth classes in community):	Assists in maintaining desired weight gain; improves muscle tone and circulation.
• Joining swim exercise groups for pregnancy (usually found at YWCAs or community centers)	
Refer to appropriate support groups for assistance in exercise programs for the pregnant woman (e.g., physical therapist, local groups that have swimming classes for pregnant women, and childbirth classes).	
If recommended intake is 2400 calories/day but 24-hour diet recall reveals a higher caloric intake:	Basic measures and teaching factors to assist in weight control.
• Recommend reduction of fat in diet (e.g., decrease amount of cooking oil used, use less salad dressing and margarine, cut excess fat off meat, and take skin off chicken before preparing).	
• Monitor size of food portions.	
• Stress appetite control with high-quality sources of energy and protein.	
Assist mothers with cultural or economic restrictions to introduce more variety into their diets.	
Stress that weight gain is the only way the fetus can be supplied with nourishment.	
Point out that added body fat will be burned and will provide necessary energy during lactation (breastfeeding).	
Assist pregnant adolescents within 3 years of menarche to plan diets that have needed additional nutrients.	Diet has to be planned to meet the growth needs of the adolescent as well as those of the fetus.
Discourage any attempts at weight reduction or dieting.	Dieting is never recommended during pregnancy because it deprives the mother and the fetus of nutrients needed for tissue growth, and because weight loss is accompanied by maternal ketosis, a direct threat to fetal well-being.[70]

(care plan continued on page 208)

NURSING ACTIONS/INTERVENTIONS WITH RATIONALES (continued from page 207)

Women's Health

ACTIONS/INTERVENTIONS	RATIONALES
A satisfactory pattern of weight gain for the average woman is: • 0 weeks of gestation 650 g (approximately 1.5 lb) • 20 weeks of gestation 4000 g (approximately 9.0 lb) • 30 weeks of gestation 8500 g (approximately 19.0 lb) • 40 weeks of gestation 12,500 g (approximately 27.5 lb)[5]	Over the course of the pregnancy, a total weight gain of 25 to 35 pounds is recommended for both nonobese and obese pregnant women. During the second and third trimesters, a gain of about 1 pound/week is considered desirable.[5]

Mental Health

Nursing actions for the Mental Health client with this diagnosis are the same as those actions in Adult Health with the following considerations:

ACTIONS/INTERVENTIONS	RATIONALES
Monitor client's taking psychotropic (especially atypical antipsychotics) medications for increased weight, blood pressure, fasting plasma glucose, and lipid profile.	Atypical antipsychotics are associated with greater metabolic dysfunction, including weight gain, changes in serum triglycerides, and glycemic control.[96]
If the client shows weight gain of 5 percent or more from baseline, consult with physician to prescribe a more weight/metabolic neutral medication.	Modest weight loss can have a significant impact on risk factors. Metabolically neutral medications have been demonstrated to improve weight and other metabolic measures.[96]
Teach the patient about this side effect of the medications, and the need to monitor his or her weight, blood sugars, and lipids.	Increases the client's sense of control.
Spend [number] minutes per day discussing client's perception of his or her weight and nutrition needs.	Change depends on the client's perception of the problem.[97]
Spend [number] minutes per day planning weight management program with client that is based on the client's perceptions of need and goals. Plan needs to include diet alterations and exercise. [Note plan here with nursing actions needed to support the plan.]	Successful weight management plans have been behavioral and included diet and exercise.[96]
• Develop, with the client, specific behavioral rewards for meeting diet and exercise goals. Note these rewards and goals with weight management plan.	Positive reinforcement increases behavior.
Consult with the nutritionist to develop a diet plan and to provide nutritional education. [Note schedule for meetings with nutritionist here, and client's plan with the assistance needed from nursing to implement the plan.]	
Consult with physical, recreational, and occupational therapy to assist client in developing an exercise and recreational activity plan.	Developing a plan that includes activities the client enjoys increases potential for continuing the activity.
Refer client to community support systems for diet and exercise. Note those resources here. Provide client with phone numbers and names of contact persons.	
Meet with client's support system to review current dietary needs and to develop a plan that can be implemented in the home.	

Gerontic Health

Nursing actions for the gerontic patient with this diagnosis are the same as those actions in Adult Health and Home Health.

Home Health/Community Health

ACTIONS/INTERVENTIONS	RATIONALES
Assist the client in identifying lifestyle changes that may be required: • Regular exercise at least three times per week, which includes stretching and flexibility exercises and aerobic activity (20 minutes) at target training rate. • Nutritional habits should include decreasing fat and simple carbohydrates, and increasing complex carbohydrates.	Knowledge and support provide motivation for change and increase the potential for positive outcomes.
Assist the client and family in identifying cues other than focus on weight and calories, such as feeling of well-being, percentage of body fat, increased exercise endurance, and better-fitting clothes.	Excess focus on the weight, as measured by the scale, and on calorie counting may increase the probability of failure and encourage the pattern of repeated weight loss followed by weight gain. This pattern results in increased percentage of body fat.
Have the client and family design personalized plan: • Menu planning • Decreased fats and simple carbohydrates, and increased complex carbohydrates • Regular, balanced exercise • Lifestyle changes	A personalized plan improves the probability of adherence to the plan.
Assist clients in identifying local resources for obtaining and ideal weight (e.g., support groups, Weight Watchers).	Support facilitates success in obtaining and maintaining ideal weight.
Assist client in modifying their environment to facilitate healthy food choices (pantry and refrigerator).	Improves probability of adherence to selected plan.
Monitor the client's ability to pay for healthy foods. Some clients may select calorie dense foods that are less expensive. Refer client to community resources for financial assistance with food as appropriate.	Improves probability of adherence to selected plan.

SWALLOWING, IMPAIRED

DEFINITION[28]

Abnormal functioning of the swallowing mechanism associated with deficits in oral, pharyngeal, or esophageal structure or function.

DEFINING CHARACTERISTICS[28]

1. Pharyngeal phase impairment
   a. Altered head position
   b. Inadequate laryngeal elevation
   c. Food refusal
   d. Unexplained fevers
   e. Delayed swallowing
   f. Recurrent pulmonary infections
   g. Gurley voice quality
   h. Nasal reflux
   i. Choking, coughing, or gagging
   j. Multiple swallowing
   k. Abnormality in pharyngeal phase by swallowing study
2. Esophageal phase impairment
   a. Heartburn or epigastric pain
   b. Acidic-smelling breath
   c. Unexplained irritability surrounding mealtime
   d. Vomitus on pillow
   e. Repetitive swallowing or ruminating
   f. Regurgitation of gastric contents or wet burps
   g. Bruxism
   h. Nighttime coughing or awakening
   i. Observed evidence of difficulty in swallowing (e.g., stasis of food in oral cavity, coughing, or choking)

j. Hyperextension of head, arching during or after meals
k. Abnormality in esophageal phase by swallow study
l. Odynophagia
m. Food refusal or volume limiting
n. Complaints of something stuck
o. Hematemesis
p. Vomiting
3. Oral phase impairment
   a. Lack of tongue action to form bolus
   b. Weak suck resulting in inefficient nippling
   c. Incomplete lip closure
   d. Food pushed out of mouth
   e. Slow bolus formation
   f. Food falls from mouth
   g. Premature entry of bolus
   h. Nasal reflux
   i. Long meals with little consumption
   j. Coughing, choking, or gagging before a swallow
   k. Abnormality in oral phase of swallow study
   l. Piecemeal deglutition
   m. Lack of chewing
   n. Pooling in lateral sulci
   o. Sialorrhea or drooling
   p. Inability to clear oral cavity

RELATED FACTORS[28]

1. Congenital deficits
   a. Upper airway anomalies
   b. Failure to thrive or protein energy malnutrition
   c. Conditions with significant hypotonia
   d. Respiratory diseases
   e. History of tube feeding
   f. Behavioral feeding problems
   g. Self-injurious behavior
   h. Neuromuscular impairment (e.g., decreased or absent gag reflex, decreased strength or excursion of muscles involved in mastication, perceptual impairment, facial paralysis)
   i. Mechanical obstruction (e.g., edema, tracheostomy tube, tumor)
   j. Congenital heart disease
   k. Cranial nerve involvement
2. Neurologic problems
   a. Upper airway anomalies
   b. Laryngeal abnormalities
   c. Achalasia
   d. Gastroesophageal reflux disease
   e. Acquired anatomic defects
   f. Cerebral palsy
   g. Internal trauma
   h. Tracheal, laryngeal, esophageal defects
   i. Traumatic head injury

j. Developmental delay
k. External trauma
l. Nasal or nasopharyngeal cavity defects
m. Oral cavity or oropharyngeal abnormalities
n. Premature infants

RELATED CLINICAL CONCERNS

1. Cerebrovascular accident
2. Any neuromuscular diagnosis (e.g., myasthenia gravis, muscular dystrophy, cerebral palsy, Parkinson's disease, Alzheimer's disease, poliomyelitis)
3. Hyperthyroidism
4. Any medical diagnosis related to decreased level of consciousness (e.g., seizures, concussions, increased intracranial pressure)
5. Tracheoesophageal problems (e.g., fistula, tumor, edema, or presence of tracheostomy tube)
6. Anxiety

 Have You Selected the Correct Diagnosis?

Impaired Oral Mucous Membrane
Impaired Swallowing implies that there is a mechanical or physiologic obstruction between the oropharynx and the esophagus. An Impaired Oral Mucous Membrane indicates that only the oral cavity is involved. Structures below the oral cavity, per se, are not affected. If liquids or solids are able to pass through the oral cavity, even though pain or difficulty might be present, there will be nothing obstructing its passage through the esophagus to the stomach. Therefore, if solids or liquids are able to pass into the stomach without crowing, coughing, or choking, the appropriate nursing diagnosis is **not** Impaired Swallowing.

Imbalanced Nutrition, Less Than Body Requirements
Certainly Imbalanced Nutrition, Less Than Body Requirements would be a consideration and probably a secondary problem to Impaired Swallowing. Choosing between the two diagnoses would be based on the related factors, with Impaired Swallowing taking priority over the Impaired Nutrition initially.

EXPECTED OUTCOME

Will be able to freely swallow [solids/liquids] by [date].

TARGET DATES

Because Impaired Swallowing can be life-threatening, the patient should be checked for progress daily. After the condition has improved, progress could be checked at 3-day intervals.

NURSING ACTIONS/INTERVENTIONS WITH RATIONALES

Adult Health

ACTIONS/INTERVENTIONS	RATIONALES
Monitor for lesions or infectious processes of the mouth and oropharynx at least once per shift.	Lesions or ulcers in the mouth promote difficulty in swallowing.
Test, before every offering of food, fluid, etc., for presence of gag reflex.	To prevent choking and aspiration.
Before offering food or fluids, test swallowing capacity with clear, sterile water **only**. Have suctioning equipment and tracheostomy tray on standby in the patient's room.	Provides equipment needed in case of aspiration or respiratory obstruction emergency.
Maintain appropriate upright position during feeding.	Gravity assists in facilitation of swallowing.
Stay with the patient while he or she tries to eat.	Basic safety measure for the patient who has difficulty in swallowing.
Be supportive to the patient during swallowing efforts.	Swallowing difficulty is very frustrating for the patient.
Teach the patient who has had supraglottic surgery an alternate method of swallowing: • Have the patient then perform a Valsalva maneuver as he or she is swallowing. • Teach at least one other family member or significant other how to support the patient in alternate swallowing, suctioning, Heimlich maneuver, etc.	Facilitates active swallowing and support for the patient as he or she begins to adapt to impaired swallowing.
Refer as needed to speech/swallow therapy and other health-care team members.	Collaboration supports a holistic approach to patient care.

Child Health

ACTIONS/INTERVENTIONS	RATIONALES
Monitor for contributory factors, especially palate formation, possible tracheoesophageal fistula, or other congenital anomalies.	A thorough assessment will best identify those patients who have greater-than-usual likelihood of swallowing difficulties due to structural, acquired, or circumstantial conditions.
Maintain the infant in upright position after feedings for at least $1^{1}/_{2}$ hours.	An upright position favors, by gravity, the digestion and absorption of nutrients, thereby decreasing the likelihood of reflux and resultant potential for choking.
Address anticipatory safety needs for possible choking: • Have appropriate suctioning equipment available. • Teach the parents CPR. • Provide parenting support for CPR and suctioning.	Usual anticipatory airway management is appropriate in long-term patient management. Education and teaching concerns can be addressed in a supportive environment, thereby reducing anxiety in event of cardiopulmonary arrest secondary to impaired swallowing.
• Assist the family to identify ways to cope with swallowing disorder (e.g., the need for extra help in feeding). Refer to health-care specialists to facilitate this, especially occupational therapist.	Appropriate individualization fosters input and respect for how to best meet needs of client in a way the family can relate.
Administer medications as ordered. Avoid powder or pill forms. Use elixirs or mix as needed.	Pills or powders may increase the likelihood of impaired swallowing in young children and infants. Appropriate mixing with fruit syrups or using manufacturer's elixir or suspension form of the drug lessens the likelihood of impaired swallowing.

(care plan continued on page 212)

NURSING ACTIONS/INTERVENTIONS WITH RATIONALES (continued from page 211)

Child Health

ACTIONS/INTERVENTIONS	RATIONALES
If training is in conjunction with tracheostomy removal, involve all the health team members to appropriately coordinate plan. [Note client's plan here with assistance needed by nursing to facilitate plan.]	Provides the most realistic and holistic plan of care.

Women's Health

The nursing actions for a woman with the nursing diagnosis of Impaired Swallowing are the same as those for Adult Health.

Mental Health

● N O T E : *The following nursing actions are specific considerations for the mental health client who has Impaired Swallowing that is caused or increased by anxiety. Refer to Mental Health nursing actions for the diagnosis of Anxiety for interventions related to decreasing and resolving the client's anxiety. If swallowing problems are related to an eating disorder, refer to Mental Health nursing actions for Imbalanced Nutrition, Less Than Body Requirements, for additional nursing actions.*

ACTIONS/INTERVENTIONS	RATIONALES
Provide a quiet, relaxed environment during meals by discussing with the client the situations that increase anxiety and excluding those factors from the situation. Provide things such as favorite music and friends or family that increase relaxation. [Note information provided by the client here, especially those things that need to be provided by the nursing staff.]	Promotes the client's control and facilitates relaxation response, thus inhibiting the sympathetic nervous system response.[27,95]
Provide medications in liquid or injectable form. [Note any special preference the client may have in presentation of medications here.]	Liquids are easier to swallow than tablets. Providing medications by injection would prevent any swallowing problems.
Teach the client deep muscle relaxation. (Refer to the Mental Health nursing actions for Anxiety for actions related to decreasing anxiety.)	Promotes client control and inhibits the sympathetic nervous system response.
Discuss with the client foods that are the easiest and the most difficult to swallow. [Note information from this discussion here. Also note time and person responsible for this discussion.]	Promotes client control.
Plan the client's most nutritious meals for the time of day he or she is most relaxed, and note that time here.	
Provide the client with high-energy snacks several times during the day. [Note snacks preferred by the client and time they are to be offered here.]	Provides additional calories in frequent small amounts.
Assign primary nurse to sit with the client 30 minutes (this can be increased to an hour as the client tolerates interaction time better) 2 times a day to discuss concerns related to swallowing. (This can be included in the time described under the nursing actions for Anxiety.) As the nurse–client relationship moves to a	Provides increased individualization and continuity of care, facilitating the development of a therapeutic relationship. The nursing process requires that a trusting and functional relationship exist between nurse and client.[95] Change depends on the client's perception of the problem.[97]

ACTIONS/INTERVENTIONS	RATIONALES
working phase, discussion can include factors that precipitated the client's focus on swallowing. These factors could be a trauma directly related to swallowing, such as an attack in which the client was choked or in which oral sex was forced.	
Teach the client and client's support system nutrition factors that will improve swallowing and maintain adequate nutrition. [Note here the names of persons the client would like included in this teaching. Also note time arranged and person responsible for this teaching here.]	Promotes long-term support for assistance with problem.

Gerontic Health

Nursing actions for the gerontic patient with this diagnosis are the same as those for Adult Health and Psychiatric Health.

Home Health/Community Health

ACTIONS/INTERVENTIONS	RATIONALES
Teach measures to decrease or eliminate Impaired Swallowing: • Principles of oral hygiene • Small pieces of food or pureed food as necessary • Aspiration precautions (e.g., eat and drink sitting up, do not force-feed or fill mouth too full, and CPR) • Proper nutrition and hydration • Use of adaptive equipment as required Teach to monitor for factors contributing to Impaired Swallowing (e.g., fatigue, obstruction, neuromuscular impairment, or irritated oropharyngeal cavity, on at least a daily basis).	Prevents or diminishes problems. Promotes self-care and provides database for early intervention.
Involve the client and family in planning, implementing, and promoting reduction or elimination of Impaired Swallowing by establishing regular family conferences to provide for mutual goal setting and to improve communication.	Goal setting and communication promote positive outcomes.
Assist the client and family in lifestyle changes that may be required: • The client may need to be fed. • Mealtimes should be quiet, uninterrupted, and at consistent times on a daily basis. • The client may require special diet and special utensils.	Knowledge and support provide motivation for change and increase the potential for a positive outcome.

THERMOREGULATION, INEFFECTIVE

DEFINITION[28]

The state in which the individual's temperature fluctuates between hypothermia and hyperthermia.

DEFINING CHARACTERISTICS[28]

1. Fluctuations in body temperature above or below the normal range
2. Cool skin
3. Cyanotic nail beds
4. Flushed skin
5. Hypertension
6. Increased respiratory rate
7. Pallor (moderate)
8. Piloerection
9. Reduction in body temperature below normal range
10. Seizures or convulsions
11. Shivering (mild)

12. Slow capillary refill
13. Tachycardia
14. Warm to touch

RELATED FACTORS[28]

1. Aging
2. Fluctuating environmental temperature
3. Trauma or illness
4. Immaturity

RELATED CLINICAL CONCERNS

1. Any infection
2. Any surgery
3. Septicemia

 Have You Selected the Correct Diagnosis?

Hyperthermia
Hyperthermia means that a person maintains a body temperature greater than what is normal for himself or herself. In Ineffective Thermoregulation, the client's temperature is changing between Hyperthermia and Hypothermia. If the temperature measurement is remaining above normal, the correct diagnosis is Hyperthermia, not Ineffective Thermoregulation.

Hypothermia
Hypothermia means that a person maintains a body temperature below what is normal for himself or herself. If the temperature is consistently remaining below normal, the correct diagnosis is Hypothermia, not Ineffective Thermoregulation.

Risk for Imbalanced Body Temperature
With this diagnosis, the patient has a potential inability to regulate heat production and heat dissipation within a normal range. The key point to remember is that a temperature abnormality does not exist yet, but the risk factors present indicate such a problem could develop. If the temperature measurements are fluctuating between hypothermia and hyperthermia, the correct diagnosis is Ineffective Thermoregulation.

EXPECTED OUTCOME

Will maintain a body temperature between 97 and 99°F by [date].

TARGET DATES

Initial target dates will be stated in terms of hours. After stabilization, an appropriate target date would be 3 days.

NURSING ACTIONS/INTERVENTIONS WITH RATIONALES

Adult Health

ACTIONS/INTERVENTIONS	RATIONALES
Monitor vital signs at least every hour on the hour. [Note times here.]	Monitors basic trends in temperature fluctuations. Permits early recognition of ineffective thermoregulation.
Maintain room temperature at all times at 72°F. Provide warmth or cooling as needed to maintain temperature in desired range; avoid drafts and chilling for the patient.	Offsets environmental impact on thermoregulation.
Reduce stress for the patient. Provide quiet, nonstimulating environment.	Assists body to maintain homeostasis. Stress could contribute to problems with thermoregulation as a result of increased basal metabolic rate.
If the patient is hypothermic, see nursing actions for Hypothermia.	Thermoregulation problems may vary from hypothermia to hyperthermia.
If the patient is hyperthermic, see nursing actions for Hyperthermia.	
Make referrals for appropriate follow-up before dismissal from hospital.	Provides long-range, cost-effective support.

Child Health

ACTIONS/INTERVENTIONS	RATIONALES
Protect the child from excessive chilling during bathing or procedures.	Evaporation and significant change of temperature for even short periods of time contribute to heat loss for the young child or infant, especially during illness.

ACTIONS/INTERVENTIONS	RATIONALES
Assist in answering the parent's or child's questions regarding temperature-monitoring procedures or administration of medications.	Appropriate teaching fosters compliance and reduces anxiety.
Assist the parents in dealing with anxiety in times of unknown causes or prognosis by allowing [number] minutes per shift for venting anxiety. [State times here.] Interview the parents specifically to ascertain anxiety.	Because the emphasis on monitoring and treating altered thermoregulation is so great, it can be easy to overlook the parents and their concerns. Specific attention must be given to ascertaining how the patient and family are feeling about all the many concerns generated.
Involve the parents and family in the child's care whenever appropriate, especially for comforting the child.	Parental involvement fosters empowerment and regaining of self-care, thereby reestablishing the likelihood for effective family coping.

Women's Health

This nursing diagnosis will pertain to women the same as it would for any other adult. The reader is referred to the Adult Health and Home Health nursing actions for this diagnosis.

Mental Health

The nursing actions for this diagnosis in the mental health client are the same as those in Adult Health.

Gerontic Health

● NOTE: *Normal changes of aging can contribute to altered thermoregulation. Age-related changes that may be associated with altered thermoregulation are a decrease in febrile response, inefficient vasoconstriction, decreased cardiac output, decreased subcutaneous tissue, diminished shivering, diminished temperature sensory perception, and diminished thirst perception. Thus, older clients are at high risk for alterations in thermoregulation, both hyperthermia and hypothermia.*

In addition to the interventions for Adult Health the following can be utilized with the older adult client:

ACTIONS/INTERVENTIONS	RATIONALES
Check on older adults often who are at risk: • During heat alerts • During cold weather • In homes without air conditioning or heating • During electrical outages or electrical service interruptions.	Primary preventive measure.
Instruct/assist the client to select proper clothing: • Layers during cold weather and lighter garments during warmer weather.	Primary preventive measure.
Monitor and record the temperature of older clients often and regularly during high risk times: • Intra- and postoperative period • When infection is present • When fluid imbalance is present	Tracks client norms and provides a mechanism for early identification of changes.
Use warmed IV solutions in older clients in the intra-/postoperative period unless hyperthermia is present.	Prevent episodes of hypothermia.

(care plan continued on page 216)

NURSING ACTIONS/INTERVENTIONS WITH RATIONALES (continued from page 215)	

Home Health

ACTIONS/INTERVENTIONS	RATIONALES
Monitor for factors contributing to Ineffective Thermoregulation (illness, trauma, immaturity, aging, or fluctuating environmental temperature).	Allows early recognition and early implementation of therapy.
Involve the client and family in planning, implementing, and promoting reduction or elimination of Ineffective Thermoregulation.	Personal involvement and input increases likelihood of maintenance of plan.
Teach the client and family early signs and symptoms of Ineffective Thermoregulation (see Hyperthermia and Hypothermia).	
Teach the client and family measures to decrease or eliminate Ineffective Thermoregulation (see Hyperthermia and Hypothermia).	
Assist the client and family to identify lifestyle changes that may be required (see Hyperthermia and Hypothermia).	Provides basic information and planning to successfully manage condition at home.

TISSUE INTEGRITY, IMPAIRED

DEFINITIONS[28]

Impaired Tissue Integrity   A state in which an individual experiences damage to mucous membrane, corneal, integumentary, or subcutaneous tissue.

  Risk for Impaired Skin Integrity   A state in which the individual's skin is at risk of being adversely altered.

  Impaired Skin Integrity   A state in which the individual has altered epidermis and/or dermis.

  Impaired Oral Mucous Membrane   Disruptions of the lips and soft tissue of the oral cavity.

DEFINING CHARACTERISTICS[28]

A. Impaired Tissue Integrity
  1. Damaged or destroyed tissue (cornea, mucous membrane, integumentary, or subcutaneous)
B. Risk for Impaired Skin Integrity*
  1. External
    a. Radiation
    b. Physical immobilization
    c. Mechanical factors (shearing forces, pressure, and restraint)
    d. Hypothermia or hyperthermia
    e. Humidity
    f. Chemical substance
    g. Excretions or secretions
    h. Moisture
    i. Extremes of age
  2. Internal

*Risk should be determined by the use of a risk assessment tool (for example, Braden Scale).

    a. Medication
    b. Skeletal prominence
    c. Immunologic factors
    d. Developmental factors
    e. Altered sensation
    f. Altered pigmentation
    g. Altered metabolic state
    h. Altered circulation
    i. Alterations in skin turgor (change in elasticity)
    j. Alterations in nutritional state (obesity, emaciation)
    k. Psychogenic
C. Impaired Skin Integrity
  1. Invasion of body structures
  2. Destruction of skin layers (dermis)
  3. Disruption of skin surfaces (epidermis)
D. Impaired Oral Mucous Membrane
  1. Purulent drainage or exudates
  2. Gingival recession with pockets deeper than 4 mm
  3. Enlarged tonsils beyond what is developmentally appropriate
  4. Smooth, atrophic, sensitive tongue
  5. Geographic tongue
  6. Mucosal denudation
  7. Presence of pathogens (per culture)
  8. Difficult speech (dysarthria)
  9. Self-report of bad taste
  10. Gingival or mucosal pallor
  11. Oral pain or discomfort
  12. Xerostomia (dry mouth)
  13. Vesicles, nodules, or papules
  14. White patches or plaques, spongy patches, or white curd-like exudate
  15. Oral lesions, lacerations, or ulcers

16. Halitosis
17. Edema (gingival or mucosal)
18. Hyperemia ("beefy-red")
19. Desquamation
20. Coated tongue
21. Stomatitis
22. Self-report of difficulty eating and/or swallowing
23. Self-report of diminished or absent taste
24. Bleeding
25. Macroplasia
26. Gingival hyperplasia
27. Fissures, cheilitis
28. Red or bluish masses (e.g., hemangioma)

RELATED FACTORS[28]

A. Impaired Tissue Integrity
1. Mechanical (pressure, shear, and friction)
2. Radiation (including therapeutic radiation)
3. Nutritional deficit or excess
4. Thermal (temperature extremes)
5. Knowledge deficit
6. Irritants
7. Chemical (including body excretions, secretions, and medications)
8. Impaired physical mobility
9. Altered circulation
10. Fluid deficit or excess

B. Risk for Impaired Skin Integrity
The risk factors also serve as the related factors.

C. Impaired Skin Integrity
1. External
   a. Hyperthermia or hypothermia
   b. Chemical substance
   c. Humidity
   d. Mechanical factors (shearing forces, pressure, restraint)
   e. Physical immobilization
   f. Radiation
   g. Extremes of age
   h. Moisture
   i. Medication
2. Internal
   a. Altered metabolic state
   b. Skeletal prominence
   c. Immunologic deficit
   d. Developmental factors
   e. Altered sensation
   f. Alterations in nutritional state (obesity, emaciation)
   g. Altered pigmentation
   h. Altered circulation
   i. Alterations in skin turgor (change in elasticity)
   j. Altered fluid status

D. Impaired Oral Mucous Membrane
1. Chemotherapy
2. Chemical (alcohol, tobacco, acidic foods, regular use of inhalers, drugs, and other noxious agents)
3. Depression
4. Immunosuppression
5. Aging-related loss of connective, adipose, or bone tissue
6. Barriers to professional care
7. Cleft lip or palate
8. Medication side effects
9. Lack of or decreased salivation
10. Trauma
11. Pathologic conditions—oral cavity (radiation to head or neck)
12. NPO status for more than 24 hours
13. Mouth breathing
14. Malnutrition or vitamin deficiency
15. Dehydration
16. Ineffective oral hygiene
17. Mechanical (ill-fitting dentures, braces, tubes [endotracheal or nasogastric], surgery in oral cavity)
18. Decreased platelets
19. Immunocompromised
20. Impaired salivation
21. Radiation therapy
22. Barriers to oral self-care
23. Diminished hormone levels (women)
24. Stress
25. Loss of supportive structures

RELATED CLINICAL CONCERNS

1. Any condition requiring immobilization of patient
2. Burns: chemical, thermal, or radiation
3. Accidents: motor vehicle, farm equipment, motorcycles, and so on
4. AIDS
5. Congestive heart failure
6. Diabetes mellitus

✔ Have You Selected the Correct Diagnosis?

Impaired Skin Integrity
If the tissue damage involves only the skin and its subcutaneous tissues, then the most correct diagnosis is Impaired Skin Integrity. Risk for Impaired Skin Integrity would be the most appropriate diagnosis if the patient is presenting a majority of risk factors for a skin integrity problem but the problem has not yet developed.

Impaired Oral Mucous Membrane
If the tissue damage involves only the oral mucous membranes, then the best diagnosis is Impaired Oral Mucous Membrane. Impaired Tissue Integrity is a higher-level diagnosis and would cover a wider range of tissue types. Impaired Oral Mucous Membrane and the two diagnoses related to Skin Integrity are more specific and exact diagnoses and should be used before Impaired Tissue Integrity **if** the problem can be definitively isolated to either the oral mucous membrane or the skin.

EXPECTED OUTCOME

Will exhibit structural intactness and normal physiological function of [skin, mucous membranes, integumentary or subcutaneous tissues] by [date].

TARGET DATES

Tissue integrity problems can begin developing within hours of a patient's admission if caution is not taken regarding turning, cleaning, and so on. Therefore, an initial target date of 2 days after admission would be most appropriate.

NURSING ACTIONS/INTERVENTIONS WITH RATIONALES

Adult Health

ACTIONS/INTERVENTIONS	RATIONALES
Ambulate to extent possible.	
Perform active or passive ROM at least once per shift at [state times here].	Stimulates circulation, which provides nourishment and carries away waste, thus reducing the likelihood of tissue breakdown.
Reduce pressure on affected skin surface by using: • Egg crate mattress • Alternating air mattress • Sheepskin • Commercial wafer barriers • Thick dressing used as pad on bony prominences	Pressure predisposes tissue breakdown.
Make sure footboard is in place for the patient to use for bracing.	
Avoid use of rubber or plastic in direct contact with the patient.	
Collaborate with dietitian regarding well-balanced diet. Assist the patient to eat as necessary.	Prevents tissue breakdown due to negative nitrogen balance.
Monitor dietary intake, and avoid irritant food and fluid intake (e.g., highly spiced food or extremes of temperature).	These factors would increase probability of oral mucous membrane problems.
Facilitate fluid intake to at least 2000 mL per 24 hours.	Maintains fluid and electrolyte balance, which is necessary for tissue repair and normal functioning.
Cleanse perineal area carefully after each urination or bowel movement. Monitor closely for any urinary or fecal incontinence.	Allowing body wastes to remain on skin promotes tissue breakdown. Incontinence would increase probability of such an event.
Teach the patient principles of good skin hygiene.	Promote self-care and self-management to prevent problem.
Administer oral hygiene at least three times a day after each meal and as needed (PRN): • Brush teeth, gums, and tongue with soft-bristled brush, sponge stick, or gauze-wrapped finger. • Floss teeth. • Rinse mouth thoroughly after brushing. Avoid commercial mouthwashes and preparations with alcohol, lemon, or glycerin. Use normal saline or oxidizing agent.	Basic care measures to maintain oral mucosa.
Administer medications as ordered and record response (e.g., topical oral antibiotics, analgesic mouthwashes). Record response within 30 minutes of administration. • Teach the patient and significant others proper oral hygiene.	

ACTIONS/INTERVENTIONS	RATIONALES
• If the patient has dentures, cleanse with equal parts of hydrogen peroxide and water.	
• Apply lubricant to lips at least every 2 hours on [odd/even] hour.	
Maintain good body hygiene. Be sure the patient has at least a sponge bath every day **unless** skin is too dry.	
Monitor for signs of infection at least daily.	Infection, through production of toxins, wastes, and so on, increases the probability of tissue damage.
Keep room temperature and humidity constant. Room temperature should be kept close to 72°F and humidity at a low level unless otherwise ordered.	Keeps skin cool and dry to prevent perspiration.
Teach the patient the impact of smoking on tissues.	Highly irritating to mucous membranes.
• Provide information on smoking cessation programs.	
• Consult with physician to provide nicotine patches and/ or gum as indicated.	
If lesions develop, cleanse area daily at [time] according to prescribed regimen.	
Protect open surface with such products as:	
• Karaya powder	
• Skin gel	
• Wafer barrier	
• Other commercial skin preparations	
Collaborate with an enterostomal therapist and physician regarding care specific to the patient (list individualized care procedures here).	
Change dressings when needed using aseptic techniques. Collaborate with health-care team regarding dressing type and use of topical agents. [Note procedure to be used for client here.]	
Teach the patient and significant others care of the wound prior to discharge.	Basic care measures for impaired skin integrity.
Avoid use of adhesive tape. If tape must be applied, use nonallergenic tape.	
Avoid use of doughnut ring.	
Use mild, unscented soap (or soap substitute) and cool or lukewarm water.	
Avoid vigorous rubbing, but do massage gently using a lanolin-based unscented lotion.	
Pat area dry.	
Monitor:	These measures would allow early detection of any complications.
• Skin surface and pressure areas at least every 4 hours at [state times here] for blanching, erythematic, temperature difference (e.g., increased warmth), or moisture.	
• Fluid and electrolyte balance. Collaborate with health-care team regarding frequency of measurement of electrolyte levels.	
Watch for signs or symptoms of edema.	
Caution the patient and assist to avoid scratching irritated areas:	Avoids further irritation of already damaged tissue.
• Apply cool compresses.	
Collaborate with health-care team regarding medicated baths (e.g., oatmeal) and topical ointments.	

(care plan continued on page 220)

NURSING ACTIONS/INTERVENTIONS WITH RATIONALES (continued from page 219)

Adult Health

ACTIONS/INTERVENTIONS	RATIONALES
Collaborate with health-care team regarding adjunct therapies (e.g., therapeutic beds, wound closure systems, or barrier lotions).	
Involve physical/occupational therapy in plan of care.	
Refer to community health agencies and other health-care providers as appropriate.	Provides on-going support and cost-effective use of available resources.

Child Health

Utilize adult health interventions with appropriate developmental adaptations with the following considerations.

ACTIONS/INTERVENTIONS	RATIONALES
Handle the infant gently; especially caution paramedical personnel regarding need for gentle handling.	The epidermis of infants and young children is thin and lacking in subcutaneous depth. Others, such as x-ray technicians, may not realize the fragile nature of skin as they carry out necessary procedures.
Place the patient on flotation pad, or if the parents choose, allow the infant or child to be held frequently (avoid placement of infant on any soft surface that presents a risk for SIDS).	Alternating surface contact and position favors circulatory return to central venous system.
Caution the patient and parents to avoid scratching irritated area: • Trim nails with appropriate scissors; receive parental permission if necessary. • Make small mitts if necessary from cotton stockinette used for precasting.	Anticipate potential injury of delicate epidermis, especially when irritation may prompt itching.
Monitor perineal area for possible allergy to diapers.	Various synthetics in diapers may evoke allergenic responses and either cause or worsen existent skin irritation.
Encourage fluids: • Infants: 250 to 300 mL/24 h • Toddler: 1150 to 1300 mL/24 h • Preschooler: 1600 mL/24 h (These are approximate ranges. The physician may order specific amounts according to the child's age and condition.)	Adequate hydration assists in normal homeostatic mechanisms that affect the skin's integrity.
Provide protection such as bandage or padding to tissue site involved.	Anticipation and protection from injury serves to limit the depth and/or degree of impaired skin integrity.
Monitor and document circulation to affected tissue via: • Peripheral arterial pulses • Blanching or capillary refill • Tissue color • Sensation to touch or temperature • Tissue general condition (e.g., bruising or lacerations) • Drainage (e.g., amount, odor, or color) • OM limitations	These factors represent basic appropriate criteria for circulatory checks. They may be added to in instances of specific concerns such as compartment syndrome associated with hand trauma.

ACTIONS/INTERVENTIONS	RATIONALES
Administer oral hygiene according to needs and status: • Special orders for postoperative cleft palate or cleft lip repair	Appropriate oral hygiene decreases the likelihood of altered integrity of surrounding tissues and is critical for care of associated oral disorders.
Teach the parents to limit time the infant sucks bottle in reclining position to prevent bottle mouth syndrome and decayed teeth.	Evidence suggests that bottle mouth syndrome is prevented by not having the infant go to sleep with bottle. Completion of feeding and removal of bottle is suggested before placing the infant in crib.
Protect the altered tissue site as needed during movement by providing support to the limb.	Provision of support and usual use of body parts favor adequate circulation and prevent further injury.
Provide ROM and ambulation as permitted to encourage vascular return. [Note specific plan for this client here.]	
Position the patient while in bed so that the head of the bed is elevated slightly and involved limb is elevated approximately 20 degrees.	Appropriate venous return is favored by resultant gravity with limb higher than heart.
Address ineffective thermoregulation, and especially protect the patient from chilling or shock due to dehydration or sepsis. Refer to care plans related to thermoregulation for detailed interventions.	In severe instances of ineffective thermoregulation or related pathology, there may not be the usual manifestations of derivations from normal. It may also be difficult to assess sensation in the young infant because of the infant's inability to provide verbal feedback.
Use restraints judiciously for involved limb or body site.	Any undue constriction or threat to circulation must be weighed appropriately in making decisions whether or not to restrain the child.
Monitor intravenous infusion and administration of medications cautiously. Avoid use of sites in close proximity to area of impaired tissue integrity.	This is usual protocol for IV therapy and must be considered paramount as IV medications or solutions pose serious threats to the veins and surrounding tissues.
Allow the patient and family time to express concerns by providing at least [number] minutes per shift for family counseling. [State times here.]	Reduces anxiety because their concerns can be made known and their feelings valued.

Teach the patient and family: [Note specific teaching plan for client here.]
• Need for follow-up care
• Signs and symptoms to be reported:
  • Increased temperature (101°F or higher)
  • Foul odors or drainage
  • Delayed healing or increase in damage site size
  • Loss of sensation or pulsation in limb or site
  • Any increase in pain
• Use of prosthetic device if indicated
• Use of aids in mobility, such as crutches or walker
• Need to avoid constrictive clothing
• Appropriate dietary needs
	Appropriate education serves to build self-confidence and effects long-term compliance with treatment and health management.

Women's Health

ACTIONS/INTERVENTIONS	RATIONALES
Monitor perineum and rectum after childbirth for injury or healing at least once per shift at [state times here]. Monitor episiotomy site for redness, edema, or hematomas each 15 minutes immediately after delivery for 1 hour, then once each shift thereafter.	Assesses basic physical condition as a basis for providing care and preventing complications.
Collaborate with physician regarding:	Provides comfort and promotes healing.

(care plan continued on page 222)

NURSING ACTIONS/INTERVENTIONS WITH RATIONALES (continued from page 221)

Women's Health

ACTIONS/INTERVENTIONS	RATIONALES
• Applying ice packs or cold pads to perineum for the first 8 to 12 hours after delivery to reduce edema and increase comfort • Warm baths twice a day at [state times here] and as necessary for pain and discomfort • Analgesics and topical anesthetics as necessary for pain and discomfort	
Teach good perineal hygiene and self-care: • Rinse perineal area with warm water after each voiding. • Pat dry gently from front to back to prevent contamination. • Apply perineal pad from front to back to prevent contamination. • Change pads frequently to prevent infection and irritation.	Promotes healing and encourages self-care.
Provide factual information on resumption of sexual activities after childbirth: • First intercourse should be after adequate healing period (usually 3 to 4 weeks). • Intercourse should be slow and easy (woman on top can better control angle, depth, and penetration).	Provides basic information to promote safe self-care.
Teach postmenopausal women the signs and symptoms of atrophic vaginitis: • Watery discharge • Burning and itching of vagina or vulva Encourage examinations (Pap smears) for estrogen levels at least annually. In collaboration with physician, encourage use as needed of: • Estrogen replacement creams or vaginal suppositories • Extra lubrication during intercourse	Provides basic information that promotes self-care and health maintenance.
Teach breastfeeding mothers about breast care. • Inspect for cracks or fissures in nipples. • Wear supportive bra (breast binder to relieve engorgement). • Shower daily; do not use soap on breast; allow to air dry. • Use lanolin-based cream (vitamin E cream, Massé Breast cream, or A and D cream) to prevent drying and cracking of nipples.	Provides basic information that assists in preventing skin breakdown and promotes self-care and successful lactation.
Enhance let-down reflex: • Nurse early and frequently. Ten minutes on each side is easier on sore nipples than nursing less frequently. • Nurse at both breasts each feeding. Switch sides to begin nursing each time (e.g., if the baby nursed first on left side at last feeding, begin on right side this time). A safety pin or small ribbon on bra strap will remind the mother which side she used first last time.	Promotes let-down reflex and successful breastfeeding.

ACTIONS/INTERVENTIONS	RATIONALES

- Change positions from one feeding to next (distributes sucking pressure).
- Check the baby's position on breast. Be certain areola is in mouth, not just nipple.
- Begin nursing on least sore side first, if possible, then switch the baby to other side.
- Apply ice to nipple just before nursing to decrease pain (fold squares, put them in the freezer and apply as needed).

Collaborate with the physician regarding analgesics as needed. Caution the patient to not take over-the-counter medication because some medications are passed to the baby via breast milk.

● N O T E : *Between the third and sixth months of pregnancy, the process of tooth calcification (hardening) begins in the fetus. What the mother consumes in her diet will affect the development of the unborn child's teeth. A well-balanced diet usually provides correct amounts of nutrients for both the mother and the child.*

Teach the patient to practice good oral hygiene at least twice a day as well as PRN:
- Each time the patient eats and, if nauseated and vomiting, vomits, the patient should clean gums and teeth.
- If the smell of toothpaste or mouth rinse makes the patient nauseated, the patient should use baking soda.

Reduce the number of times sugar-rich foods are eaten between meals.

Teach the patient to snack on fruits, vegetables, cheese, cottage cheese, whole grains, or milk.

Have the patient increase daily calcium intake to at least a total of 1.2 g of calcium per day.

Collaborate with obstetrician and dentist to plan needed dental care during pregnancy.

Assist in planning best time in pregnancy for dental visits:
- Not during the first 3 months if:
  - Previous obstetric history includes miscarriage
  - Threatened miscarriage
  - Other medical indications
  - Hypersensitive to gagging (will increase nausea and vomiting)
- Not during the last 3 months if:
  - Not able to sit in dental chair for long periods of time
  - Obstetric history of premature labor

Instruct the patient to have X-ray examinations only when it is absolutely necessary. Caution the patient to request a lead apron when having X-ray examinations.

Rationales (right column):

Promotes sense of well-being. Assists in promoting proper growth and development of the fetus, and encourages health maintenance.

Provides basic information to the patient that promotes health maintenance and increases awareness of need for self-care.

Prevents X-ray exposure to the fetus.

ADDITIONAL INFORMATION

Nursing actions for newborn health immediately follow the Women's Health nursing actions. As previously mentioned, newborn actions are included in this section because newborn care is most often administered

(care plan continued on page 224)

NURSING ACTIONS/INTERVENTIONS WITH RATIONALES (continued from page 223)

Women's Health

ACTIONS/INTERVENTIONS	RATIONALES
by nurses in the obstetric or women's health area. Focus needs to be made on the newborn simply because the newborn's oral mucous membrane problems can be easily overlooked.	
In collaboration with dentist, teach the parents the oral and dental needs of the neonate: • Use of fluoride • Proper use of pacifiers • Do not use homemade pacifiers • Use pacifiers recommended by dentist • Allowing the infant who is teething to chew on soft toothbrush (will encourage later brushing of teeth because it allows the infant to become familiar with toothbrush in mouth) • Holding on to brush • Giving brush to the infant only when an adult is present	
Teach the parents how to administer oral hygiene: • Massage and rub the infant's gums with finger daily. • Inspect oral cavity daily for hygiene and problems.	
Take the infant for first dental visit between 18 months and 2 years of age.	

Dental caries (decay) can be a result of prolonged nursing or delayed weaning:
• Do not allow the infant to nurse at breast or bottle beyond the required feeding time.
• Do not allow the infant to sleep habitually at the breast or with a bottle or pacifier in the mouth.
• Teach the neonate's parents to:
  • Avoid giving sweet liquids (soft drinks) or fruit juices in bottle.
  • Wean the child from bottle to cup soon after first birthday.
  • When continuing to nurse the infant, give water in a cup soon after the first birthday.
  • Use good handwashing techniques to prevent infection with, or reinfection of, thrush.
  • Not place the infant on sheets where the mother has been sitting.
  • Thoroughly clean breast or bottle-feeding equipment.
	Promotes good health and provides information as a basis for parental care of the infant. Assists in preventing infection.

Mental Health

Plan for adult health can provide the foundation for care with the following considerations:

ACTIONS/INTERVENTIONS	RATIONALES
Refer to Chapter 8 for stress-reduction measures and interventions for the stressors that produce psychogenic skin reactions.	

ACTIONS/INTERVENTIONS	RATIONALES
If the client is placed in restraints, monitor the integrity of skin under restraints every hour.	
Apply lanolin-based lotion and cornstarch or powder to area under restraint at least every 2 hours on [odd/even] hour and PRN.	Lubricates skin and decreases risk for breakdown.
Pad restraints with nonabrasive materials such as sheepskin.	Decreases mechanical friction against the skin, and decreases risk for breakdown.
Keep the area of restraint next to the skin clean and dry.	
Release restraints one at a time every 2 hours on [odd/even] hour and PRN. Remove restraints as soon as the client will tolerate one-to-one care without risk to self or others.	
Maintain proper movement and alignment of affected body parts.	Decreases mechanical friction on specific areas for long periods of time, thus decreasing risk for breakdown.
• Change the client's position every 2 hours on [odd/even] hour.	
• Offer the client fluids every 15 minutes. [List preferred fluids here.]	
• While the client is very agitated and physically active, provide constant one-to-one observation.	Hydration improves skin condition.
• While the limb is out of restraints, have the client move the limb through ROM.	Promotes circulation and assists in preventing the consequences of immobility.
• If the client is in four-point restraints, place him or her on side or stomach and change this position every 2 hours on [odd/even] hour.	Client safety is of primary importance. This positioning prevents aspiration by facilitating drainage of fluids away from the airway.
• Monitor skin condition of pressure areas.	
• If the client is in four-point restraints, provide one-on-one observation.	Provides supportive environment to the client.
• Continually remind the client of reason for restraint and conditions for having the restraints removed.	
• Talk with the client in a calm, quiet voice and use the client's name.	
• Use restraints that are wide and have padding. Make sure padding is kept clean and dry and free of wrinkles.	
If Impaired Tissue Integrity is the result of self-harm, place the client on one-to-one observation until the risk of future harm has diminished.	Client safety is of primary importance. Provides ongoing supervision to inhibit impulsive behavior, and encourages use of alternative coping behaviors.
Monitor self-inflicted injuries hourly for the first 24 hours for signs of infection can prevent more of infection and further damage. Note information on a flow sheet. After the first 24 hours, monitor on a daily basis.	Early identification and treatment of infection can prevent more serious damage.
Provide equipment and time for the client to practice oral hygiene at least after each meal.	Removes debris and food particles, thus reducing the risk of tissue injury.
Discuss with the client lifestyle changes to improve condition of mucous membranes, including nutritional habits, use of tobacco product, use of alcohol, maintenance of proper hydration, and effects of frequent vomiting.	Alerts the client to lifestyle patterns that increase risk for injury to oral mucous membranes. If risk factors are present, frequent assessment and increased attention to oral hygiene can decrease the risk of membrane breakdown.
Discuss with the client side effects of medications, such as antibiotics, antihistamines, phenytoin, antidepressants, and antipsychotics that contribute to alterations in oral mucous membranes.	

(care plan continued on page 226)

NURSING ACTIONS/INTERVENTIONS WITH RATIONALES (continued from page 225)

Mental Health

ACTIONS/INTERVENTIONS	RATIONALES
Teach the client to use nonsucrose candy or gum to stimulate flow of saliva.	Maintains hydration of membranes and decreases chance of breakdown.
Teach the client to avoid excessive wind and sun exposure, especially with antipsychotic drugs.	These medications can cause photosensitivity.[38]
If the client is taking antipsychotic drugs, suggest the use of a sunscreen containing PABA.	

Gerontic Health

In addition to the interventions for Adult Health, the following may be utilized with the aging client

ACTIONS/INTERVENTIONS	RATIONALES
Nursing actions for this diagnosis in the gerontic patient are essentially the same as those for Adult Health and Home Health with the following special notations: Use only superfatted, nonperfumed, mild, nondetergent, and hexachlorophene-free soap in bathing the patient.[98]	The incidence of dry skin in the older adult is increased as a result of decreased production of natural skin oils.
When drying the skin after bathing, pat the skin dry rather than rubbing, and apply lubricating lotion while the skin is still damp.	Increases the moisture level of the patient's skin. Careful attention to dry skin conditions in the older adult assists in maintaining tissue integrity for the older adult.

Home Health/Community Health

Nursing actions for this diagnosis in the home patient are essentially the same as those for Adult Health and Home Health with the following additions:

ACTIONS/INTERVENTIONS	RATIONALES
Assess resources (availability and skill of caregivers, finances, equipment) of client and refer to resources as needed.[94]	Prevention of inadequate care and subsequent complications.
Arrange interventions to meet identified psychosocial needs and goals. Follow-up should be planned in cooperation with the individual and caregiver.[94]	Individualized care is more likely to be adopted by client and caregiver.
Set treatment goals consistent with the values and lifestyle of the individual, family, and caregiver.[94]	Individualized care is more likely to be adopted by client and caregiver.
For clients who are unable to reposition themselves, caregivers should be taught to use a draw sheet to avoid shearing and skin tears.	
• Massage pressure points and bony prominences gently at least three times a day. Do not massage reddened areas.[94]	
Teach patient and caregiver signs and symptoms of tissue breakdown (e.g., redness over bony prominences, pain or discomfort in localized area, skin lesions, or itching and symptoms that require the attention of a health-care provider).	Provides data for early intervention and assists patient/caregiver to know when to seek medical attention.

ACTIONS/INTERVENTIONS	RATIONALES
Teach measures to promote tissue integrity: • Use mild laundry detergent on clothes. Double-rinse clothes, linens, and diapers if skin is sensitive. • Use sunscreen to prevent sun damage. • Avoid excessive wind and sun exposure. • Wear properly fitting shoes.	Provides knowledge and skills that will prevent or minimize skin breakdown.

REFERENCES

1. Potter, PA, and Perry, AG: Instructors' Manual for Fundamentals of Nursing: Concepts, Process, and Practice, ed 4. Mosby–Year Book, St. Louis, 1997.
2. Flynn, JM, and Heffron, PB: Nursing: From Concept to Practice, ed 2. Appleton & Lange, East Norwalk, CT, 1988.
3. Mitchell, PH, and Loustau, A: Concepts Basic to Nursing Practice, ed 3. McGraw-Hill, New York, 1981.
4. Murray, RB, and Zentner, JP: Nursing Assessment and Health Promotion Strategies Through the Life Span, ed 6. Appleton & Lange, Stamford, CT, 1997.
5. Lowdermilk, DL, and Perry, SE: Maternity and Women's Health Care, ed 8. CV Mosby, St. Louis, 2004.
6. Kemp, M, et al: Factors that contribute to pressure sores in surgical patients. Res Nurs Health 13:293, 1990.
7. Guyton, AC, and Hall, JE: Textbook of Medical Physiology, ed 9. WB Saunders, Philadelphia, 1996.
8. Schuster, CS, and Ashburn, SS: The Process of Human Development: A Holistic Life-Span Approach, ed 3. JB Lippincott, New York, 1992.
9. Korones, SB: High-Risk Newborn Infants: The Basis for Intensive Nursing Care, ed 4. CV Mosby, St. Louis, 1986.
10. Driscoll, J, and Heird, W: Maintenance fluid therapy during the neonatal period. In Winters, RW (ed): Principles of Pediatric Fluid Therapy, ed 2. Little, Brown, Boston, 1982.
11. Brandt, PA, Chinn, PE, and Smith, ME: Current Practice in Pediatric Nursing. CV Mosby, St. Louis, 1980.
12. McCrory, WW: Developmental Nephrology. Harvard University Press, Cambridge, MA, 1972.
13. Masiak, MJ, Naylor, MD, and Hayman, LL: Fluids and Electrolytes Through the Life Cycle. Appleton-Century-Crofts, East Norwalk, CT, 1985.
14. Stone, L, and Church, J: Childhood and Adolescence: A Psychology of the Growing Person. Random House, New York, 1968.
15. Young, C, et al: Body composition of pre-adolescent and adolescent girls. J Am Diabet Assoc 53:579, 1968.
16. Chinn, P, and Leitch, C: Child Health Maintenance: Concepts in Family-Centered Care, ed 2. CV Mosby, St. Louis, 1979.
17. Fishman, P: Healthy People 2000: What progress toward better nutrition? Geriatrics 51:38, 1996.
18. Stanley, M, and Beare, PG: Gerontological Nursing: A Health Promotion and Protection Approach. FA Davis, Philadelphia, 1999.
19. Barracos, A, et al: Appropriate and effective use of the NSI checklist and screens. J Am Diet Assoc 95:647, 1995.
20. Boult, C, et al: The validity of nutritional status as a marker for future disability and depressive symptoms among high-risk older adults. J Am Geriat Soc 47:995, 1999.
21. Ettinger, RL: The unique oral health needs of an aging population. Dent Clin North Am 41:633, 1997.
22. Berg, R, and Morgenstern, NE: Physiologic changes in the elderly. Dent Clin North Am 41:651, 1997.
23. Tyson, SP: Gerontological Nursing Care. WB Saunders, Philadelphia, 1999.
24. Abrams, WB (ed): The Merck Manual of Geriatrics, ed 2. Merck and Co., Whitehouse Station, NJ, 1995.
25. Hazzard, WR, et al: Principles of Geriatric Medicine and Gerontology, ed 4. McGraw-Hill, St. Louis, 1999.
26. Miller, CA: Nursing Care of Older Adults: Theory and Practice, ed 3. Lippincott, Philadelphia, 1999.
27. Gaston, NW, et al: A focus on nutrition for the elderly: It's time to take a closer look. Nurture Insights, USDA Center for Nutrition Policy and Promotion, Washington, DC, 1999.
28. Author: Nursing Diagnosis: Definitions and Classification, 2005–2006, North American Nursing Diagnosis Association, Philadelphia, 2005.
29. Portnoi, VA: Helicobacter pylori infection and anorexia of aging. Arch Intern Med 157:269, 1997.
30. Oakley, LD, and Kane, J: Personal and social illness demands related to depression. Arch Psychiatr Nurs 13:294, 1999.
31. Haber, J, et al: Psychiatric Nursing, ed 5. Addison-Wesley, Redwood City, CA, 1996.
32. Zauszniewski, J, and Rong, JR: Depressive cognitions and psychosocial functioning: A test of Beck's cognitive theory. Arch Psychiatr Nurs 13:286, 1999.
33. Kneisl, CR, Wilson, HS, and Trigoboff, E: Contemporary Psychiatric-Mental Health Nursing. Pearson Education, Upper Saddle River, NJ, 2004.
34. Verdery, RB: Clinical evaluation of failure to thrive in older people. Clin Geriatr Med 13:769, 1997.
35. Wallace, JI, and Schwartz, RS: Involuntary weight loss in elderly outpatients. Clin Geriatr Med 13:717, 1997.
36. Kimball, MJ, and Williams-Burgess, C: Failure to thrive: The silent epidemic of the elderly. Arch Psychiatr Nurs 9:99, 1995.
37. Markson, EW: Functional, social, and psychological disability as causes of loss of weight and independence in older community-living people. Clin Geriatr Med 13:639, 1997.
38. Maxmen, J, and Ward, N: Psychotropic drugs fast facts, ed 3. Norton, New York, 2002.
39. Kanusky, C: Health concerns of women in midlife. In Breslin, ET and Lucas, VA, Women's Health Nursing: Toward Evidence-Based Practice. Saunders Elsevier Science, St. Louis, 2003.
40. Gelenberg, AJ, and Bassuk, EL: The Practitioner's Guide to Psychoactive Drugs, ed 4. Plenum, New York, 1997.
41. Banks, JW: Kanistenhsera Teiakotihsnies: A Native community rekindles the tradition of breastfeeding, Lifelines 7(4):340, 2003.
42. Nelson, A, and Sethi, S: The breastfeeding experiences of Canadian Teenage Mothers, JOGNN J Obstet Gynecol Neonatal Nurs 34(5): 615, 2005.
43. Mitra, AK, Khoury, AJ, Carothers, C, and Foretich, C: The loving support breastfeeding campaign: Awareness and practices of health care providers in Mississippi, JOGNN J Obstet Gynecol Neonatal Nurs 32(6):753, 2003.
44. Chezem, J, Friesen, C, and Boettcher, J: Breastfeeding knowledge, breastfeeding confidence and infant feeding plans: Effects on actual feeding. JOGNN J Obstet Gynecol Neonatal Nurs 32:1, 40–47, 2003.
45. Lawrence, RA: Breastfeeding: A Guide for the Medical Profession, ed 5. CV Mosby, St. Louis, 1999.
46. Riordan, J, and Auerback, KG: Breast Feeding and Human Lactation, ed 2. Jones and Bartlett, Sudbury, MA, 1999.
47. Mead, LJ, et al: Breastfeeding success with preterm quadruplets. JOGNN J Obstet Gynecol Neonatal Nurs 21:221, 1992.
48. Thomas, KA: Differential effects of breast- and formula-feeding on preterm infants' sleep-wake patterns. JOGNN J Obstet Gynecol Neonatal Nurs 29:2, 2000.
49. Nichols, FH, and Zwelling, E: Maternal-Newborn Nursing: Theory and Practice. WB Saunders, Philadelphia, 1997.
50. Meier, PP, et al: Breast-feeding support services in the neonatal intensive care unit. JOGNN J Obstet Gynecol Neonatal Nurs 22:4, 338–347, 1993.

51. Meier, PP, Engstrom, JC, Mingolelli, SS, Miracle, DG, and Kiesling, S: The Rush mothers' milk club: Breastfeeding interventions for mothers with very low-birth-weight infants. JOGNN J Obstet Gynecol Neonatal Nurs 33(2):164, 2004.

52. Dennis, CL: The breastfeeding self-efficacy scale: Psychometric assessment of the short form. JOGNN J Obstet Gynecol Neonatal Nurs 32(6):734, 2003.

53. Meier, PP, and Brown, LP: State of the science: Breastfeeding for mothers and low birthweight infants. Nurs Clin North Am 31:351, 1996.

54. Author: When the Care Plan includes breastfeeding and/or Kangaroo Care, the mother and father can experience…, March of Dimes-Masimo Corporation Maternal Concepts (www.nann.org), 2005.

55. Chamblin, C: Breastfeeding after breast reduction: What nurses and moms need to know, Lifelines 10:1, 2006.

56. Ettinger, RL: The unique oral health needs of an aging population. Dent Clin North Am 41:651, 1997.

57. Wold, GH: Basic Geriatric Nursing, ed 2. CV Mosby, St. Louis, 1999.

58. Miller, CA: Nursing Care of Older Adults: Theory and Practice, ed 3. Lippincott, Philadelphia, 1999.

59. Nechyba, C, and Gunn, V: The Harriet Love Handbook, ed 16. CV Mosby, St. Louis, 2003.

60. Larsen, CE: Safety and efficacy of oral rehydration therapy for the treatment of diarrhea and gastroenteritis in pediatrics, Pediatr Nurs 26:177, 2000.

61. The Joanna Briggs Institute: Maintaining oral hydration in older people. Best Practice 5:1, 2001.

62. Wong, DL, and Perry, SE: Maternal Child Nursing Care. CV Mosby, St. Louis, 1998.

63. Teschendorf, M: Women during the reproductive years. In Breslin, ET and Lucas, VA, Women's Health Nursing: Toward Evidence-Based Practice. Saunders Elsevier Science, St. Louis, 2003.

64. Huebscher, R: Natural, alternative and complementary health care. In Breslin, ET, and Lucas, VA, Women's Health Nursing: Toward Evidence-Based Practice. Saunders Elsevier Science, St. Louis, 2003.

65. Mandeville, LK, and Troiano, N: NH: High Risk Intrapartum Nursing. JB Lippincott, Philadelphia, 1992.

66. Beland, I, and Passos, J: Clinical Nursing: Pathophysiological and Psychosocial Approaches, ed 4. Macmillan, New York, 1981.

67. Cosgray, RE, et al: The water-intoxicated patient. Arch Psychiatr Nurs 5:308, 1990.

68. Lapierre, E, et al: Polydipsia and hyponatremia in psychiatric patients: Challenge to creative nursing care. Arch Psychiatr Nurs 5:87, 1990.

69. Boyd, MA: Polydipsia in the chronically mentally ill: A review. Arch Psychiatr Nurs 5:166, 1990.

70. Nichols, FH, and Zwelling, E: Maternal-Newborn Nursing: Theory and Practice. Churchill-Livingstone, New York, 1997.

71. Orr, E: Breast feeding after a cesarean. Int J Childbirth Educ 9:26, 1994.

72. Niefert, MR, and Secat, JM: Milk yield and prolactin rise with simultaneous breast pump. Ambulatory Pediatric Association Meeting Abstracts, Washington, DC, May, 1985.

73. Neifert, MR, and Secat, JM: Lactation insufficiency: A rational approach. Birth 16:182, 1989.

74. Kavanaugh, K, et al: The rewards outweigh the efforts: Breastfeeding outcomes for mothers of preterm infants. J Hum Lactat 13:51, 1997.

75. Chezem, J, et al: Lactation duration: Influences of human milk replacements and formula samples on women employed outside the home. JOGNN J Obstet Gynecol Neonat Nurs 27:646, 1998.

76. Capili, B, and Anastasi, JK: A symptoms review: Nausea and vomiting in HIV. J Assoc Nurses AIDS Care 9:47, 1998.

77. National Institutes of Health: Acupuncture helps nausea NIH outside panel finds. Wall Street Journal, November 6, 1997, p B8.

78. Baines, MJ: Nausea, vomiting, and intestinal obstruction: ABC of palliative care. Br Med J 315:1148, 1997.

79. Henderson, CW: New guidelines for nausea and vomiting in cancer. Cancer Weekly Plus, May 24, 1999, p viii.

80. Pesko, LJ: Liquid prevents nausea, vomiting. Am Drug 214:60, 1997.

81. Simini, B: More oxygen may equal less postoperative nausea. Lancet 354:1618, 1999.

82. Voelker, R: NIH panel says more study is needed to assess marijuana's medical use. JAMA 277:867, 1997.

83. Wolfe, YL, and Chillot, R: Curb queasiness: Surprising cure for chronic nausea. Prevention 49:148, 1997.

84. Woods, A Spralla, G, and Medical Economics Company: PDR Nurses' Handbook, Montvale, NJ, 1999.

85. Eliopoulos, C: Gerontological Nursing. Lippincott, Philadelphia, 1997.

86. Staab, AS, and Hodges, AC: Essentials of Gerontological Nursing: Adaptation to the Aging Process. Lippincott, Philadelphia, 1996.

87. Metheney, N, et al: Detection of inadvertent respiratory placement of small-bore feeding tubes. Heart Lung 19:631, 1990.

88. Metheney, N, et al: Effectiveness of auscultatory method in predicting feeding tube location. Nurs Res 39:266, 1990.

89. American Dietetic Association: Position of the American Dietetic Association: Promotion of breastfeeding. J Am Diet Assoc 97:626, 1997.

90. Grams, M: Breastfeeding Source Book. Achievement Press, Sheridan, WY, 1990.

91. Garner, D, and Garfinkel, P (eds): Handbook of Treatment for Eating Disorders, ed 2. Guilford Press, New York, 1999.

92. Author: Practice guideline for the treatment of patients with eating disorders, American Psychiatric Association Workgroup on Eating Disorders. Am J Psychiatr 157:1, 2000.

93. White, J: The development and clinical testing of an outpatient program for women with bulimia nervosa. Arch Psychiatr Nurs 13:179, 1999.

94. Folkedahl, BA, and Frantz, R: Treatment of pressure ulcers. University of Iowa Gerontological Nursing Interventions Research Center, Research Dissemination Core, Iowa City, IA, 2002, www.guidelines.gov.

95. Erickson, HC, and Kinney, C: Modeling and Role-Modeling: Theory, Research, and Practice. Author, Austin, TX, 1990.

96. Meyer, J: Expert interview: Schizophrenia and the metabolic syndrome. Medscape Psychiatr Ment Health 10:2005.

97. Wright, L, and Leahey, M: Nurses and families, ed 4. FA Davis, Philadelphia, 2005.

98. Maas, M, Buckealter, K, and Hardy, M: Nursing Diagnoses and Interventions for the Elderly. Addison-Wesley Nursing, Fort Collins, CO, 1991.

4

ELIMINATION PATTERN

PATTERN DESCRIPTION

The elimination pattern focuses on bowel and bladder functioning. Although excretion also occurs through the skin and the lungs, the primary mechanisms of waste excretion are the bowel and bladder.

A problem within the elimination pattern may be the primary reason for seeking health care or may arise secondary to another health problem, such as impaired mobility. All but a very few of the other patterns or nursing diagnoses will have an ultimate impact on the elimination pattern from either a physiologic, psychological, or sociologic direction.

Included in the elimination pattern are the individual's habits in terms of excretory regularity, as well as any aids the individual uses to maintain regularity or any devices used to control either bowel or bladder incontinence.

PATTERN ASSESSMENT

1. Is there stool leakage when the client coughs, sneezes, or laughs?
   a. Yes (Bowel Incontinence)
   b. No
2. Is there involuntary passage of stool?
   a. Yes (Bowel Incontinence)
   b. No
3. Does the client take laxatives on a routine basis?
   a. Yes (Constipation, Perceived Constipation)
   b. No
4. Has the number of bowel movements decreased?
   a. Yes (Constipation)
   b. No
5. Are stools hard formed?
   a. Yes (Constipation)
   b. No
6. Does the client have to strain to have a bowel movement?
   a. Yes (Constipation)
   b. No
7. Does the client believe he or she is frequently constipated?
   a. Yes (Perceived Constipation)
   b. No
8. Does the client expect to have a bowel movement at the same time each day?
   a. Yes (Perceived Constipation)
   b. No
9. Are bowel sounds increased?
   a. Yes (Diarrhea)
   b. No
10. Has the number of bowel movements increased?
    a. Yes (Diarrhea)
    b. No
11. Does the client complain of loose, liquid stools?
    a. Yes (Diarrhea)
    b. No

12. Is there increased frequency of voiding?
    a. Yes (Urinary Incontinence; Stress Incontinence; Urge Incontinence)
    b. No (Readiness for Enhanced Urinary Elimination)
13. Is there dribbling of urine when the client laughs, coughs, or sneezes?
    a. Yes (Stress Incontinence)
    b. No (Readiness for Enhanced Urinary Elimination)[1,2]
14. Once need to void is felt, is the client able to reach the toilet in time?
    a. Yes (Readiness for Enhanced Urinary Elimination)
    b. No (Urge Incontinence; Functional Incontinence)
15. Does the client complain of bladder spasms?
    a. Yes (Reflex Incontinence; Urge Incontinence)
    b. No (Readiness for Enhanced Urinary Elimination)
16. Is there a decreased awareness of the need to void?
    a. Yes (Reflex Incontinence; Total Incontinence)
    b. No (Readiness for Enhanced Urinary Elimination)
17. Is there a decreased urge to void?
    a. Yes (Reflex Incontinence)
    b. No (Readiness for Enhanced Urinary Elimination)
18. Does the client void in small amounts?
    a. Yes (Urge Incontinence; Urinary Retention)
    b. No (Readiness for Enhanced Urinary Elimination)
19. Is there urine flow without bladder distention?
    a. Yes (Total Incontinence)
    b. No
20. Is the bladder distended?
    a. Yes (Urinary Retention)
    b. No (Readiness for Enhanced Urinary Elimination)
21. Is there decreased urine output?
    a. Yes (Urinary Retention)
    b. No (Readiness for Enhanced Urinary Elimination)

CONCEPTUAL INFORMATION

Elimination, simply defined, refers to the excretion of waste and nondigested products of the metabolic process. Elimination is essential in maintaining fluid, electrolyte, and nutritional balance of the body. A disruption in an individual's usual elimination pattern can be life-threatening, because a person cannot live long without the ability to rid his or her body of waste products.[2,3]

Elimination depends on the interrelated functioning of the gastrointestinal system, urinary system, nervous system, and skin. This chapter discusses only the lower urinary tract and gastrointestinal tract; the skin and nervous system are related to nursing diagnoses in other chapters. Also, because the nursing diagnoses related to elimination refer only to elimination and not the collection and formation of the waste materials, inclusion of other conceptual information would be confusing.

Our society has a dichotomous attitude toward elimination. A great deal of time, effort, and money is expended in designing and advertising bathrooms and aids to elimination, but to discuss elimination is considered rude.[1] Therefore, obtaining a reliable, complete elimination pattern assessment may be difficult. Added to this difficulty is the fact that each person has his or her own normal elimination habits and acceptable verbiage around elimination. Elimination is highly individualized and can be influenced by age, circadian rhythms, culture, diet, activity, stress, and a number of other factors. Elimination has elements of both involuntary and voluntary control. The mechanisms that control the production of waste materials and the neural signals that the bladder or bowel needs to be emptied are primarily involuntary. However, each person can usually control both the timing of bowel and bladder evacuation, as well as the use of abdominal and perineal muscles to assist in evacuation.

Food and fluid intake are extremely important in elimination. A fluid intake of 2000 mL per day and a food intake of high-fiber foods would, in the majority of instances, ensure an adequate elimination pattern.[3,4] Alteration in elimination may cause psychosocial problems, such as social isolation due to embarrassment, as well as physiologic problems, such as fluid and/or electrolyte imbalance.

BOWEL ELIMINATION

The lower gastrointestinal tract includes the small and large intestines. The small bowel includes the duodenum, jejunum, and ileum, and is approximately 20 feet in length and 1 inch in diameter. The large bowel includes the cecum, colon, and rectum and terminates at the anus. The large bowel is approximately 5 feet long and $2\frac{1}{2}$ inches in diameter. The small bowel and large bowel connect at the ileocecal valve.[2]

The intestines receive partially digested food from the stomach and move the food element through the lower tract, thus assisting in proper absorption of water, nutrients, and electrolytes. The intestines also provide secretory and storage functions. They secrete mucus, potassium, bicarbonate, and enzymes.

The chyme (small intestine contents) is moved by peristalsis, and the feces (large intestine contents) are propelled by mass movements that are stimulated by the gastrocolic reflex. The gastrocolic reflex occurs in response to food entering the stomach and causing distention, so mass movement occurs only a few times a day. The gastrocolic reflex occurs within 30 minutes after eating and is predominant after the first meal of the day. Therefore, the time after the first meal of the day is the most frequent occurrence bowel elimination. Other reflexes involved in elimination are the duodenocolic reflex and the defecation reflex. The duodenocolic reflex is stimulated by the distention of the duodenum as food passes from the stomach to the duodenum. The gastrocolic and duodenocolic reflexes stimulate rectal contraction and, usually, a desire to defecate. The defecation reflex occurs in response to feces entering the rectum. This reflex promotes relaxation of the internal anal sphincter, thus also promoting a desire to defecate. Extra

fluids upon morning waking potentiate the gastrocolic reflex. If the fluids are warm or contain caffeine, they will also stimulate peristalsis.[1,2]

The secretions of the gastrointestinal tract assist with food passage and further digestion. The passage rate of the contents through the intestines helps determine the absorption amount. The small intestine is responsible for about 90 percent of the absorption of amino acids, sodium, calcium chloride, fatty acids, bile salts, and water. Potassium and bicarbonate are excreted. The usual amount of time for chyme to move from the stomach to the ileocecal valve varies from 3 to 10 hours. It takes approximately 12 hours for feces to travel from the ileocecal valve to the rectum. One bowel movement may be the result of meals eaten over the past 3 to 4 days, but most of the food residue from any particular meal will have been excreted within 4 days. Passage of contents is influenced primarily by the amount of residue and the motility rate. Feces are normally evacuated on a moderately regular schedule, but it will vary from three times daily to once per week depending on the individual.

When proper absorption does not occur, necessary nutrients and electrolytes are lost for subsequent body use. Small bowel loss can cause metabolic acidosis and hypokalemia. Large bowel loss can lead to dehydration and hyponatremia.

The squatting, leaning forward position is the most supportive position for defecation because it increases intra-abdominal pressure and promotes easier abdominal and perineal muscle contraction and relaxation. Beside positioning, diet, and fluid intake, other aids to elimination include enemas and laxatives.

Enemas assist in evacuation through promotion of peristalsis, chemical irritation, or lubrication. Volume enemas—500 to 1000 mL of fluid—cause distention, which increases peristalsis. The addition of heat and soapsuds, for example, adds chemical irritation and increases peristalsis. Straight tap-water enemas should be used cautiously, because they are hypotonic and may disturb electrolyte balance. Electrolyte enemas are usually prepackaged and are hypertonic. Hypertonic enemas increase fluid amounts in the bowel through osmosis, thus slightly increasing distention and providing a relatively mild chemical irritation. Both the distention and irritation also result in increased peristalsis. Oil enemas are usually small-volume enemas (100 to 200 mL) providing lubrication as well as stool softening.[1,5]

Laxatives assist elimination by producing bulk, providing lubrication, causing chemical irritation, or softening stool. The action of laxatives ranges from harsh to mild.

Both laxatives and enemas can be abused. Persistent use of either will diminish normal reflexes so that the individual will begin to require more and more aid. The individual then establishes an aid-dependent habit just as a drug abuser does.

Although constipation and diarrhea are the two most common problems with bowel elimination, flatulence may be an associated problem. Flatus (intestinal gas) is normal.

A problem arises when the individual cannot pass the gas or when abnormally large amounts of gas are produced. Flatus is produced by swallowed air, diffusion of gases from the bloodstream to the gastrointestinal tract, carbon dioxide formed by the action of bicarbonate with hydrochloric acid or fatty acids, and bacterial decomposition of food residue. Common causes of gas problems include gas-producing foods, highly irritating foods, constipating medications such as opioids, and inactivity. The problems relate directly to the amount of gas produced and decreased motility. Increased flatus causes distention that, in turn, can cause pain, respiratory difficulty, and further problems with intestinal motility.[1]

As previously mentioned, any bowel elimination problem can ultimately be life-threatening. Any bowel elimination problem, whether constipation, diarrhea, or flatulence, that lasts more than 1 to 2 weeks in an adult, or more than 2 to 3 days for an infant or elderly person, requires immediate health care intervention.

URINARY ELIMINATION

The lower urinary tract is composed of the ureters, bladder, and urethra, which serve as storage and excretory pathways for the waste secreted by the kidneys. The ureters extend from the kidney pelvis to the trigone area in the bladder. The ureters are small tubes composed of smooth muscle that propels urine by peristalsis from the kidney to the bladder. The bladder stores the urine until it is excreted through the urethra. Between the base of the bladder and the top of the urethra is the urethral sphincter. The sphincter opens under learned voluntary control. Opening the urethral sphincter allows the urine to pass through the urethra and meatus for elimination. The female urethra is approximately 3 to 5 centimeters long, and the male urethra is approximately 20 centimeters long.[2]

In adults, the desire to void occurs when the bladder has reached a capacity of 250 to 450 mL of urine. As urine collects to the bladder capacity, the stretch receptors in the bladder muscle are activated. This stretching stimulates the voiding reflex center in the spinal cord (sacral levels two, three, and four), which sends signals to the midbrain and the pons. These stimuli result in inhibition of the spinal reflex center and pudendal nerve, which allows relaxation of the external sphincter and contraction of the bladder, and voiding occurs. The bladder is under parasympathetic control, with the learned voluntary control being guided by the cortex, midbrain, and medulla.[1,2]

The anatomically correct positions for voiding are sitting for the female and standing for the male. It is important to note that in some cultural groups the correct voiding position for the male is squatting. Either standing or squatting is anatomically correct. Difficulties arise if the male is lying down, for example, in traction or a body cast. An individual generally voids 200 to 450 mL each voiding time, and it is within normal limits to void 5 to 10 times per day. Common times for urination are on arising and before retiring. Other times will vary with habits and correspond with work breaks and availability of toilet facilities.[1,2]

Urine volume varies according to the individual and depends on normal kidney functioning, amount of fluid and food intake, environmental temperature, fluid requirements of other organs, presence of open wounds, output by other areas (skin, bowel, or respiration), and medications such as diuretics. The amount of solutes in the urine, an intact neuromuscular system, and the action of the antidiuretic hormone also influence output. A significant impact on urinary output is the opportunity to void at socially acceptable times in private.[1]

Inadequate urinary output may arise from either the kidney not producing urine (suppression) or blockage of urine flow (retention) somewhere between the kidney and external urinary meatus. Suppression may result from disease of the kidneys or other body structures and inadequate fluid intake. Retention may be either mechanical or functional in nature. *Mechanical retention* is due to anatomic blockage, such as a stricture or a calculus. *Functional retention* refers to any retention that is not mechanical and includes such areas as neurogenic problems.[2]

Urinary control relates to the integrity and strength of the urinary sphincters and perineal musculature. Inability to control urinary output often leads to social isolation due to embarrassment over control and odor. Urinary incontinence is more common than most health-care professionals realize. Studies indicate that urinary incontinence is quite common among healthy premenopausal middle-aged women.[6,7,16] These studies found no relationship between continence status, number of children, history of gynecologic surgery, smoking, physical activity, or intake of alcohol and caffeine. The studies found also that very few of these women sought treatment for this incontinence.

Bladder-retraining programs may vary according to individual hospitals and physicians. Consultation with a rehabilitation nurse clinician provides the most current and reliable information regarding a quality bladder-retraining program.[8] Two measures that may assist with incontinence are Credé's maneuver and the Valsalva maneuver. Credé's maneuver involves placing the fingertips together at the midline of the pelvic crest, then massaging deeply and smoothly down to the pubic bone. Check with the physician first, because there are contraindications, such as ureteral reflux.[5] The Valsalva maneuver involves asking the client to simulate having a bowel movement. Have the client take a deep breath, hold it, and then bear down as if expelling feces. Check with the physician first, because there are contraindications, such as glaucoma, eye surgery, and impaired circulation.[4,5]

Urine is a waste product formed as a part of body metabolism. Urine is normally produced at a rate of 30 to 50 mL per hour. Under normal circumstances, output will balance with intake approximately every 72 hours. An hourly output of less than 30 mL, a 24-hour output of 500 mL or less, or an intake–output imbalance lasting longer than 72 hours requires immediate intervention.[1,3]

DEVELOPMENTAL CONSIDERATIONS

Elimination depends on the interrelatedness of fluid intake, muscle tone, regularity of habits, culture, state of health, and adequate nutrition.[2]

INFANT

Kidney function does not reach adult levels until 6 months to 1 year of life. Nervous system control is inadequate, and renal function does not reach a mature status until approximately 1 year of life.[2] Voiding is stimulated by cold air. An infant usually voids 15 to 60 mL at each voiding during the first 24 hours of life and may void reflexively at birth. If the infant has not voided by 12 hours after birth, there is cause for concern. By the third day, the infant may void 8 to 10 times during each 24 hours, equaling about 100 to 400 mL. Urinary output is affected by the amount of fluid consumed, the amount of activity (increased activity equals less urine), and the environmental temperature (increased temperature equals less urine).[9] Uric acid crystals may be found in concentrated urine, causing a rusty discoloration to the diaper.[9]

The muscles and elastic tissues of an infant's intestines are poorly developed, and nervous system control is inadequate. Water and electrolyte absorption is functional but immature. The intestines are proportionally longer than in an adult. Although some digestive enzymes are present, they can break down only simple foods. These digestive enzymes are unable to break down complex carbohydrates or protein.

Meconium is the first waste material that is eliminated by the bowel, usually during the first 24 hours of an infant's life. After 24 hours, the characteristics of the bowel movement change as it mixes with milk. The characteristics of the stool depend on whether an infant is breastfed or bottle-fed. The breastfed infant has soft, semiliquid stools that are yellow or golden in color. The bottle-fed infant has a more formed stool that is light yellow to brown in color.

An infant may have four to eight soft bowel movements a day during the first 4 weeks of life. Flatus often accompanies the passage of stool, and there may be a sour odor to the bowel movement. By the fourth week of life, the number of bowel movements has decreased to two to four per day. By 4 months, there is a predictable interval between bowel movements.

It is common for an infant to push or strain at stool. However, if the stools are very hard or dry, the infant should be assessed for constipation. The bottle-fed infant is more prone to constipation than the breastfed infant is.

Infants sometimes suffer from what is known as *colic*, described as daily periods of distress caused by rapid, violent peristaltic waves and increased gas pressure in the rectum.[9] The cause is unknown but may have to do with the simple (rather than the complex) digestive enzymes of the infant or a decreased amount of vitamins A, K, or E. Most authorities agree that colic disappears as digestive enzymes become more complex and when normal bacterial flora accumulate.[9]

TODDLER AND PRESCHOOLER

By the time the child is 2 years of age, the kidneys are able to conserve water and to concentrate urine almost on an adult level, except under stress. The bladder increases in size and is able to hold approximately 88 mL of urine.

Nervous system and gastrointestinal maturation has occurred during infancy and the beginning of the toddler years. By the time children are 2 to 3 years of age, they are ready to control bowel and bladder functioning. Bowel elimination control is usually attained first; daytime bladder control is second; and nighttime bladder control is third. The child must be able to walk a few steps, control the sphincter, recognize and interpret that the bladder is full, and be able to indicate that he or she wants to go to the bathroom. The child must also value dryness. He or she must recognize that it is more socially acceptable to be dry than to be wet.

Parents should not attempt toilet training, even if the child is ready, if there are family or environmental stressors. Regression is normal during toilet training and, coupled with undue stress, could cause physical or psychosocial problems.

Bladder training takes time to accomplish. Both the parent and the child must have patience and not get unduly upset when accidents occur. In fact, nighttime bladder control may not be attained until age 5 to 8 years. Doctors and researchers disagree on the age at which nighttime bedwetting (enuresis) becomes a problem.[9] Parents should limit fluids at night, have the child void before going to bed, and get the child up at least once during the night to assist in attaining nighttime control.

To toilet train, the parent should watch for patterns of defecation. Eating stimulates peristaltic activity and evacuation. The child can then be taken to the toilet at the expected time after eating. The child should be told what is expected while on the toilet. Give the child enough time to evacuate the bowel, but do not have the child sit on the toilet too long, as both the child and the parent may become frustrated.

Children at this age like to please their parents. Evacuation of the bowel is a natural process and should not be approached as a dirty or unnatural one. The child should be rewarded when able to defecate, but should not be punished if unable to have a bowel movement. Children should feel proud of their accomplishments, and should not be punished or made to feel ashamed for not producing expected results.

Children usually do not need enemas or laxatives to make them regular. In fact, the artificial aids may be dangerous. Lack of parental understanding of the elimination process and child development, coupled with harsh punishment for "accidents," may lead a child to an obsessive, meticulous, and rigid personality.

Accidents can and do occur even after a child has been completely toilet trained, usually because the child ignores the defecation urge when he or she is engrossed in an activity and does not want to take the time to go to the bathroom, or when other stressors have a higher priority at that moment.

SCHOOL-AGE CHILD

The urinary system is functioning maturely by this age. The normal output is 500 mL per day. Urinary tract infections are common in girls because of improper hygiene practices. Girls should be taught to clean the perineum after elimination from front to back to avoid contamination of the urethra with gastrointestinal flora. The gastrointestinal system attains adult functional maturity during the school years. School-age children often delay defecation in order to continue with preferred activities such as play or socialization. This delay in defecation often leads to constipation.

ADOLESCENT

There are no noticeable differences in patterns of urinary elimination in this age group. The intestines grow in length and width. The muscles of the intestines become thicker and stronger.

This developmental stage is important in developing bowel habits. The teenager is engaged in developing sexuality. This group may ignore warning signals for elimination because they do not want to leave their activities or because of the close association of the anus to the teenager's developing sexual organs. In addition, if a problem arises with elimination, adolescents are reluctant to talk about it with either their peers or an adult.

YOUNG ADULT

There is no noticeable difference in patterns of elimination during this developmental period. Total urinary output for 24 hours is 1000 to 2000 mL. The rate of passage of feces is influenced by the nature of the foods consumed and the physical health of the individual. Hemorrhoids are possible in this developmental group, especially young women.

ADULT

Adequate daily fluid intake helps maintain proper elimination functions. There is a gradual decrease in the number of nephrons and therefore decreased renal functioning with age. In addition, bladder tone diminishes; thus, the adult may urinate more frequently.

Digestive enzymes (gastric acid, pepsin, ptyalin, and pancreatic enzymes) also begin to decrease. This may lead to an increasing incidence of intestinal disorders, cancer, and gastrointestinal complaints.

OLDER ADULT

Renal function is slowed by both structural and functional aging changes, mainly the decrease in the number of nephrons. Vascular sclerosing also occurs in the renal system, and this, combined with fewer nephrons, decreases available blood so that the glomerular filtration rate (GFR) becomes markedly reduced. Although the GFR reduction is still sufficient to handle normal demands, stress or illness can significantly alter the older adult's renal status.[10] Decreased concentration and dilution ability of the kidneys occurs as a result of changes in the renal tubules. Waste products are effectively processed by the kidneys, but over a longer period of time. The decreased efficiency of the kidneys makes older adults especially vulnerable to medication side effects and problems regarding drug excretion.[2]

The older man may have an enlarged prostate gland. Obstructive voiding symptoms resulting from prostatic enlargement can include hesitancy, decreased force of stream, terminal dribbling, post void fullness, and double voiding.[10] Bladder changes, resulting from loss of smooth muscle elasticity, can result in decreased bladder capacity. Uninhibited bladder contractions may interrupt bladder filling and lead to a premature urge to void. Increased residual urine and incomplete emptying of the bladder result in a higher incidence of urinary tract infections in older adults of both sexes. Bladder sonography is often helpful in determining the extent of postvoid residual urine problems.

Changes in the gastrointestinal tract include a continued decrease in digestive enzymes and questionable changes in absorption in the small intestines. The large intestine may have reduced blood flow secondary to vascular twisting, and there is debate regarding decreased motility in the colon. Problems related to constipation may occur as a result of increased tolerance for rectal distention rather than decreased motility.[2]

The link between age and constipation is often a result of many contributing factors, which can include changes in fluid intake, changes in diet, changes in mobility, environmental factors, and health factors. Older adults often drink less fluid, which slows colonic transit and reduces stool output. A decrease in fiber in the diet can lead to slowed colonic transit and decreased frequency of bowel movements. Mobility plays an important role in bowel health, as the highest risk for constipation is among those who are bedbound or chairbound.[11] Environmental factors such as reduced privacy, inaccessible toileting facilities, inappropriate facilities, and reliance on other people for assistance may also contribute to the development of constipation.[11] Anxiety, depression, and impaired cognition may also contribute to the development of constipation. Finally, many medications can contribute to constipation: opioid analgesics, anticholinergics, and antidepressants. Diuretics, hypnotics, and antipsychotics must be considered in light of their effect on genitourinary function.[12]

TABLE 4.1 NANDA, NIC, and NOC Taxonomy Linkages

GORDON'S FUNCTIONAL HEALTH PATTERN	NANDA NURSING DIAGNOSIS	NIC PRIORITY INTERVENTIONS	NOC EVALUATIONS
Elimination	Bowel Incontinence	Bowel Incontinence Care Bowel Incontinence Care: Encopresis Bowel Training	Bowel Continence Bowel Elimination Tissue Integrity: Skin & Mucous Membrane
	Constipation, Risk for, Actual, Perceived	**Actual** Bowel irritation Constipation/Impaction Management **Perceived** Bowel Management **Risk for** Constipation/Impaction Management	**Actual** Bowel Elimination Hydration Symptom Control **Perceived** Bowel Elimination Health Beliefs Knowledge: Health Behavior **Risk for** Appetite Bowel Elimination Hydration Immobility Consequences: Physiological Knowledge: Medication Medication Response Mobility Nutritional Status: Food & Fluid Intake Risk Control Risk Detection Self-Care: Non-Parenteral Medication; Toileting Symptom Control Treatment Behavior: Illness or Injury
	Diarrhea	Diarrhea Management Medication Management	Bowel Continence Bowel Elimination Electrolyte and Acid–Base Balance Fluid Balance Hydration Ostomy Self-Care Symptom Severity
	Urinary Elimination, Readiness for Enhanced	*Still in development*	Kidney Function Self-Care: Toileting Urinary Continence Urinary Elimination
	Urinary Incontinence: Functional	Prompted Voiding Urinary Habit Training	Medication Response Self-Care: Toileting Urinary Continence Urinary Elimination
	Urinary Incontinence: Reflex	Urinary Bladder Training Urinary Catheterization: Intermittent	Neurological Status: Autonomic Tissue Integrity: Skin & Mucous Membranes Urinary Continence Urinary Elimination
	Urinary Incontinence: Stress	Pelvic Muscle Exercise Urinary Incontinence Care	Urinary Continence Urinary Elimination

(table continued on page 236)

TABLE 4.1 **NANDA, NIC, and NOC Taxonomy Linkages** (continued from page 235)

GORDON'S FUNCTIONAL HEALTH PATTERN	NANDA NURSING DIAGNOSIS	NIC PRIORITY INTERVENTIONS	NOC EVALUATIONS
	Urinary Incontinence: Total	Urinary Incontinence Care	Tissue Integrity: Skin & Mucous Membrane Urinary Continence Urinary Elimination
	Urinary Incontinence: Urge	Urinary Habit Training Urinary Incontinence Care	Self-Care: Toileting Urinary Continence Urinary Elimination
	Urinary Incontinence: Urge, Risk for	Urinary Habit Training	Infection Severity Knowledge: Medication; Treatment Regimen Medication Response Neurological Status: Autonomic Risk Control Risk Detection Stress Level Urinary Continence Urinary Elimination
	Urinary Retention	Urinary Catheterization Urinary Retention Care	Urinary Continence Urinary Elimination

 APPLICABLE NURSING DIAGNOSES

BOWEL INCONTINENCE

DEFINITION[13]

Change in normal bowel habits characterized by involuntary passage of stool.

DEFINING CHARACTERISTICS[13]

1. Constant dribbling of soft stool
2. Fecal odor
3. Inability to delay defecation
4. Urgency
5. Self-report of inability to feel rectal fullness
6. Fecal staining of clothing and/or bedding
7. Recognizes rectal fullness but reports inability to expel formed stool
8. Inattention to urge to defecate
9. Inability to recognize urge to defecate
10. Red perianal skin

RELATED FACTORS[13]

1. Environmental factors (for example, inaccessible bathroom)
2. Incomplete emptying of bowel
3. Rectal sphincter abnormality
4. Impaction
5. Dietary habits
6. Colorectal lesions
7. Stress
8. Lower motor nerve damage
9. Abnormally high abdominal or intestinal pressure
10. General decline in muscle tone
11. Loss of rectal sphincter control
12. Impaired cognition
13. Upper motor nerve damage
14. Chronic diarrhea
15. Self-care deficit, toileting
16. Impaired reservoir capacity
17. Immobility
18. Laxative abuse

RELATED CLINICAL CONCERNS

1. Alzheimer's disease
2. Guillain-Barré syndrome
3. Spinal cord injury
4. Intestinal surgery
5. Gynecologic surgery

EXPECTED OUTCOME

Will have no more than one soft, formed stool per day by [date].

TARGET DATES

Target dates should be based on the individual's usual bowel elimination pattern. Incontinence may require additional retraining time and effort. Therefore, a target date 5 days from admission would be most realistic. Also remember that there must be a realistic potential that bowel continence can be regained by the client.

 Have You Selected the Correct Diagnosis?

Constipation
The problem may really be due to constipation with impaction. Incontinence may occur because some feces are leaking around the impaction site and the individual is unable to control its passage and thus appears incontinent.

Self-Care Deficit, Toileting
If the individual is unable to appropriately care for his or her evacuation needs, incontinence may result.

Diarrhea
Diarrhea relates to frequent bowel movements, but the client is aware of rectal filling and can control the feces until reaching the toilet. With incontinence, the client may not be aware of rectal filling, and the stool passage is involuntary.

NURSING ACTIONS/INTERVENTIONS AND RATIONALES

Adult Health

ACTIONS/INTERVENTIONS	RATIONALES
Check for fecal impaction on admission, and implement nursing actions for constipation if impaction is noted.	Impaction may lead to leakage of bowel contents around impacted area.[12,14]
Record each incontinent episode when it occurs as well as the amount, color, and consistency of each stool.	Assists in determining the pattern of incontinence.
Record events associated with the incontinent episode, including events both before and after the episode (i.e., activity, stress, location, people present, etc.).	Assists in determining the pattern of incontinence.
Scrutinize and/or remove factors that contribute to incontinent episodes (e.g., stress, diet, problems in accessibility to bathroom).	
Examine perianal skin integrity following each incontinent episode.	Allows early detection of any tissue integrity problems.
Keep the anal area clean and dry.	Bowel contents are damaging to the skin and predispose the patient to tissue integrity problems.
Provide emotional support for the patient through teaching, providing time for listening, etc.	The patient may find incontinence embarrassing and may try to isolate self.
Initiate bowel training at least 4 days before discharge: • Suppository 30 minutes after eating. • Toilet half-hour after suppository insertion. • Toilet prior to activity. • Stimulate defecation reflex with circular movement in rectum using gloved, lubricated finger.	Establishes consistent pattern, and conditions control of elimination.
Teach the client, beginning as soon after admission as possible:	Basic knowledge promotes understanding of condition and assists the patient to change behavior as well as empowering the patient for self-care.
• Pelvic floor muscle exercises, alternating contraction and relaxation of perineal muscles while sitting in a chair and with feet placed apart on floor [Note schedule to talk client through these here.] • Diet (i.e., role of fiber and fluids) • Use of assistive devices such as Velcro closings on clothes, pads • Perineal hygiene • Appropriate use of suppositories and antidiarrheal medications	Strengthens pelvic floor and abdominal muscles.
Refer for home health-care assistance.	

(care plan continued on page 238)

NURSING ACTIONS/INTERVENTIONS AND RATIONALES (continued from page 237)

Child Health

Nursing actions for bowel incontinence in the child are essentially the same as those for Adult Health, plus the following. Modifications need to be made for child's age and size (e.g., medication dosage and fluid amounts). Encopresis is the term noted in the literature, with a prerequisite factor identified to be that the event must occur at least once a month for at least 3 months, and the chronological or developmental age of the child must be at least 4 years.

ACTIONS/INTERVENTIONS	RATIONALES
Assess for contributory factors, especially environmental change such as a new home, birth of sibling, or change in bathrooming environment.	Allows for fullest consideration of possible etiology for the problem of bowel incontinence.
Note related abnormalities of the digestive tract including leakage secondary to bowel obstruction in infants or Hirschsprung's syndrome of mega-colon or related bowel obstruction with leakage.	Allows for fullest consideration of possible etiology for the problem of bowel incontinence.
Assess for related medical conditions such as myelomeningocele, cerebral palsy, or hypothyroidism.	Ensures consideration for fullest possible etiology of problem of bowel incontinence.
For instances of pattern of fear–pain cycles of encopresis, assess for possible disturbance in the mother–child relationship.	Emotional factors may contribute to the pattern.
Assess for stressors in the family or child's daily routine.	Stress contributes to altered bowel pattern.
Obtain a full history in order to individualize the plan of care. Identify related circumstantial factors and encourage the parents to share their thoughts regarding the problem.	Offers individualized plan of care with attention to primary factors.
Maintain a nonjudgmental attitude throughout.	Fosters open communication.
Allow for embarrassment according to age when child is expected to be self-toileting.	Communicates caring and nonjudging of behaviors.
Provide appropriate emotional support for child and family.	Offers validation of the importance of being accepted by others and how this is threatened.

Women's Health

Nursing actions and interventions in bowel incontinence in Women's Health are the same as in Adult Health, except for the following:

As women age and estrogen levels decrease, the perineal floor sometimes loses elasticity, which can lead to constipation and/or bowel incontinence if proper diet and exercise are not practiced.	Encourage women to discuss with the health care provider any problems with changes in bowel habits. Many women will not discuss these problems because of embarrassment.[16]
	Many women who have suffered uterine prolapse and pelvic relaxation with displacement of pelvic organs can be relieved only by surgical repair.[15]

Mental Health

ACTIONS/INTERVENTIONS	RATIONALES
If a pattern forms around specific events, develop plan to: • Remind the person to use the bathroom before the event. Add positive reinforcers as they remember on their own. [Note reinforcers to be used here.]	Promotes the client's perceived control, and increases potential for the client's involvement in treatment plan.[17]

Mental Health

ACTIONS/INTERVENTIONS	RATIONALES
• Alter the manner in which a specific task is performed to prevent stress. [Note alterations here.]	
• Discuss with the client alternative ways of coping with stress. (Refer to Chapter 8 for specific nursing actions related to reduction of anxiety, and Chapter 11 for specific nursing actions related to ineffective coping.)	
If assessment suggests secondary gains associated with episodes, decrease these by:	Provides negative consequences for inappropriate coping behavior.[18]
• Withdrawing social contact after an episode	
• Having the client clean him- or herself	
• Providing social contact or interactions with the client at times when no incontinence is experienced	
If not related to secondary gain, spend [number] minutes with the client after each episode to allow expression of feelings.	Verbalization of feelings in a nonthreatening environment models acceptance of feelings and positive coping behavior.[18]
Discuss with the client the effects this problem has on his or her lifestyle.	Increases the client's awareness of impact inappropriate coping behaviors have on lifestyle. Provides data for development of alternative coping, promoting the client's perceived control.[19]

Gerontic Health

● NOTE: *Incontinence is not a normal part of aging. When older adults experience incontinence, efforts should be made to both determine the cause of the incontinence and return the client to a continent state.*

In addition to the interventions for Adult Health, the following may be utilized for the aging client:

ACTIONS/INTERVENTIONS	RATIONALES
Record events associated with incontinent episode.	Assists in determining the pattern of incontinence. Older adults may have difficulty in reaching the commode or bathroom easily.
Monitor medication intake for potential to result in bowel incontinence.	Medications with a sedative effect may decrease the ability of the client to reach toilet facilities in a timely manner.
Teach toileting skills to caregivers of cognitively impaired older adults. In early dementia, labeling the bathroom and reminding the individual to toilet may result in continence.	Depending on the stage of the disease, a person with dementia may forget to toilet or have difficulty finding a bathroom that is not readily identified.

Home Health

Nursing actions for incontinence in the Home Health setting are the same as those for Adult Health, with the following additions:

ACTIONS/INTERVENTIONS	RATIONALES
Assist the client/family in identifying factors that may be contributing to the problem:	Diarrhea is a common cause of bowel incontinence. Promotes understanding of the condition and may lead to solutions.

(care plan continued on page 240)

NURSING ACTIONS/INTERVENTIONS AND RATIONALES (continued from page 239)

Home Health

ACTIONS/INTERVENTIONS	RATIONALES
• Diarrhea • Diet • Medications • Environmental issues • Fatigue • Difficulty removing clothes	
Modify the home environment as needed to facilitate continence as appropriate: • Clear the path to the bathroom. • Provide bedside commodes as needed.	
Educate the client/family on the correct use of antidiarrheal agents as needed to reduce the frequency of bowel movements.	Diarrhea is a common cause of bowel incontinence.
Monitor skin integrity for skin breakdown.	These measures prevent secondary problems from occurring as a result of the existing problem.
Educate the client/family regarding the need to keep bed linens and clothing clean and dry	These measures prevent secondary problems from occurring as a result of the existing problem.
Assess the client/family need for adult diapers, linens. Make referrals for obtaining these supplies as appropriate.	These measures prevent secondary problems from occurring as a result of the existing problem.

CONSTIPATION, RISK FOR, ACTUAL, AND PERCEIVED

DEFINITIONS[13]

Constipation   A decrease in a person's normal frequency of defecation accompanied by difficult or incomplete passage of stool and/or passage of excessively hard, dry stool.

Risk for Constipation   At risk for a decrease in a person's normal frequency of defecation accompanied by difficult or incomplete passage of stool and/or passage of excessively hard, dry stool.

Perceived Constipation   The state in which an individual makes a self-diagnosis of constipation and ensures a daily bowel movement through abuse of laxatives, enemas, and suppositories.

DEFINING CHARACTERISTICS[13]

A. Constipation
1. Change in bowel pattern
2. Bright red blood with stool
3. Presence of soft paste-like stool in rectum
4. Distended abdomen
5. Dark or black or tarry stool
6. Increased abdominal pressure
7. Percussed abdominal dullness
8. Pain with defecation
9. Decreased volume of stool
10. Straining with defecation
11. Decreased frequency
12. Dry, hard, formed stool
13. Palpable rectal mass
14. Feeling of rectal fullness or pressure
15. Abdominal pain
16. Unable to pass stool
17. Anorexia
18. Headache
19. Change in abdominal growling (borborygmi)
20. Indigestion
21. Atypical presentation in older adults (e.g., change in mental status, urinary incontinence, unexplained falls, elevated body temperature)
22. Severe flatus
23. Generalized fatigue
24. Hypoactive or hyperactive bowel sounds
25. Palpable abdominal mass
26. Abdominal tenderness with or without palpable muscle resistance

27. Nausea and/or vomiting
28. Oozing liquid stool

B. Risk for Constipation (Risk Factors)
1. Functional
   a. Habitual denial or ignoring of urge to defecate
   b. Recent environmental changes
   c. Inadequate toileting (e.g., timeliness, positioning for defecation, privacy)
   d. Irregular defecation habits
   e. Insufficient physical activity
   f. Abdominal muscle weakness
2. Psychological
   a. Emotional stress
   b. Mental confusion
   c. Depression
3. Physiologic
   a. Insufficient fiber intake
   b. Dehydration
   c. Inadequate dentition or oral hygiene
   d. Poor eating habits
   e. Insufficient fluid intake
   f. Change in usual foods and eating patterns
   g. Decreased motility of gastrointestinal tract
4. Pharmacologic
   a. Phenothiazines
   b. Nonsteroidal anti-inflammatory agents
   c. Sedatives
   d. Aluminum-containing antacids
   e. Laxative overdose
   f. Iron salts
   g. Anticholinergics
   h. Antidepressants
   i. Anticonvulsants
   j. Antilipemic agents
   k. Calcium channel blockers
   l. Calcium carbonate
   m. Diuretics
   n. Sympathomimetics
   o. Opiates
   p. Bismuth salts
5. Mechanical
   a. Rectal abscess or ulcer
   b. Pregnancy
   c. Rectal anal stricture
   d. Postsurgical obstruction
   e. Rectal anal fissures
   f. Megacolon (Hirschsprung's disease)
   g. Electrolyte imbalance
   h. Tumors
   i. Prostate enlargement
   j. Rectocele
   k. Rectal prolapse
   l. Neurologic impairment
   m. Hemorrhoids
   n. Obesity

C. Perceived Constipation
1. Expectation of a daily bowel movement with the resulting overuse of laxatives, enemas, and suppositories.
2. Expected passage of stool at same time each day.

RELATED FACTORS[13]

A. Constipation
1. Functional
   a. Habitual denial or ignoring of urge to defecate
   b. Recent environmental changes
   c. Inadequate toileting (e.g., timeliness, positioning for defecation, privacy)
   d. Irregular defecation habits
   e. Insufficient physical activity
   f. Abdominal muscle weakness
2. Psychological
   a. Emotional stress
   b. Mental confusion
   c. Depression
3. Physiologic
   a. Insufficient fiber intake
   b. Dehydration
   c. Inadequate dentition or oral hygiene
   d. Poor eating habits
   e. Insufficient fluid intake
   f. Change in usual foods and eating patterns
   g. Decreased motility of gastrointestinal tract
4. Pharmacologic
   a. Phenothiazines
   b. Nonsteroidal anti-inflammatory agents
   c. Sedatives
   d. Aluminum-containing antacids
   e. Laxative overdose
   f. Iron salts
   g. Anticholinergics
   h. Antidepressants
   i. Anticonvulsants
   j. Antilipemic agents
   k. Calcium channel blockers
   l. Calcium carbonate
   m. Diuretics
   n. Sympathomimetics
   o. Opiates
   p. Bismuth salts
5. Mechanical
   a. Rectal abscess or ulcer
   b. Pregnancy
   c. Rectal anal stricture
   d. Postsurgical obstruction
   e. Rectal anal fissures
   f. Megacolon (Hirschsprung's disease)
   g. Electrolyte imbalance
   h. Tumors
   i. Prostate enlargement

j. Rectocele
k. Rectal prolapse
l. Neurologic impairment
m. Hemorrhoids
n. Obesity
B. **Risk for Constipation**
  The risk factors are also the related factors.
C. **Perceived Constipation**
  1. Impaired thought processes
  2. Faulty appraisal
  3. Cultural or family health belief

RELATED CLINICAL CONCERNS

1. Anemias
2. Hypothyroidism
3. Hemorrhoids
4. Renal dialysis
5. Abdominal surgery

EXPECTED OUTCOME

Will return, as nearly as possible, to usual bowel elimination habits by [date].

TARGET DATES

Target dates should be based on the individual's usual bowel elimination habits. A target date 3 to 5 days from admission would be reasonable for the majority of clients.

 Have You Selected the Correct Diagnosis?

Imbalanced Nutrition, Less or More Than Body Requirements
This might be the primary nursing diagnosis. Either of these diagnoses influences the amount and consistency of the feces.

Deficient Fluid Volume
This diagnosis might also be the primary problem. The feces need adequate lubrication to pass through the gastrointestinal tract. If there is a Deficient Fluid Volume, the feces is harder, more solid, and unable to move through the system.

Diarrhea or Bowel Incontinence
Constipation can be misdiagnosed as Diarrhea or Bowel Incontinence. Diarrhea or incontinence may be a secondary condition to constipation, as semi-liquid feces may pass around the area of constipation.

Impaired Physical Mobility
This diagnosis could be the underlying cause of constipation. Decrease in physical mobility affects every body system. In the gastrointestinal tract, peristalsis is slowed, which may lead to a backlog of feces and to constipation.

Self-Care Deficit, Toileting
This diagnosis may also be the primary diagnosis. Difficulty in reaching appropriate toileting facilities and difficulty in cleansing oneself after toileting could lead to a decision to delay bowel movement, with a result of constipation.

Ineffective Individual Coping and Anxiety
These diagnoses are two psychosocial nursing diagnoses from which Constipation needs to be differentiated. Both of these psychosocial diagnoses initiate stress as an autonomic response, and the parasympathetic system stimuli (which control motility of the gastrointestinal tract) are reduced. This reduced motility may lead to constipation.

NURSING ACTIONS/INTERVENTIONS AND RATIONALES

Adult Health

ACTIONS/INTERVENTIONS	RATIONALES
Record amount, color, and consistency of feces following each bowel movement. Question the client regarding bowel movements at least once per shift. Also record if there was no bowel movement on each shift.	Basic assessment of problem severity as well as monitoring effectiveness of therapy.
Monitor and record symptoms associated with passage of bowel movement: • Any straining, pain, or headache • Any rectal bleeding or fissures	Allows early detection of additional problems.
If fecal impaction:	Prioritization of methods used to break up and remove impaction.

ACTIONS/INTERVENTIONS	RATIONALES

• Attempt digital removal using gloves and lubrication.
  • Administer oil retention enema of small volume. Have the client retain for at least 1 hour.[5]
  • Use small-volume saline enema if oil retention does not relieve impaction.
Collaborate with appropriate members of health-care team regarding additional pharmacological strategies (e.g., stool softeners, laxatives, etc.).
Measure and total intake and output every shift.
	Allows monitoring of adequate fluid intake to increase water content of feces.

Force fluids, of client's choice, to at least 2000 mL daily. Provide 8 ounces of fluid every 2 hours on [odd/even] hour beginning at awakening each morning. [Note client's preferred fluids here.]	Increases moisture and water content of feces for easier movement through intestines and anus.
Increase the client's activity to extent possible through ambulation at least three times per day while awake. [Note schedule here.]	Activity promotes stimulation of the bowel and assists in elimination.
Assist the client with implementation of stress reduction techniques at least once per shift. [Note technique to be used and schedule here.]	Promotes relaxation and can increase feces passage through the intestines.
Digitally stimulate the anal sphincter at scheduled times (usually after meals) [State times here].	Stimulates defecation reflex and urge.
Provide privacy and sufficient time for bowel elimination.	Decreases stress and promotes relaxation, which increases likelihood of bowel movement.
Help the client assume positions that facilitate bowel movements (e.g., a forward leaning position while sitting, or a semi-Fowler's position if on a bedpan).[20]	Promotes effective use of abdominal muscles, and allows gravity to assist in defecation.
Monitor anal skin integrity at least once per shift.	Straining at stool can cause splits and tears of the anal tissue.
Teach the client, starting as soon after admission as possible: • Pelvic floor muscle exercises • The importance of a bowel routine and the need to respond to the urge to defecate as soon as possible • To stimulate gastrocolic reflex through drinking prune juice or hot liquid on arising • To allow sufficient time for bowel movement and plan time for elimination • To include high-fiber foods and adequate liquid in daily diet • To avoid prolonged use of elimination aids such as laxatives and enemas • To avoid straining • To use proper perineal hygiene • To describe the relationship of diet and activity to bowel elimination	Promotes understanding of self-care needs prior to discharge.[21] Strengthens pelvic floor and abdominal muscles.
Collaborate (as deemed necessary), with the following as soon as possible after admission: • With the dietitian, regarding a high-fiber, high-roughage diet (the more food a client eats, the less laxatives the client will require) • With the physical therapist, regarding exercise program	Provides basic resources and information needed; promotes holistic approach to treatment.

(care plan continued on page 244)

NURSING ACTIONS/INTERVENTIONS AND RATIONALES (continued from page 243)

Adult Health

ACTIONS/INTERVENTIONS	RATIONALES
• With the health-care provider, regarding mild analgesics and ointments for control of pain associated with bowel movements • With the health-care provider, regarding use of stool softeners, laxatives, suppositories, and enemas • With the enterostomal therapist, regarding ostomy care (i.e., irrigations, stoma and skin care, and appliances) • With the psychiatric nurse clinician, regarding counseling for the client and family about possible underlying emotional components • With the home health nurse, regarding follow-up planning for home and usual daily activities of living with emphasis on stress, etc.	

Child Health

Nursing actions for constipation in the child are essentially the same as those for Adult Health. Modifications would be made for child's age and size, for example, medication dosage and fluid amounts. For the diagnosis of Risk for Constipation, the following actions would be appropriate:

ACTIONS/INTERVENTIONS	RATIONALES

Monitor for all possible contributory factors including:
• Hirschsprung's disease (congenital aganglionic megacolon)
• Neonatal period:
  • Failure to pass meconium in first 24 to 48 hours after birth
  • Reluctance to ingest fluids
  • Bile-stained vomitus
  • Abdominal distention
  • Intestinal obstruction
• Infancy:
  • Inadequate weight gain
  • History of constipation
  • Abdominal distention
  • Episodic diarrhea and vomiting
  • Bloody diarrhea
  • Fever
  • Severe lethargy
• Childhood:
  • Constipation
  • Ribbon-like, foul-smelling stools
  • Abdominal distention
  • Palpable fecal masses
  • History of poor appetite, poor growth
	Appropriate identification of cause of constipation in case of Hirschsprung's disease will offer appropriate treatment.

Monitor for contributing factors according to likelihood of potential for age, diet, known medical status, and developmental crisis (e.g., iron in infant formula, vitamins, known hypothyroidism, self-toileting, etc.).	Developmentally appropriate factors will assist in identification of likely essential issues.

Women's Health

Nursing actions for constipation in women are essentially the same as those for Adult Health, except for the following considerations during pregnancy:

ACTIONS/INTERVENTIONS	RATIONALES
Assist the client in identifying lifestyle adjustments that may be needed because of changes in physiologic function, or needs during experiential phases of life (e.g., during pregnancy, postpartum, and following gynecologic surgery).	Provides information needed as basis for planning care and health maintenance.
Teach the client changes that occur during pregnancy that contribute to decreased gastric motility and potential constipation:	Provides basic information for self-care during pregnancy, birthing process, and postpartum.[22]
• Fluid intake may decrease because of nausea and vomiting of early pregnancy.	
• Increased use of mother's body fluid intake to produce lactation can lead to decrease in fluid intake overall.	
• Supplemental iron during pregnancy can lead to severe constipation.	
• Fear of injury or pain upon defecation after birth can lead to constipation.	
Teach anatomic shifting of abdominal contents because of fetal growth.	Provides information as a basis for nutrition plan during pregnancy. Promotes self-care.
Teach hormonal influences (e.g., increased progesterone) on bodily functions:	
• Decreased stomach emptying time	
• Decreased peristalsis	
• Increase in water reabsorption	
• Decrease in exercise	
• Relaxation of abdominal muscles	
• Increase in flatulence	
Teach the effects of the increase in oral iron or calcium supplements on the gastrointestinal tract (e.g., constipation).	Provides basis for teaching the client plan of self-care at home, and promotes healing process.
Describe the physical changes present in the immediate postpartum period that affect the gastrointestinal tract:	
• Lax abdominal muscles	
• Fluid loss (perspiration, urine, lochia, or dehydration during labor and delivery)	
• Hunger	
Assist the client in planning diet that will promote healing, replace lost fluids, and help with return to normal bowel evacuation.	Promotes successful lactation, good self-care, and good nutrition, and provides basis for teaching care.
Instruct in the use of ointments, anesthetic sprays, sitz baths, and witch hazel compresses to relieve episiotomy pain and reduce hemorrhoids.	
Instruct in pelvic floor exercises (Kegel exercises) to assist healing and reduction of pain.	
Teach nursing mothers alternate methods of assistance with bowel evacuation other than cathartics (cathartics are expressed in breast milk).	

(care plan continued on page 246)

NURSING ACTIONS/INTERVENTIONS AND RATIONALES (continued from page 245)

Women's Health

ACTIONS/INTERVENTIONS	RATIONALES
• Prune juice • Hot liquids • High-fiber, high-roughage diet • Daily exercise	
Describe the physical changes present in the immediate postoperative period (cesarean section and gynecologic surgery) that affect the gastrointestinal tract: • Fluid loss (blood loss or dehydration as a result of NPO [nothing by mouth] status and surgery) • Decreased peristalsis • Bowel manipulation during surgery • Increased use of analgesics and anesthesia	Provides basis for teaching and planning of care. Promotes and encourages self-care.
During pregnancy:	Gastrointestinal tract motility slows because of hormones (particularly progesterone) and increased growth of uterus. Greater absorption of water causes drying of stool.
• Encourage women to drink sufficient fluids (at least eight glasses per day). • Establish regular schedule for bowel movements. • Encourage a balanced diet with appropriate amounts of fiber, fruits, and vegetables.	Constipation can be avoided by increasing fluids and fiber in the diet and regular exercise.[16]
During pregnancy the bowel is misplaced by the growing uterus and this can lead to changes in bowel elimination and function.	Education and nutritional counseling should focus on dietary advice to ensure the new mother is drinking sufficient fluids and including roughage in her diet.[22]
During the postpartum period the combination of medications used in labor and delivery, a hectic schedule, lack of sleep, as well as preoccupation with a new baby, lead to changes in elimination patterns.	The above is especially true during the postpartum period and when breastfeeding.[22]

Mental Health

Clients taking antipsychotics, antianxiety agents, and antidepressants are at risk for this diagnosis.[23] The nursing actions for Mental Health are the same as those for Adult Health. Please refer to those recommended actions.

Gerontic Health

ACTIONS/INTERVENTIONS	RATIONALES
Review medication record for drugs that may have constipation as a side effect.	Older adults receiving opioid analgesics, antidepressants, anticholinergics, or certain antacids may experience constipation due to the drug-delayed motility of waste matter through the intestine. Older adults are more likely to be on multiple medications that can result in constipation.

Gerontic Health

ACTIONS/INTERVENTIONS	RATIONALES
Collaborate with the physician regarding changes in medication to avoid the side effect of constipation.	
Collaborate with the client to increase their mobility as appropriate through: • Consultation with physical therapy • Chair exercises	Lack of exercise is associated with slowed bowel motility.
Collaborate with client and caregivers to increase fluid and fiber intake. Caution should be taken to increase fiber only when fluids are tolerated well.	Increased fluid and fiber prevent constipation. Increased fiber in the absence of adequate fluid consumption can lead to increased incidence of fecal impaction, particularly in immobile clients.
Use bulking agents with care in the aging client.	Increased fiber in the absence of adequate fluid consumption can lead to increased incidence of fecal impaction, particularly in immobile clients.
Encourage the client to establish effective bowel habits: • Taking advantage of the gastro-colic reflex but toileting after meals • Toileting at a regular time each day • Ensuring that the toilet is the correct height, using seat raisers as needed.	These habits minimize the risk of constipation.[11]
Assist the client to maintain adequate toileting facilities: • Privacy during toileting • Toilet at the correct height • Assistance with mobility as needed • Facilities to call for assistance to access toilet	These habits minimize the risk of delayed emptying which leads to constipation.[11]

Home Health

● NOTE: *Nursing actions for constipation in the Home Health setting are the same as those for Adult Health. The locus of control shifts from the nurse to the client, family, and/or caregiver.*

ACTIONS/INTERVENTIONS	RATIONALES
The nurse will teach others to complete activities.	The client and members of the family may have different ideas regarding appropriate elimination patterns.
Teach the client and family the definition of *constipation*. Determine whether the problem is perceived by the client and family because of incorrect definition or is based on physiologic dysfunction.	Nursing interventions for physiologic definition are outlined in the Adult Health nursing action. Nursing interventions for varying definitions require family involvement.
Assist the client and family in identifying lifestyle changes that may be required: • Establishment of a regular elimination routine based on cultural and individual variations • Stress management techniques • Decrease in concentrated, refined foods • Identification of any food intolerances or allergies and avoidance of those foods • Appropriate use and frequency of use of prescribed and over-the-counter medications • Physiologic parameters of constipation	Home-based care requires involvement of the family. Bowel elimination problems may require adjustments in family activities.

DIARRHEA

DEFINITION[13]

Passage of loose, fluid, unformed stools.

DEFINING CHARACTERISTICS[13]

1. Hyperactive bowel sounds
2. At least three loose stools per day
3. Urgency
4. Abdominal pain
5. Cramping

RELATED FACTORS[13]

1. Psychological
   a. High stress levels and anxiety
2. Situational
   a. Alcohol abuse
   b. Toxins
   c. Laxative abuse
   d. Radiation
   e. Tube feedings
   f. Adverse effects of medication
   g. Contaminants
   h. Travel
3. Physiologic
   a. Inflammation
   b. Malabsorption
   c. Infection process
   d. Irritation
   e. Parasites

RELATED CLINICAL CONCERNS

1. Inflammatory bowel disease (ulcerative colitis, Crohn's disease, enteritis)
2. Anemias
3. Gastric bypass or gastric partitioning surgery
4. Gastritis

EXPECTED OUTCOME

Will return to usual bowel elimination habits by [date].

TARGET DATES

Target dates should be based on the individual's usual bowel elimination habits. Thus, a target date 3 days from the day of admission would be reasonable for the majority of clients. Because diarrhea can be particularly life-threatening for infants and older adults, a target date of 2 days would not be too soon.

 Have You Selected the Correct Diagnosis?

Constipation
Diarrhea may be secondary to constipation. In instances of severe constipation or impaction, semi-liquid feces can leak around the areas of impaction and will appear to be diarrhea.

Imbalanced Nutrition, Less Than Body Requirements
If the individual is not ingesting enough food or sufficient bulk to allow feces to be well formed, diarrhea may well result.

Deficient Fluid Volume or Excess Fluid Volume
Although research has not definitely supported the impact of fluid volume on bowel elimination, it is common practice to pay attention to these diagnoses when either constipation or diarrhea is present. The general notion appears to be that the amount of fluid ingested or absorbed by the body can affect the consistency of the fecal material.

Anxiety, Self-Esteem Disturbance, or Ineffective Individual Coping
Any of these psychosocial diagnoses precipitate a stress response. Indices of stress include gastrointestinal signs and symptoms (e.g., diarrhea, vomiting, and "butterflies" in the stomach).

Disturbed Sleep Pattern
If a person's biologic clock is changed because of altered sleep–wake patterns, body responses attuned to the biologic clock will also be altered. This includes usual elimination patterns, and diarrhea may result.

NURSING ACTIONS/INTERVENTIONS AND RATIONALES

Adult Health

ACTIONS/INTERVENTIONS	RATIONALES
List here those foods that the patient has described as being irritating.	
Record amount, color, consistency, and odor following each bowel movement.	Basic monitoring of conditioning as well as monitoring of effectiveness of therapy.
Monitor weight and electrolytes at least every 2 days while diarrhea persists. [State dates here.]	Monitors fluid and electrolyte status.

ACTIONS/INTERVENTIONS	RATIONALES
Measure and total intake and output every shift.	Monitors hydration status.
Provide oral intake of fluids and bland food.	Fluid intake will assist in maintaining adequate fluid balance. Bland foods will avoid bowel stimulation.
Ensure the client can easily access bathroom facilities or bedside commode.	Helps prevent accidents and prevent embarrassment for the client.
Administer antidiarrheal medications as prescribed and document results within 1 hour after administration. For example, diarrhea decreased from one stool every 30 minutes to one stool every 2 hours.[25]	Documents effectiveness of medication.
Increase fluid intake to at least 2500 mL per day.	Maintains hydration status.
Offer fluids high in potassium and sodium at least once per hour (e.g., sports drinks).	Replaces or maintains electrolytes lost with diarrhea.
Serve fluids at tepid temperature (avoid temperature extremes).	Fluids at temperature extremes can stimulate the bowel.
List the client's fluid likes and dislikes here.	
Provide perineal skin care after each bowel movement. Inspect perianal skin integrity after each bowel movement.	Dries moisture, prevents skin breakdown, and prevents perineal infection. Monitors for skin breakdown.
If tube feedings are a causal factor, collaborate with the appropriate health-care provider regarding optimal enteral therapy.	Modification may decrease incidence of diarrhea.
Assist the client with stress reduction exercises at least once per shift; provide quiet, restful atmosphere. [Note exercises to be used and schedule here.]	Promotes relaxation and decreases stimulation of bowel.
Collaborate with the dietitian regarding low-fiber, low-residue, soft diet.	Helps identify foods that stimulate bowel and exacerbate diarrhea.
List here those foods that the client has described as being irritating.	
Teach the client: • Diet: avoiding irritating foods, including basic food pyramid groups, influence of high-fiber foods, and influence of fruits. • Fluids: maintaining intake and output balance, influence of environmental temperature, influence of activity, and influence of caffeine and milk. • Medications: caution with over-the-counter medications, those that are antidiarrheal, and those that potentiate diarrhea (e.g., antacids and antibiotics).	Increases the client's knowledge of causes, treatment, and complications of diarrhea. Promotes self-care.

Child Health

The treatment of diarrhea is obviously dictated by its severity, and the resultant effect on hydration and electrolyte balance, and is managed according to individual factors such as age, possible etiology, and status of the infant/child. As a rule, the younger the child, the more severe the effects of diarrhea. Children experiencing malnutrition, or with a compromised immune status, are typically affected more than others. Additional factors include overcrowding and potential contamination of milk.

(care plan continued on page 250)

NURSING ACTIONS/INTERVENTIONS AND RATIONALES (continued from page 249)

Child Health

ACTIONS/INTERVENTIONS	RATIONALES
Weigh diapers for urine and stools; assess specific gravity after each voiding.	A strict assessment of intake and output serves as a basis for monitoring the efficacy of the treatment and may provide a database for treatment protocol. Hydration is monitored via specific gravity as an indication of the renal ability to adjust to fluid and electrolyte imbalance.
Monitor for signs and symptoms of dehydration: • Depressed anterior fontanel in infants • Poor skin turgor • Decreased urinary output	Dehydration is extremely dangerous for the infant and requires close monitoring to offset the effects of dehydration.
Monitor signs and symptoms associated with bowel movement, including cramping, flatus, and crying.	Associated signs and symptoms serve as supportive data to follow the altered bowel function, with an emphasis on related pain or discomfort.
Provide prompt and gentle cleansing after each diaper change. For older children, offer warm soaks after each diarrheal episode.	Skin breakdown occurs in a short period of time because of frequent bowel movements and the resultant skin irritation.
• Collaborate with the physician regarding: • Frequent stooling (more than three times per shift) • Excessive vomiting • Possible dietary alterations for specific formula or diet • Monitoring electrolytes and renal function • Maintenance of intravenous (IV) fluids • Antidiarrheal medications free of opioids.	These nursing measures constitute routine measures to monitor diarrhea and its related problems. Prompt reporting and intervention decrease the likelihood of more serious complications. Oral rehydration therapy is favored when acute diarrhea occurs.

Women's Health

● N O T E : *Some women experience diarrhea 1 or 2 days before labor begins. It is not certain why this occurs, but it is thought to be due to the irritation of the bowel by the contracting uterus and the decrease in hormonal levels (estrogen and progesterone) in late pregnancy. For diarrhea that is a precursor to labor, the following action applies.*

ACTIONS/INTERVENTIONS	RATIONALES
Offer oral electrolyte solutions such as: • Gatorade® • Classic Coca-Cola® • Jell-O® • Pedialyte®	Provides nutrition, electrolytes, and minerals that support a successful labor process. Recent research has shown that women can safely eat light foods or drink fluids during labor to maintain energy and fluid balance, without harm. There was no increased vomiting in the later stages of labor than has been historically reported. However, because of other multiple variables present in the acute care setting, the authors could not provide convincing evidence to change practice.[26]

Mental Health

ACTIONS/INTERVENTIONS	RATIONALES
Monitor lithium levels when these clients present with diarrhea.	Diarrhea can be a normal side effect with the initiation of Li therapy. It is more common in toxicity. Fluid and electrolyte imbalance caused by diarrhea fluid loss can increase the risk of Li toxicity.[23]
Discuss with the client the role stress and anxiety play in this problem.	Diarrhea can be related to autonomic nervous system response to emotions.[27]
Develop with the client a stress reduction plan and practice specific interventions three times a day at [list times here].	Promotes the client's adaptive response to stress, and promotes the client's sense of control.
Refer to Chapter 8 for specific nursing actions related to the diagnosis of anxiety.	

Gerontic Health

ACTIONS/INTERVENTIONS	RATIONALES
Monitor medication intake to assess for potential side effect of diarrhea.	The older adult may be having diarrhea as a result of antibiotic therapy, use of drugs with a laxative effect, such as magnesium-based antacids, or as a sign of drug toxicity secondary to antiarrhythmics, such as digitalis, quinidine, or propranolol.
Collaborate with the physician regarding possible alterations in medications to decrease the problem of diarrhea.	
Frequently offer electrolyte-rich fluids of choice to prevent dehydration.	Provides nutrition, electrolytes, and minerals to offset or prevent dehydration.
Carefully monitor the client for early symptoms of dehydration.	

Home Health/Community Health

ACTIONS/INTERVENTIONS	RATIONALES
Teach the client and family: • How to monitor perianal skin integrity • Techniques of perianal hygiene • Techniques of maintaining fluid and electrolyte balance (see Adult Health) • Administering antidiarrheal medications	Similar to Adult Health. For Home Health, the locus of control is now the client and family, not the nurse.
Assist the client and family to set criteria to help them determine when a physician or other intervention is required (e.g., child having more than three stools in 1 day).	Provides the client and family background knowledge to seek appropriate assistance as need arises.
Assist the client and family in identifying lifestyle changes that may be required: • Avoid drinking local water when traveling in areas where water supply may be contaminated (e.g., foreign countries or streams and lakes when camping).	Behaviors to prevent recurrence of or continuation of the problem.

(care plan continued on page 252)

NURSING ACTIONS/INTERVENTIONS AND RATIONALES (continued from page 251)

Home Health/Community Health

ACTIONS/INTERVENTIONS	RATIONALES
• Practice stress management. • Avoid laxative or enema abuse. • Avoid foods that cause symptoms. • Avoid bingeing behavior.	
Assess the client/family need for adult diapers, linens. Make referrals for obtaining these supplies as appropriate.	These measures prevent secondary problems from occurring as a result of the existing problem.
Educate the client in the importance of handwashing.	To prevent the spread of microorganisms that may cause diarrhea.
Educate the client and caregivers about proper handling, cooking, and storage of food.	To prevent the spread of microorganisms that may cause diarrhea.

READINESS FOR ENHANCED URINARY ELIMINATION

DEFINITION[13]

A pattern of urinary functions that is sufficient for meeting eliminatory needs and that can be strengthened.

DEFINING CHARACTERISTICS[13]

1. The patient expresses willingness to enhance urinary elimination.
2. Urine is straw colored with no odor.
3. Specific gravity is within normal limits.
4. The amount of output is within normal limits for age and other factors.
5. The patient positions him- or herself for emptying of bladder.
6. Fluid intake is adequate for daily needs.

EXPECTED OUTCOME

Will maintain or improve current state of urinary elimination patterns by [date].

TARGET DATES

As this is a positive diagnosis with predominantly teaching interventions, appropriate target dates can be as long as 7 to 10 days with intermittent reassessment weekly.

NURSING ACTIONS/INTERVENTIONS AND RATIONALES

Adult Health

ACTIONS/INTERVENTIONS	RATIONALES
Assist the patient in devising fluid management plan including: • Adequate fluid intake • Limiting fluids proximal to bedtime	Assures adequate fluid intake for physiological needs and decreases potential for infection.
Assist the patient in identifying and managing medications and substances that potentiate urgency, have a diuretic or urinary retention effect.	Enables patient to incorporate effects of medications into devised toileting plan.
Assist the patient in creating an environment conducive to continence.	Removal of obstacles can decrease incontinent episodes by facilitating accessibility.
Obtain assistive devices as needed (e.g., bedside commode, seat adapters, safety frames).	Facilitates accessibility and safety.
Assist the patient in devising initial toileting schedule [list here]. Assist in revising plan as patient progresses.	

ACTIONS/INTERVENTIONS	RATIONALES
Assist patient in identifying appropriate bladder training program: • Pelvic muscle training program • Biofeedback • Scheduled voiding	
Follow up weekly [list dates here].	Monitors progress and allows for appropriate revision of plan.

Child Health

ACTIONS/INTERVENTIONS	RATIONALES
Assess for all possible contributory factors to consider, especially cultural influences.	Provides the most inclusive base for care.
Offer a child-oriented approach.	
Validate readiness for the toddler: • Physical • Ability to hold urine for 2 hours or more • Gross motor skills of sitting, walking, and squatting • Fine motor skills for self-removal of clothing • Mental • Recognizes cues for need to urinate • Cognitive capacity to role model others in toileting behaviors • Psychological • Expresses willingness to please parent • Capacity to self-identify wet diaper and desire to be dry	Appropriately validates realistic expectations for the child.[29,30]
Validate readiness for the caregiver(s): • Recognizes toddler's cues for readiness. • Verbalizes willingness to invest time for assisting with the urination pattern. • Verbalizes absences of major family stressors that would interfere with success of pattern (divorce, move, addition of new sibling).	
Acknowledges readiness to approximate 18 months of age with pattern for girls to exhibit earlier patterns than boys.	Validates realistic expectations.
Acknowledge cultural aspects for family.	Sensitivity to family values creates respect and provides a likelihood of success in follow-through of pattern.
Consider use of free-standing potty chair and/or transitional portable seat attached to toilet.	Provides a sense of security for child.
Practice sessions should be limited to no more than 10 minutes with parent in presence of toddler.	Ensures safety and allows for natural elimination of urine.
Praise the child for cooperative behaviors.	Offers reinforcement of learning.
Use dolls, books, or other materials for learning that are appropriate for the toddler or child.	Provides nonstressful learning at an appropriate level with greater likelihood for success.
Assist the caregiver(s) and child to identify related assistance necessary to carry out plan, especially modified equipment to augment stability of potty chair or toilet.	Satisfies individual needs to increase likelihood of safety and success in dealing with the pattern.[30,31]

(care plan continued on page 254)

NURSING ACTIONS/INTERVENTIONS AND RATIONALES (continued from page 253)

Women's Health

Interventions for Adult Health apply to women, along with the following considerations:

ACTIONS/INTERVENTIONS	RATIONALES
A thorough assessment and physical exam to determine the extent of the problem should be performed. Include in the assessment physical problems, patient's mobility, and environment.	Age-related changes of aging contribute to urinary incontinence in older women. Lack of care and assessment, as well as the patient's inability or reluctance to discuss problems with her health-care provider results in approximately 40 percent of the admissions to nursing homes.[16]
Engage the patient in bladder training: • Postpone voiding. • Urinate at timed intervals by developing a schedule of urination. • Biofeedback • Medication	Learning different techniques can result in a 50 percent reduction of incontinence in some women. "Control requires intact cognitive, neurologic and physical parameters as well as motivational and environmental factors."[30]

Mental Health

Nursing interventions for this diagnosis are the same as those for Adult Health.

Gerontic Health

In addition to the interventions for Adult Health, the following may apply to the aging client:

ACTIONS/INTERVENTIONS	RATIONALES
Maintain fluid intake:	Ensures sufficient fluid intake, but restricts fluid when activity decreases. Assists in preventing nocturia.
• Encourage fluids to at least 2000 mL per day.	Dilute urine discourages bacterial growth.
Increase client activity if client is sedentary.	Strengthens muscles and promotes kidney and bladder functioning.
Beginning on day of admission, teach the client the following exercises: • Bent-knee sit-ups • Bent-leg lifts • Contracting posterior perineal muscles as if trying to stop a bowel movement • Contracting anterior perineal muscles as if trying to stop voiding • Starting and stopping urine stream	Strengthens pelvic floor muscles.

URINARY INCONTINENCE

DEFINITIONS[13]

Urinary Incontinence The state in which the individual experiences a disturbance in urine elimination.

Functional Urinary Incontinence Inability of usually continent person to reach toilet in time to avoid unintentional loss of urine.

Reflex Urinary Incontinence An involuntary loss of urine at somewhat predictable intervals when a specific bladder volume is reached.

Stress Urinary Incontinence The state in which an individual experiences a loss of urine of less than 50 mL occurring with increased abdominal pressure.

Total Urinary Incontinence The state in which an individual experiences a continuous and unpredictable loss of urine.

Urge Urinary Incontinence   The state in which an individual experiences involuntary passage of urine occurring soon after a strong sense of urgency to void.

Risk for Urge Urinary Incontinence   Risk for involuntary loss of urine associated with a sudden, strong sensation or urinary urgency.

DEFINING CHARACTERISTICS[13]

A. Urinary Incontinence
1. Incontinence
2. Urgency
3. Nocturia
4. Hesitancy
5. Frequency
6. Dysuria
7. Retention

B. Functional Urinary Incontinence
1. May only be incontinent in early morning
2. Senses need to void
3. Amount of time required to reach toilet exceeds length of time between sensing urge and uncontrolled voiding
4. Loss of urine before reaching toilet
5. Able to empty bladder completely

C. Reflex Urinary Incontinence
1. No sensation of urge to void
2. Complete emptying with lesion above pontine micturition center
3. Incomplete emptying with lesion above sacral micturition center
4. No sensation of bladder fullness
5. Sensations associated with full bladder such as sweating, restlessness, and abdominal discomfort
6. Unable to cognitively inhibit or initiate voiding
7. No sensation of voiding
8. Predictable pattern of voiding
9. Sensation of urgency without voluntary inhibition of bladder contraction

D. Stress Urinary Incontinence
1. Reported or observed dribbling with increased abdominal pressure
2. Urinary frequency (more often than every 2 hours)
3. Urinary urgency

E. Total Urinary Incontinence
1. Constant flow of urine occurring at unpredictable times without distention, or uninhibited bladder contractions or spasms
2. Unsuccessful incontinence refractory treatments
3. Nocturia
4. Lack of perineal or bladder-filling awareness
5. Unawareness of incontinence

F. Urge Urinary Incontinence
1. Urinary urgency
2. Bladder contracture or spasm
3. Frequency (voiding more often than every 2 hours)
4. Voiding in large amounts (more than 550 mL)
5. Voiding in small amounts (less than 100 mL)
6. Nocturia (more than two times per night)
7. Inability to reach toilet in time

G. Risk for Urge Urinary Incontinence
1. Effects of medication, caffeine, alcohol
2. Detrusor hyperreflexia from cystitis, urethritis, tumor, renal calculi, and central nervous system disorders above pontine micturition center
3. Detrusor muscle instability with impaired contractility
4. Involuntary sphincter relaxation
5. Ineffective toileting habits
6. Small bladder capacity

RELATED FACTORS[13]

A. Urinary Incontinence
1. Urinary tract infection
2. Anatomic obstruction
3. Multiple causality
4. Sensory motor impairment

B. Functional Urinary Incontinence
1. Psychological factors
2. Impaired vision
3. Impaired cognition
4. Neuromuscular limitations
5. Altered environmental factors
6. Weakened supporting pelvic structures

C. Reflex Urinary Incontinence
1. Tissue damage from radiation, cystitis, inflammatory bladder conditions, or radical pelvic surgery
2. Neurologic impairment above level of sacral micturition center or pontine micturition center

D. Stress Urinary Incontinence
1. Weak pelvic muscles and structural supports
2. Overdistention between voidings
3. Incompetent bladder outlet
4. Degenerative changes in pelvic muscles and structural supports associated with increased age
5. High intra-abdominal pressure (e.g., obesity, gravid uterus)

E. Total Urinary Incontinence
1. Neuropathy preventing transmission of reflex indicating bladder fullness
2. Trauma or disease affecting spinal cord nerves
3. Anatomic (fistula)
4. Independent contraction of detrusor reflex due to surgery
5. Neurologic dysfunction causing triggering of micturition at unpredictable times

F. Urge Urinary Incontinence
1. Alcohol
2. Caffeine
3. Decreased bladder capacity (e.g., history of pelvic inflammatory disease, abdominal surgeries, or indwelling urinary catheter)
4. Increased fluids

5. Increased urine concentration
6. Irritation of bladder stretch receptors causing spasm (e.g., bladder infection)
7. Overdistention of bladder

G. Risk for Urge Urinary Incontinence

The risk factors also serve as the Related Factors.

RELATED CLINICAL CONCERNS

1. Spinal cord injury
2. Urinary tract infection
3. Alzheimer's disease
4. Pregnancy
5. Abdominal surgery
6. Prostate surgery

EXPECTED OUTCOME

Will remain continent at least 90 percent of the time by [date].

TARGET DATES

Treatment of incontinence requires training time and effort; therefore, a target date 5 days from the date of admission would be reasonable to evaluate the client's progress toward meeting the expected outcome. In addition, there must be a realistic potential that urinary continence may be regained by the client. For this reason, it would need to be qualified for use with handicapped or neurologically deficient clients according to the exact level of continence desired.

 Have You Selected the Correct Diagnosis?

Constipation
Anything in the body that creates additional pressure on the bladder or bladder sphincter may precipitate voiding. Constipation can create this additional pressure because of the increased amount of fecal material in the sigmoid colon and rectum. Incontinence may then be a direct result of constipation or fecal impaction.

Excess Fluid Volume or Deficient Fluid Volume
Because urination depends on input of the stimulus that the bladder is full and because one of the ways the body responds to excess fluid volume is by increasing urinary output, the very fact that there is excess fluid volume may result in the bladder's inability to keep up with the kidney's production of urine. Thus, incontinence may occur. Conversely, Deficient Fluid Volume can result in incontinence by eliminating the sensation of a full bladder and by decreasing the person's awareness of the sensation.

Impaired Physical Mobility
As previously stated, the individual must be able to control the sphincter, walk a few steps, recognize and interpret that the bladder is full, and be able to indicate that he or she wants to go to the bathroom. Even if the person has some control of the sphincter and has correctly recognized and interpreted the cues of a full bladder, if he or she is unable to get to the bathroom or get there in time because of mobility problems, incontinence may result. This may happen especially in a hospital.

Impaired Verbal Communication
The ability to verbally communicate the need to urinate is important. If the person is unable to tell someone or have someone understand that he or she wants to go to the bathroom, incontinence may occur.

NURSING ACTIONS/INTERVENTIONS AND RATIONALES

Adult Health

ACTIONS/INTERVENTIONS	RATIONALES
Record: • Time and amounts of each voiding • Whether voiding was continent or incontinent • The patient's activity before and after incontinent incidence	Helps determine patient's voiding pattern and monitors effectiveness of treatment.
Monitor: • At least every 2 hours on [odd/even] hour, for continence. • Weight at least every 3 days • Laboratory values (e.g., electrolytes, white blood cells [WBC], or urinalyses) • For dependent edema • Intake and output, each shift	Basic methods to monitor hydration, prevent tissue integrity problems, prevent infection, and promote comfort.

ACTIONS/INTERVENTIONS	RATIONALES
• Perineal skin integrity at least once per shift	
• For bladder distention at least every 2 hours on [odd/even] hour	
Schedule fluid intake:	Assists in predicting times of voiding. Decreases urge to void at unscheduled times.
• Avoid fluids containing caffeine and other fluids that produce a diuretic effect (e.g., coffee, grapefruit juice, and alcohol).	
• Offer 8 ounces of fluid every 2 hours on [odd/even] hour during the day.	
• Limit fluids after 6 p.m.	
Maintain bowel elimination. Monitor bowel movements, and record at least once each shift.	Fullness in bowel may exert pressure on bladder, causing bladder incontinence.
Beginning on day of admission, teach and have the patient return-demonstrate perineal skin care.	Prevents skin irritation, infection, and odor.
Respond **immediately** to the patient's request for voiding.	Immediate response may prevent an incontinent episode.
Implement scheduled voiding regimens which may include:	Voiding at scheduled intervals prevents overdistention and helps establish a voiding pattern.
• Schedule toileting every 2 hours on [odd/even] hour during the day.	
• Schedule toileting at least 30 minutes before foreseeable incontinence times.	
• Awaken the patient once during the night for voiding.	
• Verbally prompting the patient to void every 2 hours on [odd/even] hour. Praise the patient for appropriate toileting.	
Stimulate voiding at scheduled time by:	
• Assisting the patient to maintain normal anatomic position for voiding.	A normal anatomical position facilitates voiding.
• Teach trigger techniques to stimulate voiding (e.g., gently tapping over bladder or having the patient listen to dripping water).[21]	
• Using Credé's or Valsalva maneuver	
• Providing privacy	
• Providing night light and clear path to bathroom	
Implement bladder training, including gradually increasing time between voiding [Note schedule here.]	Extending time between voiding will increase volume of urine in bladder and will stretch bladder.
Implement strategies to strengthen pelvic floor muscle exercises, including Kegel exercises, biofeedback techniques, or vaginal weight training.	Strengthens pelvic floor and abdominal muscles.
Consult with the physician about the use of occlusive devices that mechanically block the leakage of urine by supporting the urethrovesical junction or occluding the urethral meatus.	
Assist the patient with stress reduction and relaxation techniques at least once per shift.	Promotes relaxation and self-control of voiding.
Collaborate with the physician regarding intermittent catheterization and obtaining postvoid residual volumes.	Prevents complications related to bladder overdistention.
Collaborate with the rehabilitation nurse clinician to establish a bladder-retraining program.	Allows establishment of a program that is current in content and procedures.

(care plan continued on page 258)

NURSING ACTIONS/INTERVENTIONS AND RATIONALES (continued from page 257)

Adult Health

ACTIONS/INTERVENTIONS	RATIONALES
Teach the patient exercises to strengthen pelvic floor muscles. Exercise should consist of 10 repetitions at least three times per day, three to four times a week. [Record date and times exercises are performed here.]	Strengthens pelvic floor muscles to better control voiding.[31]
Teach the patient the importance of maintaining a daily routine: • Voiding upon arising • Awakening self once during the night • Voiding immediately before retiring • Not postponing voiding unnecessarily	Helps establish urinary elimination pattern, and prevents overdistention of bladder.
Discuss possibilities of client regaining continence. Include discussion about techniques to facilitate socialization: • Wearing street clothes with protective pads in undergarments • Maintaining bladder-retraining program • Responding as soon as possible to voiding urge	Helps preserve self-concept and body image. Promotes compliance.
Consult with physician regarding pharmacological therapy.	
Monitor for side effects of pharmacological therapy: • Dry mouth • Constipation • Blurred vision • Dizziness	
Refer to home health care agency for follow-up.	Provides continuity of care and support system for ongoing care at home.

Child Health

Nursing actions for the child with incontinence are the same as for Adult Health, with attention to the developmental, anatomic, and physiologic parameters for age and with attention to organic potentials, including congenital malformations. Special allowance for urinary reflux or recurrent potential urinary tract infections should be made in all ages.

The definition is offered for primary enuresis as bedwetting in children who have never been dry for extended period of time, and secondary enuresis as the onset of wetting after a period of established urinary continence. Nocturnal enuresis occurs only at nighttime while diurnal enuresis occurs during both day and night. Nocturnal enuresis is more common.

Although most children with enuresis do not experience coexisting psychopathology, some children also experience developmental disorders, learning problems, or difficulties in behavior. Self-esteem is influenced according to the parental response and especially is vulnerable in harsh or punitive instances. Severe punishment for unrealistic expectations or inappropriate management of enuresis can serve as a trigger for child abuse.[29]

ACTIONS/INTERVENTIONS	RATIONALES
Assess for all possible contributing factors, including ruling out urinary tract infection, structural disorders, neurologic deficits as with myelomeningocele, and conditions with increased urinary output (diabetes mellitus or diabetes insipidus).	Offers the fullest consideration of causes to best uncover all factors.[32]

ACTIONS/INTERVENTIONS	RATIONALES
Offer psychiatric intervention as the cues arise for need for same—may be related to sexual abuse or other psychological factors.	Offers the fullest consideration to provide holism.[32]
Obtain history of wetting behavior in a nonjudgmental manner including information of toilet training and usual attempts for dealing with the behavior.	Creates a basis for open consideration of problem.[32]
Initiate or instruct caregiver(s) and child (as appropriate) on how to do a baseline record of enuresis.	Provides baseline data to determine the extent of the problem and assists in monitoring treatment.[32]
Provide assistance in chosen therapy: • Conditioning therapy includes a stimulus response conditioning often with a pad and buzzer alarm when moisture is sensed-used with a success rate of approximately 60 to 90 percent. • Retention control training is offered for enhancement of bedwetters whose functional bladder capacity was reduced. • The waking schedule training includes awakening the child during the night at intervals. This method is successful in reducing, but not eliminating incidents.	Fosters support to child and family.[32] Safeguards child from potential side effects.
Drug therapy is used more and more and may include anticholinergic agents, vasopressin analog desmopressin as a nasal spray, and other individualized combinations of modified doses for these and tricyclic antidepressants or antispasmodics. In these instances, the caregiver(s) must monitor for side effects and safeguard medications from potential overdose by other siblings.	Ensures reduction of risk from overdosage.[32]
Support child and family within a non-punitive framework during time of treatment.	Lessens sense of lost self-esteem and offers positive reinforcement without conditional acceptance of child.[32]

Women's Health

● NOTE: *The same nursing interventions pertains to Women's Health as to Adult Health. During pregnancy, the woman may occasionally experience uncontrolled voiding before reaching the toilet. This is usually caused by the overexpansion of the uterus or the pressure and weight of the baby and uterus on the bladder. This usually resolves after the delivery of the baby. Many women experience uncontrollable leakage of urine due to injury during pregnancy and childbirth. However, certain medications, such as diuretics, muscle relaxants, sedatives, and antidepressants, can contribute to urinary incontinence.*

ACTIONS/INTERVENTIONS	RATIONALES
Assist the client in identifying lifestyle adjustments that may be needed to accommodate changing bladder capacity caused by anatomic changes of pregnancy. • Teach the client to recognize symptoms of urinary tract infection (urgency, burning, or dysuria). • Teach the client how to take temperature (make sure the client knows how to read thermometer). • Instruct the client to seek immediate medical care if symptoms of urinary tract infection appear.	Bladder capacity is reduced because of enlarging uterus, displacement of abdominal contents by enlarged uterus, and pressure on bladder by enlarged uterus.

(care plan continued on page 260)

NURSING ACTIONS/INTERVENTIONS AND RATIONALES (continued from page 259)

Women's Health

ACTIONS/INTERVENTIONS	RATIONALES
Teach women Kegel exercises and pelvic floor musculature retraining.	Strengthening of pelvic floor muscles helps reduce the urge to void and prevents leakage of urine.
Encourage good hygiene and cleansing of the perineum, wiping from front to back to prevent urinary tract infections.	
Discuss the physiological changes women experience as they age that affect the bladder and can lead to incontinence. • Ability of bladder to expand decreases. • Involuntary bladder contraction increase. • Bladder outlet loses strength and resistance of pelvic floor muscles resulting in being unable to close. • Urethra shortens and weakens. • Ability to postpone voiding decreases. • Postvoiding residual volume increases.	Loss of estrogen after menopause contributes to weakening of pelvic muscle fibers. Bladder training, education, biofeedback along with medications including oral or vaginal estrogen can help alleviate some of the symptoms of incontinence.[30]
Provide a nonjudgmental, relaxed atmosphere that will encourage the woman to ask questions without embarrassment.	

Mental Health

● N O T E : *If the alteration is related to psychosocial issues and has no physiologic component, initiate the nursing actions that follow. (Refer to Adult Health for physiologically-produced problems.)*

ACTIONS/INTERVENTIONS	RATIONALES
Monitor times, places, persons present, and emotional climate around inappropriate voiding episodes.	Identifies target behaviors, and establishes a baseline measurement of behavior with possible reinforcers for inappropriate behavior.[18]
Remind the client to void before a high-risk situation or remove secondary gain process from situation.	Removes positive reinforcement for inappropriate behavior.[18]
Provide the client with supplies necessary to facilitate appropriate voiding behavior (e.g., urinal for the client in locked seclusion area).	Appropriate behavior cannot be implemented without the appropriate equipment.[18]
Inform the client of acceptable times and places for voiding and of consequences for inappropriate voiding. [Note consequences here.]	Negative reinforcement eliminates or decreases behavior.[18]
Have the client assist with cleaning up any voiding that has occurred in an inappropriate place.	Provides a negative consequence for inappropriate behavior.[18]
Provide as little interaction with the client as possible during cleanup.	Lack of social response acts as negative reinforcement.[18]
Provide the client with positive reinforcement for voiding in appropriate place and time. [List specific reinforcers for the client here.]	Positive reinforcement encourages appropriate behavior.[18]
Spend [number] minutes with the client every hour in an activity the client has identified as enjoyable; do not provide this time, or discontinue time, if the client	Interaction with the nurse can provide positive reinforcement. Withdrawing attention for inappropriate behavior provides negative reinforcement.[18]

ACTIONS/INTERVENTIONS	RATIONALES
inappropriately voids during the specified time. [List identified activities here.]	
If the client voids inappropriately [number] during a shift, he or she will spend [number] minutes (no more than 30) in time-out. Each inappropriate voiding in time-out adds 5 minutes to this time.	Negative consequences decrease or eliminate undesirable behavior.[18]
As behavior improves, add rewards for accumulated times of appropriate voiding (e.g., award a 2-hour pass for 1 day of appropriate voiding). [Record these rewards here.]	Intermittent reinforcement can render a response more resistant to extinction once it has been established.[18]

● N O T E : *Refer to Chapters 8 and 11 for interventions related to the specific alterations that would promote this coping pattern.*

Gerontic Health

Incontinence is not a normal part of aging. When older adults experience incontinence efforts should be made to both determine the cause of the incontinence and return the client to a continent state.

In addition to the interventions for Adult Health, the following may be utilized for the aging client:

ACTIONS/INTERVENTIONS	RATIONALES
Review medication record for drugs such as sedatives, hypnotics, or diuretics that may contribute to urinary incontinence.	Sedatives and hypnotics may result in a delayed response to the urge to void. Diuretic therapy, depending on dosage and time of administration, may result in an inability to reach the bathroom in a timely manner.
Assist the client/caregiver to establish a schedule for voiding.	Promotes bladder tone, helps prevent accidents from decreased sense of urge to void.
Modify the environment to facilitate continence: • Call bells within reach • Bedside commode, urinal, bedpan as appropriate in reach • Clear, unobstructed path to toileting facilities • Well lit toileting facilities	Prevents urgency incontinence due to environmental barriers.
Modify the client's garments as appropriate to facilitate continence: • Elastic waist pants rather than zippers or buttons • Pants rather than one-piece garments such as coveralls • Knee high hose rather than panty hose	Prevents urgency incontinence due to difficulty removing garments.

Home Health

● N O T E : *If this nursing diagnosis is made, it is imperative that a physician referral also be made. If referred to home care under a physician's care, it is important to maintain and evaluate response to prescribed treatments.*

ACTIONS/INTERVENTIONS	RATIONALES
Assist the client and family in identifying lifestyle changes that may be required: • Using proper perineal hygiene • Taking showers instead of tub baths • Drinking fluids to cause voiding every 2 to 3 hours to flush out bacteria • Scheduling fluid intake	Basic measures to prevent recurrence.

(care plan continued on page 262)

NURSING ACTIONS/INTERVENTIONS AND RATIONALES (continued from page 261)

Home Health

ACTIONS/INTERVENTIONS	RATIONALES
• Voiding after intercourse • Avoiding bubble baths, perfumed soaps, toilet paper, or feminine hygiene sprays • Wearing cotton underwear • Using proper handwashing techniques • Following a daily routine of voiding (see Adult Health actions) • Establishing a bladder-retraining program • Doing exercises to strengthen pelvic floor muscles Providing an environment conducive to continence: • Clear path to the bathroom • A light in the bathroom • Bedside commode as needed • Clothes that are easily removed • Wearing street clothes and protective underwear • Using an air purifier • Performing activities as tolerated • Providing unobstructed access to bathroom • Avoiding fluids that produce diuretic effect (e.g., caffeine, alcohol, or teas)	
Teach the client and family to dilute and acidify the urine by: • Increasing fluids • Introducing cranberry juice, poultry, etc., to increase acid ash	Dilute urine and acidic urine discourage bacterial growth.
Teach the client and family to monitor and maintain skin integrity: • Keep skin clean and dry. • Keep bed linens and clothing clean and dry. • Use proper perineal hygiene.	Prevents or minimizes problems secondary to incontinence.
Assist the client and family to set criteria to help them determine when a physician or other intervention is required (e.g., hematuria, fever, or skin breakdown).	Assists in preventing or minimizing further physiologic damage.
Monitor and teach the importance of appropriate medications and treatments ordered by physician.	
Refer to appropriate assistive resources as indicated.	Additional resources may be needed based on the underlying problem.
Educate the client about the importance of urinating on a regular basis, prior to urge.	Empties the bladder before stretching or distention occurs.
Assist the client in obtaining necessary personal hygiene supplies as needed (e.g., pads, diapers, linens).	Provides a sense of security.
Educate the client about prescribed medications and their possible side effects.	Promotes sense of accountability and improves compliance.

URINARY RETENTION

DEFINITION[13]

The state in which the individual experiences incomplete emptying of the bladder.

DEFINING CHARACTERISTICS[13]

1. Bladder distention
2. Small, frequent voiding or absence of urine output
3. Sensation of bladder fullness
4. Dribbling
5. Residual urine
6. Dysuria
7. Overflow incontinence

RELATED FACTORS[13]

1. High urethral pressure caused by weak detrusor
2. Inhibition of reflex arc
3. Strong sphincter
4. Blockage

RELATED CLINICAL CONCERNS

1. Benign prostatic hyperplasia
2. Hysterectomy
3. Urinary tract infection
4. Cancer

EXPECTED OUTCOME

Will void under voluntary control and empty bladder at least every 4 hours by [date].

TARGET DATES

Urinary retention poses many dangers to the client. An acceptable target date to evaluate for lessening of retention would be within 24 to 48 hours after admission.

 Have You Selected the Correct Diagnosis?

Urinary Incontinence
Overflow incontinence frequently occurs in clients whose primary problem is really retention. The bladder is overdistended in retention, and some urine is passed involuntarily because of the pressure of the retained urine on the bladder sphincter.

Self-Care Deficit, Toileting
In neurogenic bladder conditions, the bladder is chronically overdistended, resulting in urinary retention.

NURSING ACTIONS/INTERVENTIONS AND RATIONALES

Adult Health

ACTIONS/INTERVENTIONS	RATIONALES
Monitor bladder for distention at least every 2 hours on [odd/even] hour.	Monitors pattern and determines effectiveness of treatment; helps prevent complications.
Measure and record intake and output each shift.	Monitors fluid balance.
Maintain fluid intake: • Encourage fluids to at least 2000 mL per day. • Limit fluids after 6 p.m.	Ensures sufficient fluid intake, but restricts fluid when activity decreases. Assists in preventing nocturia.
Monitor: • Bowel elimination at least once per shift • Urinalysis, electrolytes, and weight at least every 3 days	Constipation may block bladder opening and lead to retention. Empty bowel facilitates free passage of urine.
Increase client activity: • Ambulate at least twice per shift while awake at [times]. • Collaborate with the physical therapist, soon after the patient's admission, regarding an exercise program.	Strengthens muscles and promotes kidney and bladder functioning.
Collaborate with the rehabilitation nurse clinician to initiate a bladder-retraining program.	Allows establishment of a program that is current in content and procedures.
Stimulate micturition reflex every 4 hours while awake at [times]: • Assist the client to assume an anatomically correct position for voiding. • Remind the client to be consciously aware of need-to-void sensations.	Helps relax sphincter and strengthens the voiding reflex.

(care plan continued on page 264)

NURSING ACTIONS/INTERVENTIONS AND RATIONALES (continued from page 263)

Adult Health

ACTIONS/INTERVENTIONS	RATIONALES
• Teach the client to assist bladder contraction: • Credé's maneuver • Valsalva maneuver • Abdominal muscle contraction • Pelvic floor muscle exercises, alternating contraction and relaxation of perineal muscles while sitting in a chair and with feet placed apart on floor.	Strengthens the pelvic floor and abdominal muscles.
Collaborate with physician regarding: • Intermittent catheterization • Pharmacological agents • Medications (e.g., urinary antiseptics or analgesics)	Relieves bladder distention, assists in scheduling voiding, and prevents infection.
Refer to home health agency as appropriate at least 2 days prior to discharge for continued monitoring.	Provides continuity of care and a support system for ongoing home care.

Child Health

●NOTE: *For infants and children less than 20 pounds, it would be necessary to calculate exact intake and output and fluid requisites according to the etiologic factors present. Attention must be paid to the child's physiologic developmental level regarding urinary control.*

ACTIONS/INTERVENTIONS	RATIONALES
Provide opportunities for the child and parents to verbalize concerns or views about body image disturbances related to urinary control and retention. Spend at least 30 minutes per shift in privacy with the child and parents to permit this verbalization.	Assists in reducing anxiety, and attaches value to the client's and parents' feelings. Promotes the development of a therapeutic relationship.[29]
Monitor parental (client as applicable) knowledge of preventive health care for the client: • Teaching and observation of urinary catheterization • Maintenance of catheters and supplies • How to obtain supplies • How to obtain a sterile culture specimen • Appropriate restraint of the infant • Potential regarding urinary control	Parental knowledge will assist in the reduction of anxiety and will provide a greater likelihood for compliance with the desired plan of care.[29]
Provide opportunities for parental participation in the care of the infant or child: • Feedings • Bathing • Monitoring intake and output. Caution for removal of too much urine* and for reporting of excessive pattern of urinary production as with diabetes insipidus. • Planning for care to include individual preferences when possible • Assisting with procedures when appropriate • Provision of safety needs • Cautious handwashing to prevent infection[33] • Appropriate emotional support	Appropriate parental involvement provides opportunities for trial care and allows the parents to practice care in a safe, supportive environment before the time of more total self-care.[29] Helps to monitor for other factors to be addressed and prevents hypovolemia, secondary to excessive removal of urine according to age/size of child.[29]

ACTIONS/INTERVENTIONS	RATIONALES
• Appropriate diversional activity and relaxation • Need for pain medication Collaborate with other health-care professionals as needed. Assist the family to identify support groups represented in the community for future needs. *Varies by size and age–get norms	Identification of support for the family will best assist them to comply with the desired plan of care while reducing anxiety and promoting self-care.[29,33]

Women's Health

Actions and rationales are the same for Adult Health except in the following situation.

ACTIONS/INTERVENTIONS	RATIONALES
Collaborate with the physician regarding intermittent catheterization.	It is not easy to catheterize a woman postpartum, nor is it desirable to introduce an added risk of infection, so every effort and support should be directed toward helping the woman to void on her own. If, however, she is unable to void or to empty her bladder, an indwelling catheter may be placed for 24 to 48 hours to rest the bladder and allow it to heal, edema to subside, and bladder and urethral tone to return.[22]

Mental Health

● N O T E : *Clients receiving antipsychotic and antidepressant drugs are at increased risk for this diagnosis.[23] Refer to Adult Health for general actions related to this diagnosis.*

ACTIONS/INTERVENTIONS	RATIONALES
Place clients receiving antipsychotic or antidepressant medication on a daily assessment for this diagnosis. Elderly clients should be evaluated more frequently if their physical status indicates.	Early intervention and treatment ensures better outcome.[23]
Monitor the bladder for distention at least every 4 hours at [times] if verbal reports are unreliable or if they indicate a voiding frequency greater than every 4 hours.	
Increase the client's activity by: • Walking with the client [number] minimum of three times per day at [list times here] • Collaborating with the physical therapist regarding an exercise program. Note the plan developed with the physical therapist here.	Activity maintains muscle strength necessary for maintenance of normal voiding patterns. (See Adult Health for specific exercises to strengthen pelvic floor muscles.)
• Placing the client in a room distant from the day area, nursing stations, and other activity if condition does not contraindicate this • Providing physical activities that the client indicates are of interest. [List those here with the time for each.]	Anxiety can increase muscle tension and therefore contribute to urinary retention.[18]
Teach deep muscle relaxation, and spend 30 minutes twice a day at [list times here] practicing this with the	Anxiety can increase muscle tension and therefore contribute to urinary retention.[18]

(care plan continued on page 266)

NURSING ACTIONS/INTERVENTIONS AND RATIONALES (continued from page 265)

Mental Health

ACTIONS/INTERVENTIONS	RATIONALES
client. Associate relaxation with breathing so that the client can eventually relax with deep breathing while attempting to void.	
Collaborate with the physician regarding catheterization and medication adjustments.	Catheterization increases the risk for infection, so every effort and support should be directed toward helping the client to void on his or her own.

Gerontic Health

● N O T E : *Obstructive voiding symptoms secondary to prostate disease include hesitancy, decreased force of stream, terminal dribbling, postvoid fullness, and double voiding. Benign prostatic hypertrophy (BPH) is the most common cause of prostatic enlargement requiring intervention. Seventy-five percent of men older than 80 years of age experience BPH and the resulting urinary symptoms.*

ACTIONS/INTERVENTIONS	RATIONALES
Collect a thorough and comprehensive history of the client's symptoms.	Assist the client and physician in determining the cause of retention.
Review the medication record for use of anticholinergic, antidepressant, and antipsychotic medications.	The use of anticholinergic, antidepressant, and antipsychotic medication can result in urinary retention as a side effect.

Home Health

● N O T E : *If this nursing diagnosis is made, it is imperative that physician referral be made. Vigorous intervention is required to prevent damage or systemic infection. If referred to home care under a physician's care, it is important to maintain and evaluate the patient's response to prescribed treatments.*

ACTIONS/INTERVENTIONS	RATIONALES
Assist the client and family in lifestyle changes that may be required: • Monitor bladder for distention. • Record intake and output. • Stimulate micturition reflex. (See Adult Health.) • Institute bladder-retraining program. • Perform exercises to strengthen pelvic floor muscles. • Use proper position for voiding. • Maintain fluid intake. • Maintain physical activity as tolerated. • Use straight catheterization.	Similar to Adult Health. Locus of control now is with the family and client.
Assist the client and family to set criteria to help them determine when a physician or other intervention is required (e.g., specified intake and output limit, pain, or bladder distention).	Knowledge will assist the client and family to seek timely interventions.
Assess the client/caregiver understanding of prescribed medications. Provide teaching as needed.	Facilitates self-care.
Refer to appropriate assistive resources as indicated.	Additional support may be required to help the client and family maintain care at home.

REFERENCES

1. Taylor C, Lillis C, and LeMone, P: Fundamentals of Nursing: The Art and Science of Nursing Care, ed 5. Lippincott, Williams & Wilkins, New York, 2005.
2. McCance, K, and Huether, S: Pathophysiology: The Biologic Basis for Disease in Adults and Children, ed 5. Mosby, St. Louis, 2005.
3. Author: Dehydration and fluid maintenance, American Medical Directors Association (AMDA), 2001.
4. Folden, SL, et al: Practice Guidelines for the Management of Constipation in Adults. Association of Rehabilitation Nurses, Glenview, IL, 2002.
5. Locke, GR, Pemberton, JH, and Phillips, SF: American Gastroenterological Association medical position statement: Guidelines on constipation. Gastroenterology 119:6, 1761, 2000.
6. Hay-Smith, EJC, et al: Pelvic floor muscle training for urinary incontinence in women. Cochrane Incontinence Group, Cochrane Database of Systematic Reviews I, 2006.
7. Mallett, VT: Female urinary incontinence: What the epidemiologic data tell us. Int J Fertil Womens Med 50:1, 12, 2005.
8. Karon, S: A team approach to bladder retraining: A pilot study. Urol Nurs 25:4, 269, 2005.
9. Freiberg, K: Annual Editions: Human Development. McGraw-Hill/Dushkin, Boston, 2005.
10. Ebersole, P, Hess, P, and Lugen, A: Toward Healthy Aging: Human Needs and Nursing Response, ed 6. Mosby, St. Louis, 2004.
11. Best Practice 3:1, 1999. (http://www.bestpractices.org/bpbriefs/)
12. Graf, C: Functional decline in hospitalized older adults. Am J Nurs 106:1, 58, 2006.
13. Author: Nursing Diagnosis: Definitions and Classification, 2005–2006. North American Nursing Diagnosis Association, NANDA International, 2005.
14. Schmelzer, M: Effectiveness of wheat bran in preventing constipation of hospitalized orthopaedic surgery patients. Orthop Nurs 9:55, 1990.
15. Fogel, CI, and Wood, NF: Health Care of Women: A Nursing Perspective, CV Mosby, St. Louis, 1981.
16. Patrick, T: Female physical development. In Breslin, ET, and Lucas, VA (eds): Women's Health Nursing: Toward Evidence-Based Practice. WB Saunders, Philadelphia, 2003.
17. Erickson, H, Tomlin, E, and Wsain, M: Modeling and Role-Modeling: A Theory and Paradigm for Nursing. Prentice-Hall, Englewood Cliffs, NJ, 1983.
18. Kneisl, C, Wilson, H, and Trigoboff, E: Contemporary Psychiatric-Mental Health Nursing, Pearson Education, Upper Saddle River, NJ, 2004.
19. Lange, N, and Tigges, BB: Nurse Practitioner 30:44, 2005.
20. Kozier, B: Fundamentals of Nursing: Concepts, Process, and Practice, ed 7. Prentice Hall Health, Upper Saddle River, NJ, 2004.
21. Smeltzer, SC, et al: Brunner & Suddarth's Textbook of Medical-Surgical Nursing, ed 10. Lippincott, Williams & Wilkins, Philadelphia, 2003.
22. Lowdermilk, DL, and Perry, SE: Maternity & Women's Care, ed 8. CV Mosby, St. Louis, 2004.
23. Maxmen, J, and Ward, N: Psychotropic Drugs Fast Facts. WW Norton, New York, 2002.
24. Management of Constipation in Older Adults. Best Practice 3(1):4, 1999.
25. Heather, C, et al: Effect of bulk forming cathartic on diarrhea in tube fed patients. Heart Lung 20:409, 1991.
26. Tranmer, JE, Hodnett, ED, Hannah, ME, and Stevens, BJ: The effect of unrestricted oral carbohydrate intake on labor process. JOGNN 34:3, 319, 2005.
27. Black, JM, and Matassarin-Jacobs, E: Medical-Surgical Nursing: Clinical Management for Continuity of Care, ed 5. WB Saunders, Philadelphia, 1997.
28. Stadtler, AC, Gorski, PA, and Brazleton, TB: Toilet training methods, clinical interventions and recommendations. Pediatrics 103:6, 1359, 1999.
29. MJ Hockenberry, Wong's Clinical Manual of Pediatric Nursing. CV Mosby, St. Louis, 2003.
30. Sellers, JB: Health care for older women. In Breslin ET, and Lucas, VA (eds): Women's Health Nursing: Toward Evidence-Based Practice. WB Saunders, Philadelphia, 2003.
31. Nygarrd, IE, and Heit, M: Stress urinary incontinence. Am Coll Obstet Gynecol 104:3, 2004.
32. Fritz, G, et al: Practice parameter for assessment and treatment of children and adolescents with enuresis. American Academy of Child and Adolescent Psychiatry (AACAP), Washington, DC, 2002.
33. Author: Evaluation and treatment of urinary tract infections in children. American Academy of Family Physicians. Wright State University School of Medicine, Dayton OH, 2005. (http://www.aafp.org//afp/980401ap?ahmed2.html)

5

ACTIVITY–EXERCISE PATTERN

PATTERN DESCRIPTION

This pattern focuses on the activities of daily living (ADLs) and the amount of energy the individual has available to support these activities. The ADLs include all aspects of maintaining self-care and incorporate leisure time as well. Because the individual's energy level and mobility for ADLs are affected by the proper functioning of the neuromuscular, cardiovascular, and respiratory systems, nursing diagnoses related to dysfunctions in these systems are included.

As with the other patterns, a problem in the activity–exercise pattern may be the primary reason for the patient entering the health-care system or may arise secondary to problems in another functional pattern. Any admission to a hospital may promote the development of problems in this area because of the therapeutics required for the medical diagnosis (e.g., bed rest) or because of agency rules and regulations (e.g., limited visiting hours).

PATTERN ASSESSMENT

1. Does the patient's heart rate or blood pressure increase abnormally in response to activity?
   a. Yes (Activity Intolerance)
   b. No
2. Does the patient have dyspnea after activity?
   a. Yes (Activity Intolerance)
   b. No
3. Does the patient have a medical diagnosis related to the cardiovascular or respiratory system?
   a. Yes (Risk for Activity Intolerance)
   b. No
4. Does the patient have a history of Activity Intolerance?
   a. Yes (Risk for Activity Intolerance, Sedentary Lifestyle)
   b. No
5. Does the patient complain of fatigue, weakness, or lack of energy?
   a. Yes (Activity Intolerance or Fatigue)
   b. No
6. Is the patient unable to maintain his or her usual routines?
   a. Yes (Fatigue or Self-Care Deficit)
   b. No
7. Does the patient report difficulty in concentrating?
   a. Yes (Fatigue)
   b. No
8. Review self-care chart. Does the patient have any self-care deficits?
   a. Yes (Self-Care Deficit [specify which area])
   b. No
9. Can the patient engage in a usual hobby while in hospital?
   a. Yes
   b. No (Deficient Diversional Activity)
10. Does the family need help with home maintenance after the patient goes home?
    a. Yes (Impaired Home Maintenance)
    b. No
11. Does the patient have health insurance?
    a. Yes
    b. No (Impaired Home Maintenance)
12. Is the patient within height and weight norm for age?
    a. Yes
    b. No (Delayed Growth and Development)
13. Can the patient perform developmental skills appropriate for age level?
    a. Yes
    b. No (Delayed Growth and Development)
14. Are there any abnormal movements?
    a. Yes (Disorganized Infant Behavior)
    b. No
15. If the patient is an infant, does he or she respond appropriately to stimuli?
    a. Yes
    b. No (Disorganized Infant Behavior)
16. Does the patient's cardiogram indicate arrhythmias?
    a. Yes (Decreased Cardiac Output)
    b. No
17. Is the patient's jugular vein distended?
    a. Yes (Decreased Cardiac Output)
    b. No
18. Are the patient's peripheral pulses within normal limits?
    a. Yes
    b. No (Decreased Cardiac Output, Ineffective Tissue Perfusion, or Risk for Peripheral Neurovascular Dysfunction)
19. Are the patient's extremities cold?
    a. Yes (Ineffective Tissue Perfusion or Risk for Peripheral Neurovascular Dysfunction)
    b. No
20. Does the patient have claudication?
    a. Yes (Ineffective Tissue Perfusion or Risk for Peripheral Neurovascular Dysfunction)
    b. No
21. Does the patient have full range of motion?
    a. Yes
    b. No (Impaired Physical Mobility or Impaired Walking)
22. Does the patient have problems moving self in bed?
    a. Yes (Impaired Bed Mobility)
    b. No
23. Does the patient have problems ambulating?
    a. Yes (Impaired Physical Mobility or Impaired Walking)
    b. No
24. Is the patient paralyzed?
    a. Yes (Risk for Disuse Syndrome)
    b. No

25. Is the patient immobilized by casts or traction?
    a. Yes (Risk for Disuse Syndrome or Risk for Peripheral Neurovascular Dysfunction)
    b. No
26. Does the patient have a spinal cord injury at T7 or above?
    a. Yes (Risk for Autonomic Dysreflexia)
    b. No
27. Does the patient have a spinal cord injury at T7 or above and paroxysmal hypertension?
    a. Yes (Autonomic Dysreflexia)
    b. No
28. Does the patient have a spinal cord injury at T7 or above and bradycardia or tachycardia?
    a. Yes (Autonomic Dysreflexia)
    b. No
29. Review the mental status examination. Is the patient exhibiting confusion or drowsiness?
    a. Yes (Impaired Gas Exchange)
    b. No
30. Review blood gas levels. Does the patient demonstrate hypercapnia?
    a. Yes (Impaired Gas Exchange or Impaired Spontaneous Ventilation)
    b. No
31. Were rales (crackles) or rhonchi (wheezes) present on chest auscultation?
    a. Yes (Ineffective Airway Clearance)
    b. No
32. Is respiratory rate increased above the normal range?
    a. Yes (Ineffective Airway Clearance or Ineffective Breathing Pattern)
    b. No
33. Is the patient on a ventilator? If yes, does the patient have restlessness or an increase from baseline of blood pressure, pulse, or respiration when weaning is attempted?
    a. Yes (Dysfunctional Ventilatory Weaning Response)
    b. No
34. Does the patient have dyspnea and shortness of breath?
    a. Yes (Ineffective Breathing Pattern, Impaired Spontaneous Ventilation, or Activity Intolerance)
    b. No
35. Is the patient exhibiting pursed-lip breathing?
    a. Yes (Ineffective Breathing Pattern)
    b. No
36. Does the patient have a history of falling?
    a. Yes (Risk for Falls)
    b. No
37. Does the patient have diminished mental status?
    a. Yes (Risk for Falls)
    b. No
38. Does the patient have difficulty in manipulating his or her wheelchair?
    a. Yes (Impaired Wheelchair Mobility)
    b. No

39. Can the patient independently transfer him- or herself from site to site?
    a. Yes
    b. No (Impaired Transfer Ability)

CONCEPTUAL INFORMATION

Several nursing diagnoses are included in this pattern that, at first glance, seem to have little relationship with each other. However, closer investigation demonstrates that there is one concept common to all of the diagnoses: immobility. Immobility, or the impulses that control and coordinate mobility, can contribute to the development of any of these diagnoses, or any of these diagnoses can ultimately lead to the development of immobility.

Mobility and immobility are end points on a continuum with many degrees of impaired mobility or partial mobility between the two points.[1] Immobility is usually distinguished from impaired mobility by the permanence of the limitation. A person who is quadriplegic has immobility, because it is permanent; a person with a long cast on the left leg has impaired mobility, because it is temporary.[2]

Mobility is defined as the ability to move freely and is one of the major means by which we define and express ourselves. The central nervous system integrates the stimuli from sensory receptor nerves of the peripheral nervous system and projection tracts of the central nervous system to respond to the internal or external environment of the individual. This integration allows for movement and expressions. A problem with mobility can be a measure of the degree of the illness or health problem of an individual.[3]

Patients with self-care deficits are most often those who are experiencing some type of mobility problem.[2] Mobility problems require greater energy expenditure, which leads to activity intolerance, deficient diversional activity, and impaired home maintenance simply because of the lack of energy or nervous system response to engage in these activities.

Problems with mobility and nervous system response also lead to other physical problems. When a person has impaired mobility or immobility, bed rest is quite often prescribed or is voluntarily sought in an effort to conserve energy. Several authors[3–5] describe the physical problems that can occur secondary to prolonged bed rest:

1. **Respiratory:** Decreased chest and lung expansion causes slower and more shallow respiration. Pooling of secretions occurs secondary to decreased respiratory effort and the effects of gravity. The cough reflex is decreased as a result of decreased respiratory effort, gravity, and decreased muscle strength. Acid–base balance is shifted, causing a retention of carbon dioxide. Respiratory acidosis causes changes in mentation: vasodilatation of cerebrovascular blood vessels and

increased cerebral blood flow, headache, mental cloudiness, disorientation, dizziness, generalized weakness, convulsions, and unconsciousness. In addition, because of the buildup of carbon dioxide in the lungs, adequate oxygen cannot be inspired, leading to tissue hypoxia.

2. **Cardiovascular:** Circulatory stasis is caused by vasodilatation and impaired venous return. Muscular inactivity leads to vein dilation in dependent parts. Gravity effects also occur. Decreased respiratory effort and gravity lead to decreased thoracic and abdominal pressures that usually assist in promoting blood return to the heart. Quite often patients have increased use of the Valsalva maneuver, which leads to increases in preload and afterload of cardiac output and, ultimately, a decreased cardiac output. Continued limitation of activity leads to decreased cardiac rate, slower circulatory volume, and arterial pressure as a result of redistribution of body fluids. Venous stasis contributes to the potential for deep venous thrombosis and pulmonary embolus. After prolonged bed rest, the normal neurovascular mechanism of the cardiovascular system that prevents large shifts in blood volume does not function adequately. When the individual who has experienced extended bed rest attempts to assume an upright position, gravity pulls an excessive amount of blood volume to the feet and legs, depriving the brain of adequate oxygen. As a result, the individual experiences orthostatic hypotension.[4]

3. **Musculoskeletal:** Inactivity causes decreased bone stress and decreased muscle tension. Osteoblastic and osteoclastic activities become imbalanced, leading to calcium and phosphorus loss. Decreased muscle use leads to decreased muscle mass and strength as a result of infrequent muscle contractions and protein loss.

4. **Metabolic:** Basal metabolic rate and oxygen consumption decrease, leading to decreased efficiency in using nutrients to build new tissues. Normally, body tissues break down nitrogen, but apparently muscle mass loss with accompanying protein loss leads to nitrogen loss and a negative nitrogen balance. Changes in tissue metabolism lead to increased potassium and calcium excretion. Decreased energy use and decreased basal metabolic rate (BMR) lead to appetite loss, which leads to a decrease in the nutrient intake necessary to offset losses.

5. **Skin:** The negative nitrogen balance previously discussed, coupled with continuous pressure on bony prominences, leads to a greatly increased potential for skin breakdown.

Immobility is not the sole causative factor of the nursing diagnoses in this pattern. Many of the diagnoses can be related to specific medical diagnoses, such as congestive heart failure, or may occur as a result of diagnoses in this pattern, for example, Delayed Growth and Development.

However, the concept of immobility does serve to point out the interrelatedness of the diagnoses.

Because fatigue plays a major role in determining the quality and amount of musculoskeletal activity undertaken, consideration of the factors that influence fatigue is an essential part of nursing assessment for the activity–exercise pattern. Fatigue might be considered in two general categories: experiential and muscular. The degree to which the individual participates in activity is significant in determining the fatigue experienced. Activities that the individual enjoys are less likely to produce fatigue than are those not enjoyed. Preferences should be considered within the framework of capacity and needs. Obviously, other factors that must be considered include the physical and medical condition of the person and his or her emotional state, level of growth and development, and state of health in general. Oxygenation needs and extrinsic factors also need to be addressed. If there is overstimulation, such as with noise, extremes of temperature, or interruption of routines, a greater amount of fatigue or disorganized behavior can be expected. Sensory understimulation with resultant boredom can also contribute to fatigue.

Fatigue can develop as a result of too much waste material accumulating and too little nourishment going to the muscles. Muscle fatigue usually is attributed to the accumulation of too much lactic acid in the muscles. Certain metabolic conditions, such as congestive heart failure, place a person at greater risk for fatigue.

DEVELOPMENTAL CONSIDERATIONS

Diet, musculoskeletal factors, and respiratory and cardiovascular mechanisms influence activity. Developmental considerations for diet are addressed in Chapter 3. The developmental considerations discussed here specifically relate to musculoskeletal, respiratory, and cardiovascular factors.

INFANT

Many things, including genetic, biologic, and cultural factors, influence physical and motor abilities. Nutrition, maturation of the central nervous system, skeletal formation, and overall physical health status, as well as amount of stimulation, environmental conditions, and consistent loving care also play a part in physical and motor abilities.[6] Girls usually develop more rapidly than do boys, although boys have a higher activity level.[6]

All muscular tissue is formed at birth, but growth occurs as the infant uses the various muscle groups. This use stimulates increased strength and function.

The infant engages in various types of play activity at various times in infancy because of developing skills and changing needs. The infant needs the stimulation of parents in this play activity to develop fully. However, parents should be aware of the dangers of overstimulation. Fatigue, inattention, and injury to the infant may result.[6]

Interruptions in the normal developmental sequence of play activities due to illness or hospitalization, for example, can have a detrimental effect on the future development of the infant or child. An understanding of the normal sequence of play development is important so that therapeutic interventions can be designed to approximate the developmental needs of the individual.

The structural description of play development focuses on the Piagetian concepts of the increasing cognitive complexity of play activities. Elementary sensorimotor-based games emerge first, with the gradual development of advanced social games in adulthood.[7]

Play activities assist in the child's development of psychomotor skills and cognitive development. Socialization skills are learned and practiced via the interaction with others during play. As the child begins to learn more about his or her body during play, he or she will incorporate more complicated gross and fine motor skills. Play is extremely valuable in the development of language and other communication skills. Play helps the individual establish control over self and the environment and provides a sense of accomplishment. Through play activities, the infant learns to trust the environment. Play also affords the child the opportunity to express emotions that would be unacceptable in other normal social situations.

Practice games begin during the sensorimotor level of cognitive development at 1 to 4 months of age, and continue with increasing complexity throughout childhood. These games include skills that are performed for the pleasure of functioning, that is, for the pleasure of practice.

Symbolic games appear later during the sensorimotor period than do practice games—at about age 12 to 18 months. Make-believe is now added to the practice game. Other objects represent elements of absent objects or persons. As previously stated, activity is influenced by respiratory and cardiovascular mechanisms.

The respiratory mechanisms, or air-conducting passages (nose, pharynx, larynx, trachea, bronchi, bronchioles, and alveoli) and lungs, of the infant are small, delicate, and immature. The air that enters the nose is cool, dry, and unfiltered. The nose is unable to filter the air, and the mucous membranes of the upper respiratory tract are unable to produce enough mucus to humidify or warm the inhaled air. Therefore, the infant is more susceptible to respiratory tract infections.[7]

In addition, the infant is a nose breather. When upper respiratory tract infections do occur, the infant is unable to clear the airways appropriately and may get into some difficulty until he or she learns to breathe through his or her mouth (at about 3 to 4 months of age). The cough of the infant is not very effective, and the infant quickly becomes fatigued with the effort.[7]

In the lungs, the alveoli are functioning, but not all alveoli may be expanded. Therefore, there is a large amount of dead space in the lungs. The infant has to work harder to exchange enough oxygen and carbon dioxide to meet body demands. The elevated respiratory rate of the infant (30 to 60 per minute) reflects this increased work. In addition, arterial blood gases of the infant may show an acid–base imbalance. The rate and rhythm of respiration in the infant is somewhat irregular, and it is not unusual for the infant to use accessory muscles of respiration. Retractions with respiration are common.

The alveoli of the infant increase in number and complexity very rapidly. By 1 year of age, the alveoli and the lining of the air passages have matured considerably.

Respiratory tract obstructions are common in this age group because of the short trachea and the almost straight-line position of the right main stem bronchus. In addition, the epiglottis does not effectively close over the trachea during swallowing. Thus, foreign objects are aspirated into the lungs.

In terms of cardiovascular development, the foramen ovale closes during the first 24 hours, and the ductus arteriosus closes after several days. The neonate can survive mild oxygen deprivation longer than an adult can. The Apgar scoring system is used to measure the physical status of the newborn and includes heart rate, color, and respiration. There is no day–night rhythm to the neonate's heart rate, but from the sixth week on, the rate is lower at night than during the day. Axillary temperature readings and age-sized blood pressure cuffs should be used to assess vital signs. The pulse is 120 to 150 beats per minute; respiration ranges from 35 to 50 per minute; and blood pressure ranges from 40 to 90 mm Hg systolic and 6 to 20 mm Hg diastolic. Vital signs become more stable over the first year. Listening for murmurs should be done over the base of the heart rather than at the apex. Breath sounds are bronchovesicular. The neonate has limited ability to respond to environmental temperature changes and loses heat rapidly. This leads to an increased basal metabolic rate (BMR) and an increased workload on the heart. Until patients reach age 7, the apex is palpated at the fourth interspace just to the left of the mid-clavicular line.

TODDLER AND PRESCHOOLER

By this age, the child is walking, running, climbing, and jumping. The toddler is very active and curious. He or she gets into everything. This helps the toddler organize his or her world and develop spatial and sensory perception.[6] It is during this period that the child begins to see him- or herself as a person separate from his or her parents and the environment. This increasing level of autonomy also presents a challenge for the caregivers. The child alternates between the security of the parents and the exciting exploration of the environment.

The toddler is fairly clumsy, but gross and fine motor coordination is improving. Neuromuscular maturation and repetition of movements help the child further develop skills.[6] Muscles grow faster than bones during these years. Safety is a major concern for children of this age. The toddler, especially, wants to do many things for him- or herself, thus testing control of self and the environment.

Bathing and Hygiene

By the age of 3, the child can wash and dry his or her hands with some wetting of clothes and can brush his or her teeth, but requires assistance to perform the task adequately. By the fourth birthday, the child may bathe him- or herself with assistance. The child will be able to bathe him or herself without assistance by the age of 5. Both parents and nurses must keep in mind the safety issues involved in bathing; the child requires supervision in selection of water temperature and in the prevention of drowning.

Dressing and Grooming

At age 18 to 20 months, the child has the fine motor skills required to unzip a large zipper. By 24 to 48 months, the child can unbutton large buttons. The child can put on a coat with assistance by age 2; the child can undress him- or herself in most situations and can put on his or her own coat without assistance by age 3. At $3^1/_2$ years the child can unbutton small buttons, and by 4 years can button small buttons. Dressing without assistance and a beginning ability to lace shoes are accomplishments of the 5-year-old. The development of fine motor skills is required for most of the tasks of dressing. It is important that the child's clothing have fasteners that are appropriate for the motor skill development. The child will require assistance with deciding the appropriateness of clothing selected; seasonal variations in weather and culturally accepted norms regarding dressing and grooming are learned by the child with assistance.

Feeding

The child can drink from a cup without much spilling by 18 months. The child will have frequent spills while trying to get the contents of a spoon into his or her mouth at this age. By 2 years of age, the child can drink from a cup; use of a spoon has improved at this age, but the child will still spill liquids (soup) from a spoon when eating. The child can eat from a spoon without spilling by $3^1/_2$ years. Accomplished use of a fork occurs at 5 years.

Toileting

By age 3, the child can go to the toilet without assistance; the child can pull pants up and down for toileting without assistance at this stage as well. The development of food preferences, preferred eating schedules and environment, and toileting behavior are imparted to the child by learning. Toileting, food, and the eating experience may also include pleasures, control issues, and learning tasks in addition to the development of the motor skills required to accomplish the task. Delays or regressions in the tasks of self-feeding may reflect issues other than a self-care deficit, for example, discipline, family coping, and role-relationships.

Physiology

During the preschool years, the child seems to have an unlimited supply of energy. However, he or she does not know when to stop and may continue activities past the point of exhaustion. Parents should provide a variety of activities for these age groups, as the attention span is short.

The lung size and volume of the toddler have now increased, and thus the oxygen capacity of the toddler has increased. The toddler is still susceptible to respiratory tract infections but not to the same extent as the infant. The rate and rhythm of respiration have decreased, and respirations average 25 to 35 per minute. Accessory muscles of respiration are used infrequently now, and respiration is primarily diaphragmatic.

The respiratory structures (trachea and bronchi) are positioned farther down in the chest now, and the epiglottis is effective in closing off the trachea during swallowing. Thus, aspiration and airway obstruction are reduced in this age group.

The respiratory rate of the preschooler is about 30 per minute. The preschooler is still susceptible to upper respiratory tract infections. The lymphatic tissues of the tonsils and adenoids are involved in these respiratory tract infections. Tonsillectomies and adenoidectomies are no longer performed "routinely." These tissues serve to protect the respiratory tract, and valid reasons must be presented to warrant their removal.

The temperature of the toddler ranges around 99°F ± 1° (orally); pulse ranges around 105 beats per minute ± 35; respirations range from 20 to 35 per minute; and blood pressure ranges from 80 to 100 mm Hg systolic and 60 to 64 mm Hg diastolic. The size of the vascular bed increases in the toddler, thus reducing resistance to flow. The capillary bed has increased ability to respond to environmental temperature changes. Lung volume increases. Breath sounds are more intense and more bronchial, and expiration is more pronounced. The toddler's chest should be examined with the child in an erect position, then recumbent, and then turned to the left side. Arrhythmias and extrasystoles are not uncommon but should be recorded.

The temperature of the preschooler is 98.6° F ± 1° (orally); pulse ranges from 80 to 100 beats per minute; respiration is 30 per minute ± 5; and blood pressure is 90/60 mm Hg ± 15. There is continued increase of the vascular bed, lung volume, and so on, in keeping with physical growth.

SCHOOL-AGE CHILD

Whereas the muscles were growing faster than the bones during the toddler and preschool years, the skeletal system is growing rapidly during these years—faster than the muscles are growing. Children may experience "growing pains" because of the growth of the long bones. There is a gradual increase in muscle mass and strength, and the body takes on a leaner appearance. The child loses his or her "baby fat," muscle tone increases, and loose movements disappear. Adequate exercise is needed to maintain strength, flexibility, and balance and to encourage muscular development.[7] Males have a greater number of muscle cells than females. Posture becomes more upright and straighter but is not necessarily influenced by exercise. Posture is a function of the strength of the back muscles and the general state of health of the child. Poor posture may be reflective of fatigue as well as skeletal defects,[7] with fatigue being exhibited by such behaviors as quarrelsomeness, crying, or lack of interest in eating. Skeletal defects such as scoliosis begin to appear during this period.

Neuromuscular coordination is sufficient to permit the school-age child to learn most skills[6]; however, care should be taken to prevent muscle injuries. Hands and fingers manipulate things well. Although children age 7 have a high energy level, they also have an increased attention span and cognitive skills. Therefore, they tend to engage in quiet games as well as active ones. Seven-year-olds tend to be more directed in their range of activities. Games with rules develop as the child engages in more social contacts. These games characteristically emerge during the operational phase of cognitive development in the school age child. These rule games may also be practice or symbolic in nature, but now the child attaches social significance and order to the play by imposing the structure of rules.

Eight-year-olds have grace and balance. Nine-year-olds move with less restlessness, their strength and endurance increase, and their hand–eye coordination is good.[6] Competition among peers is important to test out their strength, agility, and coordination. Although 10- to 12-year-old children are better able to control and direct their high energy level, they do have energetic, active, restless movements with tension release through finger drumming, foot tapping, or leg swinging.

The respiratory rate of the school-age child slows to 18 to 22 per minute. The respiratory tissues reach adult maturity, lung volume increases, and the lung capacity is proportionate to body size. The school-age child is still susceptible to respiratory tract infections. The frontal sinuses are fairly well developed by this age, and all the mucous membranes are very vulnerable to congestion and inflammation. The temperature, pulse, and respiration of the school-age child are gradually approaching adult norms, with temperature ranging from 98 to 98.6°F, pulse (resting) 60 to 70 beats per minute, and respiration from 18 to 20 per minute. Systolic blood pressure ranges from 94 to 112 mm Hg, and diastolic from 56 to 60 mm Hg. The heart grows more slowly during this period and is smaller in relation to the rest of the body. Because the heart must continue to supply the metabolic needs, the child should be advised against sustained physical activity and be watched for tiring. After age 7, the apex of the heart lies at the interspace of the fifth rib at the midclavicular line. Circulatory functions reach adult capacity. The child will still have some vasomotor instability with rapid vasodilation. A third heart sound and sinus arrhythmias are fairly common but, again, should be recorded.

ADOLESCENT

Growth in skeletal size, muscle mass, adipose tissue, and skin is significant in adolescence. The skeletal system grows faster than the muscles; thus, stress fractures may result. The large muscles grow faster than the smaller muscles, with the occasional result of poor posture and decreased coordination. Boys are clumsier than girls. Muscle growth continues in boys during late adolescence because of androgen production.[6]

Physical activities provide a way for adolescents to enjoy the stimulation of conflict in a socially acceptable way. Some form of physical activity should be encouraged to promote physical development, prevent overweight, formulate a realistic body image, and promote peer acceptance.

The respiratory rate of the adolescent is 16 to 20 per minute. Parts of the body grow at various rates, but the respiratory system does not grow proportionately. Therefore, the adolescent may have inadequate oxygenation and become more fatigued. The lung capacity correlates with the adolescent's structural form. Boys have a larger lung capacity than girls because of greater shoulder width and chest size. Boys have greater respiratory volume, greater vital capacity, and a slower respiratory rate. The boy's lung capacity matures later than the girl's. Girls' lungs mature at age 17 or 18.

The heart continues to grow during adolescence but more slowly than the rest of the body, contributing to the common problems of inadequate oxygenation and fatigue. The heart continues to enlarge until age 17 or 18. Systolic pulse pressure increases, and the temperature is the same as in an adult. The pulse ranges from 50 to 68 beats per minute; respiration ranges from 18 to 20 per minute; and blood pressure is 100 to 120/50 to 70 mm Hg. Adolescent girls have slightly higher pulse rates and basal body temperature and lower systolic pressures than boys. Hypertension incidence increases. Essential hypertension incidence is approximately equal between races for this age group.

Athletes have slower pulse rates than peers. Heart sounds are heard readily at the fifth left intercostal space. Functional murmurs should be outgrown by this time. Chest pain may arise from musculoskeletal changes, but cardiovascular pain should always be investigated. Cardiovascular problems are the fifth leading cause of death in adolescents.

More rest and sleep are needed now than earlier. The teenager is expending large amounts of energy and functioning with an inadequate oxygen supply; both these factors contribute to fatigue and lead to the need for additional rest. Parents may need to set limits. Rest does not necessarily mean sleep and can also include quiet activities.[6]

Because of the very rapid growth during this period, the adolescent may not have sufficient energy left for strenuous activities. He or she tires easily and may frequently complain of needing to sit down. Gradually the adolescent is able to increase both speed and stamina during exercise. An increase in muscular and skeletal strength, as well as the increased ability of the lungs and heart to provide adequate oxygen to the tissue, facilitates maintenance of hemodynamics and rate of recovery after exercise. The body reaches its peak of physiologic resilience during late adolescence and young adulthood. Regular physical training and an individualized conditioning program can increase both strength and tolerance to strenuous activity.

Faulty nutrition is another major cause of fatigue in the adolescent. Poor eating habits established during the school-age years, combined with the typical quick-service, quick-energy food consumption patterns of adolescents, frequently lead to anemia, which in itself can lead to activity intolerance.[7]

The adolescent may be given responsibility for assisting with the maintenance of the family home, or may be responsible for his or her own home if living independent from the family of origin. The role exploration characteristic of adolescence may lead to temporary changes in hygiene practices.

Recreational activities in adolescence often take the form of organized sports and other competitive activities. Social relationships are developed and enhanced, specific motor and cognitive skills related to a specific sport are refined, and a sense of mastery can be developed. Group activities and peer approval and acceptance are important. The adolescent responds to peer activities and experiments with different roles and lifestyles. The nurse must distinguish self-care practices that are acceptable to the peer group from those that indicate a self-care deficit.

YOUNG ADULT

Growth of the skeletal system is essentially complete by age 25. Muscular efficiency is at its peak between 20 and 30. Energy level and control of energy are high. Thereafter, muscular strength declines with the rate of muscle aging, depending on the specific muscle group, the activity of the person, and the adequacy of his or her diet.

Regular exercise is helpful in controlling weight and maintaining a state of high-level wellness. Muscle tone, strength, and circulation are enhanced by exercise. Problems arise especially when sedentary lifestyles decrease the amount of exercise available with daily activities. Caloric intake and exercise should be balanced.

Adequate sleep is important for good physical and mental health. Lack of sleep results in progressive sluggishness of both physical and cognitive functions. The major activities of individuals in this age group are work and leisure-time pursuits. The young adult should learn to balance his or her work with leisure-time activities. Getting started in a career can be very stressful and can lead to burnout if an appropriate balance is not found. Physical fitness reflects ability to work for a sustained period with vigor and pleasure, without undue fatigue, and with energy left over for enjoying hobbies and recreational activities and for meeting emergencies.[6]

Basic to fitness are regular physical exercise, proper nutrition, adequate rest and relaxation, conscientious health practices, and good medical and dental care. Regular physical fitness is a natural tranquilizer releasing the body's own endorphins, which reduce anxiety and muscular tension.

The respiratory system of the young adult has completely matured. Oxygen demand is based on exercise and activity now but gradually decreases between age 20 and 40. The body's ability to use oxygen efficiently is dependent on the cardiovascular system and the needs of the skeletal muscles.

The respiratory and cardiovascular systems change gradually with age, but the rate of change is highly dependent on the individual's diet and exercise pattern. Generally, contraction of the myocardium decreases. Maximum cardiac output is reached between the age of 20 and 30. The arteries become less elastic. The maximum breathing capacity decreases between ages 20 and 40. Cardiac and respiratory function can be improved with regular exercise. Hypertension (blood pressure 140/90 mm Hg or higher) and mitral valve prolapse syndrome are the most common cardiovascular medical diagnoses of the young adult.

ADULT

Basal metabolism rate gradually decreases. Although there is a general and gradual decline in quickness and level of activity, people who were most active among their age group during adolescence and young adulthood tend to be the most active during middle and old age. In women, there is frequently a menopausal rise in energy and activity.[8] Judicious exercise balanced with rest and sleep modify and retard the aging process. Exercise stimulates circulation to all parts of the body, thereby improving body functions. Exercise can also be an outlet for emotional tension. If the person is beginning exercises after being sedentary, certain precautions should be taken, such as increasing exercise gradually to a moderate level, exercising consistently, and avoiding overexertion. Research indicates that cardiovascular risk factors can be reduced in women by low-intensity walking.[9]

The adult is beginning to have a decrease in bone mass and a loss of skeletal height. Muscle strength and mass are directly related to active muscle use. The adult needs to maintain the patterns of activity and exercise of young adulthood and not become sedentary. Otherwise, muscles lose mass structure and strength more rapidly.

Temperature for the adult ranges from 97 to 99.6°F; pulse ranges from 50 to 100 beats per minute; respiration ranges from 16 to 20 per minute; and blood pressure is 120/80 mm Hg ± 15. Cardiac output gradually decreases, and the decreasing elasticity of the blood vessels causes more susceptibility to hypertension and cardiovascular diseases. After menopause women become as prone to coronary disease as men, so estrogen appears to be a protective agent. The BMR generally decreases. Essential and secondary hypertension and angina occur more frequently in this age group.

The lung tissue becomes thicker and less elastic with age. The lungs cannot expand as they once did, and breathing capacity is reduced. The respiratory rate may increase to compensate for the reduced breathing capacity.

The normal adult should be able to perform activities of daily living without assistance. The need for close relationships and the intimacy of adulthood can be initiated by leisure activities with identified partners or a small group of close friends (e.g., hiking, tennis, golf, or attending concerts or theaters, etc.). The middle-age adult is often interested in the personal satisfaction of diversional activities.

The adult will most likely be responsible for home maintenance as well as outside employment. Role strain or overtaxation of the adult is possible. Illness or injury to the adults in the household will significantly affect the ability of the family unit to maintain the home.

OLDER ADULT

Older adults face a gradual decline in function through the years. Age-related changes in the cardiovascular, respiratory, and musculoskeletal systems vary from person to person. Studies attempting to describe age-related system changes have faced problems in determining what changes may be age-related versus disease-induced.[11]

Changes in the older musculoskeletal system typically include decreases in bone volume and strength, decreases in skeletal muscle quality and mass, and reductions in muscle contractility.[11] After the age of 40 to 50, an incremental process of bone absorption without successful new bone formation leads to gradual bone loss.[12] This loss is greater in women, but occurs in both men and women. Tendon and ligament strength decrease with aging, and collagen stiffness and cross-linking occur. The tendon and ligament changes can result in joint range-of-motion losses of 20 to 25 percent.[11] Changes in older adults vestibular and nervous systems present a challenge to older adults attempting to maintain balance, prevent falls, and have a smooth gait.[13] Vestibular changes can impede spatial orientation. The vestibular and nervous system changes in conjunction with a slowed reaction time, increased postural sway, decreased stride, decreased toe-floor clearance, decreased arm swing, and knee and hip rotation all may impact the mobility level of older adults.[14]

Age-related changes to the respiratory system may include a decrease in lung elasticity, chest wall stiffness, diminished cough reflex, increased physiologic dead space secondary to air trapping, and nonuniform alveolar ventilation.[15] Alveolar enlargement and thinning of alveolar walls mean less alveolar surface is available for gas exchange.[16] The older adult may experience decreases in Pa_{O_2} and increases in Pa_{CO_2} because of age-related changes in the respiratory system.

Cardiovascular diseases remain the primary cause of death in the older population.[17] With aging, the cardiovascular system undergoes changes in structure and function. Left ventricular, aortic, and mitral valve thickening have an impact on cardiac contractility and systolic blood flow. Increased arterial thickness and arterial stiffening may lead to a decrease in the effectiveness of baroreceptors. Diminished baroreceptor response has an effect on the body's ability to control blood pressure with postural changes. Pacemaker cells in the sinoatrial node decrease with aging. Calcification may occur along the conduction system of the heart. Myocardial irritability leads to the potential for increased cardiac arrhythmias.[16] The ability of the cardiovascular system to respond to increased demands becomes reduced, and the older adult experiences a decrease in physiologic reserves.[16] These changes can have serious consequences when the older adult experiences physical or psychological stress. It becomes increasingly difficult for the older adult to have rapid and efficient blood pressure and heart rate changes. Vital sign ranges for older adults are similar to those for middle-age adults. There may be a slight increase in respiratory rate,[13] and blood pressure increases, especially systolic changes, are often present. Healthy older men, from age 50 onward, may experience a 5 to 8 mm Hg increase in systolic blood pressure per decade. Healthy older women, from age 40 onward, may have similar systolic changes.[18] Diastolic changes are usually minimal.

With the potential age-related changes just described, some older adults may experience changes in function. Many of the changes combined can lead to problems with energy available to cells, organs, and systems to accomplish desired activities. Health promotion efforts should focus on activity and exercise and their impact on the older adult's sense of well-being. Research in the 1990s has shown the benefits to older adults when weight training and exercise are a part of their lifestyle.[19] Older clients may need prompting and reminders to pace their activities to compensate for aging changes. The increase in leisure time associated with retirement and a lessening of occupational and child-rearing responsibilities create the opportunity for exploring other activity options.

The older adult has the developmental challenge of finding meaning in the course of the life they have lived and feeling comfort with the results of their actions and choices.[20] Strategies to support this task may take on the form of life review with the older client, promoting reminiscing, and other opportunities for the older adult to acknowledge and experience self-worth.[21]

Because of the diversity of our older population, individualized assessment is a high priority. The age-related changes cited in this section are not universal and inevitable for all older adults. Health-care providers need to be wary of stereotyping clients based on age. There are many independent older adults in our society, and the number is increasing.

TABLE 5.1 NANDA, NIC, and NOC Taxonomy Linkages

GORDON'S FUNCTIONAL HEALTH PATTERN	NANDA NURSING DIAGNOSIS	NIC PRIORITY INTERVENTIONS	NOC EVALUATIONS
Activity–Exercise	Activity, Intolerance Risk for & Actual	**Risk For** Energy Management Exercise Promotion: Strength Training **Actual** Activity Therapy Energy Management Exercise Promotion: Strength Training Self-Care Assistance: IADLs	Asthma Control Cardiac Pump Effectiveness Circulation Status Coping Energy Conservation Health Beliefs: Perceived Control Immobility Consequences: Physiological, Psycho-cognitive Knowledge: Diet, Disease Process, Prescribed Activity Mood Equilibrium Nutritional Status: Body Mass, Energy Pain: Disruptive Effects, Pain Level Respiratory Status: Gas Exchange, Ventilation Risk Control Risk Detection Symptom Control Symptom Severity
	Airway Clearance, Ineffective	Airway Management Asthma Management Cough Management Respiratory Monitoring	Knowledge: Aspiration Control Respiratory Status: Airway Patency, Gas Exchange, Ventilation
	Autonomic Dysreflexia, Risk for & Actual	Airway Management Dysreflexia Management Vital Signs Monitoring	Bowel Elimination Caregiver Home Readiness Comfort Level Infection Status Knowledge: Disease Process, Labor & Delivery, Medication Risk Control Risk Detection Thermal Regulation Tissue Integrity: Skin & Mucous Membranes Treatment Behavior: Illness or Injury Urinary Elimination Vital Signs Status
	Bed Mobility, Impaired	Bedrest Care Body Mechanics Promotion	Body Positioning: Self-Initiated Cognitive Ability Joint Movement: Active Mobility Level Muscle Function Neurological Status

GORDON'S FUNCTIONAL HEALTH PATTERN	NANDA NURSING DIAGNOSIS	NIC PRIORITY INTERVENTIONS	NOC EVALUATIONS
	Breathing Pattern Ineffective	Airway Management Asthma Management Respiratory Monitoring	Respiratory Status: Airway Patency, Ventilation Vital Signs Status
	Cardiac Output Decreased	Cardiac Care Cardiac Care: Acute Circulatory Care: Arterial Insufficiency, Mechanical Assist Devices, Venous Insufficiency Hemodynamic Regulation Shock Management	Cardiac Pump Effectiveness Circulation Status Tissue Perfusion: Abdominal Organs, Peripheral Vital Signs Status
	Disuse Syndrome, Risk for	Energy Management	Endurance Energy Conservation Immobility Consequence: Physiological, Psycho-cognitive Joint Movement: Active, Passive Mobility Level Muscle Function Neurological Status: Consciousness Pain Level Risk Control Risk Detection
	Diversional Activity, Deficient	Recreation Therapy Self-responsibility Facilitation	Leisure Participation Play Participation Social Involvement
	Dysfunctional Ventilatory Weaning Response (DVWR)	Mechanical Ventilation Mechanical Ventilatory Weaning	Respiratory Status: Gas Exchange, Ventilation Vital Signs Status
	Falls, Risk for	Body Mechanics Promotion Fall Prevention Positioning	
	Fatigue	Energy Management	Activity Tolerance Endurance Energy Conservation Nutritional Status: Energy Psychomotor Energy
	Gas Exchange Impaired	Airway Management Oxygen Therapy Respiratory Monitoring	Electrolyte & Acid–Base Balance Respiratory Status: Gas Exchange, Ventilation Tissue Perfusion: Pulmonary Vital Signs Status

(table continued on page 280)

::: TABLE 5.1 NANDA, NIC, and NOC Taxonomy Linkages *(continued from page 279)*

GORDON'S FUNCTIONAL HEALTH PATTERN	NANDA NURSING DIAGNOSIS	NIC PRIORITY INTERVENTIONS	NOC EVALUATIONS
	Growth and Development, Delayed	Developmental Care Developmental Enhancement: Adolescent, Child Nutrition Therapy Nutritional Monitoring	Child development: 1, 2, 4, 6, 12 months and 2, 3, 4 years; Preschool; Middle Childhood; Adolescence Growth Physical Aging Physical Maturation: Female; Male
	Growth, Risk for Disproportionate	Nutritional Monitoring Teaching: Infant Nutrition, Toddler Nutrition Weight Management	Appetite Body Image Child Development: 1, 2, 4, 6, 12 months and 2, 3, 4 years: Preschool; Middle Childhood; Adolescence Growth Knowledge: Infant Care; Preconception Maternal Health; Pregnancy Parenting Performance Physical Maturation: Male; Female Prenatal Health Behavior Risk Control Risk Detection Weight: Body Mass
	Home Maintenance, Impaired	Home Maintenance Assistance	Family Functioning Family Physical Environment Parenting Performance Parenting: Psychosocial Safety Role Performance Safe Home Environment Self-Care: Instrumental Activities of Daily Living (IADLs)
	Infant Behavior, Disorganized, Actual; Risk for; Readiness for Enhanced Organized	**Actual** Environmental Management Positioning	**Actual** Child Development: 1 Month; 2 Months Neurological Status Preterm Infant Organization Sleep Thermoregulation: Newborn
		Risk for Environmental Management Newborn Monitoring Positioning Surveillance	**Risk for** Child Development: 1, 2, 4, 6, 12 Months Coordinated Movement Knowledge: Infant Care; Parenting Neurological Status Preterm Infant Organization Risk Control Risk Detection Sleep Thermoregulation: Newborn

GORDON'S FUNCTIONAL HEALTH PATTERN	NANDA NURSING DIAGNOSIS	NIC PRIORITY INTERVENTIONS	NOC EVALUATIONS
		Readiness for Enhanced Organized Developmental Care Pain Management	**Readiness for Enhanced Organized** Child Development: 1 Month; 2 Months Neurological Status Sleep Thermoregulation: Newborn
	Peripheral Neurovascular Dysfunction, Risk for	Exercise Therapy: Joint Mobility Peripheral Sensation Management	Blood Coagulation Body Positioning: Self-Initiated Bone Healing Circulation Status Coordinated Movement Joint Movement: Ankle; Elbow; Hip; Knee Mobility Neurological Status Neurological Status: Cranial Sensory/Motor Function Neurological Status: Spinal Sensory/Motor Function Risk Control Risk Detection Tissue Perfusion: Peripheral
	Physical Mobility, Impaired	Exercise Therapy: Ambulation, Joint Mobility Positioning	Ambulation Ambulation: Wheelchair Balance Body Mechanics Performance Body Positioning: Self-Initiated Coordinated Movement Mobility Transfer performance
	Sedentary Lifestyle	*Still in development	*Still in development
	Self Care Deficit: Feeding, Bathing-Hygiene, Dressing/Grooming, Toileting		
	Feeding	**Feeding** Self-care Assistance: Feeding	**Feeding** Nutritional Status Nutritional Status: Food and Fluid Intake Self-Care: ADLs; Eating Swallowing Status
	Bathing/Hygiene	**Bathing** Self-care Assistance: Bathing/Hygiene	**Bathing** Ostomy Self-Care Self-Care: ADL; Bathing; Hygiene; Oral Hygiene

(table continued on page 282)

▓ TABLE 5.1 NANDA, NIC, and NOC Taxonomy Linkages (continued from page 281)

GORDON'S FUNCTIONAL HEALTH PATTERN	NANDA NURSING DIAGNOSIS	NIC PRIORITY INTERVENTIONS	NOC EVALUATIONS
	Dressing/Grooming	**Dressing** Hair Care Self-care Assistance: Dressing/Grooming	**Dressing** Self-Care: ADL; Hygiene; Dressing
	Toileting	**Toileting** Environmental Management Self-care Assistance: Toileting	**Toileting** Knowledge: Ostomy Care Ostomy Self-Care Self-Care: ADL; Hygiene; Toileting
	Ventilation, Spontaneous Impaired Tissue Perfusion, Ineffective (Specify Type)	Artificial Airway Management Mechanical Ventilation Respiratory Monitoring Resuscitation: Neonate Ventilation Assistance	Allergic Response: Systemic Mechanical Ventilation Response: Adult Respiratory Status: Gas Exchange; Ventilation Vital Signs
	Renal	**Renal** Fluid/Electrolyte Management Fluid Management Hemodialysis Therapy Hemofiltration Therapy Peritoneal Dialysis Therapy	**Renal** Circulation Status Electrolyte & Acid–Base Balance Fluid Balance Fluid Overload Severity Kidney Function Tissue Perfusion: Abdominal Organs
	Cerebral	**Cerebral** Cerebral Perfusion Promotion Intracranial Pressure (ICP) Monitoring Neurologic Monitoring Peripheral Sensation Management	**Cerebral** Cognitive Ability Neurological Status Neurological Status: Consciousness, Central Motor Control Swallowing Status Tissue Perfusion: Cerebral
	Cardiopulmonary	**Cardiopulmonary** Cardiac Care: Acute Circulatory Care: Arterial Insufficiency, Venous Insufficiency Respiratory Monitoring Shock Management: Cardiac	**Cardiopulmonary** Cardiac Pump Effectiveness Circulation Status Respiratory Status: Gas Exchange Tissue Perfusion: Cardiac; Pulmonary Vital Signs
	Gastrointestinal	**Gastrointestinal** Fluid/Electrolyte Management Gastrointestinal Intubation Nutrition Management	**Gastrointestinal** Electrolyte & Acid–Base Balance Fluid Balance Hydration Tissue Perfusion: Abdominal Organs
	Peripheral	**Peripheral** Circulatory Care: Arterial Insufficiency, Venous Insufficiency Neurologic Monitoring	**Peripheral** Circulation Status Fluid Overload Severity Tissue Integrity: Skin & Mucous Membranes Tissue Perfusion: Peripheral

GORDON'S FUNCTIONAL HEALTH PATTERN	NANDA NURSING DIAGNOSIS	NIC PRIORITY INTERVENTIONS	NOC EVALUATIONS
	Transfer Ability, Impaired	Exercise Promotion: Strength Training Self-care Assistance: Transfer	Balance Body Mechanics Performance Body Positioning: Self-Initiated Coordinated Movement Mobility Transfer Performance
	Walking, Impaired	Exercise Therapy: Ambulation	Ambulation Balance Coordinated Movement Endurance Mobility
	Wandering	Area Restriction Dementia Management Environmental Management: Safety	Fall Prevention Behavior Safe Home Environment
	Wheelchair, Mobility: Impaired	Positioning: Wheelchair	Adaptation to Physical Disability Ambulation: Wheelchair Balance Coordinated Movement Mobility Transfer Performance

 APPLICABLE NURSING DIAGNOSES

ACTIVITY INTOLERANCE, RISK FOR AND ACTUAL

DEFINITIONS[22]

Risk for Activity Intolerance   A state in which an individual is at risk of experiencing insufficient physiologic or psychological energy to endure or complete required or desired daily activities.

   Activity Intolerance   A state in which an individual has insufficient physiologic or psychological energy to endure or complete required or desired daily activities.

DEFINING CHARACTERISTICS[22]

A. Risk for Activity Intolerance (Risk Factors)
  1. Inexperience with the activity
  2. Presence of circulatory or respiratory problems
  3. History of previous intolerance
  4. Deconditioned status
B. Activity Intolerance
  1. Verbal report of fatigue or weakness
  2. Abnormal heart rate or blood pressure response to activity

  3. Electrocardiographic changes reflecting arrhythmias or ischemia
  4. Exertional discomfort or dyspnea

RELATED FACTORS[22]

A. Risk for Activity Intolerance
   The risk factors also serve as the related factors for this diagnosis.
B. Activity Intolerance
  1. Bed rest or immobility
  2. Generalized weakness
  3. Imbalance between oxygen supply and demand
  4. Sedentary lifestyle

RELATED CLINICAL CONCERNS

  1. Anemias
  2. Congestive heart failure
  3. Valvular heart disease
  4. Cardiac arrhythmia
  5. Chronic obstructive pulmonary disease (COPD)
  6. Metabolic disorder
  7. Musculoskeletal disorders

Have You Selected the Correct Diagnosis?

Impaired Physical Mobility
This diagnosis implies that an individual would be able to move independently if something were not limiting the motion. Activity Intolerance implies that the individual is freely able to move but cannot endure or adapt to the increased energy or oxygen demands made by the movement or activity.

Self-Care Deficit
Self-Care Deficit indicates that the patient has some dependence on another person. Activity Intolerance implies that the patient is independent but is unable to perform activities because the body is unable to adapt to the increased energy and oxygen demands made. A person may have a self-care deficit as a result of activity intolerance.

Ineffective Individual Coping
Persons with the diagnosis of Ineffective Individual Coping may be unable to participate in their usual roles or in their usual self-care because they feel they lack control or the motivation to do so.

Activity Intolerance, on the other hand, implies that the person is willing and able to participate in activities but is unable to endure or adapt to the increased energy or oxygen demands made by the movement or activity.

EXPECTED OUTCOME

Will participate in increased self-care activities by [date]. (Specify which self-care activities, that is, bathing, feeding, dressing, or ambulation, and the frequency, duration, or intensity of the activity.)

EXAMPLE

Will increase walking by at least 1 block each week for 8 weeks.

TARGET DATES

Appropriate target dates will have to be individualized according to the degree of activity intolerance. An appropriate range would be 3 to 5 days.

NURSING ACTIONS/INTERVENTIONS WITH RATIONALES

Adult Health

ACTIONS/INTERVENTIONS	RATIONALES
Determine current potential for desired activities, including: • Physical limitations related to illness or surgery • Factors that relate to desired activities • Realistic expectations for actualizing potential for desired activities • Objective criteria by which specific progress may be measured (e.g., distance, time, and observable signs or symptoms such as apical pulse, respiration) • Previous level of activities the patient enjoyed	Provides a baseline for planning activities and increase in activities.
Determine internal and external motivators for activities, and record here.	
Determine self-care activities the patient should assume. Increase activities as energy levels allow.	
Encourage rest as needed between activities. Assist the patient in planning a balanced rest–activity program.	Planned rest assists in maintaining and increasing activity tolerance.
Ensure the patient is getting adequate sleep. See nursing actions for Fatigue.	
Monitor and record blood pressure, pulse, and respiration before and after activities.	Vital signs increase with activity and should return to baseline within 5 to 7 minutes after activity. Maximal effort should be greater than or equal to 60 to 80 percent over the baseline.

ACTIONS/INTERVENTIONS	RATIONALES
Encourage progressive activity and increased self-care as tolerated. Schedule moderate increase in activities on a daily basis (e.g., will walk 10 feet farther each day).	Gradually increases tolerance for activities.
Assist the patient with self-care activities as needed. Let the patient determine how much assistance is needed.	Allows the patient to have some control and choice in plan; helps the patient to gradually decrease the amount of activity intolerance.
Collaborate with health-care providers regarding oxygen therapy.	Oxygen may be needed for shortness of breath associated with increased activity.
Collaborate with a physical therapist in establishing an appropriate exercise plan.	Provides most appropriate activities for the patient.
Provide for a quiet, nonstimulating environment. Limit number of visitors and length of their stay.	Determine various methods to motivate behavior.
Assure adequate dietary input, consider the patient's food preferences and consult with dietitian.	Provides adequate nutrition to meet metabolic demands.
Assist the patient in weight reduction as required.	Decreased weight requires less energy.
Teach the patient relationship between nutrition and exercise tolerance, and assist in developing a diet that is appropriate for nutritional and metabolic needs. (See Chapter 3 for further information.)	Assists the patient to learn alternate methods to conserve energy in ADLs.
Instruct the patient in energy-saving techniques of daily care (e.g., preparing meals sitting on a high stool rather than standing).	
Initiate physical therapy and/or occupational therapy early in admission.	Will deter muscle wasting and development of disuse syndrome.

Child Health

May include applicable, according to age/developmental status, the generic components of Adult Health care plan plus the following:

ACTIONS/INTERVENTIONS	RATIONALES
Monitor factors that are contributing to this problem.	Provides foundation for comprehensive approach to problem-solving.
Address relevant pre-existing issues to include issues for timing of activity, previous level of activity, current medical status and how the desired level of activity is to be attained.	A holistic approach offers the greatest likelihood for meeting the client's desired goal in the safest way possible.
*May include the pediatrician and occupational or physical therapist.	
Develop, with the child and parents, an activity plan. [Note that plan here.]	Emphasizes the role each will have for fostering the success of the plan.
Provide learning modules and practice sessions with materials suitable for the child's age and developmental capacity (e.g., dolls, videos, or pictures).	Developmentally appropriate materials enhance learning and maintain the child's attention.
Provide for continuity in care by assigning the same nurses for care during critical times for teaching and implementation.	Continuity of caregivers fosters trust in the nurse–patient relationship, which enhances learning.

(care plan continued on page 286)

NURSING ACTIONS/INTERVENTIONS WITH RATIONALES (continued from page 285)

Child Health

ACTIONS/INTERVENTIONS	RATIONALES
Modify expected behavior to incorporate appropriate developmental needs (e.g., allow for shared cards, messages, or visitors to lobby if possible for adolescent patients).	Valuing of the patient's developmental needs fosters self-esteem and serves as a reward for efforts.
Reinforce adherence to regimen with stickers or other appropriate measures to document progress.	Extrinsic rewards may help symbolize concrete progress and assist in reinforcing appropriate behaviors for achieving goals.

Women's Health

ACTIONS/INTERVENTIONS	RATIONALES
Premature Rupture of Membranes[23-25] ● N O T E : *Approach to treatment is controversial and depends on practice in your particular area.* Carefully monitor fetal heart rate to detect cord compression and/or cord prolapse. Carefully monitor for signs and symptoms of amnionitis. • Check maternal temperature every 4 h. • Evaluate for uterine tenderness at least twice a day. • Check daily leukocyte counts. • Avoid vaginal examinations. Keep the patient and partner informed, and encourage their participation in management decisions.	
Explain and provide answers to questions regarding: • Possible preterm delivery • Fetal lung maturity and possible use of corticosteroids to accelerate fetal lung maturity	Assists in reducing fears of expectant parents and increasing the likelihood of a good outcome for the pregnancy.
Provide comfort measures to decrease intolerance of bed rest: • Back or body massage • Diversional activities, such as television, reading, or handicrafts • Bedside commode (if acceptable to treatment plan)	
Preterm Labor[24-28] ● N O T E : *Although there is disagreement on the definition, the most widely used definition of preterm labor is six to eight contractions per hour or 4 contractions in 20 minutes associated with cervical change.*[25] Thoroughly explain to the patient and partner the process of preterm labor.	
Discuss options of activity allowed.	Provides the parents with information, increases motivation to continue with reduced activity, and allows informed choices

● N O T E : *This varies, and there is controversy in the literature on the value of bed rest for preterm labor; therefore, look at practice in your area.*

ACTIONS/INTERVENTIONS	RATIONALES
Discuss various treatment possibilities: • Prolonged bed rest or at least a marked reduction in activity • Intravenous volume expansion (IV therapy) • Tocolytic therapy (IV, oral, or pump) • Use of magnesium sulfate • Use of prostaglandin synthesis inhibitors such as indomethacin • Use of calcium channel blockers	
Carefully monitor those patients receiving tocolytic therapy for: • Pulmonary edema • Hypokalemia • Hyperglycemia • Shortness of breath • Chest pain • Cardiac dysrhythmia • Electrocardiographic "ischemia" changes • Hypotension	
Carefully monitor uterine contractions (strength, quality, frequency, and duration).	
Monitor fetal heart rate in association with contractions.	
Provide diversional activities for patients on bed rest.	
Refer for home monitoring and evaluation if appropriate: • Assess the patient's ability to identify contractions. • Evaluate the patient's support system at home. • Assess the patient's access to health-care provider.	Increases compliance, decreases cost, and decreases maternal stress when she can achieve treatment at home instead of in an acute care setting.

Pregnancy-Induced Hypertension (PIH)[29-32]

Explain the various screening procedures for PIH to the patient and partner:
- Blood pressure measurement
- Urine checked for protein
- Assessment of total and interval weight gain
- Signs and symptoms of sudden edema of hands and face, sudden 5-pound weight gain in 24 to 48 hours, epigastric pain, or spots before eyes or blurred vision

Discuss treatment plan with the patient and partner:
- Bed rest on either side (right or left)
- Magnesium sulfate therapy
- Reduction in noise, visual stimuli, and stress
- Careful monitoring of fetal heart rate
- Possible sonogram to determine intrauterine growth rate (IUGR)
- Good nutrition with a maximum recommended daily allowance (RDA) sodium intake of 110 to 3300 mg/day

Assess the patient's support system to determine whether the patient can be treated at home.[29-32]

Assist the family in planning for needed caretaking and housekeeping activities if the patient is at home.[29-32]

(care plan continued on page 288)

NURSING ACTIONS/INTERVENTIONS WITH RATIONALES (continued from page 287)

Women's Health

ACTIONS/INTERVENTIONS	RATIONALES
Consult with perinatalogist and visiting nurse to implement collaborative care plan.	
Ensure that the family knows procedure for obtaining emergency service.	

Uncomplicated Pregnancy

● **N O T E :** *Even though there are often no complications in pregnancy, it is not unusual, particularly during the last 4 to 6 weeks, to have activities restricted because of edema, bouts with false labor, and fatigue. This fatigue continues after the birth, when the mother and father become responsible for the care of a newborn infant 24 hours a day.*

Discuss with the expectant parents methods of conserving energy while continuing their daily activities during the last weeks of pregnancy.	
Assist the expectant mother in developing a plan whereby she can take frequent (two in the morning, two in the afternoon), short breaks during the work day to: • Retain energy and reduce fatigue. • Reduce the incident of false labor. • Increase circulation and thus reduce dependent lower limb edema and increase oxygen to the placenta and fetus.	Provides opportunity to rest throughout the day and therefore the ability to maintain as many routine activities as possible. Increases oxygen flow to the uterus and the fetus, thereby reducing the possibility of preterm labor and severe fatigue.
Assist the expectant parents to plan for the possibility of reducing the number of hours the woman works during the week. Look at the work schedule and talk with the employer about the possibilities of: • Working every other day • Working only half-day each day • Working 3 days in the middle of the week, i.e., Tuesday, Wednesday, and Thursday, thus, having a 4-day weekend to rest • Job sharing	

After Delivery

Instruct the patient in energy-saving activities of daily care: • Take care of self and baby only. • Let the partner and others take care of housework and other children. • Let the partner and others take care of the baby for a prearranged time during the day so the mother can spend quality time with the other children. • Learn to sleep when the baby sleeps. • Turn off the telephone or turn on the answering machine. • Have specific times set for visiting of friends or relatives. • If breastfeeding, partner can change the infant and bring the infant to the mother at night. (The mother does not always have to get up and go to the infant.)	A common problem with a new baby is overwhelming fatigue on the part of the mother. These measures will assist in decreasing the fatigue.

ACTIONS/INTERVENTIONS	RATIONALES
Consider taking the baby to bed with the parent.	Newest research shows that taking the baby to bed with the mother and father at night for the first few weeks[25,31]: • Allows the mother, father, and infant to get more rest. • Provides more time for the baby to nurse, and baby begins to sleep longer more quickly. • Possibly reduces the incidence of sudden infant death syndrome (SIDS) because the baby mimics the breathing patterns of the mother and father. • Promotes positive learning and acquaintance activities for the new parents. Allows the infant to feel more secure, and therefore increases infant-to-parent attachment.

Mental Health

ACTIONS/INTERVENTIONS	RATIONALES
Discuss with the client his or her perceptions of activity appropriate to his or her current capabilities.	Provides an understanding of the client's worldview so that care can be individualized and interventions developed that are acceptable to both the nurse and the client.[33]
If the client estimates a routine that far exceeds current capabilities (as with eating disorder clients or clients experiencing elated mood): • Establish appropriate limits on exercise. (The limits and consequences for not maintaining limits established should be listed here. If the excessive exercise pattern is related to an elated mood, set limits in a manner that allows the client some activity while not greatly exceeding metabolic needs until psychological status is improved.) • Begin the client slowly (e.g., with stretching exercise for 15 minutes twice a day). • Note client's goals here. • As physical condition improves, gradually increase exercise to 30 minutes of aerobic exercise once per day. • Discuss with the client appropriate levels of exercise considering his or her age and metabolic pattern. • Discuss with the client the hazards of overexercise. • Establish a reward system for clients who maintain the established exercise schedule (the schedule for the client should be listed here with the reinforcers that are to be used). • Stay with the client while he or she is engaged in appropriate exercise. • Develop a schedule for the client to be involved in an occupational therapy program to assist the client in identifying alternative forms of activity other than aerobic exercise.	Negative reinforcement eliminates or decreases behavior.[34] Because of the high energy level, elated clients need some large motor activity that will discharge energy but does not present a risk for physical harm.[35] Goals need to be achievable to promote the sense of accomplishment and positive self feelings, which will in turn increase motivation.[33] A regimen that provides positive cardiovascular fitness without risk of overexertion.[37] Overexertion can decrease benefits of exercise by increasing risk for injury.[36] Positive reinforcement encourages appropriate behavior.[34] Interaction with the nurse can provide positive reinforcement.[34] Promotes accurate perception of body size, nutrition, and exercise needs.

(care plan continued on page 290)

NURSING ACTIONS/INTERVENTIONS WITH RATIONALES (continued from page 289)

Mental Health

ACTIONS/INTERVENTIONS	RATIONALES
• Limit number of walks off the unit to accommodate client's weight, level of exercise on the unit, and physiology (the frequency and length of the walk should be listed here).	
For further information related to eating disorder clients, see Imbalanced Nutrition, Less Than Body Requirements (Chapter 3).	
If the client's expectations are much less than current capabilities (as with a depressed or poorly motivated client), implement the following actions:	Goals need to be achievable to promote sense of accomplishment and positive self feelings, which will in turn increase motivation.[33]
• Establish very limited goals that the client can accomplish (e.g., a 5-minute walk in a hallway once a day or walking in the client's room for 5 minutes). The goal established should be listed here.	
• Establish a reward system for achievement of goals (the reward program should be listed here with a list of items the client finds rewarding).	Positive reinforcement encourages appropriate behavior.[34]
• Develop a schedule for the client to be involved in an occupational therapy program (note schedule here).	Provides the client with opportunity to improve self-help skills while engaged in a variety of activities.
• Establish limits on the amount of time the client can spend in bed or in his or her room during waking hours (establish limits the client can achieve, and note limits here).	Exercise raises levels of endorphins in the brain, which has a positive effect on depression and general feeling of well-being.[35,37]
• Stay with the client during exercise periods and time out of the room until the client is performing these tasks without prompting.	Interaction with the nurse can provide positive reinforcement.[34]
• Provide the client with firm support for initiating the activity.	Attention from the nurse can provide positive reinforcement and increase the client's motivation to accomplish goal.
• Place a record of goal achievement where the client can see it, and mark each step toward the goal with a reward marker.	Provides concrete evidence of goal attainment and motivation to continue these activities that will promote well-being.
• Provide positive verbal reinforcement for goal achievement and progress.	
For further information about clients with depressed mood, refer to Ineffective Individual Coping (Chapter 11).	
Monitor effects current medications may have on activity tolerance, and teach the client necessary adjustments.	Psychotropic medications may cause postural hypotension, and the client should be instructed to change position slowly.
Schedule time to discuss plans and special concerns with the client and the client's support system. This could include teaching and answering questions. Schedule daily during initial days of hospitalization and one longer time just before discharge. Note schedule times and person responsible for this.	Recognizes the reciprocity between the client's illness and the family context.[38]

Gerontic Health

In addition to the interventions for Adult Health, the following may be utilized with aging clients.

ACTIONS/INTERVENTIONS	RATIONALES
Collaborate with the client to determine factors that contribute to activity intolerance (pain, shortness of breath). Address those factors specifically as appropriate.	Individualizes care.
Determine, with the assistance of the patient, particular time periods of highest energy, and plan care accordingly.	Maximizes potential to participate in or complete care requirements successfully.
Teach the patient to monitor pulse before, during, and after activity.	Promotes self-monitoring and provides means of determining progress across care settings.
Refer the patient to occupational therapy and physical therapy for determination of a progressive activity program.	Collaboration ensures a plan that will result in activity for maximum effect.
Establish goals that can be met in a short time frame (daily or weekly).	Provides motivation to continue program.[37]
Use positive feedback for incremental successes.	Reinforces the older adult's potential to have efforts produce positive outcomes. Enhances sense of self-efficacy.[40]
Monitor for signs of potential complications related to decreased activity level, such as problems with skin integrity, elimination complications, and respiratory problems.	Older adults are highly susceptible to the negative physiologic and psychological consequences of immobility.[40]

Home Health

● **NOTE**: *Interventions for Adult Health apply with the addition of the following interventions:*

ACTIONS/INTERVENTIONS	RATIONALES
Monitor the safety of the home environment for a client with activity intolerance. Educate client/caregiver of possible environmental modifications needed to include: • Wider doors • Lever style door handles instead of doorknobs • Bathroom rails • Removal of clutter • Functional arrangement of furniture • Flooring that facilitates use of mobility assistive devices • Phones that are readily accessible	Promotes safety.
Teach the client and family appropriate monitoring of causes, signs, and symptoms of risk for or actual activity intolerance: • Prolonged bed rest • Circulatory or respiratory problems • New activity • Fatigue • Dyspnea • Pain	Provides baseline for prevention and/or early intervention.

(care plan continued on page 292)

NURSING ACTIONS/INTERVENTIONS WITH RATIONALES (continued from page 291)	
Home Health	
ACTIONS/INTERVENTIONS	RATIONALES

ACTIONS/INTERVENTIONS	RATIONALES
• Vital signs (before and after activity) • Malnutrition • Previous inactivity • Weakness • Confusion	
Assist the client and family in identifying lifestyle changes that may be required: • Progressive exercise to increase endurance • Range of motion (ROM) and flexibility exercises • Treatments for underlying conditions (cardiac, respiratory, musculoskeletal, circulatory, etc.) • Motivation • Assistive devices as required (walkers, canes, crutches, wheelchairs, exercise equipment, etc.) • Adequate nutrition • Adequate fluids • Stress management • Pain relief • Prevention of hazards of immobility • Changes in occupations or family or social roles • Changes in living conditions • Economic concerns	Lifestyle changes require sufficient support to achieve.
Assist the client and family to set criteria to help them determine when calling a physician or other intervention is required.	Provides additional support for the client.
Monitor the client need for resources and refer appropriately. Consider possible needs such as: • Assistive devices • Mobility devices • Security devices	Provides additional support for the client.

AIRWAY CLEARANCE, INEFFECTIVE

DEFINITION[22]

Inability to clear secretions or obstructions from the respiratory tract to maintain a clear airway.

DEFINING CHARACTERISTICS[22]

1. Dyspnea
2. Diminished breath sounds
3. Orthopnea
4. Adventitious breath sounds (rales, crackles, rhonchi, and wheezes)
5. Cough, ineffective or absent
6. Sputum
7. Cyanosis
8. Difficulty vocalizing
9. Wide-eyed
10. Changes in respiratory rate and rhythm
11. Restlessness

RELATED FACTORS[22]

1. Environmental
   a. Smoking
   b. Smoke inhalation
   c. Second-hand smoke
2. Obstructed airway
   a. Airway spasm
   b. Retained secretions
   c. Excessive mucus
   d. Presence of artificial airway
   e. Foreign body in airway
   f. Secretions in the bronchi
   g. Exudate in the alveoli

3. Physiologic
   a. Neuromuscular dysfunction
   b. Hyperplasia of the bronchial walls
   c. Chronic obstructive pulmonary disease
   d. Infection
   e. Asthma
   f. Allergic airways

RELATED CLINICAL CONCERNS

1. Adult respiratory distress syndrome (ARDS)
2. Pneumonia
3. Cancer of the lung
4. Chronic obstructive pulmonary disease (COPD)
5. Congestive heart failure
6. Cystic fibrosis
7. Inhalation injuries
8. Neuromuscular diseases

 Have You Selected the Correct Diagnosis?

Ineffective Breathing Pattern
This diagnosis implies an alteration in the rate, rhythm, depth, or type of respiration, such as hyperventilation or hypoventilation. These patterns are not effective in supplying oxygen to the cells of the body or in removing the products of respiration. However, air is able to move freely through the air passages. In Ineffective Airway Clearance, the air passages are obstructed in some way.

Impaired Gas Exchange
This diagnosis means that air has been inhaled through the air passages but that oxygen and carbon dioxide are not appropriately exchanged at the alveolar–capillary level. Air has been able to pass through clear air passages, but a problem arises at the cellular level.

Deficient Fluid Volume
When fluid volume is insufficient to assist in liquefying thick, tenacious respiratory tract secretions, Deficient Fluid Volume then becomes the primary diagnosis. In this instance, the patient would be unable to expectorate the secretions effectively no matter how hard he or she tried, and Ineffective Airway Clearance would result.

Pain
If pain is sufficient to prevent the patient from coughing to clear the airway, then Ineffective Airway Clearance will result secondary to the pain.

EXPECTED OUTCOME

Will have an open, clear airway by [date].
   Respiratory rate and rhythm will be within normal limits by [date].
   Client will clear airway independently by [date].

TARGET DATES

Ineffective airway clearance is life-threatening; therefore, progress toward meeting the expected outcome should be evaluated at least on a daily basis.

ADDITIONAL INFORMATION

The various ways of measuring lung volume and capacity are summarized and defined in Table 5.2.

TABLE 5.2 Lung Capacities and Volumes

MEASUREMENT	AVERAGE VALUE, ADULT MALE RESTING (ML)	DEFINITION
Tidal volume (TV)	500	Amount of air inhaled or exhaled with each breath
Inspiratory reserve volume (IRV)	3100	Amount of air that can be forcefully inhaled after a normal tidal volume inhalation
Expiratory reserve volume (ERV)	1200	Amount of air that can be forcefully exhaled after a normal tidal volume exhalation
Residual volume (RV)	1200	Amount of air left in the lungs after a forced exhalation
Total lung capacity (TLC)	6000	Maximum amount of air that can be contained in the lungs after a maximum inspiration: TLC = TV + IRV + ERV + RV

(table continued on page 294)

TABLE 5.2 Lung Capacities and Volumes (continued from page 293)

MEASUREMENT	AVERAGE VALUE, ADULT MALE RESTING (ML)	DEFINITION
Vital capacity (VC)	4800	Maximum amount of air that can be expired after a maximum inspiration: VC = TV + IRV + ERV Should be 80% of TLC
Inspiratory capacity (IC)	3600	Maximum amount of air that can be inspired after a normal expiration: IC = TV + IRV
Functional residual capacity (FRC)	2400	Volume of air remaining in the lungs after a normal tidal volume expiration: FRC = ERV + RV

NURSING ACTIONS/INTERVENTIONS WITH RATIONALES

Adult Health

ACTIONS/INTERVENTIONS	RATIONALES
Maintain appropriate emergency equipment as dictated by the situation (e.g., suctioning apparatus).	Basic safety precautions.
Monitor respiratory rate, depth, and breath sounds at least every 4 hours.	Basic indicators of respiratory effort.
Collaborate with the health-care team in regard to obtaining arterial blood gasses.	Assists in determining changes in ventilatory status.
Initiate pulmonary toilet. Turn, cough, deep breathing every 2 hours.	
Turn every 2 hours. Perform chest physiotherapy every 2 hours while awake at [times]. Teach the family these procedures.	Facilitates postural drainage. Chest PT loosens secretions for expectoration. Teaching the family allows them to participate in care under supervision and promotes continuation of the procedure after discharge.
Maintain adequate hydration.	Inhibits formation of mucous plugs
Assure adequate pain control.	
Teach patient splinting techniques.	Increases efficacy of cough. Decreases pain that occurs with cough after surgery.
Suction as needed.	
Monitor oxygen saturation, arterial blood gases, respiratory rate, breath sounds.	Determines efficacy of plan of care and allows for adjustment of plan as necessary.
Administer medications (e.g., bronchodilator, mucolytics, and expectorants) as prescribed.	Promotes air circulation.
Assist the patient in coughing, huffing, and breathing efforts to make these more productive.	Deep breathing and diaphragmatic breathing allow for greater lung expansion and ventilation as well as a more effective cough.
Have the patient demonstrate proper coughing and breathing techniques twice a day.	

ACTIONS/INTERVENTIONS	RATIONALES
Assist the patient with clearing secretions from mouth or nose by: • Providing tissues • Using gentle suctioning if necessary	Removes tenacious secretions from airways.
Assist the patient with oral hygiene at least every 4 hours while awake at [times]: • Lubricate lips with a moisturizing agent. • Do not allow the use of oil-based products around the nose.	Oral hygiene clears away dried secretions and freshens the mouth. Oil-based products may obstruct breathing passages.
Discuss with the patient the importance of maintaining proper position to include: • Side-lying position while in bed	Facilitates expansion of the diaphragm; decreases probability of aspiration.
Promote rest and relaxation by scheduling treatments and activities with appropriate rest periods.	Avoids overexertion and worsening of condition.
Confer with appropriate consultations as needed (e.g., respiratory therapy or physical therapy). Provide for appropriate follow-up by scheduling appointments before dismissal.	Promotes cost-effective use of resources, and promotes follow-up care.

Child Health

ACTIONS/INTERVENTIONS	RATIONALES
Monitor patient factors that relate to ineffective airway clearance, including: • Feeding tolerance or intolerance • Allergens • Emotional aspects • Stressors of recent or past activities • Congenital anomalies • Parental anxieties • Infant or child temperament • Abdominal distention • Related vital signs, especially heart rate • Diaphragmatic excursion • Retraction in respiratory effort • Choking, coughing • Flaring of nares • Appropriate functioning of respiratory equipment	Provides an individualized data baseline that facilitates individualized care planning.
Provide appropriate attention to suctioning and related respiratory maintenance: • Appropriate size for catheter as needed • Appropriate administration of humidified oxygen as ordered by physician • Appropriate follow-up of blood gases • Documentation of oxygen administration, characteristics of secretions obtained by suctioning, and vital signs during suctioning, reporting apical pulse less than 70 or more than 149 beats per minute for an infant or less than 90 or more than 120 beats per minute for a young child.	Ensures basic maintenance of airway and respiratory function. Gives priority attention to the child's status and developmental level.

(care plan continued on page 296)

NURSING ACTIONS/INTERVENTIONS WITH RATIONALES (continued from page 295)

Child Health

ACTIONS/INTERVENTIONS	RATIONALES
Encourage the parent's input in planning care for the patient, with attention to individual preferences when possible.	Promotes family empowerment, and thus promotes the likelihood of more effective management of therapeutic regimen after discharge.
Provide health teaching as needed based on assessment and the child's situation.	Allows timely home care planning, family time to ask questions, practicing of techniques, etc. before discharge. Assists in reducing anxiety, and promotes continuance of the therapeutic regimen.
Plan for appropriate follow-up with health team members.	Provides for long-term support and effective management of the therapeutic regimen.
Reduce apprehension by providing comforting behavior and meeting developmental needs of the patient and family.	Sensitivity to individual feelings and needs builds trust in the nurse–patient–family relationship.
Allow for diversional activities to approximate tolerance of the child.	Realistic opportunities for diversion will be chosen based on what the patient is capable of doing and what will leave the patient feeling refreshed and renewed for having participated.
Encourage the family members to assist in care of the patient, with use of return-demonstration opportunities for teaching required skills.	Return-demonstration provides feedback to evaluate skills and serves to provide reinforcement in a supportive environment. Involvement of the parents also satisfies the emotional needs of both the parents and the child.
Provide for appropriate safety maintenance, especially with oxygen administration (no smoking), and appropriate precautions for age and developmental level.	Appropriate safety measures must be taken with the use of combustible potentials whose use outside of prescribed parameters may be toxic.
Allow ample time for parental mastery of skills identified in care of the child.	Greater success in compliance and confidence is afforded by providing ample time for skills that require mastery.

Women's Health

● N O T E : *The following nursing actions pertain to the newborn infant in the delivery room immediately following delivery. See Adult Health and Home Health for actions related to the mother.*

ACTIONS/INTERVENTIONS	RATIONALES
Evaluate and record the respiratory status of the newborn infant: • Suction and clear mouth and pharynx with bulb syringe. • Avoid deep suctioning if possible.	Basic measures to clear the newborn's airway. Deep suctioning would stimulate reflexes that could result in aspiration.
Continue to evaluate the infant's respiratory status, and act if necessary to resuscitate. Depending on the infant's response, the following nursing measures can be taken: • Administer warm, humid oxygen with a face mask. • If no improvement, administer oxygen with bag and mask.	Basic protocol for the infant who has difficulty immediately after birth.

ACTIONS/INTERVENTIONS	RATIONALES

• If no improvement, be prepared for:
  • Endotracheal intubation
  • Ventilation with positive pressure
  • Cardiac massage
  • Transport to neonatal intensive care unit	

Mental Health

Care plan for Adult Health can be utilized as a foundation with the following considerations for psychiatric clients:

ACTIONS/INTERVENTIONS	RATIONALES
Collaborate with the physician for possible use of saline gargles or anesthetic lozenges for sore throats (report all sore throats to the physician, especially if the client is receiving antipsychotic drugs and in the absence of other flu or cold symptoms).	These commonly used medications can cause blood dyscrasias that present with the symptoms of sore throat, fever, malaise, unusual bleeding, and easy bruising. Early intervention is important for patient safety.[41]
Remind the client to chew food well, and sit with the client during mealtime if cognitive functioning indicates a need for close observation. [Note any special adaptations here (e.g., soft foods, observation during meals, etc.)]	Provides safety for the client with alterations of mental status.

Gerontic Health

● N O T E : *Aging adults tend to decrease their fluid intake, which can contribute to the development of ineffective airway clearance. Consider this issue as a part of initial and ongoing assessment.*

ACTIONS/INTERVENTIONS	RATIONALES
Teach and facilitate pulmonary hygiene measures with the client and caregivers: • Coughing and deep-breathing exercises every 2 hours on [odd/even] hour • Ensuring adequate hydration (monitor intake and output) • Clearing the bronchial tree by controlled coughing • Decreasing viscosity of secretions via humidity and fluid balance • Postural drainage • Learning stress management • Ensuring adequate nutritional intake • Learning diaphragmatic breathing • Administering pain relief • Beginning progressive ambulation (avoiding fatigue) • Maintaining position so that danger of aspiration is decreased • Maintaining body position to minimize work of breathing and cleaning airway • Ensuring adequate oral hygiene • Clearing secretions from throat • Suctioning as needed	Basic pulmonary hygiene prevents further airway problems.

(care plan continued on page 298)

NURSING ACTIONS/INTERVENTIONS WITH RATIONALES (continued from page 297)

Gerontic Health

ACTIONS/INTERVENTIONS	RATIONALES
• Keeping area free of dust and potential allergens or irritants	
Provide small, frequent feedings during periods of dyspnea.	Conserves energy and promotes ventilation efforts.
Instruct the patient regarding early signs of respiratory infections (e.g., increased amount or thickness of secretions, increased cough, or changes in color of sputum produced).	Early recognition of signs of infection promotes early intervention and avoidance of severe infection.
Facilitate increased mobility, as tolerated, on a daily basis. [Note plan for this client here.]	Mobility helps increase rate and depth of respiration as well as decreasing pooling of secretions.
Teach the patient to complete prescribed course of antibiotic therapy.	Because of economic factors, patients commonly stop therapy before the designated time frame, "saving" the medication for possible future episodes.
Monitor for the use of sedative medications that can decrease the level of alertness and respiratory effort.	These medications can decrease the level of alertness and respiratory effort.
Collaborate with the physician regarding the use of cough suppressants and mucolytics.	Decreases episodes of persistent, nonproductive coughing.

Home Health/Community Health

ACTIONS/INTERVENTIONS	RATIONALES
Teach the client and family appropriate monitoring of signs and symptoms of ineffective airway clearance: • Cough (effective or ineffective) • Sputum • Respiratory status (cyanosis, dyspnea, and rate) • Abnormal breath sounds (noisy respirations) • Nasal flaring • Intercostal, substernal retraction • Choking, gagging • Diaphoresis • Restlessness, anxiety • Impaired speech • Collection of mucus in mouth	Provides for early recognition and intervention for problem.
Assist the client and family in identifying lifestyle changes that may be required: • Eliminating smoking • Treating fear or anxiety • Treating pain • Performing pulmonary hygiene: 　• Clearing the bronchial tree by controlled coughing 　• Decreasing viscosity of secretions via humidity and fluid balance 　• Postural drainage • Learning stress management	Provides basic information for the client and family that promotes necessary lifestyle changes.

ACTIONS/INTERVENTIONS	RATIONALES
• Ensuring adequate nutritional intake • Learning diaphragmatic breathing • Administering pain relief • Beginning progressive ambulation (avoiding fatigue) • Maintaining position so that danger of aspiration is decreased • Maintaining body position to minimize work of breathing and cleaning airway • Ensuring adequate oral hygiene • Clearing secretions from throat • Suctioning as needed • Keeping area free of dust and potential allergens or irritants • Ensuring adequate hydration (monitor intake and output)	
Teach the client and family purposes, side effects, and proper administration techniques of medications.	
Assist the client and family to set criteria to help them determine when calling a physician or other intervention is required.	Locus of control shifts from nurse to the client and family, thus promoting self-care.
Teach the family basic cardiopulmonary resuscitation (CPR).	
Consult with or refer to appropriate assistive resources as indicated.	Provides additional support for the client and family, and uses already available resources in a cost-effective manner.

AUTONOMIC DYSREFLEXIA, RISK FOR AND ACTUAL

DEFINITIONS[22]

Risk for Autonomic Dysreflexia Risk for life-threatening uninhibited response of the sympathetic nervous system, postspinal shock, in an individual with a spinal cord injury/lesion at T6* or above.

    Autonomic Dysreflexia Life-threatening uninhibited sympathetic response of the nervous system to a noxious stimulus after a spinal cord injury at T7 or above.

DEFINING CHARACTERISTICS[22]

A. Risk for Autonomic Dysreflexia
    An injury or lesion at T6 or above and at least one of the following noxious stimuli:
    1. Neurologic stimuli
       a. Painful or irritating stimuli below level of injury
    2. Urologic stimuli
       a. Bladder distention
       b. Detrusor sphincter dyssynergia

       c. Bladder spasm
       d. Instrumentation or surgery
       e. Epididymitis
       f. Urethritis
       g. Urinary tract infection
       h. Calculi
       i. Cystitis
       j. Catheterization
    3. Gastrointestinal stimuli
       a. Bowel distention
       b. Fecal impaction
       c. Digital stimulation
       d. Suppositories
       e. Hemorrhoids
       f. Difficult passage of feces
       g. Constipation
       h. Enema
       i. Gastrointestinal system pathology
       j. Gastric ulcers
       k. Esophageal reflux
       l. Gallstones
    4. Reproductive stimuli
       a. Menstruation
       b. Sexual intercourse

*Has been demonstrated in patients with injuries at T7 and T8.

c. Pregnancy

d. Labor and delivery

e. Ovarian cyst

f. Ejaculation

5. Musculoskeletal–integumentary stimuli

   a. Cutaneous stimulation (e.g., pressure ulcer, ingrown toenail, dressings, burns, rash)

   b. Pressure over bony prominences or genitalia

   c. Heterotrophic bone

   d. Spasm

   e. Fractures

   f. Range-of-motion (ROM) exercises

   g. Wounds

   h. Sunburn

6. Regulatory stimuli

   a. Temperature fluctuations

   b. Extreme environmental temperatures

7. Situational stimuli

   a. Positioning

   b. Drug reactions (e.g., decongestants, sympathomimetics, vasoconstrictors, narcotic withdrawal)

   c. Constrictive clothing (e.g., straps, stockings, shoes)

   d. Surgical procedure

8. Cardiac and/or pulmonary problems

   a. Pulmonary emboli

   b. Deep vein thrombus

B. Autonomic Dysreflexia

1. Pallor (below the injury)

2. Paroxysmal hypertension (sudden periodic elevated blood pressure where systolic pressure is more than 140 mm Hg and diastolic is more than 90 mm Hg)

3. Red splotches on skin (above the injury)

4. Bradycardia or tachycardia (pulse rate of less than 60 or more than 100 beats per minute)

5. Diaphoresis (above the injury)

6. Headache (a diffuse pain in different portions of the head and not confined to any nerve distribution area)

7. Blurred vision

8. Chest pain

9. Chilling

10. Conjunctival congestion

11. Horner's syndrome (contraction of the pupil, partial ptosis of the eyelid, enophthalmos, and sometimes loss of sweating over the affected side of the face)

12. Metallic taste in mouth

13. Nasal congestion

14. Paresthesia

15. Pilomotor reflex (gooseflesh formation when skin is cooled)

RELATED FACTORS[22]

A. Risk for Autonomic Dysreflexia

The risk factors also serve as the related factors.

B. Autonomic Dysreflexia

1. Bladder distention

2. Bowel distention

3. Lack of patient and caregiver knowledge

4. Skin irritation

RELATED CLINICAL CONCERNS

1. Spinal cord injury at T7 or above

 Have You Selected the Correct Diagnosis?

Decreased Cardiac Output
Dysreflexia occurs only in spinal cord–injured patients and represents an emergency situation that requires immediate intervention. Decreased Cardiac Output may be suspected because of the changes in blood pressure or arrhythmias[42,43]; but, if the patient has a spinal cord injury at T7 or above, Autonomic Dysreflexia should be considered first.

Impaired Skin Integrity
Occasionally symptoms of Autonomic Dysreflexia are precipitated by skin lesions such as pressure sores and ingrown or infected nails.[44] If the patient has a spinal cord injury at T7 or above in combination with Impaired Skin Integrity, the nurse must be extremely alert to the possible development of Autonomic Dysreflexia. In addition, one of the defining characteristics of Autonomic Dysreflexia is red splotches, which could lead to a misdiagnosis of Risk for Impaired Skin Integrity.

Urinary Retention
Dysreflexia should be suspected in patients with spinal cord injuries at T7 or above who experience bladder spasms, bladder distention, or untoward responses to urinary catheter insertion or irrigation.[44,45] Bowel distention or rectal stimulation may also lead to Dysreflexia.

EXPECTED OUTCOME

Will actively cooperate in care plan to prevent development of dysreflexia by [date].

Will verbalize understanding of the triggers of Dysreflexia by [date].

Vital signs are within normal limits by [date].

Will have noncompromised bowel and/or bladder function by [date].

TARGET DATES

Autonomic Dysreflexia is a life-threatening response. For this reason, the target date should be expressed in hours on a daily basis.

NURSING ACTIONS/INTERVENTIONS WITH RATIONALES

Adult Health

ACTIONS/INTERVENTIONS	RATIONALES
Locate source that may have triggered dysreflexia (e.g., bladder distention [76 to 90 percent of all instances], bowel distention [8 percent of all instances]),[46–48] fractures, acute abdomen, pressure ulcers, skin irritants, or other stimulation below the level of the spinal cord injury.	Finding precipitating causes prevents worsening of condition and allows further prevention of dysreflexia.
Remove the offending source. Empty bladder slowly with a straight catheter (**do not** use Credé's maneuver or tap bladder[46,47]), or manually remove impacted feces from the rectum as soon as possible. Exercise caution if symptoms worsen with digital disimpaction.	Alleviates precipitating causes.
Ensure indwelling catheter maintains patency at least every 4 hours. [Note times here.]	
Notify the health-care team regarding the administration of emergency antihypertensive therapy.	Facilitates lowering of blood pressure
Keep the patient warm; avoid chilling at all times.	Decreases sensory nervous stimulation.
Monitor intake and output every hour for 48 hours, then every 2 hours for 48 hours; then every 4 hours. [Note time schedule and dates here.]	Monitors adequate functioning of bowel and bladder, which are common causative factors for dysreflexia.
Turn the patient every 2 hours on [odd/even] hour; keep in anatomic alignment.	Alleviates potential precipitating causes.
Perform ROM (active or passive) every 4 hours while awake at [times]. Pad bony prominences.	Alleviates precipitating causes; stimulates circulation and muscular activity; decreases incidence of pressure ulcers.
Instruct the patient on isotonic exercises. Encourage the patient to perform isotonic exercises at least every 2 hours on [odd/even] hour.	Increases circulation and prevents complications of immobility.
Instruct on bladder and bowel conditioning. Monitor for bladder and bowel distention every 4 hours at [times].	Eliminates the two primary precipitating causes.
Catheterize as necessary; use rectal tube if not contraindicated to assist with flatus reduction.	Addresses potential precipitating causes.
Provide appropriate skin care each time the patient is turned. Monitor skin integrity at least once per shift at [times].	Prevents and monitors for pressure ulcers.
Ensure and educate patient regarding devising a diet that meets recommended daily requirements for nutrients, fiber, and fluids.	Assists in avoiding constipation.
Involve the family in care such as positioning, feeding, and exercising.	Assists in teaching and preparing of the family for home care.
Align the family with community resources. Make referrals as soon as possible after admission.	Provides long-range support for the patient and family.

(care plan continued on page 302)

NURSING ACTIONS/INTERVENTIONS WITH RATIONALES (continued from page 301)

Child Health

● N O T E : *Recognizing the pattern is critical as encephalopathy and shock will often ensue.*

ACTIONS/INTERVENTIONS	RATIONALES
Monitor for contributing factors, esp. bladder distention and provide intervention as needed. *Drain the bladder slowly to avoid sudden change in pressure.	Offers anticipatory guidance for plan with definitive action for most likely cause.
Administer medications as required to help control the blood pressure at appropriate levels for age and weight *Antihypertensives are administered IV initially and then PO when stabilization is reached for maintenance. Antispasmodics may also be administered.	Assists in preventing seizures, and provides appropriate intervention to maintain pressure within desired ranges.[49]
Monitor the pulse as needed and blood pressure every 5 minutes until stable. Determine parameters for the patient according to the norms for age, site, and condition.	Basic monitoring for initial indications of problem development.
Monitor the family's understanding and perception of dysreflexia. Ensure that proper attention is paid to the family's needs for support during this emergency phase.	Assists in preventing misunderstandings and in identifying learning needs.
Teach the patient, to the extent he or she is capable, and the family routine for care, including the prevention of infection (particularly urinary and integumentary).	Education enhances care and provides an opportunity for care to be practiced in a supportive environment.
Monitor for latex allergy risk because of multiple urinary catheterizations.	Frequent catheterization with latex supplies increases the risk for allergy.[49]

Women's Health

● N O T E : *The same nursing diagnosis pertains to Women's Health as to Adult Health. The following precautions should be taken when the victim is pregnant.*

ACTIONS/INTERVENTIONS	RATIONALES
Position the patient to prevent supine hypotension by: • Placing the patient on her left side if possible. • Using a pillow or folded towel under the right hip to tip to left. • If neck injury is suspected, placing the patient on a back board and then tipping the board to the left.	Keeps the weight of the uterus off the inferior vena cava.
Start an intravenous line for replacement of lost fluid volume.	The pregnant woman has 50 percent more blood volume and her vital signs may not change until there is a 30 percent reduction in circulating blood volume.
Monitor fetal status continuously. Monitor for uterine contractions at least once per hour.	Basic data needed to ensure positive outcome.

Mental Health

The expected outcomes and nursing actions for the mental health client are the same as those for the adult patient.

Gerontic Health

The nursing actions for the gerontic patient are the same as those for Adult Health.

Home Health

● **N O T E :** *The interventions listed for autonomic dysreflexia are preventive in nature. Should this condition develop in the home setting, emergency health care should be sought immediately.*

ACTIONS/INTERVENTIONS	RATIONALES
Teach the client, family, and potential caregivers measures to prevent Autonomic Dysreflexia[47–49]: • Bowel and bladder routines • Prevention of skin breakdown (e.g., turning, transfer, or prevention of incontinence) • Use and care of indwelling urinary catheter • Prevention of infection	Basic care techniques that can assist in preventing the occurrence of dysreflexia. Promotes sense of control and autonomy.
Assist the client and family in identifying signs and symptoms of Autonomic Dysreflexia[47]: • Teach the family how to monitor vital signs and how to recognize tachycardia, bradycardia, and paroxysmal hypertension.	Provides for early recognition and intervention for problem.
• Assist the client and family in identifying emergency referrals: • Physician • Emergency room • Emergency medical system	Occurrence of this diagnosis is an emergency. This information provides the family with a sense of security by providing routes to and numbers of readily available emergency assistance.
• Educate the client, family members, and potential caregivers about immediate elimination of the precipitating stimuli.	Other treatments will not be effective until the stimulus is removed.
• When an episode occurs, instruct the family and caregivers to place the head of the patient's bed to an upright position.	Decreases blood pressure and promotes cerebral venous return.
• Assist the client in obtaining necessary equipment to drain the bladder or remove impactions at home.	Allows for immediate removal of precipitating stimulus.
• Educate clients at risk for dysreflexia to be alert for signs and symptoms of Autonomic Dysreflexia during sexual encounters. Preparation for sexual intercourse should include a bowel and bladder check and disconnecting urinary drainage systems.	

(care plan continued on page 304)

NURSING ACTIONS/INTERVENTIONS WITH RATIONALES (continued from page 303)	

Home Health

ACTIONS/INTERVENTIONS	RATIONALES
Teach the patient and family appropriate uses and side effects of medications as well as proper administration of the medications.	Locus of control shifts from nurse to the client and family, thus promoting self-care.
Obtain available wallet-sized card that briefly outlines effective treatments in an emergency situation.[50] Have the client carry this card with him or her at all times. Family members must be familiar with content and location of card.	

● **N O T E :** *Labeled a Treatment Card, this card contains information related to pathophysiology, common signs and symptoms, stimuli that trigger Autonomic Dysreflexia, problems, and recommended treatment.*

BED MOBILITY, IMPAIRED

DEFINITION[22]

Limitation of independent movement from one bed position to another.

DEFINING CHARACTERISTICS[22]

1. Impaired ability to turn side to side
2. Impaired ability to move from supine to sitting or sitting to supine
3. Impaired ability to "scoot" or reposition self in bed
4. Impaired ability to move from supine to prone or prone to supine
5. Impaired ability to move from supine to long sitting or long sitting to supine

RELATED FACTORS[22]

To be developed.

RELATED CLINICAL CONCERNS

1. Any condition causing paralysis
2. Arthritic conditions
3. Major chest or abdominal surgeries
4. Malnutrition
5. Cachexia
6. Trauma
7. Depression

☑ Have You Selected the Correct Diagnosis?

Impaired Physical Mobility
Impaired Bed Mobility is a more specific diagnosis than Impaired Physical Mobility. Certainly, an individual would have both diagnoses if he or she could not change his or her position in bed. Impaired Bed Mobility would be the priority diagnosis.

Activity Intolerance
This diagnosis refers to problems that develop when a person is engaged in activities. The person with this diagnosis would be able to move freely while in bed.

Impaired Walking
This diagnosis is specific to the act of walking. This diagnosis, like Impaired Bed Mobility, could be considered a subset of Impaired Physical Mobility.

EXPECTED OUTCOME

Will freely move self in bed by [date].

TARGET DATES

Improvement in mobility will require long-term intervention; therefore, a feasible date for evaluating progress toward the outcome would be 2 weeks.

NURSING ACTIONS/INTERVENTIONS WITH RATIONALES

Adult Health

ACTIONS/INTERVENTIONS	RATIONALES
Identify and provide assistive devices (e.g., trapeze). Initiate supportive therapies: • Maintain adequate nutrient intake • Confer with physical therapy and/or occupational therapy to devise plan for muscle strengthening	Will facilitate mobility in bed.

Child Health

ACTIONS/INTERVENTIONS	RATIONALES
Monitor for contributing factors within the client's developmental capacity.	A complete ongoing assessment provides the primary database for individualization of care.
Identify priorities of basic physiologic functions to be stabilized and considered as related to movement: • Respiratory • Cardiovascular • Neurologic • Orthopedic • Urologic • Integumentary	Stabilization of basic physiologic status must be considered for tolerance and safety.
Determine need for assistive devices.	Realistic support may depend on orthotics, braces, splints, or other mechanical devices for safety.
Determine teaching needs regarding mobility for the client, family, or staff assisting with mobility activities.	Appropriate planning will offer greater likelihood of safe and consistent efforts.
Coordinate efforts for other health team members.	The nurse is best suited to provide consistent and safe planning of care with all health team members.
Determine the need for restraints of the client, and seek appropriate orders if indicated.	Appropriate attention to safety is paramount.
Provide ongoing assessment with documentation of the client's tolerance of mobility activities as often as the patient's status dictates.	Ongoing timely assessment ensures safety and prevents injury.
Provide developmentally appropriate diversional activities.	Engagement in preferred activities enhances the likelihood of cooperation by the client.
Safeguard areas of vulnerability while movement occurs, such as burns, traumatized limb, or surgical site.	Caution to entire body will best help prevent further injury.
Honor the child's ability to safely carry out activities as appropriate.	Supports autonomy.[49]

Women's Health

The nursing actions for Women's Health are the same as those for Adult Health.

(care plan continued on page 306)

NURSING ACTIONS/INTERVENTIONS WITH RATIONALES (continued from page 305)

Mental Health

Refer to Adult Health for interventions and rationales related to this diagnosis.

Gerontic Health

ACTIONS/INTERVENTIONS	RATIONALES
Consult with occupational therapist and physical therapist for adaptive equipment to support the client while in bed (such as trapeze, transfer enabler, and foam support blocks).	Facilitates mobility efforts the client may be able to support.[51]
Ensure that adaptive equipment is maintained in proper functioning order.	Ensures that safety needs are met.
Implement pressure-reducing devices, such as therapeutic mattresses or mattresses with removable sections, to prevent problems with skin integrity.	Older adults are at high risk for pressure ulcers because of skin fragility, changes in sensation, and altered nutrition.[52]
Schedule turning and position changes according to the client's tolerance to pressure. (Determined for each individual based on general condition and risk for pressure ulcer development.)	Depending on the individual client's health status, turning at the usually prescribed interval of q 2 h may not be sufficient to reduce risk for pressure ulcers.[52]
Initiate ROM interventions (active or passive) on a daily basis.	Maintains joint mobility and prevents contractures.[53]

Home Health

ACTIONS/INTERVENTIONS	RATIONALES
Assist the client in obtaining necessary durable medical equipment to facilitate independent movement and assisted movement (e.g., over-bed trapeze, hospital bed with siderails, and sliding board).	
Educate the client, family, and caregivers in the correct use of equipment to facilitate independent movement and assisted movement (e.g., over-bed trapeze, hospital bed with siderails, and sliding board).	
Instruct the caregivers in the proper use of draw sheets to reposition the client rather than dragging the client or using poor body mechanics to assist in repositioning.	Minimizes risk of injury to both the client and caregiver.
Assist the client in obtaining necessary supplies to prevent thrombus formation due to immobility, such as thromboembolic stockings or pneumatic devices.	Prevents deep vein thrombosis.
Encourage ROM exercises to promote strength.	Improves circulation and motor tone.
Teach the client regarding proper body mechanics.	Prevents further injury.
As the client begins to progress in his or her efforts toward independent mobility, the nurse provides minimal assistance from the weak side, supporting the unaffected side.	Promotes independence while protecting from further injury.

BREATHING PATTERN, INEFFECTIVE

DEFINITION[22]

Inspiration and/or expiration that does not provide adequate ventilation.[21]

DEFINING CHARACTERISTICS[22]

1. Decreased inspiratory and/or expiratory pressure
2. Decreased minute ventilation
3. Use of accessory muscles to breathe
4. Nasal flaring
5. Dyspnea
6. Altered chest excursion
7. Shortness of breath
8. Assumption of three-point position
9. Pursed-lip breathing
10. Prolonged expiration phase
11. Increased anterior–posterior chest diameter
12. Respiratory rate (infants, <25 or >60; ages 1 to 4, <20 or >30; ages 5 to 14, <15 or >25; adults [age 14 or older], <11 or >24)
13. Depth of breathing (infants, 6 to 8 mL/kg; adults, tidal volume [VT] 500 mL at rest)
14. Timing ratio
15. Orthopnea
16. Decreased vital capacity

RELATED FACTORS[22]

1. Hyperventilation
2. Hypoventilation syndrome
3. Bone deformity
4. Pain
5. Chest wall deformity
6. Anxiety
7. Decreased energy or fatigue
8. Neuromuscular dysfunction
9. Musculoskeletal impairment
10. Perception or cognition impairment
11. Obesity
12. Spinal cord injury
13. Body position
14. Neurologic immaturity
15. Respiratory muscle fatigue

RELATED CLINICAL CONCERNS

1. Chronic obstructive or restrictive pulmonary disease
2. Pneumonia
3. Asthma
4. Acute alcoholism (intoxication or overdose)
5. Congestive heart failure
6. Chest trauma
7. Myasthenia gravis

 Have You Selected the Correct Diagnosis?

Ineffective Airway Clearance
Ineffective Airway Clearance means that something is blocking the air passage, but when air gets to the alveoli, there is adequate gas exchange. In Ineffective Breathing Pattern, the ventilatory effort is insufficient to bring in enough oxygen or to get rid of sufficient amounts of carbon dioxide. However, air is able to freely move through the air passages.

Impaired Gas Exchange
This diagnosis indicates that enough oxygen is brought into the respiratory system, and the carbon dioxide that is produced is exhaled, but there is insufficient exchange of oxygen and carbon dioxide at the alveolar–capillary level. There is no problem with either the ventilatory effort or the air passageways. The problem exists at the cellular level.

EXPECTED OUTCOME

Will demonstrate an effective breathing pattern by [date] as evidenced by (specify criteria here, for example, normal breath sounds, arterial blood gases within normal limits, no evidence of cyanosis).

TARGET DATES

Evaluation should be made on an hourly basis, because this diagnosis has the potential to be life-threatening. After the patient has stabilized, target dates can be spaced further apart.

NURSING ACTIONS/INTERVENTIONS WITH RATIONALES

Adult Health

ACTIONS/INTERVENTIONS	RATIONALES
Perform nursing actions to maintain airway clearance. (See Ineffective Airway Clearance; enter those orders here.)	Maintains a patent airway for gas exchange.

(care plan continued on page 308)

NURSING ACTIONS/INTERVENTIONS WITH RATIONALES (continued from page 307)

Adult Health

ACTIONS/INTERVENTIONS	RATIONALES
Maintain appropriate attention to relief of pain and anxiety via positioning and administration of medications as prescribed.	
Raise head of bed 30 degrees or more if not contraindicated.	Allows gravity to assist in lowering the diaphragm, and provides greater chest expansion.
Instruct in diaphragmatic deep breathing and pursed-lip breathing.	Promotes lung expansion and slightly increases pressure in the airways, allowing them to remain open longer.
Reduce pain, fear, and anxiety.	These can cause altered breathing patterns (e.g., hyperventilation).
Exercise caution with use of drugs that cause respiratory depression.	
Position patient in semi-Fowler's position.	Promotes lung expansion.
Encourage the patient's mobility as tolerated (see Impaired Physical Mobility).	Promotes tolerance for activities and helps with lung expansion and ventilation.
Instruct the patient in effects of smoking, air pollution, etc., prior to discharge, on breathing pattern.	Knowledge will assist the patient to avoid harmful environments and to protect him- or herself from the effects from such activities.
Provide teaching based on needs of the patient and family regarding: • Illness • Procedures and related nursing care • Implications for rest and relief of anxiety secondary to respiratory failure • Advocacy role	Reduces anxiety; starts appropriate home care planning; assists the family in dealing with health-care system.

Child Health

The adult health-care plan can be implemented as developmentally appropriate with the following considerations:

ACTIONS/INTERVENTIONS	RATIONALES
Determine possible contributing factors.	Facilitates comprehensive care planning.
Maintain appropriate emergency equipment in an accessible place. (Specify actual size of endotracheal tube for the infant, child, or adolescent, tracheotomy set size, and suctioning catheters or chest tube for size of the patient.)	Standard accountability for emergency equipment and treatment is basic to patient care and especially so when risk factors are increased.
Allow at least 5 to 15 minutes per shift for the parents and child to verbalize concerns related to illness.	Appropriate time for venting may be hard to determine, but efforts to do so demonstrate valuing of patient and family needs and serve to reduce anxiety.
Determine perception of illness by the patient and parents.	How the parents and child see (perceive) the patient's problem provides meaningful data that serve to ensure sensitivity in care and provides information regarding teaching needs. Provides cues to questions regarding continued implementation of therapeutic regimen.

ACTIONS/INTERVENTIONS	RATIONALES
Include the parents in the care of the child as appropriate, to include comfort measures, assisting with feeding, and the like.	Parental involvement is critical in maintaining emotional bonds with the child. Also augments sense of contributing to the child's care, with opportunities for mastering the skills in a supportive environment.
Collaborate with appropriate health team members as needed.	Appropriate coordination of services will best meet the patient's needs with attention to the patient's individuality.

Women's Health

ACTIONS/INTERVENTIONS	RATIONALES
Assist the patient and significant other in identifying lifestyle changes that may be required to prevent Ineffective Breathing Pattern during pregnancy (e.g., stopping smoking or avoiding crowds during influenza epidemics).	Increased cardiovascular fitness supports increased respiratory effectiveness.
Develop exercise plan for cardiovascular fitness during pregnancy.	
Teach the patient to avoid wearing constrictive clothing during pregnancy.	Any constriction contributes to further breathing difficulties, and breathing becomes more difficult as the expanding uterus and abdominal contents press against the diaphragm.[54]
Teach and encourage the patient to practice correct breathing techniques for labor.	Assists in preventing hyperventilation.
During the latter stages of pregnancy, encourage the patient to: • Walk up stairs slowly. • Lie on left or right side, to get more oxygen to the fetus. • Position herself in bed with pillows for optimum comfort and adequate air exchange. • Take frequent rest breaks during the workday.	During this stage, the chest cavity has less room to expand because of the enlarging uterus.[55] Often edema of the latter stage of pregnancy causes "stuffy" noses and full sinuses.
Carefully monitor maternal respiration during the laboring process.	Analgesics and anesthesia can cause maternal hypoxia and reduce fetal oxygen.
If prolonged decrease in fetal heart tone (FHT) immediately prior to delivery, administer pure oxygen (10 to 12 L/min) to the mother before delivery and until cessation of pulsation in cord.	
Evaluate and record the respiratory status of the newborn infant: • Determine the 1-minute Apgar score. • Suction and clear mouth and pharynx with bulb syringe. • Avoid deep suctioning if possible.	Basic care measures to ensure effective respiration in the newborn infant.
Dry excess moisture off the infant with towel or blanket.	Helps stimulate the infant; prevents evaporative heat loss.
Stimulate (if necessary), using firm but gentle tactile stimulation: • Rubbing up and down spine • Flicking heel	

(care plan continued on page 310)

NURSING ACTIONS/INTERVENTIONS WITH RATIONALES (continued from page 309)

Women's Health

ACTIONS/INTERVENTIONS	RATIONALES

Place the infant in warm environment:
• Place the infant under radiant heat warmer.
• Place the infant next to the mother's skin
• Cover the infant's head with a stocking cap.
• Cover both the mother and infant with a warm blanket.
Determine and record the 5-minute Apgar score.
 	
Continue to evaluate the infant's respiratory status and be prepared to act if necessary to resuscitate. Depending on the infant's response, the following nursing measures can be taken:
• Administer warm, humid oxygen with face mask.
• If no improvement, administer oxygen with bag and mask.
• If no improvement, be prepared for:
  • Endotracheal intubation
  • Ventilation with positive pressure
  • Cardiac massage
  • Transport to neonatal intensive care unit
	Basic protocol to care for the newborn who has respiratory problems.

Mental Health

● N O T E : *The following orders are for Ineffective Breathing Pattern Related to Anxiety. When the diagnosis is related to physiologic problems, refer to Adult Health nursing actions.*

ACTIONS/INTERVENTIONS	RATIONALES
Monitor causative factors.	Provides information on the client's current status so interventions can be adapted appropriately.
Place the client in a calm, supportive environment.	Anxiety is contagious, as is calm. A calm, reassuring environment can communicate indirectly to the client that the situation is safe and that the nurse can assist him or her in mobilizing their internal resources, thus facilitating the client's sense of control.
Maintain a calm, supportive attitude, reassuring the client that you will assist him or her in maintaining control.	
Give the client clear, concise directions.	Anxiety can decrease the client's ability to focus on and understand a complex presentation of information.
Have the client maintain direct eye contact with nurse. Modulate based on the client's ability to tolerate eye contact. Should not be done in a manner that appears to "stare the client down."	Communicates interest in the client, and assists the client in tuning out extraneous stimuli.
Instruct the client to take slow, deep breaths. Demonstrate breaths to the client, and practice with the client. Provide the client with constant, positive reinforcement for appropriate breathing patterns.	Helps stimulate relaxation response.
Remain with the client until the episode is resolved.	Reassures the client of safety and security.
If the client does not respond to the attempts to control breathing, have the client breathe into a paper bag.	Rebreathing air with higher carbon dioxide (CO_2) content slows the respiratory rate.

ACTIONS/INTERVENTIONS	RATIONALES
Distract the client from focus on breathing by beginning a deep muscle relaxation exercise that starts at the client's feet.	Interrupts pattern of thought that reinforces anxiety and therefore increases breathing difficulties.
Use successful resolution of a problematic breathing episode as an opportunity to teach the client that he or she can gain conscious control over breathing and that these episodes are not out of his or her control.	Promotes the client's self-esteem and perceived control; also provides positive reinforcement for adaptive coping behaviors.
Teach the client and significant others proper breathing techniques, to include: • Maintaining proper body alignment • Using diaphragmatic breathing (see Ineffective Airway Clearance for information on this technique) • Use of deep muscle relaxation before the onset of ineffective breathing pattern begins	Promotes perceived control and adaptive coping behaviors. Provides information that will facilitate positive reinforcement from the support system, increasing the probability for the success of the behavior change.[56]
Practice with the client diaphragmatic breathing twice a day for 30 minutes. [Note practice times here.]	Enhances relaxation response.
Develop a plan with the client for initiating slow, deep breathing when an ineffective breathing pattern begins.	Early recognition of problematic situations facilitates the client's ability to gain control and utilize adaptive coping behaviors.
Identify with the client the situations that are most frequently associated with the development of ineffective breathing patterns, and assist him or her in practicing relaxation in response to these situations 1 time a day for 30 minutes. [NOTE time of practice session here.]	Positive imagery promotes positive psychophysiologic responses and enhances self-esteem, which promotes the possibility for a positive outcome.[36]

Gerontic Health

ACTIONS/INTERVENTIONS	RATIONALES
Monitor respiratory rate, depth, effort, and lung sounds every 4 hours around the clock.	Minimum database needed for this diagnosis.
Because of age-related "air trapping," have the patient focus on improving expiratory effort. Instruct the patient to inhale to the count of 1 and exhale for 3 counts.[57]	Decreased alveoli and decreased elasticity lead to air trapping, which results in hyperinflation of lungs.
Collaborate with occupational therapy and respiratory therapy regarding other measures to enhance respiratory function.	Occupational therapist can teach the patient less energy-expanding means to complete activities of daily living. Respiratory therapist can assist the patient and family in learning how to perform pulmonary toileting at home.
In the event of a chronic Ineffective Breathing Pattern, refer the patient to a support group such as those sponsored by the American Lung Association.	Provides long-term support for coping with problems; provides updated information; provides role modeling from other group members.
Instruct in relaxation techniques (e.g., guided imagery or progressive muscle relaxation, to reduce stress).	May assist in decreasing the episodes of acute breathing problems in those with chronic Ineffective Breathing Pattern.
Where applicable, monitor for knowledge of proper medication use, especially if inhalers are a part of the therapy.	Maximum benefit may be derived from proper drug administration and usage. Inhalers may be difficult to operate because of physical problems and lack of information regarding proper usage.

(care plan continued on page 312)

NURSING ACTIONS/INTERVENTIONS WITH RATIONALES (continued from page 311)

Home Health

● N O T E : *If this diagnosis is suspected when caring for a patient in the home, it is imperative that a physician referral be obtained immediately. If the patient has been referred to home health care by a physician, the nurse will collaborate with the physician in the treatment of the patient.*

ACTIONS/INTERVENTIONS	RATIONALES
Teach the client and family appropriate monitoring of signs and symptoms of Ineffective Breathing Pattern: • Cough • Sputum production • Fatigue • Respiratory status: cyanosis, dyspnea, rate • Lack of diaphragmatic breathing • Nasal flaring • Anxiety or restlessness • Impaired speech	Provides for early recognition and intervention for problem.

Assist the client and family in identifying lifestyle changes that may be required in assisting to prevent ineffective breathing pattern:
• Stopping smoking
• Prevention and early treatment of lung infections
• Avoidance of known irritants and allergies
• Practicing pulmonary hygiene:
  • Clearing bronchial tree by controlled coughing
  • Decreasing viscosity of secretions via humidity and fluid balance
• Clearing postural drainage
• Treatment of fear, anxiety, anger, depression, thorax trauma, or narcotic overdoses
• Adequate nutritional intake
• Stress management
• Adequate hydration
• Breathing techniques (diaphragmatic, pursed lips)
• Progressive ambulation
• Pain relief
• Preventing hazards of immobility
• Appropriate use of oxygen (dosage, route, and safety factors)
	Provides basic information for the client and family that promotes necessary lifestyle changes.

Teach the patient and family purposes, side effects, and proper administration techniques of medication.	
Assist the client and family to set criteria to help them determine when calling a physician or other intervention is required.	Locus of control shifts from nurse to the client and family, thus promoting self-care.
Teach the family basic CPR.	

CARDIAC OUTPUT, DECREASED

DEFINITION[22]

Amount of blood pumped by the heart is inadequate to meet metabolic demands of the body.

DEFINING CHARACTERISTICS[22]

1. Altered heart rate and/or rhythm
   a. Arrhythmias (tachycardia, bradycardia)
   b. Palpitations
   c. Electrocardiographic (ECG) changes
2. Altered preload
   a. Jugular vein distention
   b. Fatigue
   c. Edema
   d. Murmurs
   e. Increased or decreased central venous pressure (CVP)
   f. Increased or decreased pulmonary artery wedge pressure (PAWP)
   g. Weight gain
3. Altered afterload
   a. Cold and/or clammy skin
   b. Shortness of breath and/or dyspnea
   c. Prolonged capillary refill
   d. Decreased peripheral pulses
   e. Variations in blood pressure readings
   f. Increased or decreased systemic vascular resistance (SVR)
   g. Increased or decreased pulmonary vascular resistance (PVR)
   h. Skin color change
4. Altered contractility
   a. Crackles
   b. Cough
   c. Orthopnea or paroxysmal nocturnal dyspnea
   d. Cardiac output <4 L/min
   e. Cardiac index <2.5 L/min
   f. Decreased ejection fraction, stroke volume index (SVI), and left ventricular stroke work index (LVSWI)
   g. S_3 or S_4 sounds
5. Behavioral and emotional factors
   a. Anxiety
   b. Restlessness

RELATED FACTORS[22]

1. Altered heart rate and/or rhythm
2. Altered stroke volume
   a. Altered preload
   b. Altered afterload
   c. Altered contractility

RELATED CLINICAL CONCERNS

1. Congestive heart failure
2. Myocardial infarction
3. Valvular heart disease
4. Inflammatory heart disease (e.g., pericarditis)
5. Hypertension
6. Shock
7. Chronic obstructive pulmonary disease (COPD)

 Have You Selected the Correct Diagnosis?

Ineffective Tissue Perfusion
Decreased Cardiac Output relates specifically to a heart malfunction, whereas Ineffective Tissue Perfusion relates to deficits in the peripheral circulation that have cellular-level impact. Tissue perfusion problems may develop secondary to Decreased Cardiac Output, but can also exist without cardiac output problems.[59] In either diagnosis, close collaboration will be needed with medical practitioners to ensure the best possible interventions for the patient.

EXPECTED OUTCOME

Will exhibit no signs or symptoms of decreased cardiac output by [date].

TARGET DATES

Because the nursing diagnosis Decreased Cardiac Output is so life-threatening, progress toward meeting the expected outcomes should be evaluation at least daily for 3 to 5 days. If significant progress is demonstrated, then the target date can be increased to three-day intervals. Patients who develop this diagnosis should be referred to a medical practitioner immediately and transferred to a critical care unit.

ADDITIONAL INFORMATION

Cardiac output (CO) refers to the amount of blood ejected from the left ventricle into the aorta per minute. Cardiac output is equivalent to the stroke volume (SV), which is the amount of blood ejected from the left ventricle with each contraction, times the heart rate (HR), or the number of beats per minute:

$$CO = SV \times HR$$

The average amount of cardiac output is 5.6 L per minute. This amount varies according to the individual's amount of exercise and body size.

Cardiac output is dependent on the relationship between stroke volume and the heart rate. Cardiac output is maintained by compensatory adjustment of these two variables. If the rate slows, the time for ventricular filling (diastole) increases. This allows for an increase in the preload and a subsequent increase in stroke volume. If the stroke volume falls, the heart rate increases to compensate. Preload, contractility, and afterload affect stroke volume.

Preload refers to the amount of stretching of the myocardial fibers. The fibers stretch as a result of the increase in the volume of blood delivered to the ventricles during diastole. The degree of myocardial stretch before contraction is preload. Preload is determined by the venous return and ejection fraction (amount of blood left in the ventricle at the end of systole). Prolonged excessive stretching leads to a decrease in cardiac output.

Contractility is a function of the intensity of the actinomycin linkages. Increased contractility increases ventricular emptying and results in increased stroke volume. Contractility can be increased by sympathetic stimulation or by administration of such substances as calcium and epinephrine.

Afterload is the amount of tension developed by the ventricle during contraction. The amount of peripheral resistance predominantly determines the amount of tension. An excessive increase in the afterload reduces stroke volume and cardiac output.

The heart rate is predominantly influenced by the autonomic nervous system, through both the sympathetic and parasympathetic nervous systems. The sympathetic fibers can increase both rate and force, whereas the parasympathetic fibers act in an opposite direction. Other factors such as the central nervous system pressoreceptor reflexes, cerebral cortex impulses, body temperature, electrolytes, and hormones also affect the heart rate, but the autonomic nervous system keeps the entire system in balance.[58]

NURSING ACTIONS/INTERVENTIONS WITH RATIONALES

Adult Health

ACTIONS/INTERVENTIONS	RATIONALES
Place on cardiac monitor and continuously monitor cardiac rhythm and rate.	Allows for assessment of contributors to decreased cardiac output.
Collaborate with the health-care team regarding various tests including ABGs, cardiac enzymes, chemistries, echocardiograms, EKGs, and hemodynamic monitoring.	Additional baseline data needed for accurate monitoring of condition.
Administer oxygen, maintenance intravenous fluid (MIVF) and medications as prescribed, and monitor effects.	Enhances myocardial perfusion and decreases workload.
Measure urinary output hourly. Measure and record intake and total at least every 8 hours.	Can give additional data about renal perfusion and fluid volume balance.
Weigh daily at [time] and in same weight clothing.	Helps determine changes in fluid volume.
Provide adequate pain control.	
Provide adequate rest periods: • Schedule at least one 5-minute rest after any activity.	Decreases stress on already stressed circulatory system.
Limit visitors and visiting time. Explain the need for restriction to the patient and significant others. If the presence of significant other promotes rest, allow them to stay beyond time limits.	
Collaborate with dietitian regarding dietary restrictions when developing plan of care, and reinforce prior to discharge (e.g., sodium, fluids, calories, and cholesterol).	These dietary factors can compromise cardiac output.
Collaborate with occupational therapist and the family regarding diversional activities. Refer to: • Physical therapist for home exercise program • Home health	Promotes collaboration and holistic care.

Child Health

This pattern represents a life-threatening status, which demands immediate attention.

ACTIONS/INTERVENTIONS	RATIONALES
Assess for all possible contributing factors, especially known underlying cardiac anomaly.	Provides realistic basis for plan of care.
Provide in-depth monitoring and documentation related to the following:	These factors constitute the basic measures utilized in monitoring for decompensation of cardiac status. Closely related are respiratory function, hydration status, and hemodynamic status.
• Ventilator, if applicable:	
• If continuous positive airway pressure (CPAP), adjust setting according to the physician order	
• Peak pressure as ordered	
• O$_2$ percentage desired as ordered	
• Intake and output hourly and as ordered. Notify the physician if below 10 mL/h or as specified for size of the infant or child	
• Excessive bleeding. If in postoperative status, notify the physician if more than 50 mL/h or as specified.	
• Tolerance of feedings	
• Notify the physician for:	
• Premature ventricular contractions (PVCs) or other arrhythmias	
• Limits of pulse, respiratory rate, output criteria as specified for the individual patient	
• Use caution in the administration of medications as ordered, especially digoxin:	
• Have another RN check the dose and medication order.	
• Validate and document the heart rate to be greater than the specified lower limit parameter (e.g., 100 for an infant) or as ordered per pediatric cardiologist or intensivist before administering.	
• Document if the medication is withheld because of heart rate.	
• Monitor for signs and symptoms of toxicity (e.g., vomiting).	
• Ensure potassium maintenance. Collaborate with the physician regarding frequency of serum potassium measurement, and immediately report results.	
• Maintain digitalizing protocol.	
• Make sure that the parents understand the patient's status and treatment.	
• Monitor the patient's response to suctioning, x-ray exam, or other procedures.	
Ensure availability of a crash cart and emergency equipment as needed, to include:	Standard nursing care includes availability and appropriate use of equipment and medications in event of cardiac arrest. Anticipation for need of equipment with a child in high-risk status is required.
• Cardiac or emergency drugs	
• Defibrillator	
• Ambu bag (pediatric or infant size)	
• Appropriate suctioning equipment	

(care plan continued on page 316)

NURSING ACTIONS/INTERVENTIONS WITH RATIONALES (continued from page 315)

Child Health

ACTIONS/INTERVENTIONS	RATIONALES
Allow time for the parents to voice concern on a regular basis. Set aside 10 to 15 minutes per shift for this purpose.	Verbalization of concerns helps reduce anxiety. Attempting to set aside time for this verbalization demonstrates the value it holds for the patient's care.
Encourage parental input in care, such as with feeding, positioning, and monitoring intake and output as appropriate.	Parental input assists in meeting the emotional needs of both the parents and child, and supports the care given by health care personnel. This action also allows for learning essential skills in a supportive environment.
Encourage the patient, as applicable, to participate in care.	Self-care enhances sense of autonomy and empowerment.
Allow for sensitivity to time in understanding of diagnosis. The seemingly abstract nature of underlying cardiac physiology, especially in noncyanotic heart disease, can be confusing.	Abstract aspects of an illness often prove more difficult to grasp. Congenital cardiac anomalies are often complex in nature, which requires health-care personnel to use consistent terms and offer appropriate aids to depict key issues of anatomy.
Support the parents in usual appropriate coping mechanisms.	Emotional security may be afforded by encouragement of usual coping mechanisms for age and developmental status.
Maintain appropriate technique in dressing change (asepsis and cautious handwashing).	Standard care requires universal precautions, which minimize risk factors for infection.
Limit visitors in immediate postoperative status as applicable.	Visitation may prove overwhelming to all when unlimited in immediate postoperative period. Remember that numerous nursing–medical therapies must be attended to during this time also.
Help reduce patient and parental anxiety by touching and allowing the patient to be held and comforted.	Comforting allows the parent and child to feel more secure and decreases feelings of intimidation the parents might experience from seeing numerous pieces of equipment and activity. Human caring helps offset perceptions of impersonal high tech.
Provide teaching with sensitivity to patient and parental needs regarding equipment, procedures, or routines (e.g., use a doll for demonstration with a toddler).	Individualized teaching with appropriate aids will most likely serve to reinforce desired learning and enlist the patient's cooperation.
Encourage the parents to meet other parents of similarly involved cardiac patients.	Sharing with similarly involved clientele or families affords a sense of unity, hope, and affirmation of the future far beyond what nurses or others may offer.
Address the need for the parents to continue with ADLs with confidence regarding knowledge of restrictions in the child's status.	Aim should be for normalcy within parameters dictated by the child's condition. Strive to refrain the family from labeling the child or encouraging the child to become a "cardiac cripple."

Women's Health

● N O T E : *Caution the patient never to begin a new vigorous exercise plan while pregnant. Teach the patient to exercise slowly, in moderation, and according to the individual's ability. A good rule of thumb is to use moderation and, with the consent of the physician, continue with the pre-pregnant established exercise plan. Most professionals discourage aerobics and hot tubs or spas because of the heat. It is not known at this time if overheating by the mother is harmful to the fetus.*

ACTIONS/INTERVENTIONS	RATIONALES
Assist the patient with relaxation techniques.	Assists in stress reduction.
Assist in developing an exercise plan for cardiovascular fitness during pregnancy. Some good exercises are: • Swimming • Walking • Bicycling • Jogging (If the patient has done this before and is used to it, jogging is probably not harmful, *but* remember that during pregnancy joints and muscles are more susceptible to strain. If the patient feels pain, fatigue, or overheating, she should slow down or stop exercise.)	Assists in increasing cardiovascular fitness during pregnancy.
Refer the patient to support groups that understand the physiology of pregnancy and have developed exercise programs based on this physiology, such as swimming classes for pregnant women at the local YWCA, childbirth education classes, or exercise videotapes specifically directed and produced for use during pregnancy.	
Teach the patient and significant others how to avoid "supine hypotension" during pregnancy (particularly the later stages).	The expanded uterus causes pressure on the large blood vessels.
Prior to the start of labor, encourage the patient to attend childbirth education classes to learn how to work with her body during labor.	
During the second stage of labor[59–61]: • Allow the patient to assume whatever position aids her in the second stage of labor (i.e., upright, squatting, kneeling position, the use of birth balls, etc.). • Provide the patient with proper physical support during the second stage of labor. This support might include allowing the partner or support person to sit or stand beside her and support her head or shoulders, or behind her supporting her with his or her body. The partner might also stand in front of her, allowing her to lean on his or her neck. The patient may also use a birthing bed or chair, pillows, over-the-bed table, or bars.	
Do not urge the woman to "push, push" or to hold breath during the second stage of labor. Allow the woman to bear down with her contractions at her own pace: • Encourage spontaneous bearing down only if fetal head has not descended low enough to stimulate Ferguson's reflex. • Encourage the mother to push when she feels the urge and to rest between contractions.[62]	Avoids straining and the Valsalva maneuver.[62]

(care plan continued on page 318)

NURSING ACTIONS/INTERVENTIONS WITH RATIONALES (continued from page 317)

Women's Health

ACTIONS/INTERVENTIONS	RATIONALES
• Discourage prolonged maternal breath-holding (longer than 6 to 8 seconds) during pushing. • Assist the mother to accomplish four or more pushing efforts per contraction. • Support the mother's efforts in pushing, and validate the normalcy of sensations and sounds the mother is verbalizing. (These sounds may include grunting, groaning, and exhaling during the push or breath-holding less than 6 seconds.)	Breath-holding involves the Valsalva maneuver. Increased intrathoracic pressure due to a closed glottis causes a decrease in cardiac output and blood pressure. The fall in pressure causes a decrease in placental perfusion, causing fetal hypoxia.[54,62,63]

Mental Health

ACTIONS/INTERVENTIONS	RATIONALES
Monitor risk factors: • Medications • Past history of cardiac problems • Age • Current condition of the cardiovascular system • Weight • Exercise patterns • Nutritional patterns • Psychosocial stressors	Early identification and intervention helps ensure better outcome.
Monitor every [number] hours (depends on level or risk, can be anywhere from 2 to 8 hours) the client's cardiac functioning. [list times to observe here]: • Vital signs • Chest sounds • Apical–radial pulse deficit • Mental status	Basic database for further intervention.
Report alterations to the physician.	
If acute situation develops, notify the physician and implement adult health nursing actions.	
If the client's condition or other factors necessitate the client's remaining in the mental health area beyond the acute stage, refer to adult health nursing actions for care on an ongoing basis. This is not recommended because of the lack of equipment and properly trained staff to care for this situation on most specialized care units.	

Adult Health

ACTIONS/INTERVENTIONS	RATIONALES
If the client is placed on the unit while in the rehabilitation stage of this diagnosis, implement the following nursing actions: (Discuss with the client and other health-care providers current rehabilitation schedule, and record special consideration here.)	Promotes the client's perceived control and supports self-care activities.

ACTIONS/INTERVENTIONS	RATIONALES
Provide appropriate rest periods following activity. This varies according to the client's stage in rehabilitation. Most common times of needed rest are after meals and after any activity. [Note specific limits here.]	Prevents excessive stress on the cardiovascular system, and prevents fatigue.
Assist the client with implementation of exercise program. List types of activity, time spent in activity, and times of activity here. Also list special motivators the client may need, such as a companion to walk for 30 minutes three times a day at [times].	Promotes cardiovascular strength and well-being.
Provide diet restrictions (e.g., low-sodium, low-calorie, low-fat, low-cholesterol, or fluid restrictions).	Decreases dietary contributions to increased risk factors.
Monitor intake and output each shift.	Medications can affect fluid balance, and excessive fluid can increase demands on the cardiovascular system.
Monitor for and teach the client to assess for: • Potassium loss (muscle cramps) • Chest pain • Dyspnea • Sudden weight gain • Decreased urine output • Increased fatigue	Increases the client's perceived control, and promotes early recognition and treatment of problem.
Monitor risk factors, and assist the client in developing a plan to reduce these (e.g., smoking, obesity, or stress). Refer to appropriate nursing diagnosis for assistance in developing interventions.	Increases the client's perceived control, and decreases risk for further damage to the cardiovascular system.
Spend 30 minutes twice a day teaching the client deep muscle relaxation and practicing this process. [List times here.]	Relaxation decreases stress on the cardiovascular system.
Discuss with the patient's support system the lifestyle alterations that may be required.	
Develop stress reduction program with the client, and provide necessary environment for implementation. This could include massage therapy, meditation, aerobic exercise as tolerated, hobbies, or music. [Note specific plan here.]	Enhances possibility for continuation of behavior change.[56]

Gerontic Health

In addition to the interventions for Adult Health, the following may be utilized in aging clients.

ACTIONS/INTERVENTIONS	RATIONALES
Monitor the older adult for atypical signs of pain, such as alterations in mental status, anxiety, or decreasing functional capacity.	Older adults may experience physiologic and psychological alterations that affect their response to pain.[64]

(care plan continued on page 320)

NURSING ACTIONS/INTERVENTIONS WITH RATIONALES (continued from page 319)

Gerontic Health

ACTIONS/INTERVENTIONS	RATIONALES
Monitor for possible side effects of diuretic therapy.	Older adults may have excessive diuresis on normal diuretic dosage.
Review the health history for liver or kidney disease in patients on diuretic therapy.	To avoid complications, dosages of diuretics may need to be adjusted in those with pre-existing kidney or hepatic disease.
Whenever possible, give diuretics in the morning.	Decreases problems with nocturia and consequent distributed sleep–rest pattern or risk for injury from falls.
Teach proper medication usage (e.g., dosage, side effects, dangers related to missed doses, and food/drug interactions).	Basic safety for medication administration.
Teach patients who are on potassium-wasting diuretics: • The need for potassium replacement • Foods that are high in potassium (e.g., bananas) • Signs and symptoms of potassium depletion	
Assist the patient and/or family to determine environmental conditions that may need to be adapted to promote energy.	Assists in conservation of energy and balancing oxygen demands with resources.

Home Health

● NOTE: *If this diagnosis is suspected when caring for a client in the home, it is imperative that a physician referral be obtained immediately. If the client has been referred to home health care by a physician, the nurse will collaborate with the physician in the treatment of the client.*

ACTIONS/INTERVENTIONS	RATIONALES

Teach the patient and significant others:
• Risk factors (e.g., smoking, hypertension, or obesity)
• Medication regimen (e.g., toxicity or effects)
• Need to balance rest and activity
• Monitoring of:
  • Weight daily
  • Vital signs
  • Intake and output
• When to contact health-care personnel:
  • Chest pain
  • Dyspnea
  • Sudden weight gain
  • Decreased urine output
  • Increased fatigue
• Dietary adaptations, as necessary:
  • Low sodium
  • Low cholesterol
  • Caloric restriction
  • Soft foods
	Provides for early recognition and intervention for problem.

ACTIONS/INTERVENTIONS	RATIONALES
Assist the patient and family in identifying lifestyle changes that may be required: • Eliminating smoking • Cardiac rehabilitation program • Stress management • Weight control • Dietary restrictions • Decreased alcohol • Relaxation techniques • Bowel regimen to avoid straining and constipation • Maintenance of fluid and electrolyte balance • Changes in role functions in the family • Concerns regarding sexual activity • Monitoring activity and responses to activity. ● N O T E : *Level of damage to left ventricle should be determined before exercise program is initiated.*[66] • Providing diversional activities when physical activity is restricted. (See Deficient Diversional Activity.) • Pain control	Provides basic information for the client and family that promotes necessary lifestyle changes.
Teach the family basic CPR.	Locus of control shifts from nurse to the client and family, thus promoting self-care.
Teach the client and family purposes and side effects of medications and proper administration techniques.	
Teach the client and family to refrain from activities that increase the demands on the heart (e.g., snow shoveling, lifting, or Valsalva maneuver).	
Assist the client and family to set criteria to help them determine when calling a physician or other intervention is required.	
Consult with or refer to appropriate assistive resources as indicated.	Provides additional support for the client and family, and uses already available resources in a cost-effective manner.

DISUSE SYNDROME, RISK FOR

DEFINITION[22]

A state in which an individual is at risk for deterioration of body systems as the result of prescribed or unavoidable musculoskeletal inactivity.

DEFINING CHARACTERISTICS[22]

None listed.

RISK FACTORS[22]

1. Severe pain
2. Mechanical immobilization
3. Altered level of consciousness
4. Prescribed immobilization
5. Paralysis

RELATED FACTORS[22]

The risk factors are also the related factors.

RELATED CLINICAL CONCERNS

1. Cerebrovascular accident
2. Fractures
3. Closed head injury
4. Spinal cord injury or paralysis
5. Rheumatoid arthritis
6. Amputation
7. Cerebral palsy

Have You Selected the Correct Diagnosis?

Activity Intolerance
This diagnosis implies that the individual is freely able to move but cannot endure or adapt to the increased energy or oxygen demands made by the movement or activity.

Impaired Physical Mobility
With this diagnosis, the individual could move independently if something was not limiting the motion. Impaired Physical Mobility could very well be a predisposing factor to Risk for Disuse Syndrome.

EXPECTED OUTCOME

Will exhibit no signs or symptoms of disuse syndrome by [date].

TARGET DATES

Disuse syndrome can develop rapidly after the onset of immobilization. The initial target date, therefore, should be no more than 2 days.

NURSING ACTIONS/INTERVENTIONS WITH RATIONALES

Adult Health

ACTIONS/INTERVENTIONS	RATIONALES
According to the patient's status, determine realistic potential: • Cognition • Mobility, head control, positioning • Communication, receptive and expressive, verbal or nonverbal • Augmentive aids for daily living	Improves planning and allows for setting of more realistic goals and actual levels of functioning with regard to general physical condition.
Turn and anatomically position the patient. Perform active and passive ROM (range of motion) exercises to all joints at least twice a shift while awake. [State times here.]	Promotes circulation, prevents venous stasis, and helps prevent thrombosis.
Demonstrate and have the patient return-demonstrate isotonic exercises.	Helps avoid syndrome; offsets complications of immobility.
Arrange daily activities with appropriate regard for rest as needed.	
Maintain adequate nutrition and fluid balance on daily basis.	Provides fluid and nutrient necessary for activity.
Monitor the patient and family for perceived and actual health teaching needs, including: • Equipment required for the patient's care • Signs or symptoms to be reported to physician • Medication administration, instructions, and side effects • Plans for follow-up	Initiates appropriate home care planning.
Refer to Impaired Physical Mobility for additional nursing actions.	

Child Health

ACTIONS/INTERVENTIONS	RATIONALES
Assist the family in development of an individualized plan of care to best meet the child's potential.	The family is the best source for individual preferences and needs as related to what daily living for the child involves.

ACTIONS/INTERVENTIONS	RATIONALES
Assist the family in identification of factors that will facilitate progress as well as those factors that may hinder progress in meeting the child's potentials. List those factors here, and assist the family in planning how to offset factors that hinder progress and encourage factors that facilitate progress.	Identifies learning needs and reduces anxiety. Fosters a plan that can be adhered to if all involved participate in its development. Empowers the family.
Facilitate both patient and family ventilation of feelings that may relate to disuse problem by scheduling of 15 to 20 minutes each nursing shift for this activity.	Ventilation of feelings assists in reducing anxiety and promotes learning about condition.
Assist the family in identification of the support system for best possible follow-up care.	Promotes coordination of care and cost-effective use of already available resources.

Women's Health

This nursing diagnosis will pertain to women the same as to adults. Refer to nursing actions for Risk for Activity Intolerance to meet the needs of women with the diagnosis of Risk for Disuse Syndrome.

Mental Health

● N O T E : *The nursing actions in this section reflect the Risk for Disuse Syndrome related to mental health, including use of restraints and seclusion. If the inactivity is related to a physiologic or physical problem, refer to the Adult Health nursing actions.*

ACTIONS/INTERVENTIONS	RATIONALES
Attempt all other interventions before considering immobilizing the client. (See Risk for Violence in Chapter 9 for appropriate actions.)	Promotes the client's perceived control and self-esteem.[65]
Carefully monitor the client for appropriate level of restraint necessary. Immobilize the client as little as possible while still protecting the client and others.	Client safety is of primary importance while maintaining, as much as possible, the client's perceived control and self-esteem.
Obtain necessary medical orders to initiate methods that limit the client's physical mobility.	Provides protection of the client's rights. This should be done in congruence with the state's legal requirements.
Carefully explain to the client, in brief, concise language, reasons for initiating the intervention and what behavior must be present for the intervention to be terminated.	High levels of anxiety interfere with the client's ability to process complex information. Maintains relationship and promotes the client's perceived control.
Attempt to gain the client's voluntary compliance with the intervention by explaining to the client what is needed and with a "show of force" (having the necessary number of staff available to force compliance if the client does not respond to the request).	Communicates to the client that staff has the ability to maintain control over the situation, and provides the client with an opportunity to maintain perceived control and self-esteem.
Initiate forced compliance only if there is an adequate number of staff to complete the action safely. (See Risk for Violence in Chapter 9 for a detailed description of intervention with forced compliance.)	Staff and client safety are of primary importance.

(care plan continued on page 324)

NURSING ACTIONS/INTERVENTIONS WITH RATIONALES (continued from page 323)

Mental Health

ACTIONS/INTERVENTIONS	RATIONALES
Secure the environment the client will be in by removing harmful objects such as accessible light bulbs, sharp objects, glass objects, tight clothing, metal objects, or shower curtain rods.	Provides a safe environment by removing objects the client could use to impulsively harm self.
If the client is placed in four-point restraints, maintain one-to-one supervision.	Promotes client safety and communicates maintenance of relationship while meeting security needs.
If the client is in seclusion or in bilateral restraints, observe the client at least every 15 minutes, or more frequently if he or she is agitated. [List observation schedule here.]	Ensures client safety.
Leave a urinal in the room with the client or offer toileting every hour.	Meets the client's physiologic needs and communicates respect for the individual.
Offer the client fluids every 15 minutes while he or she is awake.	
Discuss with the client his or her feelings about the initiation of immobility, and review at least twice a day the kinds of behavior necessary to have immobility discontinued. [Note behaviors here.]	Promotes the client's regaining control, and clearly provides the client with alternative behaviors for coping.
When checking the client, let him or her know you are checking by calling him or her by name and orienting him or her to day and time. Inquire about the client's feelings, and implement necessary reality orientation.	Promotes a sense of security, and provides information about the client's mental status that will provide information for further interventions.
Provide meals at regular intervals in paper containers, providing necessary assistance. [Amount and type of assistance required should be listed here.]	Meets physiologic needs while maintaining client safety.
If the client is in restraints, remove restraints at least every 2 hours, one limb at a time. Have the client move limbs through a full ROM and inspect for signs of injury. Apply lubricants such as lotion to area under restraint to protect from injury.	Maintains adequate blood flow to the skin and prevents breakdown. Maintains joint mobility and prevents contractures and muscle atrophy.
Pad the area of the restraint that is next to the skin with sheepskin or other nonirritating material.	Protects skin from mechanical irritation from the restraint.
Check circulation in restrained limbs in the area below the restraint by observing skin color, warmth, and swelling. The restraint should not interfere with circulation.	Early assessment and intervention prevent long-term damage.
Change the client's position in bed every 2 hours on [odd/even] hour. Have the client cough and deep breathe during this time.	Protects skin from ischemic and shearing pressure damage. Promotes normal clearing of airway secretions.
Place the body in proper alignment to prevent complications and injury. Use pillows for support if the client's condition allows.	
If the client is in four-point restraints, place him or her on the stomach or side or elevate the head of the bed.	Prevents aspiration or choking.

ACTIONS/INTERVENTIONS	RATIONALES
Place the client on intake and output monitoring to ensure that adequate fluid balance is maintained.	Promotes normal hydration, which prevents thickening of airway secretions and thrombus formation.[66]
Have the client in seclusion move around the room at least every 2 hours on [odd/even] hour. During this time, initiate active ROM and have the client cough and take deep breaths.	Assesses the client's risk for the development of orthostatic hypotension.
Administer medications as ordered for agitation.	
Monitor blood pressure before administering antipsychotic medications.	
Have the client change position slowly, especially from lying to standing.	The combination of immobility and antipsychotic medications can place the client at risk for the development of orthostatic hypotension. Slowing position change allows time for blood pressure to adjust and prevents dizziness and fainting.
Assist the client with daily personal hygiene.	Gives the client a sense of control.
Have the environment cleaned on a daily basis.	Communicates respect for the client.
Remove the client from seclusion as soon as the contracted behavior is observed for the required amount of time. (Both of these should be very specific and listed here. See Risk for Violence in Chapter 9 for detailed information on behavior change and contracting specifics.)	Promotes the client's perception of control, and provides positive reinforcement for appropriate behavior.
Schedule a time to discuss this intervention with the client and his or her support system. Inform the support system of the need for the intervention and about special considerations related to visiting with the client. This information must be provided with consideration of the support system before and after each visit.	Promotes family understanding, and optimizes potential for positive client response.[56]

Gerontic Health

In addition to the interventions for Adult Health, the following may be utilized for the aging client.

ACTIONS/INTERVENTIONS	RATIONALES
Monitor for iatrogenesis, especially in the case of institutionalized elderly.	Although the regulations of the Omnibus Bill Reconciliation Act (OBRA) require the least-restrictive measures and ideally restraint-free care, older adults in long-term care may be placed at risk for disuse syndrome secondary to geri-chairs, use of wheelchairs, and lack of properly functioning or fitted adaptive equipment. In addition, there may be reluctance to prescribe occupational therapy or physical therapy because of costs.
Advocate for older adults to ensure that inactivity is not based on ageist perspectives.	Health-care providers may be reluctant to ensure early mobilization in older patients, especially the old-old clientele.
In the event of impaired cognitive function, remind the patient of need for and assist the patient (or caregiver) in mobilizing efforts.	Prompting may encourage increased activity and decreased risk for disuse.

(care plan continued on page 326)

NURSING ACTIONS/INTERVENTIONS WITH RATIONALES (continued from page 325)

Home Health

ACTIONS/INTERVENTIONS	RATIONALES
Teach the client and family appropriate monitoring of causes, signs, and symptoms of Risk for Disuse Syndrome: • Prolonged bed rest • Circulatory or respiratory problems • New activity • Fatigue • Dyspnea • Pain • Vital signs (before and after activity) • Malnutrition • Previous inactivity • Weakness • Confusion • Fracture • Paralysis	Provides for early recognition and intervention for problem.
Assist the client and family in identifying lifestyle changes that may be required: • Progressive exercise to increase endurance • ROM and flexibility exercise • Treatments for underlying conditions (cardiac, respiratory, musculoskeletal, circulatory, neurologic, etc.) • Motivation • Assistive devices as required (walkers, canes, crutches, wheelchairs, ramps, wheelchair access, etc.) • Adequate nutrition • Adequate fluids • Stress management • Pain relief • Prevention of hazards of immobility (e.g., antiembolism stockings, ROM exercises, position changes) • Changes in occupations, family, or social roles • Changes in living conditions • Economic concerns • Proper transfer techniques • Bowel and bladder regulation	Provides basic information for the client and family that promotes necessary lifestyle changes.
Teach the client and family the purposes and side effects of medications and proper administration techniques (e.g., anticoagulants or analgesics). Assist the client and family to set criteria to help them determine when calling a physician or other interventions are required.	The locus of control shifts from the nurse to the client and family, thus promoting self-care.
Consult with, or refer to, appropriate resources as indicated.	Provides additional support for the client and family, and uses already available resources in a cost-effective manner.

DIVERSIONAL ACTIVITY, DEFICIENT

DEFINITION[22]

The state in which an individual experiences a decreased stimulation from or interest or engagement in recreational or leisure activities.[22]

DEFINING CHARACTERISTICS[22]

1. Usual hobbies cannot be undertaken in hospital.
2. Patient's statements regarding boredom. (Wishes there was something to do or read, etc.)

RELATED FACTORS[22]

1. Environmental lack of diversional activity, as in:
   a. Long-term hospitalization
   b. Frequent lengthy treatments

RELATED CLINICAL CONCERNS

Any medical diagnosis that could be connected to the related factors.

 Have You Selected the Correct Diagnosis?

Activity Intolerance
If the nurse observes or validates reports of the patient's inability to complete required tasks because of insufficient energy, then Activity Intolerance is the appropriate diagnosis, not Deficient Diversional Activity.

Impaired Physical Mobility
When the patient has difficulty with coordination, range of motion, or muscle strength and control or has activity restrictions related to treatment, the most appropriate diagnosis is Impaired Physical Mobility. Deficient Diversional Activity is quite likely to be a companion diagnosis to Impaired Physical Mobility.

Social Isolation
This diagnosis should be considered if the patient demonstrates limited contact with community, peers, and significant others. When the patient talks of loneliness rather than boredom, Social Isolation is the most appropriate diagnosis.

Disturbed Sensory Perception
This diagnosis would be the best diagnosis if the patient is unable to engage in his or her usual leisure time activities as a result of loss or impairment of one of the senses.

EXPECTED OUTCOME

Will assist in designing and implementing a plan to overcome deficient diversional activity by [date].

Participates in one leisure activity [number] times by [date].

Identifies resources necessary to implement action plan by [date].

TARGET DATES

Planning and accessing resources will require a moderate amount of time. A reasonable target date would be within 2 to 3 days.

NURSING ACTIONS/INTERVENTIONS WITH RATIONALES

Adult Health

ACTIONS/INTERVENTIONS	RATIONALES
Dialogue with the patient regarding lack of interest.	Helps the patient identify feelings and begin to deal with them.
Gradually involve the patient, to the extent possible, in more daily self-care activities.	Increases self-worth and adequacy.
Rearrange environment as needed: • Provide ample light. • Place the bed near a window. • Schedule activities throughout the day • Provide radio, television set, DVDs, reading material, or CDs. Ensure access. • Provide clear pathway for wheelchair, ambulations, etc.	Facilitates environmental stimulation.
Provide change of environment at least twice a day at [times] (e.g., out of room).	Creates change.

(care plan continued on page 328)

NURSING ACTIONS/INTERVENTIONS WITH RATIONALES (continued from page 327)

Adult Health

ACTIONS/INTERVENTIONS	RATIONALES
Encourage significant others to assist in increasing diversional activity by: • Bringing books, games, or hobby materials • Visiting more frequently • Encouraging other visitors	Reinforces "normal" lifestyle, and encourages feelings of self-worth.
Provide for appropriate adaptations in equipment or positioning to facilitate desired diversional activity.	
Provide for scheduling of diversional activity at a time when the patient is rested and without multiple interruptions.	
Consider alternate therapies (e.g., pet therapy).	
Refer the patient to individual health-care practitioners who can best assist with problem.	

Child Health

ACTIONS/INTERVENTIONS	RATIONALES
Monitor the patient's potential for activity or diversion according to: • Attention span • Physical limitations and tolerance • Cognitive, sensory, and perceptual deficits • Preferences for gender, age, and interests • Available resources • Safety needs • Pain	Provides essential database for planning desired and achievable diversion.
Facilitate parental input in planning and implementing desired diversional activity plan.	Helps ensure that the plan is attentive to the child's interests, thus increasing the likelihood of the child's participation.
Allow for peer interaction when appropriate through diversional activity.	Involvement of peers serves to foster self-esteem and meets developmental socialization needs.
Consult with the play therapist and plan for introduction of play therapy here.	Specialists facilitate the development of client-specific plans of care in complex situations.[49]

Women's Health

● N O T E : *The following refers to women placed on restrictive activities because of threatened abortions, premature labor, multiple pregnancy, or pregnancy-induced hypertension.*

ACTIONS/INTERVENTIONS	RATIONALES
Encourage the family and significant others to participate in the plan of care for the patient.	Promotes socialization, empowers the family, and provides opportunities for teaching.

ACTIONS/INTERVENTIONS	RATIONALES
Encourage the patient to list lifestyle adjustments that need to be made as well as ways to accomplish these adjustments.	Basic problem-solving technique that encourages the patient to participate in his or her care. Will increase understanding of the current condition.
Teach the patient relaxation skills and coping mechanisms.	
Maintain proper body alignment with use of positioning and pillows.	
Provide diversional activities:	Provides a variety of options to offset deficit.
• Hobbies (e.g., needlework, reading, painting, or television)	
• Job-related activities as tolerated (that can be done in bed) (e.g., reading, writing, or telephone conferences)	
• Activities with children (e.g., reading to the child, painting or coloring with the child, allowing the child to "help" the mother such as bringing water to the mother or assisting in fixing meals for mother)	
• Encourage help and visits from friends and relatives (e.g., visit in person, telephone visit, help with childcare, or help with housework).	

Mental Health

ACTIONS/INTERVENTIONS	RATIONALES
Determine the source of deficient diversional activity. Is the nursing unit appropriately stimulating for the level or type of clients, or is the problem the client's perceptions?	Recognizes the impact of physical space on the client's mood.
Nursing Unit–Related Problems	
Develop a milieu therapy program:	Promotes here-and-now orientation and interpersonal interactions.
• Include seasonal activities for clients, such as parties, special meals, outings, or games. Post schedule of activities in client care areas. Enlist clients in activity planning.	Role models for clients skills in developing and initiating diversional activities.
• Alter the unit environment by changing pictures, adding appropriate seasonal decorations, updating bulletin boards, and cleaning and updating furniture.	Enhances the aesthetics of the environment and has a positive effect on the client's mood.[35]
• Alter the mood of the unit with bright colors, seasonal flowers, or appropriate music.	Colors and sounds affect the client's mood.[33]
• Develop group activities for clients, such as team sports; Ping-Pong; bingo games; and activity planning, meal planning, meal preparation, current events discussion, book discussion, exercise, or craft groups.	Provides opportunities to build social skills, explore different types of activities, and learn alternative methods of coping.
• Decrease emphasis on television as a primary unit activity.	Television does not provide opportunities for learning alternative coping skills and decreases physical activity.
• Provide books, newspapers, records, tapes, and craft materials.	These resources assist the client in meeting belonging needs by facilitating interaction with others on the unit and the world around him or her.

(care plan continued on page 330)

NURSING ACTIONS/INTERVENTIONS WITH RATIONALES (continued from page 329)

Mental Health

ACTIONS/INTERVENTIONS	RATIONALES
• Use community service organizations to provide programs for clients.	Provides varied sensory stimulation.
Collaborate with the occupational therapist for ideas regarding activities and supplies. Note schedule for these activities here.	
Collaborate with the physical therapist regarding physical exercise program.	
Client Perception–Related Problems	
Discuss with the client past activities, reviewing those that have been enjoyed and those that have been tried and not enjoyed.	Promotes the client's sense of control.
List activities that the client has enjoyed in the past, with information about what keeps the client from doing them at this time.	
Monitor the client's energy level, and develop an activity that corresponds to the client's energy level and physiologic needs. For example, a manic client may be bored with playing cards, and yet physiologic needs require less physical activity than the client may desire, so an appropriate activity would address both these needs. [Note client's activity plan here.]	Promotes development of alternative coping behaviors by assisting the client in choosing appropriate activities.
Develop with the client a plan for reinitiating a previously enjoyed activity. [Note that plan here.]	Promotes the client's sense of control.
Develop time in the daily schedule for that activity. [Note that time here.]	
Relate activity to enjoyable time, such as a time for interaction with the nurse alone or interaction with other clients in a group area.	Interaction can provide positive reinforcement for engaging in the activity.
Provide positive verbal feedback to the client about his or her efforts at the activity.	Positive verbal reinforcement encourages appropriate coping behaviors.
Assist the client in obtaining necessary items to implement activity, and list necessary items here.	Facilitates appropriate coping behaviors.
Develop a plan with the client to attempt one new activity—one that has been interesting for him or her but that he or she has not had time or direction to pursue. [Note plan and rewards for accomplishing goals here.]	Promotes the client's perceived control, and provides positive reinforcement for the behavior.
Have the client set realistic goals for activity involvement (e.g., one cannot paint like a professional in the beginning).	Promotes the client's strengths and self-esteem.
Discuss feelings of frustration, anger, and discomfort that may occur as the client attempts a new activity.	Verbalization of feelings and thoughts provides opportunities for developing alternative coping strategies.
Frame mistakes as positive tools of learning new behavior.	Promotes the client's strengths.

Gerontic Health

In addition to the interventions for Adult Health, the following can be utilized for the aging client.

ACTIONS/INTERVENTIONS	RATIONALES
Assess the client's level of activity prior to illness/hospitalization.	Establishes a baseline and allows for realistic goal setting and intervention.
Provide at least 10 to 15 minutes per shift, while the patient is awake, to engage in reminiscing with the patient.	Increases self-esteem, and focuses on strengths the patient has developed over his or her lifetime.[67]

Home Health

ACTIONS/INTERVENTIONS	RATIONALES
Monitor factors contributing to deficient diversional activity.	Provides database for prevention and/or early intervention.
Involve the client and family in planning, implementing, and promoting an increase in diversional activity via: • Family conference • Mutual goal setting • Communication	Involvement improves motivation and improves the outcome.
Assist the client and family in lifestyle adjustments that may be required: • Time management • Work, family, social, and personal goals and priorities • Rehabilitation • Learning new skills or games • Development of support systems • Stress management techniques • Drug and alcohol use issues	Provides basic information for the client and family that promotes necessary lifestyle changes.
Refer the patient to appropriate assistive resources as indicated.	Provides additional support for the client and family, and uses already available resources in a cost-effective manner.

DYSFUNCTIONAL VENTILATORY WEANING RESPONSE (DVWR)

DEFINITION[22]

A state in which a patient cannot adjust to lowered levels of mechanical ventilator support, which interrupts and prolongs the weaning response.[21]

DEFINING CHARACTERISTICS[22]

1. Mild DVWR
   a. Warmth
   b. Restlessness
   c. Slight increased respiratory rate from baseline
   d. Queries about possible machine malfunction
   e. Expressed feelings of increased need for oxygen
   f. Fatigue
   g. Increased concentration on breathing
   h. Breathing discomfort
2. Moderate DVWR
   a. Slight increase from baseline blood pressure <20 mm Hg
   b. Baseline increase in respiratory rate <5 breaths per minute
   c. Slight increase from baseline heart rate <20 beats per minute

d. Pale, slight cyanosis
e. Slight respiratory accessory muscle use
f. Inability to respond to coaching
g. Inability to cooperate
h. Apprehension
i. Color changes
j. Decreased air entry on auscultation
k. Diaphoresis
l. Eye widening, "wide-eyed look"
m. Hypervigilence to activities

3. Severe DVWR
a. Deterioration in arterial blood gases from current baseline
b. Respiratory rate increases significantly from baseline
c. Increase from baseline blood pressure >20 mm Hg
d. Agitation
e. Increase from baseline heart rate >20 beats per minute
f. Paradoxical abdominal breathing
g. Adventitious breath sounds
h. Cyanosis
i. Decreased level of consciousness
j. Full respiratory accessory muscle use
k. Shallow, gasping breaths
l. Profuse diaphoresis
m. Discoordinated breathing with the ventilator
n. Audible airway secretion

RELATED FACTORS[22]

1. Physiologic
   a. Inadequate nutrition
   b. Sleep pattern disturbance
   c. Uncontrolled pain or discomfort
   d. Ineffective airway clearance
2. Psychological
   a. Patient-perceived inefficacy about the ability to wean
   b. Powerlessness
   c. Anxiety (moderate or severe)
   d. Knowledge deficit of the weaning process and patient role
   e. Hopelessness
   f. Fear
   g. Decreased motivation
   h. Decreased self-esteem
   i. Insufficient trust of the nurse
3. Situational
   a. Uncontrolled episodic energy demands or problems
   b. Adverse environment (noisy, active environment, neg-ative events in the room, low nurse–patient ratio, extended nurse absence from bedside, or unfamiliar nursing staff)
   c. History of multiple unsuccessful weaning attempts
   d. History of ventilator dependence >1 week
   e. Inappropriate pacing of diminished ventilator support
   f. Inadequate social support

RELATED CLINICAL CONCERNS

1. Closed head injury
2. Coronary bypass
3. Respiratory arrest
4. Cardiac arrest
5. Cardiac transplant

☑ Have You Selected the Correct Diagnosis?

Ineffective Breathing Pattern
In this diagnosis, the patient's respiratory effort is insufficient to maintain the cellular oxygen supply. This diagnosis would contribute to the patient's being placed on ventilatory assistance; however, DVWR occurs after the patient has been placed on a ventilator and efforts are being made to re-establish a regular respiratory pattern. The key difference is whether or not a ventilator has been involved in the patient's therapy.

Impaired Gas Exchange
This diagnosis refers to the exchange of oxygen and carbon dioxide in the lungs or at the cellular level. This probably has been a problem for the patient and is one of the reasons the patient was placed on a ventilator. DVWR would develop after the patient has received treatment for the impaired gas exchange via the use of a ventilator.

EXPECTED OUTCOME

Will be weaned from the ventilator by [date]. Patient will demonstrate progressively longer intervals off ventilator [target intervals in terms of hours]
   Will maintain

TARGET DATES

Initial target dates should be in terms of hours as the patient is going through the weaning process. As the patient improves, the target date could be expressed in increasing intervals from 1 to 3 days.

NURSING ACTIONS/INTERVENTIONS WITH RATIONALES

Adult Health

ACTIONS/INTERVENTIONS	RATIONALES
Collaborate with the health-care team to devise a plan for ventilatory weaning and explain the weaning procedure.	Psychologically prepares patient for weaning process.
Initiate supportive measures:	
• Ensure that nutrient intake supports energy requirements for spontaneous breathing.	
• Provide ample rest periods.	Ensures patient has adequate energy stores to assume work of breathing.
• Initiate measures to minimize bronchial secretions. See nursing actions for Ineffective Airway Clearance.	Interference with gas exchange will adversely affect the weaning process.
Limit activity prior to removing the patient off the ventilator.	Nursing activity and/or visitors can increase patient energy expenditure, leaving less energy for ventilatory weaning.
Limit use of medications that cause respiratory depression.	
Monitor for signs and symptoms of inability to tolerate weaning process, including abdominal breathing, increased respiratory effort, decreasing oxygen saturation, tachycardia, and tachypnea. Stop the weaning process before the patient becomes exhausted.	Essential monitoring for efficacy of the weaning process.
Gradually increase times off the ventilator as tolerated.	
Allow the patient to rest overnight on the ventilator.	Allows for periods of rest.
Document times and length of time the patient is able to stay off the ventilator.	Essential for monitoring progress.
If the patient is unable to wean while still in the hospital, initiate referral to pulmonary rehabilitation program as soon as feasible.	Coordinates team efforts and allows sufficient planning time for home care.

Child Health

ACTIONS/INTERVENTIONS	RATIONALES
Monitor for contributing factors[68]: • Pathophysiologic health concerns (e.g., infections, anemia, fever, or pain) • Previous respiratory history, especially risk indicators of reactive airway disease and bronchopulmonary dysplasia • Previous cardiovascular history, especially risk indicators such as increased or decreased pulmonary blood flow associated with congenital deficits • Previous neurologic status • Recent surgical procedures • Current medication regimen • Psychological and emotional stability of the parents as well as the child	Provides a database that will assist in generating the most individualized plan of care.

(care plan continued on page 334)

NURSING ACTIONS/INTERVENTIONS WITH RATIONALES (continued from page 333)

Child Health

ACTIONS/INTERVENTIONS	RATIONALES
Collaborate with the physician, respiratory therapist, and other health-care team members to determine respiratory parameters that suggest readiness to begin the weaning process[69]: • Spontaneous respirations for age (e.g., rate or depth) • Oxygen saturations in normal range for condition (e.g., spontaneous tidal volume of 5 mL/kg body weight, vital capacity per Wright) Respirometer of 10 mL/kg body weight, effective oxygenation with positive end-expiratory pressure (PEEP) of 4 to 6 centimeters of H_2O. An exception to the norms would exist if the infant has transposition of the great vessels. • Blood gases in normal range • Stable vital signs • Parental or patient anxiety regarding respirator • Patient's facial expression and ability to rest • Resolution of the precipitating cause for intubation and mechanical support • Tolerance of suctioning and use of Ambu bag • Central nervous system and cardiovascular stability • Nutritional status, muscle strength, pain, drug-induced respiratory expression, or sleep deprivation	Specific ventilator-related criteria offer the best decision-making support for determining the best plan of ventilator weaning.

● N O T E : *Oxygen saturation, blood gases, and vital signs may be abnormal secondary to chronic lung damage with accompanying hypoxemia and hypercapnia, but the pH may be normal with metabolic compensation for chronic respiratory acidosis. In this instance, acceptable ranges would be defined.*

Provide constant one-to-one attention to the patient, and focus primarily on cardiorespiratory needs. Have CPR backup equipment readily available.	Hierarchy of needs for oxygenation must be met for all vital functions to be effective in homeostasis. Anticipatory safety for a patient on a ventilator demands backup equipment in case of failure of the current equipment.
Monitor the anxiety levels of the patient and family at least once per shift.	Expression of feelings will assist in monitoring family concerns and help reduce anxiety.
Monitor patient-specific parameters during actual attempts at weaning: • Arterial blood gases • Vital signs • Chest sounds • Pulse oximetry • Chest X-ray exam • Hematocrit	Assists in further planning for weaning.
Provide teaching as appropriate for the patient and family, with emphasis on the often slow pace of weaning.	Assessment and individualized learning needs allow appropriate focus on the patient. Explanation regarding the slow pace encourages a feeling of success rather than failure when each session does not meet the same time limits as the previous session.

ACTIONS/INTERVENTIONS	RATIONALES
Provide attention to rising related emotional problems secondary to the association of ventilators with terminal life support.	With the need to implement intubation and ventilation, there can arise a myriad of concerns regarding the patient's prognosis.
Refer the patient for long-term follow-up as needed.	Fosters long-term support and coping with care at home.
Administer medications as ordered with appropriate attention to preparation for weaning (e.g., careful use of paralytic agents or narcotics).	The best chance for successful weaning includes appropriate consciousness, no respiratory depression, and adequate neuromuscular strength. Special caution must be taken in positioning the patient receiving neuromuscular blocking agents so that dislocation of joints does not occur.[70]
Maintain a neutral thermal environment.	Altered oxygenation and metabolic needs occur in instances of hyperthermia and hypothermia.
Provide the parents the option to participate in care as permitted.	Family input offers emotional input and security for the child in times of great stress, thereby allowing for growth in parental–child coping behaviors.
Communicate with the infant or child using age-appropriate methods (e.g., an infant will enjoy soft music or a familiar voice, whereas an older child may be able to use a small magic slate or point to key terms).	Effective communication serves to allow for expression of or reception of messages of cares or concerns, thereby acknowledging the value of the patient.

Women's Health

The nursing actions for Women's Health clients with this diagnosis are the same as those for Adult Health.

Mental Health

This diagnosis is not appropriate for the mental health care unit.

Gerontic Health

In addition to the interventions for Adult Health, the following may be utilized for the aging client:

ACTIONS/INTERVENTIONS	RATIONALES
Monitor the patient for presence of factors that make weaning difficult, such as[71]: • Poor nutritional status • Infection • Sleep disturbances • Pain • Poor positioning • Large amounts of secretions • Bowel problems	These factors can significantly contribute to a delay in the weaning process.
Ensure that communication efforts are enhanced by the proper use of sensory aids such as eyeglasses, hearing aids, or adequate light, decreased noise level in room, speaking in a low-pitched tone of voice, and facing the patient when speaking. If written instructions are used, make sure they are brief, jargon-free, printed or written in dark ink, and printed or written in large letters.	Effective communication is critical to the success of weaning efforts. Lack of information or misinterpreted information may result in increased anxiety and decreased weaning success.

(care plan continued on page 336)

NURSING ACTIONS/INTERVENTIONS WITH RATIONALES (continued from page 335)

Gerontic Health

ACTIONS/INTERVENTIONS	RATIONALES
Maintain same staff assignments whenever possible.[72]	Facilitates communication, and decreases anxiety and fear caused by unfamiliarity with caregivers.
Contract with the patient for short-term and long-term weaning goals, providing reinforcements and rewards for progress. Use wall chart or diary to record progress.	

Home Health

Clients are discharged to the home health setting with ventilators; however, the nursing care required is the same as those actions covered in Adult Health and Gerontic Health.

FALLS, RISK FOR

DEFINITION[22]

Increased susceptibility to falling that may cause physical harm.

DEFINING CHARACTERISTICS[22]

1. Adults
   a. Demographics
      (1) History of falls
      (2) Wheelchair use
      (3) Age 65 or older
      (4) Female (if elderly)
      (5) Lives alone
      (6) Lower limb prosthesis
      (7) Use of assistive devices
   b. Physiologic
      (1) Presence of acute illness
      (2) Postoperative conditions
      (3) Visual difficulties
      (4) Hearing difficulties
      (5) Arthritis
      (6) Orthostatic hypotension
      (7) Sleeplessness
      (8) Faintness when turning or extending neck
      (9) Anemias
      (10) Vascular disease
      (11) Neoplasms (i.e., fatigue or limited mobility)
      (12) Urgency and/or incontinence
      (13) Diarrhea
      (14) Decreased lower extremity strength
      (15) Postprandial blood sugar changes
      (16) Foot problems
      (17) Impaired physical mobility
      (18) Impaired balance
      (19) Difficulty with gait
      (20) Unilateral neglect
      (21) Proprioceptive deficits
      (22) Neuropathy
   c. Cognitive
      (1) Diminished mental status (e.g., confusion, delirium, dementia, impaired reality testing)
   d. Medications
      (1) Antihypertensive agents
      (2) Angiotensin-converting enzyme (ACE) inhibitors
      (3) Diuretics
      (4) Tricyclic antidepressants
      (5) Alcohol use
      (6) Antianxiety agents
      (7) Hypnotics or tranquilizers
      (8) Narcotics
   e. Environment
      (1) Restraints
      (2) Weather conditions (e.g., wet floors or ice)
      (3) Throw or scatter rugs
      (4) Cluttered environment
      (5) Unfamiliar, dimly lit rooms
      (6) No antislip material in bath and/or shower
2. Children
   a. Younger than 2 years of age
   b. Male gender when younger than 1 year of age
   c. Lack of autorestraints
   d. Lack of gate on stairs
   e. Lack of window guard
   f. Bed located near window
   g. Unattended infant on bed, changing table, or sofa
   h. Lack of parental supervision

RELATED FACTORS[22]

The risk factors also serve as related factors.

RELATED CLINICAL CONCERNS

1. Vertigo
2. Osteoporosis
3. Hypotension
4. Recent history of anesthesia
5. Cataracts or glaucoma
6. Cerebrovascular insufficiency
7. Epilepsy

 Have You Selected the Correct Diagnosis?

Risk for Injury
This diagnosis is a broader diagnosis than Risk for Falls. Certainly, a fall would increase the likelihood of injury, but making the specific diagnosis of Risk for Falls as a primary problem allows more specific focus on prevention.

Impaired Physical Mobility
This diagnosis is a contributing factor to falls. Again, Risk for Falls would be a more specific diagnosis.

EXPECTED OUTCOME

Will have experienced no falls by [date].

TARGET DATES

A patient with this diagnosis would need to be checked at least hourly. After some of the risk factors have been alleviated, an appropriate target date would be 5 days.

NURSING ACTIONS/INTERVENTIONS WITH RATIONALES

Adult Health

● N O T E : *Assessment of risk factors for falls is an important element in prevention of falls. Risk factors associated with falls include a history of falls, fear of falling, bowel and bladder incontinence, cognitive impairment, dizziness, functional impairment, medications, medical problems, and environmental risks. Hospitalization or illness of the otherwise healthy adult often results in increased risk for falls. Chronically ill adults often experience these risk factors.*[73]

ACTIONS/INTERVENTIONS	RATIONALES
Keep the bed in the lowest position.	Lessens the distance of a fall.
Remove hazards from the environment.	Safety and security.
Place the patient in a room close to the nurses' station.	Allows for close visualization of patient.
Assess nutrition and elimination needs at least every 2 hours.	
Exercise caution with medications including sedatives, hypnotics, narcotics, or diuretics.	May precipitate disorientation or contribute to disequilibrium.
Keep frequently used items within reach.	Avoids reaching and becoming off balance.[74]
Provide slip-resistant surfaces in the bathroom tub or shower; raise toilet seats.	
Ensure that there are grab bars in bathroom or in the room; ensure that handrails are installed in halls.	
Involve the patient in identifying ways to prevent falls.	Empowers the patient to take an active role in his or her own health care.
Use protective alarm sensors as necessary.	Identifies when the patient is outside safety limits.[74]
Use alternatives to physical or chemical restraints, including continuous caretaker.	Lessens independence and may lead to more falls.[75]
Educate the family on fall prevention strategies.	Empowers the family to become a part of caregiving.
Refer to the Gerontic and Home Health Nursing Care Plans.	

(care plan continued on page 338)

NURSING ACTIONS/INTERVENTIONS WITH RATIONALES (continued from page 337)

Child Health

ACTIONS/INTERVENTIONS	RATIONALES
Identify all contributing factors, including: • Neurologic • Musculoskeletal • Cardiovascular • Cognitive • Developmental • Environmental • Situational • Pharmacologic • Medical	A holistic approach provides a thorough database to provide individualized care.
Ensure safety in the environment on an ongoing basis.	Risk is reduced by anticipatory safety measures.
Provide teaching to the client, family, and health team members based on specific content per plan.	Standardization and shared plan will afford the best chance for attainment of goal with empowerment of others to provide appropriate assistance.
Provide transfer of principles of prevention to alternate settings as required per daily activities of living (e.g., playroom, dining area, etc.).	Offers validation of the importance of principles of safety that can be applied in the future as needed.
Maintain ongoing surveillance for potential changes.	Constant anticipatory safety needs are mandatory.
Determine the need for post-hospitalization teaching regarding preventive or related data.	Provides appropriate time for questions or concerns prior to dismissal.
Administer medications, treatments, or related care in a manner that permits the best likelihood for noninterference in usual mobility.	Clustering of care and appropriate attention to timing of medications or treatments will best afford safety and lessen risk.
Ensure adequate lighting on a 24-hour basis.	Safety needs include appropriate lighting, especially at night or in times of darkness.
Ensure availability of assistive devices as required per client (e.g., corrective lenses, braces, helmet, etc.).	Appropriate augmentation as needed will prevent likelihood of falls.

Women's Health

The nursing interventions for this diagnosis in Women's Health are the same as those for Adult Health and Gerontic Health.

Mental Health

The nursing interventions for this diagnosis in Mental Health are the same as those for Adult Health and Gerontic Health.

Gerontic Health

● N O T E : *Aging adults are at high risk for falls due to the prevalence of common fall risk factors among this age group. Common risk factors for falls include muscle weakness, history of falls, gait or balance deficits, use of assistive devices, visual deficits, arthritis, impaired activities of daily living, depression, cognitive impairment, and age older than 80 years. (National Guidelines Clearinghouse, http://www.guidelines.gov)*

ACTIONS/INTERVENTIONS	RATIONALES
Perform fall risk assessment on all older clients, appropriate to the caregiving site.	Risk factors for falls in older clients are multifactorial and site-specific assessment tools help target factors (such as equipment, structures, furnishings, personnel issues) that may increase fall potential.
All older persons should be asked at least once a year about falls.	
All older persons who report a single fall should be observed as they stand up from a chair without using their arms, walk several paces, and return (Get Up and Go Test). Those demonstrating no difficulty or unsteadiness need no further assessment. Persons with difficulty or demonstrated unsteadiness performing this test require further assessment. (National Guidelines Clearinghouse, http://www.guidelines.gov)	
Older persons who have recurrent falls or risk for falls should be offered long-term exercise and balance training. (National Guideline Clearinghouse, http://www.guidelines.gov)	Promotes strength and balance needed to prevent falls.
Persons who have fallen should have their medications reviewed and altered or stopped as appropriate. Particular attention should be given to persons taking four or more medications and those taking psychotropic medications. (National Guidelines Clearinghouse, http://www.guidelines.gov)	Removes a potential risk factor for future falls.
Instruct client to use assistive devices as a part of a comprehensive program for falls prevention.[73]	Assistive devices alone are not adequate to prevent falls.
Carefully monitor the client's cardiovascular status and address issues such as syncope and dysrhythmias.[73]	Falls that have a cardiac cause may be amenable to treatment of the cardiac condition (pacing, medication changes).
Carefully assess the client's visual system and collaborate with the health-care team to address any remediable visual abnormalities.[73]	Visual changes are associated with a higher rate of falls.
Avoid the use of restraints as a falls prevention method.	The use of restraints has not been demonstrated to prevent falls and may contribute to client injury.[73]
Ensure that any sensory adaptive equipment is available and properly functioning. [Note equipment needed for client here.]	Visual and auditory deficits can affect balance.[14]
Consult with occupational therapist and physical therapist for balance, gait, transfer, and strength assessment and training as needed.	The factors listed have been identified as having an impact on the potential for falls in older adults.[19]
Review drug list to evaluate any medication-associated risks, such as diuretics, antihypertensives, sedatives, psychotropics, and hypoglycemic drugs.	These medications have been shown to increase the incidence of falls in older adults.[76]
Develop a teaching plan for the client and/or caregiver to reduce fall potential based on risk factors present.	Raises awareness of fall potential and strategies needed to reduce risks.

(care plan continued on page 340)

NURSING ACTIONS/INTERVENTIONS WITH RATIONALES (continued from page 339)

Home Health/Community Health

ACTIONS/INTERVENTIONS	RATIONALES
Assess the home for hazards: • Throw rugs • Electrical cords • Uneven floor surfaces • Raised thresholds • Slick floors • Animals	Basic safety measures.
Modify the home to reduce or eliminate hazards: • Skid-proof surfaces in showers and on stairs. • Mark uneven areas and stairs. • Eliminate throw rugs and cords. • Install safety rails in halls, stairs, and bathrooms.	The items listed are primary hazards.
Assess client-related factors that increase risk for falls: • Poorly fitting shoes • Medications that increase sedation or contribute to dizziness • History of falls • Inner ear infections or disorders	Basic safety measures.
Educate the client and family about reducing client-related factors that increase the risk for falls: • Medication effects or side effects • Changing position slowly to reduce risk • Acquire properly fitting, nonskid footwear	
Utilize night lights in dark areas.	
Reduce or eliminate clutter in traffic areas.	
Refer the client and family to an emergency response service as appropriate.	To provide rapid response should a fall occur.
Utilize gates to keep pets isolated if they pose a risk for falls.	
Request a physical therapy consult as appropriate to improve muscle strength and gait.	
Request a physical therapy consult to ensure the correct use of assistive devices.	To prevent injury before it occurs.

FATIGUE

DEFINITION

An overwhelming sustained sense of exhaustion and decreased capacity for physical and mental work at usual level.[22]

DEFINING CHARACTERISTICS[22]

1. Inability to restore energy even after sleep
2. Lack of energy or inability to maintain usual level of physical activity
3. Increase in rest requirements
4. Tired
5. Inability to maintain usual routines
6. Verbalization of an unremitting and overwhelming lack of energy
7. Lethargic or listless
8. Perceived need for additional energy to accomplish routine tasks
9. Increase in physical complaints
10. Compromised concentration
11. Disinterest in surroundings, introspection
12. Decreased performance
13. Compromised libido

14. Drowsy
15. Feelings of guilt for not keeping up with responsibilities

RELATED FACTORS[22]

1. Psychological
   a. Boring lifestyle
   b. Stress
   c. Anxiety
   d. Depression
2. Environmental
   a. Humidity
   b. Lights
   c. Noise
   d. Temperature
3. Situational
   a. Negative life events
   b. Occupation
4. Physiologic
   a. Sleep deprivation
   b. Pregnancy
   c. Poor physical condition
   d. Disease states
   e. Increased physical exertion
   f. Malnutrition
   g. Anemia

RELATED CLINICAL CONCERNS

1. Acquired immunodeficiency syndrome (AIDS)
2. Hyper- or hypothyroidism
3. Cancer

4. Menopause
5. Depression
6. Anemia

✔ Have You Selected the Correct Diagnosis?

Disturbed Sleep Pattern
Fatigue is defined as a sense of exhaustion and decreased capacity for mental work regardless of adequate sleep. In this sense, Fatigue may be considered an alteration in quality, not quantity, of sleep, and is subjective.

Decreased Cardiac Output
Decreased oxygenation to the muscles, brain, and so on could result in a sense of fatigue.

Imbalanced Nutrition, Less Than Body Requirements
Decreased nutrition will ultimately lead to decreased muscle mass and decreased energy, which will result in Fatigue.

EXPECTED OUTCOME

Will have decreased complaints of fatigue by [date].
   Will resume performance of normal routine for [number] minutes/hours by [date].

TARGET DATES

Fatigue can have far-reaching impact. For this reason, the initial target date should be set at no more than 4 days.

NURSING ACTIONS/INTERVENTIONS WITH RATIONALES

Adult Health

ACTIONS/INTERVENTIONS	RATIONALES
Collaborate with the diet therapist for in-depth dietary assessment and planning. Monitor the patient's food and fluid intake daily.	Adequate, balanced nutrition assists in reducing fatigue.
Identify contributory factors on a daily basis at [time].	Assists in identifying causative factors, which then can be treated.
Carefully plan activities of daily living (ADLs) and daily exercise schedules with input from the patient. Determine how to best foster future patterns that will maintain optimal sleep–rest patterns.	Realistic schedules based on the patient's input promote participation in activities and a sense of success.

(care plan continued on page 342)

NURSING ACTIONS/INTERVENTIONS WITH RATIONALES (continued from page 341)

Adult Health

ACTIONS/INTERVENTIONS	RATIONALES
Instruct the patient in stress reduction techniques. Have the patient return-demonstrate at least once a day through the day of discharge.	Mental and physical stress contribute greatly to a sense of fatigue.
Provide frequent rest periods. Schedule at least 30 minutes of rest after any strenuous activity.	Allows the patient to gradually increase strength and tolerance for activities.
Assist the patient with self-care as needed. Plan gradual increase in activities over several days.	
Promote rest at night: • Warm bath at bedtime • Warm milk at bedtime • Back massage	
Avoid sensory overload or sensory deprivation. Provide diversional activities.	Sensory stimulation can deplete energy stores; diversional activities help prevent overload or deprivation by focusing the patient's concentration on an activity he or she personally enjoys.
Limit visitation as necessary.	
Address issues that will interfere with sleep, including pain.	
Educate the patient to avoid activities that will interfere with sleep or reduce quality of sleep (consumption of alcohol or stimulants, or exercising close to bedtime).	
Refer to local exercise center for assistance with regular exercise plan.	Regular exercise decreases fatigue.

Child Health

ACTIONS/INTERVENTIONS	RATIONALES
Develop, with patient and parents, a plan to best address contributory factors as determined by verbalized perceptions of fatigue (may be related to parents' perceptions). [Note plan here.]	Parents are best able to describe objective behaviors that offer cues to fatigue factors, especially when the patient cannot speak or describe his or her feelings. When the plan is developed in collaboration with the client and family there is a greater probability of success.[49]
Provide daily feedback and positive reinforcement regarding progress, and reassess the child's and the family's perception of fatigue. [Note those things that are reinforcing to the child here.]	Because of the ever-changing fatigue factors, close attention to progress will aid in a sense of mastery and objectify concerns.
Ensure safety needs according to the child or infant's age and developmental capacity.	Standard accountability is to provide for safety needs with special attention to the child's age, developmental capacity, parental education, compliance, etc.
Collaborate with other members of the health-care team as indicated, especially pediatrician, pediatric cardiologist, dietician, and physical therapist.	Offers input from team members to safeguard the client's progress.

Women's Health

ACTIONS/INTERVENTIONS	RATIONALES
During pregnancy, schedule rest periods during the day.	Realistic planning to offer brief rest periods during the day.
Find restful area, and get away from the work area to rest 5 to 10 minutes with feet propped above the abdomen, once in the morning and once in the afternoon.	
During lunch, leave the work area to rest 10 to 15 minutes lying on the left side or with feet propped above the abdomen.	
Have the patient research the possibility of split time or job sharing at work during pregnancy.	
Teach the patient relaxation techniques.	Techniques induce a restful state and can be used for short periods of rest as well as more extended periods of rest.
Teach the patient to use music of preference during rest periods.	Assists with relaxation.
Plan for at least 6 to 8 hours of sleep during the night. (See Disturbed Sleep Pattern, Chapter 6, for nursing actions to promote sleep.)	
Involve significant others in discussion and problem-solving activities regarding lifestyle changes needed to reduce fatigue.	The family can assume more responsibilities to assist in increasing rest time for the patient.
After delivery, identify a support system that can assist the patient with infant care and household duties.	Assists in alleviating fatigue related to trying to manage household as always as well as trying to care for a new baby.
Learn to rest and sleep when the infant sleeps.	Conserves energy and increases amount of time available for rest.
Plan daily activities to alleviate unnecessary steps and to allow for frequent rest periods.	
• If bottle-feeding, prepare formula for 24 hours at a time.	
• If breastfeeding, let spouse get up at night and bring the baby to the mother.	
• If breastfeeding, sleep with the baby in bed.	The baby begins to feed for longer periods and begins to sleep longer more quickly. Both the mother and infant get more rest.
• Prepare extra when cooking meals for the family, and freeze extra for future meals (e.g., prepare big batch of stew or spaghetti on one day, and freeze portions for future meals).	
Plan return to work on a gradual basis (e.g., work part-time for the first 2 weeks, gradually increasing time at work until full-time by end of 4 weeks).	Provides gradual return to activities, and decreases likelihood of fatigue.

(care plan continued on page 344)

NURSING ACTIONS/INTERVENTIONS WITH RATIONALES (continued from page 343)

Mental Health

● **N O T E :** *All goals established for the nursing actions should be achievable and adjusted as the client's condition changes.*

ACTIONS/INTERVENTIONS	RATIONALES
Schedule time by which the client must be out of bed and dressed. [Note time here.] Initially this goal may be limited to the client getting out of bed without dressing.	Provides goal the client can achieve, and enhances self-esteem.
Assist the client with grooming activities. [Note here the degree of assistance needed as well as any special items needed.]	Promotes the client's sense of control, and enhances self-esteem.
While assisting the client with grooming activities, teach performance of tasks in energy-efficient ways (e.g., placing all necessary items in one place before grooming is begun).	Promotes the client's control by providing increased opportunity for self-care.
Provide the client with appropriate rewards for accomplishing established goals (Note special goals here with the reward for achievement of goal). Establish rewards with client input.	Positive reinforcement encourages appropriate behavior.
Establish time for the client to rest during the day. Initially this will be more frequent and diminish as the client's condition changes. [Note times and duration of rest periods here.]	Meets physiologic need for rest. Also provides the client with an opportunity for perceived control in determining when these rest periods should be provided.
Walk with the client on unit [number] minutes [number] times a day.	Promotes cardiorespiratory fitness, and promotes self-esteem by providing a goal the client can meet. Interaction with the nurse can provide positive reinforcement for this activity.
Have the client identify pleasurable activities that cannot be performed because of fatigue.	Promotes positive orientation by connecting the client with images of past pleasures, and provides material for developing positive imaging.
Identify one pleasurable activity, and develop a gradually escalating plan for client involvement in this activity. Provide rewards for accomplishment of each step in this plan.	Promotes positive orientation by providing the client with positive goal to work toward. This will increase motivation. Positive reinforcement encourages behavior.
Provide the client with foods that are high in nutritional value and are easy to consume.	Meets physiologic needs for nutrition in a manner that conserves energy.
Talk with the client 30 minutes twice a day. Topics for this discussion should include: • Client's perception of the problem • Identification of thoughts that support the feeling of fatigue • Identification of thoughts that decrease feelings of fatigue • Identification of unrealistic goals • Client's evaluation of and attitudes toward self	Promotes the client's sense of control by providing time for his or her input into the plan of care on a daily basis; also provides positive reinforcement through social interaction with the nurse and verbal feedback about accomplishments.

ACTIONS/INTERVENTIONS	RATIONALES
• Identification of circumstances in the client's environment that support continuing feelings of fatigue (e.g., family stressors or secondary gain from fatigue) • Identification of the client's accomplishments	
After the client has verbalized the effects negative thoughts have on feelings and behavior, teach the client how to stop negative thoughts and replace them with positive thoughts.	Cognitive maps impact feelings and behavior. When cognitive maps are used inappropriately, they can promote maladaptive thinking, behaving, and feeling. Recognition of dysfunctional maps provides the client with the opportunity for developing positive orientation and adaptive cognitive maps.[37]
Reward the client for positive self-statements with informative positive verbal reinforcement.	Positive reinforcement encourages appropriate behavior.
Assign the client tasks on the unit, and provide positive reinforcement for task accomplishment. [Note task assigned and reward established here.]	
Involve the client in group activity with other clients for [number] minutes [number] times a day.	Interaction with peers provides opportunities to increase social network, learn problem-solving strategies, and test perceptions of self and experiences with peers.
Meet with the client and client's family to evaluate interaction patterns and provide information that would assist them in assisting the client.	Family support enhances probability of behavior changes being maintained after discharge.
Have the client identify those factors that will maintain a feeling of well-being after discharge, and develop a specific behavioral plan for implementing them. [Note plan here.]	Reinforces behavior change and new coping skills, while providing positive feedback and enhancing self-esteem.[37]

Gerontic Health

ACTIONS/INTERVENTIONS	RATIONALES
Review medications for side effects or possible drug interactions.	Many medications can contribute to the sensation of fatigue, particularly cardiac and antihypertensive medications, high-dose or replacement corticosteroids, antivirals, antifungals, and immune therapy.[73]
Collaborate with the health-care team in assessing the patient for depression.	Depression is often underreported and undertreated in older adults.
Collaborate with the health-care team in assessing thyroid function and hormone levels.	Alterations in thyroid function and hormone levels can lead to fatigue.
Monitor for activities that interrupt the patient's sleep pattern, such as taking vital signs, daily weights, or treatments.	Environmental noises and inattention to the patient's usual sleep pattern may result in sleep fragmentation.
Carefully assess sleep patterns and sleep hygiene and make recommendations for improvement as needed.	Sleep deprivation can lead to fatigue.
Avoid bedrest when possible.	Bedrest and sedentary lifestyle can contribute to fatigue.
Collaborate with the health-care team to provide graded aerobic exercise.	Graded aerobic activity offers benefit in cases of fatigue.[73]
Plan care activities around periods of least fatigue.	Gives attention to the patient's circadian rhythm.

(care plan continued on page 346)

NURSING ACTIONS/INTERVENTIONS WITH RATIONALES (continued from page 345)

Home Health/Community Health

ACTIONS/INTERVENTIONS	RATIONALES
Assist the patient and family in identifying risk factors pertinent to the situation: • Chronic disease (e.g., arthritis, cancer, or heart disease) • Medications • Pain • Role strain	Provides additional support for the client and family, and uses already available resources in a cost-effective manner.
Teach the client and family measures to enhance capacity for physical and mental work: • Use of assistive devices as appropriate (wheelchairs, crutches, canes, walkers, adaptive eating utensils, etc.) • Maintain sufficient pain control. • Provide a safe environment to reduce physical barriers to mobility (throw rugs, stairs, blocked pathways, etc.) and decrease potential for accidents. • Provide balance of work and recreational activities. • Assess client/family need for in-home support and provide referrals as needed to appropriate community resources such as tutors, Meals on Wheels, housekeeping assistance, daily hygiene assistance.	Promotes self-care and safety.

GAS EXCHANGE, IMPAIRED

DEFINITION[22]

Excess or deficit in oxygenation and/or carbon dioxide elimination at the alveolar–capillary membrane.

DEFINING CHARACTERISTICS[22]

1. Visual disturbances
2. Increased carbon dioxide
3. Tachycardia
4. Hypercapnia
5. Restlessness
6. Somnolence
7. Irritability
8. Hypoxia
9. Confusion
10. Dyspnea
11. Abnormal arterial blood gases
12. Cyanosis (in neonate only)
13. Abnormal skin color (pale, dusky)
14. Hypoxemia
15. Hypercarbia
16. Headache upon awakening
17. Abnormal rate, rhythm, and depth of breathing
18. Diaphoresis
19. Abnormal arterial pH
20. Nasal flaring

RELATED FACTORS[22]

1. Ventilation perfusion imbalance
2. Alveolar–capillary membrane changes

RELATED CLINICAL CONCERNS

1. Chronic obstructive pulmonary disease (COPD)
2. Congestive heart failure
3. Asthma
4. Pneumonia
5. Pulmonary tuberculosis

 Have You Selected the Correct Diagnosis?

Ineffective Airway Clearance
This diagnosis means that something is blocking the air passage but that, when and if air gets to the alveoli, there is adequate gas exchange. In Impaired Gas Exchange, the air (oxygen) that reaches the alveoli is not sufficiently diffused across the alveolar–capillary membrane.

Ineffective Breathing Pattern
This diagnosis suggests that the rate, rhythm, depth, and type of ventilatory effort are insufficient to bring in enough oxygen or get rid of sufficient amounts of carbon dioxide. These gases are sufficiently exchanged

at the alveoli-circulatory membrane, but the pattern of ventilation makes breathing ineffective.

Decreased Cardiac Output
In this diagnosis, the heart is not pumping a sufficient amount of blood through the lungs to take up enough oxygen or release enough carbon dioxide to meet the body requirements. There is no impairment in the gas exchange, but there is not enough circulating blood to combine with sufficient amounts of oxygen to supply the body's needs.

EXPECTED OUTCOME

Will demonstrate improved blood gases and vital signs by [date]. Note initial blood gas measurements and vital signs here.

TARGET DATES

Because of the extreme danger of Impaired Gas Exchange, progress should be evaluated at least every 8 hours until the client has stabilized. Thereafter, target dates at 3 to 5 days are acceptable.

NURSING ACTIONS/INTERVENTIONS WITH RATIONALES

Adult Health

ACTIONS/INTERVENTIONS	RATIONALES
Perform nursing actions to maintain effective airway clearance. (See Ineffective Airway Clearance for nursing actions, and enter those actions here.)	Clearing airways of secretions improves ventilation–perfusion relationship.
Analyze lab work including arterial blood gases and hemoglobin and hematocrit.	Will provide integral information to determine deficits in capacity and effect of oxygen delivery.
Position the patient to optimize gas exchange:	
• Raise head of bed to 30 degrees or more if not contraindicated.	Facilities chest expansion.
• Position the patient with the "good lung down."	
• Collaborate with the health-care team regarding prone positioning.	Promotes gas exchange and with alveolar recruitment.
Maintain adequate nutrition. Collaborate with diet therapist regarding several small meals per day rather than three large meals.	Decreases energy demand for digestion, and prevents constriction of chest cavity as a result of a full stomach.
Have the patient practice exercises such as incentive spirometer or pursed lipped breathing once every hour while the patient is awake.	Promotes alveolar open.
Provide teaching regarding respiratory exercises:	
• Assume a sitting position with back straight and shoulders relaxed.	
• Use conscious, controlled deep-breathing techniques that expand diaphragm downward (abdomen should rise).	
• Breathe in deeply through the nose, hold for 2 to 3 seconds, and then breathe out slowly through pursed lips. Abdomen will sink down with the exhalation.	
Assist with postural drainage and chest physiotherapy. Teach these exercises to significant other.	
Administer bronchodilators and mucolytic agents as prescribed.	
Collaborate with the health-care team regarding monitoring of blood gases.	Pco_2, Po_2, and O_2 saturation are indicators of the efficiency of gas exchange.
Turn every 2 hours on [odd/even] hour. Encourage the patient's mobility to the extent tolerated without dyspnea.	Position changes modify ventilation–perfusion relationships and enhance gas exchange.

(care plan continued on page 348)

NURSING ACTIONS/INTERVENTIONS WITH RATIONALES (continued from page 347)

Adult Health

ACTIONS/INTERVENTIONS	RATIONALES
Provide for periods of activity and rest.	Conserves energy needed for breathing and decreased oxygen consumption.
Discuss with the patient the effects smoking has on the respiratory system, and refer the patient to a stop smoking group if the patient is motivated to stop smoking. If the patient is not motivated to stop smoking, instruct the patient not to smoke 15 minutes before meals and physical activity.	Smoking, or passive smoke for the nonsmoker, greatly increases the risk for development of respiratory and cardiovascular diseases. Smoking immediately before eating or exercise causes vasoconstriction, leading to decreased gas exchange, and compounding the condition.
Review the patient's resources and home situation regarding long-term management of Impaired Gas Exchange before discharge. Refer to appropriate community resources.	Initiates appropriate home care planning and long-range support for the patient and family.

Child Health

ACTIONS/INTERVENTIONS	RATIONALES
Monitor contributing factors, especially current medical status and respiratory demands.	
Ensure availability of emergency equipment as appropriate: • Ambu bag • Endotracheal tube appropriate for age and size of infant (3.5) • Suctioning unit and catheters: infant, 5 or 8 Fr; child, 8 or 10 Fr • Crash cart with appropriate drugs • Defibrillation unit with guidelines • O_2 tank (check amount of oxygen left) • Tracheostomy sterile set • Sterile chest tube tray	Basic emergency preparedness.
Provide for parental input in planning and implementing care (e.g., comfort measures, assisting with feedings, and daily hygienic measures).	Parental involvement provides emotional security for the child's parents; offers empowerment and allows practicing of care techniques in a supportive environment.
Allow at least 10 to 15 minutes per shift for the family to verbalize concerns regarding the child's status and changes. Encourage the parents to ask questions as often as needed.	Assists in reducing anxiety, and provides teaching opportunity.
Collaborate with related health-care team members as needed.	Promotes coordination of care without undue duplication and fragmentation of care.
While the child is still in the hospital, provide opportunities for the parents and child to master essential skills necessary for long-term care, such as suctioning.	Learning of essential skills is enhanced when opportunities for practice are allowed in a safe, secure environment. Compliance is also fostered.
Schedule parents and family for CPR training well before dismissal from hospital. [Note time and responsible person here.]	Anticipatory need for CPR should better prepare parents and other family members in the event of pulmonary arrest. Having this basic knowledge will assist in reducing anxiety regarding home care.

ACTIONS/INTERVENTIONS	RATIONALES
Facilitate the parents' use of the support system to aid in coping with illness and hospitalization.	Reliance on others should afford the parents some degree of relief from constant worry based on the likelihood of primary needs with a chronically ill child.
Allow for sibling visitation as applicable within institution or specific situation.	Sibling visitation enhances the opportunity for family coping and growth. Provides moral support to both siblings.
Administer medications that are ordered. Monitor for variable response in child especially antibiotics, corticosteroids (inhaled and IV).	Provides anticipatory guidance with safe administration of medications.
Teach the child and family about needs for follow-up care and protection from triggering events, including exposure to respiratory infections.	Reinforces need for realistic plan of follow-up and anticipatory prevention.
Refer to appropriate community agencies for support after discharge. [Note those referral agencies here.]	Offers support to child and family.

Women's Health

● N O T E : *This nursing diagnosis will pertain to women the same as in any other adult. The following nursing actions focus only on the fetal–placental unit during pregnancy. Placental function is totally dependent on maternal circulation; therefore, any process that interferes with maternal circulation will affect the oxygen consumption of the placenta and, in turn, the fetus.*

ACTIONS/INTERVENTIONS	RATIONALES
Assist the patient in developing an exercise plan during pregnancy.	Increases cardiovascular fitness, and therefore increases oxygenation and nutrition to placenta and fetus.
Teach the patient and significant others how to avoid "supine hypotension" during pregnancy (particularly during the later stages):	
• Lying on right or left side to reduce pressure on vena cava	
• Taking frequent rest breaks during the day	
Assist the patient in identifying lifestyle adjustments that may be needed because of changes in physiologic function or needs during pregnancy:	
• Stop smoking.	
• Reduce exposure to secondhand smoke.	
• Avoid lying in the supine position.	
• Take no drugs unless advised to do so by physician.	
Identify underlying maternal diseases that will affect the fetal–placental unit during pregnancy:	These disorders have direct impact on the gas exchange in the fetal–placental unit.
• Maternal origin:	
• Maternal hypertension	
• Drug addiction	
• Diabetes mellitus with vascular involvement	
• Sickle cell anemia	
• Maternal infections	
• Maternal smoking	
• Hemorrhage (abruptio placentae or placenta previa)	

(care plan continued on page 350)

NURSING ACTIONS/INTERVENTIONS WITH RATIONALES (continued from page 349)

Women's Health

ACTIONS/INTERVENTIONS	RATIONALES
• Fetal origin: • Premature or prolonged rupture of membranes • Intrauterine infection • RH disease • Multiple pregnancy	

Mental Health

In addition to the nursing interventions for Adult Health, the following interventions apply to specific Mental Health situations:

ACTIONS/INTERVENTIONS	RATIONALES
If the client is demonstrating alterations in mental status, assess for increased hypoxia.	The central nervous system is particularly sensitive to impaired gas exchange because of its reliance on simple sugar metabolism for energy production.[66]
Observe the client for signs of respiratory infection.	Infection will increase mucus production, which decreases airway clearance.[66]
Protect the client from respiratory infection by: • Maintaining proper humidity in the environment. • Observe the client closely for signs and symptoms of respiratory infection. If infection is present, and the client is sharing a room, move the roommate to another room. • Arrange staff assignments so that staff who care for clients with infections are not also caring for clients who are free of infection. • Keeping the client away from crowds. • Assisting the client in obtaining appropriate immunizations against influenza. • Having the client inform staff of signs or symptoms of respiratory infection when the earliest symptoms appear. • Keeping environment as free of respiratory irritants as possible (e.g., dust, allergens, or pollution). • Provide the client with equipment required to maintain adequate oxygenation. [Note that equipment and special adaptations here.] • Collaborate with respiratory therapy to provide client education about proper use of the equipment.	Prevents further injury to a system that is stressed, and promotes airway patency.
Discuss with the client the effects of alcohol and other depressant drugs on the respiratory system. Refer to a drug-abuse recovery program as necessary.	The sedative effects of some drugs decrease airway clearance, increasing the risk for the development of infection. Diffusion is also decreased with chronic alcoholism.[77]
Collaborate with physician regarding supplemental vitamins, especially thiamine, if the impaired gas exchange is secondary to alcohol abuse.	Thiamine is essential for the conversion of glucose to metabolically useful forms. Nerve cell function depends on this glucose. This compensates for the nutritional deficits that result when nutritional calories are replaced by alcohol.[78]

ACTIONS/INTERVENTIONS	RATIONALES
Spend [number] minutes [number] times a day with the client discussing feelings and reactions to current situation. As feelings are expressed, begin to explore lifestyle changes with the client. Refer to Ineffective Individual Coping (Chapter 11) and Powerlessness (Chapter 8) for specific care plans related to coping styles.	Promotes the client's sense of control by facilitating understanding of factors that contribute to maladaptive coping behaviors.
Develop with the client a plan for gradually increasing physical activity. (See Activity Intolerance for specific behavioral interventions.)	Improves cardiorespiratory functioning, thus improving gas exchange.

Gerontic Health

ACTIONS/INTERVENTIONS	RATIONALES
Ensure that oxygen delivery system is properly functioning and fits well. Avoid face mask if the patient is emaciated. Check proper positioning of nasal cannula (prongs turned inward), and ensure that all oxygen is humidified.	Basic care standards.
Monitor skin color, mental status, and vital signs every 2 hours on [odd/even] hour.	
Check oxygen flow and amount every 4 hours around the clock at [times].	The patient may increase the liter flow during acute episodes of impaired gas exchange and cause respiratory system depression with retention of carbon dioxide.
Monitor for potential carbon dioxide narcosis (e.g., changes in level of consciousness, changes in oxygen and carbon dioxide blood gas levels, flushing, decreased respiratory rate, and headaches). This is especially important for a patient on long-term oxygen therapy.[58]	
Teach the patient and family the signs and symptoms of carbon dioxide narcosis, especially those on long-term oxygen therapy.	Decreases potential for carbon dioxide narcosis.

Home Health

● N O T E : *If this diagnosis is suspected when caring for a client in the home, it is imperative that a physician referral be obtained immediately. If a physician has referred the client to home health care, the nurse will collaborate with the physician in the treatment of the client. Preliminary research[77] indicates that women with chronic bronchitis or chronic obstructive pulmonary disease (COPD) cannot walk as far as men. Activity should be planned according to tolerance, keeping in mind gender differences. There is no doubt that better control of dyspnea is a pressing need, with research[79] indicating that a client's subjective report of health status is a better predictor of level of functioning than is objective measure of the lung function.*

ACTIONS/INTERVENTIONS	RATIONALES
Teach the client and family appropriate monitoring of signs and symptoms of Impaired Gas Exchange:	Provides for early recognition and intervention for problem.

(care plan continued on page 352)

NURSING ACTIONS/INTERVENTIONS WITH RATIONALES (continued from page 351)

Home Health

ACTIONS/INTERVENTIONS	RATIONALES
• Pursed-lip breathing • Respiratory status: cyanosis, rate, dyspnea, or orthopnea • Fatigue • Use of accessory muscles • Cough • Sputum production or change in sputum production • Edema • Decreased urinary output • Gasping	
Assist the client and family in identifying lifestyle changes that may be required:	Provides basic information for the client and family that promotes necessary lifestyle changes.
Prevention of Impaired Gas Exchange: Stopping smoking, prevention or early treatment of lung infections, avoidance of known irritants and allergens, obtaining annual influenza and pneumonia immunizations. • Pulmonary hygiene: clearing bronchial tree by controlled coughing, decreasing viscosity of secretions via humidity and fluid balance, and postural drainage • Daily activity as tolerated (remove physical barriers to mobility/activity) • Breathing techniques to decrease work of breathing (diaphragmatic, pursed lips, or sitting forward) • Adequate nutrition intake • Appropriate use of oxygen (dosage, route of administration, safety factors). Ensure that the patient and caregiver understand the risks associated with smoking in the presence of supplemental oxygen. • Stress management • Limiting exposure to upper respiratory infections • Avoiding extreme hot or cold temperatures • Keeping area free of animal hair and dander or dust • Assistive devices required (oxygen, nasal cannula, suction, ventilator, etc.) • Adequate hydration (monitor intake and output)	
Teach the client and family purposes, side effects, and proper administration technique of medications.	To promote adequate self-care and to prevent complications from untoward medication side effects.
Assist the client and family to set criteria to help them determine when calling a physician or other intervention is required (e.g., change in skin color, increased difficulty with breathing, increase or change in sputum production, or fever).	To promote adequate self-care and facilitate timely acquisition of professional health care as needed.
Teach the family basic CPR.	Basic safety measure.
Assess the client/family need for additional resources and refer to community resources, as appropriate.	Provides additional support for the client and family, and uses already available resources in a cost-effective manner.

GROWTH AND DEVELOPMENT, DELAYED; DISPROPORTIONATE GROWTH, RISK FOR; DELAYED DEVELOPMENT, RISK FOR

DEFINITIONS[22]

Delayed Growth and Development   The state in which an individual demonstrates deviations in norms from his or her age group.

   Risk for Disproportionate Growth   At risk for growth above the 97th percentile, or below the 3rd percentile for age, crossing two percentile channels; or disproportionate growth.

   Risk for Delayed Development   At risk for delay of 25 percent or more in one or more of the areas of social or self-regulatory behaviors, or cognitive, language, gross, or fine motor skills.

DEFINING CHARACTERISTICS[22]

A. Delayed Growth and Development
   1. Altered physical growth
   2. Delay or difficulty in performing skills (motor, social, or expressive) typical of age group
   3. Inability to perform self-care or self-control activities appropriate to age
   4. Flat affect
   5. Listlessness
   6. Decreased responses

B. Risk for Disproportionate Growth
   1. Prenatal
      a. Congenital or genetic disorders
      b. Maternal nutrition
      c. Multiple gestation
      d. Teratogen exposure
      e. Substance use or abuse
      f. Infection
   2. Individual
      a. Infection
      b. Prematurity
      c. Malnutrition
      d. Organic and inorganic factors
      e. Caregiver and/or individual maladaptive feeding behaviors
      f. Anorexia
      g. Insatiable appetite
      h. Chronic illness
      i. Substance abuse
   3. Environmental
      a. Deprivation
      b. Teratogen
      c. Lead poisoning
      d. Poverty
      e. Violence
      f. Natural disasters

   4. Caregiver
      a. Abuse
      b. Mental illness
      c. Mental retardation
      d. Severe learning disability

C. Risk for Delayed Development
   1. Prenatal
      a. Maternal age less than 15 or greater than 35 years
      b. Substance abuse
      c. Infections
      d. Genetic or endocrine disorders
      e. Unplanned or unwanted pregnancies
      f. Lack of, late, or poor prenatal care
      g. Inadequate nutrition
      h. Illiteracy
      i. Poverty
   2. Individual
      a. Prematurity
      b. Seizures
      c. Congenital or genetic disorders
      d. Positive drug screening test
      e. Brain damage (e.g., hemorrhage in postnatal period, shaken baby, abuse, accident)
      f. Vision impairment
      g. Hearing impairment or frequent otitis media
      h. Chronic illness
      i. Technology-dependent
      j. Failure to thrive
      k. Inadequate nutrition
      l. Foster or adopted child
      m. Lead poisoning
      n. Chemotherapy
      o. Radiation therapy
      p. Natural disaster
      q. Behavioral disorder
      r. Substance abuse
   3. Environmental
      a. Poverty
      b. Violence
   4. Caregiver
      a. Abuse
      b. Mental illness
      c. Mental retardation or severe learning disability

RELATED FACTORS[22]

A. Delayed Growth and Development
   1. Prescribed dependence
   2. Indifference
   3. Separation from significant others
   4. Environmental and stimulation deficiencies
   5. Effects of physical disability
   6. Inadequate caretaking
   7. Inconsistent responsiveness
   8. Multiple caretakers

B. Risk for Disproportionate Growth
The risk factors also serve as the related factors.
C. Risk for Delayed Development
The risk factors also serve as the related factors.

RELATED CLINICAL CONCERNS

1. Hypothyroidism
2. Failure to thrive syndrome
3. Leukemia
4. Deficient growth hormone
5. Personality disorders
6. Schizophrenic disorders
7. Substance abuse
8. Dementia
9. Delirium

 Have You Selected the Correct Diagnosis?

Disturbed Sensory Perception
This diagnosis should be considered when blindness, deafness, or neurologic impairment is present. Assisting the patient to adapt to these problems could resolve any developmental problems.

Impaired Physical Mobility
When physical disabilities are present, they can definitely impact growth and development. In this example, Impaired Physical Mobility and Delayed

Growth and Development would be companion diagnoses.

Imbalanced Nutrition, Less Than Body Requirements
Lack of essential vitamins and minerals will also show a direct link to Delayed Growth and Development. Assessment should be implemented for both diagnoses.

The nursing diagnoses grouped under Self-Perception and Self-Concept Pattern, Role-Relationship Pattern, and Coping-Stress Tolerance Pattern should also be considered when alterations in growth and development are present.

EXPECTED OUTCOME

Will return, as nearly as possible, to expected growth and development parameter for [specify exact parameter] by [date].

TARGET DATES

Assisting in modifying Delayed Growth and Development factors will require significant time; therefore, an initial target date of 7 to 10 days would be reasonable for evaluating progress.

NURSING ACTIONS/INTERVENTIONS WITH RATIONALES

Adult Health

● N O T E : *Nursing actions for this diagnosis are varied and complex and incorporate nursing actions associated with other nursing diagnoses. For example, the patient may have either a total self-care deficit or a deficit in hygiene, grooming, feeding, or toileting. For an adult, any of these would be an alteration in growth and development. Therefore, it would be appropriate to include the nursing actions associated with these nursing diagnoses in the nursing actions for Delayed Growth and Development.*

An adult is generally able to find or initiate diversional and social activities. However, if the adult does not participate in diversional or social activities, it could indicate Delayed Growth and Development. Therefore, the nursing actions associated with Deficient Diversional Activity and Social Isolation would be appropriate to be included in the nursing actions for Delayed Growth and Development.

ACTIONS/INTERVENTIONS	RATIONALES
In general, the nurse should provide adequate opportunities for the patient to be successful in whatever task he or she is attempting.	Success increases motivation.
Reward and reinforce success, however minor. Downplay relapses. Allow the patient to be as independent as possible.	Increases self-esteem and active participation in care.
Have consistent, nonjudgmental, caring people in the caregiving role.	Caring people instill confidence in a patient and willingness to try new tasks.
Work collaboratively with other health-care professionals and with the patient and family in developing a plan of care.	Facilitates development of a plan that all will use consistently.

Child Health

ACTIONS/INTERVENTIONS	RATIONALES
Monitor and teach the parents to monitor the child's growth and development status. Determine what alterations there are (i.e., delays or precocity).	As a rule, single assessments are not as revealing in growth and development parameters as are serial, longitudinal patterns. Parental involvement offers a more thorough monitoring, fosters their involvement with the child, and empowers the family.
Determine what other primary health-care needs exist, especially brain damage or residuals of brain damage.	In instances of brain damage or retardation, it is often difficult to get an accurate assessment of cognitive capability. The general health of the patient will often influence, to a major degree, what alteration in cognitive functioning exists (e.g., sickle cell anemia with resultant infarcts to major organs such as the brain).
Identify, with the child or the parents, realistic goals for growth and development.	A plan of care based on individual needs, with parental input, better reflects holistic care and increases probability of effective home management of problem.
Collaborate with related health-care team members as necessary. [Note those providers involved here with a plan for their involvement.]	Collaboration is required for meeting the special long-term needs for activities of daily living.
Identify anticipatory safety for the child related to Delayed Growth and Development (e.g., ingestion of objects, falls, or use of wheelchair). [Note special safety adaptations that are needed for this child here.]	These children may be large physically because of chronologic age, and there is a possibility of overlooking the developmental or mental age.
Teach parents special diet necessitated by a metabolic disorder (e.g., various enzymes lacking).	Appropriate diet can assist in preventing further deterioration or be essential to replace lacking vitamins, enzymes, or other nutrients.
Refer the child and parents to appropriate community resources to assist in fostering growth and development, such as the early childhood intervention services.	Offering early intervention assists in fostering development, while preventing tertiary delays.
Assist the parents to provide for learning needs related to future development, including identification of schools for developmentally delayed children.	Appropriate match of services to needs enhances the child's development to the highest level possible.
Refer the child and parents to state and national support groups such as National Cerebral Palsy Association.	Support groups assist in empowerment and advocacy at local, state, and national levels.
Provide the patient and family with long-term follow-up appointments before discharge.	Promotes implementation of management regimen, and provides anticipatory resources and checkpoint for the patient and family.

Women's Health

● N O T E : *The same nursing diagnosis pertains to Women's Health as to Adult Health. The following nursing actions pertain only to women with reproductive anatomic abnormalities. The mother does need to be aware of the normal growth patterns in order to assess the health and development of her child. See Child Health.*

ACTIONS/INTERVENTIONS	RATIONALES
Obtain a thorough sexual and obstetric history, especially noting recurrent miscarriages in the first 3 months of pregnancy.	Provides a basic database for determining therapy needs.
Collaborate with the physician regarding assessment for infertility.	

(care plan continued on page 356)

NURSING ACTIONS/INTERVENTIONS WITH RATIONALES (continued from page 355)

Women's Health

ACTIONS/INTERVENTIONS	RATIONALES
Refer to a gynecologist for further testing if primary amenorrhea is present.	
Encourage the patient to verbalize her concerns and fears.	Decreases anxiety. Allows an opportunity for teaching, and allows correction of any misinformation.
Encourage communication with significant others to identify concerns and explore options available.	Provides a base for teaching and long-range counseling.

Mental Health

● N O T E : *If anorexia nervosa is the underlying cause for growth risk, refer to the Mental Health care plan for the diagnosis Imbalanced Nutrition, Less Than Body Requirements, for the appropriate intervention.*

ACTIONS/INTERVENTIONS	RATIONALES
Provide a quiet, nonstimulating environment, or an environment that does not place additional stress on an already overwhelmed coping ability.	Too little or too much sensory input can result in a sense of disorganization and confusion and result in dysfunctional coping behaviors.[35]
Sit with the client [number] minutes [number] times per day at [list specific times] to discuss current concerns and feelings.	Attention from the nurse can enhance self-esteem. Expression of feelings can facilitate identification and resolutions of problematic coping behaviors.
Provide the client with familiar or needed objects. These should be noted here.	Promotes the client's sense of control by providing an environment in which the client feels safe and secure.
Discuss with the client perceptions of self, others, and the current situation. This should include the client's perceptions of harm, loss, or threat. Assist the client in altering perception of these situations so they can be seen as challenges or opportunities for growth rather than threats.	Provides positive orientation, which improves self-esteem and provides hope for the future.
Provide the client with an environment that will optimize sensory input. This could include hearing aids, eyeglasses, pencil and paper, decreased noise in conversation areas, and appropriate lighting. These interventions should indicate an awareness of sensory deficit as well a sensory overload, and the specific interventions for the client should be noted here (e.g., place hearing aid in when the client awakens, and remove before bedtime).	Appropriate levels of sensory input promote contact with the reality of the environment, which facilitates appropriate coping.
Provide the client with achievable tasks, activities, and goals (these should be listed here). These activities should be provided with increasing complexity to give the client an increasing sense of accomplishment and mastery.	Provides positive reinforcement, which enhances self-esteem and provides motivation for working toward the next goal.

ACTIONS/INTERVENTIONS	RATIONALES
Communicate to the client an understanding that all coping behavior to this point has been his or her best effort and asking for assistance at this time is not failure. Explain that a complex problem often requires some outside assistance in resolution. (This will assist the client in maintaining self-esteem and diminish feelings of failure.)	Promotes positive orientation, which enhances self-esteem and promotes hope.
Provide the client with opportunities to make appropriate decisions related to care at his or her level of ability. This may begin as a choice between two options and then evolve into more complex decision making. It is important that this be at the client's level of functioning so confidence can be built with successful decision-making experiences.	Promotes the client's perception of control, which promotes self-esteem.
Provide constructive confrontation for the client about problematic coping behavior. (See Wilson and Kneisl[32] for guidelines on constructive confrontation.) The kinds of behavior identified by the treatment team as problematic should be listed here.	Provides opportunities for the client to question aspects of behavior that can promote a desire to change.
Provide the client with opportunities to practice new kinds of behavior either by role playing or by applying them to graded real-life experiences.	Provides opportunities to practice new behavior in a safe environment where the nurse can provide positive feedback for gradual improvement of coping strategies. This increases the probability for the success of the new behavior in real-life situations, which in turn serves as positive reinforcement for behavior change.
Provide positive social reinforcement and other behavioral rewards for demonstration of adaptive behavior. (Those things that the client finds rewarding should be listed here with a schedule for use. The kinds of behavior that are to be rewarded should also be listed.)	Positive reinforcement encourages appropriate behavior.
Assist the client in identifying support systems and in developing a plan for their use.	Support systems can provide positive reinforcement for behavior change, increasing the opportunities for the client's success enhancing self-esteem.
Assist the client with setting appropriate limits on aggressive behavior by (see Risk for Violence, Chapter 9, for detailed nursing actions if this is an appropriate diagnosis):	Excessive environmental stimuli can increase a sense of disorganization and confusion.
• Decreasing environmental stimulation as appropriate. (This might include a secluded environment.)	
• Providing the client with appropriate alternative outlets for physical tension. (This should be stated specifically and could include walking, running, talking with a staff member, using a punching bag, listening to music, or doing a deep muscle relaxation sequence. These outlets should be selected with the client's input.)	Promotes a sense of control, and teaches constructive ways to cope with stressors.
Meet with the client and support system to provide information on the client's situation and to develop a plan that will involve the support system in making changes that will facilitate the client's movement to age-appropriate behavior. [Note this plan here.]	Enhances opportunities for success of the treatment plan.
Refer to appropriate assistive resources as indicated.	

(care plan continued on page 358)

NURSING ACTIONS/INTERVENTIONS WITH RATIONALES (continued from page 357)

Gerontic Health

Nursing interventions provided in the Adult Health and Home Health sections for this diagnosis may be enhanced for the older client with the addition of the following actions.

ACTIONS/INTERVENTIONS	RATIONALES
Provide opportunities for clients to reflect on their strengths and life accomplishments through activities such as life review, reminiscing, and oral or written autobiographies.	Promotes ability to obtain perspective on life experiences.[80] Provides potential for enhancing life satisfaction.[80]
Consult with the physician for potential assessment and treatment of depression.	Depression often goes undetected in older adults and may negatively impact their ability to effectively cope with losses and to positively appraise their current situation.[80]
Ask older clients what tasks of aging they have defined for themselves.	Promotes discussion of the older adult's expectations.[81]

Home Health

ACTIONS/INTERVENTIONS	RATIONALES
Monitor for factors contributing to Delayed Growth and Development.	Provides a database for prevention and/or early intervention.
Involve the client and family in planning, implementing, and promoting reduction or correction of the delay in growth and development: • Family conference • Mutual goal setting • Communication	Involvement improves motivation and improves the outcome.
Teach the client and family measures to prevent or decrease delays in growth and development: • Explain expected norms of growth and development with anticipatory guidance. If the caretakers realize, for example, that the newborn begins to roll over by 2 to 4 months or that the 2-year-old can follow simple directions, then appropriate environmental and learning conditions can be provided to protect the child and to promote optimal development. • Alert the parents to signs and symptoms of alterations in growth and development that may require professional evaluation (e.g., delay in language skills, delay in crawling or walking, or delay in growth below 50 percent on growth chart). • Teach parents how to recognize developmental milestones and their expected/associated behaviors and how to discipline effectively without violence. • Provide guidance on developmentally appropriate nutrition (e.g., how to introduce finger foods to toddlers, how to monitor calorie intake for expected developmental stage, and how to ensure a balanced diet).	Locus of control shifts from nurse to the client and family, thus promoting self-care.
Assist the client and family to identify lifestyle changes that may be required: • Care for handicaps (e.g., blindness, deafness, or musculoskeletal or cognitive deficit)	Provides basic information for the client and family that promotes necessary lifestyle changes.

ACTIONS/INTERVENTIONS	RATIONALES
• Proper use of assistive equipment • Adapting to need for assistance or assistive equipment • Determining criteria for monitoring the client's ability to function unassisted • Time management • Stress management • Development of support systems • Learning new skills • Work, family, social, and personal goals and priorities • Coping with disability or dependency • Development of consistent routine • Mechanism for alerting family members to the need for assistance • Providing appropriate balance of dependence and independence	
Assess the client/caregiver need for assistive equipment or supplies and assist the client and family to obtain assistive equipment as required (depending on alteration present and its severity): • Adaptive equipment for eating utensils, combs, brushes, etc. • Straw and straw holder • Wheelchair, walker, motorized cart, or cane • Bedside commode or incontinence undergarments • Hearing aid • Corrective lenses • Dressing aids: dressing stick, zipper pull, button hook, long-handled shoehorn, shoe fasteners, or Velcro closures • Bars and attachments and benches for shower or tub • Handheld shower device • Medication organizers • Magnifying glass • Raised toilet seat	Assistive equipment improves function and increases the possibilities for self-care.
Assess the client/family need for in home assistance (daily hygiene, housework, meal delivery services) and refer to community resources as appropriate.	Provides additional support for the client and family, and uses already available resources in a cost-effective manner.
Assist the client or caregivers in obtaining prescribed medications, and ensure that they understand doses, administration times, therapeutic effects, and possible side effects.	Promotes adherence to the therapeutic regimen.
If the client is a child, the nurse can serve as a liaison between the school nurse, family, and primary physician to monitor effectiveness of therapy and to provide anticipatory guidance for family members.	Provides continuity of care.
Instruct the client as appropriate and the caregivers to maintain a consistent home environment (e.g., schedules, parenting, and goal setting). The home environment should be free of distractions when it is necessary for the client to perform tasks.	Consistency can promote success and focus on the strengths of the client.
Refer clients and family members for counseling, special training (e.g., parenting classes), or support groups as necessary.	Helps develop healthier self-esteem and positive coping strategies.

HOME MAINTENANCE, IMPAIRED

DEFINITION[22]

Inability to independently maintain a safe growth-promoting immediate environment.[21]

DEFINING CHARACTERISTICS[22]

1. Objective
   a. Overtaxed family members, for example, exhausted, anxious
   b. Unwashed or unavailable cooking equipment, clothes, or linen
   c. Repeated hygienic disorders, infestations, or infections
   d. Accumulation of dirt, food wastes, or hygienic wastes
   e. Disorderly surroundings
   f. Presence of vermin or rodents
   g. Inappropriate household temperature
   h. Lack of necessary equipment or aids
   i. Offensive odors
2. Subjective
   a. Household members express difficulty in maintaining their home in a comfortable fashion.
   b. Household members describe outstanding debts or financial crises.
   c. Household members request assistance with home maintenance.

RELATED FACTORS[22]

1. Individual or family member disease or injury
2. Unfamiliarity with neighborhood resources
3. Lack of role modeling
4. Lack of knowledge
5. Insufficient family organization or planning
6. Impaired cognitive or emotional functioning
7. Inadequate support systems
8. Insufficient finances

RELATED CLINICAL CONCERNS

1. Dementia problems, such as Alzheimer's disease
2. Rheumatoid arthritis
3. Depression
4. Cerebrovascular accident
5. Acquired immunodeficiency syndrome (AIDS)

 Have You Selected the Correct Diagnosis?

Activity Intolerance
If the nurse observes or validates reports of the patient's inability to complete required tasks because of insufficient energy, then Activity Intolerance would be the more appropriate diagnosis.

Deficient Knowledge
The problem with home maintenance may be due to the family's lack of education regarding the care needed and the environment that is essential to promote this care. If the patient or family verbalizes less-than-adequate understanding of home maintenance, then Deficient Knowledge is the more appropriate diagnosis.

Disturbed Thought Process
If the patient is exhibiting impaired attention span; impaired ability to recall information; impaired perception, judgment, and decision making; or impaired conceptual and reasoning ability, the most proper diagnosis would be Disturbed Thought Process. Most likely, Impaired Home Management would be a companion diagnosis.

Ineffective Individual Coping or Compromised or Disabled Family Coping
Suspect one of these diagnoses if there are major differences between reports by the patient and the family of health status, health perception, and health care behavior. Verbalizations by the patient or the family regarding inability to cope also require looking at these diagnoses.

Interrupted Family Processes
Through observing family interactions and communication, the nurse may assess that Interrupted Family Processes should be considered. Poorly communicated messages, rigidity of family functions and roles, and failure to accomplish expected family developmental tasks are a few observations to alert the nurse to this possible diagnosis.

EXPECTED OUTCOME

Will demonstrate alterations necessary to reduce Impaired Home Maintenance by [date].

Will describe a plan to improve household safety by [date].

Describes plan for allocation of family responsibilities to maintain home in a safe comfortable condition by [date].

TARGET DATES

Target dates will depend on the severity of the Impaired Home Maintenance. Acceptable target dates for the first evaluation of progress toward meeting this outcome would be 5 to 7 days.

NURSING ACTIONS/INTERVENTIONS WITH RATIONALES

Adult Health

A nurse in an acute care facility might receive enough information while the patient is hospitalized to make this nursing diagnosis. However, nursing actions specific for this diagnosis will require implementation in the home environment; therefore, the reader is referred to the Home Health nursing actions for this diagnosis.

Child Health

ACTIONS/INTERVENTIONS	RATIONALES
Monitor risk factors of or contributing factors to Impaired Home Maintenance, to include: • Addition of a family member (e.g., birth) • Increased burden of care as a result of the child's illness or hospitalization • Lack of sufficient finances • Loss of family member (e.g., death) • Hygienic practices • History of repeated infections or poor health management • Offensive odors	Provides primary database for intervention.
Identify ways to deal with home maintenance alterations with assistance of applicable health team members.	Coordinated activities will be required to meet the entire range of needs related to improving problems with home maintenance.
Allow for individual patient and parental input in plan for addressing home maintenance issues.	Parental input offers empowerment and attaches value to family preferences. This in turn increases the likelihood of compliance.
Monitor educational needs related to illness and the demands of the situation (e.g., mother who must attend to a handicapped child and six other children with various school appointments, health care appointments, etc.)	Monitoring of educational needs balanced with the home situation will best provide a base for intervention.
Provide health teaching with sensitivity to the patient and family situation (e.g., seeming inability to manage with overwhelming demands of the child's need for care, such as a premature infant or a child with cerebral palsy who has feeding difficulties).	Teaching to address identified needs reduces anxiety and promotes self-confidence in ability to manage.
Provide 10 to 15 minutes each 8-hour shift as a time for discussion of patient and family feelings and concerns related to health management.	Setting aside times for discussion shows respect and assigns value to the patient and family.
Provide the patient and family with information about support groups in the community. Arrange contact with groups that would provide the most support before discharge.	Support groups empower and facilitate family coping.
If the infant is at risk for sudden infant death syndrome (SIDS) by nature of prematurity or history of previous death in family, assist parents in learning about alarms and monitoring respiration, and institute CPR teaching.	When risk factors for pulmonary arrest are present as, for example, for a SIDS infant, family members will be less anxious if they are taught CPR techniques and given opportunities to rehearse and master these techniques.
Refer to community and primary care providers for follow-up after discharge from the hospital.	Follow-up plans provide a means of further evaluation for progress in coping with home maintenance. Ideally, actual home visitation allows the best opportunity for monitoring goal achievement.

(care plan continued on page 362)

Women's Health

ACTIONS/INTERVENTIONS	RATIONALES
Assist the client to describe her perception or understanding of home maintenance as it relates to her lifestyle and lifestyle decisions. Include stress-related problems and effects of environment: • Allow the patient time to describe work situation. • Allow the patient time to describe the home situation. • Encourage the patient to describe how she manages her responsibilities as a mother and a working woman. • Encourage the patient to describe her assets and deficits as she perceives them. • Encourage the patient to list lifestyle adjustments that need to be made. • Monitor identified possible solutions, modifications, etc., designed to cope with each adjustment. • Teach the client relaxation skills and coping mechanisms.	Provides a database needed to plan changes that will increase ability in home maintenance.
Consider the patient's social network and significant others: • Identify significant others in the patient's social network. • Involve significant others if so desired by the patient in discussion and problem-solving activities regarding lifestyle adjustments.	
Encourage the patient to get adequate rest: • Take care of self and baby only. • Let significant others take care of the housework and other children. • Learn to sleep when the baby sleeps. • Have specific, set times for friends or relatives to visit. • If breastfeeding, significant other can change the infant and bring the infant to the mother at night so that the mother does not always have to get up for the infant. Or the mother can sleep with the infant. • Cook several meals at one time for the family and freeze them for later use. • Prepare baby formula for a 24-hour period and refrigerate for later use. • Freeze breast milk, emptying the breast after the baby eats; significant other can then feed the infant one time at night so the mother can get adequate, uninterrupted sleep. • Put breast milk into a bottle and directly into the freezer: 　• Milk can be added each time breasts are pumped until the needed amount is obtained. 　• Milk can be frozen for 6 weeks if needed. 　• To use, milk should be removed from the freezer and allowed to thaw to room temperature. 　• Once thawed, must be used within a 12- to 24-hour period. **Do not refreeze.**	Fatigue can be a major contributor to impaired home maintenance. Both the parents and infant get more rest. The baby begins to nurse longer and sleep for longer periods of time.

Mental Health

ACTIONS/INTERVENTIONS	RATIONALES
Discuss with the client his or her concerns about returning home.	Promotes the client's sense of control, which enhances self-esteem.
Develop with the client and significant others a list of potential home maintenance problems.	Promotes the client's and support system's sense of control, which increases the willingness of the client to work on goals.
Teach the client and family tasks that are necessary for home care. [NOTE tasks and teaching plan here.]	Provides opportunities for positive reinforcement of approximation of goal achievement.
Provide time to practice home maintenance skills, at least 30 minutes once a day. Medication administration could be evaluated with each dose by allowing the client to administer own medications. The times and types of skills to be practiced should be listed here.	
If financial difficulties prevent home maintenance, refer to social services or a financial counselor.	
If the client has not learned skills necessary to cook or clean home, arrange a time with occupational therapist to assess for ability and to teach these skills. Support this learning on unit by [check all that apply]: • Having the client maintain own living area. • Having the client assist with the maintenance of the unit (state specifically those chores the client is responsible for). • Having the client assist with the planning and preparation of unit meals when this is a milieu activity. • Having the client clean and iron own clothing.	Provides opportunities to practice new skills in a safe environment and to receive positive reinforcement for approximation of goal achievement.
If special aids are necessary for the client to maintain self successfully, refer to social services for assistance in obtaining these items.	
If the client needs periodic assistance in organizing self to maintain home, refer to homemaker service or other community agency.	
If meal preparation is a problem, refer to community agency for Meals-on-Wheels, or assist the family with preparing several meals ahead of time or exploring nutritious, easy ways to prepare meals.	
Determine with the client a list of rewards for meeting the established goals for achievement of home maintenance, and then develop a schedule for the rewards. [Note the reward schedule here.]	Positive reinforcement encourages the maintenance of new behavior.
Assess the environment for impairments to home maintenance, and develop with the client and family a plan for resolving these difficulties (e.g., recipes that are simplified and written in large print to make them easier to follow).	
Provide appropriate positive verbal reinforcers for accomplishment of goals or steps toward the goals.	Positive reinforcement encourages maintenance of new behaviors.
Utilize group therapy once a day to provide: • Positive role models • Peer support • Realistic assessment of goals	

(care plan continued on page 364)

NURSING ACTIONS/INTERVENTIONS WITH RATIONALES (continued from page 363)	

Adult Health

ACTIONS/INTERVENTIONS	RATIONALES
• Exposure to a variety of problem solutions • Socialization and learning of social skills Refer to a home health agency for continued support after discharge. • Provide the client and family with contact information for the agency so that a relationship can be established before discharge.	This will increase the potential for community follow-up after discharge.

Gerontic Health

Nursing actions for Adult and Home Health are appropriate for the older adult. The nurse may provide information on resources that target the elderly, such as the area Agency on Aging; local support groups for people with chronic illnesses; and city, county, or state resources for the elderly.

Home Health/Community Health

ACTIONS/INTERVENTIONS	RATIONALES
Monitor factors contributing to Impaired Home Maintenance (items listed under related factors section).	Provides database for prevention and/or early intervention.
Involve the patient and family in planning, implementing, and promoting reduction in the Impaired Home Maintenance: • Family conference • Mutual goal setting • Communication • Family members given specified tasks as appropriate to reduce the Impaired Home Maintenance (shopping, washing clothes, disposing of garbage and trash, yard work, washing dishes, meal preparation, etc.)	Involvement improves motivation and improves the outcome.
Assist the patient and family in lifestyle adjustments that may be required: • Hygiene practices—obtaining assistance from family members, friends, or community agencies may be required. • Elimination of drug and alcohol use—refer the client to sources of assistance such as Alcoholics Anonymous, physicians who specialize in treatment of substance abuse, or support groups. • Stress management techniques – teach client stress management techniques and refer as needed to community resources for stress management (support groups, therapists). • Family and community support systems—refer the client/family to community resources. • Removal of hazardous environmental conditions, such as improper storage of hazardous substances, open heaters and flames, breeding areas for mosquitoes or mice, or congested walkways.	Provides basic information for the client and family that promotes necessary lifestyle changes.

ACTIONS/INTERVENTIONS	RATIONALES
• Proper food preparation and storage—teach the client/family safety measures for food preparation and storage, assist client to obtain materials to facilitate safe food handling when indicated.	
Assess the client/family's need for additional assistive resources and refer to appropriate community agencies as indicated.	Provides additional support for the client and family, and uses already available resources in a cost-effective manner.

INFANT BEHAVIOR, DISORGANIZED, RISK FOR AND ACTUAL, AND READINESS FOR ENHANCED ORGANIZED

DEFINITION[22]

Risk for Disorganized Infant Behavior Risk for alteration and modulation of the physiologic and behavioral systems of functioning, that is, autonomic, motor, state, organizational, self-regulatory, and attention–interaction systems.

DEFINING CHARACTERISTICS[22]

Risk for Disorganized Infant Behavior (Risk Factors)

1. Invasive or painful procedures
2. Lack of containment or boundaries
3. Oral or motor problems
4. Prematurity
5. Pain
6. Environmental overstimulation

DEFINITION[22]

Disorganized Infant Behavior Disintegrated physiologic and neurologic responses to the environment.

DEFINING CHARACTERISTICS[22]

A. Regulatory Problems
  1. Inability to inhibit startle response
  2. Irritability
B. State-Organization System
  1. Active–awake (fussy, worried gaze)
  2. Diffuse/unclear sleep, state-oscillation
  3. Quiet–awake (staring, gaze aversion)
  4. Irritable or panicky crying
C. Attention–Interaction System
  1. Abnormal response to sensory stimuli (e.g., difficult to soothe, inability to sustain alert status)
D. Motor System
  1. Increased, decreased, or limp tone
  2. Finger splay, fisting or hands to face
  3. Hyperextension of arms and legs
  4. Tremors, startles, twitches
  5. Jittery, jerky, uncoordinated movement
  6. Altered primitive reflexes

E. Physiological
  1. Bradycardia, tachycardia, or arrhythmias
  2. Pale, cyanotic, mottled, or flushed color
  3. Time-out signals (e.g., gaze, grasp, hiccough, cough, sneeze, sigh, slack jaw, open mouth, tongue thrust)
  4. Oximeter reading: Desaturation
  5. Feeding intolerances (aspiration or emesis)

RELATED FACTORS[22]

A. Prenatal
  1. Congenital or genetic disorders
  2. Teratogenic exposure
B. Postnatal
  1. Malnutrition
  2. Oral/motor problems
  3. Pain
  4. Feeding intolerance
  5. Invasive/painful procedures
  6. Prematurity
C. Individual
  1. Illness
  2. Immature neurologic system
  3. Gestational age
  4. Postconceptual age
D. Environmental
  1. Physical environment inappropriateness
  2. Sensory inappropriateness
  3. Sensory overstimulation
  4. Sensory deprivation
E. Caregiver
  1. Cue misreading
  2. Cue knowledge deficit
  3. Environmental stimulation contribution

DEFINITION[22]

Readiness for Enhanced Organized Infant Behavior A pattern of modulation for the physiologic and behavioral systems of functioning, that is, autonomic, motor, state, organizational, self-regulatory, and attention–interaction systems, in an infant that is satisfactory but that can be improved, resulting in higher levels of integration in response to environmental stimuli.

DEFINING CHARACTERISTICS[22]

1. Definite sleep–wake states
2. Use of some self-regulatory behaviors
3. Response to visual or auditory stimuli
4. Stable physiologic measures

RELATED FACTORS[22]

1. Pain
2. Prematurity

RELATED CLINICAL CONCERNS

1. Hospitalization
2. Any invasive procedure
3. Prematurity

4. Neurologic disorders
5. Respiratory disorders
6. Cardiovascular disorders

EXPECTED OUTCOME

Will return to more organized behavioral response by [date].
    Will demonstrate [Note defining characteristic here] within normal developmental limits by [date].

TARGET DATES

Disorganized infant behavior is very tiring, physically and emotionally, to both the infant and parents. Therefore, the initial target date should be within 24 hours of the diagnosis. As the infant's behavior becomes more organized, target dates can be increased in increments of 72 hours.

NURSING ACTIONS/INTERVENTIONS WITH RATIONALES

Adult Health

For this diagnosis, the Child Health nursing actions serve as the generic actions. This diagnosis would probably not arise on an adult health care unit.

Child Health

ACTIONS/INTERVENTIONS	RATIONALES
Monitor for all possible contributing factors related to the infant's status, including: • Prenatal course • Birth history and Apgar scores • Known medical diagnoses • All genetically relevant data • Actual description of problem/triggering cues • Treatment modalities (monitors, medications, special equipment, and/or special care related)	Inclusion of all contributing factors will result in an individualized plan of care.
Determine both the mother's and father's (parental) perception of the infant's status.	Ultimate responsibility will be better assumed by the caregiver if planning is long term and considers parental input.
Spend [number] minutes per shift with parents discussing their concerns and feelings about infants status	Opportunities to express concerns and gain knowledge will enhance coping.
Identify specific parameters (according to etiologic or known cause of problem) for appropriate management of infant; i.e., laboratory ranges (arterial blood gases) and respiratory rate, as applicable. [Note client specific plan for management of these parameters here.]	Treatment of condition will be enhanced with a specific, individualized plan of care. Inclusion of early childhood developmental specialist, occupational therapist, physical therapist, dietitian, home health nurse, and others as required will offer essential specialized care.
Evaluate parental capacity to assume caregiving role of the infant by: • Asking the parent to verbalize special care the infant requires	Anticipatory planning will enhance likelihood of adequate timing and gradual relinquishment of care to the parents or, when necessary, other primary caregivers.

ACTIONS/INTERVENTIONS	RATIONALES
• Observing the parent in care behaviors while still in hospital setting for appropriateness (e.g., feeding, handling, or as necessary, giving medications, suctioning, etc.)	
• Assessing problem-solving skills related to the infant's care (i.e., when to call for assistance)	
• Risk factor analysis of total 24-hour care of the infant	
• Ability to identify the infant's cues	
• Ability to respond to the infant's cues	
• Ability to handle, emotionally and otherwise, demands of the infant's status	
• Verbalization of expected prognosis or developmental potential	
• Evidence of realistic planning for respite care backup after discharge from hospital	
Spend [number] minutes per shift discussing a plan of care with parents. Note status of plan development here and update as planning progresses, noting assistance needed from staff to facilitate the implementation.	
Provide anticipatory care, including positioning, in planning for feedings, if necessary, with safety-mindedness as dictated by the infant's status, including possibility of cardiac or respiratory arrest.	Appropriate anticipation of possible cardiac or respiratory arrest and/or related dysfunction of vital functions will best identify degree of physiologic support required to sustain the infant.
Provide stimulation only as tolerated by the infant, to include minimal gentle touching, decreased sound, decreased light, decreased strong chemical odors, and gentle suctioning of oropharynx as necessary. [Note special adaptations for this client.]	Protection of the infant from undue environmental stressors during acute phase will decrease the possibility of increased levels or length of time when disorganized behavior is present.
Support the infant in basic physiologic needs as required, including:	Support of adaptive potentials may help restore patterns of organized behavior or at least maintain a more enhanced organized behavior pattern with individualized allowances as a basis for determining effective care.
• Dietary needs (by mouth [p.o.]), gastrostomy tube, hyperalimentation, etc.)	
• Respiratory functioning or maintenance (O_2, tracheotomy, endotracheal + ventilation + pulmonary toileting)	
• Urinary/elimination (self-toileting, diapering, Foley catheter)	
• Cardiac homeostasis (self-regulatory, medication, pacemaker, monitoring)	
• Neuromuscular requisites (positioning in alignment, protection from injury in event of seizure, use of splints, special equipment for adaptive needs, administration of seizure medications if needed)	
• Communication augmentation (close and continuous observation, interpretation of cues, adaptive aids ranging from musical toys to developmentally appropriate interactive toys)	
• Tolerance of stimulation (satisfactory oxygen saturation, ability to rest at intervals, etc.)	

(care plan continued on page 368)

NURSING ACTIONS/INTERVENTIONS WITH RATIONALES (continued from page 367)

Child Health

ACTIONS/INTERVENTIONS	RATIONALES
Readiness for Enhanced Organized Infant Behavior	
Monitor for all factors contributing to disorganized behavior that can be controlled (e.g., sounds, sights, and other stimuli). Note client-specific factors here.	Inclusion of all contributing factors will most likely offer potential to influence the infant's behavior on an individualized basis.
Develop a plan for identifying adaptation behaviors for evaluating effectiveness of current treatment and redefinition.	Ongoing evaluation will serve the purpose of substantiation of progress and thereby define enhancement behaviors and patterns.
Once enhancement behaviors are identified, redefine plan of care to best incorporate client goals.	

● N O T E : *Case management becomes an issue of paramount importance with a need to keep the family updated as changes occur. Also, in event of compromise and/or ultimate death, there should be consideration for:*

• Spiritual Distress, Risk For
• Anticipatory Grieving
• Parent, Infant, Child Attachment, Impaired, Risk for

Also, it could be that this infant requires long-term care with allowance for acute exacerbations made worse by underlying disorganized infant behavior.

Women's Health

● N O T E : *This diagnosis will relate to the delivery room and the immediate postpartum period (48 to 72 hours). For further clarification beyond this period, see Child Health.*

ACTIONS/INTERVENTIONS	RATIONALES
Monitor the infant's cardiovascular and respiratory system by use of Apgar score, at 1 and 5 minutes after birth.	Apgar score is an indicator of the infant's condition at birth and provides a baseline for determining the need for appropriate interventions and neonatal resuscitation.
Prepare for neonatal resuscitation by having all equipment and supplies ready. Be prepared to support neonatal staff, if available, and/or pediatrician. Support and reassure the parents by keeping them informed of the infant's condition.	If there is a compromised infant, then it is appropriate for the nurse in the delivery room to support and assist the neonatal staff in stabilizing the infant. If no neonatal staff is available, the labor–delivery staff needs to be well versed in neonatal stabilization and resuscitation.
Support the parents of the ill neonate by being available to listen and answer questions.	Parents often need to verbalize what they have been told by the neonatologist and the NICU staff. This helps them cope and can provide clarification of any information they have been given. The nurse who listens can correct inaccurate perceptions and keep NICU staff informed of the parents' understanding so they can better understand and provide support where the mother and family are physically and emotionally stressed.
Act as a liaison between neonatal intensive care unit (NICU) and the parents, assisting both parties by clarifying and explaining.	

ACTIONS/INTERVENTIONS	RATIONALES
Accompany and/or transport the patient to NICU the first time, to provide guidance and support, as well as introducing him or her to the NICU staff.	
If the infant is transported to another hospital, keep the mother informed by establishing contact with the NICU staff.	
Obtain pictures of the infant and telephone numbers so the mother can call and talk with NICU staff.	
Monitor and document the infant's physiologic parameters during periods of reactivity:	Utilizing every opportunity to teach new parents about their newborn increases confidence and infant caretaking activities.
• Assist new parents in utilizing the normal periods of reactivity in the neonate to begin breastfeeding and the parent–infant attachment process.	
• Perform a complete physical assessment of the newborn, documenting findings in an organized manner (usually head to toe).	
• Note and inform the parents of aspects of normal newborn appearance, especially noting such items as milia, normal newborn rash, or "stork bites."	
• Explain the importance of thermoregulation, voiding patterns, and neurologic adaptations during the immediate newborn period.	
• Practice good handwashing techniques before touching the newborn, and explain to the parents the importance of this in preventing infection.	
• Monitor the infant for ability to feed (breast or bottle), intake, output, and weight loss or gain.	
• Encourage parent participation in the care and observation of the infant.	
• Be available to answer questions and demonstrate techniques of baby care to new parents.	
Prevent heat loss by immediately drying the infant and laying him or her on a warmed surface (best place is skin-to-skin with the mother).	Drying decreases the incidence of iatrogenic hypothermia in the newborn. (Infant's temperature can drop as much as 4.7°F in the delivery room.)[82]
Immediate Postpartum Period	
Perform a gestational age assessment, and compare the infant's gestational age and weight. Based upon this examination, determine whether infant is[83]:	Gestational age and the size (AGA, SGA, LGA) of the infant can affect the transition to extrauterine life.
• Average for gestational age (AGA)	
• Small for gestational age (SGA)	
• Large for gestational age (LGA)	
Review the mother's prenatal and labor–delivery histories for factors that would interfere with the normal transitional physiologic process by the neonate, such as metabolic disorders (diabetes, etc.) and/or use of medications, both therapeutic and abusive.	The use of drugs during labor or prenatally, and maternal diseases such as diabetes may inhibit the thermoregulatory and cardiovascular responses or respiratory effort.[83]
Continue to monitor the infant's vital signs frequently.	

(care plan continued on page 370)

NURSING ACTIONS/INTERVENTIONS WITH RATIONALES (continued from page 369)

Mental Health

● N O T E : *Mental health interventions for this diagnosis would focus on family support.*
Refer to the following diagnoses for care plans:
  Management of Therapeutic Regimen (Family), Ineffective
  Caregiver Role Strain
  Family Coping, Compromised or Disabled
  Family Coping, Readiness for Enhanced

Parenting, Impaired or Risk for
The practitioner should review the definition and defining characteristics of these diagnoses to determine which one relates to those characteristics being demonstrated by the infant's family and/or support system.

Gerontic Health

This diagnosis would probably not be used in Gerontic Health.

Home Health

ACTIONS/INTERVENTIONS	RATIONALES
Assist the client and family in lifestyle changes that may be required. Provide for: • Supportive environment • Consistent care provider • Appropriate stimulation • Control of pain—teach the caregiver to recognize signs of pain, and appropriate pain management actions, to include safe use of prescribed analgesics. • Understanding of normal growth and development—teach the caregiver normal developmental milestones and their associated behaviors.	Home-based care requires involvement of the family. Disorganized infant behavior can disrupt family schedules. Adjustment in family activities may be required.
Assist the family to set criteria to help them determine when additional intervention is required (e.g., change in baseline physiologic measures).	Provides the family with background knowledge to seek appropriate assistance as need arises.
Assess the client/caregiver need for assistive resources and refer to appropriate community agencies.	Additional assistance may be required for the family to care for the infant. Use of readily available resources is cost effective.

PERIPHERAL NEUROVASCULAR DYSFUNCTION, RISK FOR

DEFINITION[22]

A state in which an individual is at risk of experiencing a disruption in circulation, sensation, or motion of an extremity.

DEFINING CHARACTERISTICS[22]

1. Trauma
2. Vascular obstruction
3. Orthopedic surgery
4. Fractures
5. Burns
6. Mechanical compression, for example, tourniquet, cast, brace, dressing, or restraint
7. Immobilization

RELATED FACTORS[22]

The risk factors also serve as the related factors for this risk diagnosis.

RELATED CLINICAL CONCERNS

1. Fractures
2. Buerger's disease
3. Thrombophlebitis
4. Burns
5. Cerebrovascular accident

 Have You Selected the Correct Diagnosis?

Ineffective Tissue Perfusion
Ineffective Tissue Perfusion is an actual diagnosis and indicates that a definite problem has developed. Risk for Peripheral Neurovascular Dysfunction indicates

that the patient is in danger of developing a problem if appropriate nursing measures are not instituted to offset the problem development.

EXPECTED OUTCOME

Will develop no problems with peripheral neurovascular function by [date].

TARGET DATES

Initial target dates should be stated in hours. After the patient is able to be more involved in self-care and prevention, the target date can be expressed in increments of 3 to 5 days.

NURSING ACTIONS/INTERVENTIONS WITH RATIONALES

Adult Health

ACTIONS/INTERVENTIONS	RATIONALES
Assess skin integrity, especially areas affected by devices that may affect peripheral neurovascular function (e.g., restraints, traction, or casts) every 2 hours on [odd/even] hour.	Allows intervention before skin breakdown occurs.
Perform color, movement, sensation (CMS) checks to potential trouble areas (e.g., circumferential burns, cardiac catheterization, fractures) at least every 2 hours.	
Assist the patient with ROM exercise every 2 hours on [odd/even] hour.	Increases circulation and maintains muscle tone and movement.
Instruct the patient regarding isometric and isotonic exercises. Have the patient exercise every 4 hours while awake at [times].	
Keep extremities warm.	Promotes circulation.
Turn every 2 hours on [odd/even] hour.	Prevents sustained pressure on any pressure point.
Monitor the patient's understanding of the effects of smoking, or if nonsmoker, the effects of passive smoke on peripheral circulation.	Smoking constricts peripheral circulation, leading to increased problems with peripheral neurologic and vascular functioning.
Refer to physical therapy as necessary.	

Child Health

ACTIONS/INTERVENTIONS	RATIONALES
Determine exact parameters to be used in monitoring risk concerns (e.g., if the patient is without sensation in specific levels of anatomy, document what the known deficits are: High level of myelomeningocele, lumbar 4, with apparent sensation in peroneal site). [Note client specific adaptations here.]	Specific parameters for assessment of neurodeficits can guide caregivers in choosing the best precautionary treatment.[49]

(care plan continued on page 372)

NURSING ACTIONS/INTERVENTIONS WITH RATIONALES (continued from page 371)

Child Health

ACTIONS/INTERVENTIONS	RATIONALES
Carry out treatments with attention to the neurologic deficits (e.g., using warm pads for a child unable to perceive heat would require constant attention for signs or symptoms of burns).	Common safety measure.
Provide teaching according to the patient and family needs, especially with regard to safety. [Note client specific teaching plan here.]	Appropriate assessment will best foster learning and help prevent injury.[49]
Include the family in care and use of equipment (e.g., braces, etc.).	Family involvement assuages the child's emotional needs and empowers the parents.
Refer to appropriate community agencies for follow-up.[49]	Long-term follow-up validates the need for rechecking and offers a time to reassess progress in goal attainment or altered patterns.
Teach the patient (as developmentally appropriate) and family administration of medications especially anticoagulation agents as low-dose heparin.[49]	Provides anticipatory guidance in safe administration of medications.[49]

Women's Health

● NOTE: *Women are at risk for thrombosis in the lower extremities during pregnancy and the early postpartum period. Because of decreased venous return from the legs, compression of large vessels supplying the legs during pregnancy, and during pushing in the second stage of labor, patients need to be continuously assessed for this problem.[84]*

ACTIONS/INTERVENTIONS	RATIONALES
Closely monitor the patient at each visit and teach patient to self-monitor size, shape, symmetry, color, edema, and varicosities in the legs.	Knowledge of the problem and its causative factors can assist in planning and carrying out good health habits during pregnancy. This knowledge can assist in preventing thrombotic complications during pregnancy.
Encourage the patient to walk daily during the pregnancy and to wear supportive hosiery.	
Assist the patient to plan a day's schedule during pregnancy that will allow her time to rest. The schedule should also include several times during the day for her to elevate her legs.	
Encourage the patient to use a small stool when sitting (e.g., at desk to keep feet elevated and less compression on upper thighs and knees).	
In the event thrombophlebitis develops: • Monitor legs for stiffness, pain, paleness, and swelling in the calf or thigh every 4 hours around the clock.	Basic assessment for early detection of complications.
• Place the patient on strict bedrest with the affected leg elevated.	Basic safety measure to avoid dislodging of clots.
Provide analgesics as ordered for pain relief, and assess for effectiveness within 30 minutes of administration.	
Place a bed cradle on the bed.	Keeps pressure of bed linens off the affected leg.

ACTIONS/INTERVENTIONS	RATIONALES
Administer and monitor the effects of anticoagulant therapy as ordered. Collaborate with the physician regarding the frequency of laboratory examinations to monitor clotting factors.	
● N O T E : *Breastfeeding mothers who are taking heparin can continue to breastfeed. Breastfeeding mothers who are taking dicumarol should **stop** breastfeeding, because it is passed to the infant in breast milk.*	
Do not rub, massage, or bump affected leg. Handle with care when changing linens or giving bath.	Basic safety measures to avoid dislodging clots.
Assist the family to plan for care of the infant; include the mother in planning process.	Assist the patient and family in coping with illness. Promotes effective implementation of home care. Provides support and teaching opportunity.
Encourage verbalizations of fears and discouragement by the mother and family.	

Mental Health

The mental health client with this diagnosis requires the same type of nursing care as the adult client. A review of the nursing actions for Activity Intolerance, Impaired Physical Mobility, and Ineffective Tissue Perfusion would also be of assistance.

Gerontic Health

ACTIONS/INTERVENTIONS	RATIONALES
Avoid the use of restraints if at all possible.	Restraint use in older adults can lead to physical and mental deterioration, injury, and death.[85]
Monitor restraints, if used, at least every 2 hours on [odd/even] hour. Release restraints, and perform ROM exercises before reapplying.	Frequent monitoring decreases the injury risk.

Home Health

Nursing actions for the home health client with this diagnosis are the same as those for the Adult Health client.

PHYSICAL MOBILITY, IMPAIRED

DEFINITION[22]

A limitation in independent purposeful physical movement of the body on one or more extremities

DEFINING CHARACTERISTICS[22]

1. Postural instability during performance of routine activities of daily living
2. Limited ability to perform gross motor skills
3. Limited ability to perform fine motor skills
4. Uncoordinated or jerky movements
5. Limited range of motion
6. Difficulty turning
7. Decreased reaction time
8. Movement-induced shortness of breath
9. Gait changes (e.g., decreased walk-spread, difficulty initiating gait, small steps, shuffles feet, exaggerated lateral position sway)
10. Engages in substitutions for movement (e.g., increased attention to other's activity, controlling behavior, focus on pre-illness or disability activity)
11. Slowed movement
12. Movement-induced trauma

RELATED FACTORS[22]

1. Medications
2. Prescribed movement restrictions
3. Discomfort

4. Lack of knowledge regarding value of physical activity
5. Body mass index above 75th age-appropriate percentile
6. Sensoriperceptual impairments
7. Neuromuscular impairment
8. Pain
9. Musculoskeletal impairment
10. Intolerance to activity or decreased strength and endurance
11. Depressive mood state or anxiety
12. Cognitive impairment
13. Decreased muscle strength, control, and/or mass
14. Reluctance to initiate movement
15. Sedentary lifestyle, or disuse or deconditioning
16. Selective or generalized malnutrition
17. Loss of integrity of bone structure
18. Developmental delay
19. Joint stiffness or contracture
20. Limited cardiovascular endurance
21. Altered cellular metabolism
22. Lack of physical or social environmental supports
23. Cultural beliefs regarding age-appropriate activities

RELATED CLINICAL CONCERNS

1. Fractures that require casting or traction
2. Rheumatoid arthritis
3. Cerebrovascular accident
4. Depression
5. Any neuromuscular disorder

 Have You Selected the Correct Diagnosis?

Activity Intolerance
This diagnosis implies that the individual is freely able to move but cannot endure or adapt to the increased energy or oxygen demands made by the movement or activity. Impaired Physical Mobility indicates that an individual would be able to move independently if something were not limiting the motion.

Impaired Physical Mobility
This diagnosis also needs to be differentiated from the respiratory (Impaired Gas Exchange and Ineffective Breathing Pattern) and cardiovascular (Decreased Cardiac Output and Ineffective Tissue Perfusion) nursing diagnoses. Mobility depends on effective breathing patterns and effective gas exchange between the lungs and the arterial blood supply. Muscles have to receive oxygen and get rid of carbon dioxide for contraction and relaxation. Because oxygen is transported and dispersed to the muscle tissue via the cardiovascular system, it is only logical that the respiratory and cardiovascular diagnoses could impact mobility.

Imbalanced Nutrition, More or Less Than Body Requirements
Nutritional deficit would indicate that the body is not receiving enough nutrients for its metabolic needs. Without adequate nutrition, the muscles cannot function appropriately. With More Than Body Requirements, mobility may be impaired simply because of the excess weight. In someone who is grossly obese, range of motion is limited, gait is altered, and coordination and tone are greatly reduced.

EXPECTED OUTCOME

Will verbalize plan to increase strength and endurance by [date].

Will demonstrate ability to [note target mobility behavior here] with assistance by [date].

Will demonstrate ability to [note target mobility behavior here] unaided by [date].

TARGET DATES

These dates may be short term or long term, based on the etiology of the diagnosis. An acceptable first target date would be 5 days.

*Suggested Functional Level Classification
0 = Completely independent
1 = Requires use of equipment or device
2 = Requires help from another person, for assistance, supervision, or teaching
3 = Requires help from another person and equipment service
4 = Dependent, does not participate in activity
(Code adapted by NANDA.) [106]

NURSING ACTIONS/INTERVENTIONS WITH RATIONALES

Adult Health

ACTIONS/INTERVENTIONS	RATIONALES
Educate the patient regarding proper use of assistive devices	
Provide progressive mobilization as tolerated. Schedule increased mobilization on a daily basis.	Maintains muscle tone and prevents complications of immobility.

ACTIONS/INTERVENTIONS	RATIONALES
Medicate for pain as needed, especially before activity. Exercise caution with medications that effect sensorium.	Pain interferes with ability to ambulate by inhibiting muscle movement.
Perform ROM exercises (passive, active, and functional) every 2 hours on [odd/even] hour.	Increases circulation, maintains muscle tone, and prevents joint contractures.
Maintain proper body alignment at all times; support extremities with pillows, blankets, towel rolls, or sandbags.	Prevents flexion contractures and progression of complications.
Implement measures to prevent falls, such as keeping bed in low position, wearing appropriately fitting shoes or nonskid slippers.	Basic safety measures.
Devise strategies for strength training.	
Maintain adequate nutrition.	Provides nutrients for energy, and prevents protein loss due to immobility.
Observe for complications of immobility (e.g., constipation, muscle atrophy, decubitus ulcers).	Allows early detection and prevention of complications.
Include the patient and family or significant other in carrying out plan of care.	Allows time for practice under supervision. Increases likelihood of effective management of therapeutic regimen.
Initiate physical therapy and/or occupational therapy as soon as feasible.	

Child Health

ACTIONS/INTERVENTIONS	RATIONALES
Monitor alteration in mobility each 8-hour shift according to: • Actual movement noted and tolerance for the movement • Factors related to movement (e.g., braces used, progress in use) • Situational factors (e.g., previous status, current health needs, or movement permitted) • Pain • Circulation check to affected limb • Change in appearance of affected limb or joint	Provides the primary database for an individualized plan of care.
Include related health team members in care of the patient as needed. [Note plan for their involvement here.]	The nurse is in the prime position to coordinate health team members to best match needs and resources.
Consider patient and family preferences in planning to meet desired mobility goals. [Note special adaptations needed to incorporate family/patient preferences here.][49]	Consideration of preferences increases likelihood of plan success.
Facilitate participation of family members, especially the parents, in care of the patient according to needs and situation (feeding, comfort measures). [Note patient/family specific adaptations here.]	Involving the family in care serves to enhance their skills in care required at home.

(care plan continued on page 376)

NURSING ACTIONS/INTERVENTIONS WITH RATIONALES (continued from page 375)

Child Health

ACTIONS/INTERVENTIONS	RATIONALES
Provide diversional activities appropriate for age and developmental level. [Note those activities preferred by client here.]	Diversional activity, when appropriately planned, serves to refresh and relax the patient
Maintain appropriate safety guidelines according to age and developmental guidelines.	Basic requirements for maintaining standards of care.
Monitor traction or related equipment in use (e.g., weights hanging free or rope knots tight).	Ensures therapeutic effectiveness of equipment, and provides for safety issues related to these interventions.
Monitor patient and family needs for education regarding the patient's situation and any future implications. [Note plan for family education here.]	Allows timely planning for home care, and allows practice of care in a supportive environment.
Monitor intake and output to ensure adequate fluid balance for each 24-hour period.	Strict intake and output will assist in monitoring hydration status, which is crucial for healing and circulatory adequacy.
Address related health issues appropriate for the patient and family.	Appropriate attention to related health issues fosters holistic care (e.g., the child may need braces, but may also have need for healing, or speech followup secondary to meningitis, and developmental delays).[49]

Women's Health

● NOTE: *The following nursing actions apply to those women placed on restrictive activities because of threatened abortions, premature labor, multiple pregnancy, or pregnancy-induced hypertension.*

ACTIONS/INTERVENTIONS	RATIONALES
Facilitate the participation of the family and significant others in the plan of care for the patient.	
When resting in bed, have the patient rest in the left lateral position as much as possible.	Prevents supine hypotension, and allows adequate renal and uterine perfusion.
Encourage the patient to list lifestyle adjustments that will need to be made.	
Teach the patient relaxation skills and coping mechanisms.	Decreases anxiety and muscle tension.
Facilitate adequate protein intake. [Note special needs here.]	Replaces protein lost because of decreasing muscle contraction during immobility.
Maintain proper body alignment with use of positioning and pillow.	
Provide diversionary activities (e.g., hobbies, job-related activities that can be done in bed, or activities with children).	Decreases anxiety and reduces muscle tension. Provides appropriate amounts of activity without danger to pregnancy.
Facilitate help and visits from friends and relatives: • Visit in person • Telephone visit • Help with child care • Help with housework	

Mental Health

ACTIONS/INTERVENTIONS	RATIONALES
● N O T E : *The following actions and interventions are related to imposed restrictions. This includes seclusion and restraint.*	
Attempt all other interventions before considering immobilizing the client as an intervention. (See Risk for Violence, Chapter 9, for appropriate nursing actions.)	Promotes the client's sense of control and supports self-esteem.
Carefully monitor the client for appropriate level of restraint necessary. Immobilize the client as little as possible while still protecting the client and others.	
Obtain necessary medical orders to initiate methods that limit the client's physical mobility.	
Carefully explain to the client in brief, concise language reasons for initiating this intervention, and what behavior must be present for the intervention to be terminated.	Excessive stimuli can increase confusion. Provides the client with sense of control.
Attempt to gain the client's voluntary compliance with the intervention by explaining to the client what is needed and with a "show of force" (have the necessary number of staff available to force compliance).	Promotes the client's sense of control and safety, which promotes self-esteem.
Initiate forced compliance only if there is an adequate number of staff to complete the action safely. (See Risk for Violence, Chapter 9, for a detailed description of intervention with forced compliance.)	Client and staff safety are of primary concern.
Secure the environment the client will be in by removing harmful objects such as accessible light bulbs, sharp objects, glass objects, tight clothing, and metal objects such as clothes hangers or shower curtain rods.	Prevents injury by protecting the client from impulsive actions of self-harm.
If the client is placed in four-point restraints, maintain one-to-one supervision.	Client safety is primary concern.
If the client is in seclusion or bilateral restraints, observe the client at least every 15 minutes, more frequently if agitated [List observation schedule here.]	
Leave the urinal in room with the client, or offer toileting every hour.	
Offer the client fluids every 15 minutes.	Maintains adequate hydration.
Discuss with the client his or her feelings about the initiation of immobility, and review with him or her again, at least twice a day, the behavior necessary to have immobility discontinued.	Exploration of feelings in an accepting environment helps the client identify and explore maladaptive coping behaviors. Promotes the client's sense of perceived control.
When checking the client, let him or her know you are checking by calling him or her by name and orienting him or her to day and time. Inquire about the client's feelings, and implement necessary reality orientation.	Promotes perceived control and promotes an environment of trust.
Provide meals at regular intervals on paper containers, providing necessary assistance. [Amount and type of assistance required should be listed here.]	Meets biophysical needs while providing consistency in a respectful manner, which promotes self-esteem and trust.

(care plan continued on page 378)

NURSING ACTIONS/INTERVENTIONS WITH RATIONALES (continued from page 377)

Mental Health

ACTIONS/INTERVENTIONS	RATIONALES
If the client is in restraints, remove restraints at least every 2 hours, one limb at a time. Have the client move limb through a full ROM and inspect for signs of injury. Apply lubricants such as lotion to area under restraint to protect from injury.	Promotes normal circulation and motion, which prevents injury to the limb.
Pad the area of the restraint that is next to the skin with sheepskin or other nonirritating material.	Protects skin from mechanical irritation.
Check circulation in restrained limbs in the area below the restraint by observing skin color, warmth, and swelling. Restraint should not interfere with circulation.	Early assessment and intervention prevents serious injury.
Change the client's position in the bed every 2 hours on [odd/even] hour.	Prevents disuse syndrome.
Place body in proper alignment. Use pillows for support if the client's condition allows.	Prevents complications and injury.
If the client is in four-point restraints, place him or her on stomach or side.	Prevents aspiration or choking.
Place the client on intake and output monitoring.	Ensures that adequate fluid balance is maintained.
Have the client in seclusion move around the room at least every 2 hours on [odd/even] hour, and during this time initiate active ROM.	Prevents complications of immobility.
Administer medications as ordered for agitation.	Medications reduce anxiety and facilitate interaction with others.
Monitor blood pressure before administering antipsychotic medications.	Psychotropic medications can cause orthostatic hypotension.
Assist the client with daily personal hygiene (record time for this here).	Communicates positive regard for the client by the nurse, which facilitates the development of positive self-esteem.
Have environment cleaned on a daily basis.	Promotes sanitary conditions and provides an orderly environment, which can decrease the client's disorganization and confusion.
Review with the client the purpose for restraint or seclusion as required, and discuss alternative kinds of behavior that will express feelings without threatening self or others.	Promotes the client's sense of control by providing him or her with behavioral alternatives and establishing clear limits.
Remove the client from seclusion as soon as the contracted behavior is observed for the required amount of time (both of these should be very specific and listed here). (See Risk for Violence, Chapter 9, for detailed information on behavior change and contracting specifics.)	Provides positive reinforcement for appropriate coping behavior, and promotes the client's sense of control.
Schedule time to discuss this intervention with the client and his or her support system. Inform support system of the need for the intervention and about special considerations related to visiting with the client. This information must be provided with consideration of client confidentiality. Plan to spend at least 5 minutes with the members of the support system before and after each visit.	Support system understanding and support of treatment goals has a positive effect on client outcome.

ACTIONS/INTERVENTIONS	RATIONALES
Arrange consultations with appropriate resources after the client is released from mobility limitations to assist the client with developing alternative coping behavior. This could include a physical therapist, an occupational therapist, or a social worker.	Facilitates the development of trust as well as respect for the client, which can have a positive effect on the client's self-esteem.

● N O T E : *The following interventions are related to restrictions due to psychogenic causes.*

* If restrictions are due to anxiety, refer to Chapter 8 and the diagnosis of Anxiety.
* If restrictions are due to depressed mood, implement the following interventions:
  * Sit with the client for [number] minutes [number] times per shift. Initially these times will be brief but frequent (e.g., 5 minutes per hour).

ACTIONS/INTERVENTIONS	RATIONALES
• Establish clear expectations for these interactions (e.g., the client is not expected to talk, it is okay for these times to be spent in silence).	Communicates respect for the client, and facilitates the client's perception of control.
Explain to the client in simple concrete terms the positive effects of physical activity on mood. [Note person responsible for this teaching here.]	Physical activity can stimulate endorphin production, which has a positive effect on mood.
Talk with the client about activities they have enjoyed in the past.	Promotes a positive expectational set based on past positive experiences.
Develop with the client a program for increasing physical activity. Note that contact here. Also note rewards for accomplishing goals (e.g., will walk from bed to door once per hour). If accomplished, the client can remain in bed during visiting hours. Activities can increase as the client masters each step.	Promotes the client's sense of control. Positive reinforcement encourages behavior and enhances self-esteem.
Provide positive verbal reinforcement for accomplishing tasks.	Positive recognition from significant others enhances self-esteem.
Recognize the client's perceptions about the difficulty of physical activity in the initial stages of recovery.	Communicates acceptance of the client, and facilitates the development of a trusting relationship.
Pair physical activity with situations the client finds rewarding. Note these situations here (e.g., walking with the client to get a cup of coffee. This pairs walking with two things the client finds rewarding: time with the nurse and coffee).	Promotes positive expectational set by pairing physical exercise with a positive stimulus.
Have the client identify perceived barriers to increased physical activity. Note those here and develop with the client plan for reducing these. [Note plan here.]	Promotes the client's sense of control and increases the client's commitment to the plan because he or she has contributed to the plan.
Teach support system importance of the client's increasing physical activity, and have them identify ways they could assist with this. Note here the person responsible for this, and record the plan when it is developed.	Support system involvement increases the probability for positive outcome.

(care plan continued on page 380)

NURSING ACTIONS/INTERVENTIONS WITH RATIONALES (continued from page 379)

Gerontic Health

In addition to the interventions for Adult Health, the following may be utilized with the aging client.

ACTIONS/INTERVENTIONS	RATIONALES
Monitor for complications of immobility such as: • Orthostatic hypotension • Thrombosis • Urinary tract infections • Constipation	Normal aging changes in combination with immobility can leave the older adult at increased risk for complications.[86]
Assess the client for depression and treat appropriately.	Depression can contribute to sedentary lifestyle and resulting immobility.
Observe the patient for Valsalva maneuver (increased intrathoracic pressure induced by forceful exhalation against a closed glottis) when he or she is changing position, pushing a wheelchair, or toileting.	Valsalva maneuver can produce increased pulse rate and increased blood pressure. This adversely affects patients with cardiovascular disorders, which may lead to their choosing not to engage in physical activity.[86]
Monitor for behavioral changes that may result from decreased sensory stimulation or decreased socialization (e.g., depression, hostility, confusion, or anxiety).	Psychological changes not addressed may increase problems of physical mobility and lead to prolonged periods of immobility.
Observe when increasing mobility, transferring, or during early ambulation stage for the risk for falls.	Older adults may be at risk for falls secondary to orthostatic blood pressure changes or problems with balance, especially after prolonged periods of immobility.
Teach the client to perform isometric muscle contraction (i.e., tightening of muscle group as hard as possible and then relaxing the muscle).	Isometric contraction helps maintain muscle strength, which can decrease with immobility as much as 5 percent per day.[86]
Collaborate with health-care team to provide supervised flexibility and range of motion exercises for client.	Maintain muscle strength.

Home Health

ACTIONS/INTERVENTIONS	RATIONALES
Assist the patient and family in identifying risk factors pertinent to the situation: • Immobility • Malnourishment • Confusion or lethargy • Physical barriers • Neuromuscular deficit • Musculoskeletal deficit • Trauma • Pain • Medications that affect coordination and level of arousal • Debilitating disease (cancer, stroke, diabetes, muscular dystrophy, multiple sclerosis, arthritis, etc.) • Depression • Lack of or improper use of assistive devices • Casts, slings, traction, IVs, etc. • Weather hazards	Locus of control shifts from nurse to the client and family, thus promoting self-care.

ACTIONS/INTERVENTIONS	RATIONALES
Teach the client and family measures to promote physical activity: • Use of assistive devices (wheelchairs, crutches, canes, walkers, prostheses, adaptive eating utensils, devices to assist with activities of daily living, etc.) • Providing safe environment (reducing barriers to activity such as throw rugs, furniture in pathway, electric cords on floor, doors, or steps) • Maintaining skin integrity • Use of safety devices (ramps, lift bars, tub rails, tub or shower seat) • Proper transfer techniques	
Assist the patient and family in identifying lifestyle changes that may be required: • Alteration in living space (ramps, assistive devices, etc.) • Changes in role functions • Range of motion exercises • Positioning and transferring techniques • Pain control • Progressive activity • Use of assistive devices • Prevention of injury • Maintenance of skin integrity • Assistance with activities of daily living • Special transportation needs • Financial concerns	Provides basic information for the client and family that promotes necessary lifestyle changes.
Assess the client/family need for assistance with obtaining assistive devices, or in home assistance with ADLs, cooking, and housework. Refer to community agencies providing needed services.	Provides additional support for the client and family, and uses already available resources in a cost-effective manner.

SEDENTARY LIFESTYLE

DEFINITION[22]

Reports a habit of life that is characterized by a low physical activity level.

DEFINING CHARACTERISTICS[22]

1. Chooses a daily routine lacking physical exercise.
2. Demonstrates physical deconditioning.
3. Verbalizes preference for activities low in physical activity.

RELATED FACTORS[22]

1. The risk factors also serve as the related factors for this diagnosis.
2. Deficient knowledge of health benefits of physical exercise
3. Lack of training for accomplishment of physical exercise

4. Lack of resources (time, money, companionship, facilities)
5. Lack of motivation
6. Lack of interest

EXPECTED OUTCOME

Will participate in increased physical activity by [date]. (Specify which activity: walking, swimming, chair exercises, and the frequency, duration, or intensity of the activity.)

EXAMPLE

Will increase walking by at least one block each week for 8 weeks.

TARGET DATES

Appropriate target dates will have to be individualized according to the degree of deconditioning. An appropriate range would be 3 to 5 days.

NURSING ACTIONS/INTERVENTIONS WITH RATIONALES

Adult Health

ACTIONS/INTERVENTIONS	RATIONALES
Collaborate with primary care provider to ensure that patient has no medical conditions precluding the initiation of an exercise plan.	Ensures that physical activity will be initiated safely.
Engage the patient in a dialogue to determine perception of barriers and patient preferred activities that would promote lifestyle change	Change is dependent on patient's perception of the problem.
Provide teaching to convey pertinent benefits that would enhance patient's health status. [Note specific teaching plan for this client here.]	Gives the patient a rationale for lifestyle change.
Collaborate with the patient to establish realistic goals for increasing activity. Note client goals here.	
Discuss simple methods that do not involve financial investment: walking in the neighborhood, parking car farther from destination, taking stairs, and moderate yard work.	Conveys to patient that finances are not a realistic barrier to exercise and provide easy access with minimal lifestyle change.
Advise patient regarding safety precautions (e.g., starting in moderation and not in extreme temperatures).	Promotes safety.
Underscore the importance of gradual introduction into exercise routine. Teach the patient about indicators of overexertion: shortness of breath, chest pain, and dizziness.	
Have the patient maintain weekly journal of activity including type, frequency, and response.	Provides tangible feedback to the patient and tracks progress and need for change.
Collaborate with patient and physical therapy or rehabilitation specialist to devise appropriate program with increasing intensity.	Promotes sense of ownership in program.

Child Health

ACTIONS/INTERVENTIONS	RATIONALES
Monitor for contributing factors, especially current medical status and potential limitations imposed.	Provides a realistic basis for plan of care.
Develop, with the client and family, specific goals for activity.	Creates a measurable goal.
Identify strategies to attain the goal.	Provides a realistic plan.
Involve other health team members as appropriate, including pediatrician, pediatric cardiologist, or other primary care provider, nutritionist, occupational or physical therapist, and child life specialist.	Offers safe and appropriate plan to match the child's potential.
Establish need for supervision and equipment essential in event of untoward response to exercise or activity *May include halter monitoring or peak flow meter assessment.	Provides anticipatory planning in the event of an untoward response during activity.
Determine a mutually satisfactory way to reward the child for participation. [Note that plan here.]	Satisfies reinforcement with likelihood for continued success with plan.

ACTIONS/INTERVENTIONS	RATIONALES
Discuss with child and family values related to increased activity vs. rationale for not remaining sedentary.	Allows for likelihood of exploring lifelong values to assist in maintenance of health.
Develop peer activities mutually agreed upon by child and parents to assist in support of desired activities.	Allows for child's input within parental framework to consider peer interaction with resultant likelihood to continue activity.

Women's Health

● N O T E : *Women's lifestyles will be the same as for Adult Health with the following notations:*

ACTIONS/INTERVENTIONS	RATIONALES
Living—A Five-Step Program (American College of Sports Medicine: 1998); 1. Get moving, quantity of cardiovascular exercise 2. Get in the zone–quality of cardiovascular exercise 3. Strength Training Assessment (excellent to prevent bone loss) 4. Nutrition and Exercise[104]	Statistics show that 55% of American adults have been classified as obese, and 58 million Americans are diagnosed as "clinically obese." This factor, along with stress and a sedentary lifestyle is leading to millions of Americans becoming progressively disabled, losing their ability to perform such basic functions as getting in and out of a car or chair.[104]
Assist the client to plan, start, and maintain an exercise program that fits their life-stage. Be certain that when planning an exercise program, you (1) consider the woman's experiences, (2) make no assumptions based on popular literature, and (3) look at what is meaningful interaction for the woman.[104]	Women go through five stages of change as they adopt an exercise regimen: (1) precontemplation, (2) contemplation, (3) preparation, (4) action, and (5) maintenance. When most women reach the maintenance stage and exercise has become a routine part of their life, they feel a sense of empowerment and well-being.[104]
Poverty remains one of the major factors affecting women's health. Sixty percent of chronic diseases are preventable, and exercise is becoming known as having the greatest benefit to prevent chronic diseases.	Lifestyle choices such as nutritious diet, regular exercise, and avoidance of smoking will help prevent the majority of chronic diseases.[87]
Biological changes in cardiovascular, respiratory, and musculoskeletal systems plus inactivity place women at risk for disability.[88]	Researchers report that 30 to 60 percent of the general population does not do any physical activity, and 42 percent of those who are 65 and older state they lead sedentary lives.[88]

Mental Health

ACTIONS/INTERVENTIONS	RATIONALES
Spend [number] minutes discussing with client his or her perception of lifestyle and experiences with increased activity and exercise. Identify what he or she thinks is most important about the current situation.	Helps determine aspects of the client's cognitive appraisal that could impact learning.[34]
Determine the client's current physical abilities. This can be done in collaboration with his or her primary care provider.	
Provide feedback to the client about discrepancies in current behavior and stated values/goals.	Presents an opportunity to review with the client how behavior change will facilitate goal achievement.[89]
Provide the client with arguments for and against change.	If the client is resistant to change, this places the nurse in a neutral position and prevents the client pushing back in non-growth-promoting directions.[89]

(care plan continued on page 384)

NURSING ACTIONS/INTERVENTIONS WITH RATIONALES (continued from page 383)

Mental Health

ACTIONS/INTERVENTIONS	RATIONALES
Contribute positive outcomes and successes to the client. • Use these successes to demonstrate to the client that he or she has the resources to change their behavior.	Promotes self-efficacy. Builds confidence in ability to change.[89]
Include the client in decisions about change and progress toward changes.	Promotes self-efficacy.[89]
Develop, with the client, a specific plan for change. [Note that plan here and the support needed from staff to implement the plan.]	
Provide positive, informative verbal reinforcement for goal attainment.	Positive reinforcement promotes behavior change.[34]
Develop, with the client, a specific plan for maintaining these changes after discharge. • Provide the client with a written plan to take with him or her.	

Gerontic Health

ACTIONS/INTERVENTIONS	RATIONALES
Monitor current potential for activities, including: • Activities of interest • Physical limitations • Realistic expectations for goal achievement • Objective criteria by which specific progress may be measured (e.g., distance, time) • Previous activities the patient enjoyed	Provides baseline for planning activities and increase in activities.
Assess community resources for exercise (e.g., walking tracks, indoor pools, and church activity centers) and refer the client to facilities that are nearby or that match the client's interests.	Assists the client in utilizing existing resources.
Teach client about various ways to increase activity: • Walking • Graduated Walking • Bicycling • Swimming Include education about safety with each type of activity.	Assists the client in making informed decisions.
Teach the client safety measures to consider when increasing activity: • Always check with a physician before starting an exercise program. • Stop and consult a health-care professional if pain or unusual symptoms occur (e.g., chest pain, palpitations, irregular heart beat, dizziness, light headedness, nausea, vomiting, extreme fatigue, pale or splotchy skin, "cold sweat")	Promotes safety.

ACTIONS/INTERVENTIONS	RATIONALES
• Start in small increments and increase as tolerated • Avoid exercising for 2 hours after a large meal and do not eat for 1 hour after exercising. • Include warmup and cool down exercises. • Use proper equipment and clothing • Wear comfortable rubber soled shoes and loose clothing. • Avoid exercising in extreme heat or cold.[90]	

Home Health/Community Health

ACTIONS/INTERVENTIONS	RATIONALES
Monitor current potential for activities, including: • Activities of interest • Physical limitations • Realistic expectations for goal achievement • Objective criteria by which specific progress may be measured (e.g., distance, time) • Previous activities the patient enjoyed	Provides a baseline for planning activities and increase in activities.
Assess community resources for exercise (e.g., walking tracks, indoor pools, and church activity centers) and refer the client to facilities that are nearby or that match the client's interests.	Assists the client in utilizing existing resources.
Teach the client about various ways to increase activity: • Walking • Graduated Walking • Bicycling • Swimming	Assists the client in making informed decisions.
Include education about safety with each type of activity.	
Teach the client safety measures to consider when increasing activity: • Always check with a physician before starting an exercise program. • Stop and consult a health-care professional if pain or unusual symptoms occur (e.g., chest pain, palpitations, irregular heart beat, dizziness, light-headedness, nausea, vomiting, extreme fatigue, pale or splotchy skin, "cold sweat"). • Start in small increments and increase as tolerated. • Avoid exercising for 2 hours after a large meal and do not eat for 1 hour after exercising. • Include warmup and cool down exercises. • Use proper equipment and clothing. • Wear comfortable rubber soled shoes and loose clothing. • Avoid exercising in extreme heat or cold.[90]	Promotes safety.

SELF-CARE DEFICIT (FEEDING, BATHING-HYGIENE, DRESSING-GROOMING, TOILETING)

DEFINITION[22]

An impaired ability to perform or complete feeding, bathing-hygiene, dressing-grooming, or toileting activities for oneself.

DEFINING CHARACTERISTICS[22]

A. Feeding Self-Care Deficit
1. Inability to swallow food
2. Inability to prepare food for ingestion
3. Inability to handle utensils
4. Inability to chew food
5. Inability to use assistive devices
6. Inability to get food onto utensil
7. Inability to open containers
8. Inability to manipulate food in mouth
9. Inability to ingest food safely
10. Inability to bring food from a receptacle to the mouth
11. Inability to complete a meal
12. Inability to ingest food in a socially acceptable manner
13. Inability to pick up cup or glass
14. Inability to ingest sufficient food

B. Bathing-Hygiene Self-Care Deficit
1. Inability to get bath supplies
2. Inability to wash body or body parts
3. Inability to obtain or get to water source
4. Inability to regulate temperature or flow of bath water
5. Inability to get in and out of bathroom
6. Inability to dry body

C. Dressing–Grooming Self-Care Deficit
1. Inability to choose clothing
2. Inability to use assistive devices
3. Inability to use zippers
4. Inability to remove clothes
5. Inability to put on socks
6. Inability to put clothing on upper body
7. Impaired ability to put on or take off necessary items of clothing
8. Impaired ability to obtain or replace articles of clothing
9. Inability to maintain appearance at a satisfactory level
10. Inability to put clothing on lower body
11. Inability to pick up clothing
12. Inability to put on shoes

D. Toileting Self-Care Deficit
1. Inability to manipulate clothing
2. Unable to carry out proper toilet hygiene
3. Unable to sit or rise from toilet or commode
4. Unable to flush toilet or commode

RELATED FACTORS[22]

A. Feeding Self-Care Deficit
1. Weakness or tiredness
2. Severe anxiety
3. Neuromuscular impairment
4. Pain
5. Perceptual or cognitive impairment
6. Discomfort
7. Environmental barriers
8. Decreased or lack of motivation
9. Musculoskeletal impairment

B. Bathing–Hygiene Self-Care Deficit
1. Decreased or lack of motivation
2. Weakness or tiredness
3. Severe anxiety
4. Inability to perceive body part or spatial relationship
5. Perceptual or cognitive impairment
6. Pain
7. Neuromuscular impairment
8. Musculoskeletal impairment
9. Environmental barriers

C. Dressing-Grooming Self-Care Deficit
1. Decreased or lack of motivation
2. Pain
3. Severe anxiety
4. Perceptual or cognitive impairment
5. Neuromuscular impairment
6. Musculoskeletal impairment
7. Discomfort
8. Environmental barriers
9. Weakness or tiredness

D. Toileting Self-Care Deficit
1. Environmental barriers
2. Weakness or tiredness
3. Decreased or lack of motivation
4. Severe anxiety
5. Impaired mobility status
6. Impaired transfer ability
7. Musculoskeletal impairment
8. Neuromuscular impairment
9. Pain
10. Perceptual or cognitive impairment

RELATED CLINICAL CONCERNS

1. Cerebrovascular accident
2. Spinal cord injury
3. Dementia
4. Depression
5. Rheumatoid arthritis

 Have You Selected the Correct Diagnosis?

Activity Intolerance
This diagnosis implies that the individual is freely able to move but cannot endure or adapt to the increased

energy or oxygen demands made by the movement or activity. Activity Intolerance can be a contributing factor to the development of self-care deficits.

Impaired Physical Mobility

This diagnosis is quite often a contributing factor to the development of Self-Care Deficit. It is probable that any time a patient has Impaired Physical Mobility, he or she will also have some degree of Self-Care Deficit.

Disturbed Thought Process

If the patient is exhibiting impaired attention span; impaired ability to recall information; impaired perception, judgment, and decision making; or impaired conceptual and reasoning ability, the most proper diagnosis would be Disturbed Thought Process. Most likely, Self-Care Deficit would be a companion diagnosis.

Ineffective Individual Coping or Compromised or Disabled Family Coping

Suspect one of these diagnoses if there are major differences between reports by the patient and the family of health status, health perception, and health care behavior. Verbalizations by the patient or the family regarding inability to cope also require looking at these diagnoses.

Interrupted Family Processes

Through observing family interactions and communication, the nurse may assess that Interrupted Family Processes should be considered. Poorly communicated messages, rigidity of family functions and roles, and failure to accomplish expected family developmental tasks are a few observations to alert the nurse to this possible diagnosis.

EXPECTED OUTCOME

Will return-demonstrate, with 100 percent accuracy, [specify] self-care by [date].

TARGET DATES

Overcoming a self-care deficit will take a significant investment of time; however, 7 days from the date of diagnosis would be appropriate to check for progress.

NURSING ACTIONS/INTERVENTIONS WITH RATIONALES

Adult Health

● N O T E : *Self-care deficits range from a total self-care deficit to very specific areas of self-care deficits, such as bathing-hygiene or feeding. The nursing actions presented are general in nature and would need to be adapted to fit the exact self-care deficit of the individual. Collaboration with a rehabilitation nurse clinician and/or review of rehabilitation literature would be excellent sources for current and specific nursing actions related to a patient's particular self-care deficit. Review of the nursing actions for Urinary Incontinence, Activity Intolerance, Impaired Physical Mobility, Impaired Skin Integrity, and Imbalanced Nutrition will also be helpful.*

ACTIONS/INTERVENTIONS	RATIONALES
Provide an environment that facilitates self-care: • Arrange food or furniture that addresses visual deficits. • Obtain assistive devices such as raised toilet seats or shower seats, buttonhooks, angled extension comb and brush. • Place items within reach.	
Provide extra time for giving daily care, and include: • Teaching • Return-demonstration of self-care activities • Emotional support	Instills trust, avoids overwhelming the patient, facilitates self-motivation, and allows immediate feedback on self-care.
Provide privacy and safety for the patient to practice self-care.	Avoids embarrassment for the patient, provides basic safety, and allows practice under closely supervised situation.
Remind the patient to wear corrective appliances (e.g., braces, prostheses, or eyeglasses).	Promotes self-care by offsetting present limitations.

(care plan continued on page 388)

NURSING ACTIONS/INTERVENTIONS WITH RATIONALES (continued from page 387)	

Adult Health

ACTIONS/INTERVENTIONS	RATIONALES
Provide positive reinforcement for each self-care accomplishment.	Increases self-esteem and motivation.
Perform ROM exercises, or assist the patient with every 4 hours while the patient is awake at [times].	Maintains muscle tone and joint mobility.
Assist the patient and significant others in planning measures to overcome or adapt to self-care deficits: • Gradual increments in self-care responsibility (e.g., getting up in chair independently before ambulating to bathroom by self) • Self-care assistive devices (e.g., helping hand)	Promotes timely home care planning and encourages participation in care.
Place a visual aid in the room to help document progress.	Visually documents success.
Monitor: • Vital signs every 4 hours while the patient is awake at [times]. • Ambulation: Increase, to extent possible.	Allows evaluation of progress and assist in determining physiologic impact of progress.
Monitor bowel and bladder elimination at least once daily at [time].	Baseline data that assist in determining bowel functioning pattern.
Establish bowel- and bladder-retraining programs as necessary. (See Bowel Incontinence and Urinary Incontinence, Chapter 4.)	Provides basic education, practice, and reinforcement that facilitate the patient's control of these functions.
Collaborate with dietitian regarding diet (e.g., foods to facilitate self-feeding).	Promotes self-care, and provides motivation to continue striving for improvement.
Refer the patient to community support services.	Provides for long-term support.
Make a home health referral to assist significant others to adapt home environment, as soon as feasible: • Nonskid rugs • Ramps • Handrails • Safety strips in tub and shower	Provides time to adapt home for basic safety measures.

Child Health

Adult Health care plan can provide the foundation for care of children with the following adaptations/considerations:

ACTIONS/INTERVENTIONS	RATIONALES
Monitor the patient's and parents' potential for self-care measures appropriate to age and developmental factors.	Provides a database for an individualized plan of care.
Allow the patient and parents to participate in planning for care when possible to help ensure best compliance. [Note plan for including the family here.]	Enhances satisfaction, and increases the likelihood that care will be continued after discharge from hospital.
Teach the appropriate skills necessary for self-care in the child's terms, with sensitivity to developmental needs for practice, repetition, or reluctance. [Note client-specific plan here.]	Individualized teaching best affords reinforcement of learning. Sensitivity to special need attaches value to the patient and family's needs.
Provide opportunities that will enhance the child's confidence in performing self-care. [Note plan for this client here.]	Confidence in self-care will enhance self-esteem.

Women's Health

● N O T E : *These activities relate to the new mother, their self care, and care of infant during the first postpartum days. Other activities will apply to women the same as Adult Health, Gerontic Health, and Home Health.*

ACTIONS/INTERVENTIONS	RATIONALES
Encourage the patient to list lifestyle adjustments that need to be made.	Promotes gradual assumption of self-care while avoiding overwhelming the patient with activities that must be accomplished.
Encourage progressive activity and increased self-care as tolerated: • Ambulation • Bathing • Body image and early postpartum exercises • Bowel care • Breast care • Perineal care	
Encourage the patient to get adequate rest: • Take care of self and baby only. • Let significant other take care of the housework and other children. • Learn to sleep when the baby sleeps. • Have specific, set times for friends or relatives to visit. • If breastfeeding, significant other can bring the infant to the mother at night (the mother doesn't have to get up every time for the infant).	
Provide quiet, supportive atmosphere for interaction with the infant.	Promotes attachment.
Instruct the patient in infant care, and have her return-demonstrate: • Bathing 　• **Never** leave the infant or small child alone in bath. 　• Bathe the infant in a small area (the kitchen sink is good) for the first few weeks. 　• Use a warm area in the house. 　• Use an area convenient for the mother. 　• Be sure the area is not drafty. 　• Never run water directly from the faucet onto the infant; always test with a forearm before placing the infant in water (water should be warm, but not too hot). • Cord care 　• Clean the cord with alcohol and cotton swabs when changing diapers. 　• Clean around the base of the cord. 　• Leave the cord alone until it drops off. 　• Alert the mother that there will be a small amount of spotting (bleeding) at the cord site when it drops off. • Clothing 　• To determine whether the infant is warm enough, feel the infant's chest or back with hand; never judge the infant's body temperature by feeling the infant's hands or feet.	Basic teaching measures for care of newborn.

(care plan continued on page 390)

NURSING ACTIONS/INTERVENTIONS WITH RATIONALES (continued from page 389)

Women's Health

ACTIONS/INTERVENTIONS	RATIONALES

• Use a mild detergent when laundering the infant's clothing
• Diapering
• Cloth diapers
• Disposable diapers
• Cleaning of the infant when changing diapers
• Circumcision care—Yellen clamp (metal clamp)
  • Gently wash the penis with water to remove urine and feces.
  • Reapply fresh, sterile Vaseline gauze around glans.
  • It is best to use cloth diapers until completely healed (approximately 7 to 10 days).
• Circumcision care—plastic bell
  • Gently wash the penis with water to remove urine and feces.
  • **Do not** apply petrolatum gauze.
  • Leave the plastic circle on the penis alone until tissue heals and circle falls off.
• Taking the baby's temperature and reading a thermometer:
  • Axillary
  • Rectal
Explain infant alert and rest states and how the caretaker can best use these states to interact with the infant.
	Promotes attachment.

Mental Health

ACTIONS/INTERVENTIONS	RATIONALES
Determine the client's optimum level of functioning and note here.	This information assists in establishing realistic goals.
Develop behavioral short-term goals by: • Listing those activities the client can assume • Breaking these activities into their component parts • Determining how much of each activity the client could successfully complete, and listing achievable activities here with goal achievement dates • Discussing expectations with the client	Goal accomplishment provides positive reinforcement and enhances self-esteem.
Keep instructions simple.	Inappropriate levels of sensory stimuli can contribute to the client's sense of disorganization and confusion.
Provide support to the client during tasks by: • Spending time with the client while he or she is completing the task. • Having all items necessary to achieve task readily available. • Assisting the client in focusing on the task at hand. • Providing positive verbal feedback as each step of the task is achieved.	Interaction with the nurse can be a source of positive reinforcement. Increases the possibility for the client to complete the task successfully. Positive feedback encourages behavior.

ACTIONS/INTERVENTIONS	RATIONALES
Keep the environment uncluttered, presenting only those items necessary to complete the task in the order needed.	Inappropriate levels of sensory stimuli can contribute to the client's sense of disorganization and confusion.
Develop a reward schedule for achievement of goals. Discuss possible rewards with the client, and list the things the client finds rewarding here with the goal to be achieved to gain the reward.	Promotes the client's sense of control. Positive feedback encourages behavior.
Schedule adequate time for the client to accomplish task (depressed client may need 2 hours to bathe and dress). [Note the client's schedule here.]	Communicates acceptance of the client, which facilitates the development of trust and self-esteem.
Decrease environmental stimuli to the degree necessary to assist the client in focusing on task. [Note the client's adaptations here.]	Promotes the client's sense of control.
Present ADLs on a regular schedule and note that schedule here. This schedule should be developed in consultation with the client.	
Spend [number] minutes with the client twice a day discussing feelings and reactions to current progress and expectations. Times for this and person responsible for this activity should be listed here.	Expression of feelings in a safe environment can facilitate problem identification and the development of coping strategies.
Allow the client to perform activities even though it might be easier at times for staff to complete the task for the client.	Communicates trust, and promotes the client's sense of control.
Communicate expectations and goals to all staff members.	Promotes consistency in the treatment, and communicates respect for the client.
Discuss with the family and other support systems and the client the plan and goals. Spend at least 5 minutes with the family after each visit to answer questions and explain treatment plan.	Increases potential for success of treatment plan.
Have members of support system identify how they can assist the client in achieving established goals.	
Spend time with the client discussing alternative ways of coping with the frustration that may occur while attempting to reach established goals.	Promotes the client's sense of control when encountering these difficulties. Successful coping will promote positive self-esteem.
Collaborate with the occupational therapist or physical therapist regarding special adaptations needed to assist the client with task accomplishment (e.g., exercises to increase muscle strength when muscles have not been used for a period of time).	
Monitor effects medications might have on goal achievement, and collaborate with the physician regarding problematic areas.	
Develop goals and schedules with the client, communicating that he or she does have responsibility and control in issues related to care.	
Discuss with the client and significant others the things that will facilitate continuance of self-care at home, and develop a plan that will assist the client in obtaining necessary items.	Facilitates the development of positive coping strategies, and increases potential for success when the client returns home. Successful accomplishment of this transition promotes positive self-esteem.
Refer to community resources as necessary for continued support.	

(care plan continued on page 392)

NURSING ACTIONS/INTERVENTIONS WITH RATIONALES (continued from page 391)

Gerontic Health

In addition to the interventions for Adult Health, the following may be utilized with the aging client.

ACTIONS/INTERVENTIONS	RATIONALES
Teach self-monitoring skills such as maintaining a journal or diary to record what factors may increase the self-care deficit.	Encourages the patient to identify areas that may need improvement or changes in lifestyle.[91]
Contract with the patient for achievement of specific incremental goals, and provide rewards or reinforcements when goals are met.	Enhances motivation to increase self-care.

Home Health

ACTIONS/INTERVENTIONS	RATIONALES
Monitor factors contributing to self-care deficit of [specify]. This includes items in the related factors section.	Provides a database for prevention and/or early intervention.
Involve the client and family in planning, implementing, and promoting reduction of the specific self-care deficit: • Family conference • Mutual goal setting • Communication	Involvement improves motivation and improves the outcome.
Assist the client and family to obtain assistive equipment as required: • Raised toilet seat • Adaptive equipment for eating utensils, combs, brushes, etc. • Rocker knife • Suction device under plate or bowl • Wrist or hand splints • Blender, crock pot, or microwave • Long-handled reacher (helping hand) • Box on seat of chair • Raised ledge on utility board • Straw and straw holder • Washcloth with soap • Wheelchair, walker, motorized cart, or cane • Bedside commode, incontinence undergarments • Bars and attachments and benches for shower or tub • Hand-held shower device • Long-handled sponge • Shaver holder • Medication organizers and magnifying glass • Diet supplements • Hearing aid • Corrective lenses	Assistive equipment improves function and increases the possibilities for self-care.

ACTIONS/INTERVENTIONS	RATIONALES
• Dressing aids: dressing stick, zipper pull, buttonhook, long-handled shoehorn, shoe fasteners, or Velcro closures	
Teach the client and family signs and symptoms of overexertion: • Pain • Fatigue • Confusion • Decrease or excessive increase in vital signs • Injury	Planning activities around physical capabilities prevents further reduction in self-care capacity.
Assist the client and family in lifestyle adjustments that may be required: • Proper use of assistive equipment • Adapting to need for assistance or assistive equipment • Determining criteria for monitoring the client's ability to function unassisted • Time management • Stress management • Development of support systems • Learning new skills • Work, family, social, and personal goals and priorities • Coping with disability or dependency • Providing environment conducive to self-care privacy, pain relief, social contact, and familiar and favorite surroundings and foods • Prevention of injury (falls, aspiration, burns, etc.) • Monitoring of skin integrity • Development of consistent routine • Mechanism for alerting family members to need for assistance	Provides basic information for the client and family that promotes necessary lifestyle changes.
Refer the patient to appropriate assistive resources as indicated.	Provides additional support for the client and family, and uses already available resources in a cost-effective manner.

SPONTANEOUS VENTILATION, IMPAIRED

DEFINITION[22]

A state in which the response pattern of decreased energy reserves results in an individual's inability to maintain breathing adequate to support life.[21]

DEFINING CHARACTERISTICS[22]

1. Dyspnea
2. Increased metabolic rate
3. Increased pCO_2
4. Increased restlessness
5. Increased heart rate
6. Decreased tidal volume
7. Decreased pO_2
8. Decreased cooperation
9. Apprehension
10. Decreased SaO_2
11. Increased use of accessory muscles

RELATED FACTORS[22]

1. Respiratory muscle fatigue
2. Metabolic factors

RELATED CLINICAL CONCERNS

1. Chronic obstructive pulmonary disease (COPD)
2. Asthma
3. Closed head injury
4. Respiratory arrest
5. Cardiac surgery
6. Adult respiratory distress syndrome (ARDS)

Have You Selected the Correct Diagnosis?

Ineffective Breathing Pattern
In this diagnosis, the patient's respiratory effort is insufficient to maintain the cellular oxygen supply. Both diagnoses would contribute to the patient being placed on ventilatory assistance; however, Impaired Spontaneous Ventilation is a more life-threatening, critical diagnosis than just an Ineffective Breathing Pattern. The major difference would be the criticalness of the patient's condition.

Impaired Gas Exchange
This diagnosis refers to the exchange of oxygen and carbon dioxide in the lungs or at the cellular level. Both this diagnosis and Impaired Spontaneous

Ventilation demonstrate this characteristic, but Impaired Spontaneous Ventilation is of a more critical nature than impairment.

EXPECTED OUTCOME

Blood gases will return to normal range by [date].

TARGET DATES

Because of the life-threatening potential of this diagnosis, initial target dates will need to be stated in terms of hours. After the patient's condition has improved and stabilized, the target date can be increased in increments of 1 to 3 days.

NURSING ACTIONS/INTERVENTIONS WITH RATIONALES

Adult Health

ACTIONS/INTERVENTIONS	RATIONALES
Monitor ventilator, ventilator settings, and patient response to therapy at least hourly.	Ensures correct functioning of equipment.
Provide sedation if needed.	Allows therapeutic effect of ventilation by preventing the patient from working against ("bucking") the ventilator.
Monitor lab work and other data including oxygen saturation, arterial blood gases, and lung sounds.	Monitors the effectiveness of therapy.
Implement actions that support adequate gas exchange. See nursing actions for Impaired Gas Exchange	
Provide adequate hydration. Monitor and document intake and output at least every shift, total every 24 hours. Weigh the patient daily at same time and in same-weight clothing.	Avoids fluid-volume deficit, assists in liquefying secretions, and prevents development of pulmonary edema.
Plan the activity–rest schedule on a daily basis. Allow at least 2 hours of uninterrupted rest during the day.	Conserves energy and promotes REM (rapid eye movement) sleep.
Review the patient's resources and support systems for management of a ventilator at home.	Initiates timely home care planning.
Reassure the patient's family while the patient is on ventilator.	
Collaborate with respiratory therapists as needed.	Ensures coordination of care.

Child Health

ACTIONS/INTERVENTIONS	RATIONALES
Determine parameters for respiratory status: • Range of acceptable rate, rhythm, and quality of respiration • Limits for apnea monitor setting.[92] The settings should be set for a range of safety according to age-related norms:	A specific respiratory assessment will help individualize the need plan of care.

ACTIONS/INTERVENTIONS	RATIONALES
• Neonates: 30–60 • Infants: 25–60 • Toddlers: 24–40 • Preschoolers: 22–34 • Adolescents: 12–16 • Arterial blood gases • Oxygen saturation levels • Respiratory testing (e.g., pneumogram) • Other indicators of respiratory function (e.g., cyanosis, mottling, diminished pulses, listless behavior, poor feeding, or vital signs)	
Provide one-to-one care for infants and children at risk for apnea or pulmonary arrest.	In high-risk respiratory patients, the possibility of arrest should be planned for. Identification of the actual arrest is a major factor in successful resuscitation.
Keep emergency medications and equipment (Ambu bag, airway, suctioning equipment, crash cart, ventilator, and oxygen) in close proximity.	Success in appropriate treatment of pulmonary arrest requires anticipatory planning with standard treatment modalities according to the American Heart Association guidelines and Pediatric Advanced Life Support guidelines.
Administer medication as ordered, being careful in administration of medications that might affect respirations (e.g., narcotics, bronchodilators, or vasoconstrictors). Monitor blood levels for therapeutic parameters of aminophylline–theophylline. Report levels above or below the desired range.	Anticipatory planning for the possibility of respiratory depression or arrest will lessen the likelihood of actuality in many instances and serve to allow for more success in treatment of these problems. If neuromuscular blocking agents are utilized, exercise caution in positioning because of the possibility of dislocation.[70,93]
Spend [number] minutes per shift with the family. During this time, focus on their concerns about the patient's respiratory status.	Verbalization of concerns helps reduce anxiety and provides subjective data for assessment and an opportunity for teaching.
Allow parental input as an option when it is realistic.	Parental involvement provides emotional security for the child and reinforces parental coping.
Carry out teaching according to inquiries by the patient or family. [Note special teaching needs here.]	Individualized learning is facilitated when it is directed toward stated needs.
Check level of consciousness (responsiveness) at least every 30 minutes.	Decreased responsiveness is indicative of onset of respiratory failure.
Monitor and document episodes of crying that result in apnea or loss of usual color for prolonged periods (15 seconds or more).	Breath-holding or crying may seem to cause hypoxia, but often there are underlying causes. Attention to underlying cause can be carried out, but vigilance for possible arrest is necessary.
Exercise caution in feeding or offering fluids.	Possible aspiration is likely if the infant is apneic, unable to suck well, or has problems swallowing.
Monitor for contributing factors to problem: • Central nervous system status • Airway • Chest wall • Respiratory muscles • Lung tissue	Alteration in any aspect of respiratory anatomy will affect adequate ventilation.
ADDITIONAL INFORMATION: Be aware of the major nursing considerations involved in the legal regulations related to brain death determination in children in the event of a decision to withhold or cease use of the ventilator for the purpose of determining brain death.	

(care plan continued on page 396)

NURSING ACTIONS/INTERVENTIONS WITH RATIONALES (continued from page 395)

Women's Health

The nursing actions for Women's Health are the same as those for Adult Health.

Mental Health

● N O T E : *If the client develops this diagnosis while being cared for in a mental health unit, he or she should immediately be transferred to an intensive care unit or adult health unit. A mental health unit is not equipped to handle this type of emergency.*

Gerontic Health

ACTIONS/INTERVENTIONS	RATIONALES
Monitor for iatrogenic reactions to medications.	Medication reactions may decrease respiratory drive and effort.
Observe for signs and symptoms of sleep-pattern disturbance.	Decreased rest secondary to sleep-pattern disturbances further diminishes physiologic reserves in older patients.[94]

Home Health

N O T E : *Should the home health client develop this diagnosis, the nurse should immediately have the client transferred to an acute care setting for the proper care.*

TISSUE PERFUSION, INEFFECTIVE (SPECIFY TYPE: RENAL, CEREBRAL, CARDIOPULMONARY, GASTROINTESTINAL, PERIPHERAL)

DEFINITION[22]

A decrease in oxygen resulting in failure to nourish the tissues at the capillary level.[21]

DEFINING CHARACTERISTICS[22]

1. Renal
   a. Altered blood pressure outside of acceptable parameters
   b. Hematuria
   c. Oliguria or anuria
   d. Elevation in blood urea nitrogen (BUN) and/or creatinine ratio
2. Cerebral
   a. Speech abnormalities
   b. Changes in pupillary reactions
   c. Extremity weakness or paralysis
   d. Altered mental status
   e. Difficulty in swallowing
   f. Changes in motor response
   g. Behavioral changes
3. Cardiopulmonary
   a. Altered respiratory rate outside of acceptable parameters
   b. Use of accessory muscles
   c. Capillary refill greater than 3 seconds
   d. Abnormal arterial blood gases
   e. Chest pain
   f. Sense of "impending doom"
   g. Bronchospasms
   h. Dyspnea
   i. Arrhythmias
   j. Nasal flaring
   k. Chest retraction
4. Gastrointestinal
   a. Hypoactive or absent bowel sounds
   b. Nausea
   c. Abdominal distention
   d. Abdominal pain or tenderness
5. Peripheral
   a. Edema
   b. Altered skin characteristics (hair, nails, and moisture)
   c. Weak or absent pulses

d. Skin discoloration
e. Skin temperature changes
f. Altered sensations
g. Claudication
h. Blood pressure changes in extremities
i. Bruits
j. Delayed healing
k. Diminished arterial pulsations
l. Skin color pale on elevation, color does not return on lowering leg

RELATED FACTORS[22]

1. Hypovolemia
2. Interruption of arterial flow
3. Hypervolemia
4. Interruption of venous flow
5. Mechanical reduction of venous and/or arterial blood flow
6. Hypoventilation
7. Impaired transport of oxygen across alveolar and/or capillary membrane
8. Mismatch of ventilation with blood flow
9. Decreased hemoglobin concentration in blood
10. Enzyme poisoning
11. Altered affinity of hemoglobin for oxygen

RELATED CLINICAL CONCERNS

1. Thrombophlebitis
2. Amputation reattachment
3. Varicosities
4. Diabetes mellitus
5. Cardiac infections
6. Anemia
7. Myocardial infarction
8. Coronary artery disease
9. Kawasaki's disease
10. Congestive heart failure
11. Congenital cardiac anomalies
12. Coronary artery aneurysm

 Have You Selected the Correct Diagnosis?

Decreased Cardiac Output
Ineffective Tissue Perfusion relates to deficits in the peripheral circulation with cellular impact. Decreased Cardiac Output relates specifically to a heart malfunction. Tissue perfusion problems may develop secondary to decreased cardiac output but can also exist without cardiac output problems.[105]

EXPECTED OUTCOME

Signs or symptoms of Ineffective Tissue Perfusion (note defining characteristics for this client here, e.g., pulse pressure, pulses, skin color, blood pressure) will be within normal limits by [date].

TARGET DATES

A maximum target date would be 2 days from the date of admission because of the dangers involved. A patient who develops this diagnosis should be referred to a medical practitioner immediately.

ADDITIONAL INFORMATION

Perfusion is the movement of blood to and from a body part. Adequate perfusion determines cell survival and depends on an adequate pump and vascular volume, as well as adequate functioning of the precapillary sphincters. The adequacy of these structures is affected by, among others, vasomotor, metabolic, and neural factors.[58,95]

The basic function of the cardiovascular system is to transport water, oxygen, nutrients, and hormones to the cells and to remove carbon dioxide, waste products, and heat from the cells. The size of the blood vessels decreases along the length of the arterial system, which increases resistance to fluid flow. To perfuse the cells adequately, the mean arterial blood pressure is maintained within a relatively narrow range by such regulatory systems as the baroreceptors, sympathetic nerves, and the cardiac branch of the vagus nerve.[58,95]

NURSING ACTIONS/INTERVENTIONS WITH RATIONALES

Adult Health

ACTIONS/INTERVENTIONS	RATIONALES
Adequate tissue perfusion is contingent on, among other factors, maintaining adequate fluid volume and adequate cardiac output. See nursing actions in these areas to ensure these areas are being met.	
If situation allows, facilitate early ambulation	
Ensure DVT prophylaxis has been implemented.	

(care plan continued on page 398)

NURSING ACTIONS/INTERVENTIONS WITH RATIONALES (continued from page 397)

Adult Health

ACTIONS/INTERVENTIONS	RATIONALES
Address and remove any physical or chemical factors that interfere with circulation.	
Implement measures to optimize adequate cerebral perfusion:	Maintains cerebral perfusion.
• Avoid undue elevations of ICP, maintain cerebral perfusion pressure	
• Implement actions to avoid vasospasm including administration of appropriate medications and HHH therapy as prescribed by the health-care team	
• Maintain blood pressure within prescribed therapeutic range as determined by health-care team	
Collaborate with the health-care team regarding medications that can improve perfusion such as vasopressors and positive inotropes.	
Implement strategies that decrease myocardial oxygen consumption (e.g., negative chronotropes).	
Maintain euthermia.	
Assure that areas susceptible to pressure are addressed (e.g., casts, endotracheal tube pilot balloon).	
Assess circulation to sites distal to temporary equipment (e.g., venous access devices, IABP).	To monitor for adverse effects of large venous devices.
Interpret data including lab work, hemodynamic monitoring, ICP	Determines efficacy of therapy and need for alternation of plan of care.

Child Health

ACTIONS/INTERVENTIONS	RATIONALES
Perform appropriate monitoring and documentation for contributory factors to include:	Provides basic database to ascertain progress and to individualize plan of care.
• Circulatory monitoring of anatomic site or general signs and symptoms related to peripheral pulses	
• Apical pulse, blood pressure, temperature, and respiration (monitor at least every hour or as ordered, and check cardiac monitor if applicable)	
• Intake and output every hour	
• Nausea or vomiting	
• Constipation or diarrhea	
• Tolerance of feeding	
• Pain or discomfort	
• Skin color and temperature; any integrity problems	
• Circulatory pattern: Notify the physician for any change in the pattern that suggests lack of oxygenation (e.g., cyanosis, arterial blood gas results, or decreased pulses).	
• Appropriate functioning of equipment, such as ventilator, arterial line, or intravenous pump	
• Maintenance of intravenous line for administration of fluids	

ACTIONS/INTERVENTIONS	RATIONALES
• Positional demands • Pain or discomfort • Sensory input appropriate for age and developmental status • Fluid and electrolytes Collaborate with other health-care providers as needed. [Note special needs of collaboration here.]	Coordination and implementation of plan of care may involve numerous professionals according to the cause of alteration and the treatment modalities available.
Provide for appropriate availability of resuscitative equipment, including: • Ambu bag • Crash cart for pediatrics with drugs and defibrillator • Appropriate respiratory intubation equipment	Basic emergency preparedness.
Allow for parental and child health teaching needs by allowing 10 to 15 minutes per 8-hour shift for verbalization of concerns. [Note special teaching needs here.]	Verbalization of health-related concerns may serve as cues for teaching needs and also serves to reduce anxiety.
Allow for parental participation in care of the child at appropriate level (e.g., giving comfort measures or assisting with feeding).	Parental involvement in care puts the child at ease and provides self-esteem and empowerment for the parents.
Provide rest by scheduling procedures together with ample time between activities. Note the routine for this client here.	Appropriate attention to rest needs helps prevent further metabolic demands on already less than ideal homeostasis scenario. Consistency increases the sense of security.
Allow patient and parental preferences in plan of care. Note those preferences here.	Individualization shows value attached to parents' input.
Deal with appropriate related factors associated with ineffective tissue perfusion (e.g., minimizing crying by anticipating needs).	All efforts to lessen workload on heart and respiratory system will assist in preventing further decompensation.
Provide appropriate safety for age (e.g., keeping siderails up or positioning as ordered).	Safety is a standard part of care and ought to be planned for according to health status, age, and development.
Maintain proper use of equipment, such as Clinitron bed, or special K-pads.	Assists circulation.
Provide for appropriate follow-up via scheduled appointments after hospitalization. [Note follow-up plan here.]	Encourages consistency in long-range care. Demonstrates how to schedule appointments, and provides support for parents.
Provide the patient with teaching appropriate to needs of illness and family (e.g., if activities and daily care are to be modified, consider use of pulse oximeter to monitor perfusion, and explain how to do circulatory checks after cast application). [Note teaching plan here.]	Assists in reducing anxiety, and facilitates home management of care.
Ensure that the parents have been certified in CPR before the child is dismissed from hospital.	Basic need for home care when perfusion problem is present.

● NOTE: *A major effort will be that of follow-up with appropriate specialized care to include pediatric cardiology and, as needed, other expertise to anticipate a long course of therapy. Care is focused on early diagnosis, especially in instances of congenital cardiac anomaly (e.g., simple coronary artery malformation versus that associated with other related physiologic malformation of the heart and vasculature). A specific concern is Kawasaki's disease, with a residual concern of coronary artery aneurysm. Periodic echocardiography is mandated for those individuals.*

(care plan continued on page 400)

NURSING ACTIONS/INTERVENTIONS WITH RATIONALES (continued from page 399)

Women's Health

● N O T E : *In instances of decreased coronary tissue perfusion, the women's health client should immediately be transferred to a coronary care unit.*

ACTIONS/INTERVENTIONS	RATIONALES
Assist the patient in identifying lifestyle adjustments that may be needed because of changes in physiologic function or needs during experiential phases of life (e.g., pregnancy, birth, postpartum and related to gynecology): • Avoid prolonged sitting, sitting with crossed legs, or standing. • Develop exercise plan for cardiovascular fitness during pregnancy. • Avoid wearing constrictive clothing. • Maintain a balanced diet with adequate hydration. • Avoid constipation and bearing down to prevent hemorrhoids.	Decreases factors that could lead to decreased perfusion of oxygen to uterus, placenta, and fetus.
Monitor the patient for signs of pregnancy-induced hypertension (PIH): • Prenatal weight • Blood pressure • Presence of edema • Proteinuria • Pre-eclampsia • Headaches • Visual changes such as blurred vision • Increased edema of face and pitting edema of extremities • Oliguria • Hyperreflexia • Nausea or vomiting • Epigastric pain • Eclampsia • Convulsions • Coma	Allows early intervention to avoid perfusion problems and development of complications.
Monitor for edema: • Swelling of hands, face, legs, or feet. • **Caution:** The patient may have to remove rings. • The patient may need to wear loose shoes or a bigger shoe size. • Schedule rest breaks during day when the patient can elevate legs. • When the patient is lying down, he or she should lie on the left side to promote placental perfusion and prevent compression of vena cava. In collaboration with physician (as appropriate): • Check intake and output (urinary output not less than 30 mL/h or 120 mL/4 h).	Provides early warning of perfusion problems, and promotes early intervention.

ACTIONS/INTERVENTIONS	RATIONALES
• Use magnesium sulfate ($MgSO_4$) and hydralazine hydrochloride (Apresoline) therapy according to physician order. Have antidote for $MgSO_4$ (calcium gluconate) available at all times during $MgSO_4$ therapy. • Assess deep tendon reflexes (DTR). • Check respiratory rate, pulse, and blood pressure at least every 2 hours on [odd/even] hour. • Evaluate for possibility of seizures. • Limit the amount of noise in the patient's environment. • Monitor fetal heart rate and well-being.	
Provide quiet, nonstimulating environment for the patient.	Reduces anxiety and promotes rest. Both measures will assist in maintaining peripheral circulation by avoiding vasoconstriction.
Provide the patient and family factual information and support as needed.	Reduces anxiety and provides teaching opportunity.
Monitor and teach the patient to monitor and report any signs of PIH immediately: • Rapid rise in blood pressure • Rapid weight gain • Marked hyperreflexia, especially transient or sustained ankle clonus • Severe headache • Visual disturbances • Epigastric pain • Increase in proteinuria • Oliguria, with urine output of less than 30 mL/h • Drowsiness	Allows early detection of problem and more rapid intervention.
In collaboration with dietitian: • Obtain nutritional history. • Provide a high-protein diet (80–100 grams of protein). • Provide low-sodium diet (not more than 6 grams daily or less than 2.5 grams daily).	Dietary measures that assist in controlling blood pressure.
Oral Contraceptive Therapy	
Monitor for factors that contraindicate use of oral birth control. • Family history of stroke, diabetes, or reproductive cancer • History of thromboembolic disease or vascular problems, hypertension, hepatic disease, and smoking • Presence of any breast disease, nodule, or fibrocystic disease	These factors promote side effects and untoward effects from birth control pills.

Mental Health

● NOTE: *The nursing actions in this section reflect alteration in tissue perfusion related to the cerebral and peripheral vascular systems, because these are the systems most commonly affected in the mental health setting.*

(care plan continued on page 402)

NURSING ACTIONS/INTERVENTIONS WITH RATIONALES (continued from page 401)

Mental Health

ACTIONS/INTERVENTIONS	RATIONALES
Check on orthostatic hypotension by taking blood pressure while the client is lying down, then taking blood pressure just after the client stands or sits up (provide support for the client to prevent injury from a fall).	Psychotropic medications can predispose the client to orthostatic hypotension.
Monitor the client's mental status. If compromised, provide information in a clear, concise manner.	
Discuss with the client causes of decreased cerebral blood flow.	Assists in explaining reasons for therapies to the client.
Have the client get out of bed slowly by: • Sitting up • Swinging legs over edge of bed • Resting in this position for at least 2 minutes • Standing up slowly • Walking slowly	Allows time for cardiovascular system to adapt, thus preventing fainting or dizziness due to orthostatic hypotension.
Teach the client to avoid situations in which he or she changes position quickly (e.g., bending over to pick something up off the floor or standing quickly from a sitting position).	
Have the client supported while changing positions that cause vertigo until problem is resolved.	
Assist the client in getting in and out of the bathtub.	
Collaborate with physician regarding alterations in medications.	Promotes changing to a medication that would not interfere with perfusion.
If situation persists, have the client: • Sleep sitting up or with head elevated. • Use elastic stockings that are waist high. • Apply stockings while the client is still in bed. • Have the client raise legs for several minutes. • Apply stockings slowly and evenly. • Remove stockings after the client is lying down at least every 8 hours.	Provides external support for venous system.
Develop with the client a plan for daily exercise that is very modest (e.g., walking the length of the hall for 15 minutes twice a day for 3 days, then increasing distance and time gradually until the client is walking for 30 minutes twice a day). [Note the client's exercise regimen here.]	Improves cardiovascular strength. Assists in maintaining muscle tone, which assists in supporting the venous circulation.
Develop with the client a reward schedule for implementing exercise plan. [List rewards and the reward schedule here.]	
Provide the client with positive verbal support for goal accomplishment.	
Do not allow the client to participate in unit activities that could produce injury until the condition is resolved (e.g., cooking or using sharp objects while standing).	Basic safety measures.

ACTIONS/INTERVENTIONS	RATIONALES
Discuss with the client the effects of alcohol and smoking on blood flow, and assist him or her to develop alternative coping behavior if necessary. [Note plan for this here.]	
Provide decaffeinated beverages for the client. Consult with the dietary department about this adaptation.	
Increase the client's fluid intake during times of increased loss, such as exercise or periods of anxiety. Instruct the client in the need for this.	
Observe the client carefully after injecting medications that have a high potential for producing hypotension. This is especially true for clients who are very agitated and physically active.	Basic measure to offset the possibility of falling secondary to orthostatic hypotension.
Inform the client of need to change position slowly after injecting medication.	
Teach the client and support system about over-the-counter medications that alter blood flow (e.g., cold medications, antihistamines, or diet pills).	
Monitor peripheral pulses on affected limbs every 8 hours at [times].	
Avoid, and teach the client to avoid, pressure in points on affected limbs to include: • Changing position frequently when sitting or lying down • Avoiding pressure in the area behind the knee • Not crossing legs while sitting • Making sure shoes fit properly and do not rub feet • Elevating feet when sitting to reduce pressure on backs of legs	Avoids compromising circulation by pressure or constriction.
Keep feet clean and dry, and teach the client to do the same by assessing foot condition once a day at [time]. This assessment should include: • Washing feet • Checking for sores, reddened areas, and blisters • Keeping toenails trimmed and caring for ingrown nails • Applying lotion to feet • Rubbing reddened areas if the client does not have a history of emboli • Applying clean, dry socks • Teaching significant others to assist with foot care of the elderly client • Keeping limbs warm (but **do not** use external heating sources such as heating pads or hot-water bottles)	Avoids lower extremity skin integrity problems and possible infection with the resultant impact on circulation.
Develop with the client an exercise program, and note that program here. Begin slowly, and gradually increase time and distance (e.g., walk for 15 minutes 2 times per day for 1 week). This should be increased until the client is walking 1 mile in 30 to 45 minutes three times a week.	Promotes normal venous return.

(care plan continued on page 404)

NURSING ACTIONS/INTERVENTIONS WITH RATIONALES (continued from page 403)

Mental Health

ACTIONS/INTERVENTIONS	RATIONALES
Instruct the client to discontinue exercise if: • Pulse does not return to resting rate within 3 minutes after exercise. • Shortness of breath continues for more than 10 minutes after stopping exercise. • Fatigue is excessive. • Muscles are painful. • The client experiences dizziness, pain in the chest, lightheadedness, loss of muscle control, or nausea.	Client safety is of primary importance.
Encourage the client's exercise by: • Walking with him or her • Determining things that the client would find rewarding and supplying these as goals are achieved • Providing positive verbal support as goals are achieved [Note the client's specific reward system here.]	
Monitor the client's nutritional status, and refer to nutritionist for teaching if necessary.	
Discuss with the client the effects of smoking on peripheral blood flow, and assist him or her in decreasing or eliminating this by: • Referring the client to a stop-smoking group • Encouraging him or her not to smoke before meals or exercise • Decreasing amount smoked per day	Nicotine causes vasospasm and vasoconstriction.
Discuss special needs with the client and support system before discharge.	Increases probability of the client's behavior change being maintained after discharge.
Refer the client to community agencies to provide ongoing care as needed.	

Gerontic Health

In addition to the interventions for adults, the following may be utilized for aging clients.

ACTIONS/INTERVENTIONS	RATIONALES
Monitor for signs of dyspnea, chronic fatigue, behavioral changes, or evidence of acute cerebral insufficiency.	Older clients with decreased cardiac perfusion often present with these symptoms.
Plan physical activities, such as hygiene, meals, and ambulation, with rest periods.	Decreases cardiac workload.
Instruct in use of oxygen, if prescribed.	Supplemental oxygen may be prescribed to help decrease cardiac workload.
Teach the client relaxation methods to help decrease anxiety.	Decreasing anxiety helps decrease the release of catecholamines. An increase in catecholamines results in increased cardiac workload.

Home Health

● **N O T E :** *If this diagnosis is suspected when caring for a client in the home, it is imperative that a physician referral be obtained immediately. If a physician has referred the client to home health care, the nurse will collaborate with the physician in the treatment of the client.*

ACTIONS/INTERVENTIONS	RATIONALES
Teach the client and family appropriate monitoring of signs and symptoms of alteration in tissue perfusion: • Pulse (lying, sitting, and standing) • Skin temperature and turgor • Edema • Motor status • Sensory status • Blood pressure (lying, sitting, standing, and pulse pressure) • Respiratory status (dyspnea, cyanosis, and rate) • Weight fluctuations • Urinary output • Leg pain with walking	Provides database for prevention and/or early intervention.
Assist the client and family in identifying lifestyle changes that may be required: • Eliminating smoking • Decreasing caffeine • Decreasing alcohol • Avoiding over-the-counter medications • Protecting skin and extremities from injury due to decreased sensation (burns, frostbite, etc.) • Protecting skin from pressure injury (making frequent position changes and using sheepskin for pressure areas and foot cradle) • Improving arterial blood flow (keeping extremities warm, elevating head and chest, avoiding crossing legs or sitting for long periods of time, wiggling fingers and toes every hour, and performing ROM exercises) • Performing exercise program as tolerated • Improving venous blood flow (elevating extremity, using antiembolus stockings, and avoiding pressure behind knees) • Performing skin and foot care • Decreasing cholesterol and saturated fat intake • Performing diversional activities as needed • Practicing stress management	Provides basic information for the client and family that promotes necessary lifestyle changes.
Teach the family basic CPR.	Basic safety measure.
Teach the client and family purposes, side effects, and proper administration technique of medications.	Promotes safe adherence to the therapeutic regimen.
Assist the client and family to set criteria to help them determine when a physician or other intervention is required.	Locus of control shifts from nurse to the client and family, thus promoting self-care.
Assess the client/family need for assistive resources and refer to community agencies that provide such resources.	Provides additional support for the client and family, and uses already available resources in a cost-effective manner.

TRANSFER ABILITY, IMPAIRED

DEFINITION[22]

Limitation of independent movement between two nearby surfaces.[21]

DEFINING CHARACTERISTICS[22]

1. Impaired ability to transfer from bed to chair and chair to bed
2. Impaired ability to transfer on or off a toilet or commode
3. Impaired ability to transfer in and out of tub or shower
4. Impaired ability to transfer between uneven levels
5. Impaired ability to transfer from chair to car or car to chair
6. Impaired ability to transfer from chair to floor or floor to chair
7. Impaired ability to transfer from standing to floor or floor to standing

RELATED FACTORS[22]

To be developed.

RELATED CLINICAL CONCERNS

1. Arthritis
2. Paralysis
3. Neuromuscular diseases

4. Amputation
5. Fractures

 Have You Selected the Correct Diagnosis?

Impaired Physical Mobility
Certainly anyone who had Impaired Transfer Ability would also have Impaired Physical Mobility. The inability to transfer from one site to another would need to be resolved before Impaired Physical Mobility could be resolved.

Ineffective Management of Therapeutic Regimen, Individual
A patient who cannot transfer himself or herself from one site to another could well have difficulty with managing a therapeutic regimen. However, the patient will never be able to manage the therapeutic regimen until the problem with transfer ability is resolved.

EXPECTED OUTCOME

Will independently transfer self by [date].

TARGET DATES

Resolving this diagnosis requires an extended length of time. An appropriate initial evaluation date would be 7 to 10 days after the date the diagnosis is made.

NURSING ACTIONS/INTERVENTIONS WITH RATIONALES

Adult Health

ACTIONS/INTERVENTIONS	RATIONALES
Devise and implement a strength training regimen in conjunction with physical therapist. • Devise a daily schedule. • Provide adequate periods of rest • Provide patient with implements to increase strength (e.g., resistance bands, weights)	Adequate strength is integral to movement between surfaces.
Provide the patient with assistive devices that enhance ability to transfer (e.g., trapeze, crutches, raised toilet seats, hand rails).	Facilitates transfer.
Provide the patient with appropriate accessories including non-skid slippers, appropriate fitting shoes, gloves.	Ensures safety during transfer.
Ensure that area to which the patient is transferring is appropriately prepared.	Reduces obstacles and ensures safety during transfer.
Utilize appropriate number of personnel to assist patient.	
Ensure that patient has adequate nutritional intake to support muscle development.	
Refer the patient to nutrition services or devise weight loss plan if weight is the limiting factor.	

ACTIONS/INTERVENTIONS	RATIONALES
Educate the patient about working with limitations and gradually increasing activity as physical ability allows.	Gives patient realistic purview of progress through plan of care.
Refer to rehabilitation facility as appropriate and as soon as feasible.	

Child Health

ACTIONS/INTERVENTIONS	RATIONALES
Determine all contributing factors, to include: • Neuromuscular • Cardiovascular • Pulmonary • Cognitive • Developmental • Situational	All possible factors are considered in providing a holistic database for individualization.
Determine augmentative devices, personnel, or environmental needs and have these available before transfer. [Note the client's special needs here.]	Appropriate support ensures safety.
Determine the client's level of proprioception.	Prerequisite for each maneuver to increase likelihood of success.
Determine strength and ability to coordinate body movements well in advance of attempted maneuver.	Pre-assessment helps ensure safety needs are met.
Schedule transfer activities in a timely manner when possible. [Note the time needed for the client to perform activity here.]	Time to adjust and slowly incorporate concept of transfer will be best afforded in a leisure vs. crisis time frame.
Determine readiness for taking on task of transfer.	Validation of readiness offers empowerment and a sense of control in attempt.
Determine need for teaching the client, family, or other caregivers how to assist in transfer activities. [Note teaching plan here.]	Teaching with focus on learner's needs will most likely ease anxiety and afford consistency in safe manner.
Determine a reward system to fit developmental status of the client for appropriate attainment of goal. [Note those rewards and situations to be rewarded here.]	Provides reinforcement of desired behavior.
Schedule group teaching of transfer activities. [Note schedule here.]	Group behavior offers peer support.
Determine need for adaptations related to the patient's changing status and environmental needs. (Home and school vs. hospital)	Principles of safety may be altered yet upheld for changes that occur.
Allow sufficient time for teaching and mastery of transfer if discharge may occur within short period of time. [Note teaching plan and schedule here.]	Early teaching with plan for dismissal results in greater likelihood of attainment and may be reason to keep patient until satisfied.

Women's Health

The nursing actions for Women's Health are the same as those for Adult Health.

(care plan continued on page 408)

NURSING ACTIONS/INTERVENTIONS WITH RATIONALES (continued from page 407)

Mental Health

The nursing actions for the mental health client are the same as those for Adult Health.

Gerontic Health

The nursing actions for Gerontic Health are the same as those for Adult Health.

Home Health/Community Health

The nursing actions for Home/Community Health are the same as those for Adult Health with the following additions:

ACTIONS/INTERVENTIONS	RATIONALES
Educate the client, family, and potential caregivers about the following: • Using proper body mechanics • Maintaining a clear wheelchair path	Assists in avoiding injury.
Assist the client in obtaining and proper use of a sliding board.	Facilitates a safe transfer.
Assist the client in developing a schedule for range of motion exercises.	To maintain and build muscle strength.
Refer clients for a home physical therapy consult to help them maximize their ability to safely use a wheelchair at home and to have assistive devices appropriate for the home environment.	

WALKING, IMPAIRED

DEFINITION[22]

Limitation of independent movement within the environment on foot.[21]

DEFINING CHARACTERISTICS[22]

1. Impaired ability to climb stairs
2. Impaired ability to walk required distances
3. Impaired ability to walk on an incline or decline
4. Impaired ability to walk on uneven surfaces
5. Impaired ability to navigate curbs

RELATED FACTORS[22]

To be developed.

RELATED CLINICAL CONCERNS

1. Arthritis
2. Chronic obstructive pulmonary disease
3. Cerebrovascular accident
4. Neuromuscular disorders
5. Amputation involving lower extremities

 Have You Selected the Correct Diagnosis?

Impaired Physical Mobility
Impaired walking could be considered to be a subset of Impaired Physical Mobility and is a more specific diagnosis. If the patient is having difficulty only with walking and not other aspects of mobility, such as moving in bed and getting up and down in sitting, then Impaired Walking is the most correct diagnosis.

Activity Intolerance
This diagnosis relates more to feeling fatigued or weakness while performing activities. Again, Activity Intolerance is a broader diagnosis than Impaired Walking.

EXPECTED OUTCOME

Will independently walk by [date].

TARGET DATES

Activities to facilitate walking with ease require weeks. An appropriate evaluation target date would be 1 to 2 weeks from the day of admission.

NURSING ACTIONS/INTERVENTIONS WITH RATIONALES

Adult Health

ACTIONS/INTERVENTIONS	RATIONALES
Determine the appropriate equipment and pattern based on your assessment, and the goals of treatment.	
Remove items in the area that may interfere with ambulation.	To maintain a safe environment.
Explain and demonstrate the gait pattern for the patient; ask the patient to describe the pattern, how it is to be performed, and what he or she is expected to do.	To verify that he or she truly understands and comprehends your instructions.
Be sure the patient is wearing appropriate footwear; **do not** allow the patient to ambulate while wearing slippers, loosely fitting shoes, or while not wearing shoes.	These conditions can lead to patient insecurity and injury as a result of a fall.
Monitor the patient's physiologic responses to ambulation frequently, and evaluate his or her vital signs, general appearance, and mental alertness during the activity. Compare your findings to normal values to determine the patient's reaction to the activity.	
See nursing actions related to impaired physical mobility for a plan of care that supports improvement of walking.	
Collaborate with Physical Therapy as needed.	To assist in planning the ambulation activities.

Child Health

ACTIONS/INTERVENTIONS	RATIONALES
Monitor for all contributing factors including: • Orthopedic • Neurologic • Developmental • Situational	A complete assessment provides primary database for individualization.
Monitor readiness for weight-bearing. Note exact limits of activity with reliance on limbs, both lower and upper.	Validation of status of limbs and their capacity for weight-bearing is critical for safety and non-injury before ambulation is considered.
Assess for need for assistive devices or personnel for walking activity.	Appropriate augmentive aids help ensure safe activity.
Determine teaching needs for the client, family, or related assistants. [Note teaching plan here.]	Specific data for safety and likelihood of success is paramount for all involved to feel empowered.
Provide posture-appropriate alignment during walking activities.	Lessens likelihood of related injury to spine or limbs.
Provide appropriate cautionary information when assistance is required for the patient's walking. State when, what must be done, and with whom to meet prerequisite walking behaviors.	Ensures likelihood of safe walking with appropriate attention to limit setting to reinforce importance of plan.
Coordinate health-care team members and scheduling of walking activities. [Note collaboration plan here as well as assistance needed from nursing staff to implement plan.]	The nurse is in the best position to provide safe and consistent care with total patient needs in mind.

(care plan continued on page 410)

NURSING ACTIONS/INTERVENTIONS WITH RATIONALES (continued from page 409)

Child Health

ACTIONS/INTERVENTIONS	RATIONALES
Provide safe environment, free of clutter or equipment, to degree possible.	Lessens the likelihood for barriers or obstacles to free path.
Schedule medications to enhance success in walking activities. [Note schedule here.]	According to nature of medication, onset of action, half-life, side effects, or untoward effects, the best likelihood for walking without undesired effects is upheld.
Seek assistance from Occupational and/or Physical Therapy to facilitate progress in walking activities.	Periodic regular assessment with appropriate health team members provides appropriate validation for safe walking.
Determine an appropriate reward system according to the patient's developmental capacity. [Note plan here.]	Reinforces desired behavior.
Provide opportunities for group teaching of walking activity as appropriate for the child's developmental level.	Peer pressure and interaction offers diversionary stimulus to perform desired activity.
If equipment is required, offer artistic opportunities for the client to decorate same per developmental interest.	Self-expression provides a sense of identity for the client.
Determine need for discharge planning well before actual event. [Note plan and person responsible for coordinating this activity here.]	Prior planning permits sufficient time to safely master walking protocol in a supportive environment.
Discuss with the child and family a plan for adapting mobility needs to school or other regular activities.	Anticipation of usual events of daily living to be reincorporated in advance will lessen likelihood of unsafe or unsuccessful attempts to adapt lifestyle.

Women's Health

The nursing actions for Women's Health are the same as those for Adult Health.

Mental Health

The nursing actions for the mental health client are the same as those for Adult Health.

Gerontic Health

In addition to the interventions for Adult Health, the following may be utilized with the aging client:

ACTIONS/INTERVENTIONS	RATIONALES
Collaborate with the physical therapist for assessment and treatment plan to improve walking ability.	Physical therapists are health-care professionals specializing in problems related to the lower extremities and ambulation skills.
Ensure that any adaptive or assistive equipment (such as braces, footwear, or eyeglasses) fit correctly and are properly functioning.	Reduces potential for injuries when the client is walking.
Promote interdisciplinary team member communication to ensure that plan of care is consistently applied.	Ensures continuity of care across disciplines and care settings.

ACTIONS/INTERVENTIONS	RATIONALES
Monitor and report symptoms as needed from medications (e.g., antihypertensives, diuretics, or psychotropics) with side effects such as lightheadedness, or orthostatic blood pressure changes that may affect the client's ambulatory ability.	Older adults may require medication adjustments to decrease side effects that have a deleterious effect on ambulation ability and safety.[96,97]
Encourage client participation in a walking program, if available in care setting.	Promotes the client's physical and psychological well-being.
Teach the client and/or caregivers to check for environmental aids (e.g., handrails) or barriers (poorly fitting shoes, shiny floor surfaces, or cluttered pathways) to walking.	Emphasizes safety focus prior to onset of activity.
Promote use of activity programs, if available, that support the goal of increasing walking ability in clients (e.g., Senior Olympic activities, exercises to promote lower extremity strengthening, or enhanced trunk control and balance abilities).[97]	Provides increased opportunities for older adults to practice skills to enhance walking ability.

Home Health

ACTIONS/INTERVENTIONS	RATIONALES
Educate the client, family, and potential caregivers about the following: • Using proper body mechanics to avoid injury • Maintaining a clear walking path • Installation of rails in the home to assist the client as he or she ambulates • Eliminating throw rugs and cords that cross walking paths, because they increase the risk of falls • The correct use of assistive devices • Ensuring that all assistive devices are set to the correct height Assist the client in obtaining necessary durable medical equipment (e.g., crutches or walkers). Refer the client for a home physical therapy consult to help maximize his or her ability to safely ambulate at home and to have assistive devices appropriate for the home environment.	

WANDERING

DEFINITION[22]

Meandering, aimless, and/or repetitive locomotion, frequently incongruent with boundaries, limits, or obstacles that expose the individual to harm.[21]

DEFINING CHARACTERISTICS[22]

1. Frequent or continuous movement from place to place, often revisiting the same destination(s)
2. Persistent locomotion in search of "missing" or unattainable persons or places
3. Haphazard locomotion
4. Locomotion into unauthorized or private spaces
5. Locomotion resulting in unintended leaving of the premises
6. Long periods of locomotion without an apparent destination
7. Inability to locate significant landmarks in a familiar setting
8. Fretful locomotion or pacing
9. Locomotion that cannot easily be dissuaded or redirected
10. Following behind or shadowing a caregiver's locomotion

11. Trespassing
12. Hyperactivity
13. Scanning, seeking, or searching behaviors
14. Periods of locomotion interspersed with periods of nonlocomotion, for example, sitting, standing, or sleeping
15. Getting lost

RELATED FACTORS[22]

1. Cognitive impairment, specifically memory and recall deficits, disorientation, poor visuoconstructive (or visuospatial) ability, language (primarily expressive) defects
2. Cortical atrophy
3. Premorbid behavior; for example, outgoing, sociable personality, premorbid dementia
4. Separation from familiar people and places
5. Sedation
6. Emotional state, especially frustration, anxiety, boredom, or depression (agitated)
7. Physiologic state or need; for example, hunger, thirst, pain, urination, or constipation
8. An over- or understimulating social or physical environment
9. Time of day

RELATED CLINICAL CONCERNS

1. Dementia
2. Neurologic diseases impacting the brain
3. Head injuries

4. Medication side effects; for example, analgesics, sedatives, or hypnotics
5. Hyperthermia

 Have You Selected the Correct Diagnosis?

Disturbed Thought Process
A disturbance in thought processing could well lead to wandering; however, Wandering is a specific physical behavior. Disturbed Thought Process is more specific to cognition.

Impaired Memory
Impaired Memory could also contribute to wandering, but again, Wandering is a specific physical behavior. Impaired Memory refers specifically to the mental behavior of remembering.

EXPECTED OUTCOME

Will have decrease in number of episodes of wandering by [date].

Will participate in [number] diversional activities per [day/hour].

Environment will promote client safety (note specific adaptations here, e.g. locked doors, client tracking device) by [date].

TARGET DATES

Wandering needs to be monitored on a daily basis; however, a target date of 5 days would be appropriate for initial evaluation of progress.

NURSING ACTIONS/INTERVENTIONS WITH RATIONALES

Adult Health

ACTIONS/INTERVENTIONS	RATIONALES
Review current medications, both prescription and over-the-counter.	May have adverse effects or interactions.
Clear a safe area. Eliminate clutter or other hazards.	Safety is the primary concern for patients who may wander.
Consider the use of weight alarm sensors or other types of alert sensors on the bed, chair, or wheelchair.	Alarm will sound when the patient exceeds safety limits.[98]
Have patient ID in clothes, on a bracelet or necklace, or wallet ID card.	Assists in identifying the wandering patient.
Refer the family to the Alzheimer's Association Safe Return Program: (800) 272-3900.	
Please refer to the Gerontic Health and Home Health Care plans for additional nursing actions.	

Child Health

This diagnosis, according to its definition and defining characteristics, would not be appropriate for Child Health.

Women's Health

Interventions for a Women's Health client with this diagnosis would be the same as the interventions given in Adult Health and Gerontic Health.

Mental Health

The mental health client with this diagnosis would require the same interventions as those given in Adult Health and Gerontic Health.

Gerontic Health

● N O T E : *Wandering, a behavior noted in clients with dementia, remains a perplexing activity for study and nursing interventions. Current research is attempting to describe and design assessments and nursing interventions for various types of wandering behavior.[94] With this need for further investigation in mind, the following actions are based on keeping clients safe, providing an outlet for stress and anxiety reduction, and providing environmental cues for clients. Nursing interventions should be adapted to meet the needs of the individual client who wanders. Some clients may favorably respond to interventions such as touch or music, whereas others may not. All clients should be thoroughly assessed for possible underlying cognitive dysfunction using the Folstein Mini Mental State Exam (MMSE) or a similar tool. In addition, a thorough assessment of the client's functional status should be conducted to establish a baseline and safety precautions.*

ACTIONS/INTERVENTIONS	RATIONALES
Determine the pattern of wandering and share observations with caregivers[95] (e.g., the client wanders at certain times of day or evening, or after visits from family or friends).	Knowledge of patterns can prompt caregivers to anticipate need for activities or personal attention.
Monitor for possible causes of wandering and address them as appropriate. Wandering can be caused by environmental stimuli or a lack of stimuli, feelings of loneliness or separation, situational insecurity, boredom or fear, sleep disorder, anxiety, or unmet physical needs such as hunger or pain.	
Monitor for expression of intent "I'm going home now" and expression of the loss of a valued adult role, "The children need me now."	
Modify the environment to provide adequate rest, safety, and sleep for the client.	Eliminate possible precipitators of wandering.
Evaluate the patient's response to medications and collaborate with the health-care team to adapt the medication regimen as needed.	Some medications may increase the risk for falls in the client who wanders.
Provide the patient with essential sensory aids (glasses, hearing aids).	Prevents possible sensory confusion that can lead to wandering and prevents falls when wandering occurs.

(care plan continued on page 414)

NURSING ACTIONS/INTERVENTIONS WITH RATIONALES (continued from page 413)

Gerontic Health

ACTIONS/INTERVENTIONS	RATIONALES
Avoid physical and chemical restraints.	These do not stop the urge to wander and may exacerbate the urge to wander. These measures may contribute to client injury.
Schedule and maintain a regular toileting schedule. [Note the client's schedule here.]	Eliminate possible precipitators of wandering.
Provide information to all staff that a patient is a wanderer. Develop a mechanism for identification, and a plan to follow if a wanderer is missing. [Note that plan here.]	Prevention of injury related to wandering.
Use grid like markings in front of doorways.	May prevent the client from exiting due to a change in visual cues.
Ensure that the client has ID bracelet or necklace listing his or her name and an emergency telephone number.[98]	Provides means of identification if the client becomes lost.
Monitor the environment for possible safety hazards (e.g., toxic solutions or plants, electrical hazards, fire risks, or firearms).[99]	Decreases environmental injury risk.
Have poison control number available in the event of ingestion of unsafe products.	Decreased cognition may result in the client ingesting toxic substances.
Encourage community-dwelling caregivers to enroll the client in the Alzheimer's Association Safe Return Program.	Provides organized response if the client becomes lost.
Ensure that there is an updated client photograph available.	Assists in identification efforts. As dementia progresses, there may be marked changes in the client's appearance.
Discourage access to exits by using electronic keypad alarm systems on doors.	Provides audible alarm if door is opened without using the correct code.
Depending on care setting, promote group walking activity in early afternoon or after evening meals.[100]	Offers outlet for socializing and meeting the client's activity and exercise needs.
Based on client preference, use music for 20 to 30 minutes before periods when the client is known to become increasingly agitated.	Music has been shown to reduce or eliminate agitation in some clients affected with dementia.[101]
Incorporate slow-stroke massage for brief periods (10 to 20 minutes) to the client's neck, shoulders, and back in early morning or late afternoon.	Slow-stroke massage has been helpful with some dementia clients in reducing the frequency and severity of agitation and the onset of aggressive behaviors.[102]
Use familiar items, pictures, and furniture in the client's surroundings.	Familiar objects may provide a sense of comfort for the client.
Use distractions such as preferred activities, food, or fluids to provide rest periods for the client.	Clients may not be able to recognize onset of fatigue when wandering.
Remove items from environment, such as coats, hats, or keys, that may trigger wandering.	Decreases stimulus for leaving the site.
Disguise doors by painting them the same color as the wall surface.	Difficult for the client to identify as an exit area.
Place fabric strips attached to door frames or stop signs on doors to prevent the client from entering areas that are "off limits."	Signs or fabric strips often serve as deterrents to clients who wander.
Use pictures and universal symbols for bathrooms, dining areas, or room identification.	Wanderers may no longer have ability to read and interpret signs for these areas.

ACTIONS/INTERVENTIONS	RATIONALES
Arrange furniture areas where clients wander, to encourage resting spots.	Provides cues to clients for rest periods.
Arrange repetitive activities for the client, such as linen folding, rocking, or paper work, if the client is engaged in "lapping type wandering" and showing signs of fatigue.[101]	The client has opportunity for repetitive movement with less energy expended.
Consider offering food, fluids, toileting, or pain medication when the client initiates wandering episodes, if this seems to be a need pattern for the client.[103]	Clients with decreased or absent verbal communication skills may be unable to articulate these basic needs to caregivers.

Home Health

ACTIONS/INTERVENTIONS	RATIONALES
Consult with and/or refer the patient to assistive resources such as caregiver support groups, as needed.	Utilization of existing services is an efficient use of resources.
When wandering is related to inappropriate responses to cues, adapt the environment to change the cues: • Cover doorknobs. • Remove keys that are in a visible location. • Remove knobs from the oven and stove.	May help prevent episodes of wandering and subsequent injury.
Ensure that the environment is as safe as possible when wandering occurs: • Remove knobs from the oven and stove. • Alert neighbors that the client may wander, and inform them about actions to take when the client is found wandering.	To prevent injury in the event of wandering by the client.
Provide the client with an ID bracelet indicating numbers where caregivers can be reached.	To minimize the time the client is away from caregivers in the event of wandering.
Assist the client and caregiver in obtaining alarm systems to indicate when doors have been opened.	To alert the caregiver if the client begins to wander.

WHEELCHAIR MOBILITY, IMPAIRED

DEFINITION[22]

Limitation of independent operation of wheelchair within environment.[21]

DEFINING CHARACTERISTICS[22]

1. Impaired ability to operate manual or power wheelchair on even or uneven surface
2. Impaired ability to operate manual or power wheelchair on an incline or decline
3. Impaired ability to operate wheelchair on curbs

RELATED FACTORS[22]

To be developed.

RELATED CLINICAL CONCERNS

1. Fracture
2. Paralysis
3. Neuromuscular disorders
4. Nutritional deficiencies

 Have You Selected the Correct Diagnosis?

Impaired Physical Mobility
Impaired Wheelchair Mobility could be considered as a subset of Impaired Physical Mobility. Certainly a patient who has Impaired Wheelchair Mobility would also have Impaired Physical Mobility. Impaired Wheelchair Mobility would need to be resolved before Impaired Physical Mobility.

Activity Intolerance
If the patient can tolerate only minimal activities before having problems, then Activity Intolerance would be the priority diagnosis. Only after Activity Intolerance has been resolved would the nurse be able to effectively intervene for Impaired Wheelchair Mobility.

EXPECTED OUTCOME

Will complete wheelchair mobility training program by [date].

Will demonstrate ability to maneuver wheelchair as necessary to complete activities of daily living by [date].

TARGET DATES

Resolution of this diagnosis may vary from weeks to months. An appropriate initial evaluation target date would be 1 to 2 weeks after the date the diagnosis was established.

NURSING ACTIONS/INTERVENTIONS WITH RATIONALES

Adult Health

ACTIONS/INTERVENTIONS	RATIONALES
Collaborate with Physical Therapy as needed.	To assist in planning activities to improve the patient's ability to independently operate a wheelchair within the environment.
Reinforce instructions from physical therapy.	
Assist the patient with strengthening exercises as appropriate. [Note assistance needed here.]	
Assist the patient with functional wheelchair activities as needed. [Note assistance needed here.]	
Facilitate the patient's participation in his or her own care as much as possible.	

Child Health

ACTIONS/INTERVENTIONS	RATIONALES
Determine contributing factors to best consider child's assistive needs that would facilitate their reaching highest potential of functioning.	A full assessment of contributing factors offers the most holistic approach to determining the degree of assistance needed.
Identify priorities of basic functions (e.g., breathing, airway maintenance, cardiovascular endurance, tolerance of positioning, proprioception, and neuromuscular coordination).	Basic physiologic functioning must be provided for if the movement is to be successful and not bring about alterations to basic functions.
Define limitations of tolerance for positioning, movement, and ideal plan for mobility.	Critical thresholds will assist in defining reasonable likelihood for success.
Determine equipment or assistive equipment needed.	Stabilization and use of appropriate assistive devices offer likelihood of success without injury.
Anticipate safety needs and environmental considerations related to safety needs.	Anticipatory safety is inherent in all mobility endeavors and serves to prevent injury.
According to maternal and infant or maternal and child dyad or caregiver status, decide who will assist in mobility activities.	Caregiver input serves to put the infant or child at ease with likelihood of success, plus provides an important opportunity for sense of input by the patient.
Assess for medication implications for movement timing and best potential for desired effects in relation to mobility, freedom of undesired effects, or contraindication of related treatments.	The best likelihood for desired effects will be related to appropriate medication correlation, with related mobility or position.
Establish a plan for each 8-hour period to include the maneuvers to be carried out, equipment or personnel needed, and critical thresholds to be attended to as dictated per patient's status (i.e., pulse oximeter level above [specify], pulse range [specify], etc). [Note child's plan here.]	Regular scheduled movement with attention to prescribed assessments, documentation, and awareness of thresholds assists in maintaining the client's stable status.

ACTIONS/INTERVENTIONS	RATIONALES
Document critical thresholds and report to the physician as ordered.	Ongoing assessment and appropriate reporting of critical thresholds will maintain desired stability of the client and provide basis for setting limits or increasing limits.
Determine outcomes according to previous baseline or desired level of activity. (May require sub-goals over a longer period of time.) [Note child's goals here.]	If it takes a period of time more than 3 to 4 days, sub-goals will better reflect the incremental change or gradual attainment of a greater goal.
Coordinate mobility activities as necessary with appropriate health team members, to include physical therapy, occupational therapy, child life specialist, etc.	Each person's input is best utilized in a manner of patient-centered planning to afford optimum likelihood of success and not tire the patient, vs. fragmented, duplicated, or less than individualized efforts for mobility.
Schedule meetings between child/family and others who are successfully managing mobility issues (as developmentally appropriate).	Role modeling significantly enhances learning.
Refer to community agencies and groups that can continue support for client and family. If use of a wheelchair will be long term, this could include wheelchair sports teams, and adults in the community who are successfully living with similar mobility concerns.	Role modeling enhances learning, and community support enhances self-esteem and decreases sense of isolation.

Women's Health

The nursing actions for Women's Health are the same as those for Adult Health.

Mental Health

The nursing actions for the mental health client are the same as those for Adult Health.

Gerontic Health

ACTIONS/INTERVENTIONS	RATIONALES
Obtain consultation with occupational and physical therapists to determine treatment plan for the client.	Occupational and physical therapists are health-care professionals best suited to evaluate the client and design treatment regimen.
Check wheelchair for proper fit for the client (adequate seat width, appropriate armrest height, and level of footrests).	Proper fit enhances the client's ability to control wheelchair.
Provide positive feedback when the client correctly manipulates wheelchair.	Positive feedback encourages the desired behavior.
Ensure environment where the client is active is accessible by wheelchair (e.g., width of door frames, table height, ramps, and curb cuts present in walkways).	Adapted environment supports wheelchair use.
Promote interdisciplinary communication to ensure that treatment plan is followed.	Clearly described and communicated treatment goals assist caregivers in providing care and feedback.
Review with the client and/or caregiver teaching plan for wheelchair use.	Provides opportunities to evaluate learning and address any questions related to wheelchair use.

(care plan continued on page 418)

NURSING ACTIONS/INTERVENTIONS WITH RATIONALES (continued from page 417)

Home Health

ACTIONS/INTERVENTIONS	RATIONALES
Educate the client, family, and potential caregivers about the following: • Using proper body mechanics to avoid injury • Maintaining a clear wheelchair path	
Assist the client in developing a schedule for range of motion exercises.	To maintain and build muscle strength.
Refer the client for a home physical therapy consult.	To help maximize his or her ability to safely use a wheelchair at home and to have assistive devices appropriate for the home environment.

REFERENCES

1. Potter, PA, and Perry, AG: Instructor's Manual for Use with Fundamentals of Nursing: Concepts, Process, and Practice, ed 4. Mosby–Year Book, St. Louis, 1997.
2. Kelly, MA: Nursing Diagnosis Source Book. Appleton-Century-Crofts, East Norwalk, CT, 1985.
3. Mitchell, PH: Motor status. In Mitchell, PH, and Loustau, A (eds): Concepts Basic to Nursing, ed 3. McGraw-Hill, New York, 1981.
4. Lentz, M: Selected aspects of deconditioning secondary to immobilization. Nurs Clinics North Am 16:729, 1980.
5. Pardue, N: Immobility. In Flynn, JM, and Heffron, PB (eds): Nursing: From Concept to Practice, ed 2. Appleton & Lange, East Norwalk, CT, 1988.
6. Murray, RB, and Zentner, JP: Health Assessment and Promotion Strategies Through the Life Span, ed 6. Appleton & Lange, Stamford, CT, 1997.
7. Schuster, CS, and Asburn, SS: The Process of Human Development: A Holistic Life-Span Approach, ed 3. Lippincott, Philadelphia, 1992.
8. Noble, E: Essential Exercises for the Childbearing Year, ed 3. Houghton Mifflin, Boston, 1988.
9. Duncan, J, Gordon, N, and Scott, C: Women walking for health and fitness: How much is enough? JAMA 266:3295, 1991.
10. Lakatta, EG: Circulatory function in younger and older humans. In Hazzard, WR (ed): Principles of Geriatric Medicine and Gerontology, ed 4. McGraw-Hill, St. Louis, 1999.
11. Loeser, RF, and Delbono, O: Aging and musculoskeletal system. In Hazzard, WR (ed): Principles of Geriatric Medicine and Gerontology, ed 4. McGraw-Hill, St. Louis, 1999.
12. Luggen, A, and Meiner, S: NGNA Core Curriculum for Gerontological Nursing, ed 2. CV Mosby, St. Louis, 2001.
13. Abrams, WB (ed): The Merck Manual of Geriatrics, ed 2. Merck Research Laboratories, Whitehouse Station, NJ, 1995.
14. Kane, RL (ed): Essentials of Clinical Geriatrics, ed 4. McGraw-Hill, St. Louis, 1999.
15. Enright, PL: Aging of the respiratory system. In Hazzard, WR (ed): Principles of Geriatric Medicine and Gerontology, ed 4. McGraw-Hill, St. Louis, 1999.
16. Miller, CA: Nursing Care of Older Adults: Theory and Practice, ed 3. Lippincott, Philadelphia, 1999.
17. Stanley, M: Congestive heart failure in the elderly. Geriatr Nurs 20:180, 1999.
18. Pearson, JD: Age-associated changes in blood pressure in a longitudinal study of healthy men and women. J Gerontol 52A:M177, 1997.
19. Butcher, DM: Preserving mobility in older adults. West J Med 167:258, 1997
20. Papalia, DE, and Olds, SW: Human Development, ed 7. McGraw-Hill, Burr Ridge, IL, 1998.
21. Moore, SL: Aging and meaning in life: Examining the concept. Geriatr Nurs 21:27, 2000.
22. North American Nursing Diagnosis Association: Nursing Diagnosis: Definitions and Classification, 2005–2006. Author, Philadelphia, 2005.
23. Buckley, K, and Kulb, NW: High Risk Maternity Nursing Manual, ed 2. Williams & Wilkins, Baltimore, 1993.
24. Creasy, RK, and Resnik, R: Maternal-Fetal Medicine, ed 4. WB Saunders, Philadelphia, 1999.
25. Gabbe, SG, Niebyl, JR, and Simpson, JL: Obstetrics: Normal and Problem Pregnancies, ed 3. Churchill-Livingstone, New York, 1996.
26. Maloni, JA: Preventing preterm birth: Evidence-based interventions shift toward prevention, Lifelines 4:26, 2000.
27. Eganhouse, DJ, and Burnside, SM: Nursing assessment and responsibilities in monitoring the preterm pregnancy. J Obstet Gynecol Neonatal Nurs 21:355, 1992.
28. Fuchs, A, Fuchs, F, and Stubblefield, PG: Preterm Birth: Causes, Prevention, and Management, ed 2. McGraw-Hill, New York, 1993.
29. Knuppel, RA, and Drukker, JE: High Risk Pregnancy: A Team Approach, ed 2. WB Saunders, Philadelphia, 1993.
30. Mandeville, LK, and Troiano, NH: High-Risk and Critical Care Intrapartum Nursing, ed 2. Lippincott, Philadelphia, 1999.
31. Lowdermilk, DL, and Perry, SE: Maternity and Women's Health Care, ed 8, CV Mosby, St. Louis, 2004.
32. Kidner, MC, and Flanders-Stepans, MB: A model for the HELLP syndrome: The maternal experience. JOGNN J Obstet Gynecol Neonatal Nurs 33:44,. 2004.
33. Erickson, HC, and Kinney, CK: Modeling and Role-Modeling: Theory, Research and Practice. Society for Advancement of Modeling and Role-Modeling, Austin, TX, 1990.
34. Kneisl, CR Wilson, JS, and Trigoboff, E: Contemporary Psychiatric-Mental Health Nursing,. Pearson Education, Upper Saddle River, NJ, 2004.
35. Haber, J, et al: Comprehensive Psychiatric Nursing, ed 5. Mosby–Year Book, St. Louis, 1997.
36. Dossey, BM, Keegan L, and Guzzetta, CE: Holistic Nursing: A Handbook for Practice, ed 3. Aspen, Gaithersburg, MD, 2000.
37. Clark, C: Wellness Practitioner: Concepts, Research and Strategies, ed 2. Springer, New York, 1996.
38. Wright, LM, and Leahey, M: Nurses and Families: A Guide to Family Assessment and Intervention, ed 4. FA Davis, Philadelphia, 2005.
39. Resnick, B: Motivating older adults to perform functional activities. J Gerontol Nurs 24:25, 1998.
40. Resnick, B: Efficacy beliefs in geriatrics. J Gerontol Nurs 24:34. 1998.
41. Maxmen, J, and Ward, N: Psychotropic Drugs Fast Facts, ed 3, WW Norton, New York, 2002.
42. Forrest, G: Atrial fibrillation association with autonomic dysreflexia in patients with tetraplegia. Arch Phys Med Rehabil 72:592, 1991.
43. Pine, A, Miller, S, and Alonso, J: Atrial fibrillation associated with autonomic dysreflexia. Am J Phys Med Rehabil 70:271, 1991.
44. Lindan, R, et al: Incidence and clinical features of autonomic dysreflexia in patients with spinal cord injury. Paraplegia 18:285, 1980.

45. Earnhardt, J, and Frye, B: Understanding dysreflexia. Rehabil Nurs 9:28, 1986.
46. Ceron, GE, and Rakowski-Reinhardt, AC: Action stat! Autonomic dysreflexia. Nursing 91 21:33, 1991.
47. Trop, C, and Bennett, C: Autonomic dysreflexia and its urological implications. J Urol 146:1461, 1991.
48. Finocchiaro, DN, and Herzfeld, ST: Understanding autonomic dysreflexia. Am J Nurs 90:56, 1990.
49. Hockenberry, MJ: Wong's Essentials of Pediatric Nursing, ed 7. CV Mosby, St. Louis, 2006.
50. Drayton-Hargrove, S, and Reddy, M: Rehabilitation and the long term management of the spinal cord impaired adult. Nurs Clin North Am 21:599, 1986.
51. Capezuti, E: Individualized interventions to prevent bed-related falls and reduce siderail use. J Gerontol Nurs 25:26, 1999.
52. Eliopoulos, C: Gerontological Nursing, ed 4. Lippincott, Philadelphia, 1997.
53. Easton, KL: Gerontological Rehabilitation Nursing. WB Saunders, Philadelphia, 1999.
54. Association of Women's Health, Obstetric, and Neonatal Nurses: Second Stage Labor Nursing Management Protocol. Author, Washington, DC, 1994.
55. Andrews, CM, and Chranowski, M: Maternal position, labor, and comfort. Appl Nurs Res 3:7, 1990.
56. Gilliss, C, et al: Toward a Science of Family Nursing. Addison-Wesley, Menlo Park, CA, 1989.
57. Eliopoulos, C: Manual of Gerontologic Nursing. CV Mosby, St. Louis, 1995.
58. Kavanagh, J, and Riegger, M: Assessment of the cardiovascular system. In Phipps, WJ, et al (eds): Medical-Surgical Nursing: Concepts and Clinical Practice, ed 6. Mosby, St. Louis, 1999.
59. Adenhold, KJ, and Roberts, JE: Phases of second stage labor. J Nurse Midwifery 36:267, 1991.
60. Golay, J, Vedam, S, and Sorger, L: The squatting position for the second stage of labor: Effects on labor and on maternal and fetal well-being. Birth 20:73, 1993.
61. Thomson, AM: Pushing techniques in the second stage of labor. J Adv Nurs 18:171, 1993.
62. Minato, JF: Is it time to push? Examining rest in second-stage labor. Lifelines 4: 21, 2001.
63. Mayberry, LJ, et al: Labor and fetal well-being. Lifelines 3:28, 2000.
64. Harkins, SW, and Scott, RB: Pain and presbyalgos. In Birren, JE (ed): Encyclopedia of Gerontology: Age, Aging, and the Aged. Academic Press, San Diego, 1996.
65. Kneisl, C, Wilson, H, and Trigoboff, E: Contemporary Psychiatric-Mental Health Nursing. Upper Saddle River, NJ: Pearson Education.
66. Beland, IL, and Passos, JY: Clinical Nursing: Pathophysiological and Psychosocial Approaches, ed 4. Macmillan, New York, 1981.
67. Osborn, CL: Reminiscence: When the past erases the present. J Gerontol Nurs 15:6, 1989.
68. Richless, C: Current trends in mechanical ventilation. Crit Care Nurse 11:41, 1991.
69. Hazinski, MF: Nursing Care of the Critically Ill Child, ed 2. CV Mosby, St. Louis, 1992.
70. Department of Health and Human Services: Executive Summary: Guidelines for the Diagnosis and Management of Asthma. Author, Washington, DC, 1991.
71. Norton, LC, and Neureuter, A: Weaning the long-term ventilator dependent patient: Common problems and management. Crit Care Nurse 9:42, 1989.
72. Knebel, AR: Weaning from mechanical ventilation: Current controversies. Heart Lung 20:47, 1991.
73. Author: NGC - National Guideline Clearinghouse Quality Report. http://www.guideline.gov, 2005.
74. McConnell, EA: Wandering and fall prevention. Nursing 27:8, 1997.
75. Tideiksaar, R: Falls in Older Persons: Prevention and Management. Health Professions Press, Baltimore, 1998.
76. Steinwig, KK: The changing approach to falls in the elderly. Am Fam Physician 56:1815, 1998.
77. Thompson, C: Gender differences in walking distances of people with lung disease. Appl Nurs Res 1:141, 1989.
78. Black, JM: Medical-Surgical Nursing: Clinical Management for Continuity of Care, ed 5. WB Saunders, Philadelphia, 1997.
79. Lee, R, Grayder, J, and Ross, E: Effectiveness of psychological well-being, physical status and social support on oxygen dependent COPD patients' level of functioning. Res Nurs Health 14:323, 1991.
80. Stanley, M, and Beare, PG: Gerontological Nursing: A Health Promotion and Protection Approach, ed 2. FA Davis, Philadelphia, 1999.
81. Ebersole, P, and Hess, P: Toward Healthy Aging: Human Needs and Nursing Response, ed 5. CV Mosby, St Louis, 1998.
82. Kenner, C, Brueggemeyer, A, and Gunderson, LP: Comprehensive Neonatal Nursing: A Physiologic Perspective, ed 2. WB Saunders, Philadelphia, 1998.
83. Nichols, FH, and Zwelling, E: Maternal-Newborn Nursing: Theory and Practice. Churchill-Livingstone, New York, 1997.
84. Wong, DL, and Perry, SE: Maternal-Child Nursing Care. CV Mosby, St. Louis, 1998.
85. Strumpf, NE, and Evans, LK: The ethical problems of prolonged physical restraint. J Gerontol Nurs 17:27, 1991.
86. Mobily, PR, and Kelley, LS: Factors of immobility. J Gerontol Nurs 17:5, 1991.
87. Breslin, E: Women's health: Challenges and Opportunities. In Breslin, ET, and Lucas, VA (eds): Women's Health Nursing; Toward Evidence-Based Practice. Elsevier, St. Louis, 2003.
88. Sellers, JB: Health care for older women. In Breslin, ET, and Lucas, VA (eds): Women's Health Nursing; Toward Evidence-Based Practice. Elsevier, St. Louis, 2003.
89. Author: Motivational interviewing: An approach to counseling for behavior change attracts growing interest. Harvard Ment Health Lett 21:5, 2005.
90. Stanhope, M, and Knollmueller, R: Handbook of Public and Community Health Nursing Practice. CV Mosby, St. Louis, 2001.
91. Penn, C: Promoting independence. J Gerontol Nurs 14:14, 1988.
92. Wong, DL: Whaley and Wong's Nursing Care of Infants and Children, ed 6. CV Mosby, St. Louis, 1999.
93. Author: Evidence based clinical practice guideline for managing an acute exacerbation of asthma. Cincinnati Children's Hospital Medical Center—Hospital/Medical Center. 1998 July 20, 1998 (revised September 3, 2003), 21 pp.
94. Fulmer, T, and Walker, K: Lessons from the elder boom in ICUs. Geriatr Nurs 11:120, 1990.
95. Cunningham, S: Circulatory and fluid-electrolyte status. In Mitchell, PH, and Loustau A (eds): Concepts Basic to Nursing, ed 3. McGraw-Hill, New York, 1981.
96. Koroknay, VJ: Maintaining ambulation in the frail nursing home resident: A nursing administered walking program. J Gerontol Nurs 21:18, 1995.
97. Galindo-Ciocon, DJ: Gait training and falls in the elderly. J Gerontol Nurs 21:11, 1995.
98. McConnell, EA: Wandering and fall prevention. Nursing 27:8, 1997.
99. Algase, DL: Wandering: A dementia-compromised behavior. J Gerontol Nurs 25:17, 1999.
100. Gerdner, LA: Individualized music intervention protocol. J Gerontol Nurs 25:10, 1999.
101. Holmberg, SK: A walking program for wanderers: Volunteer training and development of an evening walkers' group. Geriatr Nurs 18:160, 1997.
102. Rowe, M, and Alfred, D: The effectiveness of slow-stroke massage in diffusing agitated behaviors in individuals with Alzheimer's disease. J Gerontol Nurs 25:22, 1999.
103. Schweiger, JL, and Huey, RA: Alzheimer's disease: Your role in the caregiving equation. Nursing 29: 34, 1999.
104. Miller, E: Exercise and Fitness for Women. In Breslin, ET, and Lucas, VA (eds): Women's Health Nursing; Toward Evidence-Based Practice. Elsevier, St, Louis, 2003.
105. Doenges, ME, Moorhouse, MF, and Murr, AC: Nurses' Pocket Guide: Diagnoses with Interventions and Rationales, ed 9. FA Davis, Philadelphia, 2004.
106. Jones, E, et al: Patient Classification for Long Term Care Users' Manual. HEW, Publication No. HRA-74-3107, November, 1974.

6

SLEEP–REST PATTERN

PATTERN DESCRIPTION

The sleep–rest pattern includes relaxation in addition to sleep and rest. The pattern is based on a 24-hour day and looks specifically at how an individual rates or judges the adequacy of his or her sleep, rest, and relaxation in terms of both quantity and quality. The pattern also looks at the patient's energy level in relation to the amount of sleep, rest, and relaxation described by the patient as well as any sleep aids the patient uses.

PATTERN ASSESSMENT

1. Does the patient report a problem falling asleep?
   a. Yes (Disturbed Sleep Pattern)
   b. No (Readiness for Enhanced Sleep)
2. Does the patient report interrupted sleep?
   a. Yes (Disturbed Sleep Pattern)
   b. No (Readiness for Enhanced Sleep)
3. Does the patient report long periods without sleep, resulting in daytime malaise?
   a. Yes (Sleep Deprivation Pattern)
   b. No (Readiness for Enhanced Sleep)

CONCEPTUAL INFORMATION

A person at rest feels mentally relaxed, free from anxiety, and physically calm. *Rest* need not imply inactivity, and inactivity does not necessarily afford rest. Rest is a reduction in bodily work that results in the person's feeling refreshed and with a sense of readiness to perform activities of daily living (ADLs).

Sleep is a state of rest that occurs for sustained periods at a deeper level of consciousness. The reduced consciousness during sleep provides time for essential repair and recovery of body systems. Sleep is as essential to our bodies as good nutrition and exercise. Sleep is considered one of the major components to our health, performance, safety, and quality of life.[1] A person who sleeps has temporarily reduced interaction with the environment. Sleep restores a person's energy and sense of well-being and lets him or her function in a safe, efficient, and effective manner.

Studies have confirmed that sleep is a cyclical phenomenon. The most common sleep cycle is the 24-hour day–night cycle. This 24-hour cycle is also referred to as the *Circadian Biological Clock,* which regulates the timing of sleep and wakefulness.[1,2] In general, light and darkness govern the 24-hour circadian rhythm. Additional factors that influence the sleep–wake cycle of the individual are biologic, such as hormonal and thermoregulation cycles. Most individuals attempt to synchronize activity with the demands of modern society. The two specialized areas of the brain that control the cyclical nature of sleep are the *reticular activating system* in the brain stem, spinal cord, and cerebral cortex and the *bulbar synchronizing portion* in the medulla. These two systems function intermittently by activating and suppressing the higher centers of the brain.[2]

After falling asleep, a person passes through a series of stages that afford rest and recuperation physically, mentally, and emotionally. In stage 1, the individual is in a relaxed, dreamy state, and is aware of his or her surroundings. In stages 2 and 3, there is progression to deeper levels of sleep in which the individual becomes unaware of his or her surroundings but wakens easily. In stage 4, there is profound sleep characterized by little body movement and difficult arousal. Stage 4 restores and allows the body to rest. Stages 1 through 4 are known as *non–rapid eye movement* (*NREM*) sleep. NREM sleep accounts for 75 percent of an 8-hour night's sleep. Stage 5 is called *rapid eye movement* (*REM*) sleep. REM sleep accounts for 25 percent of an 8-hour night's sleep and is the stage in which dreaming occurs. Other characteristics of REM sleep are irregular pulse, variable blood pressure, muscular twitching, profound muscular relaxation, and an increase in gastric secretions.[2,3] After REM sleep, the individual progresses back through stages 1, 2, and 3 again.

Sleep patterns and characteristics vary and change over the life cycle. A person's age, general health status, culture, and emotional well-being dictate the amount of sleep he or she requires. On the whole, older persons require less sleep, whereas young infants require the most sleep. As the nurse assesses the patient's needs for sleep and rest, he or she makes every effort to individualize the care according to this sleep–rest cycle. A major emphasis is to provide patient education regarding the influence of disease process on sleep–rest patterns.

Reports of the occurrence of excessive and pathologic sleep most commonly relate to narcolepsy and hypersomnia.[2,3] *Narcolepsy* is characterized by an attack of irresistible sleep of brief duration with "auxiliary" symptoms. In sleep paralysis, the narcoleptic patient is unable to speak or move and breathes in a shallow manner. Auditory or visual hypnagogic hallucinations may occur. *Cataplexy,* a brief form of narcolepsy, is an abrupt and reversible decrease or loss of muscle tone and is most often elicited by emotion. The attacks may last several seconds and almost go undetected, or they may last as long as 30 minutes with muscular weakness being evident. In the initial stage of the attack, consciousness remains intact.[2,3]

Hypersomnia, in contrast, is characterized by daytime sleepiness and sleep states that are less imperative and of longer duration than those in narcolepsy. Often, a deepening and lengthening of night sleep is also noted. Sleep apnea and the Kleine–Levin syndrome are two examples of the hypersomnia disorders.[2,3]

Sleep apnea may occur in patients with a damaged respiratory center in the brain, brain stem infarction, drug intoxication (barbiturates, tranquilizers, etc.), bilateral cordotomy, and/or Ondine's curse syndrome. Patients with the typical pickwickian syndrome show marked obesity and associated alveolar hypoventilation, sleep apnea, and hypersomnia. Several forms of this condition may exist without obesity. One such syndrome is Ondine's curse syndrome, which involves the loss of the automaticity of breathing and manifests during sleep as a recurrent apnea. Another is the Kleine–Levin syndrome, which is associated with periods of hypersomnia accompanied by bulimia or polyphagia and mental disturbances. A cyclic hypersomnia is also reported that is related to the premenstrual periods. The typical syndrome—pickwickian—is rare, whereas the atypical variants seem more common.[3]

Various factors influence a person's capability to gain adequate rest and sleep.[4,5] For the home setting, it is appropriate for the nurse to assist the patient in developing behavior conducive to rest and relaxation. In a healthcare setting, the nurse must be able to provide ways of promoting rest and relaxation in a stressful environment. Loss of privacy, unfamiliar noises, frequent examinations, tiring procedures, and a general upset in daily routines culminate in a threat to the client's achievement of essential rest and sleep.

DEVELOPMENTAL CONSIDERATIONS

In general, as age increases, the amount of sleep per night decreases. The length of each sleep cycle—active (REM) and quiet (NREM)—changes with age. For adults, there is no particular change in the actual number of hours slept, but there is a change in the amount of deep sleep and light sleep. As a person ages, the amount of deep sleep decreases and the amount of light sleep increases. This helps explain why the older patient wakens more easily and spends time in sleep throughout the day and night. REM sleep decreases in amount from the time of infancy (50 percent) to late adulthood (15 percent). The changes in sleep pattern with age development are[7]:

Infant: Awake 7 hours; NREM sleep, 8.5 hours; REM sleep, 8.5 hours

Age 1: Awake 13 hours; NREM sleep, 7 hours; REM sleep, 4 hours

Age 10: Awake 15 hours; NREM sleep, 6 hours; REM sleep, 3 hours

Age 20: Awake 17 hours; NREM sleep, 5 hours; REM sleep, 2 hours

Age 75: Awake 17 hours; NREM sleep, 6 hours; REM sleep, 1 hour

INFANT

The development of sleep and wakefulness can be traced to intrauterine life. A gestational age of 36 weeks seems to be a landmark, for it is at this time that the behavioral states in the fetus and preterm infant begin to take on a more mature character. The joining of physiologic variables results in identification of recurrent behavioral states with various parameters. Term birth leads to a number of profound changes, especially in respiratory regulation, but more evidence suggests that continuity of development, rather than discontinuity, prevails.[7]

The newborn begins life with a regular schedule of sleep and activity that is evident during periods of reactivity. For the first hour, infants born of unmedicated mothers spend 60 percent of the time in the quiet, alert state and only 10 percent of the time in the irritable, crying states. Six distinct sleep–activity states for the infant have been noted: (1) deep sleep, (2) light sleep, (3) drowsiness, (4) quiet alert, (5) active alert, and (6) crying.[7,8]

After 1 month of age, sleep and wakefulness change dramatically, as do a large number of physiologic variables. This period of central nervous system (CNS) reorganization (with a likely increased vulnerability) is immediately followed by a short transient interval at 3 months of age in which play and wakefulness—and, within it, the basic rest–activity cycle–show excessive regularity. This regularity may carry its own risk.

The study of mobility has proved worthwhile in detecting the origin of the basic rest–activity cycle in the fetus. Neonatologists, who deal with the immature infant, often use mobility in prognosis.

Apneas during sleep are common in normal infants and occur most often during the newborn period, with a marked decrease in the first 6 months of life. Long apneas, lasting longer than 15 seconds, are not usually observed during sleep in laboratory conditions. Obstructive apneas of 6 to 10 seconds are also rarely observed. However, in laboratory studies, paradoxical breathing is observed in neonates, and periodic breathing is associated with REM sleep in normal infants.[7,9]

Infants found not breathing by parents are usually rushed to the hospital. Causes for life-threatening apnea to be investigated include congenital conditions, especially cardiac disease or arrhythmias; cranial, facial, or other conditions affecting the anatomy of the airway; infections such as sepsis, meningitis, pneumonia, botulism, and pertussis; viral infections such as respiratory syncytial virus; metabolic abnormalities; administration of sedatives; seizures; and chronic hypoxia. If these causes are ruled out, the infant is diagnosed as having "apnea of infancy." Sleep studies, with polygraph recordings, are required. The term *near-miss sudden infant death syndrome* (near-miss SIDS) implies the child is found limp, cyanotic, and not breathing and would have died had caretakers not intervened. Because the relationship of the near miss SIDS event to SIDS is speculative, *apnea of infancy* is the preferred term.[9,10]

Obstructive and central apnea identification, hypopnea, prolonged expiration, apnea and reflux, and apnea and cardiac arrhythmia are the current issues being studied in trying to solve this problem. For any infant-related apnea, hospitalization, with special observation for all possible contributing factors and close monitoring of cardiac and respiratory function, is recommended. Attention must be given to parents for the extreme anxiety this problem creates.

The newborn and young infant spends more time in REM sleep than adults do. As the infant's nervous system develops, the infant will have longer periods of sleep and wakefulness that become more regular. At approximately 8 months of age, the infant goes through the stage of separation anxiety with potentially altered sleep patterns. Teething, ear infections, or other disorders affect sleep patterns. Respirations are quiet, with minimal activity noted during deep sleep. The infant sleeps an average of 12 to 16 hours per day.

TODDLER AND PRESCHOOLER

The toddler needs approximately 10 to 12 hours of sleep at night, with an approximate 2-hour nap in the afternoon. The percentage of REM sleep is 25 percent. Rituals for preparation for sleep are important, with bedtime associated as separation from family and fun. Quiet time to gradually unwind, a favorite object for security, and a relatively consistent bedtime are suggested. Nightmares may begin to occur because of magical thinking.

The preschooler sleeps approximately 10 to 12 hours per day. Dreams and nightmares may occur at this time, and resistance to bedtime rituals is also common. Unwinding or slowing down from the many activities of the day is recommended to lessen sleep disturbances. Actual attempts to foster relaxation by mental imaging at this age have proved successful. The percentage of REM sleep is 20 percent.

Special needs may be prompted for the toddler during hospitalization. When at all possible, a parent's presence should be encouraged throughout nighttime to lessen fears. Limit-setting with safety in mind is also necessary for the toddler because of his or her surplus of energy and the desire for constant activity. The preschooler may be at risk for fatigue. Sleep may not be necessary at naptime, but rest without disturbance is recommended to supplement night sleep and to prevent fatigue.

SCHOOL-AGE CHILD

The school-age child seems to do well without a nap and requires approximately 10 hours of sleep per day, with REM sleep being approximately 18.5 percent. Individualized rest needs are developed by this age, with a reliable source being the child who can express his or her feelings about rest or sleep. Health status would also determine to a great extent how much sleep the child at this age requires. Permission to stay up late must be weighed against the potential upset to routine and demands of the next day. When bedtime is assigned a status, peer pressure and power issues may ensue.

When the school-age child alters the usual routines of sleep and rest, fatigue may result. Attempts should be made to maintain usual routines even when school is not in session to best maintain the usual sleep–rest pattern.

ADOLESCENT

Irregular sleep patterns seem to be the norm for the adolescent as a result of high activity levels and usual peer-related activities. There may be a tendency to overexertion, which is made more pronounced by the numerous physiologic changes that create increased demands on the body. Fatigue may occur during this time. On average, the adolescent sleeps approximately 8 to 10 hours per day, with REM sleep comprising 20 percent.

Rest may be necessary to supplement sleep. Supplementing sleep with rest serves to assist in preventing illness or the risk of illness. Extracurricular activities may also need to be prioritized.

ADULT

An adult sleeps approximately 8 hours per day, with REM sleep comprising 22 percent. Sleep patterns may be subject to the demands of young infants or children in the household or after-hours professional and social activities.

The adult may be at high risk for fatigue because of increasing role expectations, especially in caring for a new baby. Sleep deprivation can adversely affect the ability to cope with the many expectations the adult may feel.

Research has shown that women of all ages have higher rates of sleep disturbance than men do. Some speculation has occurred that relates this to the reproductive lives of women and hormonal changes. It is well documented that the psychosocial and hormonal changes that accompany pregnancy lead to sleep disturbances.[6] That sleep deprivation occurs during the postpartum period is a well-known fact. A new baby does not allow a mother uninterrupted sleep for approximately 4 to 6 weeks after birth.[8,11,12]

Sleep disturbance seen in women who are experiencing perimenopausal and menopausal symptoms is often related to declining estrogen levels. "Disrupted sleep is one of the earliest effects on the brain of decreasing levels of estrogen."[11] Sometimes these sleep changes begin as early as 8 to 10 years before menses cease, and research has proved that sleep deprivation not only causes suppression of the immune system but is also a major factor in causing persistent fatigue.

OLDER ADULT

As adults age, they are more likely to report sleeping difficulties. As many as 50 percent of people age 65 and older complain of sleep problems on a regular basis. Complaints often include sleeping less, frequent nighttime awakening, waking too early in the morning, and napping in the daytime.[13,14] The proportion of REM sleep may vary from 20 to 25 percent; however, deep sleep (stage 4 NREM sleep) is decreased. There is no clinical evidence showing that older adults require less sleep, but evidence exists showing that older adults sleep less and sleep less well.[15] Obstructive sleep apnea, periodic limb movement disorder, and restless leg syndrome are common sleep disorders found in the older population.[16] Circadian rhythm changes with aging can cause changes in the older adult's sleep–wake cycle that result in poor nighttime sleep and increased daytime napping.

Sleep pattern disturbances in the elderly may occur as a result of undiagnosed depression or medication-induced sleep problems. Other risk factors interfering with sleep may include unrelieved pain, alcohol use, lack of daytime activity, nocturia, or medical conditions such as dementia.[17] Older adults involved in caregiving for people with dementia are at risk for developing sleep deprivation as the dementia progresses.[2,3,18] Institutionalized older adults may report problems with sleeping if their usual sleep pattern does not coincide with the facility schedule.

Individualized attention to sleep and potential fatigue is critical to prevent further decreases in activity and changes in self-worth for older adults. Fatigue plays a major role in determining the quality and amount of musculoskeletal activity engaged in by the elderly. Poor sleep may affect rehabilitation potential, alertness, safety, and psychological comfort. Examining factors that may influence fatigue is an essential part of the assessment for the sleep–rest pattern.

 APPLICABLE NURSING DIAGNOSES

SLEEP DEPRIVATION

DEFINITION

Prolonged periods of time without sleep (sustained, natural, periodic suspension of relative consciousness).[19]

DEFINING CHARACTERISTICS[19]

1. Daytime drowsiness
2. Decreased ability to function
3. Malaise
4. Tiredness
5. Lethargy
6. Restlessness
7. Irritability
8. Heightened sensitivity to pain
9. Listlessness
10. Apathy
11. Slowed reaction
12. Inability to concentrate
13. Perceptual disorders (e.g., disturbed body sensation, delusions, and feeling afloat)
14. Hallucinations
15. Acute confusion
16. Transient paranoia
17. Agitated or combative
18. Anxious
19. Mild, fleeting nystagmus
20. Hand tremors

RELATED FACTORS[19]

1. Prolonged physical discomfort
2. Prolonged psychological discomfort

•••
••• TABLE 6.1 NANDA, NIC, and NOC Taxonomic Linkages
•••

GORDON'S FUNCTIONAL HEALTH PATTERN	NANDA NURSING DIAGNOSIS	NIC PRIORITY INTERVENTIONS	NOC EVALUATIONS
Sleep–rest Pattern	Sleep Deprivation	Sleep Enhancement	Concentration Mood Equilibrium Sleep Rest
	Sleep Pattern, Disturbed	Sleep Enhancement	Mood Equilibrium Person Well-being Sleep Rest Well-Being
	Sleep, Readiness for Enhanced	*Still in development*	Comfort Level Pain Control Rest Sleep

3. Sustained inadequate sleep hygiene
4. Prolonged use of pharmacologic or dietary antiso-
   porifics
5. Aging-related sleep stage shifts
6. Sustained circadian asynchrony
7. Inadequate daytime activity
8. Sustained environmental stimulation
9. Sustained unfamiliar or uncomfortable sleep environment
10. Non–sleep-inducing parenting practices
11. Sleep apnea
12. Periodic limb movement (e.g., restless leg syndrome
    and nocturnal myoclonus)
13. Sundowner's syndrome
14. Narcolepsy
15. Idiopathic central nervous system hypersomnolence
16. Sleepwalking
17. Sleep terror
18. Sleep-related enuresis
19. Nightmares
20. Familial sleep paralysis
21. Sleep-related painful erections
22. Dementia

RELATED CLINICAL CONCERNS

1. Colic
2. Hyperthyroidism
3. Anxiety
4. Chronic obstructive pulmonary disease
5. Pregnancy; postpartum period
6. Pain
7. Alzheimer's disease

 Have You Selected the Correct Diagnosis?

Ineffective Individual Coping
Patients sometimes use sleep as an avoidance mechanism and will report "not getting enough sleep" when
in fact there is no sleep deprivation. A review of the
number of hours of sleep would indicate the patient is
getting a sufficient amount of sleep.

Fatigue
The patient will talk about lack of energy and difficulty
in maintaining his or her usual activities. However,
assessment documents that this fatigue exists regardless of the amount of sleep.

Disturbed Sleep Pattern
Sleep Deprivation refers specifically to a decreased
amount of sleep; Disturbed Sleep Pattern refers to
multiple problems with sleeping. Disturbed Sleep
Pattern could, if not resolved, result in Sleep
Deprivation.

EXPECTED OUTCOME

Will sleep, uninterrupted, for at least 6 to 8 hours per night
by [date].

● N O T E : *The actual hours of uninterrupted sleep will
depend on the patient's age and developmental level.*

TARGET DATES

The suggested target date is no less than 2 days after the date
of the diagnosis and no more than 5 days. This length of
time will allow for initial modification of the sleep pattern.

NURSING ACTIONS/INTERVENTIONS WITH RATIONALES	
Adult Health	
ACTIONS/INTERVENTIONS	RATIONALES
Avoid coffee or cola, which contain caffeine, from late afternoon on.	Caffeine is a stimulant that interferes with sleep.
Avoid over-the-counter pain relievers that contain caffeine from late afternoon on.	
Avoid cold medicines that contain pseudoephedrine and phenylpropanolamine from late afternoon on.	Pseudoephedrine and phenylpropanolamine as well as other adrenergics act as stimulants.[20,22]
Avoid alcohol at night.	Alcohol interferes with substances in the brain that allow for continuous sleep.[22]
Adjust the timing of diuretics to avoid nighttime trips to the bathroom.	Waking to go to the bathroom will interfere with sleep.
Check for other prescription drugs taken to determine whether they may interfere with sleep patterns (e.g., antidepressants, thyroid medication, etc.)	Side effects of some prescriptions include sleep pattern disturbances.
Avoid eating a heavy meal late at night. However, a small snack such as warm milk or chamomile tea may be relaxing.	Heavy meals increase stomach acid and intestinal stimu- lation. A light snack may allay hunger pains.[20]

ACTIONS/INTERVENTIONS	RATIONALES
Consider herbal solutions such as valerian. However, watch for side effects such as headaches, nausea, blurred vision, heart palpitations, and paradoxically, excitability and restlessness. Do not take concurrently with other sleep aids or alcohol.	Reduces the time it takes to get to sleep but does not seem to reduce the number of times people wake in the night.
Assess the patient's mattress and pillow. Is it too hard or soft? Does it offer enough support?	The mattress is an important component of restful sleep.
Check for mild iron deficiency. Vitamin E may also help with restless leg syndrome.	Even a low–normal iron level may cause restless leg syndrome.
Teach the patient to try relaxation techniques such as meditation, counting your breaths, slowly tensing and relaxing muscles, guided imagery, etc. just before bedtime.	
Encourage the patient to exercise earlier in the day rather than at night.	Exercise stimulates the body.
Counsel the patient to not "take problems to bed." He or she should sit quietly in a chair for a few minutes before going to bed and think about all those things that have worried him or her during the day.	Helps clear the patient's mind, order his or her problems, and set his or her plans for the next day.[20]

Child Health

ACTIONS/INTERVENTIONS	RATIONALES
Determine all possible contributing factors that may impact sleep deprivation (including situational, environmental, or those related to another medical condition).	Provides a database for individualization of care.
Stabilize factors that can be stabilized to minimize contributing factors*: • Clustering activities to not disturb unnecessarily. • Providing as near to normal routine for sleep for the client, with attention to developmental needs (as noted in under Conceptual Information).	Affords a better picture of actual causative factors for sleep deprivation with attention to anticipatory needs.
Consider reassessment on an ongoing basis for disruptive contributing factors.	In a short period of time there may be significant changes to consider for accurate sleep assessment.
Based on assessments, develop a restructured plan for sleep allowance by eliminating, to degree possible, all factors identified to be barriers to sleep.	Restructuring may afford sleep and awake cycles to recur.
Determine teaching needs of the client, parents, and/or caregivers.	Specific knowledge regarding sleeping and waking cycles facilitates individualized match of needs for clients and caregivers.[7,8]
Reevaluate measures to define the optimum likelihood for sleep to occur as desired.	Possible growth and developmental phases may be required for appropriate reestablishment of cycles.
Implement appropriate nursing measures as noted for sleep disturbance as applicable.	Once major factors are stabilized, basic maneuvers to encourage sleep may be afforded per prior successful plan with allowance for updated developmental needs.
Monitor for caregiver frustration in attempts to deal with sleep deprivation secondary to caregiver role strain.	Parents will often be subject to sleep deprivation of the infant or child.

(care plan continued on page 428)

NURSING ACTIONS/INTERVENTIONS WITH RATIONALES (continued from page 427)

Child Health

ACTIONS/INTERVENTIONS	RATIONALES
Assist the parents in identification of ways to deal with sleep deprivation of the infant or child.	Empowerment for possible solutions offers growth potential as parents and acknowledges potential need of caregiver.[7,24]
Reassure the parents or, if applicable, the child, of the likelihood for regular sleep pattern to be reestablished with sufficient time and allowance for recycling.	Ability to cope with problem is increased when individuals believe problem is manageable.
Determine effect sleep deprivation may have over time, monitoring every 8 hours to note related alterations, with attention to basic physiologic parameters as indicated per the client's condition and needs.	Related physiologic alterations often ensue related to sleep deprivation.
Monitor for mental and cognitive capacity, with attention to subjective or behavioral changes.	Identification of related onset of interference in usual mental or behavioral domain will help minimize greater disturbance of the client's status.
Ensure safety needs are met at all times.	Altered sleep and wake cycles may alter usual proprioception or cognitive ability.[7,24]

*In instances of nightmares, offer safety and reassurance to child.

Women's Health

Nursing actions for the Women's Health client with this diagnosis are the same as those actions for Adult Health with the following exceptions:

ACTIONS/INTERVENTIONS	RATIONALES
Assess the client for feelings of sleepiness or drowsiness during the day.	Disruptive sleep patterns can lead to problems with memory and are associated with daytime drowsiness, fatigue, feeling "foggy" mentally along with disturbances in memory, concentration, and libido.
If the client is reporting perimenopausal symptoms and disturbances in memory at any age, but particularly in the 30s, 40s, and 50s, refer to the physician for hormonal evaluation.[12]	As estrogen levels drop, the brain responds with bursts of adrenalin-type chemicals that arouse one from sleep. Prolonged periods of sleep disruption can be a cause of biochemical changes, which can lead to chronic fatigue and depression.[11,12]
Provide the patient/client with suggestions to adapt to the newborn infant's sleep–wake cycle during the first 2 to 4 weeks postpartum: • Turn off pagers and phones during sleep times. • Rest and/or sleep when the baby sleeps. Plan with the partner to take turns during the night to get the baby (partner can bring the baby to the mother for breastfeeding, which helps the mother to fall asleep again faster).	Research has shown that the most critical period for sleep disturbance is the first 2 to 6 weeks postpartum. If the new mother does not experience some relief and assistance, it could very easily lead to sleep deprivation, chronic fatigue, and depression.[8,25]

Mental Health

ACTIONS/INTERVENTIONS	RATIONALES
Collaborate with the physician and pharmacist to assess for physiologic and pharmacologic factors that contribute to wakefulness.	Sleep disorders, such as sleep apnea, and certain medical conditions can contribute to sleep deprivation by disruption of normal sleep patterns.[26–28]

ACTIONS/INTERVENTIONS	RATIONALES
Assess the client's use of caffeine, alcohol, tobacco, and other substances. (This can be accomplished with a sleep journal.)	Use of certain chemicals can contribute to sleep disturbance by increasing central nervous system stimulation.[28]
Assess the client for changes in normal activity patterns. (This can be accomplished with a sleep journal.)	Changes in environmental conditions can contribute to sleep disturbance. Exercise close to bedtime can cause stimulation and make it difficult to begin sleep. Irregular daily cycles can interfere with sleep patterns. Also, the client's perceived sleep time may differ from the actual time.[28]
Sit with the client for [number] minutes each shift to discuss current stressors.	Emotional stressors can increase anxiety and decrease the client's ability to relax sufficiently to sleep normally.[27]
Spend 30 minutes each shift in the first 24 hours to review with the client the strategies he or she has used to improve sleep. Validate and normalize the client's responses. [Note persons responsible for this here.]	Understanding the client's perception of the situation of past solutions facilitates change. Decreases feelings of isolation and creates the perception of a manageable problem.[20,21]
Develop with the client a plan to limit caffeine-containing beverages and nicotine 4 hours before bedtime. [Note that plan here.]	Caffeine and nicotine stimulate the central nervous system.[28]
Develop with the client a plan for positive reinforcement for accomplishing the goals established. [Note the behaviors to reward and the rewards here.]	Positive reinforcement strengthens desired behaviors.[28]
Develop an exercise schedule. [Note schedule and type of exercise here.] Arrange schedule so the client is not exercising just before bedtime.	Exercise promotes normal daytime fatigue and facilitates normal sleep patterns.
Spend [number] minutes [times a day] assisting the client with problem solving at least 2 hours before bedtime.	Concerns not addressed in a constructive manner can contribute to nighttime wakefulness. Stress before bedtime can inhibit normal sleep.[31]
Establish a bedtime routine with the client. [Note the client's routine here.]	Routine promotes relaxation.[28]
Provide a light, high-carbohydrate snack before bedtime. [Note the client's preference here.]	Hunger can interfere with normal sleep patterns. Carbohydrates increase tryptophan, which facilitates the development of serotonin. Serotonin promotes sleep.[28]

Gerontic Health

ACTIONS/INTERVENTIONS	RATIONALES
Teach the older adult or caregiver to maintain his or her daily schedule of rising, resting, and sleeping.	Avoid further changes in circadian rhythm.
Encourage the older adult to use progressive muscle relaxation as a strategy to promote sleep.	Progressive muscle relaxation has been found to be an effective nonpharmacologic intervention to improve sleep onset and quality in older adults.[32]
Provide caregivers with information on community resources, stress management, and ways to reduce disruptive behaviors when caring for people with dementia.	Assists caregivers in reducing sense of isolation and stress.[18]
Consult with the physician for possible evaluation of sleep disorder.	Because sleep problems are assumed to be normal aging by elderly and health-care professionals, sleep disorders are often not evaluated or treated.[13]

(care plan continued on page 430)

Home Health/Community Health

● N O T E : *The Adult Health interventions also apply to the Home Health/Community Health client with the following additions:*

ACTIONS/INTERVENTIONS	RATIONALES
Maintain client safety: • Ensure that the client does not attempt to drive while sleep deprived. • Ensure that the client does not try to cook while sleep deprived. • Ensure that the caregiver is not sleep deprived while trying to care for the patient or administering medications.	Basic safety measures.
Reinforce in writing any client education that occurs while the client is sleep deprived.	Ensures that the content is available for review as needed.
Manage pain quickly and effectively.	Pain can contribute to further sleep deprivation, and the client experiences a heightened sensation of pain when sleep deprived.
Identify predisposing factors. Eliminate identified factors that contribute to the present sleep deprivation and/or that place the client at risk for exacerbation of existing problems: • Pain or other symptoms that are not properly managed • Environmental disturbances, such as outside lights or noises • Frequent interruptions during normal sleep times	
Assess the client's emotional stressors and provide referrals as needed for counseling or other community resources, such as support groups.	
The use of prescription or over-the-counter medications, such as the following, may disrupt sleep: • Hypnotics • Diuretics • Antidepressants and stimulants • Alcohol • Caffeine • Beta-adrenergic blockers • Benzodiazepines • Narcotics • Anticonvulsants	
Assist the client/family in modifying the home environment to facilitate effective sleep patterns: • Good ventilation • Quality mattress • Quiet sleep environment or soft "white" noise, if preferred • Dark sleep environment with soft night lights, if preferred • Where possible, the bedroom should be used for sleeping only. • Work, television viewing, studying, and other activities should be done in other rooms.	To facilitate effective sleep patterns

ACTIONS/INTERVENTIONS	RATIONALES
Assist the client/family in developing an activity plan to facilitate effective sleep patterns: • Exercise 2 or more hours before bedtime. • Engage in enjoyable exercise. • Avoid excess fatigue. • Avoid excess sleep on weekends or holidays to prevent alterations in the normal sleep cycle.	To facilitate effective sleep patterns
Assist the client/family in developing an eating/diet plan to facilitate effective sleep patterns: • Avoid large, heavy meals at night. • Avoid caffeine in the evening. • Identify food allergies and avoid allergens. • Maintain a normal, healthy body weight.	To facilitate effective sleep patterns
Encourage self-care, exercise, and activity, as appropriate, based on medical diagnosis and client condition.	Sleep and rest patterns are stabilized by a balance of activity and exercise.

SLEEP PATTERN, DISTURBED

DEFINITION[19]

Time-limited disruption of sleep (natural, periodic suspension of consciousness) amount and quality.

DEFINING CHARACTERISTICS[19]

1. Prolonged awakenings
2. Sleep maintenance insomnia
3. Self-induced impairment of normal pattern
4. Sleep onset longer than 30 minutes
5. Early morning insomnia
6. Awakening earlier or later than desired
7. Verbal complaints of difficulty falling asleep
8. Verbal complaints of not feeling well rested
9. Increased proportion of stage one sleep
10. Dissatisfaction with sleep
11. Less than age-normal total sleep time
12. Three or more nighttime awakenings
13. Decreased proportion of stages three and four sleep (e.g., hyporesponsiveness, excess sleepiness, and decreased motivation)
14. Decreased proportion of REM sleep (e.g., REM rebound, hyperactivity, emotional lability, agitation and impulsivity, and atypical polysomnographic features)
15. Decreased ability to function

RELATED FACTORS[19]

1. Psychological
   a. Ruminative presleep thoughts
   b. Daytime activity pattern
   c. Thinking about home
   d. Body temperature
   e. Temperament
   f. Dietary
   g. Childhood onset
   h. Inadequate sleep hygiene
   i. Sustained use of antisleep agents
   j. Circadian asynchrony
   k. Frequent changing sleep–wake schedule
   l. Depression
   m. Loneliness
   n. Frequent travel across time zones
   o. Daylight or darkness exposure
   p. Grief
   q. Anticipation
   r. Shift work
   s. Delayed or advanced sleep phase syndrome
   t. Loss of sleep partner, life change
   u. Preoccupation with trying to sleep
   v. Periodic gender-related hormonal shifts
   w. Biochemical agents
   x. Fear
   y. Separation from significant others
   z. Social schedule inconsistent with chronotype
   aa. Aging-related sleep shifts
   bb. Anxiety
   cc. Medications
   dd. Fear of insomnia
   ee. Maladaptive conditioned wakefulness
   ff. Fatigue
   gg. Boredom
2. Environmental
   a. Noise
   b. Unfamiliar sleep furnishings
   c. Ambient temperature, humidity
   d. Lighting
   e. Other-generated awakening
   f. Excessive stimulation

g. Physical restraint
h. Lack of sleep privacy or control
i. Nurse for therapeutics, monitoring, or laboratory tests
j. Sleep partner
k. Noxious odors

3. Parental
   a. Mother's sleep–wake pattern
   b. Parent–infant interaction
   c. Mother's emotional support

4. Physiologic
   a. Urinary urgency
   b. Wet
   c. Fever
   d. Nausea
   e. Stasis of secretions
   f. Shortness of breath
   g. Position
   h. Gastroesophageal reflux

RELATED CLINICAL CONCERNS

1. Colic
2. Hyperthyroidism
3. Anxiety
4. Depression
5. Chronic obstructive pulmonary disease
6. Any postoperative state
7. Pregnancy; postpartum period

EXPECTED OUTCOME

Will verbalize decreased number of complaints regarding loss of sleep by [date].

TARGET DATES

The suggested target date is no less than 2 days after the date of diagnosis and no more than 5 days. This length of time will allow for initial modification of the sleep pattern.

NURSING ACTIONS/INTERVENTIONS AND RATIONALES

Adult Health

ACTIONS/INTERVENTIONS	RATIONALES
Teach relaxation exercises as needed.	Decreases sympathetic response and decreases stress.
Suggest sleep-preparatory activities, such as quiet music, warm fluids, and decreased active exercise at least 1 hour before scheduled sleep time. Provide a high-carbohydrate snack.	These winding-down activities promote sleep. Carbohydrates stimulate secretion of insulin. Insulin decreases all amino acids but tryptophan. Tryptophan in larger quantities in the brain increases production of serotonin, a neurotransmitter that induces sleep.[1,33]
Provide warm, noncaffeinated fluids after 6 P.M.; limit fluids after 8 P.M.	Warm drinks are relaxing. Limiting fluid reduces the chance of mid-sleep interruption to go to the bathroom.
Assist to bathroom or bedside commode, or offer bedpan at 9 P.M.	The urge to void may interrupt the sleep cycle during the night. Voiding immediately before going to bed lessens the probability of this occurring.
Schedule all patient therapeutics before 9 P.M.	Promotes uninterrupted sleep.
Maintain room temperature at 68 to 72°F.	Environment temperature that is the most conducive to sleep.
Notify operator to hold telephone calls starting at 9 P.M.	Promotes uninterrupted sleep.
Ensure adherence, as closely as possible, to the patient's usual bedtime routine.	Follows the patient's established pattern; promotes comfort and allows the patient to wind down.
Close door to room; and limit traffic into room beginning at least 1 hour before scheduled sleep time.	Reduces environmental stimuli.[5]
Administer required medication (e.g., analgesics or sedatives, after all daily activities and therapeutics are completed). Monitor effectiveness of medication 30 minutes after time of administration.	Promotes action and effect of medication; allows evaluation of medication effectiveness; and provides data for suggesting changes in medication, if needed.
Give a back massage immediately after administering medication. If no medications are needed, give back massage after toileting.	Relaxes muscles and promotes sleep.
Place the patient in preferred sleeping position; support position with pillows.	Promotes the patient's comfort, and follows the patient's usual routine.
Ascertain whether the patient would like a night light.	Promotes sense of orientation in an unfamiliar environment.

ACTIONS/INTERVENTIONS	RATIONALES
Once the patient is sleeping, place a "do not disturb" sign on the door.	Promotes uninterrupted sleep.
Increase exercise and activity during day as appropriate for the patient's condition.	Promotes a regular diurnal rhythm.
When appropriate, discuss reasons for the sleep pattern disturbance and teach appropriate coping mechanisms.	Promotes adaptation that can increase sleep.

Child Health

ACTIONS/INTERVENTIONS	RATIONALES
Give a warm bath 30 minutes to 1 hour before scheduled sleep time.	Promotes relaxation, and provides quiet time as a part of the sleep routine.
Feed formula, or a snack of protein and simple carbohydrate (no fats), 15 to 30 minutes before scheduled sleep time.	In young infants and small children, a sense of fullness and satiety, without difficulty in digestion, promotes sleep without the likelihood of upset or disturbances.
Implement usual bedtime routine: • Rocking • Patting • Child cuddling with favorite stuffed animal • Using special blanket	A structured approach to setting limits while honoring individual preference. Provides security and promotes sleep.
Read a calm, quiet story to the child immediately after putting to bed.	Reading allows a passive, meaningful enjoyment that occupies the attention of the young child while creating a bond between the caretaker and child. Serendipitous relaxation often follows.
Provide environment conducive to sleep, such as: • Room temperature of 74 to 78°F • Soft, relaxing music • Night light	Lack of unpleasant stimuli will provide sensory rest, as well as a chance to tune out need for cognitive–perceptual activity.
Restrict loud physical activity at least 2 to 3 hours before scheduled sleep time.	Overstimulating physical activity may signal the central nervous system to activate bodily functions.
Schedule therapeutics around sleep needs. Complete all therapeutics at least 1 hour before scheduled sleep time.	The nurse's valuing of the sleep schedule will convey respect for the importance of sleep to the patient and family.
Assist the parents with defining and standardizing a general waking and sleeping schedule.	Parents will be able to cope better with developmental issues given the knowledge and opportunity to inquire about sleep-related issues. It is reported that limit setting with confidence by parents is the most effective way to develop healthy patterns of sleep when no related health problems exist.
Teach the parents and child appropriate, age-related relaxation techniques (e.g., imagination of the "most quiet place game" and other imaging techniques).	Improves parents' coping skills in dealing with common developmental issues that affect sleep.
Discuss with the parents the difference between inability to sleep and fears related to developmental crises: • Infant and toddler—Separation anxiety • Preschooler—Fantasy versus reality • School-age—Ability to perform at expected levels • Adolescent—Role identity versus role diffusion	
Ensure the child's safety according to developmental and psychomotor abilities (e.g., infant placed on side or back; no plastic, loose-fitting sheets; and bedrails to prevent falling out of bed).	Basic safety standards for infants and children.

(care plan continued on page 434)

NURSING ACTIONS/INTERVENTIONS AND RATIONALES (continued from page 433)

Women's Health

ACTIONS/INTERVENTIONS	RATIONALES
Assist the patient in scheduling rest breaks throughout day.	Knowledge and proper planning can help the patient reduce fatigue during pregnancy and the immediate postpartum period.[8,34]
Review daily schedule with the patient, and assist the patient to adjust her sleep schedule to coincide with the infant's sleep pattern.	Knowledge of life changes can help in planning and implementing mechanisms to reduce fatigue and sleep disturbance.
Identify a support system that can assist the patient in alleviating fatigue.	
Assist the patient in identifying lifestyle adjustments that may be needed because of changes in physiologic function or needs during experiential phases of life (e.g., pregnancy, postpartum, or menopause):	During the immediate postpartum period, 2 to 4 weeks after birth, it is important for the mother to adjust her sleep cycle to the infant's if at all possible, in order to get enough rest and sleep.[8]
• Possible lowering of room temperature	During perimenopause and menopause try such things as avoiding caffeine, alcohol, and nicotine; and exercising, but not too close to bedtime. About an hour before going to bed engage in a relaxing, nonalerting activity, do not drink or eat too much, and maintain a quiet, dark, and preferably cool but comfortable, sleep environment.[1,12]
• Layering of blankets or covers that can be discarded or added as necessary	
• Practicing relaxation immediately before scheduled sleep time	
• Establishing a bedtime routine (e.g., bath, food, fluids, or activity)	
Involve significant others in discussion and problem-solving activities regarding life-cycle changes that are affecting work habits and interpersonal relationships (e.g., hot flashes, pregnancy, or postpartum fatigue).	
Teach the patient to experiment with restful activities when she cannot sleep at night rather than lying in bed and thinking about not sleeping.	
Discuss with women the following to assess sleep pattern disturbance:	
• Do they have an irregular sleep–wake pattern?	
• Do they have problems falling asleep at night?	
• Do they regularly wake up several times at night and have difficulty falling back asleep?	
• Do they feel sleepy or drowsy during the day?	
Assess for snoring, jerky movements during sleep, or stoppage of breathing during sleep. (Can assess in sleep lab or question the client's sleeping partner.)	
Collaborate with the woman's physician, and recommend an evaluation of hormone levels and/or further evaluation of sleep disorders.	For women in midlife, restless sleep with several awakenings may be one of the earliest indicators of declining estrogen. Sleep apnea can lead to sexual dysfunction, major depression, high blood pressure, chronic fatigue, problems with memory and concentration during the day, and potentially a heart attack.[11,12]

Mental Health

ACTIONS/INTERVENTIONS	RATIONALES
Provide only decaffeinated drinks during all 24 hours.	Caffeine stimulates the central nervous system.
Spend [amount] minutes with the client in activity of the client's choice at least twice a day.	Increases mental alertness and activity during daytime hours.
Provide appropriate positive reinforcement for achievement of steps toward reaching a normal sleep pattern.	Positive reinforcement encourages behavior.
Talk the client through deep muscle relaxation exercise for 30 minutes at 9 P.M.	Facilitates relaxation and disengagement from the activities and thoughts of the day to prepare the client both physically and mentally for sleep.
Sit with the client for [amount] minutes three times a day in a quiet environment, and provide positive reinforcement for the client's accomplishments.	Positive reinforcement encourages calm behavior and enhances self-esteem.
● N O T E : *This is for clients with increased activity.*	
Go to the client's room and walk with him or her to the group three times a day.	Stimulates wakefulness during daytime hours, and facilitates the area development of a trusting relationship.
Spend time out of the room with the client until he or she demonstrates ability to tolerate 30 minutes of interaction with others.[35]	Stimulates wakefulness during daytime hours.
● N O T E : *This is for clients with depressed mood.*	
Spend 30 minutes with the client discussing concerns 2 hours before bedtime.	Facilitates problem-solving during daytime hours at a time when normal sleep patterns will not be disturbed.

Gerontic Health

ACTIONS/INTERVENTIONS	RATIONALES
Collaborate with the physician and pharmacist, if a sleeping medication is prescribed, to ensure that the drug is one that minimally interferes with the normal sleep cycle.	This ensures that the older adult has as natural a sleep pattern as possible.
Assess for the presence of physical causes of interrupted sleep and provide referrals as needed: • Prostatic hypertrophy leading to nocturia. • Prescription medications that may interrupt normal sleep patterns (beta-blockers are commonly used in elderly clients and can cause nightmares and insomnia). • Recent losses or grief can lead to altered sleep patterns. • Some cardiac disorders can lead to orthopnea.	
Monitor for the presence of pain prior to bedtime and if the patient is found awake frequently during the night.	Untreated pain may prevent the onset of sleep and interrupt the individual's usual sleep pattern.
Monitor for symptoms of depression,[36] especially if the older adult reports waking very early in the morning with an inability to fall back to sleep, and is experiencing feelings of anxiety on awakening.	Depression is frequently underreported and undertreated in older adults.

(care plan continued on page 436)

NURSING ACTIONS/INTERVENTIONS AND RATIONALES (continued from page 435)

Home Health

ACTIONS/INTERVENTIONS	RATIONALES
Involve the client and family in planning, implementing, and promoting restful environment and sleep routine: • Coordinate family activities and the client's sleep needs to maximize both schedules. • Request that visits and calls be at specified times so that sleep time is not interrupted. • Provide favorite music, pillows, bedclothes, teddy bears, etc. • Support usual bedtime routine as much as possible in relation to medical diagnosis and the client's condition. • Assist the client with maintaining a consistent bedtime routine as necessary.	Household involvement is important to ensure the environment is conducive for sleep and rest.

Provide client/family teaching about medications that may disrupt normal sleep patterns:
• Hypnotics
• Diuretics
• Antidepressants and stimulants
• Alcohol
• Caffeine
• Beta-adrenergic blockers
• Benzodiazepines
• Narcotics
• Anticonvulsants

Assist the client/family in modifying the home environment to facilitate effective sleep patterns:
• Good ventilation
• Quality mattress
• Quiet sleep environment or soft "white" noise, if preferred
• Dark sleep environment with soft night lights, if preferred
• Where possible the bedroom should be used for sleeping only. Work, television viewing, studying, and other activities should be done in other rooms.
• Unplug telephone in room, or adjust volume control on bell.

Assist the client/family in developing an activity plan to facilitate effective sleep patterns:
• Exercise 2 or more hours before bedtime.
• Engage in enjoyable exercise.
• Avoid excess fatigue.
• Avoid excess sleep on weekends or holidays to prevent alterations in the normal sleep cycle.

Assist the client/family in developing an eating/diet plan to facilitate effective sleep patterns:
• Avoid large, heavy meals at night.
• Avoid caffeine in the evening.
• Identify food allergies and avoid allergens.
• Maintain a normal, healthy body weight.

ACTIONS/INTERVENTIONS	RATIONALES
Maintain pain control via appropriate medications, body positioning, and relaxation. Narcotics can suppress REM sleep and lead to increased daytime sleepiness.	Pain disturbs or prevents sleep and rest.
Encourage self-care, exercise, and activity as appropriate and based on medical diagnosis and client condition.	Sleep–rest patterns are stabilized by a balance of activity and exercise.

SLEEP, READINESS FOR ENHANCED

DEFINITION[19]

A pattern of natural, periodic suspension of consciousness that provides adequate rest, sustains a desired lifestyle, and can be strengthened.

DEFINING CHARACTERISTICS[19]

1. Expresses willingness to enhance sleep.
2. Amount of sleep and REM sleep is congruent with developmental needs.
3. Expresses a feeling of being rested after sleep.
4. Follows sleep routines that promote sleep habits.
5. Occasional or infrequent use of medications to induce sleep.

RELATED CLINICAL CONCERNS

1. Long work hours or shift in work hours
2. Environmental impacts of modern living
3. Jet lag
4. Driving while fatigued
5. Life changes that affect one's sleep patterns and/or characteristics

☑ Have You Selected the Correct Diagnosis?

Fatigue
The patient will complain of lack of energy and being tired during the day, as well as having difficulty in maintaining his or her usual activities. However, assessment documents that this fatigue exists regardless of the amount of sleep.

Health-Seeking Behaviors
The patient will tell the health-care provider that they need assistance with sleep, whether with medication or a change in environment, when in actuality the patient documents adequate sleep for age and life cycle.

Ineffective Coping
Patient complains of inability to cope related to lack of sleep, when in reality, there is another factor of worry, fear, or lifestyle which is interfering with patient's sleep patterns.

EXPECTED OUTCOME

The client will sleep at least (number) hours in 24 hours by (date).
The client will demonstrate effective sleep habits by (date).

TARGET DATES

Since this is a positive diagnosis, target dates should be 1 to 2 days after diagnosis.

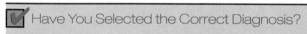

NURSING ACTIONS/INTERVENTIONS WITH RATIONALES

Adult Health

ACTIONS/INTERVENTIONS	RATIONALES
Collaborate with patient to develop sleep schedule	
Assist patient in developing environment that promotes restful sleep. Note that plan here.	
Have patient identify actions that enhance and deter restful sleep.	
Devise schedule to gradually taper reliance on sleep medications.	
Have patient keep journal about sleep pattern. Review weekly.	Allows identification of progress of plan of care and alterations as necessary

(care plan continued on page 438)

NURSING ACTIONS/INTERVENTIONS AND RATIONALES (continued from page 437)

Child Health

ACTIONS/INTERVENTIONS	RATIONALES
Assess for all contributory factors, especially evidence for pattern of sleep, which are appropriate for developmental age and status.	Provides realistic base for plan.
Foster current daily regimen with specific attention to continuing plan for sleep routine.	Values current need for sleep and success in attainment of desired plan for adequate rest.
Provide opportunity for development of mutually agreeable ongoing guidelines for caregiver(s) and/or child, as appropriate, to continue to monitor sleep patterns with best practice to attain desired sleep.[37]	Provides anticipatory guidance for plan.
Offer instructions according to caregiver(s) baseline knowledge of sleep, especially regarding aids to sleep, need for maintenance of schedule, and routine for sleep.	Provides a realistic basis for teaching and likelihood of follow-up for plan.
Offer resources according to infant or child's age/developmental status.	Provides appropriate anticipatory guidance for realistic expectations.
Warn caregiver(s) of dangers of co-sleeping and of risk for SIDS for young infants.[37]	Offers safe anticipatory guidance.[7,37] Childcare programs outlines what should be included in the safe sleep policy (http://www.healthychildcare.org/pdf/SIDSchildcaresafesleep.pdf)

Women's Health

Women's Health will follow the same interventions and rationales as does Adult Health, Home Health, and Gerontic Health, except for the following:

ACTIONS/INTERVENTIONS	RATIONALES
Assess sleeping arrangements of childbearing couples, particularly after the birth of the new baby. Be sensitive to cultural diversity and family sleeping habits. Assess lifestyle changes that the addition of a new baby brings to the household	A through assessment of sleeping arrangements, cultural influences, sleeping habits of the parents, presence of pets in the household, and any additional lifestyle changes that have occurred since the arrival of the new baby will allow the health care provider to make suggestions and help the couple plan. This planning will help the couple to maintain their sleep patterns and promote enhanced readiness for sleep.[7,8,25]

Assist women who are approaching midlife and experiencing perimenopause and menopause plan and learn methods of continuing to maintain healthy sleep patterns. Some tips to share are:
• Avoid shift work if possible, especially switching shifts at work on a routine basis.
• Avoid caffeine, alcohol, and nicotine.
• Exercise, but not too close to bedtime.
• Avoid naps.
• About an hour before going to bed:
  • Engage in a relaxing, nonalerting activity.
  • Do not drink or eat too much.
• Maintain a quiet, dark, and preferably cool, but comfortable sleep environment.
	Women who are aware of their life-cycles and know what to expect can better plan and implement changes in their environment that will help them maintain good sleeping habits. That will prevent sleep problems and promote optimal sleep and show enhanced readiness for sleep.[1,11,12,14–16]

ACTIONS/INTERVENTIONS	RATIONALES
• Keep a sleep diary to identify your sleep habits and patterns. • Layer blankets, so that you can take them off or put them on if you are experiencing "hot flashes." • Keep the bedroom cool and use only for sleep (do not watch television in bed).	

Mental Health

Spend [number] minutes [number] times a day discussing with client his or her perceptions of current sleep patterns. [Note the schedule of these meetings here.]	Change is dependent on the client's perception of the problem.[37]
Develop, with the client, a plan for addressing his or her needs for sleep enhancement.	
• Utilize information about sleep hygiene to guide client in plan development (See information on sleep hygiene in Sleep Deprivation care plan).	
[Note the client's plan here with information about the assistance needed from nursing for goal achievement.]	
Develop, with the client, a plan for rewarding positive behavior change.	Positive reinforcement encourages behavior change.[29,37]
[Note the plan for rewarding behavior here.]	

Home Health/Community Health

ACTIONS/INTERVENTIONS	RATIONALES
Provide the client/family teaching about medications that may disrupt normal sleep patterns: • Hynotics • Diuretics • Antidepressants and stimulants • Alcohol • Caffeine • Beta-adrenergic blockers • Benzodiazepines • Narcotics • Anticonvulsants	To prevent sleep problems.
Assist the client/family in modifying the home environment to facilitate effective sleep patterns: • Good ventilation • Quality mattress • Quiet sleep environment or soft "white" noise, if preferred • Dark sleep environment with soft night lights, if preferred • Where possible the bedroom should be used for sleeping only. Work, television viewing, studying, and other activities should be done in other rooms.	To facilitate effective sleep patterns

(care plan continued on page 440)

NURSING ACTIONS/INTERVENTIONS WITH RATIONALES (continued from page 439)

Home Health/Community Health

ACTIONS/INTERVENTIONS	RATIONALES
Assist the client/family in developing an activity plan to facilitate effective sleep patterns: • Exercise 2 or more hours before bedtime. • Engage in enjoyable exercise. • Avoid excess fatigue. • Avoid excess sleep on weekends or holidays to prevent alterations in the normal sleep cycle.	To facilitate effective sleep patterns
Assist the client/family to develop an eating/diet plan to facilitate effective sleep patterns: • Avoid large, heavy meals at night. • Avoid caffeine in the evening. • Identify food allergies and avoid allergens. • Maintain a normal, healthy body weight.	To facilitate effective sleep patterns

REFERENCES

1. McGovern, J: The Basics of Sleep. Unpublished presentation, Milwaukee, WI, 2005.
2. Lavie, P, Malhotra, A, Pillar, G, and Dunitz, M: Sleep Disorders: Diagnosis, Management and Treatment: A Handbook for Clinicians. Martin Dunitz, London, 2002.
3. Hayter, J: The rhythm of sleep. Am J Nurs 80: 457, 1980.
4. Courtenay, WH: Behavioral factors associated with disease, injury, and death among men: Evidence and implications for prevention. Int J Men Health 1:281, 2002.
5. Babisch, W: Noise and health. Environ Health Perspect 113:14, 2005.
6. Lee, K: Rest status. In Mitchell, PH, and Loustau, A (eds): Concepts Basic to Nursing, ed 3. McGraw-Hill, New York, 1981.
7. Hockenberry, MJ. Wong's Clinical Manual of Pediatric Nursing, ed 6. CV Mosby, St. Louis, 2004.
8. Lowdermilk, DL, and Shannon, EP: Maternity and Women's Health Care, ed 8. CV Mosby, St. Louis, 2004.
9. Guilleminault, C: Sleep and Its Disorders in Children. Raven Press, New York, 1987.
10. Task Force on Sudden Infant Death Syndrome. Pediatrics 116: 1245, 2005.
11. Vliet, EL: Screaming to Be Heard: Hormonal Connections Women Suspect and Doctors Ignore. M. Evans and Co., New York, 1995.
12. Kanusky, C: Health Concerns of Women in Midlife. In Breslin, ET, and Lucas, VA (eds): Women's Health Nursing: Toward Evidence-Based Practice. Saunders, St. Louis, 2003.
13. Ancoli-Israel, S: Sleep problems in older adults: Putting myths to bed. Geriatrics 52:20, 1997.
14. Sellers, JB: Health care for older women. In Breslin, ET, and Lucas, VA (eds): Women's Health Nursing: Toward Evidence-Based Practice. WB Saunders, St. Louis, 2003.
15. Bundlie, SR: Sleep in aging. Geriatrics 53:41, 1998.
16. Beck-Little, R, and Weinrick, SP: Assessment and management of sleep disorders in the elderly. J Gerontol Nurs 24:21, 1998.
17. Miller, CA: Nursing Care of Older Adults: Theory and Practice, ed 3. Lippincott, Philadelphia, 1999.
18. McCurry, SM: Successful behavioral treatment for reported sleep problems in elderly caregivers of dementia patients: A controlled study. J Gerontol 53:122, 1998.
19. Author: Nursing Diagnosis: Definitions and Classification, 2005–2006, North American Nursing Diagnosis Association, NANDA International. 2005.
20. Stevenson, J, and Murphy, PM: Slumber, jack: 20 knockout tactics guaranteed to help you sleep. Men's Health 10:34, 1995.
21. Schmetzer, AD: The medicines for insomnia. Ann Am Psychother Assoc 7(2):30, 2004.
22. Courtenay, WH: Behavioral factors associated with disease, injury, and death among men: Evidence and implications for prevention. J Men's Studies 9(1):81, 2000.
23. What to swallow (or avoid) for better sleep. Tufts U Health Nutr Lett 17: 1999.
24. Clinical practice guideline: Diagnosis and management of childhood obstructive sleep apnea syndrome. April, NGC: 002431, American Academy of Pediatrics-Medical Specialty Society, 2002.
25. Yamazaki, A, Lee, KA, Kennedy, HP, and Weiss, SJ: Sleep-wake cycles, social rhythms, and sleeping arrangement during Japanese childbearing family transition. JOGNN J Obstet Gynecol Neonatal Nurs 34(3):342, 2005.
26. Yantis, M: Identifying depressing as a symptom of sleep apnea. J Psychosoc Nurs 37:28, 1999.
27. McFarland, G, Wasli, E, and Gerety, E: Nursing Diagnoses and Process in Psychiatric Mental Health Nursing, ed 3. Lippincott, Philadelphia, 1997.
28. Townsend M: Psychiatric Mental Health Nursing: Concepts of Care, ed 3. FA Davis, Philadelphia, 2000.
29. Kneisl, C, Wilson, H, and Trigoboff, E: Contemporay Psychiatric-Mental Health Nursing, Pearson Education, Upper Saddle River, NJ, 2004.
30. McCloskey, J, and Bulechek, G: Nursing Interventins Classification, ed 2. Mosby-Year Book, St. Louis, 1996.
31. Floyd, JA: Sleep promotion in adults. Annu Rev Nurs Res 17:27, 1999.
32. Driskell, JE, and Mullen, B: The efficacy of naps as a fatigue counter-measure: A meta-analytic integration. Human Factors 47:1122, 2005.
33. Fisch, R, et al: The Tactics of Change: Doing Therapy Briefly. Jossey-Bass, San Francisco, 1982.
34. Keane, SM, and Stella, S: Recognizing depression in the elderly. J Gerontol Nurs 15:21, 1990.
35. Author: Practice parameters for using polysomnography to evaluate insomnia: An update: American Academy of Sleep Medicine—Professional Association. NGC: A 003292, 2003.
36. Author: Safe sleep for my grandbaby: Did you know that guidelines for safe sleep have changed since your children were babies? The American Academy of Pediatrics (http://www.sidsalliance.org), 2005.
37. Wright, L, and Leahey, M: Nurses and Families, ed 4. FA Davis, Philadelphia, 2005.

7

COGNITIVE-
PERCEPTUAL PATTERN

PATTERN DESCRIPTION

Rationality, the ability to think, has often been described as the defining attribute of humans. Thus, the cognitive–perceptual pattern becomes the essential premise for all other patterns used in the practice of nursing. Because it deals with the adequacy of the sensory modes and adaptations necessary to negate inadequacies in the cognitive functional abilities, any failure in recognizing alterations in this pattern will hamper assessment and intervention in all the other patterns. The nurse must be aware of the cognitive–perceptual pattern as an integral and important part of holistic nursing.

The cognitive–perceptual pattern deals with thought, thought processes, and knowledge as well as the way the patient acquires and applies knowledge. A major component of the process is perceiving. *Perceiving* incorporates the interpretation of sensory stimuli. Understanding how a patient thinks, perceives, and incorporates these processes to best adapt and function is paramount in assisting him or her to return to or maintain the best health state possible. Alterations in the process of cognition and perception are an initial step in any assessment.

In addition, the nurse–patient relationship identifies human response as a major premise for the nursing process. Ultimately, then, it is this very notion of thought and learning potential that facilitates the self-actualization of humans.

PATTERN ASSESSMENT

1. Does intracranial pressure fluctuate after a single activity?
   a. Yes (Decreased Intracranial Adaptive Capacity)
   b. No
2. Does the patient have a problem with appropriate responses to stimuli?
   a. Yes (Confusion)
   b. No
3. Does the patient have a problem with fluctuating levels of consciousness (in the presence of inappropriate responses to stimuli)?
   a. Yes (Acute Confusion)
   b. No (Chronic Confusion)
4. Does the patient indicate difficulty in making choices between options for care?
   a. Yes (Decisional Conflict [Specify])
   b. No (Readiness for Enhanced Knowledge)
5. Is the patient delaying decision making regarding care options?
   a. Yes (Decisional Conflict [Specify])
   b. No (Readiness for Enhanced Knowledge)
6. Has the patient been disoriented to person, place, and time for more than 3 months?
   a. Yes (Impaired Environmental Interpretation Syndrome)
   b. No

7. Can the patient respond to simple directions or instructions?
   a. Yes (Readiness for Enhanced Knowledge)
   b. No (Impaired Environmental Interpretation Syndrome)
8. Does the patient indicate lack of information regarding his or her problem?
   a. Yes (Deficient Knowledge [Specify])
   b. No (Readiness for Enhanced Knowledge)
9. Can the patient restate the regimen he or she needs to follow for improved health?
   a. Yes
   b. No (Deficient Knowledge [Specify])
10. Can the patient remember events occurring within the past 4 hours?
    a. Yes
    b. No (Impaired Memory)
11. Review the mental status examination. Is the patient fully alert?
    a. Yes
    b. No (Disturbed Thought Process or Disturbed Sensory Perception)
12. Does the patient or his or her family indicate that the patient has any memory problems?
    a. Yes (Disturbed Thought Process)
    b. No
13. Review sensory examination. Does the patient display any sensory problems?
    a. Yes (Disturbed Sensory Perception [Specify])
    b. No
14. Does the patient use both sides of his or her body?
    a. Yes
    b. No (Unilateral Neglect)
15. Does the patient look at, and seem aware of, the affected body side?
    a. Yes
    b. No (Unilateral Neglect)
16. Does the patient verbalize that he or she is experiencing pain?
    a. Yes (Acute Pain; Chronic Pain)
    b. No
17. Has the pain been experienced for more than 6 months?
    a. Yes (Chronic Pain)
    b. No (Acute Pain)
18. Does the patient display any distraction behavior (moaning, crying, pacing, or restlessness)?
    a. Yes (Pain)
    b. No

CONCEPTUAL INFORMATION

A person who is able to carry out the activities of a normal cognitive-perceptual pattern experiences conscious thought, is oriented to reality, solves problems, is able to perceive via sensory input, and responds appropriately in carrying out the usual activities of daily living in the fullest level of functioning. All these functions rely on a healthy nervous system containing receptors to detect input accurately, a brain that can interpret the information correctly, and transmitters that can transport decoded information. Bodily response is also a basic requisite to respond to the sensory and perceptual demands of the individual.

Cognition is the process of obtaining and using knowledge about one's world through the use of perceptual abilities, symbols, and reasoning. For this reason, it includes the use of human sensory capabilities to receive input about the environment. Cognition usually leads to *perception*, which is the process of extracting information in such a way that the individual transforms sensory input into meaning. Cognition incorporates knowledge and the process used in its acquisition; therefore, ideas (concepts of mind symbols) and language (verbal symbols) are two tools of cognition. Learning may be considered the dynamic process in which perceptual processing of sensory input leads to concept formation and change in behavior. Cognitive development is highly dependent on adequate, predictable sensory input.

There are two general approaches to contemporary cognitive theory. The information-processing approach attempts to understand human thought and reasoning processes by comparing the mind with a sophisticated computer system that is designed to acquire, process, store, and use information according to various programs or designs.

The second approach is based on the work of the Swiss psychologist Jean Piaget, who considered cognitive adaptation in terms of two basic processes: assimilation and accommodation. *Assimilation* is the process by which the person integrates new perceptual data or stimulus events into existing schemata or existing patterns of behavior. In other words, in assimilation, a person interprets reality in terms of his or her own model of the world based on previous experience. *Accommodation* is the process of changing the model the individual has of the world by developing the mechanisms to adjust to reality. Piaget believed that representational thought originates not in a social language but in unique symbols that provide a foundation later for language acquisition.[1]

American psychologist Jerome Bruner broadened Piaget's concept by suggesting that the cognitive process is affected by three modes. The *enactive mode* involves representation through action, the *iconic mode* uses visual and mental images, and the *symbolic mode* uses language.[1]

Cognitive dissonance is the mental conflict that takes place when beliefs or assumptions are challenged or contradicted by new information. The unease or tension the individual may experience as a result of cognitive dissonance usually results in the person's resorting to defense mechanisms in an attempt to maintain stability in his or her conception of the world and self.

In a broad sense, thinking activities may be considered internally adaptive responses to intrinsic and extrinsic stimuli. The thought processes serve to express inner impulses, but they also serve to generate appropriate goal-seeking behavior by the individual. Perceptual processes enhance this behavior as well.

Perception is the process of extracting information in such a way that the individual transforms sensory input into meaning. The senses, which serve as the origin of perceptual stimuli, are as follows:

1. Exteroceptors (distance sensors)
   a. Visual
   b. Auditory
2. Proprioceptors (near sensors)
   a. Cutaneous (skin senses that detect and communicate, or transducer, changes in touch, e.g., pressure, temperature, and pain)
   b. Chemical sense of taste
   c. Chemical sense of smell
3. Interoceptors (deep sensors)
   a. Kinesthetic sense that senses changes in position of the body and motions of the muscles, tendons, and joints
   b. Static or vestibular sense that senses changes related to maintaining position in space and the regulation of organic functions such as metabolism, fluid balance, and sensual stimulation

It is important to note that because perceptual skill processing is an internal event, its presence and development are inferred by changes in overt behavior. For full appreciation of the cognitive–perceptual pattern, it is also necessary to understand the normal physiology of the nervous system.

DEVELOPMENTAL CONSIDERATIONS

INFANT

The full-term newborn has several sensory capacities. The neonate should have a pupillary reflex in response to light and a corneal reflex in response to touch. At birth, the sensory myelination is best developed for hearing, taste, and smell.

Vision. Structurally, the eye is not completely differentiated from the macula. The newborn has the capacity to fixate momentarily on a bright or moving object held within 8 inches and in the midline of the visual field. By approximately 4 months of age, the infant is capable of 20/200 visual acuity. Binocular fixation and convergence to near objects is possible by approximately 4 months of age. In a supine position, the infant can follow a dangling toy from the side to past midline.

Hearing. The neonate is capable of detecting a loud sound of approximately 90 decibels and reacts with a startle. At birth, all the structural components of the ear are fully developed. However, the lack of cortical integration and full myelination of the neural pathways prevents specific response to sound. The infant will usually search to locate sounds. By approximately 15 months of age, the infant is beginning to acquire eye–hand coordination and is capable of accommodation to near objects. Of concern at this age would be any abnormalities noted in any of these tasks plus rubbing of eyes, self-rocking, or other self-stimulating behavior. By approximately 2 months, the infant will turn to the appropriate side when a sound is made at ear level. By approximately 20 months, the infant will localize sounds made below the ear. A cause for concern might be failure to be awakened by loud noises or abnormal findings in any of the previously mentioned responses. Speech or the uttering of sounds by age 6 to 8 months would also be a component.

Smell. Smell seems to be a factor in breastfed infants' response to the mother's engorgement and leaking. Newborns will turn away from strong odors such as vinegar and alcohol. By approximately 6 to 9 months, the infant associates smell with different foods and familiar people of his or her circle of activity. The infant also avoids strong, unpleasant odors.

Taste. The newborn responds to various solutions with the following facial reflexes:

1. A tasteless solution elicits no facial expression.
2. A sweet solution elicits an eager suck and look of satisfaction.
3. A bitter liquid produces an angry, upset expression.

By 1 year of age, the infant shows marked preferences, with similar responses to different flavors, as did the young neonate.

Touch. At birth, the neonate is capable of perception of touch, and the mouth, hands, and soles of the feet are the most sensitive. There is increasing support for the notion that touch and motion are essential to normal growth and development.

By 1 year of age, the infant has a preference for soft textures over rough, grainy textures. The infant relies on the sense of touch for comforting. Over-response or under-response to stimuli, for example pain, is a cause for concern.

Proprioception. At birth, the infant is limited in perceiving itself in space, because this requires deep myelination and total integration of cortical activity. There is momentary head control. In general, referral to more exacting neurologic reflexes of the neonate will provide in-depth supplementary data. In essence, primitive reflexes, which are protective in nature, serve to assist the neonate in adjustment to extrauterine life and identification of congenital anomalies. A critical appreciation of organic and operational synergy for the central nervous system is necessary as sensory deficits are considered.

By approximately 3 months of age, the infant will, when suspended in a horizontal prone position with the head flexed against the trunk, reflexively draw up the legs. This is known as the *Landau reflex.* It remains present until approximately 12 to 24 months of age. Another related reflex is the *parachute reflex,* in which the infant, on being suspended in a horizontal prone position and suddenly thrust downward, will place hands and fingers forward as an attempt to protect him- or herself from falling. This reflex appears at approximately 7 months and persists indefinitely.

The neonate responds with total body reaction to a painful stimulus. The primitive reflexes demonstrate this, especially the *Moro,* or *startle, response* to sudden loss of support or loud noises. The neonate is dependent on others for protection from pain. The mother of a newborn is most often the person who assumes this task, along with the father and other primary caregivers. For this reason, management of pain must also include the parents. Distraction, for example, a pacifier, is useful in dealing with painful stimuli.

The infant gradually offers localized reaction in response to pain at approximately 6 to 9 months of age. Still, the cognitive abilities of the infant remain limited with respect to pain. Often a physical tugging of the painful body part proves to be the clue of pain for the infant, as with an earache. The infant is incapable of offering cooperation in procedures and must be physically restrained, because he or she is largely incapable of resisting painful stimuli. Crying and irritability may also be manifestations of pain, particularly when the nurse is certain other basic needs have been attended to.

If chronic pain comes to be a way of life for the infant soon after birth or before much development has occurred, there may be alterations in any subsequent development. In some instances, infants adapt and develop high tolerances for pain.

The neonate is dependent on others for appropriate care and health maintenance. Values for health care are being formed through this provision of care by others. The infant will gradually continue to learn values of health care. Safety becomes an ongoing concern, as has been previously acknowledged. Parents or primary caregivers assume this responsibility. The infant is capable of object permanence but cannot be expected to remember abstract notions.

The neonate subjected to hypoxia in the perinatal period is at risk for possible future developmental delays. Apgar scores are typically used as criteria, in addition to neurologic reflexes. Seizures during the neonatal period must also be followed up. In a general sense, the premature infant of less than 37 weeks' gestation should also be considered at risk for developmental delays. It is paramount that close examination be performed for basic primitive reflexes and general neonatal status as well as identification of any genetic syndromes or congenital anomalies.

The infant gradually incorporates symbols and interacts with the world through primary caregivers. Any major delays in development should be cause for further close follow-up. Sensory-perceptual deficiencies may indeed bring about impaired thought processes.

TODDLER AND PRESCHOOLER

Binocular vision is well established by now. The toddler can distinguish geometric shapes and can demonstrate beginning depth perception. Marked strabismus should be treated at this time to prevent amblyopia. The toddler can begin to name colors.

Smell, taste, and touch all become more related as the toddler initially sees an object and handles it while enjoying, via all the senses, what it is to "know." Regression to previous tactile behavior for comfort is common in this group, as exemplified by a preference for being patted and rocked to sleep during times of stress, such as illness. Concerns by this time would be for secondary deficits in development that may arise. There is also a great concern for the toddler who shows greater response to movement than to sound or who avoids social interaction with other children. By this time, speech should be sufficiently developed to validate a basic sense of the toddler's ability to use symbols. Proprioception is not perfected, but "toddling" represents a major milestone. Falls are common at this age.

There is an even greater incorporation of sensory activity in sequencing for the preschooler, in whom major myelination for the most part is fully developed. There is refinement of eye–hand coordination, and reading readiness is apparent. Visual acuity begins to approach 20/20, and the preschooler will know colors. Before age 5, the child should be screened for amblyopia; after age 5, there is minimal potential for development of amblyopia. Language becomes more sophisticated and serves to provide social interaction. By this age, the child will remember and exercise caution regarding potential dangers, such as hot objects.

The toddler may regress to previous behavior levels with physical resistance in response to painful stimuli. This will be especially true with invasive procedures. On occasion, a toddler may demonstrate tolerance for painful procedures on the basis of understanding benefits offered, for example, young children with a medical diagnosis of leukemia. This is not the usual case, however. Temper tantrums, outbursts, and avoidance of painful stimuli describe the usual behavior of the toddler. When the toddler must deal with chronic pain, he or she may regress to previous behavior as a means of coping.

The preschooler views any invasive procedure as mutilation and attempts to withdraw in response to pain. The preschooler cries out in pain and will express feelings in his or her own terms as descriptors of pain. The interpretation of pain is influenced greatly by the parental and familial value systems. In severe pain, the potential for regression to previous behavior is high. The nurse should be aware that fears of abandonment, death, or the unknown would be brought out by pain for this age group. Also, the effect the pain has on others may serve to further frighten the child.

Play is an ideal noninvasive means of assessment. Difficulties in gait, balance, or the use of upper limbs in symmetry with lower limbs should be noted, as well as related holistic developmental components including speech, motor, cognitive, perceptual, and social components. Allowance should be made for regression to prior patterns as needed in times of stress, such as illness and hos-

pitalization. If a deficit exists, parents should be encouraged to continue appropriate follow-up and intervention.

The preschooler may be aware of how he or she is different from peers, although egocentrism continues. Of importance is the mastery of separation from parents for increasing periods of time. The likelihood of sibling integration should be considered also. At this time, a known neglect of one side of the body may be problematic, as the child may rebel and fail to comply with desired therapy.

The toddler gradually learns to care for him- or herself and is strongly influenced by the family's value system. There is capacity for expression of beginning thoughts.

The preschooler has a capacity for magical thinking and enjoys role-play of the parent of the same sex. At this age, beginning resistance to parental authority is common, and the child is still egocentric in thought. This makes it difficult to apply universal understanding of use of language and symbols for children of this age; for example, death may be perceived as "sleep."

By this age, there should be a general notion of the cognitive capacity of the child. The child explores the world in a meaningful fashion and still relies closely on primary caregivers. If there are marked delays, they should be monitored with a focus on maintaining optimum functioning with developmental sequencing.

The preschooler will enjoy activity and is beginning to enjoy learning colors, using words in sentences, and gradually forming relationships with persons outside the immediate family. If there are delays, they should continue to be monitored. By now, major deficits in cognition become more obvious.

SCHOOL-AGE CHILD

The school-age child has a significant ability to perform logical operations. More complete myelination and maturation enhance the basic physiologic functioning of the central nervous system. Generally, the school-age child can establish and follow simple rules. There is self-motivation with a gradual grasp of time in a more abstract nature. The concept of death is recognized as permanent.

The school-age child begins to interpret the experience of pain with a cognitive component—the cause or source of pain, as well as implications for possible recurrence. The child in this developmental category will attempt to hold still as needed, with an appearance of bravery. Expression of the experience of pain is to be expected by a school-age child. If the school-age child is particularly shy, special attempts should be made to establish a trusting relationship to best manage pain. A major fear is loss of control. The nurse must consider the need to completely evaluate chronic pain. In some instances, it may signal other altered patterns, especially a distressed family or inability to cope. Lower performance in school can be an indicator of chronic pain. Also, the nurse should be aware of the increased complexity required for activities of daily living (ADLs). The child of this age may feel negative about him- or herself if he or she is unable to perform as peers do. The importance of group activities cannot be over-stressed.

The school-age child will blossom with a sense of accomplishment. When school does not bring success, frustration follows. It is mandatory that caution be exercised in assessing for deficits versus behavioral manifestations of not liking school.

ADOLESCENT

Vision. Acuity of 20/20 is reached by now. Squinting should be investigated, as should any symptoms of prolonged eyestrain.

Hearing. Further investigation should be done on any adolescent who speaks loudly or who fails to respond to loud noises.

Touch. Over- or under-reaction to painful stimuli is a cause for further investigation.

Taste. The adolescent may prefer food fads for a length of time, but concern is appropriate if the adolescent overuses spices, especially salt or sugar, or complains of foods not "tasting as they used to."

Smell. The adolescent should distinguish a full range of odors. The nurse should be concerned if the adolescent is unresponsive to noxious stimuli.

Proprioception. There may be temporary clumsiness associated with growth spurts. The nurse should be concerned if he or she observes patterns of deteriorating gross and fine motor coordination and ataxia.

By now the adolescent is capable of formal operational thought and is able to move beyond the world of concrete reality to abstract possibilities and ideas. Problem solving is evident with inductive and deductive capacity. There is an interest in values, with a tendency toward idealism. Attention must be given to the adolescent's sensitivity to others and potential for rejection if body image is altered. Of particular importance at this time are sports and peer-related activities. As feelings are explored more cautiously, there is a tendency to draw into oneself at this stage. There may be major conflicts over independence when self-care is not possible.

The adolescent fears mutilation and attempts to deal with pain as an adult might. Self-control is strived for, with allowance for capitalization on gains from pain. Sexuality factors of role performance enter into this group as pain occurs. As with the adult, an attempt to discover the cause and implication of the pain is made. The adolescent experiencing chronic pain will be at risk for abnormal peer interaction and may potentially endure altered self-perception.

The adolescent will most often remain steady in cognitive functioning if there are no major emotional or sensory problems. Of concern at this age would be substance abuse that could impair thought processes.

ADULT AND OLDER ADULT

Vision. The adult is capable of 20/20 vision with a gradual decline in acuity and accommodation after approximately 40 years of age. There is a tendency toward farsightedness. Color discrimination decreases in later ages, with green and blue being the major hues affected. Depending on the cause, there is a great potential for the use of corrective aids. In examples of degenerative processes, such is not the case, as with macular degeneration. Eventually depth perception and peripheral vision are also affected. There may also be sensitivity to light, as with cataract formation. The nurse should be alert for all etiologic components, especially the retinopathy associated with diabetic alterations.

Hearing. The adult has sensitivity to accurately discriminate 1600 different frequencies. There should be equal sensation of sounds for the left and right ear. The Rinne test may be done to validate air and bone conduction via a tuning fork. The Weber test may be used to assess lateralization. Equilibrium assessment provides data regarding the vestibular branch.

With time, the acuity of what is heard gradually diminishes, with detection of high-pitched frequencies especially affected. The nurse should be concerned with a lack of response to loud noises and increased volume of speech, and should be alert to cues of decreased hearing, such as cupping of the hand on the "better" ear or leaning sideways to catch the conversation on the "better" side.

Smell. There may be a gradual deterioration in sensitivity for smell after approximately age 60, although for the most part the sense of smell remains functional in the absence of organic disease. There may be altered gastrointestinal enzyme production, which ultimately interferes with usual perception of smells.

Taste. The ability to taste is well differentiated in adulthood. Sweet and sour can be detected bilaterally. Concern may be raised if the client states the sense of taste has diminished or changed. There is a gradual loss of acuity in taste as aging occurs in later life. This is due in part to decreased enzymatic production and utilization in digestive processes. Over-salting or -spicing of foods may serve as a clue to this loss of taste sensation. The use of dentures may also affect the sensation of taste and enjoyment of food.

Touch. The adult is able to discriminate on a wide range of tactile stimuli, including pressure, temperature, texture, and pain or noxious components. With aging, there is a decrease in subcutaneous fat, loss of skin turgor, increase in capillary fragility, and a decrease in conduction of impulses. All these changes influence the sense of touch, with a loss of acuity in aging.

Proprioception. The adult is well coordinated and has a keen sense of perception of his or her body in space. There are multiple protective mechanisms that aid in maintaining balance. Typically, even with eyes closed, the individual is able to stand and maintain balance.

By now the tolerance and threshold one has for pain is well established. The individual has learned various ways to cope with pain, and thus may be equipped with a more stable base from which to respond. Paradoxically, the adult may experience unresolved conflicts of previous development levels as well. For this reason, the required change may be subject to associated changes as pain and its response affect the multiple demands of daily living by the adult.

The adult is equipped to solve problems and apply principles to everyday living. There is emphasis on seeking a lifetime mate who is able to satisfy basic companionship needs. There may be difficulties in accepting life's challenges as parents or as adults juggling the many necessary roles. There is, in later life, a gradual decline in problem-solving capacity, which may be exaggerated by illness.

Allowing for potential decrease in bodily perception and functioning with age must be considered. As assessment is carried out, focus should be on risk factors such as chronic illness, financial deficits, resolution of ego integrity versus despair, and obvious etiologic components. The nurse should assist the patient to maintain self-care, as the patient desires.

With aging, there is a gradual loss of balance, perhaps most related to the concurrent vascular changes. For this reason proprioceptive data may provide an immediate basis for safety needs of the geriatric client.

In the absence of adversity, the adult enjoys the daily challenges of living. If coping is altered for whatever reason, a risk for impaired thought process exists. With aging there are potential risks for impaired thought processes. In addition, there may be potential risks for some regarding degenerative brain and central nervous system disorders, which also include impaired thought processes. Two concerns for older adults related to altered thought processes are dementia and delirium or acute confusional states.

TABLE 7.1 NANDA, NIC, and NOC Taxonomic Linkages

GORDON'S FUNCTIONAL HEALTH PATTERN	NANDA NURSING DIAGNOSIS	NIC PRIORITY INTERVENTIONS	NOC EVALUATIONS
Cognitive–Perceptual Pattern	Adaptive Capacity, Intracranial, Decreased	Cerebral Edema Management Cerebral Perfusion Promotion Intracranial Pressure (ICP) Monitoring Neurologic Monitoring	Neurological Status Neurological Status: Consciousness Seizure Control Tissue Perfusion: Cerebral
	Confusion, Acute and Chronic	**Acute** Delirium Management Delusion Management	**Acute** Cognitive Orientation Distorted Thought Self-Control Information Processing Neurological Status: Consciousness
		Chronic Dementia Management Dementia Management: Bathing Mood Management	**Chronic** Cognition Cognitive Orientation Decision-Making Distorted Thought Self-Control Identity Information Processing Memory Neurological Status: Consciousness
	Decisional Conflict (Specify)	Decision-Making Support	Decision-Making Information Processing Participation in Health Care Decisions Personal Autonomy
	Environmental Interpretation	Dementia Management	Cognitive Orientation

(table continued on page 448)

TABLE 7.1 NANDA, NIC, and NOC Taxonomic Linkages *(continued from page 447)*

GORDON'S FUNCTIONAL HEALTH PATTERN	NANDA NURSING DIAGNOSIS	NIC PRIORITY INTERVENTIONS	NOC EVALUATIONS
	Syndrome, Impaired	Dementia Management: Bathing	Concentration Fall Prevention Behavior Memory Neurological Status: Consciousness Safe Home Environment
	Knowledge (Specify), Readiness for Enhanced	*Still in Development	Knowledge: Body Mechanics; Breastfeeding; Cardiac Disease Management; Child Physical Safety; Conception Prevention; Diabetes Management; Diet; Disease Process; Energy Conservation; Fall Prevention; Fertility Promotion; Health Behavior; Health Promotion; Health Resources; Illness Care; Infant Care; Infection Control; Labor and Delivery; Medication; Ostomy Care; Parenting; Personal Safety; Postpartum Maternal Health; Preconception Maternal Health; Pregnancy; Prescribed Activity; Sexual Functioning; Substance Use Control; Treatment Procedure(s); Treatment Regimen
	Knowledge, Deficient (Specify)	Parent Education: Adolescent, Childrearing Family, Infant, Teaching: Disease Process, Foot Care, Individual, Infant Nutrition, Infant Safety, Infant Stimulation, Perioperative, Prescribed Activity/Exercise, Prescribed Diet, Prescribed Medication, Procedure/Treatment, Psychomotor Skill, Safe Sex, Sexuality, Toddler Nutrition, Toddler Safety, Toilet Training	Knowledge: Body Mechanics, Breastfeeding, Cardiac Disease Management, Child Physical Safety, Conception Prevention, Diabetes Management, Diet, Disease Process, Energy Conservation, Fertility Promotion, Health Behavior, Health Promotion, Health Resources, Illness Care, Infant Care, Infection Control, Labor & Delivery, Medication, Ostomy Care, Parenting, Personal Safety, Postpartum Maternal Health, Preconception Maternal Health, Pregnancy, Prescribed Activity, Sexual Functioning, Substance Use Control, Treatment Procedure(s), Treatment Regimen
	Memory, Impaired	Memory Training Dementia Management Environmental Management: Safety	Cognition Cognitive Orientation Concentration Memory Neurological Status Neurological Status: Consciousness

GORDON'S FUNCTIONAL HEALTH PATTERN	NANDA NURSING DIAGNOSIS	NIC PRIORITY INTERVENTIONS	NOC EVALUATIONS
	Pain, Acute and Chronic	**Acute** Analgesic Administration Pain Management Patient-Controlled Analgesia (PCA) Assistance Sedation Management	**Acute** Comfort Level Pain Control Pain Level Stress Level
	Chronic	**Chronic** Analgesic Administration Pain Management Patient-Controlled Analgesia (PCA) Assistance Environmental Management: Comfort	**Chronic** Comfort Level Depression Level Pain: Adverse Psychological Response Pain Control Pain: Disruptive Effects Pain Level
	Sensory Perception, Disturbed (Specify: Visual, Auditory, Kinesthetic, Gustatory, Tactile, Olfactory)	**Visual** Communication Enhancement: Visual Deficit Environmental Management **Auditory** Communication Enhancement: Hearing Deficit **Kinesthetic** Body Mechanics Promotion	**Visual** Sensory Function: Vision Vision Compensation Behavior **Auditory** Communication: Receptive Hearing Compensation Behavior Sensory Function: Hearing **Kinesthetic** Balance Body Positioning: Self-Initiated Coordinated Movement Sensory Function: Proprioception
		Gustatory Nausea Management Nutrition Management **Tactile** Lower Extremity Monitoring Peripheral Sensation Management Teaching: Foot Care **Olfactory** Environmental Management Nutrition Management	**Gustatory** Appetite Nutritional Status: Food & Fluid Intake Sensory Function: Taste & Smell **Tactile** Sensory Function: Cutaneous **Olfactory** Appetite Nutritional Status: Food & Fluid Intake Sensory Function: Taste & Smell
	Thought Processes, Disturbed	Delusion Management Dementia Management Environmental Management: Safety	Cognition Cognitive Orientation Concentration Decision-Making Distorted Thought Self-Control Identity Information Processing Memory Neurological Status: Consciousness

(table continued on page 450)

TABLE 7.1 **NANDA, NIC, and NOC Taxonomic Linkages** *(continued from page 449)*

GORDON'S FUNCTIONAL HEALTH PATTERN	NANDA NURSING DIAGNOSIS	NIC PRIORITY INTERVENTIONS	NOC EVALUATIONS
	Unilateral Neglect	Unilateral Neglect Management Environmental Management: Safety	Adaptation to Physical Disability Body Positioning: Self-Initiated Coordinated Movement

APPLICABLE NURSING DIAGNOSES

ADAPTIVE CAPACITY, INTRACRANIAL, DECREASED

DEFINITION[2]

Intracranial fluid dynamic mechanisms that normally compensate for increases in intracranial volumes are compromised, resulting in repeated disproportionate increases in intracranial pressure (ICP) in response to a variety of noxious and nonnoxious stimuli.

DEFINING CHARACTERISTICS[2]

1. Repeated increases in ICP of greater than 10 mm Hg for more than 5 minutes following any of a variety of external stimuli
2. Baseline ICP equal to or greater than 10 mm Hg
3. Disproportionate increase in ICP following single environmental or nursing maneuver stimulus
4. Elevated P2 ICP waveform
5. Volume pressure response test variation (volume: pressure ratio greater than 2, pressure–volume index less than 10)
6. Wide amplitude ICP waveform

RELATED FACTORS[2]

1. Decreased cerebral perfusion pressure less than or equal to 50 to 60 mm Hg
2. Sustained increase in ICP greater than or equal to 10 to 15 mm Hg
3. Systemic hypotension with intracranial hypertension
4. Brain injuries

RELATED CLINICAL CONCERNS

1. Head injury
2. Cerebral ischemia
3. Cranial tumors
4. Hydrocephalus
5. Cranial hematomas

6. Arteriovenous formation
7. Vasogenic or cytotoxic cerebral edema
8. Hyperemia
9. Obstruction of venous outflow

 Have You Selected the Correct Diagnosis?

Ineffective Protection
This diagnosis is typically associated with immune disorders or clotting disorders. However, maladaptive stress response and general neurosensory alterations are also associated with Ineffective Protection. Decreased Intracranial Adaptive Capacity is a specific diagnosis related to intracranial fluid dynamic mechanisms.

Excess Fluid Volume
This diagnosis refers to the overall fluid in the body. Body fluid may be normal in Decreased Intracranial Adaptive Capacity. However, the intracranial fluid volume and pressure are abnormal.

Ineffective Tissue Perfusion
This diagnosis defines a decrease in nutrition and oxygenation at the cellular level due to a deficit in capillary blood supply and may be a companion diagnosis to Decreased Intracranial Adaptive Capacity, depending on the cerebral perfusion pressure and the secondary physiologic cellular damage brought on by the brain injury.

EXPECTED OUTCOME

Will have ICP (Intracranial Adaptive Capacity) within normal range by [date].

TARGET DATES

Decreased Intracranial Adaptive Capacity is a life-threatening condition, and should have target dates in terms of hours. After stabilization, the time frame may be moved to 48-hour increments.

NURSING ACTIONS/INTERVENTIONS WITH RATIONALES

Adult Health

ACTIONS/INTERVENTIONS	RATIONALES
Perform neurologic assessments at least q1h, including the Glasgow Coma Scale, pupillary response, and strength. Also trend VS, ICP, and cerebral perfusion pressure (CPP) at a similar frequency.	Allows for continuous monitoring of the patient's condition and allows for early detection of complications and capacity for the adaptive response.
Implement measures that decrease susceptibility for elevated ICP:	
• Minimize environmental stimuli (light, sounds, and visitors).	Minimizes fluctuations in ICP and CPP.[3]
• Elevate head of bed 0 to 30 degrees. Institute measures to keep head and neck in a neutral position (e.g., use of a towel roll).	Promotes venous drainage from the head.[4]
• Avoid hip flexion of more than 90 degrees.	
• Give medications for pain and agitation as needed.	Agitation can elevate ICP.
• Maintain euthermia.	Hyperthermia increases cellular metabolism and subsequently ICP. Hypothermia may elicit shivering, which also will increase O_2 consumption and ICP.
• Interpret arterial blood gases and collaborate with respiratory therapy to ensure ventilator settings are appropriate.	Hypercapnia can increase ICP.
• Initiate an appropriate bowel regimen.	Straining or Valsalva can increase ICP.
Collaborate with the health-care team regarding therapy to guard against vasospasm including hypervolemic, hypertensive, and hemodilutional therapy.	
Collaborate with the health-care team regarding pharmacological therapy including antiseizure medications, calcium channel blockers, pain control, etc.	
Analyze lab work including electrolytes, complete blood count, serum osmolality and coagulation studies.	Provides insight into fluid–volume balance, progress in plan of care, and need for alterations.
Suction cautiously as needed.	Integral to facilitating gas exchange. Caution must be used as suctioning can cause increase in ICP.[5–7]
Cluster nursing intervention and minimize stimulation.	Many activities including coughing, sneezing, vomiting, bathing, pain, dressing change, agitation, spontaneous movement, can increase ICP[6,8,9]
Collaborate with the health-care team regarding target fluid volume status:	Ensures therapeutic goals are achieved related to adequate cerebral perfusion, minimizing hypoperfused areas, and minimizing vasospasm.
• Manage external ventricular drainage systems or monitoring devices according to the standard of care.	

Child Health

ACTIONS/INTERVENTIONS	RATIONALES
Monitor for factors contributing to altered intracranial pressure including medical/physiologic deviation and related issues, especially positioning, treatments, medications, suctioning, ventilation, etc.	Thorough evaluation for contributing factors allows for early detection of complications.
Carry out thorough neurologic assessment according to the degree of stimulation and movement permitted per the infant's or child's status.	Deviations from norms will assist in differential workup and expedite treatment plan.

(care plan continued on page 452)

NURSING ACTIONS/INTERVENTIONS WITH RATIONALES (continued from page 451)

Child Health

ACTIONS/INTERVENTIONS	RATIONALES
Maintain the head of bed at greater than 30 degrees, with the head in line with the body, and, ideally, not positioned from side to side unless specified. (Avoid use of pillows under the patient's head.) Recheck every 1 to 2 hours.	Neutral body alignment will assist in stabilizing the intracranial adaptation.
Offer a calm, supportive environment with attention to safety of airway maintenance, side rails up with padding, and availability of emergency equipment according to the infant's or child's needs.	Few stimuli will enhance the infant's or child's likelihood of rest during acute phase, while anticipatory safeguarding will minimize further injury.
Develop a daily plan of care that best matches the developmental capacity of the infant or child, yet allows for possible regression. [Note plan here.]	Previous skills may not be able to be remastered, or altered temporarily because of illness in the pediatric client.
Incorporate parental input in the daily plan of care as appropriate. [Note parent preferences here.]	Family will feel valued, and their input will assist in providing some familiarity to the infant or child and lessen effects of multiple caregivers.
Offer time (30 minutes each shift and as needed) for parents to ventilate feelings regarding the infant's or child's status.	Assists in reducing anxiety, and offers cues regarding parental concerns.
Assess caregiver(s) knowledge level for care of the infant or child.	Provides a realistic base for teaching needs.
Provide appropriate teaching regarding equipment, procedures, surgery, etc. [Note teaching plan here.]	Knowledge allows for acceptance.
Offer gentle massage, and monitor carefully skin integrity and tissue perfusion, especially when the condition lasts more than 2 days.	Likelihood of skin breakdown increases when repositioning is limited.
Check for potential untoward effects of medications, and exercise caution in appropriate dilution for IV administration.	Likelihood of interaction increases with three or more medications, and inappropriate administration may likewise cause side effects.
Maintain ongoing communication with the family to offer updates on the infant's or child's condition.	Trust in caregivers will be enhanced if the family can be kept abreast of activities on an ongoing basis.
Encourage the parents to bring the infant's or child's favorite blanket, small toy, or security object if possible.	Familiar favored objects offer a sense of security in an otherwise foreign setting, thereby reducing stress.
Arrange for appropriate follow-up, including home health, physical therapy, or neurology, especially when there may be a ventricular peritoneal (V–P) shunt. For example, including when to notify primary care provider for possible infection or malfunction.	Appropriate referral will foster long-term continued regimen and offer goals over time.[10,11]

Women's Health

For Women's Health, see Adult Health, except for the following interventions:

ACTIONS/INTERVENTIONS	RATIONALES
Hypertensive Disorders of Pregnancy	Gestational hypertensive disorders, including pre-eclampsia and eclampsia, and chronic hypertension complicate pregnancy.[13]

ACTIONS/INTERVENTIONS	RATIONALES
Place on continuous intensive monitoring (cardiac and fetal). Observe blood pressure, urine output, reflexes, headache, visual problems, irritability/changes in affect, and epigastric pain.[7,8]	The reason for difficulty in diagnosing hypertension has been a lack of standardization in blood pressure measurement. It is important for the health care provider to establish a baseline and monitor throughout the pregnancy.[12,13]
Progression from pre-eclampsia to severe pre-eclampsia to eclampsia can occur.	Monitor maternal parameters: Pre-eclampsia—usually occurs after the 20th week of pregnancy, gestational hypertension plus presence of proteinuria. Severe pre-eclampsia—systolic 160 mmHg Diastolic blood pressure 110 mmHg, plus proteinuria, plus oliguria, cerebral or visual disturbances, hepatic involvement, thrombocytopenia and pulmonary or cardiac involvement. Eclampsia—onset of seizure activity or coma with no history of existing pathology.[13]
To prevent progression to eclampsia: • Place in a darkened, quiet environment, to decrease external stimuli. • Constantly monitor signs and symptoms of progression of disease.	Reduction of external stimuli can reduce or prevent convulsions in these patients. They need the reduction of light to lessen eye pain and headache.
Place padded tongue blade at head of bed. Suction equipment and oxygen should be available, and emergency medication tray and emergency birth pack should be accessible.	Seizure precautions and medications close at hand to use quickly. As this disease can progress quickly, even when every precaution is taken.[13]
Carefully monitor magnesium sulfate (MgSO$_4$) levels, if appropriate, for therapeutic dose and/or toxicity.	Often lethargy and confusion are the result of MgSO$_4$ therapy for eclampsia.
Monitor fetal heart tone (FHT). Assist the patient in orientation to time and place. Do not allow the patient to ambulate alone. Provide assistance. Provide a bedside commode.	These patients feel out of control, lethargic, and confused and cannot remember what has just been said to them as a result of both the convulsion and the medication. They need specific direction and a lot of support and understanding.
HELLP Syndrome: laboratory diagnosis for variant of severe preeclampsia that involves hepatic dysfunction: Hemolysis (H) Elevated liver enzymes (EL) Low platelets (LP)	Associated with increased risk for both mother and fetus, as well as adverse outcomes. Increased risk for placenta abruption, renal failure, preterm birth and fetal or maternal death.[13,14]

Newborn

Carefully assess the newborn for cranial injury.

Carefully examine the infant's skull. Note the anterior and posterior fontanels. Be especially alert for a bulging anterior fontanel indicative of:
• Increased intracranial pressure
• Major hemorrhage
• Hydrocephalus

(care plan continued on page 454)

NURSING ACTIONS/INTERVENTIONS WITH RATIONALES (continued from page 453)

Mental Health

The nursing actions for Mental Health for this diagnosis are the same as the actions presented in the Adult Health section.

Gerontic Health

ACTIONS/INTERVENTIONS	RATIONALES
Maintain the head in a neutral position, even while the patient is side-lying.	Prevents increases in pressure from flexion or extension of the head.

● **N O T E :** *Nursing interventions found in the Adult Health section are appropriate to this age group. Caution must be used because of the potential for problems regarding hydration, hypothermia, pupillary reaction, deficits related to eye surgery, and risk for sensory deprivation with decreased activity.*

Home Health

See Adult Health care plan. If the patient with this diagnosis is living in the home, professional home care will be required.

CONFUSION, ACUTE AND CHRONIC

DEFINITIONS[2]

Acute Confusion Abrupt onset of a cluster of global, transient changes and disturbances in attention, cognition, psychomotor activity, level of consciousness, and/or sleep–wake cycle.

Chronic Confusion Irreversible, long-standing and/or progressive deterioration of intellect and personality characterized by decreased ability to interpret environmental stimuli and decreased capacity for intellectual thought processes and manifested by disturbances of memory.

DEFINING CHARACTERISTICS[2]

A. Acute Confusion
1. Lack of motivation to initiate and/or follow through with goal-directed or purposeful behavior
2. Fluctuation in psychomotor activity
3. Misperception
4. Fluctuation in cognition
5. Increased agitation or restlessness
6. Fluctuation in level of consciousness
7. Fluctuation in sleep–wake cycle
8. Hallucination

B. Chronic Confusion
1. Altered interpretation or response to stimuli
2. Clinical evidence of organic impairment
3. Progressive and/or long-standing cognitive impairment
4. Altered personality
5. Impaired memory (short term and long term)

6. Impaired socialization
7. No change in level of consciousness

RELATED FACTORS[2]

A. Acute Confusion
1. Older than 60 years of age
2. Alcohol abuse
3. Delirium
4. Dementia
5. Drug abuse

B. Chronic Confusion
1. Multi-infarct dementia
2. Korsakoff's psychosis
3. Head injury
4. Alzheimer's disease
5. Cerebral vascular accident

RELATED CLINICAL CONCERNS

1. Head injury
2. Cerebral vascular accident
3. Alzheimer's disease
4. Chemical abuse
5. Dementia

 Have You Selected the Correct Diagnosis?

Disturbed Sensory Perception
An alteration in one of the senses could create a short-term confusion that is correctable. If a sensory deficit is found, the most correct diagnosis is Disturbed Sensory Perception.

Disturbed Thought Process
The individual has a problem with cognitive operation and engages in nonreality thinking. Other functioning is normal. Confusion causes problems in both mental and physical functioning.

Impaired Memory
This diagnosis is related to memory only. Other cognitive functioning may be normal.

EXPECTED OUTCOMES

1. If acute, will be oriented ×3 (person, place, and time) by [date].

2. If chronic, family/support system will identify [number] measures to maintain the client's optimal functioning by [date].
3. If chronic, will demonstrate no signs/symptoms [note client-specific signs of anxiety] in current living situation by [date].

TARGET DATES

For acute confusion, an appropriate target date would be 72 hours after admission. Chronic confusion may be permanent, but the family should be able to learn appropriate intervention techniques within 72 hours.

NURSING ACTIONS/INTERVENTIONS WITH RATIONALES

Adult Health

ACTIONS/INTERVENTIONS	RATIONALES
Identify self and the patient by name at the beginning of each interaction.	Memory loss necessitates frequent orientation to person, time, and environment.
Speak slowly and in short, clear, concrete, simple sentences and words.	Allows time for information processing, and avoids use of complex statements and abstract ideas.
Periodically orient and/or reorient the patient to the environment.	Helps alleviate anxiety brought on by changing levels of orientation, and helps meet safety needs of the patient.
When the patient is delusional, focus on underlying feelings and reinforce reality (have clocks, calendars, etc., on the wall). Do not argue with the patient.	Recognizing and/or acknowledging feelings may decrease the patient's anxiety, and give him or her a sense of being understood. Arguing may increase the patient's anxiety and reinforce intensity delusions.[15]
When hallucinations and/or illusions are present, reinforce reality and attempt to identify underlying feelings or environmental stimuli.	False and/or distorted sensory experiences are common in confused states. To help decrease anxiety, focus on feelings underlying these experiences while calmly reinforcing reality.[15]
If the patient becomes aggressive, focus on underlying feelings and attempt to refocus interaction on topics more acceptable and/or less threatening to the patient.	Focusing on feelings increases the patient's feelings of being understood, and discussing nonthreatening topics increases the patient's sense of competency and self-esteem.
Keep the patient's room well lighted. Maintain a calm environment.	Decreases possibility of environmental sensory misrepresentations, and helps meet patient safety needs. Patients with confusion are experiencing increased levels of anxiety and can become physically and mentally exhausted. Promoting rest often means controlling environmental stimuli that contribute to the confusion.
Encourage the patient to wear and use personal devices (eyeglasses or hearing aids).	These items increase accuracy of visual and auditory perceptions.
During abusive episodes, ignore insults and focus on underlying feelings. Set limits on behavior if physically abusive.	Projection of fear and anger onto persons in the environment is common in confused states. Arguing with or becoming defensive escalates the situation and adds to the patient's fear and anger.

(care plan continued on page 456)

NURSING ACTIONS/INTERVENTIONS WITH RATIONALES (continued from page 455)

Adult Health

ACTIONS/INTERVENTIONS	RATIONALES
Teach the family about the patient's condition and how to interact more effectively with the patient; i.e., provide ongoing orientation to surroundings and happenings within the family.	Assists the family in understanding changes in the patient's orientation, cognition, and behavior. Increases the family's sense of competency in relating to the patient.
Recognize family responses to the patient's condition, and teach about reasons for condition and how to respond during acute episodes.	Family members often feel anxious and helpless about the patient's behavior. Teaching reasons for the patient's condition and how to respond decreases anxiety and may help decrease the patient's confusion.
Refer to psychiatric-mental health clinical nurse specialist (CNS). Make other referrals to community agencies as needed, i.e., Alzheimer's support group, adult day care, Meals-on-Wheels, etc.	The psychiatric-mental health CNS has the expertise to collaborate with the adult health nurse to plan nursing interventions for the patient that will help the patient and nursing staff deal with chronic confusion in the acute care setting.

Child Health[11,16]

Although intended for the population older than 60 years of age, confusion may occur in younger people as well, as a result of similar causes. Uncertainty may be greater regarding potential for recovery because of age, exact cause of problem, and so on.

ACTIONS/INTERVENTIONS	RATIONALES
Acute Monitor for potential contributory factors, especially as applicable: • Prenatal influences, i.e., drugs, sepsis • Previous health status • Known conditions, whether or not requiring treatment • Triggering event, trauma, surgery, emotional event • Daily routine or alterations	A thorough assessment offers the best basis for identification and treatment of confusion.
Determine with the parents previous patterns of development, and develop daily plan of care within capacity offered by the infant's or child's status.	Parents are best able to provide previous development capacity cues within level of comfort for the infant or child, thus enhancing likelihood of sense of security for all.
Identify current plan of care to best suit the infant's or child's capacities with input from all members of the health-care team, especially the parents.	Best holistic plan of care reflects expertise of all which best know and interact with the infant or child.
Offer treatment within developmentally appropriate framework of the infant or child.	In all situations there is greater likelihood of success in care when the infant or child is approached from developmentally appropriate stance to afford a sense of security.
Provide a safe and calm environment with stimuli best suited to the infant's or child's needs.	An environment that is safe and developmentally appropriate provides freedom from injury while allowing the infant or child to recover.
Offer the parents realistic plans for the infant or child with frequent updates.	Parents will better be able to trust and accept the infant's or child's status and caregivers when trusting relationships are based on communication that is honest and forthright.

ACTIONS/INTERVENTIONS	RATIONALES
Provide 30 minutes each shift for the parents to ventilate feelings about the infant or child.	Helps reduce anxiety, and offers cues to parental concerns.
Identify discharge and follow-up needs with attention to all members of the health-care team.	Support for the parents upon the family's return to home will help maintain plan for care and thereby attain therapeutic goals.
Chronic	
Offer resources for support groups and advocacy interest opportunities.	Specific support groups will assist the parents in dealing with situation represented by the infant's or child's status.
Explore specific patterns of daily care needs and how best to offer care within domain of resources available.	Realistic demands will best direct care according to time and constraints.
Note risk for caregiver role strain due to demands over time.	

Women's Health

See nursing actions for Adult Health.

Mental Health

ACTIONS/INTERVENTIONS	RATIONALES
Acute	
● N O T E : *Mental health clients at risk for this diagnosis include:*	
Patients taking the following substances: lithium, antianxiety agents, anticholinergics, phenothiazine, barbiturates, methyldopa, disulfiram, alcohol, cocaine, amphetamines, opiates, and hallucinogenics.	*Compendium of psychotropic drugs-fast reference for health-care provider.*[17]
Patients experiencing drug withdrawal, electroconvulsive therapy (ECT) treatments, dementia, dissociative disorders, mood disorders, and thought disorders, and elderly clients with acute infections such as urinary tract infections.	
Place the client in an environment with appropriate stimuli. Note level of stimulation and alterations in environmental stimuli here. For example, specific objects in the environment that stimulate illusions should be removed; appropriate lighting, clocks and calendars, and holiday decorations should be used. Refer to day, date, and other orienting information during each interaction with the client.	Increases patient safety and promotes orientation.[18,19]
Assign the client a room that provides opportunities for careful observation but is not a chaotic environment.	Promotes client safety and decreases environmental stimuli. High levels of stimuli can increase confusion and hyperactivity.[17,20,21]
Place identifying information on the patient and the patient's room. Utilize the patient's preferred name in each interaction. [Note that name here.]	Promotes safety and orientation.

(care plan continued on page 458)

NURSING ACTIONS/INTERVENTIONS WITH RATIONALES (continued from page 457)

Mental Health

ACTIONS/INTERVENTIONS	RATIONALES
Remove harmful objects from the environment. This could include objects in walkways, cords, belts, and raised bedrails or other restraining devices. During periods of increased agitation, one-to-one observation should be instituted.	Protects the client from falls and accidental injury. Clients attempting to free themselves can fall or be injured on the restraints.[18] Promotes client safety.
Assign primary care nurse each shift. [Note those persons here.]	Promotes client orientation by providing familiar environment.[19,20]
Communicate with the client using a moderate rate of speech and simple sentences without many questions. Allow time for responding, and avoid indefinite pronouns.	Decreases ambiguity, prevents information overload, and provides the time necessary for the client to process information, which preserves self-esteem, decreases anxiety, and improves orientation.[22]
Observe every [number] minutes. Inform the client of this schedule, and provide the client with written information as necessary. Provide this schedule in written form, i.e., written on a white board in the client's room. [Note information necessary for the client here.]	Promotes client safety. Provides opportunities to reorient the client to here and now and to ensure client comfort.[21] Promotes the client's sense of control.
Replace the use of physical restraints with one-to-one observation, comfort measures, recliners, appropriate physical activity, visual barriers, secure unit, lower bed or bed on floor. [Note here those interventions specific to this client.][18]	Promotes safety and the client's self-esteem by maintaining personal control and dignity. Frequent use of restraints can encourage clients to assume a passive approach to avoid further restraint or as an adaptation to daily use of restraints. At times, physical restraints may increase agitation.[18,21,23]
If physical restraints are used, check circulation at least every 15 minutes, remove restraint from one limb at a time at least every 2 hours, and provide ROM, opportunities to void, nourishment, brief clear explanations about the purpose of the restraint, and information about when they will be removed during each interaction.	Promotes client safety, sense of personal control, and self-esteem.[19,24] Promotes physical comfort, which decreases agitation.
Utilize touch as appropriate to the client. [Note the client's preferences here.]	Clients' touch preferences are very personal. Some clients may find it comforting, whereas others may perceive it as an intrusion and respond with increased agitation.[21]
Administer antipsychotic medication only if neurologic status indicates that this will not increase confusion.	Antipsychotic medications can increase confusion. These medications can also produce orthostatic hypotension, increasing the client's fall risk.[17,18]
Provide daily routine that closely resembles the client's normal schedule. [Note that schedule here.]	Promotes orientation; increases the client's sense of personal control.
Provide whatever aids the client needs to adequately perceive the environment (hearing or vision). [Note necessary aids here and location for storing when not in use by the client.]	Promotes orientation to the environment and sense of personal control.
Assess mental status through normal interactions with the client. Do not use formal mental status examinations unless absolutely necessary. [Note method and schedule for assessment here.]	Repeated questioning can increase the client's confusion, and inability to answer questions may have negative impact on self-esteem.[19,24]

ACTIONS/INTERVENTIONS	RATIONALES
Limit the client's choices, and provide information or direction in brief, simple sentences. Note the level of the client's ability to process information here (e.g., the client can choose between two items). Support optimal cognitive functioning by: [Note here those interventions to be used with this client.]	Increases orientation while preserving the client's self-esteem. Large amounts of information provided at one time can increase confusion and agitation.[19,21]
• Responding to the client's confused verbalizations (delusions, hallucinations, confabulations, illusions, etc.) in a calm manner	Increased anxiety can increase confusion and agitation.[19,21]
• Utilizing refocusing and/or responding to the feelings underlying the content to respond to confused verbalizations	Maintains self-esteem, relieves anxiety, and orients to present reality.[25]
• Utilizing "I" messages rather than arguments to reorient when necessary.	Meets the client's esteem needs by communicating respect while providing orientation.[19,24,25] Promotes here-and-now orientation.[19]
• Providing clothing that is appropriate to time of day and situation (e.g., night clothes at night and street clothes during the day)	
• Scheduling participation in groups that provide opportunities to remember, review current events, discuss seasonal activities, and socialize. [Note here the schedule and appropriate groups for this client.]	Promotes here-and-now orientation. Provides opportunities to maintain current cognitive skills.[19,25]
• Providing measures that promote rest and sleep. [Note here those measures that are specific for this client with schedule for implementation.]	Inadequate sleep can increase confusion and disorientation.[19]
Provide clear feedback on appropriate behavior. Refer to Risk for Violence if the client is at risk for violent behavior toward self or others. Assess expectations for being realistic with the client's abilities. [Note limits to be set here with specific consequences for unwanted behaviors and specific reinforcers for desired behaviors.]	Positive reinforcement encourages behavior. Realistic goals increase opportunities for success, providing positive reinforcement and enhancing self-esteem.
Provide support system with information about the client and how to best approach the client. Note here the information to be provided and responsible person.	Provides support system with positive coping strategies that enhance the client's functioning.

Chronic

● N O T E : *Mental health clients at risk for this diagnosis include those with Alzheimer's disease, Korsakoff's psychosis, and AIDS dementia. In addition to those interventions for acute confusion, the following interventions are included. It is important to remember that the primary difference between these two diagnoses is the irreversibility of the cognitive deficits in this diagnosis. It is also important to assess the client for depression, because depression can appear as those illnesses that are related to this diagnosis, especially in elderly clients.*

Maintain familiar environment:	
• Provide objects from the client's home environment, to include pictures, personal bedding, personal clothing, music, and other special objects with personal meaning. Note those objects important to the client here, with the nursing actions necessary to maintain the objects.	Promotes orientation while promoting sense of safety and security.[22]
• Label room with name in large letters and a familiar picture or item.	Maintains orientation while promoting a sense of personal control by maintaining independence.[19,24]

(care plan continued on page 460)

NURSING ACTIONS/INTERVENTIONS WITH RATIONALES (continued from page 459)

Mental Health

ACTIONS/INTERVENTIONS	RATIONALES
• Provide the same room for the entire hospital stay. Assign primary care personnel. [Note those persons here.]	Maintains orientation by providing continuity of surroundings and staff familiar with the client's needs, perspective, and treatment plan. Excessive stimulation can exacerbate cognitive or behavioral problems.
• Provide structured daily routines, and note the client's routine here. This should parallel prehospital routine as much as possible.	Promotes orientation by providing familiarity.[18,26]
Provide opportunities for the client to be involved in reminiscence, remotivation, current events, socialization, and other groups as appropriate by providing the client with assistance needed to get to the groups. [Note the client's group schedule here, with the assistance needed from nursing staff.]	Provide opportunities for clients to interact using current cognitive skills, which helps decrease anxiety, maintain dignity, and prevent further deterioration and withdrawal.[25]
Spend [number] minutes [number] times a day discussing the client's past experiences. This activity can be facilitated with music, family photographs, and other items that elicit memories. Note the client's response to this activity, and if it appears to increase stress, discontinue. The process of this interaction is to provide positive cognitive reframes of past experiences.	Promotes positive reorientation, maintains the client's dignity, and promotes positive self-esteem. It is important to note that some clients may have a great deal of difficulty coping with past experiences. If this process increases anxiety, the activity should be discontinued, because high levels of anxiety can increase confusion.
Identify and control underlying causes or triggers of increased cognitive and behavioral problems. This could include limiting visitors or certain topics of conversation, increasing rest or providing rest periods during the day, and ensuring adequate hydration. [Note the special adaptations here.]	Preserves the client's dignity and sense of control.[26] Each of these factors can decrease the client's ability to cope.
Utilize nonconfrontational approaches for dealing with behavior extremes. This could include changing the client's context, responding to the feelings being expressed, or meeting comfort needs. [Note here those responses that are most effective for the client.]	Maintains the client's dignity, and recognizes the limitations of cognitive abilities.[26]
Spend [number] minutes [number] times a day with the client doing activities (this should be some activity the client enjoys and that provides an opportunity for success).	Positive environmental cues from staff have been shown to decrease problematic behaviors in these clients.[27]
Spend [number] minutes [number] times a day involved in [type] exercise with the client. (Choose an exercise the client enjoys and that involves large motor activity if at all possible.)	Increased physical activity decreases wandering behavior and improves the client's rest.[23,27]
Retrieve and divert the client when wandering behavior presents risk or takes her or him into unobserved areas.	Decreases the client's wandering behaviors.[27]
Schedule meetings with the primary care provider before discharge to teach effective behavior management techniques and develop a plan for care at home. This should include respite for the caregiver. [Note plan here.]	Facilitates support for caregivers and prevents caregiver "burnout".[19]
Refer to community agencies that will facilitate ongoing care. [Note agencies here.]	

Gerontic Health

● N O T E : *Aging clients may experience age-related changes in memory to include forgetting specific details but remembering them later, ability to learn new information with some difficulty in information retrieval, a general awareness of memory impairment, and memory impairment that does not affect daily life. Causes of confusion should be ruled out upon identification of new onset confusion. Causes may include metabolic diseases, infection, neoplasm, drug side effects, nutritional deficiencies, and cerebrovascular injury. Alzheimer dementia is possible with new onset confusion and should be ruled out as well.*

Goals for clients with confusion may not necessarily need to include reversal of confusion. Rather, assisting the confused client and caregiver to feel safe, comfortable and in control is a worthy goal.

ACTIONS/INTERVENTIONS	RATIONALES
Review pertinent laboratory work for possible imbalances.	Acute confusion may be related to changes in electrolytes, glucose, or drug levels.
Obtain medication list from the client or family of all prescribed and over-the-counter (OTC) medications used by the client.	Medications are a frequent precipitant for acute confusion, especially in the very young or old.
Decrease extraneous audible–visual input. Provide low-stimuli environment.	Decreases sensory overload and need to cope with a complex and noisy environment.
Provide orienting cues to the physical layout of the care site (such as universal symbols for the bathroom, eating area, and the client's room).	Promotes independence.
Provide personalized surroundings (familiar pictures, clothing, or mementos).	Promotes identification with self.
Use a client photograph to identify personal space.	Increases connectedness with self. Provides sense of belonging.
Address the client by preferred name at each contact.	Reinforces sense of self.
Introduce self by name at each contact.	Provides sense of the familiar.
Arrange for the family or significant others to be available during periods of increased anxiety or agitation.	Provides for familiar person in the care setting.
Use name and orienting cues in conversations.	Enhances sense of self and connectedness.
Provide physical contact and/or comfort along with verbal interactions.	Decreases anxiety generated when trying to cope with threatening environment. Assists the client in sorting out environment and setting.
Explore and explain briefly equipment used in care.	Decreases fearfulness.
Use familiar objects for activities such as glasses or cups for fluids rather than styrofoam cups or paper or plastic cartons.	Decreases complexity of coping with the unfamiliar.
Assign consistent caregivers.	Provides sense of security.
Limit choices to two in situations where the client must make decisions such as dressing or eating.	Decreases stress of too many choices.
Provide positive feedback for independent function.	Promotes self-esteem.
Ensure quiet time or rest periods during the day.	Decreases stress.
Approach and work with the client in an unhurried manner.	Sense of urgency associated with speed perceived as threatening.
Provide information in simple sentences, and allow time for the client to process information.	Decreases complexity.

(care plan continued on page 462)

Gerontic Health

ACTIONS/INTERVENTIONS	RATIONALES
If repetition is needed, repeat information in the exact manner as originally stated.	Allows for processing of information.
Encourage participation in failure-free activities such as singing, exercise, or uncomplicated crafts.	Enhances self-esteem.
Monitor mental status for changes at least daily and every shift in acute care setting.	
Monitor for increased confusion related to new medication usage.	

Chronic (Often Alzheimer dementia)

ACTIONS/INTERVENTIONS	RATIONALES
Retrieve and divert the client when wandering behavior presents risk or takes her or him into unobserved areas.	Decreases the client's wandering behaviors.[27]
Assess for expression of intent, "I'm going home now," and the expression of loss of a valued adult role, "The children need me now."[28]	
Modify the environment to provide adequate rest, safety, and sleep for the client.[28]	Eliminate possible preciptators of confusion.
Provide client with essential sensory aides such as glasses, dentures, and hearing aids.	Prevents possible sensory confusion.[28]
Avoid chemical and physical restraints.	These can increase confusion and agitation. These do not stop the urge to wander and may exacerbate the urge to wander by decreasing the client's perception of safety. These measures may contribute to client injury.[28]
Schedule and maintain a regular toileting schedule. [Note schedule here.]	Eliminate possible precipitators of confusion and wandering.
Provide information to all staff that a client is a wanderer. Develop a mechanism for identification and a plan to follow if a wandering client is missing.[28]	Prevention of injury related to wandering.
Use grid-like markings in front of doorways.	May prevent a client from exiting due to a change in visual cues.[28]

Home Health

● N O T E : *Onset of acute confusion may be an emergency requiring immediate referral for care.*

ACTIONS/INTERVENTIONS	RATIONALES
Rule out possible causes of confusion: • Drugs • Hypoxia • Pain or discomfort • Full bladder or urinary tract infection • Bowel impaction • Infection (particularly pulmonary or urinary). Keep in mind that elder clients may not exhibit typical signs of infection. • Alcohol or benzodiazepine withdrawal • Extreme anxiety	Understanding the cause of confusion determines the best intervention.

ACTIONS/INTERVENTIONS	RATIONALES
Offer explanation and support to the family members and caregivers.	Confusion is difficult to cope with at home and can be distressing to family members.
Encourage the family members and caregivers to maximize communication with the client during lucid intervals. Critical information should be exchanged during these times.	Some effective communication can still occur if the client experiences lucid intervals.
Help the family members and caregivers identify and cope with impending death if confusion is occurring in the last hours of life. Terminal confusion, a condition common to impending death, is best treated with morphine, chlorpromazine, and scopolamine.[29]	Understanding the cause of confusion determines the best intervention.

Assist the client and family in identifying lifestyle changes that may be required:
• Treatment or prevention of underlying problem (substance abuse, infection, pain, or nutritional deficits)
• Providing for rest periods
• Providing safe environment
• Providing environmental cues to orient the patient (e.g., clocks, calendars, photos, familiar objects).
• Provide assistive resources as required to include:
  • Glasses
  • Hearing aids
  • Clocks with large numbers
• Family response to changing behavior and mental status of the affected person
	Home-based care requires involvement of the family. Acute confusion disrupts family schedules and role relationships. Adjustments in family activities and roles may be required.
	
	Decreased vision or hearing acuity may contribute to confusion.

Assist the family to set criteria to help them determine when additional intervention is required, for example, change in baseline behavior.	Provides the family with background knowledge to seek appropriate assistance as need arises.
Refer the patient to appropriate assistive resources as indicated.	Additional assistance may be required for the family to care for the acutely confused person. Use of readily available resources is cost-effective.

DECISIONAL CONFLICT (SPECIFY)

DEFINITION[2]

The state of uncertainty about course of action to be taken when choice among competing actions involves risk, loss, or challenge to personal life values.[2]

DEFINING CHARACTERISTICS[2]

1. Verbalization of undesired consequences of alternative actions being considered
2. Verbalized uncertainty about choices
3. Vacillation between alternative choices
4. Delayed decision making
5. Verbalized feeling of distress while attempting a decision
6. Self-focusing
7. Physical signs of distress or tension (e.g., increased heart rate, increased muscle tension, restlessness)
8. Questioning personal values and beliefs while attempting a decision

RELATED FACTORS[2]

1. Support system deficit
2. Perceived threat to value system
3. Multiple or divergent sources of information
4. Lack of relevant information
5. Unclear personal values or beliefs
6. Lack of experience or presence of interference with decision making

RELATED CLINICAL CONCERNS

1. Any surgery causing body image change
2. Any illness carrying a potential terminal prognosis
3. Any chronic disease
4. Dementia

5. Traumatic events (natural disasters, significant personal loss)

 Have You Selected the Correct Diagnosis?

Anxiety
Anxiety is considered to be a feeling of threat that may not be known by the person as a specific causative factor. In Decisional Conflict, the patient knows the options but cannot decide between specifics.

Deficient Knowledge
In Deficient Knowledge, the client does not have the information to make a decision. In Decisional Conflict, the information is known.

Ineffective Individual Coping
This diagnosis is closely related in that adaptive behavior and problem-solving abilities are not able to meet the demands of the client's needs. Ineffective

Individual Coping and Decisional Conflict may very well be companion diagnoses.

EXPECTED OUTCOME

Will verbalize at least one concrete personal decision by [date].

Identifies [number] of resources needed to facilitate decision-making by [date].

Identifies [number] of alternatives by [date].

TARGET DATES

Value clarification, belief examination, and learning decision-making processes will require a considerable length of time and will require much support. Therefore, target dates in increments of weeks would be most appropriate.

NURSING ACTIONS/INTERVENTIONS WITH RATIONALES

Adult Health

ACTIONS/INTERVENTIONS	RATIONALES
Engage the patient in discussions regarding his or her perception of the problem and information that lends to conflict.	
Assist the patient to develop problem-solving processes. Help the patient verbalize alternatives and advantages and disadvantages of solutions. Help the patient realistically appraise situations and set realistic short-term objectives daily.	Assists the patient to learn to use the problem-solving process.
Assist the patient in identifying values as necessary. Acknowledge the patient's values.	Helps the patient focus on what is important to self in decision making rather than being concerned about pleasing others.
Refer to the psychiatric nurse clinician as needed.	A nurse specialist may be better able to help the patient focus on the underlying process.

Child Health

ACTIONS/INTERVENTIONS	RATIONALES
Determine who will intervene on behalf of the infant or child: parents or appointed legal guardian. [Note that person here.]	For legal and ethical reasons, it is essential to clarify when the parent(s) are unable to assume the parental role and obligations and to make this fact known to all involved in the child's care. It is likewise essential for all caregivers to know who is the legal guardian or spokesperson.

ACTIONS/INTERVENTIONS	RATIONALES
In instances of conflicting decision makers, ensure that the child's rights are protected according to legal statutes.	Irrespective of conflicts in decision making, the infant or child is entitled to appropriate care. In extreme cases of conflict, a state or local judge may appoint guardians or foster parents to assume decision making regarding health matters. In other instances (e.g., withholding suggested treatment because of religious beliefs), individual statutes, and precedents must be sought by the parties involved.
Ensure that appropriate documentation is carried out according to situational needs.	Legal documentation according to health care decisions and related matters is to be carried out as standard care, with attention to the mandates of the institution regarding appropriate paper forms to complete.
Although the child may be ill equipped or unable to participate fully in decision-making, facilitate developmentally appropriate involvement of the child in decision-making. In these interactions, teach the child decision-making skills.	Early involvement in decision making fosters safe support for the child, thereby increasing the likelihood of learning effective coping behaviors. Will also empower the child and foster a positive self-image.
Be certain that choices or options indeed exist when the child is allowed to exercise decision-making.	Preferences and individualization will be realistically valued when there is choice or options in the care plan. It is unethical to indicate there are choices when none exist (e.g., medication cannot be given by any other route but intramuscular).
Provide behavioral reinforcement that best fosters learning with appropriate follow-up when the child is involved in decisional conflict. [Note behaviors to be reinforced and reinforcers here.]	Appropriate reinforcement will serve to enhance learning and assist the patient in growth in decision-making.
Explore with the child and support system potential long-term residual effects related to specific decisional conflict for the child or family.	Decision making often has far-reaching effects (e.g., in early childhood, values of a lifetime are formulated). Appropriate regard to this fact should guide all involved in this aspect of child-rearing and supportive aspects of health care.[30]

Women's Health
Unwanted Pregnancy

ACTIONS/INTERVENTIONS	RATIONALES
Provide an atmosphere that encourages the patient to view her options in the event of an unwanted pregnancy. Assure the patient of confidentiality.	Provides information that allows the patient to make an informed choice.[45]
Give clear, concise, complete information to the patient, describing the choices available to her: • Carrying the pregnancy and keeping the infant • Adoption of the infant • Abortion	
Discuss the advantages and disadvantages of each option with the patient.	
Encourage the patient to discuss beliefs and practices in a nonthreatening atmosphere, and include significant others in the conversation and decision as the patient desires.	

(care plan continued on page 466)

NURSING ACTIONS/INTERVENTIONS WITH RATIONALES (continued from page 465)

Women's Health

ACTIONS/INTERVENTIONS	RATIONALES
Refer the patient to the proper agency for guidance and treatment.	
Discuss and review with the patient the different methods of birth control.	Provides information and support to assist the patient in planning future pregnancies.[31]
Assess the patient's ability to correctly use the different methods of birth control.	
Provide factual information, listing the advantages and disadvantages of each method.	
Provide the patient information on obtaining her method of choice.	
Explore with the patient and significant other their views on children and family.	

Women's Health

Less-Than-Perfect Infant

● N O T E : *Families faced with the birth of a child with congenital anomalies or developmental defects experience decisional conflict and great confusion about choices that need to be made. Often there is a sense of urgency, because decisions need to be made quickly to save the life of the infant. Many times the infant was delivered by cesarean section, and it is the mother's partner who, alone, must often make crucial decisions that could affect the family and the life of the infant. Parents experience not only confusion, fear, guilt, and helplessness, but also feelings of inadequacy as parents.*

ACTIONS/INTERVENTIONS	RATIONALES
Provide accurate information to the parents as soon as possible.	Provides information and supportive environment that helps the parents make decisions.[32,33]
Stillborn or Fetal Demise	
Let the parents see and hold the infant if at all possible.	Promotes bonding and provides comfort for both the parents and infant.
Support the parents in their grieving process for the loss of the perfect infant, and perhaps the death of the infant.[34,35]	
Keep the parents informed continuously, and encourage the health-care team to talk to them often.	
Contact significant persons, of the parents' choice, who can come and be of support to them.[36]	
Give the parents a private place to be with their support persons.	
Encourage the parents to visit the infant in the neonatal intensive care unit (NICU) as often as possible.	
Collaborate with NICU staff to plan activities that allow the mother and infant to spend as much time together as much as possible.	
Refer to support groups and agencies as needed for follow-up care when leaving hospital.[37,38]	Support is essential in resolving decisional conflict.

Mental Health

● N O T E : *The client who is experiencing a decisional conflict is faced with confusion about alternative solutions. When assisting these clients, the nurse should be careful not to connote the client's confusion negatively. Various authors[39–41] have supported the positive role confusion plays in the change process. Erickson[39] frequently encouraged confusion as a way to distract the conscious mind and allow the unconscious to develop solutions. It is from this theoretical base that the following interventions are developed.*

ACTIONS/INTERVENTIONS	RATIONALES
Assure the client that the difficulty he or she is experiencing in decision-making is positive in that it has placed him or her in a position to look for new creative solutions. If he or she were not experiencing this difficulty, he or she might be tempted to remain in the same old problem solution set.	Promotes positive orientation, self-worth, and hope.
Assist the client in reducing the pressure of time on making a decision.	
Have the client explain the time he or she has given him- or herself to make a decision. Asking the client the following question may assist in this process: "What is the worst that will happen if a decision is not made right now?"	Provides time to develop alternative problem solutions, and decreases stress on the client.
Sit with the client for [number] minutes twice per day to discuss the information and perceptions she or he has regarding the current situation and possible solutions. As the client explores the situation, the remaining interventions can be added to these discussions.	Aids in understanding the client's perception of the situation.
Have the client explore feelings related to the choices and the information related to the choices. This process may extend over several days. The client may be reluctant to verbalize negative feelings related to certain choices if a trusting relationship has not yet been developed with the nurse.	The client's cognitive style and feelings about the situation affect his or her appraisal of both the situation and possible solutions.[42]
Have the client discuss how significant others think and feel about the various choices. Have the client evaluate the impact of the feelings of significant others on his or her decision-making process.	Support system involvement increases the probability of positive outcomes.
Have the client fantasize an ideal choice.	Accesses creative problem solutions that bypass the client's self-imposed limits.
Have the client construct a list of solutions (at least 20) that would produce the ideal choice. (These solutions are not to be evaluated at this time.) Encourage the client to develop some unrealistic solutions. This may be promoted by asking the client what he or she might tell a friend to do in this situation or by having the client generate three magic-wish solutions (e.g., "If you had a magic wand, what would you do to resolve this situation?")	
Sort through developed list with the client generating solutions from the ones listed. At this time, the client can begin to combine and eliminate ideas after evaluation. Carefully evaluate each solution before it is eliminated. What appears to be a bizarre solution can become useful when altered or combined with another idea.	

(care plan continued on page 468)

NURSING ACTIONS/INTERVENTIONS WITH RATIONALES (continued from page 467)

Mental Health

ACTIONS/INTERVENTIONS	RATIONALES
As each idea is evaluated, provide all information necessary to evaluate the idea.	Aids in assessing the client's commitment to each possible solution.
Explore the client's thoughts and feelings about each idea.	
Remind the client that there are no perfect answers and that each of us makes the best choice that can be made at the time.	Promotes positive orientation, self-worth, and hope for the future.
Remind the client that if a choice that is made does not resolve the problem, alternative solutions can then be tried.	Promotes positive orientation.
Remind the client that a solution that does not work provides more information about the problem that can be used in developing future solutions.	
Meet with the client and support system to allow the support system to be a part of the decision-making process, if appropriate.	Support system involvement increases the probability of positive outcome.
Discuss with the client and support system any secondary gains from not making a decision.	Assesses for positive reinforcement for not resolving problem.
Once a decision is made, have the client develop a behavioral plan for implementation. [Note that plan here.]	Having a plan to cope with the anticipated situations promotes a perception of greater control over future situations and increases the probability of the client's enacting new coping behaviors.

Gerontic Health

In addition to the following interventions, the interventions for Adult Health can be applied to the aging client. Decision-making capacity is defined as possessing a set of values and goals, being able to communicate and understand information, and having the ability to reason and deliberate about one's choices.[43] The mere presence of aging should not imply impaired decision-making capacity. In the absence of dementia, older adults are usually capable of adequate decision-making independently or with assistance.

ACTIONS/INTERVENTIONS	RATIONALES
Discuss with the patient prior examples of Decisional Conflict and their outcomes.	Emphasizes ability to problem solve, and reinforces successes.
Assess for the presence of dementia	May affect the client's ability to make sound decisions.
Assess for the presence of legal documents granting durable power of attorney for health care in new clients.	Surrogate decision makers may already be in place.

Home Health

ACTIONS/INTERVENTIONS	RATIONALES
Teach the client and family measures to decrease Decisional Conflict: • Providing appropriate health information • Joining a support group • Clarifying values • Performing stress reduction activities	Appropriate knowledge and values clarification between the client and family will reduce conflict.

ACTIONS/INTERVENTIONS	RATIONALES
• Seeking spiritual or legal assistance as needed • Identifying useful sources of information	
Assist the client and family in identifying risk factors pertinent to the situation: • Lack of knowledge • Developmental or situational crisis • Role confusion • Excess stress • Excess stimuli	Early identification of risk factors provides opportunity for early intervention.
Answer questions about a terminal diagnosis and prognosis with honesty and sensitivity.	Develops trusting relationship, and helps clients make well-informed decisions.
Consult with or refer the patient to appropriate assistive resources as indicated.	Use of the network of existing community services provides for effective utilization of resources.

ENVIRONMENTAL INTERPRETATION SYNDROME, IMPAIRED

DEFINITION[2]

Consistent lack of orientation to person, place, time, or circumstances over more than 3 to 6 months, necessitating a protective environment.

DEFINING CHARACTERISTICS[2]

1. Chronic confusional state
2. Consistent disorientation in known and unknown environments
3. Loss of occupation or social functioning from memory decline
4. Slow in responding to questions
5. Inability to follow simple direction, instructions
6. Inability to concentrate
7. Inability to reason

RELATED FACTORS[2]

1. Depression
2. Huntington's disease
3. Dementia (e.g., Alzheimer's disease, multi-infarct dementia, Pick's disease, AIDS, alcoholism, Parkinson's disease)
4. Alcoholism
5. Parkinson's disease

RELATED CLINICAL CONCERNS

See Related Factors.

 Have You Selected the Correct Diagnosis?

There are several diagnoses that interface with this diagnosis (e.g., Impaired Memory, Disturbed Thought Process, or Confusion). This diagnosis refers to a long-term problem (3 to 6 months) that results in the patient's having to be admitted to a protective environment. This diagnosis predominantly relates to an end result of the other diagnoses.

EXPECTED OUTCOME

Will have decreased episodes of environmental confusion by [date].

Identifies [self, environment, month, significant other] by [date].

Caregivers verbalize [number] environmental safety measures needed by [date].

TARGET DATES

This is a long-term diagnosis, so an appropriate target date would be expressed in terms of weeks or months.

NURSING ACTIONS/INTERVENTIONS WITH RATIONALES

Adult Health

● N O T E : *These Actions/Interventions and Rationales are essentially the same as those for Chronic Confusion.*

(care plan continued on page 470)

NURSING ACTIONS/INTERVENTIONS WITH RATIONALES (continued from page 469)

Adult Health

ACTIONS/INTERVENTIONS	RATIONALES
Identify self and the patient by name at each interaction.	Short-term memory loss necessitates frequent orientation to person, time, and environment.
Speak slowly and clearly in short, simple words and sentences.	Allows time for information processing, and avoids use of complex statements and abstract ideas.
When the patient is delusional, focus on underlying feelings and reinforce reality (have clocks, calendars, etc. on the wall). Do not argue with the patient.	Recognizing and acknowledging feelings may decrease the client's anxiety and give a sense of being understood. Arguing may increase the patient's anxiety and reinforce intensity delusions.[44]
If the patient becomes aggressive, focus on underlying feelings and attempt to refocus interaction on topics more acceptable and/or less threatening to the patient.	Focusing on feelings increases the patient's feelings of being understood, and discussing nonthreatening topics increases the patient's sense of competency and self-esteem.
Keep the patient's room well lighted. Maintain a calm environment.	Decreases possibility of environmental sensory misrepresentations, and helps meet patient safety needs.
Teach the family about the patient's condition and how to interact more effectively with the patient; i.e., provide ongoing orientation to surroundings and happenings within the family.	Assists the family in understanding changes in the patient's orientation, cognition, and behavior. Increases the family's sense of competency in relating to the patient.
Refer to psychiatric–mental health CNS. Make other referrals to community agencies as needed, i.e., Alzheimer's support group, adult day care, Meals-on-Wheels, etc.	The psychiatric-mental health CNS has the expertise to collaborate with the adult health nurse to plan nursing interventions for the patient that will help the patient and nursing staff deal with chronic confusion in the acute care setting.

Child Health

This diagnosis may present in children also. If so, the same basic plan of care as that of adults should be implemented, with attention to safe, developmentally appropriate interventions.

ACTIONS/INTERVENTIONS	RATIONALES
Monitor for parental–infant reciprocity to determine nature of parent–infant or parent–child relationship.	Reciprocity will offer cues as to what match does or does not exist in the relationship.
When there may be a genetic concern, offer appropriate counseling.	When a genetic component exists, there is an obligation for present and futuristic planning by all involved.
Offer [number] minutes each shift for the parents to ventilate specific concerns regarding the infant or child.	Offers reduction in anxiety, plus an opportunity to note parental concerns.
Explore all contributing factors, especially underlying medical status or deviation in behavior.	Provides a comprehensive base for plan.
Provided environmental adaptations to protect from self-injury. [Note those adaptations necessary here.]	Provides anticipatory safety.
Provide routine of care with attention to caregiver(s) input.	Values parental input.
Seek assistance from primary care health team members, especially pediatric psychiatrist, child life specialist, and pediatrician, as appropriate.	Satisfies need for special care.

Women's Health

See Adult Health nursing actions.

Mental Health

ACTIONS/INTERVENTIONS	RATIONALES
Monitor the client's level of anxiety and refer to Anxiety (Chapter 8) for detailed interventions related to this diagnosis.	Increased anxiety can negatively impact memory and orientation and contribute to further deficits.
Place the client in an environment with appropriate stimuli. Note level of stimulation and alterations in environmental stimuli here; i.e., specific objects in the environment that stimulate illusions should be removed, and appropriate lighting, clocks, calendars, and holiday decorations should be provided. Refer to day, date, and other orientating information during each interaction with the client.	Increases patient safety and promotes orientation.
Place identifying information on the patient and the patient's room. Utilize the client's preferred name in each interaction. [Note that name here.]	Provides safety and promotes orientation.
Remove harmful objects from the environment. This could include objects in walkways, cords, belts, and raised bedrails or other restraining devices. Note here special precautions for this client.	Protects the client from falls and accidental injury.
Assign primary care nurse each shift. Note those persons here.	Promotes client orientation by providing familiar environment.
Observe every [number] minutes. Inform the client of this schedule, and provide the client with written information as necessary. Note information necessary for the client here. If the client is depressed, this observation may be increased because of increased risk for self-harm. Refer to Risk for Violence (Chapter 9) for specific interventions.	Promotes client safety. Provides opportunities to reorient the client to here and now and to ensure client comfort. Promotes the client's sense of control.
Provide daily routine that closely resembles the client's normal schedule. [Note that schedule here.]	Promotes orientation, and increases the client's sense of personal control and orientation.
Assess mental status through normal interactions with the client. Do not use formal mental status examinations unless absolutely necessary. [Note here method and schedule for assessment.]	Repeated questioning can increase the client's confusion, and inability to answer questions may have negative impact on self-esteem.
Limit the client's choices, and provide information or direction in brief, simple sentences. [Note here the level of the client's ability to process information (e.g., the client can choose between two items).]	High levels of stimulation can increase confusion, and inability to make choices may have negative impact on the client's self-esteem.
Keep initial interactions short but frequent. Speak to the client in brief, clear sentences. [Note frequency and length of interactions here.]	Too much information can increase the client's confusion and disorganization.
Utilize "I" messages, rather than argument, to reorient when necessary.	Meets the client's esteem needs by communicating respect while providing orientation. Promotes here-and-now orientation.
Respond to confused verbalizations by responding to the feelings being expressed.	Maintains self-esteem, relieves anxiety, and orients to present reality.

(care plan continued on page 472)

NURSING ACTIONS/INTERVENTIONS WITH RATIONALES (continued from page 471)

Mental Health

ACTIONS/INTERVENTIONS	RATIONALES
When the client's ability to tolerate more complex situations increases, schedule his or her participation in groups that provide opportunities to remember, review current events, discuss seasonal activities, and socialize. [Note here the schedule and appropriate groups for this client.]	Promotes here-and-now orientation. Provides opportunities to maintain current cognitive skills.
Provide clear feedback on appropriate behavior. Set behavior goals that the client can achieve. [Note here the behaviors that are to be rewarded and the rewards that are to be given.]	Positive reinforcement encourages behavior. Realistic goals increase opportunities for success, providing positive reinforcement and enhancing self-esteem.
Spend [number] minutes [number] times a day involved in exercise with the client. (Choose exercise the client enjoys and that involves large motor activity if at all possible.) [Note the specific activity here.]	Improves rest and increases natural endorphins.
Spend [number] minutes [number] times per week providing information to the client's support system. Note specific information to be provided and person responsible for this activity here.	Family and client involvement enhances effectiveness of intervention and promotes community support.
Refer to community agencies that will provide ongoing monitoring of client's condition and support for caregivers.	

Gerontic Health

In addition to the following interventions, the interventions for Adult Health can be applied to the aging client.

ACTIONS/INTERVENTIONS	RATIONALES
Review mental status examination to identify areas of strengths and needs.	Depending on examination used, may indicate the client's ability to read, interpret symbols, or process simple versus complex instructions.
Survey current environment for potential unsafe areas.	Correcting unsafe areas decreases potential for client injury.
Adapt the environment to decrease risk for injury (e.g., access to exits, thermal injury potential, or ingestion of harmful substances).	
Instruct the caregiver in environmental adaptations to provide protective environment.	
Use labeling or pictorial symbols to indicate specific areas or conveniences (such as universal symbols for food or restrooms or pictures to indicate the client's room).	Assists the client to interpret environment.
Ensure identification of the client (ID bracelet or necklace).	Provides means of identification in the event the client leaves the care setting.
Provide conversational cues to person, place, and time.	Presents information in a nonthreatening manner.
Retrieve and divert the client when wandering behavior presents risk or takes her or him into unobserved areas.	Decreases the client's wandering behaviors.[27]

ACTIONS/INTERVENTIONS	RATIONALES
Assess for expression of intent, "I'm going home now," and the expression of loss of a valued adult role, "The children need me now."[28]	
Modify the environment to provide adequate rest, safety, and sleep for the client.[28]	Eliminate possible preciptators of confusion.
Provide client with essential sensory aides such as glasses, dentures, and hearing aids.	Prevents possible sensory confusion.[28]
Avoid chemical and physical restraints.	These can increase confusion and agitation. These do not stop the urge to wander and may exacerbate the urge to wander by decreasing the client's perception of safety. These measures may contribute to client injury.[28]
Schedule and maintain a regular toileting schedule. [Note schedule here.]	Eliminate possible precipitators of confusion and wandering.
Provide information to all staff that a client is a wanderer. Develop a mechanism for identification and a plan to follow if a wandering client is missing.[28]	Prevention of injury related to wandering.
Use grid like markings in front of doorways.	May prevent a client from exiting due to a change in visual cues.[28]

Home Health

In addition to the following interventions, the interventions for Adult Health can be applied with the home health client.

ACTIONS/INTERVENTIONS	RATIONALES
Assist the client and family in identifying lifestyle changes that may be required: • Provide a consistent care provider. • Provide for consistent daily schedule with structured activities. • Have the client wear identification bracelet; put name in clothing. • Provide safe environment. • Provide environmental cues to orient the patient (e.g., clocks or calendars).	Home-based care requires involvement of the family. Impaired interpretation of the environment disrupts family schedules and role relationships. Adjustments in family activities and roles may be required.
• Provide assistive resources as required.	Decreased vision or hearing acuity may contribute to confusion.
• Monitor family response to changing behavior and mental status of the affected person.	
Assist the family to set criteria to help them determine when additional intervention is required; for example, help them to recognize signals indicating a change in their ability to maintain a safe environment.	Provides the family with background knowledge to seek appropriate assistance as need arises.
Offer support to the caregivers and family members: • Teaching about management of behavior • Self-care strategies • Community resources	Promotes adaptive coping.
Refer to appropriate assistive resources as indicated.	Additional assistance may be required for the family to care for the family member with Impaired Environmental Interpretive Syndrome.

KNOWLEDGE, DEFICIENT (SPECIFY)

DEFINITION[2]

Absence or deficiency of cognitive information related to specific topic.[2]

DEFINING CHARACTERISTICS[2]

1. Verbalization of the problem
2. Inappropriate or exaggerated behaviors (e.g., hysterical, hostile, agitated, or apathetic)
3. Inaccurate follow-through of instruction
4. Inaccurate performance of test

RELATED FACTORS[2]

1. Cognitive limitation
2. Information misinterpretation
3. Lack of exposure
4. Lack of interest in learning
5. Lack of recall
6. Unfamiliarity with information resources

RELATED CLINICAL CONCERNS

1. Any diagnosis that is entirely new to the patient
2. Mental retardation
3. Post head injury
4. Depression
5. Dementia
6. Chronic illness that client is having difficulty managing

 Have You Selected the Correct Diagnosis?

Noncompliance
In Noncompliance, the patient can return-demonstrate skills accurately or verbalize the regimen needed, but does not follow through on the care.

Disturbed Thought Process
This diagnosis would be evident by lack of immediate recall on return-demonstration rather than inaccurate or limited demonstration and recall.

Powerlessness
This diagnosis would be reflected by statements such as "How will this help?", "I have no control over this," "I have to rely on others" rather than statements related to "I don't really understand," "I'm not really sure how," or "Is this right?"

Ineffective Health Maintenance
Ineffective Health Maintenance may include Deficient Knowledge, but is broader in scope and includes such aspects as limited resources and mobility factors.

EXPECTED OUTCOME

Will return-demonstrate [specific knowledge deficit activity] by [date].

TARGET DATES

Individual learning curves vary significantly. A target date ranging from 3 to 7 days could be appropriate based on the individual's previous experience with this material, education level, potential for learning, and energy level.

NURSING ACTIONS/INTERVENTIONS WITH RATIONALES

Adult Health

ACTIONS/INTERVENTIONS	RATIONALES
Identify how the patient perceives the impact of the situation.	
Identify the patient's best methods for learning.	
Initiate teaching when patient is most amenable to receiving information (rested, reduced anxiety, pain relief, etc.)	
Provide relevant information only.	Adult learning principles indicate that adult learners better relate to information that is directly pertinent to their situation.
Provide an environment conducive to learning.	
Design teaching plan specific to the patient's deficit area and specific to the patient's level of education. Include significant others in teaching sessions. [Note specific plan here.]	Provides new knowledge based on the patient's perceived needs. Individuals learn in their own way and in their own time frame. Motivates learning and provides support and reinforcement for learning.

ACTIONS/INTERVENTIONS	RATIONALES
Explain each procedure as it is being done, and give the rationale for procedure and the patient's role.	Incorporates another teaching method; reduces anxiety, thus promoting learning.
Provide positive reinforcement as often as possible for the patient's progress.	Reinforces learning achieved and promotes positive orientation.
Have the patient restate, in his or her own words, cognitive materials during teaching session. Have repeat on each subsequent day until discharge.	Repeated practice of a behavior internalizes and personalizes the behavior.[44]
Ensure that basic needs are taken care of before and immediately after teaching sessions.	Prevents distractions during teaching session due to basic needs not being met.
Pace teaching according to the patient's rate of learning and preference during teaching session.	Considers the patient's learning style and ability to process new information.
Provide the patient with ample opportunity to ask questions.	
Collaborate with and refer the patient to appropriate assistive resources.	Coordinates team approach to health and provides means to follow up and reinforce learning.

Child Health

ACTIONS/INTERVENTIONS	RATIONALES
Determine whether there are ambiguities in the minds of the parents or child.	Clarification and verification will ensure a greater likelihood of understanding and valuing aspects critical to patient teaching.
Identify the learning capacity for the patient and family.	Realistic capacity for learning should be a primary factor in patient teaching, because it serves as one major parameter in expectations of learning.
Determine the scope and appropriate presentation for the patient and family based on previous actions, plus developmental crises for each. **Do not** overwhelm the patient. [Note adaptations needed based on client need.]	Developmental needs of all involved will best serve as an essential framework for teaching the patient and family. Potentials and capacity for use of all the sensory-perceptual aspects of cognition should be explored and used to ensure the best opportunity for effective teaching.
Evaluate the effectiveness of the teaching-learning experience by: • Brief verbal discourse to provide concrete data • Brief written examination to show progress • Observation of skills critical for care (e.g., change of dressing according to sterile technique) • Allowing the child to perform skills in general fashion with use of dolls	Evaluation is an indicator of both teaching effectiveness and learning. It serves as another essential aspect of patient teaching, with the appropriate focus on individualization, by pointing out areas needing reteaching.

Women's Health

ACTIONS/INTERVENTIONS	RATIONALES
Teach normal physiologic changes the new mother can expect postpartum: • Lochia flow • Breast changes	Provides information to assist new mothers in postpartum adaptation and transition to motherhood.[46,47]

(care plan continued on page 476)

NURSING ACTIONS/INTERVENTIONS WITH RATIONALES (continued from page 475)

Women's Health

ACTIONS/INTERVENTIONS	RATIONALES
• Breastfeeding: Engorgement, comfort measures, clothing, positions for mother and infant comfort and hygiene (see actions for the Nutrition diagnoses in Chapter 3). • Non-breastfeeding: Suppression of lactation (medications, clothing such as tight-fitting bra, and comfort measures); importance of holding the baby while bottle-feeding (*NEVER* prop *bottle* and do burp the baby often); formulas (different kinds and preparation). • Perineum and rectum: episiotomy, hemorrhoids, hygiene, medications, and comfort measures	Stress during the postpartum period is physical, intrapersonal and interpersonal, research suggests that breastfeeding can reduce stress by protecting the mother from environmental stimuli.[48] Breast binding should be discontinued as a means of lactation suppression as research shows that supportive bras are more effective.[49]
Demonstrate infant care to new parents: • Bathing • Feeding • Cord care • Holding, carrying, etc. • Safety • Sleep–wake states of the infant	Assists new parents in adapting to parenting role. Allows the parents to practice new skills in a nonthreatening environment and seek clarification from an informed source.[50–54]
Provide quiet, supportive atmosphere for interaction with the infant to allow the parent to: • Become acquainted with infant • Practice caretaking activities such as breastfeeding or formula feeding • Begin integration of the infant into the family	Promotes positive learning experience for the mother, father, and baby.[50–54]
Discuss infant care, taking into consideration age and cultural differences of the parents: • Teenagers: Involve significant others. Have the mother return-demonstrate infant care. Refer to support systems such as Young Parent Services and church groups. • First-time older mothers: Allow verbalization of fears. Involve significant others. Provide encouragement.	
Adjust teaching to take into consideration different cultural caretaking activities, such as preventing the evil eye in the Hispanic culture, or the mother not holding the baby for several days immediately after birth in some Far Eastern Indian cultures.	
Demonstrate newborn skills to the parents. Utilize different assessment skills to teach the parents about their newborn's capabilities—gestational age assessment, physical examination of newborn, or Brazelton Neonatal Assessment Scale (sleep–wake states).	
Encourage the parents to hold and talk to the newborn.	Helps the parents gain confidence when caring for the newborn. Provides opportunity for nurse to teach and reinforce teaching.[50–54]
Discuss different methods of birth control and the advantages and disadvantages of each method:	Informs the new mother (parents) of choices in birth control methods, and gives them the opportunity to ask questions.

ACTIONS/INTERVENTIONS	RATIONALES
• Chemical: spermicides and pills • Mechanical: condom, diaphragm, intrauterine device (IUD) • Behavioral: abstinence, temperature-ovulation-cervical mucus (Billing's method), or coitus interruptus • Sterilization: vasectomy, tubal ligation, or hysterectomy	
Discuss signs and symptoms of perimenopausal and menopausal changes with the woman: hot flashes, perspiration, and/or chilly sensations; numbness or tingling of skin; insomnia or restlessness; interrupted sleep; feelings of irritability, anxiety, or apprehension; feeling depressed or unhappy; sensations of dizziness or swimming in the head; feeling of weariness of mind and body associated with desire for rest; joint or muscle pain; headaches; quickening or acceleration of heartbeat; and sensation of "crawly skin" (feels like insects creeping over skin).[55–57]	Clients who are informed and active participants in their own health decisions, in collaboration with the health care provider who can provide a screening of hormone levels, can relieve some of the symptoms of menopause.

Mental Health

ACTIONS/INTERVENTIONS	RATIONALES
Ask the client about previous learning experiences in general and about those related to the current area of concern (e.g., has the client learned that he or she is a poor learner, that he or she does not have the intellectual ability to learn the type of information that is currently required, or that the smallest mistake in the activity to be learned could be fatal?)	Helps determine aspects of the client's cognitive appraisal that could impact learning.
Monitor the client's current level of anxiety. If level of anxiety will inhibit learning, assist the client with anxiety reduction. (Refer to Anxiety in Chapter 8 for detailed interventions.)	Severe anxiety and impaired cognitive functioning can decrease the client's ability to attend to the environment in a manner that facilitates learning.
Determine what the client thinks is most important in the current situation.	The client's cognitive appraisal can impact his or her willingness to attend to the information. This is especially true of adult learners. Change is dependant on the client's perception of the problem.[58]
Assist the client in meeting those needs that represent lower-level needs on Maslow's hierarchy so attention can be focused on the area of learning to be addressed (e.g., if the client is concerned that children are not being cared for while he or she is hospitalized, he or she may not be able to focus on learning). [List the needs to be met here.]	Promotes attention to learning. Reduces anxiety.
Sit with the client for [number] minutes 2 times each day to discuss the following (each discussion point can be added as appropriate to the client's situation):	Facilitates client change and understanding by addressing the client's perceptions of need. When information is presented when the client is ready in a way that is meaningful for the client, it has greater impact.[58,59]
• Have the client describe those issues that are most important for them to address.	Change is dependant on client's perception of the problem.[58]

(care plan continued on page 478)

NURSING ACTIONS/INTERVENTIONS WITH RATIONALES (continued from page 477)

Mental Health

ACTIONS/INTERVENTIONS	RATIONALES
• Provide all information in a format that is meaningful to the client. This includes careful selection of language and of the information provided.	
• Provide successive information based on client's response to previous information presented.	
Provide positive, informative verbal reinforcement for the client's efforts to learn. [Note here those statements that are reinforcing for this client.]	Positive reinforcement increases behavior.
Establish learning goals with the client that ensure success. [Note those goals here.]	Success provides positive reinforcement and promotes continued learning efforts.
Establish time to include significant others in the learning experiences. During this interaction, address the concerns of these support systems. [Note schedule here and those to be included.]	A change in one part of the system affects the whole system. If the intervention is developed with the input of significant others, then it has meaning to this support system.[58,59]
Include the client in group learning experiences (e.g., medication groups).	Provides the client with opportunity to learn from others and to discuss new coping behaviors in a safe environment.
Refer client and support system to community agencies that will provide ongoing support for learning. [Note those agencies here.]	

Gerontic Health

In addition to the following interventions, the interventions for Adult Health can be applied to the aging client.

● N O T E : *Aging clients are able to learn new material readily but may experience difficulty with information retrieval. This should be considered when teaching elderly clients.*

ACTIONS/INTERVENTIONS	RATIONALES
Determine current knowledge base by interviewing the patient and have the patient state current knowledge regarding condition.	Provides a stepping-stone to pieces of information that may be incorrect or lacking.
Ensure that glasses and hearing aids, if needed, are functioning and used.	Enhances communication process.
Encourage the patient to set the pace of the teaching sessions.[59]	Assists in keeping sessions focused on the patient's ability to acquire new information.
Monitor for fatigue.	Fatigue interferes with concentration and thus decreases learning.
Present small pieces of information in each session.	Avoids overwhelming the patient. Promotes learning.
Use examples that can be related to the individual's life and lifestyle.	Adds realism to information, and makes transferring of information easier.
Determine whether there is increased anxiety during teaching sessions (e.g., watch body language). If so, use relaxation techniques prior to session.	Anxiety decreases concentration and ability to learn.
Use audiovisual aids that are appropriate for the individual in regard to print size, colors, volume, and tone pitch.	Promotes visual and sensory input according to the individual's needs.
Use repetition with positive feedback for correct responses.	Reinforces learning and allows evaluation of learning.

Home Health

● N O T E : *Many of the interactions between clients, families, and the nurse during the course of home health care are related to health education. Proper assessment by the nurse of the potential for or actual knowledge deficit is imperative. The nurse should use techniques based on learning theory to design teaching interventions that will be appropriate to the situation at hand. These techniques include, but are not limited to, using teaching materials that match the readiness of the participant, repeating the material using several senses, reinforcing the learner's progress, using a positive and enthusiastic approach, and decreasing barriers to learning, for example, language, pain, or physical illness.*

ACTIONS/INTERVENTIONS	RATIONALES
Teach the client and family measures to reduce knowledge deficit by seeking the following information and learning conditions: • Information regarding disease process • Rationale for treatment interventions • Techniques for improving learning situation [motivation, teaching materials that match cognitive level of participants, reduction of discomfort (e.g., control of pain and use of familiar surroundings)] • Enhancement of self-care capabilities • Written materials to supplement oral teaching (i.e., written materials that are appropriate to cognitive level and to self-care management) • Addressing client and family questions	Conditions that support learning will decrease deficit. Provides the client and family with necessary information.
Coordinate the teaching activities of other health care professionals who may be involved. Reinforce the teaching of ROM by the physical therapist, for example.	Coordination reduces duplication and enhances planning. Provides an opportunity for health care professionals to clarify any conflicting information before sharing it with the client.
Involve the client and family in planning, implementing, and promoting reduction in knowledge deficit: • Family conference • Mutual goal setting • Communication • Family members responsible for specific tasks or information	Involvement improves motivation and improves the outcome.
Consult with or refer to assistive resources as indicated.	Use of the network of existing community services provides for effective utilization of resources.

KNOWLEDGE, READINESS FOR ENHANCED

DEFINITION[2]

The presence of acquisition of cognitive information related to a specific topic is sufficient for meeting health related goals and can be strengthened.

DEFINING CHARACTERISTICS[2]

1. Expresses an interest in learning
2. Explains knowledge of the topic
3. Behaviors congruent with expressed knowledge
4. Describes previous experiences pertaining to the topic

 Have You Selected the Correct Diagnosis?

Knowledge, Deficient
Deficient Knowledge is utilized when the client currently does not have the knowledge necessary to manage a health care situation or meet desired health-care goals.

Knowledge, Readiness for Enhanced
Readiness for Enhanced Knowledge would be the correct diagnosis when the client has sufficient information to meet health-care goals but has a desire/need to have this information enhanced.

EXPECTED OUTCOME

The client will verbalize enhanced knowledge of [topic] by [date].

TARGET DATES

Since this is a positive diagnosis involving teaching as a primary intervention a target date of 1 to 2 days after diagnosis is preferred.

NURSING ACTIONS/INTERVENTIONS WITH RATIONALES

Adult Health

ACTIONS/INTERVENTIONS	RATIONALES
Collaborate with the patient to identify areas that require further development. Set realistic and achievable goals.	
Refer the patient to reliable health resources.	
Provide the patient with requested information [Note information needed and plan for presentation here.]	
Meet with the patient [weekly/daily] to evaluate progress and need for adaptation of plan.	

Child Health

ACTIONS/INTERVENTIONS	RATIONALES
Determine learning needs and focus on developmentally appropriate method. [Note method to be used for this child here.]	Ensures realistic approach for child and parents.
Determine goals for health-related requisite knowledge with inclusion of parents.	Sets relevant focus for learning.
Provide appropriate tools and models for teaching. For example, flow meter for asthmatic training, or insulin, syringes, and guidelines for plan for diabetes client and family.	Offers realistic opportunity for practice in supportive environment
Monitor for follow-up. Use appropriate technique to accurately ascertain required information. For example, how to perform peak flow meter demo or administer accurate dosage of insulin subcutaneously with aseptic technique.	Validates appropriate knowledge and application.
Teach the patient and family when to seek assistance or to report to primary care pediatrician.	Offers anticipatory guidance.
Facilitate adaptation of plan for long-term needs with specific attention to possible school nursing assistance or a setting other than home.	Provides realistic planning of health plan.
Provide opportunities to meet with other children experiencing similar health-care needs.	Engenders a sense of peer support to afford a sense of shared affiliation.
Assist in identification of how the usual daily routine may be maintained with incorporation of essential health-care regimen.	Provides realistic anticipatory planning.
Provide reinforcement for success in meeting goals and compliance with the expected health-care regimen. [Note reinforcement plan for this client here.]	Values and enhances learning with empowerment for future success.

Women's Health

These would be the same as for Adult Health except for the following:

ACTIONS/INTERVENTIONS	RATIONALE
Women teach other women, and have been viewed as healers throughout history.	Research has shown that women are more open to alternative methods of health and healing.[60]
Provide women with information about tests and screenings that will prevent health-care problems.	Women will seek out information and care for their health-care needs.[61]

Mental Health

Refer to nursing interventions for Knowledge, Deficient, Mental Health to assist client in addressing knowledge needs.

Gerontic Health

ACTIONS/INTERVENTIONS	RATIONALES
Determine the client's priorities and preferred learning style.	Allow the nurse to focus on what is relevant to client and provide teaching that is best received by the client.
Monitor physical changes that may impact learning (visual changes, hearing loss, memory impairment).	This allows the nurse to make needed accommodations when teaching.
Assist the patient in setting realistic goals for learning.	Client will not become discouraged by unrealistic goals.
Provide an environment conducive to learning: • Maintain a comfortable temperature. • Ensure the client is not hungry, in pain, or sleepy. • Have a family member present if desired or needed. • Use real equipment when possible to facilitate understanding. • Keep the session short, factual, and to the point. • Use common vocabulary and avoid the use of medical jargon.	Maximizes the effectiveness of teaching and learning.
Provide referral as needed to include: • Enterostomal therapist • Dietician • Physical therapy • Occupational therapy	Use of the interdisciplinary team facilitates most comprehensive and accurate information and assistance for the client.
Utilize adult teaching principles during educational sessions: • Focus on information that is important to the client. • Use teaching materials that appeal to many types of learners (visual, auditory, kinesthetic).	Maximizes the effectiveness of teaching and learning.

Home Health/Community Health

ACTIONS/INTERVENTIONS	RATIONALES
Spend [number] minutes per shift to discuss the client's priorities and preferred learning style.	Allow the nurse to focus on what is relevant to client and provide teaching that is best received by the client.
Monitor physical changes that may impact learning (visual changes, hearing loss, memory impairment).	This allows the nurse to make needed accommodations when teaching.

(care plan continued on page 482)

NURSING ACTIONS/INTERVENTIONS WITH RATIONALES (continued from page 481)

Home Health/Community Health

ACTIONS/INTERVENTIONS	RATIONALES
Assist the patient in setting realistic goals for learning.	Client will not become discouraged by unrealistic goals.
Provide an environment conducive to learning: • Minimize distractions in the home (phones, persons coming in and out). • Maintain a comfortable temperature. • Ensure that the client is not hungry, in pain, or sleepy. • Have a family member present if desired or needed. • Use real equipment when possible to facilitate understanding. Have equipment that will be in the home delivered prior to the teaching learning session to ensure that the client is able to use the equipment. • Keep the session short, factual, and to the point. • Use common vocabulary and avoid the use of medical jargon. • Leave written materials in the home when possible. • Leave a phone number for the client to call should further questions arise.	Maximizes the effectiveness of teaching and learning.
Provide referral as needed to include • Enterostomal therapist • Dietician • Physical therapy • Occupational therapy	Use of the interdisciplinary team facilitates most comprehensive and accurate information and assistance for the client.
Utilize adult teaching principles during educational sessions: • Focus on information that is important to the client. • Use teaching materials that appeal to many types of learners (visual, auditory, kinesthetic).	Maximizes the effectiveness of teaching and learning.
Refer the client to community resources as appropriate: • Support groups for clients and families • Educational web resources	Utilizing existing resources facilitates success and is time and cost efficient.

MEMORY, IMPAIRED

DEFINITION[2]

Inability to remember or recall bits of information or behavioral skills.*

DEFINING CHARACTERISTICS[2]

1. Inability to recall factual information
2. Inability to recall recent or past events
3. Inability to learn or retain new skills or information
4. Inability to determine whether a behavior was performed
5. Observed or reported experiences of forgetting
6. Inability to perform a previously learned skill
7. Forgets to perform a behavior at a scheduled time

RELATED FACTORS[2]

1. Fluid and electrolyte imbalance
2. Neurologic disturbances
3. Excessive environmental disturbances
4. Anemia
5. Acute or chronic hypoxia
6. Decreased cardiac output

RELATED CLINICAL CONCERNS

1. Hypoxia
2. Anemia
3. Congestive heart failure
4. Alzheimer's disease

*Impaired memory may be attributed to pathophysiologic or situational causes that are either temporary or permanent.

5. Cerebral vascular accident
6. Dementia

 Have You Selected the Correct Diagnosis?

This diagnosis is very similar to other diagnoses in this pattern; for example, Confusion and Disturbed Thought Process. However, this diagnosis relates specifically to memory problems.

EXPECTED OUTCOME

Will verbalize recall of [immediate information/recent information/remote information] by [date].

TARGET DATES

For some patients, this may be a permanent problem, so dates would be stated in terms of weeks and months. For other patients, it would be appropriate to check for progress within 3 days.

NURSING ACTIONS/INTERVENTIONS WITH RATIONALES

Adult Health

ACTIONS/INTERVENTIONS	RATIONALES
Identify self and the patient by name at each interaction.	Memory loss necessitates frequent orientation to person, time, and environment.
Support and reinforce the patient's efforts to remember bits of information or behavioral skills.	Reinforcing the patient's efforts at remembering can decrease anxiety levels and perhaps help with further recovery. Placing unrealistic expectations on the patient can increase anxiety, frustration, and feelings of help-lessness.
Observe for improvement or deterioration in memory based on the suspected or confirmed underlying medical diagnosis.	Memory impairment due to some reversible physiologic problem should improve as the condition becomes resolved. Memory impairment due to irreversible physiologic-physical problems generally will not improve and will likely deteriorate over time.
Teach the family about the patient's condition and how to respond to the patient's loss of memory.	Assists the family in understanding underlying cause(s) for memory impairment. Increases the family's sense of competency in relating to the patient during periods of memory loss

Child Health

Same as Adult Health within developmental capacity for infant or child, and safety-mindedness in all aspects.

ACTIONS/INTERVENTIONS	RATIONALES
Determine all who may need to be involved to best support the infant or child in situations where actual known level of involvement may not be clear.	Ambiguous unknowns present frustration for all involved, so it is best to establish most complete team to manage care to foster holistic approach.
Offer 30 minutes each shift and as needed for the parents to express concerns.	Reduces anxiety and offers insight into parental concerns.
Offer appropriate advocacy on behalf of the infant or child when the parents are unable to offer this component.	Child advocacy will best protect the child's interests when the parents cannot.

Women's Health

Same as Adult Health except for magnesium sulfate therapy specific to pregnancy-induced hypertension. For midlife women, the actions and interventions are the same as those given for perimenopausal and menopausal life periods in Deficient Knowledge, Sleep Deprivation, and Disturbed Sleep Pattern.

(care plan continued on page 484)

NURSING ACTIONS/INTERVENTIONS WITH RATIONALES (continued from page 483)

Mental Health

ACTIONS/INTERVENTIONS	RATIONALES
Monitor the client's level of anxiety, and refer to Anxiety (Chapter 8) for detailed interventions related to this diagnosis.	Anxiety can increase the client's confusion and disorganization.
Speak to the client in brief, clear sentences.	Too much information can increase the client's confusion and disorganization, increasing memory problems.
Interact with the client for [number] minutes every [number] minutes. Begin with 5-minute interactions and gradually increase the length of interactions.	Time of interaction should be guided by the client's attention span.
Be consistent in all interactions with the client.	Facilitates the development of a trusting relationship, and meets the client's safety needs.
Initially, place the client in an area with little stimulation.	Inappropriate levels of sensory stimuli can contribute to the client's sense of disorganization and confusion, increasing memory problems.
Orient the client to the environment, and assign someone to provide one-to-one interaction while the client orients to unit.	Promotes the client's safety needs while promoting the development of a trusting relationship.
Do not argue with the client about inaccurate memory of situations (e.g., the client insisting he or she has not eaten when he or she has just finished a meal). Inform the client in a matter-of-fact manner that this is not your experience of the situation.	Communicates acceptance of the client and promotes self-esteem.
Provide orientation information to the client as needed. Specify here what information this client needs (e.g., name on room, calendar, clock, written daily schedule, or information provided in written form in a notebook or on a white board).	Facilitates maintenance of self-esteem and memory.
Utilize reflection of the last statement made by the client in conversations.	Facilitates memory within conversation.
Establish a daily schedule for the client, and provide a written copy to him or her or post a copy of the daily schedule in an obvious location in the milieu. [Note the client's specific schedule here.]	Decreases anxiety and promotes consistency.
Spend [number] minutes [number] times a day reviewing with the client concerns about memory and developing memory techniques. These could include visual imagery, mnemonic devices, memory games, association techniques, making lists, rehearsing information, or keeping a journal about activities.	Associating information from various senses enhances memory by providing meaningful links. Written material provides prompts.
Practice memory techniques with the client [number] minutes 2 times a day. [Note specific techniques to be practiced.]	Practice improves performance and integrates behavior into the client's coping strategies.
Spend [number] minutes following an activity discussing the activity to provide the client with an opportunity to practice remembering.	Opportunities to use memory enhance memory.

ACTIONS/INTERVENTIONS	RATIONALES
Provide positive verbal reinforcement to the client for accomplishing task progress.	Positive feedback encourages behavior.
Sit with the client each morning and develop a list of the day's activities. Review this list each evening.	Provides practice with memory techniques.
Schedule the client for groups that provide opportunities to utilize memory. These could be current event groups, reminiscence groups, or life review groups. Note the client's group schedule(s) here, as well as the assistance needed from staff to get the client to the group(s).	Provides opportunities for the client to practice using memory, which enhances memory.
Spend [number] minutes each week discussing the client's coping strategies with support system. Note here person responsible and time for this discussion.	Support system reactions impact the client.

Gerontic Health

In addition to the following interventions, the interventions for Adult Health can be applied to the aging client.

● NOTE: *Aging clients may experience age related changes in memory to include forgetting specific details but remembering them later, ability to learn new information with some difficulty in information retrieval, a general awareness of memory impairment, and memory impairment that does not affect daily life.*

ACTIONS/INTERVENTIONS	RATIONALES
Introduce self with each client contact.	Promotes comfort for the client to identify caregiver.
Use the client's preferred name in course of conversations.	Provides orienting cue to the client's identity.
Request photographs and names of significant others from the family or caregiver.	Provides information about the client and point of reference while providing care.
Maintain consistency in environment.	Decreases need to cope with change on a frequent basis.
Document any appliances client requires (prostheses, eyeglasses, hearing aids, cane, or walker).	Provides a record of needed equipment that the client may not be able to recall.
Ensure permanent identification of all appliances required by the client.	Assists in keeping equipment available to the client, and eliminates potential of using incorrect assistive devices.
Maintain consistent routine of care.	Provides sense of the familiar.
Avoid arguments over forgetful behavior.	Promotes client self-esteem, and decreases potential for escalating anxiety related to the memory loss.
Omit statements or questions that emphasize memory loss such as "Don't you remember eating breakfast?" or "Do you know who came to see you this morning?"	Promotes client self-esteem, and decreases potential for escalating anxiety related to the memory loss.
In congregate social or living situations, introduce clients prior to group activities.	Fosters social skills and interactions.
Monitor solid and liquid intake on a daily basis.	Memory loss may prevent the client from obtaining adequate nutrition or fluid intake.
Document responses to medications, and note any changes in memory associated with medications.	Some medications may have side effects that in the older client promote amnesia. This problem can occur especially with long-acting benzodiazepines and hypnotics.
Administer mental status examination on a semiannual basis unless the client is receiving medication to enhance memory.	Monitors memory function and may assist in identifying changing strengths. Increased frequency recommended if the client is taking memory-improving medication.
Monitor for changes in activities of daily living (ADLs) ability and for performance of ADLs without prompting.	If memory loss is progressive, ADL skills will decrease over time and increased assistance will be needed.

(care plan continued on page 486)

NURSING ACTIONS/INTERVENTIONS WITH RATIONALES (continued from page 485)

Gerontic Health

ACTIONS/INTERVENTIONS	RATIONALES
Use distraction techniques if the memory-impaired client becomes increasingly agitated or aggressive in the care setting.	Distraction can allow time for the client to forget cause of agitation.
Educate the caregiver to recognize signs of personal stress when caring for the client with impaired memory.	Decreases potential for caregiver burnout.
Provide the caregiver information on available respite services.	Decreases potential for caregiver burnout.
Monitor the patient for changes in elimination patterns.	The memory-impaired client may not be able to report changes in bowel or bladder function.

Home Health

● NOTE: *If this is an acute development, immediate referral is required.*

ACTIONS/INTERVENTIONS	RATIONALES
Assist the client and family in lifestyle adjustments that may be necessary: • Provide a safe environment. • Structure teaching methods and interventions to the person's ability. • Explain to the family the changes from their usual roles required in caring for the patient.	Home-based care requires involvement of the family. Impaired memory can disrupt family schedules and role relationships. Adjustments in family activities and roles may be required.
Assist the family to set criteria to help them determine when additional intervention is required (e.g., explain how to recognize change in baseline behavior).	Provides the family with background knowledge to seek appropriate assistance as need arises.
Refer to appropriate assistive resources as indicated. • Support groups for caregivers • Support groups for persons with similar problems • Home care assistance	Additional assistance may be required for the family to care for the person with impaired memory. Use of readily available resources is cost-effective.
Teach the client and family memory involvement tasks, such as reminiscence and memory practice exercises.	Structured memory tasks can increase the client's functional ability.
Teach the client and family compensation strategies (e.g., daily planner or checklists).	Compensation strategies can increase the client's functional ability.

PAIN, ACUTE AND CHRONIC

DEFINITIONS[2]

Acute Pain Unpleasant sensory and emotional experience arising from actual or potential tissue damage, or described in terms of such damage (International Association for the Study of Pain). Sudden or slow onset of any intensity from mild to severe, with an anticipated or predictable end, and a duration of less than 6 months.

Chronic Pain Unpleasant sensory and emotional experience arising from actual or potential tissue damage, or described in terms of such damage (International Association for the Study of Pain). Sudden or slow onset of any intensity from mild to severe, constant or recurring, without anticipated or predictable end and a duration of longer than 6 months.

DEFINING CHARACTERISTICS[2]

A. Acute Pain
1. Verbal or coded report
2. Observed evidence

3. Antalgic positioning to avoid pain
4. Protective gestures
5. Guarding behavior
6. Facial mask
7. Sleep disturbance (eyes lack luster, beaten look, fixed or scattered movement, or grimace)
8. Self-focus
9. Narrowed focus (altered time perception, impaired thought process, or reduced interaction with people and environment)
10. Distraction behavior (pacing, seeking out other people and/or activities, or repetitive activities)
11. Autonomic responses (diaphoresis; changes in blood pressure, respiration, pulse; pupillary dilation)
12. Autonomic change in muscle tone (may span from listless to rigid)
13. Expressive behavior (restlessness, moaning, crying, vigilance, irritability, or sighing)
14. Changes in appetite and eating

B. **Chronic Pain**
1. Weight changes
2. Verbal or coded report or observed evidence of protective behavior, guarding behavior, facial mask, irritability, self-focusing, restlessness, depression
3. Atrophy of involved muscle group
4. Changes in sleep pattern
5. Fatigue
6. Fear of reinjury
7. Reduced interaction with people
8. Altered ability to continue previous activities
9. Sympathetic-mediated responses (temperature, cold, changes of body position, or hypersentivity)
10. Anorexia

RELATED FACTORS[2]

A. **Acute Pain**
1. Injury agents (biologic, chemical, physical, psychological)
B. **Chronic Pain**
1. Chronic physical or psychosocial disability

RELATED CLINICAL CONCERNS

1. Any surgical diagnosis
2. Any condition labeled chronic, for example, rheumatoid arthritis
3. Any traumatic injury
4. Any infection
5. Anxiety or stress
6. Fatigue

 Have You Selected the Correct Diagnosis?

There are no other nursing diagnoses that are easily confused with this diagnosis. Many of the other nursing diagnoses will serve as companion diagnoses and may have pain as a contributing factor to that diagnosis. For example, an individual with chronic pain may be exhausted from trying to deal with the pain and have a companion diagnosis of Fatigue, or may be using alcohol or street drugs in an attempt to ease the pain and would have the companion diagnosis of Ineffective Individual Coping.

EXPECTED OUTCOME

Will describe [number] of methods to facilitate pain control by [date].

Will report a decrease in pain on a 0 to 10 scale by [date].

Will demonstrate the use of one nonanalgesic method to prevent or control pain by [date].

TARGET DATES

Since uncontrolled pain affects a client's ability to ambulate and heal properly, both short- and long-term goals for pain management are appropriate. Acute pain should be reduced within hours. Long term, pain should be managed so that a patient's pain rating is at a level that is acceptable to them, generally less than 3 on a 0 to 10 scale.

NURSING ACTIONS/INTERVENTIONS WITH RATIONALES

Adult Health

ACTIONS/INTERVENTIONS	RATIONALES
Monitor for pain at least every 2 hours on [odd/even] hour. Utilize appropriate method of assessment (e.g., numeric pain scales, behavior assessment).	Pain is subjective in nature, and only the patient can fully describe it.
Teach the patient to report pain as soon as it starts. Allow the patient to describe the pain in detail to include aggravating factors, relieving factors, type of pain (burning, tingling, throbbing).	Pain is more readily controlled when it is treated early. Treating pain at first report prevents the client from experiencing a "roller coaster" effect of pain relief alternating with pain elevation.

(care plan continued on page 488)

NURSING ACTIONS/INTERVENTIONS WITH RATIONALES (continued from page 487)

Adult Health

ACTIONS/INTERVENTIONS	RATIONALES
Administer pain medication as prescribed. Reassess and document amount of pain relief within 30 minutes after administration. Devise alternate methods for pain relief in conjunction with other health-care team members if pain is not relieved. [Note that plan here.]	Response to pain and pain medication is unique to each patient.
Consider continuous dosing (e.g., continuous drip or PCA for patients with consistent pain).	Avoids a roller coaster effect in pain relief.
Consider alternative methods including massage, biofeedback, progressive relaxation, or guided imagery. [Note methods to be used with client here.]	
Turn at least every 2 hours on [odd/even] hour. Maintain anatomic alignment with pillows or other padded support.	Helps stimulate circulation. Alignment helps prevent pain from malposition and enhances comfort.
Provide calm, quiet environment.	Promotes action and effect of medication by providing decreased stimuli.
Monitor vital signs at least every 4 hours while awake at [times].	Detects early changes that might indicate pain.
Monitor the sleep–rest pattern. Promote rest periods during day and at least 8 hours sleep each night. (See nursing actions for Disturbed Sleep Pattern, Chapter 6.)	Fatigue may contribute to an increased pain response, or pain can contribute to interrupted sleep.
Check bowel elimination at least once per shift.	Immobility caused by pain may decrease the parasympathetic stimulation to the bowel. Many analgesics have constipation as a side effect.
Allow time for the patient to discuss fears and anxieties related to pain by scheduling at least 15 minutes once per shift to visit with the patient on one-to-one basis.	Just as pain is unique to the individual, so is the pain control intervention. Discussions with the patient provide collaboration and increase the patient's compliance. Decreases feeling of powerlessness, and initiates basic teaching regarding control of pain.
Collaborate with health-care team regarding use of transcutaneous electrical nerve stimulation (TENS).	Collaboration promotes the best approach to pain management.
Teach the patient and significant others: • Cause of pain • Common and expected side effects of analgesics • The low rate of addiction when narcotics are used for pain • The importance of maintaining round-the-clock dosing for continuous pain and preventive dosing for expected pain • Avoiding and minimizing pain • Splinting • Gradual increase in activities • Use of alternative noninvasive techniques (See previous nursing action.) • Combining techniques (e.g., medication with relaxation technique)	Knowledge assists the patient in feeling like an active participant on the health team. Decreases sense of powerlessness. Promotes effective pain management.
Refer the patient to or collaborate with other health-care professionals.	Collaboration promotes the best long-range plan for management of pain.

ADDITIONAL INFORMATION

Keep current on comparative doses of analgesics, true effect of so-called potentiators, and noninvasive means of pain relief. Do not worry about a patient becoming addicted. With the average length of stay of 3 to 5 days, it is doubtful addiction could occur. Current research in this area shows an extremely low rate of addiction due to medication administration in a health-care setting. The same research indicates that we undermedicate, rather than overmedicate, for pain. Undermedication is particularly true in the case of infants, children, and older adults. See the Department of Health and Human Services Guidelines[60] for a discussion of this research as well as further information on pain control.

Child Health

ACTIONS/INTERVENTIONS	RATIONALES
Monitor for contributory factors to pain at least every 1 to 2 hours, or according to need. • Physical injury or surgical incision • Stressors • Fears • Knowledge deficit • Anxieties • Fatigue • Description of exact nature of pain, whether per the McGill, Elkind or faces by Wong pain assessment tool • Vital signs—many consider pain to be a fifth vital sign. • Response to medication • Meaning of pain to the child and family	Provides the essential database for planning and modification of planning.
Provide appropriate support in management of pain for the patient and significant others by: • Validation of the pain • Maintaining self-control to extent feasible • Providing education to deal with pain and assist the patient and family to talk about the pain experience by allowing at least [number] minutes per shift for such ventilation and education at [times]. [Note topics to be addressed for this client here.] • Allowing the parents to be present and participate in comforting of the patient; assisting the child and parents to develop a plan of care that addresses individual needs and is likely to result in a better coping pattern (particularly for chronic pain). [Note client's plan here.] • Appropriate diversional activities for age and developmental level *Collaborate with child life specialist to identify appropriate activities. • Attention to controlling external stimuli such as noise and light • Use of relaxation techniques appropriate for the child's capacity. (This could include visual imagery of favorite places or comforting situations.) • Appropriate follow-up of pain tolerance and response to medication as ordered.	Validation and support of the patient and family will serve to show value and respect for the individual's health need. Maintains basic standards of care. Ventilation reduces anxiety, and parental involvement enhances coping skills.
Facilitate provision of pain medication by least invasive and most effective. Insist on appropriate and prompt mode for relief of pain.	Utilize least invasive and most individually safe, effective and appropriate mode of pain relief for child.

(care plan continued on page 490)

Child Health

ACTIONS/INTERVENTIONS	RATIONALES

If IV route is utilized, monitor for respiratory and blood pressure depression every 10 minutes × 6 at [times].

Monitor intake and output for decrease as a result of hypomotility or spasm.

Give appropriate emotional support during painful procedures or experiences:
- Provide explanations at the child's level of openness and honesty.
- Use puppets to demonstrate the procedure.
- Explain to the parents that even if the child cries excessively, their presence is encouraged.
- Comfort child before, during, and after procedure.
- Reward the child for positive behavior according to developmental need (e.g., stars on a chart). [Note rewards to be used here.]
- Facilitate parents and child sharing feelings about the painful experience while providing care.

Collaborate with or refer the patient to appropriate health-care team members.

Teach the patient and family ways to follow up at home or school with needed pain regimen:
- Appropriate timing of medication
- Appropriate administration of medication
- Not to substitute acetaminophen for aspirin in arthritis
- Contact the school nurse with the plan of care

Monitor for side effects of medications such as decreased peristalsis, GI bleed, and respiratory depression.

Develop daily plans for pain management that meet the child's individual needs. [Note that plan here.]

Develop several contingency pain control plans. Note plans for this client here.

● **N O T E :** *Chronic pain is going to recur; therefore, there is a need for long-term follow-up. This follow-up is especially critical because chronic pain places the patient at risk for developmental delays and altered quality of life.*

Women's Health

Gynecologic Pain

● **N O T E :** *A significant amount of the pain experienced by women is associated with the pelvic area and the reproductive organs. Determining the origin of the pain is one of the most difficult tasks facing nurses dealing with the gynecologic patient. An organic explanation for pain is never found in approximately 25 percent of women. Because of the close association with the reproductive organs, gynecologic pain can be extremely frightening, can connote social stigma, affect the perception of the feminine role, cause anger and guilt, and totally dominate the woman's existence. "Pain is culturally more acceptable in certain parts of the body and may elicit more sympathy than pain in other sites."*[31,62]

ACTIONS/INTERVENTIONS	RATIONALES
Identify factors in the patient's lifestyle that could be contributing to pain.	Provides the database to adequately assess pain and determine the underlying cause.
Record accurate menstrual cycle and obstetric, gynecologic, and sexual history, being certain to note problems, previous pregnancies, descriptions of previous labors, previous infections or gynecologic problems, and any infections as a result of sexual activities.	
Assist the client to describe her perception of pain as it relates to her.	
Include dysmenorrhea pain pattern, being certain to determine whether the pain occurs before, during, or after menstruation.	
Monitor disturbance of the client's daily routine as a result of pain. Have the patient describe the location of the pain (e.g., lower abdomen, legs, breast, or back).	
Have the patient describe any edema, especially "bloating" at specific times during the month.	
Have the patient describe the onset and character of the pain (e.g., mild or severe cramping).	
Ascertain whether the pain is associated with nausea, vomiting, or diarrhea.	
Identify any precipitating factors associated with pain (e.g., emotional upsets, exercise, or medication).	This information can assist in pinpointing source of pain and devising a plan of care.
Assist the patient in identifying various methods of pain relief, including exercise (pelvic rock), biofeedback, relaxation, and medication (analgesics and antiprostaglandins).	Individualizes pain control and provides options for the patient.

Women's Health

Labor Pain and Nursing

ACTIONS/INTERVENTIONS	RATIONALES
Labor	
Encourage the patient to describe her perception of labor pain related to her previous laboring experiences.	Providing information about the laboring process helps the patient cope with the pain of labor.[13,31,63]
Provide factual information about the laboring process.	
Refer the patient to childbirth preparation group (e.g., Lamaze groups).	
Describe methods of coping with labor pain (e.g., relaxation, imaging, breathing, medication, hydrotherapy, or ambulation).	
Provide support during labor.	
Encourage involvement of significant others as support during labor process.	
Postpartum	
Encourage the patient to describe her perception of pain associated with the postpartum period.	

(care plan continued on page 492)

NURSING ACTIONS/INTERVENTIONS WITH RATIONALES (continued from page 491)

Women's Health

ACTIONS/INTERVENTIONS	RATIONALES
Provide information for pain relief (e.g., Kegel exercises, sitz baths, or medications).	
Explain etiology of "afterbirth pains" to involution of uterus.	Knowing the source of pain increases the patient's sense of control.
Explain the relationship of breastfeeding to involution and uterine contractions.	
Assist the patient in putting on a supportive bra.	
Encourage early, frequent breastfeedings to enhance let-down reflex.	
Support the patient and provide information on correct breastfeeding techniques, such as changing positions from one feeding to next to distribute sucking pressure and prevent sore nipples.	Knowledge of how to lessen discomfort during breastfeeding contributes to successful or effective breastfeeding.
Check the baby's position on the breast; be certain the areola is in mouth and not just the nipple.	
Provide warm, moist heat for relief of engorged breasts.	Demonstrates to the patient various pain relief methods.
Provide analgesics for discomfort of engorged breasts.	
Pump after the infant nurses until the breast is emptied.	
Encourage the patient to nurse on least sore side first to encourage let-down reflex.	
Apply ice to nipple just before nursing to decrease pain.	

Mental Health

● N O T E : *Pain in the mental health client should be carefully assessed for physiologic causes. The following interventions are for pain associated with psychological factors or chronic pain. For chronic pain, they are used in conjunction with physiologic interventions. Refer to Adult Health nursing actions for physiologic pain management strategies.*

ACTIONS/INTERVENTIONS	RATIONALES
Monitor the nurse's response to the client's perception of pain. If the nurse has difficulty understanding or coping with the client's expression of pain, he or she should discuss these feelings with a colleague in an attempt to resolve the concerns.	The nurse's response to the client can be communicated and have an effect on the client's level of anxiety, which can then affect the pain response.
Note any recurring patterns in the pain experience, such as time of day, recent social interactions, or physical activity. If a pattern is present, begin a discussion of this observation with the client.	Initiates the client's awareness of this pattern, and allows the nurse to assess the client's perception of this observation.
Determine effects pain has had on the client's life, including role responsibilities, financial impact, cognitive and emotional functioning, and family interactions.	Assesses meaning of pain to the client's amount of anxiety associated with the pain and possible benefits of pain in the client's life. Change depends on the client's perception of the problem.[58]
Review the client's beliefs and attitudes about the role pain is assuming in the client's life. If pain is very important to the client's definition of self, assure the client that you are not requiring him or her to give up	If pain is assuming an important role, then it might be difficult for the client to "give up" all of the pain, and this should be considered in all further interventions.[49,50]

ACTIONS/INTERVENTIONS	RATIONALES
the pain by indicating that you are only interested in that pain that causes undue discomfort or by indicating that this client's pain is special and that it would be difficult, if not impossible, for the health care team to get rid of it.	
Spend brief, goal-directed time with the client when he or she is focusing conversation on pain or pain-related activities.	Decreases positive reinforcement for the client's focus on pain and diminishes secondary gain for pain.
Schedule a time with the client when he or she is not complaining about pain. List this schedule here. Focus on special activities in which the client is involved or follow-up on a non–pain-related conversation the client seemed to enjoy.	Provides positive feedback to the client about an aspect of himself or herself that is not pain related.
Find at least one non–pain-related activity the client enjoys that can be the source of positive interaction between the client and others, and encourage client participation in this activity with positive reinforcement (list client-specific positive reinforcers here along with the activity).	Reinforcement encourages a positive behavior and improves self-esteem.
Discuss with the client alternatives for meeting personal need currently being met by pain. You may need to refer the client to another, more specialized care provider if this is a problem of long standing or if the client demonstrates difficulty in discussing these concerns. Refer to the self-esteem diagnoses (Chapter 8) for specific interventions related to perceptions of self.	
Develop with the client a plan to alter those factors that intensify the pain experience. For example, if the pain increases at 4 P.M. each day and the client associates this with his boss's daily visit at 5 P.M., then the plan might include limiting the visits from the boss or having another person present when the boss visits. [List specific interventions here.]	The social milieu can change the basic quality of the pain experience.
Develop with the client plan for learning relaxation techniques, and have the client practice technique 30 minutes two times a day at [times]. Remain with the client during practice session to provide verbal cues and encouragement as necessary. These techniques can include: • Meditation • Progressive deep muscle relaxation • Visualization techniques that require the client to visualize scenes that enhance the relaxation response (such as being on the beach or having the sun warm the body) • Biofeedback • Prayer • Autogenic training	These techniques decrease anxiety.
Monitor interaction of analgesic with other medications the client is receiving, especially antianxiety, antipsychotic, and hypnotic drugs. Collaborate with pharmacist and physician to maintain adequate pain control.	These medications may potentiate one another.

(care plan continued on page 494)

NURSING ACTIONS/INTERVENTIONS WITH RATIONALES (continued from page 493)

Mental Health

ACTIONS/INTERVENTIONS	RATIONALES
Review the client's history for indication of illicit drug use and the effects this may have on the client's tolerance to analgesics.	The client may have developed a cross-tolerance for these drugs.
If the client is to be withdrawn from the analgesic, discuss the alternative coping methods and how they will assist the client with the process. Assure the client that support will be provided during this process. Help the client identify those situations that will be most difficult, and schedule one-to-one time with the client during these times.	Promotes perception of control, and decreases anxiety.
• Develop plan with client for management of pain without analgesics. [Note patients plan here.]	
If the client demonstrates altered mood, refer to Ineffective Individual Coping (Chapter 11) for interventions.	
Consult with occupational therapy to assist the client in developing diversional activities. [Note time for these activities here as well as a list of special equipment that may be necessary for the activity.]	Decreases conscious awareness of pain, thus decreasing the pain experience.
Consult with physical therapy to develop exercise routines that will facilitate pain management. [Note support needed from nursing to facilitate exercise plan.]	
Involve the client in group activities by sitting with him or her during a group activity, such as a game, or assign the client a responsibility for preparing one part of a unit meal. Begin with activities that require little concentration, and then gradually increase the task complexity.	Alters the client's perception of the pain.
Consult with physician for possible referral for use of hypnosis in pain management.	
Sit with the client and the family during at least two visits to assess family interactions with the client and the role pain plays in family interaction.	
Discuss with the client the role of distraction in pain management, and develop a list of those activities the client finds distracting and enjoyable. These could include listening to music, watching television or special movies, or physical activity. Develop with the client a plan for including these activities in the pain management program, and list that plan here.	Provides other pain relief options for the client.
Discuss with the client the role that exercise can play in pain management, and develop an exercise program with the client. This should begin at or below the client's capabilities and could include a 15-minute walk twice a day or 10 minutes on a stationary bicycle. [Note the plan here, with the type of activity, length of time, and time of day it is to be implemented.]	Exercise encourages release of natural endorphins.
Provide positive reinforcement to the client for implementing the exercise program by spending time with	Positive reinforcement encourages repeating the behavior and enhances self-esteem.

ACTIONS/INTERVENTIONS	RATIONALES
the client during the exercise, providing verbal feedback, and allowing the client the rewards that have been developed. These rewards are developed with the client. [Note reward schedule to be used here.]	
Monitor family and support system understanding of the pain and perceptions of the client. If they demonstrate the attitude that interaction with the client is closely linked with the pain, then develop a plan to include them in the experiences described here. List that plan here. Consider referral to a clinical specialist in mental health nursing or a family therapist to assist the family in developing non–pain-related interaction patterns.	Assists the family in normalizing and in moving away from a pain-focused identity.
Provide ongoing feedback to the client or support system about progress.	
Refer to outpatient support systems, and assist with arranging for the client to contact these systems before discharge.	Long-term support enhances the likelihood of effective home management.

Gerontic Health

In addition to the following interventions, the interventions for Adult Health can be applied to the aging client.

ACTIONS/INTERVENTIONS	RATIONALES
Acute Pain	
Ask the client about the presence of pain using a 0 to 10 scale, word descriptor scale, faces scale, or pain thermometer at least every 2 hours.	Pain is often underreported or minimized. Asking and using a scale facilitates reporting and understanding of pain intensity.
For clients with cognitive impairment, assessment of behaviors and family or caregiver observations should be used to assess for pain.	Early identification of pain facilitates effective treatment.[64]
Abstain from the use of placebos.	The use of placebos is unethical and impairs the trust relationship between client and nurse.[64]
Opioids for episodic pain (non-recurring) should be prescribed as needed, rather than round the clock. (NGC, Retrieved February 8, 2006 from http:// www.guidelines.gov)	Prevention of overuse.
Assess the client often and regularly for breakthrough pain: • End of dose failure • Incident pain • Spontaneous, unpredictable pain and titrate dose accordingly	Maintain adequate pain control.
Titrate medications in the older client carefully, considering the propensity for drug accumulation, drug interactions, and side effects.[64]	Pharmocokinetics and pharmacodynamics are affected by the aging process.
Assess clients taking opioid analgesics regularly and often for alterations in bowel function and treat constipation as needed. Anticipate slowed bowel motility when starting an opioid analgesic and begin preventive stool softeners concurrently.[64]	Opioid analgesics consistently cause slowing in bowel motility and subsequent constipation.

(care plan continued on page 496)

NURSING ACTIONS/INTERVENTIONS WITH RATIONALES (continued from page 495)

Gerontic Health

ACTIONS/INTERVENTIONS	RATIONALES
Medicate every 4 to 6 hours rather than on an as needed (PRN) basis for the first 48 to 72 hours, especially postoperatively.[65]	Enhances pain control, and thus promotes early mobility, which decreases the potential for postoperative complications.
Collaborate with physician to prescribe medications other than meperidine, talwin, methadone, and darvon, if a narcotic analgesic is required.	These medications are more likely to cause side effects such as confusion and psychotic behavior when given to the older adult.[66]
When beginning a new medication for pain, start with the lowest dose and increase slowly as needed.[66]	Older adults often respond differently to pain medications than younger adults.
Investigate the patient's beliefs regarding pain. Does he or she consider pain a punishment? Does he or she think that having to take pain medication signals severe illness or a potential for dying?[67]	May be a barrier to seeking pain relief.
Teach the patient to report pain as soon as it occurs, especially if medication order is PRN.	Pain is more easily controlled when treated early. Patient may not realize that medication won't be given on a scheduled basis.
Avoid presenting self in a hurried manner.	Older adults are less likely to report pain if caregiver is rushed.[67]

Chronic Pain

Explore with the patient how he or she has managed chronic pain in the past.	Assists in determining what measures were of significant or of little help.
Determine use of distraction in helping the patient cope with chronic pain.[65]	Music, humor, and relaxation techniques can provide temporary respite from discomfort.
Monitor skin status when thermal interventions are used, such as ice or heat packs.	Changes in sensation may result in thermal injury if not closely monitored.
In the presence of chronic pain, depression may also exist. Screen for depression.[64]	Chronic pain is exhausting physically and mentally.

Home Health

ACTIONS/INTERVENTIONS	RATIONALES
Teach the client and family measures to promote comfort: • Proper positioning • Appropriate use of medications (e.g., narcotics as ordered, nonnarcotic analgesics, anti-inflammatories) • Knowledge regarding source of pain or of disease process • Self-management of pain and of care as much as is appropriate • Relaxation techniques • Therapeutic touch • Massage (if not contraindicated) • Distraction • Breathing techniques • Heat or cold treatments (if not contraindicated) • Regular activity and exercise • Planning and goal setting	Involvement of the client and family promotes comfort and decreases self-reported pain and analgesic use.[65]

ACTIONS/INTERVENTIONS	RATIONALES
• Biofeedback • Yoga or tai chi • Imagery or hypnosis • Group or family therapy	
Teach the client and family factors that decrease tolerance to pain and methods for decreasing these factors: • Lack of knowledge regarding disease process or pain control methods • Lack of support from significant others regarding the severity of the pain	Reducing these factors can increase the tolerance to pain.[66]
• Fear of addiction or fear of loss of control. • Fatigue • Boredom • Improper positioning	Addiction occurs very infrequently in clients medicated for legitimate pain.[64]
Involve the client and family in planning, implementing, and promoting reduction in pain: • Family conference • Mutual goal setting • Communication • Support for the caregiver	Involvement improves motivation and improves outcome.
Assist the client and family in lifestyle adjustments that may be required: • Occupational changes • Family role alterations • Comfort measures for chronic pain • Financial situation • Responses to pain (mood, concentration, or ability to complete activities of daily living) • Coping with disability or dependency • Mechanism for altering need for assistance • Providing appropriate balance of dependence and independence • Stress management • Time management • Obtaining and using assistive equipment (e.g., for arthritis) • Regular, rather than as-needed, schedule of pain medication	Lifestyle changes require changes in behavior.
Teach the client and family purposes, side effects, and proper administration techniques of medications.	Provides necessary information for safe self-care.
Consult with or refer to appropriate assistive resources as indicated.	Use of the existing community services network provides effective utilization of resources.

SENSORY PERCEPTION, DISTURBED (SPECIFY: VISUAL, AUDITORY, KINESTHETIC, GUSTATORY, TACTILE, OLFACTORY)

DEFINITION[2]

Change in the amount or patterning of incoming stimuli accompanied by a diminished, exaggerated, distorted, or impaired response to such stimuli.[2]

DEFINING CHARACTERISTICS[2]

1. Poor concentration
2. Auditory distractions
3. Change in usual response to stimuli
4. Restlessness
5. Reported or measured change in sensory acuity
6. Irritability
7. Disoriented in time, in place, or with people
8. Change in problem-solving abilities

9. Change in behavior pattern
10. Altered communication patterns
11. Hallucinations
12. Visual distortions

RELATED FACTORS[2]

1. Altered sensory perception
2. Excessive environmental stimuli
3. Psychological stress
4. Altered sensory reception, transmissions, and/or integration
5. Insufficient environmental stimuli
6. Biochemical imbalances for sensory distortion (e.g., illusions or hallucinations)
7. Electrolyte imbalance
8. Biochemical imbalance

RELATED CLINICAL CONCERNS

1. Any neurologic diagnosis
2. Glaucoma or cataracts
3. Intensive care unit patient
4. Psychosis
5. Substance abuse
6. Toxemia

 Have You Selected the Correct Diagnosis?

Disturbed Thought Process
Disturbed Thought Process refers to a patient's cognitive abilities, whereas Disturbed Sensory Perception relates to just the sensory input–output.

Self-Care Deficit
Certainly sensory perception problems could result in self-care deficits; however, one diagnosis refers to ability to care for the self, whereas the other focuses on response to sensory input.

EXPECTED OUTCOME

Will identify and initiate at least two adaptive ways to compensate for [specific sensory deficit] by [date].

TARGET DATES

Assisting the patient in dealing with an uncompensated sensory deficit is a long-term process. Also, the patient may never accept the deficit but can be helped to adapt to the deficit. Therefore, an appropriate target date would be no sooner than 5 to 7 days from the date of diagnosis.

NURSING ACTIONS/INTERVENTIONS WITH RATIONALES

Adult Health

ACTIONS/INTERVENTIONS	RATIONALES

Check safety factors frequently:
• Siderails
• Uncluttered room
• Lighting: Dim at night, increased during day, and nonglare
• Environment arranged to assist in compensating for specific deficit
  • Orient to room
  • Provide calm, nonthreatening environment
	Basic safety measures.

Place bedside table and over-the-bed table in same position each time and within easy reach. Ascertain which items the patient wants on these tables and where the items are to be placed. Place items in same place each time.	Maintains consistency of environment, which facilitates the patient's comfort and decreases anxiety.
Have significant others bring familiar items from home.	Enhances physical and psychological comfort.
Promote consistency in care (e.g., same nurse, as near same routine as possible).	Decreases unessential stimuli. Inspires trust. Reinforces the patient's own routine.
Follow the patient's own routine as much as possible (e.g., bath, bedtime, meals, and grooming. Pace activities to the patient's preference). [Note client preferences here.]	Promotes comfort and empowers the patient.
Provide reality orientation as necessary:	Reinforces reality.

ACTIONS/INTERVENTIONS	RATIONALES
• Keep clock and calendar in room. • Touch the patient frequently. • Check orientation to person, time, and place at least once per shift. • Listen carefully. Collaborate with occupational therapist regarding appropriate diversionary activity. [Note recommendations here with support needed for implementation.]	Provides stimuli.

Auditory Deficit

Enhance communication by speaking in low tones when interacting with the patient.	Allows for alteration in hearing high-frequency sounds. High-frequency tones are lost first.
• Do not shout when talking with the client.	Shouting accentuates vowel sounds while decreasing consonant sounds.
• Decrease background noise as much as possible when talking with the client.	Avoids confusion, and increases the patient's ability to localize sounds.
• Stand where the client can watch your lips when you are speaking to him or her.	
Allow the patient extended time to respond to verbal messages.	Allows for understanding and interpretation of message.
Use visual cues as much as possible to enhance verbal messages.	Utilizes alternative communication methods.
• Provide message board to use with the patient.	
Teach the patient and family proper maintenance of hearing aid.	Promotes proper functioning of hearing aid.
• Replace batteries in hearing aids and clean earwax for ear mold of hearing aid as necessary	

Visual Deficit

Assure that glasses or other visual aids are available and placed proximal to patient.	Facilitates the patient's use of equipment, and assists in preventing damage or loss of equipment.
Provide written information in large-print or audio recorded format.	
Provide telephone dials and other equipment necessary that have large numbers on nonglare surfaces. List here special equipment that is necessary for this patient and when the patient may need it so it can be provided at appropriate times.	
Identify the patient's room with large numbers or the patient's name in large print.	
Provide large-screen television and pictures with large, colorful images.	Larger images are easier for the patient to interpret.
Provide nonglare work surfaces.	
Identify stairs and door frames with contrasting tape or paint.	Increases visual acuity. Basic safety measure.
Verbally address the patient when entering the patient's proximity, and approach the patient from the front.	Makes the patient aware of presence.
Do not alter the patient's physical environment without telling him or her of the changes.	Promotes consistency in environment, which improves safety.
Teach the patient and family proper maintenance of eyeglasses and other prosthesis.	Ensures proper functioning and prevents scratching of lenses.

(care plan continued on page 500)

NURSING ACTIONS/INTERVENTIONS WITH RATIONALES (continued from page 499)

Adult Health

ACTIONS/INTERVENTIONS	RATIONALES
Teach the patient and family methods to improve environmental safety.	
Assist the patient with activities of daily living (ADLs) as necessary. List the activities that require assistance here, along with the type of assistance that is needed (e.g., assisting the patient to eat to extent necessary [feed totally or cut up food and open packages]).	Allows the patient to be as independent as possible.
Touch and Kinesthesia Deficit	
Provide safe environment:	Basic safety measures.
• Remove sharp objects from the patient's environment.	
• Protect the patient from exposure to excessive heat and cold.	Basic safety measures to prevent accidental burns.
Teach patient to utilize visualization as a method to assess for injury and method for compensation for decrease in tactile response.	
Have the patient change position every 2 hours on [even/odd] hour.	Promotes circulation, and relieves pressure on bony prominences.
Monitor condition of skin every 4 hours at [times]. Note any alteration in integrity. Teach the patient to visually inspect skin on a daily basis.	Guards against skin breakdown.
Assist the patient in determining whether clothing is fitting properly without abrading the skin.	
Perform and teach adequate foot care on a daily basis to include: [Note schedule here and teaching plan.]	
• Bathing feet in warm water	
• Applying moisturizing lotion	
• Trimming nails as needed	
• Checking skin for abrasions or reddened areas	
Assist the patient with care of affected body parts.	Prevents unilateral neglect, and provides cues for the patient.
Assist the patient with ADLs (note type and amount of assistance needed here).	Promotes self-care through demonstrating care to the patient.
Refer the patient to occupational therapy for assisting with learning new self-care behavior.	
Olfactory Deficit	
Teach patient to utilize other senses to adapt to deficit including visualization, color and texture assessments.	
Determine effect the smell deficit has on the patient's appetite, and work with dietitian to make meals visually appealing.	Assists to compensate for loss of smell.
Provide for appropriate follow-up appointments before dismissal. [Note referral plan here.]	Providing specific appointments lessens the confusion about the specifics of appointments and increases the likelihood of subsequent follow-through.

Child Health

ACTIONS/INTERVENTIONS	RATIONALES
Determine how the parent and child perceive the deficit addressed by setting aside adequate time (30 minutes) each shift for discussion and listening.	Appropriate attention to both subjective as well as objective data is required to best plan care.
Facilitate follow-up evaluation for any suspected sensory deficits of infants and young children. [Note plan for follow-up here.]	Preventing or minimizing secondary and tertiary deficits is enhanced by appropriate attention to sensory perception follow-up.
Provide safe environment according to sensory deficit and the child's developmental capacity. [Note special adaptations for client here.]	Sensory deficits and developmental capacity increase the risk of accidents.
Initiate plans for discharge immediately to provide time for building confidence in the performance of necessary self-care tasks.	Adequate practice time in a nonjudgmental situation allows positive feedback and corrective action. Lessens anxiety and performance pressures. Increases confidence in giving care at home.
Provide attention to family coping as it may relate to the deficit: • Monitoring of usual dynamics • Identification of impact on the parents and siblings • Presence of mental deficits • Values regarding the deficit • Support systems	A child with sensory perception problems and the interventions necessary to deal with these problems place strain on the family. Promoting coping will lessen the strain on the family while increasing the likelihood that the child's needs are met.
Review for appropriate immunization, especially rubella, mumps, and measles.	In the event of early deficits, the likelihood exists for the need to modify the schedule of immunization. This is too often overlooked and will then place the infant or child at unnecessary risk for infectious diseases.
In the presence of ear infections, exercise caution regarding use of ototoxic medications.	Treatment for chronic infections with antibiotics by several practitioners must be carried out with precaution to prevent potential side effects.
Correlate medical history for potential risk factors such as chronic middle ear infections, upper respiratory infections, or allergies.	Contributory factors to the pattern of health must be pursued with openness to all possible causes.
Provide appropriate sensory stimulation for age, beginning slowly so as not to overload child. [Note special adaptations for this client here.]	Appropriate sensory stimulation will favor gradual progress in development.
Deal with other contributory factors such as nutrition, illness, or effects from behavioral disorders or medications.	Related factors must be considered in total health of the infant or child with altered sensory–perceptual pattern.
Include the parents in plans for rehabilitation whenever possible by: • Using basic plan for care • Adapting intervention as required for the child • Supporting them in their role • Pointing out opportune times for interaction • Informing them of appropriate safety precautions for the child's age and situation • Encouraging gentle handling and comforting of the infant	Inclusion of the parents provides an opportunity for learning essential skills and enhances security of the infant or child. All efforts contribute to empowerment and potential growth of the family unit.
Provide continuity in staffing for nursing care of the child and family.	Continuity provides trust and opportunities for reinforcement of learning.

(care plan continued on page 502)

NURSING ACTIONS/INTERVENTIONS WITH RATIONALES (continued from page 501)

Child Health

ACTIONS/INTERVENTIONS	RATIONALES
In instances of a handicapped child, provide appropriate attention to developing sequencing to best actualize potential offered.	Appropriate introduction of new skills or reinforcement of existent patterns will favor progress.
Especially note, on follow-up, the home environment for nurturing aspects and support systems.	The home to which the infant or child will go may require reasonable adaptation to foster appropriate resources.

Women's Health

ACTIONS/INTERVENTIONS	RATIONALES
Vision	
Monitor the patient for signs of pregnancy-induced hypertension (PIH).	Knowledge of signs of visual disturbances associated with PIH can assist the patient in seeking early treatment.[13,14]
Monitor for signs and symptoms of preeclampsia (e.g., headaches, visual changes such as blurred vision, increased edema of face, oliguria, hyperreflexia, nausea or vomiting, and epigastric pain).[13,14]	
Teach the patient the importance of reporting these signs and symptoms, because they can be precursors to eclampsia.	
Smell	
Be aware of the patient's tendency during early pregnancy to experience morning sickness, i.e., nausea and vomiting.	
In collaboration with dietitian:	
• Obtain dietary history.	
• Assist the patient in planning diet that will provide adequate nutrition for her and her fetus's needs.	
Teach methods for coping with gastric upset, nausea, and vomiting:	Knowledge can assist the patient in planning actions to decrease incidences of nausea and vomiting and assist in preventing dehydration and possibly hospitalization.
• Eating bland, low-fat foods	
• Increasing carbohydrate intake	
• Eating small, frequent meals	
• Having dry crackers or toast before getting out of bed	
• Taking vitamins and iron with snack before going to bed	
• Supplementing diet with high-protein liquids (e.g., soups or eggnog)	
Touch During Pregnancy	
Be aware of the expectant mother's sensitivity to extraneous touching:	Assists the mother to know that her feelings are normal.
• Shyness	
• Protectiveness of unborn child	
• Uterine sensitivity during pregnancy and particularly during labor	
Maternal Touch	
Encourage visual and tactile contact between the mother and infant as soon as possible.	Provides time for beginning attachment process between the mother and infant.

ACTIONS/INTERVENTIONS	RATIONALES
Provide an atmosphere conducive to continual mother–infant contact.	
Delay newborn eye treatment for 1 hour, so that the baby can see the mother's face.	
Kinesthesia	
Be aware of the expectant mother's increased vulnerability related to physical size of body in third trimester: • Protectiveness of unborn child • Heavy movement • Possible slowed reflexes • Tires easily	Reassures mothers that this is a temporary state.
Assist in and out of furniture that is too low and difficult to get up from.	
Encourage correct body mechanics when lying down or sitting up.	
Encourage to wear seat belt when traveling in automobile. (Shoulder belts are best.)	Provides for safety measures for the mother and fetus.

Mental Health

ACTIONS/INTERVENTIONS	RATIONALES
Monitor the client's neurologic status as indicated by current condition and history of deficit (e.g., if deficit is recent, assessment would be conducted on a schedule that could range from every 15 minutes to every 8 hours). Note the frequency and times of checks here. If checks are to be very frequent, then it might be useful to keep a record of these checks on a flow sheet.	Client safety is of primary importance. Early recognition and intervention can prevent serious alterations.
If deficit is determined to result from a psychological rather than a physiologic dysfunction, refer to Ineffective Individual Coping, Disturbed Body Image, Anxiety, and Chronic Low or Situational Low Self-Esteem for detailed nursing actions.	Client safety is of primary importance.

● NOTE: *A comprehensive physical examination and other diagnostic evaluations should be completed before this determination is made. Each of these deficits can be symptoms of severe physiologic or neurologic dysfunction and should be approached with this understanding, especially in a mental health environment where the clients may be assigned without careful assessment. This is a great risk for the client who has a history of mental health problems.*

If deficit is related to a physiologic dysfunction, attend to needs resulting from the identified sensory deficit in a matter-of-fact manner, providing basic care and having the client do the majority of the care. (See Adult Health interventions for additional care.)	Provides positive reinforcement for adaptive coping behaviors.
If deficit is related to a psychological dysfunction, spend [number] minutes every hour with the client in an activity that is not related to the sensory deficit. If the client begins to focus on the deficit, terminate the interaction.	Promotes the client's sense of control, and increases self-esteem. Provides positive reinforcement for positive coping behaviors and removes social reinforcement for negative coping behaviors.[19]

(care plan continued on page 504)

Mental Health

ACTIONS/INTERVENTIONS	RATIONALES
Spend [number] minutes twice a day discussing with the client the effects the deficit will have on his or her life and developing alternative coping behavior. Note times for conversations here. If the family is involved in the client's care, they should be included on a planned number of these interactions.	
Refer to appropriate mental health professional if the client is going to require long-term assistance in adapting to the deficit or if current emotional adaptation becomes complicated.	
Discuss with the client and support system the necessary alterations that may be necessary in the home environment to facilitate daily living activities.	Promotes the client's sense of control.

Auditory or Visual Alterations[68–71]

ACTIONS/INTERVENTIONS	RATIONALES
Observe for signs of hallucinations (intent listening for no apparent reason, talking to someone when no one is present, muttering to self, stopping in mid-sentence, or unusual posturing). When these symptoms are noted, engage the client in here-and-now, reality-oriented conversation or involve the client in here-and-now activity.	Interrupts patterns of hallucinations.
Initiate touch only after warning the client that you are going to touch him or her.	The client may perceive touch as a threat and respond in an aggressive manner.
Communicate acceptance to the client to encourage the sharing of the content of the hallucination.	Provides information on the content of the hallucination so early intervention can be initiated when content suggests harm to the client or others.
If hallucinations place the client at risk for self-harm or harm to others, place the client on one-to-one observation or in seclusion.	Client and staff safety are of primary importance.
If the client is placed in seclusion, interact with the client at least every 15 minutes.	Provides reality orientation, and assists the client in controlling the hallucinations.
Have the client tell staff when hallucinations are present or when they are interfering with the client's ability to interact with others.	Early intervention promotes the client's sense of safety and control.
Maintain environment in a manner that does not enhance hallucinations (e.g., television programs that validate the client's hallucinations, abstract art on the walls, wallpaper with abstract designs, or designs that enhance imagination).	High levels of environmental stimuli can increase the client's disorganization and confusion.
Teach the client to control hallucinations by: • Checking ideas out with trusted others • Practicing thought stopping by singing to self, telling the voices to go away (This can be done quietly to self, or by asking the voices to come back later, but not to talk now.) • Telling the voices to go away, using headphones to listen to music, watching TV, or wearing ear plug in one ear.	Promotes the client's sense of control, and enhances self-esteem. Provides control of auditory alterations.[72]

ACTIONS/INTERVENTIONS	RATIONALES
When the client is not constantly experiencing alterations, engage him or her in a group that addresses management of these alterations.	Facilitates interaction, self-management, and monitoring of symptoms, and instills hope.[72]
When the client is responding to hallucinations, respond to the feelings expressed in the client's communication.	
Respond to the client with "I" statements ("I do not see or hear that") when they request validation of hallucinations. Do not argue with client's experience.	Provides indirect confrontation of their experience. Preserves self-esteem while indicating that nurse does not experience the same stimuli.[73]
Talk with the client about ways to distract him- or herself from the hallucinations, such as physical exercise, playing a game or a craft that takes a great deal of concentration. [Note those activities preferred by the client here.]	
When signs of the client's hallucinating are present, assist the client in initiating those activities or other control behaviors that have been identified by the client as useful.	Reinforces new coping behaviors, and increases the client's perceived control.
As the client's condition improves, primary nurse will assist the client to identify onset of hallucinations and situations that facilitate their onset.	Facilitates the development of alternative coping behaviors.
As difficult situations are identified, primary nurse can begin working with the client on alternative ways of coping with these situations. (Note alternative coping behaviors selected by the client here.) Use relaxation techniques to manage anxiety that focus on concrete directions and do not include open-ended visualizations for clients who are currently experiencing sensory perceptual alterations.	Promotes the client's sense of control and self-esteem.
Refer the client and support system to appropriate support systems in the community (e.g., Compeer). [Contact local mental health association for programs in your community.]	Establishes continuity of responses and support for the client after discharge.
Arrange time with significant others to provide education about sensory–perceptual alterations and appropriate responses to them.	Client outcomes are improved when support systems are provided education and included in discharge planning.[14,28]

Gerontic Health

The nursing actions for the gerontic patient with this diagnosis are the same as those for the Adult Health patient.

Home Health

ACTIONS/INTERVENTIONS	RATIONALES
Teach the client and family measures to prevent sensory deficit: • Use of protective gear (e.g., goggles, sunglasses, earplugs, or special clothing in hazardous conditions to prevent radiation, sun, or chemical burns)	Family and client involvement in basic safety measures enhances the effectiveness of preventive measures.

(care plan continued on page 506)

NURSING ACTIONS/INTERVENTIONS WITH RATIONALES (continued from page 505)

Home Health

ACTIONS/INTERVENTIONS	RATIONALES
• Prevention of injuries to eyes, ears, skin, nose, and tongue • Prevention of nutritional deficiencies • Close monitoring of medications that may be toxic to the eighth cranial nerve • Correct use of contact lenses • Prevention of fluid and electrolyte imbalances	
Involve the client and family in planning, implementing, and promoting correction or compensation for sensory deficit [specify] by [date]: • Family conference • Mutual goal setting • Communication (e.g., use of memorabilia and audio-tapes or videotapes provided by family members to stimulate in cases of impaired communication)[72]	Involvement improves motivation. Communication and mutual goals increase the probability of positive outcomes.
Assist the patient and family in lifestyle adjustments that may be required: • Assistance with activities of daily living • Adjustment to and usage of assistive devices (e.g., hearing aid, corrective lenses, or magnifying glass) • Providing safe environment (e.g., protect kinesthetically impaired individuals from burns) • Stopping substance abuse • Changes in family and work role relationships • Techniques of communicating with the individual with auditory or visual impairment • Providing meaningful stimulation • Special transportation needs • Special education needs	Lifestyle changes require change in behavior. Self-evaluation and support facilitate these changes.
Consult with or refer to appropriate assistive resources as indicated.	Use of existing community services provides for effective utilization of resources.

THOUGHT PROCESS, DISTURBED

DEFINITION[2]

A state in which an individual experiences a disruption in cognitive operations and activities.

DEFINING CHARACTERISTICS[2]

1. Cognitive dissonance
2. Memory deficit or problems
3. Inaccurate interpretation of environment
4. Hypovigilance
5. Hypervigilance
6. Distractibility
7. Egocentricity
8. Inappropriate, nonreality-based thinking

RELATED FACTORS[2]

To be developed.

RELATED CLINICAL CONCERNS

1. Dementia
2. Neurologic diseases affecting the brain
3. Head injuries
4. Medication overdose, for example, digitalis, sedatives, or narcotics
5. Major depression
6. Bipolar disorder, manic or depressive or mixed
7. Schizophrenic disorders
8. Dissociative disorders
9. Obsessive–compulsive disorders
10. Paranoid disorder

11. Delirium
12. Eating disorders

 Have You Selected the Correct Diagnosis?

Disturbed Sensory Perception
This diagnosis refers to deficits or overloads in sensory input. If the patient is having difficulty with sight, hearing, or any of the other senses, then a confused patient might well be the result. Double-check the pattern assessment to be sure sensory deficit is not the primary problem.

Ineffective Health Maintenance
The diagnosis of Disturbed Thought Process might well contribute to Ineffective Health Maintenance. In this case, Disturbed Thought Process and Ineffective Health Maintenance would be companion diagnoses.

EXPECTED OUTCOME

Describes [number] of strategies to manage distorted thoughts by [date].
   Will engage in reality based conversation for [number] minutes [number] times per day by [date].
   Will be oriented to person, place, and time by [date].

TARGET DATES

A target date of 3 to 5 days is reasonable for this long-range problem.

NURSING ACTIONS/INTERVENTIONS WITH RATIONALES

Adult Health

ACTIONS/INTERVENTIONS	RATIONALES
Monitor at least every 4 hours while awake: • Vital signs • Neurologic status, particularly for signs and symptoms of ICP • Mental status • Laboratory values for metabolic alkalosis, hypokalemia, increased ammonia levels, or infection	Assists in determining pathophysiologic causes for Disturbed Thought Process.
Consistently provide a safe, calm environment: • Provide siderails on bed. • Keep the room uncluttered. • Reorient the client at each contact. • Reduce extraneous stimuli (e.g., limit noise and visitors, and reduce bright lighting). • Use touch judiciously. • Prepare for all procedures by explaining simply and concisely. • Provide good lighting. • Have the family bring clock, calendar, and familiar objects from home.	Basic safety measures and reinforcement of reality.
Design communications according to the patient's best means of communication (e.g., writing, visuals, or sound): • Give simple, concise directions. • Listen carefully. • Present reality consistently. • Do not challenge illogical thinking.	Enhances communication and quality of care.
Facilitate the patient's use of prosthetic or assistive devices (e.g., eyeglasses, dentures, hearing aid, or walker).	Increases sensory input and reinforces reality.
Provide consistent approach in nursing care and routine. [Note routine for this client here.]	Inspires trust, reinforces reality, decreases sensory stimuli, and provides memory cues.

(care plan continued on page 508)

NURSING ACTIONS/INTERVENTIONS WITH RATIONALES (continued from page 507)

Adult Health

ACTIONS/INTERVENTIONS	RATIONALES
Facilitate self-care to the extent possible. [Note patient's abilities here.]	Increases self-esteem, forces reality check, decreases powerlessness, and provides a means of evaluating the patient's status.
Involve significant others in care, and include in teaching sessions. [Note teaching plan here.]	Provides social support and consistency in management.
Refer to and collaborate with appropriate assistive resources.	Provides for long-term support and a more holistic approach to care.
Collaborate with psychiatric nurse clinician and rehabilitation nurse specialist.	Collaboration provides the best plan of care.

Child Health

ACTIONS/INTERVENTIONS	RATIONALES
Monitor cognitive capacity according to age and developmental capacity.	Basic data needed to plan individualized care.
Note discrepancies in chronologic age and mastery of developmental milestones.	
Provide ongoing reality orientation by encouraging the family to visit, and by emphasizing time, personal awareness, and gradual resumption of daily routine to degree possible.	As the patient attempts to reorient, it is helpful that date, time, and specific concrete planning, hour by hour, are offered. The infant should be reintroduced to data, in a calm manner, that will assist in regaining some control over the environment and in regaining the previous functioning level so that he or she can continue to progress.
Provide safety based on developmental needs. [Note client specific adaptations here.]	Disturbed Thought Process serves as a high-risk factor for all involved. It would be a reasonable standard of care to increase all anticipatory safety efforts.
Facilitate family member's expressions of concerns for the child's condition by allowing [number] minutes each shift for discussion.	Promotes ventilation, which helps reduce anxiety and offers insight into thoughts about the patient's condition.
Provide for primary health needs, including administration of medications, comfort measures, and control of environment to aid in the child's adaptation.	Attention to regular health needs must also be considered as the whole person is considered.
Structure the room in a manner that befits the child's needs.	Keeping the environment adapted to personal needs will facilitate care, minimize the chance for accidents, and demonstrate the needed structure.
*Keep room free of clutter with clear path for special needs.	
Allow for ample rest and sleep periods according to developmentally appropriate guidelines. Note specific adaptations for this client here.	Rest is a key and essential consideration to provide optimal potential for cognitive–perceptual functioning.
Monitor for altered coping and role performance.	All contributing factors must be explored to ensure meeting the patient's needs.
Assist the family with discharge plans with referral to community resources.	Improves family adjustment and coping by assisting in preparing for home needs. Empowerment then permits them the opportunity for growth in coping skills and parenting.

ACTIONS/INTERVENTIONS	RATIONALES
If institutionalization is required, assist the family in learning about related issues, such as visitation, medical records maintenance, prognosis, and risk factors.	Planning provides the means for coping and adjusting to the move with an opportunity for clarification. Provides advocacy for the patient and family.
Allow for culturally unique aspects in management of care (e.g., respect for visitation on religious holidays, family wishes for diet, and bathing).	Increases individuation and satisfaction with care. Shows respect for the family's values. Enhances nurse–patient relationship.
Provide for appropriate follow-up by making appointments for next clinic visits.	Follow-up arrangements for clinic visits enhance the likelihood of follow-up and demonstrate the importance of this follow-up care.
Allow the family members opportunities for learning necessary care and mastery of content for long-term needs, such as resolution of conflicts related to institutionalization or respite care and prognosis.	Anticipating learning needs serves to minimize crises related to the child's condition.

Women's Health

This nursing diagnosis will pertain to the woman the same as any other adult, with the following exception. For midlife women, the nursing actions and interventions are the same as those given in Deficient Knowledge, Sleep Deprivation, and Disturbed Sleep Pattern under the headings perimenopausal and menopausal life periods.

Mental Health

ACTIONS/INTERVENTIONS	RATIONALES
Monitor the client's level of anxiety, and refer to Anxiety (Chapter 8) for detailed interventions related to this diagnosis.	Too much information can increase the client's confusion and disorganization. The amount of time devoted to interaction should be guided by the client's attention span.[73]
Speak to the client in brief, clear sentences.	
Keep initial interactions short but frequent. Interact with client for [number] minutes every 30 minutes. Begin with 5-minute interactions and gradually increase the times of interactions.	Facilitates the development of a trusting relationship.
Assign the client a primary care nurse on each shift to assume responsibility for gaining a relationship of trust with the client.	Facilitates the development of a trusting relationship.
Be consistent in all interactions with the client.	Facilitates the development of a trusting relationship, and meets the client's safety needs.
Set limits on inappropriate behavior that increases the risk of the client or others being harmed. [Note the limits here as well as revisions to the limits.]	Client and staff safety are of primary importance.
Initially place the client in an area with little stimulation.	Inappropriate levels of sensory stimuli can contribute to client's sense of disorganization and confusion.
Orient the client to the environment, and assign someone to provide one-to-one interaction while the client orients to unit.	Promotes the client's safety needs while facilitating the development of a trusting relationship.
Do not make promises that cannot be kept.	Facilitates the development of a trusting relationship.
Inform the client of your availability to talk with him or her; do not pry or ask many questions.	Communicates acceptance of the client, which facilitates the development of trust and self-esteem.

(care plan continued on page 510)

NURSING ACTIONS/INTERVENTIONS WITH RATIONALES (continued from page 509)

Mental Health

ACTIONS/INTERVENTIONS	RATIONALES
Do not argue with the client about delusions; inform the client in a matter-of-fact way that this is not your experience of the situation (e.g., "I do not think I am angry with you.")	Argument may reinforce the client's need to maintain the delusional system and interferes with the development of a trusting relationship.
Recognize and support the client's feelings (e.g., "You sound frightened.")	Focuses on the client's real feelings and concerns.
Respond to the feelings being expressed in delusions or hallucinations.	
Initially have the client involved in one-to-one activities; as condition improves, gradually increase the size of the interaction group. [Note current level of functioning here.]	High levels of environmental stimuli may increase confusion and disorganization.
Have the client clarify those thoughts you do not understand. Do not pretend to understand that which you do not.	Facilitates the development of a trusting relationship, and prevents inadvertent support of the delusional thinking.
Do not attempt to change delusional thinking with rational explanations.	This may encourage the client to cling to these thoughts.
After listening to delusion once, do not engage in conversations related to this material or focus conversations on this material.	Decreases the possibility of supporting or reinforcing the delusion.
Focus conversations on here-and-now content related to real things in the environment or to activities on the unit.	Facilitates the client's contact with reality.[69]
Do not belittle or be judgmental about the client's delusional beliefs.	Protects the client's self-esteem.
Avoid nonverbal behavior that indicates agreeing with delusional beliefs.	Decreases the possibility of supporting or reinforcing the delusion.
When the client's behavior and anxiety level indicate readiness, place the client in small-group situations. **Do not put clients who are actively hallucinating in groups.** The client will spend [number] minutes in group activities [number] times a day. (Time and frequency will increase as the client's ability to cope with these situations improves.)	Provides feedback about delusional beliefs from peers.
Develop a daily schedule for the client that encourages focus on "here and now" and is adapted to the client's level of functioning so that success can be experienced. Note daily schedule here.	Facilitates the client's contact with reality. Promotes positive self-image.
Assign the client meaningful roles in unit activities. Provide roles that can be easily accomplished by the client to provide successful experiences. [Note client responsibilities here.]	Facilitates the client's contact with reality. Promotes positive self-image.
Primary nurse will spend [number] minutes with the client twice a day to discuss the client's feelings and the effects of the delusions on the client's life. (Number of minutes and the degree of exploration of the client's feelings will increase as the client develops relationship with nurse.)	Assists in the development of alternative coping behaviors.

ACTIONS/INTERVENTIONS	RATIONALES
Provide rewards to the client for accomplishing task progress on the daily schedule. These rewards should be ones the client finds rewarding.	Positive feedback encourages productive behavior.
Spend [number] minutes twice a day walking with the client. This should start at 10-minute intervals and gradually increase. This can be replaced by any physical activity the client finds enjoyable. A staff member should be with the client during this activity to provide social reinforcement to the client for accomplishing the activity.	Facilitates the development of a trusting relationship. Social interaction provides positive reinforcement. Helps increase daytime wakefulness, promoting a normal sleep–wake cycle.
Arrange a consultation with the occupational therapist to assist the client in developing or continuing special interests.	Increases daytime wakefulness, maintaining a normal sleep-rest cycle.
Monitor delusional beliefs for potential of harming self or others.	Patient and staff safety are of primary concern.
Note any change in behavior that would indicate a change in the delusional beliefs that could indicate a potential for violence.	Patient and staff safety are of primary concern.
If the client is placed in seclusion, interact with the client at least every 15 minutes.	Provides reality orientation, and assists the client with controlling hallucinations and delusions.
Maintain environment that does not stimulate the client's delusions (e.g., if the client has delusions related to religion, limit discussions of religion and religious activity on unit to very concrete terms). Limit interaction with persons who stimulate delusional thinking.	Excessive environmental stimuli can increase confusion and disorganization.
The primary nurse will assist the client in identifying signs and symptoms of increasing thought disorganization and in developing a plan to cope with these situations before they get out of control. This will be done in the regularly scheduled interaction times between the primary nurse and the client.	Promotes the client's sense of control, and enhances self-esteem.
As the client's condition improves, primary nurse will assist the client to identify onset delusions with periods of increasing anxiety.	Facilitates the client's developing alternative coping behaviors.
As connection is made between thought disorder and anxiety, the client will be assisted to identify specific anxiety-producing situations and learn alternative coping behaviors. See Anxiety (Chapter 8) for specific interventions.	Promotes the client's sense of control, and enhances self-esteem.
Teach client strategies to manage the thoughts that precede increases in anxiety by: • Linking increase in anxiety to dysfunctional thinking • Thought stopping techniques (wearing rubber band on wrist and snapping it when negative thoughts occur) • Rehearse changes in self-talk that would decrease anxiety (replace words like should, never, and always with more reality based thinking). Refer to resources on Cognitive therapy for more techniques.[19]	
Refer the client to outpatient support systems, and assist with making arrangements for the client to contact these before discharge.	Facilitates the client's reintegration into the community.

(care plan continued on page 512)

NURSING ACTIONS/INTERVENTIONS WITH RATIONALES (continued from page 511)

Gerontic Health

● N O T E : *Problems related to Disturbed Thought Process with older adults may present themselves in various ways. Two conditions, dementia and delirium, are considered here. Irreversible dementia, such as Alzheimer's or multi-infarct dementia, is usually progressive, gradual in onset, of long duration, and has a steady downward course. Delirium, or acute confusional state, presents with acute onset, is of short duration, and has a fluctuating course and is often reversible with treatment.[74] Nursing interventions vary depending on the cause of the Disturbed Thought Process.*

ACTIONS/INTERVENTIONS	RATIONALES
Dementia	
Conduct a thorough assessment and collaborate with the health-care team to treat possible etiologies of dementia: metabolic diseases, toxin exposure, infection, neoplasm, drug side effects, nutritional deficiencies, degenerative neurologic disease, cerebral vascular injury.	To facilitate treatment of the primary problem.
Offer immediate attention with supportive and symptomatic care.	Prevent further disturbed thought processes.
Assure continuity of care personnel.	Facilitates feelings of safety by client, allows for early identification of changes in client mental status.
Support sensory function in all stages of dementia by using assistive devices such as glasses, hearing aids, and dentures.	Minimizes sensory sources of disturbed thought processes.
Maintain safe environment. Avoid leaving solutions, equipment, or medications near the patient that could result in injury through misuse or ingestion.	Basic preventive measure.
Provide a consistent environment and schedule but remain flexible.	Prevents exacerbation of disturbed thought processes.
Communicate with the client using verbal or nonverbal strategies as appropriate for the stage of dementia.	Clients with middle stage Alzheimer disease often have difficulty understanding or expressing verbally. Late-stage Alzheimer's clients often lose their ability to communicate verbally.
Monitor environment to prevent overstimulating the patient with light, sounds, and frequent activity. Support sensory function in all stages of dementia by using assistive devices such as glasses, hearing aids, and dentures.	With dementia, the patient has a reduced threshold for stress.
Provide appropriate environmental cues and limit inappropriate environmental cues.	
For example, when preparing a client to bathe, place towels and clean clothing in a visible location. This provides an environmental cue for the activity of bathing.	
• Limit the client's exposure to cues such as keys, oven knobs, or cooking utensils if they stimulate the client to engage in activities that are not appropriate or safe.	
Schedule activities that are of short duration (usually 20-minute sessions). [Note client's schedule here.]	Prevents stresses on an individual already suffering from attention deficits and anxiety.
Use short sentences and clear directions when communicating with the patient.	Allows processing of basic information without distraction.

ACTIONS/INTERVENTIONS	RATIONALES
Determine self-care abilities that are intact, and encourage continued participation in these activities.	Provides stimulation and sense of pride. Promotes physical activity.
Monitor food and fluid intake to determine that nutritional status is adequate.	
Provide consistent staff.	Reduces anxiety.
Refer the family to local Alzheimer's and related disease support groups.	Provides long-term support.
Delirium	
Monitor for conditions that can induce delirium.	Certain factors such as electrolyte imbalance, preoperative dehydration, unanticipated surgery, intraoperative hypotension, postoperative hypothermia, and a large number of medications have been found to be associated with acute confusional states in older adults.[75,76]
Provide orienting information to the patient as often as necessary.	Provides information to the patient about the current situation, and assists in reducing anxiety and confusion.
Provide sensory stimulation such as bathing, touching, and back massages.	Assists in restoring the patient's sense of body image.[77]

Home Health

In addition to the following interventions, the interventions for Adult Health can be applied to the home health client.

ACTIONS/INTERVENTIONS	RATIONALES
Teach the client and family to monitor for signs and symptoms of Disturbed Thought Process: • Poor hygiene • Poor decision making or judgment • Regression in behavior • Delusions • Hallucinations • Changes in interpersonal relationship • Distractibility	Basic monitoring that allows for early intervention.
Involve the client and family in planning, implementing, and promoting appropriate thought processing: • Family conference • Mutual goal setting • Communication	Involvement improves cooperation and motivation, thereby increasing the probability of an improved outcome.
Assist the client and family in lifestyle adjustments that may be necessary: • Providing safety and prevention of injury • Frequent orientation to person, place, and time • Providing reality testing and patient verification • Assisting in working through alterations in role functions in family or at work • Stopping substance abuse • Facilitating family communication • Setting limits • Learning new skills • Decreasing risk for violence • Preventing suicide • Explaining possible chronicity of disorder	

(care plan continued on page 514)

NURSING ACTIONS/INTERVENTIONS WITH RATIONALES (continued from page 513)

Home Health

ACTIONS/INTERVENTIONS	RATIONALES
• Referring the client to community resources for financial assistance • Reducing sensory overload • Teaching stress management • Teaching relaxation techniques • Referring the client and family to support groups	
Assist the client and family to set criteria to help them determine when professional intervention is required.	Early identification of issues requiring professional evaluation will increase the probability of successful interventions.
Teach the client and family purposes, side effects, and proper administration techniques for medications.	Provides necessary information for the client and family that promotes safe self-care.
Consult with or refer to appropriate assistive resources as required.	Efficient and cost-effective use of community resources.

UNILATERAL NEGLECT

DEFINITION[2]

Lack of awareness and attention to one side of the body.[2]

DEFINING CHARACTERISTICS[2]

1. Consistent inattention to stimuli on an affected side
2. Does not look toward affected side
3. Positioning and/or safety precautions in regard to the affected side
4. Inadequate self-care
5. Leaves food on plate on the affected side

RELATED FACTORS[2]

1. Effects of disturbed perceptual abilities, for example, hemianopsia
2. Neurologic illness or trauma
3. One-sided blindness

RELATED CLINICAL CONCERNS

1. Cerebrovascular accident
2. Glaucoma
3. Blindness secondary to diabetes mellitus

4. Spinal cord injury
5. Amputation
6. Ruptured cerebral aneurysm
7. Brain trauma

 Have You Selected the Correct Diagnosis?

Disturbed Sensory Perception
This diagnosis refers to a problem with receiving sensory input and interpretation of this input. Unilateral Neglect could be, as indicated by the related factors, an outcome of this disturbance in sensory input and/or perception of this input.

EXPECTED OUTCOME

Performs self-care of all body parts by [date].
    Verbalizes plan to address self-care deficits by [date].
    Identifies [number] of needs for assistance by [date].

TARGET DATES

A target date between 5 and 7 days would be appropriate to evaluate initial progress.

NURSING ACTIONS/INTERVENTIONS WITH RATIONALES

Adult Health

ACTIONS/INTERVENTIONS	RATIONALES
Ensure patient safety. Raise siderails on affected side.	Provides basic safety.
Assist patient in self-care	
Adapt environment deficiency, place items on unaffected side.	

ACTIONS/INTERVENTIONS	RATIONALES
Frequently remind the patient to attend to both sides of his or her body.	Repetition improves brain processing.
Consult with physical and occupational therapy to facilitate patient's awareness of and articulate sensations on neglected side. [Note support from nursing needed here.]	Increases brain's awareness of neglected side.
Assist the patient with ROM exercises to neglected side of body every 4 hours while awake at [times]. Teach the extent of movement of each joint on the neglected side of body.	Increases brain's awareness of neglected side, and maintains muscle tone and joint mobility.
Help the patient position neglected side of body in a similar way as attended side of body whenever position is changed.	
Refer to rehabilitation nurse clinician.	Collaboration provides a more holistic plan of care, and rehabilitation nurse will have most up-to-date knowledge regarding this diagnosis.

Child Health

See nursing actions under Disturbed Sensory Perception in addition to those listed here.

ACTIONS/INTERVENTIONS	RATIONALES
Allow 30 minutes every shift for the patient and family to express how they perceive the unilateral neglect.	Ventilation of feelings is paramount in understanding the effect the problem has on the patient and the family; it is also critical as a means of evaluating needs.
Determine how the unilateral neglect affects the usual expected behavior or development for the child.	Previous and/or current developmental capacity may be affected by the unilateral neglect depending on the degree of severity. To be able to judge the best means of therapy requires these data to be considered (e.g., does the child use the affected hand as a helper, or not try to use it at all?)
Monitor for presence of secondary or tertiary deficits.	Identification of primary deficits should alert all to monitor for possible secondary and tertiary deficits to minimize further sequelae, which can be treated early.
Establish, with family input, appropriate anticipatory safety guidelines that are based on the unilateral neglect and the developmental capacity of the child.	Safety needs and measures must reflect the developmental capacity of the child and slightly beyond it. There is a special need to structure the environment to allow for appropriate exploratory behavior while maintaining safety without overprotection.
Stress appropriate follow-up prior to dismissal from hospital with appropriate time frame for the family.	Arrangement for follow-up increases the likelihood of compliance and shows the importance of follow-up.

Women's Health

This nursing diagnosis will pertain to women the same as any other adult.

Mental Health

Nursing interventions for this diagnosis are those described in Adult Health.

(care plan continued on page 516)

NURSING ACTIONS/INTERVENTIONS WITH RATIONALES (continued from page 515)

Geronic Health

The interventions for Adult Health can be applied to the aging client.

Home Health

In addition to the following interventions, the interventions for Adult Health can be applied to the home health client.

ACTIONS/INTERVENTIONS	RATIONALES
Monitor for factors contributing to Unilateral Neglect (e.g., disturbed perceptual abilities, neurologic disease, or trauma).	This action provides the database needed to identify interventions that will prevent or diminish Unilateral Neglect.
Involve the client and family in planning, implementing, and promoting reduction in effects of Unilateral Neglect: • Schedule family conferences (e.g., to discuss concerns family members have). • Encourage the family's ideas for addressing the concern. • Set mutual goals (e.g., establish two measures to offset the effect of unilateral neglect). Be sure roles for the participants are identified. • Maintain communication. • Provide support for the caregiver (e.g., plan respite time for the primary caregiver). Alternate caregivers are identified and trained.	Family involvement is important to ensure success. Communication and mutual goals improve the outcome.
Teach the client and family measures to decrease effects of Unilateral Neglect: • Active and passive ROM exercises • Ambulation with assistive devices (canes, walkers, or crutches) • Objects placed within field of vision and reach • Assistive eating utensils • Assistive dressing equipment • Safe environment (e.g., objects removed from area outside field of vision)	These actions diminish the negative effects of Unilateral Neglect.
Assist the family and client to identify lifestyle changes that may be required: • Change in role functions • Coping with disability or dependency • Obtaining and using assistive equipment • Coping with assistive equipment • Maintaining safe environment	Lifestyle changes require changes in behavior. Self-evaluation and support facilitate these changes.
Consult with appropriate assistive resources as indicated.	Appropriate use of existing community services is effective use of resources.

REFERENCES

1. Murray, RB, and Zentner, JP: Health Assessment and Promotion Strategies Through the Life Span, ed 6. Appleton & Lange, Norwalk, CT, 1997.
2. North American Nursing Diagnosis Association: Nursing Diagnosis: Definitions and Classification, 2005–2006. Author, Philadelphia, 2005.
3. Eisenhart, K: New perspectives in the management of adults with severe head injury. Crit Care Nurs Q 17:1, 1994.
4. Walleck, CA: Preventing secondary brain injury. AACN Clin Issues Crit Care Nurs 3:19, 1992.
5. Hickey, JV: The Clinical Practice of Neurological and Neurosurgical Nursing, ed 4. JB Lippincott, Philadelphia, 1997.
6. Kerr, M, et al: Head-injured adults: Recommendations for endotracheal suctioning. J Neurosci Nurs 25:86, 1993.

7. Crosby, LJ, and Parsons, LC: Cerebrovascular response of closed head-injured patients to a standardized endotracheal tube suctioning and manual hyperventilation procedure. J Neurosci Nurs 24:40, 1992.

8. Rising, CJ: The relationship of selected nursing activities to ICP. J Neurosci Nurs 25:302, 1993.

9. Barsevick, A, and Llewellyn, J: A comparison of the anxiety-reducing potential of two techniques of bathing. Nurs Res 31:22, 1982.

10. Author: Part I. Guidelines for the management of severe traumatic brain injury. In: Management and prognosis of severe traumatic brain injury. (2) Update notice. Guidelines for the management of severe traumatic brain injury: Cerebral perfusion pressure. American Association of Neurological Surgeons—Medical Specialty Society, Brain Trauma Foundation—Disease Specific Society. 2000 (revised 2003). 165 pages. National Guidelines Clearinghouse: 003020.

11. Hockenberry, MJ: Wong's Essentials of Pediatric Nursing, ed 7. CV Mosby, St. Louis, 2006.

12. Moss, SW: The power to terrify: Eclampsia in 19th-Century American Practice. JOGNN J Obstet Gynecol Neonatal Nurs 31:5, 514, 2002.

13. Lowdermilk, DL, and Perry, SE: Maternity and Women's Health Care, ed 8. CV Mosby, St. Louis, 2004.

14. Kidner, MC, and Flanders-Stepans, MB: A model for the HELLP syndrome: The maternal experience. JOGNN J Obstet Gynecol Neonatal Nurs 33(1):44, 2004.

15. Varacarolis, EM: Foundations of Psychiatric–Mental Health Nursing, ed 3. WB Saunders, Philadelphia, 1998.

16. Author, The Agency for Healthcare Research and Quality in the United States, Clinical practice guidelines, abstracts, http://www.guideline.gov 2006.

17. Maxmen, JS: Psychotropic Drugs Fast Facts, ed 3. WW Norton, New York, 2002.

18. Mahoney, DF: Analysis of restraint free nursing homes. Image 33:155, 1995.

19. Kneisl, C, Wilson, H, and Trigoboff, E: Contemporary Psychiatric–Mental Health Nursing. Pearson Education, Upper Saddle River, NJ, 2004.

20. McCloskey, J, Dochterman, J, and Bulechek, G: Nursing Interventions Classification, ed 4. CV Mosby, St. Louis, 2004.

21. Weinrich, S, et al: Agitation: Measurement, management, and intervention Res Arch Psychiatr Nurs 9:251, 1994.

22. Roberto, K, et al: Communication patterns between caregivers and their spouses with Alzheimer's disease: A case study. Arch Psychiatr Nurs 12:202, 1998.

23. Sullivan-Marx, E: Delirium and physical restraint in the hospitalized elderly. Image 26:295, 1994.

24. Erickson, H, Tomlin, E, and Swain, M: Modeling and Role Modeling: Theory, Practice and Research. Society for the Advancement of Modeling and Role-Modeling, Austin, TX, 1990.

25. Hall, E: The role of oxygen radicals in traumatic injury: Clinical implications. J Emerg Med 11:31, 1993.

26. Harvath, TA, et al: Dementia-related behaviors. J Psychosoc Nurs 33:35, 1994.

27. Goldsmith, SM, Hoeffer, B, and Rader, J: Problematic wandering behavior in the cognitively impaired elderly. J Psychosoc Nurs 33:6, 1994.

28. Veterans Administration, DOD (2004). Management of Persons with Psychoses. National Guideline Clearing House, 2006.

29. Kaye, P: Notes on Symptom Control in Hospice and Palliative Care. Hospice Education Institute, Essex, CT, 1990.

30. Zyzanski, S, and Kodish, E: Committee on Bioethics, American Academy of Pediatrics, Informed consent, parental permission, and assent in pediatric practice. 95:314, 2006.

31. Teschendorf, M: Women during the reproductive years. In Breslin, ET, and Lucas, VA (eds): Women's Health Nursing: Toward Evidenced-Based Practice. Saunders, Philadelphia, 2003.

32. Krause, KD, and Younger, VJ: Nursing diagnoses as guidelines in the care of the neonatal ECMO patient. J Obstet Gynecol Neonatal Nurs 21:176, 1992.

33. Cox, BE: What if? Coping with unexpected outcomes. Childbirth Instructor 1:24, 1991.

34. Parkman, SE: Helping families to say good-bye. MCN Am J Matern Child Nurs 17:14, 1992.

35. Ryan, PF, Cote-Arsenault, D, and Sugarman, LL: Facilitating care after perinatal loss: A comprehensive checklist. J Obstet Gynecol Neonatal Nurs 20:385, 1991.

36. Ladebauche, P: Unit-based family support groups: A reminder. MCN: Am J Matern Child Nurs 17:18, 1992.

37. Cote-Arsenault, D, and Mahlangu, N: Impact of perinatal loss on the subsequent pregnancy and self: Women's experiences. JOGNN J Obstet Gynecol Neonatal Nurs 28:274, 1999.

38. DeMontigny, F, Beauder, L, and Duman, L: A baby has died: The impact of perinatal loss on family social networks. JOGNN J Obstet Gynecol Neonatal Nurs 28:151, 1999.

39. Erickson, MH: The Practical Applications of Medical and Dental Hypnosis. Brunner & Mazel, New York, 1990.

40. Keeney, BP: Aesthetics of Change. Guilford Press, New York, 1983.

41. Watzlawick, P, Weakland, J, and Fisch, R: Change. WW Norton, New York, 1974.

42. Aguilera, DC: Crisis Intervention: Theory and Methodology, ed 8. CV Mosby, St. Louis, 1998.

43. Black, HC: Black's Law Dictionary, ed 6. West Publishing, St. Paul, MN.

44. Creasia, JL, and Parker, B: Conceptual Foundations of Professional Nursing Practice, ed 2. Mosby–Year Book, St. Louis, 1996.

45. Simmonds, KE, and Likis, FE: Providing options counseling for women with unintended pregnancies. JOGNN J Obstet Gynecol Neonatal Nurs 34(3):373, 2005.

46. Nelson, AM: Transition to motherhood. JOGNN J Obstet Gynecol Neonatal Nurs 32(4):465, 2003.

47. Martell, LD: Postpartum women's perceptions of the hospital environment. JOGNN J Obstet Gynecol Neonatal Nurs 32(4):478, 2003.

48. Groer, MW, Davis, MW, and Hemphill, J: Postpartum stress: Current concepts and the possible protective role of breastfeeding. JOGNN J Obstet Gynecol Neonatal Nurs 31(4):411, 2002.

49. Swift, K, and Janke, J: Breast binding…Is it all that it's wrapped up to be? JOGNN J Obstet Gynecol Neonatal Nurs 32(3):332, 2003.

50. Bowman, KG: Postpartum learning needs. JOGNN J Obstet Gynecol Neonatal Nurs 34(4):438, 2005.

51. Buist, A, Morse, CA, and Durkin S: Men's adjustment to fatherhood: Implications for obstetric health care. JOGNN J Obstet Gynecol Neonatal Nurs 32(2):172, 2003.

52. de Montigny, F, and Lacharite, C: Fathers' Perceptions of the immediate postpartal period. JOGNN J Obstet Gynecol Neonatal Nurs 33(3):328, 2004.

53. St. John, W, Cameron, C, and McVeigh, C: Meeting the challenge of new fatherhood during the early weeks. JOGNN J Obstet Gynecol Neonatal Nurs 34(2):180, 2005.

54. Matthey, S, Morgan, M, Healey, L, Barnett, B, Kavanagh, DJ, and Howie, P: Postpartum issues for expectant mothers and fathers. JOGNN J Obstet Gynecol Neonatal Nurs 31(4):428, 2002.

55. Vliet, EL: Screaming to be Heard: Hormonal Connections Women Suspect and Doctors Ignore. M. Evans and Co., New York, 1995.

56. Lindsay, SH: Menopause naturally: Exploring alternatives to traditional HRT. Lifelines 3:32, 1999.

57. Learn, CD, and Higgins, PG: Harmonizing herbs: Managing menopause with help from Mother Earth. Lifelines 3:39, 1999.

58. Wright, L, and Leahey, M: Nurses and families: A guide to family assessment and intervention, ed 4. F.A. Davis, Philadelphia, 2005.

59. Newfield, S, Lewis, D, and Newfield, N: Facilitating lifestyle change: An approach to patient education. Unpublished, 2000.

60. Huebscher, R: Natural, Alternative, and Complementary Health Care. In Breslin, ET, and Lucas, VA (eds): Women's Health Nursing: Toward Evidence-Based Practice. WB Saunders, St. Louis, 2003.

61. Burns, M: Screening and Diagnostic Tests. In Breslin, ET, and Lucas, VA (eds): Women's Health Nursing: Toward Evidence-Based Practice. WB Saunders, St. Louis, 2003.

62. Fogel, CI, and Woods, NF: Health Care of Women: A Nursing Perspective. CV Mosby, St. Louis, 1981.

63. Hinz, M, and Leick, M: Identifying the five most common nursing diagnoses utilized in labor and delivery, unpublished presentation, 14th Biennial Conference on Nursing Diagnosis, Orlando, Florida, April 8, 2000.

64. Author: Database of Clinical Practice Guidelines, The Agency for Healthcare Research and Quality in the United States, http://www.guideline.gov, 2006.

65. Maas, M, Buckwalter, KC, and Hardy, MA: Nursing Diagnosis and Interventions for the Elderly. Addison-Wesley, Redwood City, CA, 1991.

66. Ferrell, B, and Ferrell, B: Easing the pain. Geriatric Nursing 11:175, 1990.

67. Hofland, S: Elder beliefs: Blocks to pain management. J Gerontol Nurs 18:19, 1992.

68. Haber, J, et al: Comprehensive Psychiatric Nursing, ed 5. Mosby–Year Book, St. Louis, 1997.

69. Puskar, KR, et al: Psychiatric nursing management of medication-free psychotic patients. Arch Psychiatri Nurs 4:78, 1990.

70. Townsend, M: Nursing Diagnosis in Psychiatric Nursing, ed 5. FA Davis, Philadelphia, 2001.

71. Schwartz, MS, and Shockley, EL: The Nurse and the Mental Patient. Russell Sage Foundation, New York, 1956.

72. Buccheri, R, et al: Auditory hallucinations in schizophrenia. Journal Psychosocial Nursing 34:12, 1996.

73. Dochtermann, McCloskey, J, and Bulechek, G: Nursing Interventions Classification, cd 4. Mosby–Ycar Book, St. Louis, 2004.

74. Gomez, G, and Gomez, E: Dementia? Or delirium? Geriatr Nurs 11:136, 1989.

75. Foreman, M: Complexities of acute confusion. Geriatric Nurs 11:136, 1990.

76. Bowman, AM: The relationship of anxiety to development of post operative delirium. J Gerontol Nurs 18:24, 1992.

77. Faraday, K, and Berry, M: The nurse's role in managing reversible confusion. J Gerontol Nurs 15:17, 1989.

8

SELF-PERCEPTION AND SELF-CONCEPT PATTERN

PATTERN DESCRIPTION

As the nurse interacts with the client, the most important knowledge the client contributes is self-knowledge. It is this understanding, most often labeled "self-concept," that determines the individual's manner of interaction with others. One's self-concept is composed of beliefs and attitudes about the self, including perception of abilities (cognitive, affective, or physical), body image, identity, self-esteem, and general emotional pattern.[1] An individual's behavior is affected not only by experiences prior to interactions with the health-care system, but also by interactions with the health-care system.

PATTERN ASSESSMENT

1. Does the patient express concern the regarding current situation?
   a. Yes (Anxiety or Fear)
   b. No
2. Can the patient identify the source of concern?
   a. Yes (Fear)
   b. No (Anxiety)
3. As a result of this admission, will the patient going have a change in body structure or function?
   a. Yes (Disturbed Body Image)
   b. No
4. Does the patient verbalize a change in lifestyle as a result of this admission?
   a. Yes (Disturbed Body Image)
   b. No
5. Does the patient express fear about dying?
   a. Yes (Death Anxiety)
   b. No
6. Does the patient express worries about the impact of his or her death on his or her family and/or friends?
   a. Yes (Death Anxiety)
   b. No
7. Does the patient verbalize a negative view of self?
   a. Yes (Situational Low Self-Esteem)
   b. No (Readiness for Enhanced Self-Concept)
8. Does the patient believe he or she can deal with the current problem that led to this admission?
   a. Yes
   b. No (Situational Low Self-Esteem)
9. Does the patient or his or her family indicate that the self-negating impression is a long-standing (several years) problem?
   a. Yes (Chronic Low Self-Esteem)
   b. No (Situational Low Self-Esteem)
10. Does the patient question who he or she is or verbalize lack of an understanding regarding his or her role in life?
   a. Yes (Disturbed Personal Identity)
   b. No (Readiness for Enhanced Self-Concept)
11. Does the patient appear passive or verbalize passivity?
   a. Yes (Hopelessness)
   b. No
12. Does the patient demonstrate decreased verbalization and/or flat affect?
   a. Yes (Hopelessness)
   b. No
13. Does the patient have a problem with physical or social isolation?
   a. Yes (Risk for Loneliness)
   b. No (Readiness for Enhanced Self-Concept)
14. Has the patient recently suffered the loss of a significant other?
   a. Yes (Risk for Loneliness)
   b. No
15. Does the patient verbalize lack of control?
   a. Yes (Powerlessness)
   b. No
16. Is the patient participating in care and decision making regarding care?
   a. Yes (Readiness for Enhanced Self-Concept)
   b. No (Powerlessness)

CONCEPTUAL INFORMATION

Definition of the self and of a self-concept has been an issue of debate in philosophy, sociology, and psychology for many years, and many publications are available on this topic.[2] The complexity of the problem of defining self is compounded by the knowledge that external observation provides only a superficial glimpse of the self, and introspection requires that the "knower" knows himself or herself so that information actually gained is self-referential. In spite of these problems, the concept continues to be pervasive in the literature and in the universal experience of "self" or "not self." Intuitively one would say, of course, "There is a self because I have experiences separate from those around me; I know where I end and they begin." The importance of self is also emphasized by the language in the multitude of self-referential terms such as self-actualization, self-affirmation, ego-involvement, and self-concept.

Cognitive neuroscientists have utilized brain imaging during various self-referential tasks to understand the process of experiencing the self. This research has linked specific areas of the brain with activities of self-reference.[3] The medial prefrontal cortex is one area that demonstrates the most activity when thinking about the self. It is hypothesized that this area links multiple self-knowledge systems in the brain.[3] Clearly, the neurological response is different when one is thinking of the self, and this process changes as we develop a better self-concept.[4] The understandings evolving from cognitive neuroscience provide a map to the intricacies of self-knowledge, which can inform client care.

Some of the basic neuroscience understandings with implications for intervening with human responses related to self-perception are related to the awareness of one's own body. This is the foundational understanding of the self, to know where the physical self begins and ends. The process of knowing this occurs when the neuro command to move a body part is issued. At this point two signals are sent, one to the body part that needs to be moved, and one to the part of the brain that monitors movement. The monitoring process predicts the action experience. If the prediction does not match what is experienced, and the difference cannot be reconciled, then the brain processes this as not caused by the self.[4] Difficulties in making this link could result in a disturbed body image or delusional thinking. The client, in search of an explanation for his or her experience, could conclude that someone or something outside of him- or herself is controlling his or her actions. Continued research in cognitive neuroscience will increase understanding about how to facilitate the development of self-knowledge links and assist in refining nursing interventions.

Neuroscientists recognize that humans have developed a uniquely complex sense of self. The evolution of this complexity may have been a response to living in complex social networks.[4] This connection between the brain and social networks reflects the circular causal model of systems/cybernetics that provides the theoretical foundation for the research.[3] In that circular wholistic perspective, the sociological understandings of the development of the self must also be considered.

Turner[5] addresses society's need for the individual to conceptualize the self-as-object. Recognizing the self-as-object allows society to place responsibility, which becomes a very valuable asset in maintaining social control and social order. This returns us to the initial problem of what the self is and how we can understand others' selves and ourselves.[6] In this section, the assumption is made that self-concept refers to the individual's subjective cognitions and evaluations of self; thus, it is a highly personal experience. This indicates that the self is a personal construct and not a fact or hard reality. It is further assumed that the individual will act, as stated earlier, in congruence with the self-concept. This conceptualization is consistent with the authors who will be discussed, and with the assumptions utilized in psychological research.[6] It is also important to recognize that language assists in developing a concept. This becomes crucial when thinking about the concept of self in English, because the English language comes from a tradition of Cartesian dualism that does not express integrated concepts well. Often it will appear that the information presented is separating the individual into various parts, when, in fact, an integrated whole is being addressed. For example, James[7] talks about an "I" and a "Me." If these terms were taken at face value, it would appear that the individual is being divided into multiple parts, when, in fact, an integrated whole is being discussed. The words describe patterns of the whole person. Unless otherwise stated, it can be assumed that the concepts presented in this book reflect on the individual as an integrated whole.

Symbolic interaction theory provides a basis for understanding the self. James[7] and Mead[8] developed the foundation for the self in this theoretical model. James outlines the internal working of the self with his concepts of "I" and "Me." "I" is the thinker or the state of consciousness. "Me" is what the "I" is conscious of, and includes all of what people consider theirs. This "Me" contains three aspects: the "material me," the "social me," and the "spiritual me."[6] The self-construction outlined by Mead[8] indicates that there is the "knower" part of the self and that which the "knower" knows. Mead conceptualizes the thoughts themselves as the "knower" to resolve the metaphysical problem of who the "I" is. In Mead's writings, the consciousness of self is a stream of thought in which the "I" can remember what came before and continues to know what was known. Mead[8] expressly addresses the development of these memories and how they affect one's behavior.

Mead[8] describes the self-concept as evolving out of interactions with others in social contexts. This process begins at the moment of birth and continues throughout a lifetime. The definition of self can occur only in social interactions, for one's own self exists only in relation to other selves. The individual is continually processing the reactions of others to his or her actions and reactions. This processing is taking place in a highly personalized manner, for the information is experienced through the individual's selective attention, which is guided by the current needs that are struggling to be expressed. This results in an environment that is constructed by one's perceptions. Mead's conceptualization leads to an interesting feedback process in that we can only perceive self as we perceive others perceive us. This continues to reinforce the idea that the self-concept is highly personalized.

Many authors[5,7,8] have addressed the process of developing a concept of self. The model developed by Harry Stack Sullivan[9] is presented here because it is consistent with the information presented in the symbolic interaction literature, and is used as the theoretical base in much of the nursing literature.

Sullivan[9] describes the self-concept as developing in interactions with significant others. Sullivan sees development of the self-concept as a dynamic process resulting from interpersonal interactions that are directed toward meeting physiologic needs. This process has its most obvious beginnings with the infant and becomes more complex as the individual develops. This increasing complexity results from the layering of experiences that occurs in the developing individual. The biologic processes become less and less important in directing the individual the further away from birth one is and as the importance of interpersonal interaction increases. The initial interpersonal interaction is between the infant and the primary caregivers. An infant expresses discomfort with a cry and the "parenting one" responds. This response, whether tender or harsh, begins to influence the infant's beliefs about herself or himself, as well as the world in general. If the interaction does not provide the infant with a feeling of security, anxiety results and interferes with the progress toward other life goals. Sullivan makes a distinction between the inner experience and the outer event and describes three modes of understanding experience.

The first developmental experience is the *prototaxic mode*. In this mode, the small child experiences self and the universe as an undifferentiated whole. At 3 to 4 months, the child moves into the parataxic mode. The *parataxic mode* presents experiences as separated but without recognition of a connectedness or logical sequence. Finally, the individual enters the *syntaxic mode*, in which consensual validation is possible. This allows for events and experiences to be compared with others' experiences and for establishment of mutually understandable communication instead of the autistic thinking that has characterized the previous stages.[10,11]

As one experiences the environment through these three modes of thought, the self-system or self-concept is developed. Sullivan conceptualized three parts of the self. The part of the self that is associated with security and approval becomes the "good me," whereas that which is within one's awareness, but is disapproved of, becomes the "bad me." The "bad me" could include those feelings, needs, or desires that stimulate anxiety. Those feelings and understandings that are out of awareness are experienced as "not me." These "not me" experiences are not nonexistent but are expressed in indirect ways that can interfere with the conduct of the individual's life.[9,10]

As the social sciences adopted a cybernetic worldview, this theoretical perspective has been applied to developing a concept of self. Glasersfeld[12] spoke of the self as a relational entity that is given life through the continuity of relating. This relating provides the intuitive knowledge that our experience is truly ours. It reflects the perspective of knowing presented at the beginning of this section.

Watts[13] describes what many authors feel is the self, as it can be understood through a cybernetic worldview. Self is the whole, for it is part of the energy that is the universe and cannot be separated. "At this level of existence 'I' am immeasurably old; my forms are infinite and their comings and goings are simply the pulses or vibrations of a single and eternal flow of energy." In this view, an individual is connected to every other living being in the universe. This places the self in a unique position of responsibility. The self then becomes responsible to everything because it is everything. This conceptual model resolves the issue of responsibility to society without relying on an individual self to whom responsibility is assigned.

Although the conceptual model represented here by Watts[13] fits with current theoretical models being utilized in nursing and the social sciences, it is not congruent with the experience of most persons in Western society. This limits its usefulness when working with clients in a clinical setting. It is presented here to provide practitioners with an alternative model for themselves.

Stake[14,15] developed an instrument to measure self-perception. Knowledge of the factors contributing to the development of the self-perception can assist in the formulation of interventions focused on improving perceptions of self. Five facets that contribute to a positive perception of self emerged from Stake's[15] research: task accomplishment, power, giftedness, likeability, and morality. The characteristics of task accomplishment include perceptions of having good work habits and the ability to manage and complete tasks efficiently. Perceptions of personal power include having strength, toughness, and the ability to influence others. Perceiving oneself as having special natural aptitudes and talents provides the foundation for the facet of giftedness. Seeing oneself as pleasant and enjoyable to be with constitutes the characteristic of likeability. Morality is made up of factors that indicate the individual perceives himself or herself as having qualities valued as good and virtuous. Additional facets have been added to these basic foundations.[16,17] These factors include perceptions about physical appearance, behavioral conduct and job, and athletic and scholastic competence.

Integration of theory and research related to self-concept indicates that positive self-perceptions evolve in a positive nurturing environment. Factors that contribute to the success of this environment include positive support for decision making; warm acceptance; positive, informative praise; promotion of self-efficacy; a sense of belonging and purpose; and the development of positive social skills.[18]

The complex interaction of facets that evolve into the self-concept is an ongoing process occurring throughout the individual's life. This process can be impacted by life events, including illness,[19,20] that impinge on any of the identified factors, whether positively or negatively.

The Search Institute[21] has developed, as a result of their research, a list of 40 assets that support the development of young people. If these assets are compared with the facets necessary to build a positive self-concept, many parallels can be identified. The 40 assets are divided into internal and external. The four general external asset categories are support, empowerment, boundaries and expectations, and constructive use of time. The internal asset categories include commitment to learning, positive values, social competencies, and positive identity. These eight general categories are further divided into assets that are more specific. The assets of positive identity, empowerment, positive values, and social competencies are similar to the concepts of likeability, power, and morality discussed in the self-concept literature.

The Search Institute[21] has found that the more assets the young person has, the fewer his or her high-risk behaviors. Specific behaviors for nurturing the development of each asset have been identified. These asset development guidelines provide concrete direction facilitating the development of self-concept-enhancing experiences in the young person's life. Specific asset-building behaviors are discussed in the next section under each developmental age to provide practitioners with direction in supporting the development of positive perceptions of self.

Sidney Jourard[22] provides direction for interventions related to an individual's self-concept. The healthy self-concept allows individuals to play roles they have satisfactorily played while gaining personal satisfaction from this role enactment. This person also continues to develop and maintain a high level of physical wellness. This high level of wellness is achieved by gaining knowledge of oneself through a process of self-disclosure. Jourard[22] states that, "If self-disclosure is one of the means by which healthy personality is both achieved and maintained, we can also note that such activities as loving, psychotherapy, counseling, teaching and nursing, all are impossible—without the disclosure of the client."

Elaboration of this thought reveals that for the nurse to effectively meet the needs of the client, an understanding of the client's self must be achieved. This understanding must go beyond the interpretation of overt behavior, which is an indirect method of understanding, and access the client's understanding of self through the process of self-disclosure.

Dufault and Martocchio[23] present a conceptual model for hope that also provides a useful perspective for nursing intervention. Hope is defined as multidimensional and process-oriented. Hopelessness is not the absence of hope but is the product of an environment that does not activate the process of hoping. Vaillot[24] supports the view presented by Dufault and Martocchio with the existential philosophical perspective that hope arises from relationships and the beliefs about these relationships. One believes that help can come from the outside of oneself when all internal resources are exhausted. Hopelessness arises in an environment where hope is not communicated. This model supports nursing interventions from a systems theory perspective, because it validates the ever-interacting system, the whole. In this perspective, the nurse, as well as the client, contributes to the "hopelessness," and thus the responsibility of nurturing hope is shared.[23–27]

DEVELOPMENTAL CONSIDERATIONS

INFANT

In general, the sources of anxiety begin in a very narrow scope with the infant and broaden out as he or she matures. Initially the relationship with the primary caregiver is the source of gratification for the infant, and disruptions in this relationship result in anxiety. As one matures, needs are met from multiple sources, and therefore the sources of anxiety expand. Specific developmental considerations are described in the paragraphs that follow.

The primary source of anxiety for the infant appears to be a sense of "being left." This response begins at about 3 months. Sullivan,[9] as indicated earlier, would contend that the infant could experience anxiety even earlier with any disruption in having needs met by the primary caregiver. At age 8 to 10 months, separation anxiety peaks for the first time. At 5 to 6 months, the infant begins to demonstrate stranger anxiety. Primary symptoms include disruptions in physiologic functioning and could include colic, sleep disorders, failure to thrive syndrome, and constipation with early toilet training. Stranger anxiety and separation anxiety may be demonstrated with screaming, attempting to withdraw, and refusing to cooperate. Both stranger anxiety and separation anxiety are normal developmental responses, and should not be considered pathologic as long as they are not severe or prolonged, and if the parental response is appropriately supportive of the infant's needs.

Fear is a normal protective response to external threats and will be present at all ages. It becomes dysfunctional at the point that it is attached to situations that do not present a threat, or when it prevents the individual from responding appropriately to a situation. Thus, it is important that children have certain fears to protect them from harm. The hot stove, for example, should produce a fear response to the degree that it prevents the child from touching the stove and being injured. Fear is a learned response to situations, and children learn this response from their caregivers. Thus, it becomes the caregivers' responsibility to model and teach appropriate fear. If a mother cannot tolerate being left alone in the house at night with her children, her children will learn to fear being in this situation. When this home is located in a low-crime area with supportive neighbors and appropriate locks, fear becomes an inappropriate response, and the children may be affected by it for a lifetime.

Various developmental stages have characteristic fears associated with them. In the mind of the child, these characteristic fears present threats, so the fears can be seen both as a source of fear and as a source of anxiety. The characteristic fears result from strong or noxious environmental stimuli such as loud noises, bright lights, or sharp objects against the skin. The response to fears produces physiologic symptoms. The most immediate and obvious response of the child is crying and pulling away from the stressful object or situation.

Erickson[28] indicated that he thought hope evolved out of the successful resolution of this first developmental stage, basic trust versus mistrust. Hope was perceived by Erickson to be a basic human virtue. The type of environment that has been identified as promoting the development of this basic trust is warm and loving, where there is respect and acceptance for personal interests, ideas, needs, and talents.[25] Several environmental conditions have been associated with early childhood and are seen as increasing the perceptions consistent with hopelessness. These conditions are economic deprivation, poor physical health, being raised in a broken home or a home where parents have a high degree of conflict, having a negative perception of parents, or having parents who are not mentally healthy. From an existential perspective, Lynch[29] identified five areas of human existence that can produce hopelessness. If these areas are not acknowledged in the developmental process, the individual is at greater risk of frustration and hopelessness because hope is being intermingled with a known area of hopelessness. The five areas that Lynch identified are death, personal imperfections, imperfect emotional control, inability to trust all people, and personal areas of incompetence. This supports Erickson's contention that hope evolves out of the first developmental stage, because these basic areas of hopelessness are issues related primarily to the resolution of trust and mistrust. It should be remembered that previously resolved or unresolved developmental issues must be renegotiated throughout life.

Each developmental stage has a set of specific etiologies and symptom clusters related to hopelessness. Because the relationship between self-concept strength and degree of hopefulness is seen as a positive link, many of the etiologies and symptoms of hopelessness at the various developmental stages are similar to those of self-esteem disturbances.[30]

As conceptualized by Erickson,[28] infancy is the primary age for developing a hopeful attitude about life. If the infant does not experience a situation in which trust in another can be developed, then the base of hopelessness has begun. Thus, if the infant experiences frequent change in caregivers, or has a caregiver who does not meet the basic needs in a consistent and warm manner, the infant will become hopeless. Research[29] has indicated that children who have been raised in an environment of despair are at greater risk for experiencing hopelessness. Symptoms of hopelessness in infants resemble infant depression or failure to thrive. Because symptoms in infants are a general response, the diagnosis of Hopelessness must be considered equally with other diagnoses that produce similar symptom clusters, such as Powerlessness and Ineffective Coping.

One's perceptions of place in the larger system and of influence in this system begin at birth. These perceptions are developed through interactions with those in the immediate environment and continue throughout life with each new interaction in each new experience. Thus, the child learns from primary caregivers that his or her expressions of need may or may not have an effect on those around him or her and also learns what must be done to have an effect. If the caregiver responds to the earliest cries of the infant, a sense of personal influence has begun. The two areas that consistently influence one's perceptions of influence are discipline and communication styles.

Implementation of discipline in a manner that provides the child with a sense of control over the environment while teaching appropriate behavior can produce a perception of mutual system influence. Harsh, over-controlling methods can produce the perception that the child does not have any influence in the system if acting in a direct manner. This produces an indirect influencing style. An example of indirect influence is the child who always becomes ill just before his parents leave for an evening on the town. The parents, out of concern for the child, decide to remain at home and thus never have time together as a couple. Authoritarian styles of interaction can also produce perceptions of powerlessness in adults in unfamiliar environments. If the hospital staff acts in an authoritarian manner, the client may develop perceptions of powerlessness.

Double-bind communication can place the individual in a position of feeling that "no matter what action I take, it appears to be wrong," and also can produce a perception of powerlessness. They are "damned if they do and damned if they don't." If the individual cannot influence this system in a direct manner, again, indirect behavior patterns are chosen. Bateson[30] proposes that this is the process behind the symptom cluster identified as schizophrenia. This suggests that if the child is continually placed in the position of being wrong no matter what he or she has done, the child could develop the perception that his or her position is one of powerlessness and carry this attitude with him or her throughout life.

Infants have a need for consistent response to having physiologic needs met, and the most important relationship becomes that with the "parenting one." If this relationship is disrupted and needs are not met, symptoms related to infant depression or failure to thrive could communicate a perception related to powerlessness.

It is important to remember that self-concept, including body image, is developed throughout life. For the infant, the primary source of developing self-concept and body image is physical interaction with the environment. This includes both the environment's response to physical needs and the body's response to environmental stimuli.

Some behaviors that build assets in the infant and toddler include playing with the child at eye level; exposing the child to positive values by modeling sharing and being nice to others; reading to the child; providing a safe, caring, stimulating environment; and communicating to the child that he or she is important by spending time with him or her.[31]

These behaviors have the strongest impact on the infant when they are provided in an environment of consistent relationships and respect. Consideration of the child's preferences and abilities nurtures positive self-knowledge.[32]

TODDLER AND PRESCHOOLER

The basic sources of anxiety remain the same as for the infant. Separation anxiety appears to peak again at 18 to 24 months, and stranger anxiety peaks again at 12 to 18 months. Loss of significant others is the primary source of anxiety at this age. In addition to the physiologic responses already mentioned, the child may demonstrate anxiety by motor restlessness and regressive behavior. The preschooler can begin to tolerate longer periods away from the parenting one and enjoys having the opportunity to test his or her new abilities. Lack of opportunity to practice independent skills can increase the discomfort of this age group. Increased anxiety can be seen in regressive behavior, motor restlessness, and physiologic response.

Sources of anxiety can include concerns about the body and body mutilation, death, and loss of self-control. These concerns can be expressed in the ways previously discussed, as well as with language and dramatic play, as language abilities increase. This could include playing out anxiety-producing situations with dolls or other toys. This play can assume a very aggressive nature. The anxieties of the day can also be expressed in dreams and result in nightmares or other sleep disturbance.

In this age group, fears evolve from real environmental stimuli and from imagined situations. Typical fears of specific age groups are fear of sudden loud noise (2 years), fear of animals (3 to 4 years), fear of the dark (4 to 5 years), and fear of the dark and of being lost (6 years). Symptoms of fears include regressive behavior, physical and verbal cruelty, restlessness, irritability, sleep disturbance, dramatic play around issues related to the fear, and increased physical closeness to the caregiver.

Alterations to the body or its functioning place a child at this age at the greatest risk of experiencing hopelessness. If the child experiences a difference between self and other or is ashamed about body functioning, in a nonsupportive environment, hopelessness can develop. A specific issue encountered at this stage is toilet training. If the child is placed in a position of being required to gain control over bowel and bladder functions before the ability to physically master these functions has developed, the child can experience hopelessness in that he or she truly cannot make his or her body function in the required manner. Peer interactions are also important at this time because they foster the beginnings of trust in someone other than the "mothering" one, thus understanding that hope can be gained elsewhere.

Struggle between self-control and control by others becomes the primary psychosocial issue. If appropriate expansion of self-control is encouraged, the child will develop perceptions related to mutual systemic influence. This appropriate support is crucial if the child is to develop a perception of a personal role in the social system. If this struggle for self-control is thwarted, the child can express themes of over control in play or become overly dependent on the primary caregiver and withdraw completely from new situations and learning.

For the preschooler, there is a continuation and refinement of a sense of personal influence. Varying approaches are explored, and a greater sense of what can be achieved is developed. One of the primary sources of anxiety during this stage is loss of self-control. Symptoms of difficulties in this area include playing out situations with personal influence as a theme and aggressive play.

Sources of the self-concept perceptions are the responses of significant others to exploration of new physical abilities and to the toddler's place in these relationships. The primary concept of self is related to physical qualities, motor skills, sex type, and age. A concept of physical differences and of physical integrity is developed. Thus, situations that threaten the toddler's perception of physical wholeness can pose a threat. This would include physical injury. Toilet training poses a potential threat to the successful development of a positive self-concept or body image. Failure at training could produce feelings of personal incompetence or of the body being shameful.

In the preschooler, physical qualities, motor skills, sex type, and age continue to be the primary components of self-concept. Peers begin to assume greater importance in self-perceptions. Physical integrity continues to be important, and physical difference can have a profound effect on the preschool child.

Actions that build assets in the preschooler include playing and talking to them on eye level; asking them to talk with you about things they have seen; working with them to use words to express themselves; reading to them; taking them to community events, museums, and cultural events; modeling for them how to behave; providing a supportive family life; providing clear rules and consequences; involving child in creative activities; modeling expectation that others will do things well; valuing expressions of caring; assisting the child to learn the difference between truth and lying; assisting the child to make simple choices and decisions; and helping the child to learn how to deal nonviolently with challenges and frustrations.[27] With growing sense of self independent of others, positive responses to their increased competencies facilitates the development of a positive perception of self.[32]

SCHOOL-AGE CHILD

Typically, fears are aroused by strange noises such as ghosts and imagined phantoms; natural elements such as fire, water, or thunder (6 years); not being liked or being late for school (7 years); and personal failure or inadequacy (8 to 10 years). Symptoms of these fears include physical symptoms of autonomic stimulation, increased verbalization, withdrawal, aggression, sleep disturbance, or needing to repeat a specific task many times.

Concerns about imagined future events produce the anxieties of the school-age child. The specific concern varies with the developmental age. Young school-age children demonstrate concerns related to the unknowns in their environment, such as dark rooms, and natural elements, such as fire or tornadoes. Older school-age children have anxieties related to personal inadequacies. Preadolescence brings increasing concerns about the valuation of peers and concerns about the acceptance of peers. Expression of anxiety can occur in the ways discussed in the previous level, with the addition of increased verbalization and compulsive behavior such as repeating a specific task many times.

Peers' perceptions of the individual assume a role in the development of attitudes related to personal hopefulness and influence within the larger social system. This is built on the perceptions achieved during earlier stages of development. The sense of a strong peer group can produce perceptions of help coming from the outside as long as the child thinks and believes along with the group, but can produce perceptions of exaggerated personal influence. Problems at this developmental stage can be demonstrated by withdrawal, daydreaming, increased verbalizations of helplessness and hopelessness, angry outbursts, aggressive behavior, irritability, and frustration.

Self-perception expands to include ethnic awareness, ambition, ideal self, ordinal position, and conscience. There is increasing awareness of self as different from peers. Peers become increasingly important in developing a concept of self, and there is increased comparison of real to ideal self.

Behaviors that can build assets in this age group include exposing the child to caring environments and role models outside the family; providing the child with useful, age-appropriate roles; providing clear and appropriate boundaries and expectations; promoting involvement in creative activities; promoting involvement with positive learning experiences; exposing the child to values that include caring, honesty, and appropriate responsibility; and providing the child opportunities to make age-appropriate decisions.[31]

ADOLESCENT

The developmental theme that elicits anxiety in this age group revolves around the development of a personal identity. This is facilitated by peer relationships, which can also be the source of anxiety. Expression of this anxiety can occur in any of the ways previously discussed and with aggressive behavior. This aggression can take both verbal and physical forms. A certain amount of "normal" anxiety is experienced as the adolescent moves from the family into the adult world. Anxiety is considered abnormal only if it violates societal norms and is severe or prolonged. Parental education and support during this development crisis can be crucial.

Peer relationships, independence, authority figures, and changing roles and relationships can contribute to fears for adolescents. Expression of these fears produces cognitive and affective symptoms. These symptoms could include difficulties with attention and concentration, poor judgment, alterations in mood, and alterations in thought content.

The cognitive development of adolescents would suggest that their perceptions of situations are guided by hypothetical–deductive thought, and as a result they could develop reasonable models of hopefulness. This cognitive process occurs in conjunction with a lack of a variety of life experience and self-discipline and with a heightened state of emotionality. This can result in a situation in which the immediate goal can overshadow future consequences or possibilities. An adolescent who appears very hopeful when cognitive functioning is not overwhelmed by emotions can be filled with despair when involved in a very emotional situation. Consideration of this ability is important when caring for this age group. It is important to distinguish problem behavior from normal behavior and mood swings. Kinds of behavior that could indicate problems in this area include withdrawal and increased or amplified testing of limits. Situations that affect the peer group hope can place the adolescent at great risk.

Again, issues of dependence–independence assume a primary role. The focus of this struggle is dependence on peers and independence from family. The challenge for adolescents becomes achieving what Erickson and Kinney[32] refer to as "affiliated individuation." This requires that they learn how to be dependent on support systems while maintaining their independence from these same support systems and feeling accepted in both positions.

Body image becomes a crucial area of self-evaluation because of changing physical appearance and heightened sexual awareness. This evaluation is based on the cultural ideal as well as that of the peer group. Perceived personal failures are often attributed to physical differences.

The importance of a positive self-concept for adolescents is highlighted by research that indicates a complex relationship between self-concept, psychological adjustment, and behavior. Most significant is the consistent finding that low self-concept leads to a greater incidence of delinquency. This relationship appears to be strongest with factors that are associated with the moral–ethical self-concept.[33] Theoretical explanations for this phenomenon consider the behavior as a method for balancing the negative view of self or as part of a cycle of punishment resulting in shame, guilt, and expulsion rather than reconstruction.[33] This link between self-concept and the complex of behaviors termed delinquency increases the importance of providing adolescents with asset-building experiences. Assets important for adolescents include family love and support, parent involvement in schooling, positive family communication, caring school environment, useful community roles, safe community environment, clear rules and consequences, positive adult role models, participation in creative activities, involvement in community activities, spending most evenings at home, positive learning experiences, development of planning and decision-making skills, development of interpersonal skills, development of a sense of personal power, a sense of purpose, and a positive view of the future.[31] Specific asset-building behaviors can include asking teens for their opinion or advice, helping teens to contribute to their communities, encouraging them to assume leadership roles in addressing issues that are of concern to them, talking with teens about their goals, providing challenging learning opportunities, providing increasing opportunities for teens to make their own decisions, celebrating their accomplishments, providing listening time, learning their names, and asking them about their interests.[34]

ADULT

Changes in role and relationship patterns generate the fears specific to these age groups. These could include parenthood, marriage, divorce, retirement, or death of a spouse. Fear expression in these age groups produces cognitive and affective symptoms similar to those described for the adolescent.

A specific developmental crisis can produce a perception of hopelessness and powerlessness. The situations that place the adult at risk are marriage, pregnancy, parenthood, and divorce.

Concerns about role performance assume an important role in self-perceptions. Perceived failures in meeting role expectations can produce negative self-evaluation. The number of roles a person has assumed and the personal, cultural, and support system value placed on the identified roles determine the threat that negative evaluation of performance can be to self-perception. Cultural value and personal identity formation determine the degree to which body image remains important in providing a positive evaluation of self. The adult endows unique significance to various body parts. This valuing process is personal and is often not in personal awareness until there is a threat to the part.

OLDER ADULT

As the older adult continues to age, he or she faces numerous challenges to self-perception and self-concept. Roles may change secondary to retirement or loss of significant others, such as a spouse or child. Financial resources may become limited or fixed as a result of illness, retirement, or loss of spouse.[35] Chronic illness that necessitates a decrease in social interactions or increased dependence on others, and the resulting loss of control, has a negative impact on self-esteem for some elderly.[36]

Negative societal feedback, such as ageism, sends a message to older adults that they are somehow no longer valuable to the society. In the face of these decremental losses, it is necessary to consider what health-care professionals can do to assist the older adult in maintaining a positive regard for self.

TABLE 8.1 NANDA, NIC, and NOC Taxonomic Linkages

GORDON'S FUNCTIONAL HEALTH PATTERN	NANDA NURSING DIAGNOSIS	NIC PRIORITY INTERVENTIONS	NOC EVALUATIONS
Self Perception and Self-Concept Pattern	Anxiety	Anxiety Reduction Calming Technique Coping Enhancement	Anxiety Level Anxiety Self-Control Concentration Coping Hyperactivity Level
	Body Image, Disturbed	Body Image Enhancement Coping Enhancement Self-Esteem Enhancement	Adaptation to Physical Disability Body Image Child Development: Adolescence Self-Esteem
	Death Anxiety	Dying Care Spiritual Support	Acceptance: Health Status Anxiety Self-Control Comfortable Death Dignified Life Closure Fear Self-Control Psychosocial Adjustment: Life Change Spiritual Health
	Fear	Anxiety Reduction Coping Enhancement Security Enhancement	Fear Level Fear Level: Child Fear Self-Control
	Hopelessness	Hope Instillation Decision-Making Support Emotional Support Energy Management Support System Enhancement	Depression Self-Control Hope Mood Equilibrium Psychomotor Energy Quality of Life Will to Live

(table continued on page 528)

TABLE 8.1 NANDA, NIC, and NOC Taxonomic Linkages (continued from page 527)

GORDON'S FUNCTIONAL HEALTH PATTERN	NANDA NURSING DIAGNOSIS	NIC PRIORITY INTERVENTIONS	NOC EVALUATIONS
	Loneliness, Risk for	Family Integrity Promotion Socialization Enhancement Visitation Facilitation	Adaptation to Physical Disability Communication Family Functioning Family Integrity Family Social Climate Grief Resolution Immobility Consequences: Psycho-Cognitive Leisure Participation Loneliness Severity Psychosocial Adjustment: Life Change Risk Control Risk Detection Social Interaction Skills Social Involvement Social Support
	Personal Identity, Disturbed	Decision-Making Support Self-Esteem Enhancement	Distorted Thought Self-Control Identity Self-Mutilation Restraint
	Powerlessness, Risk for and Actual	**Actual** Self-Esteem Enhancement Self-Responsibility Facilitation	**Actual** Family Participation in Professional Care Health Beliefs Health Beliefs: Perceived Ability to Perform; Perceived Control; Perceived Resources Hope Participation: Health Care Decisions Personal Autonomy Self-Esteem
		Risk for Self-Esteem Enhancement Self-Responsibility Facilitation	**Risk for** Abuse Recovery Status Anxiety Level Anxiety Self-Control Decision-Making Depression Level Depression Self-Control Fear Level Fear Self-Control Health Beliefs Health Beliefs: Perceived Ability to Perform; Perceived Control; Perceived Resources Immobility Consequences: Psycho-Cognitive Information Processing

GORDON'S FUNCTIONAL HEALTH PATTERN	NANDA NURSING DIAGNOSIS	NIC PRIORITY INTERVENTIONS	NOC EVALUATIONS
			Participation in Health Care Decisions Personal Autonomy Risk Control Risk Detection Self-Esteem Social Interaction Skills Social Involvement Social Support Stress Level
	Self-Concept, Readiness for Enhanced	*Still in development*	Abuse Recovery Status Body Image Personal Autonomy Self-Esteem
	Self-Esteem: Chronic Low, Situational Low, and Situational Low, Risk for	**Chronic Low** Self-Esteem Enhancement **Situational Low** Self-Esteem Enhancement **Situational Low, Risk for** Self-Esteem Enhancement	**Chronic Low** Depression Level Personal Autonomy Quality of Life Self-Esteem **Situational Low** Adaptation to Physical Disability Grief Resolution Psychosocial Adjustment: Life Change Self-Esteem **Situational Low, Risk for** Abuse Recovery Status Abuse Recovery: Emotional; Financial; Physical; Sexual Adaptation to Physical Disability Body Image Child Development: Adolescence Coping Grief Resolution Neglect Recovery Psychosocial Adjustment: Life Change Risk Control Risk Detection Role Performance Self-Esteem
	Self-Mutilation, Risk for and Actual	**Actual** Behavior Management-Self Harm Counseling Environmental Management Safety Impulse Control Training Wound Care	**Actual** Identity Impulse Self-Control Self-Mutilation Restraint

(table continued on page 530)

⣿⣿ TABLE 8.1 NANDA, NIC, and NOC Taxonomic Linkages *(continued from page 529)*

GORDON'S FUNCTIONAL HEALTH PATTERN	NANDA NURSING DIAGNOSIS	NIC PRIORITY INTERVENTIONS	NOC EVALUATIONS

		Risk for
		Anger Control Assistance
		Behavior Management
		  Self-Harm
		Environmental
		  Management: Safety
			Risk for
			Abuse Recovery Status
			Abuse Recovery:
			  Emotional, Physical,
			  Sexual
			Anxiety Level
			Distorted Thought Self-
			  Control
			Impulse Self-Control
			Mood Equilibrium
			Risk Control
			Risk Detection
			Self-Mutilation Restraint
			Substance Addiction
			  Consequences

 APPLICABLE NURSING DIAGNOSES

ANXIETY

DEFINITION⁴⁰

A vague uneasy feeling of discomfort or dread accompanied by an autonomic response; the source is often nonspecific or unknown to the individual; a feeling of apprehension caused by anticipation of danger. It is an alerting signal that warns of impending danger and enables the individual to take measures to deal with threat.

DEFINING CHARACTERISTICS⁴⁰

1. Behavioral
   a. Diminished productivity
   b. Scanning and vigilance
   c. Poor eye control
   d. Restlessness
   e. Glancing about
   f. Extraneous movement (e.g., foot shuffling and hand and arm movements)
   g. Expressed concerns due to change in life events
   h. Insomnia
   i. Fidgeting
2. Affective
   a. Regretful
   b. Irritability
   c. Anguish
   d. Scared
   e. Jittery
   f. Overexcited
   g. Painful and persistent increased helplessness
   h. Rattled

   i. Uncertainty
   j. Increased wariness
   k. Focus on self
   l. Feelings of inadequacy
   m. Fearful
   n. Distressed
   o. Worried, apprehensive
   p. Anxious
3. Physiologic
   a. Voice quivering
   b. Increased respiration (sympathetic)
   c. Urinary urgency (parasympathetic)
   d. Increased pulse (sympathetic)
   e. Pupil dilation (sympathetic)
   f. Increased reflexes (sympathetic)
   g. Abdominal pain (parasympathetic)
   h. Sleep disturbance (parasympathetic)
   i. Tingling in extremities (parasympathetic)
   j. Increased tension
   k. Cardiovascular excitation (sympathetic)
   l. Increased perspiration
   m. Facial tension
   n. Anorexia (sympathetic)
   o. Heart pounding (sympathetic)
   p. Diarrhea (parasympathetic)
   q. Urinary hesitancy (parasympathetic)
   r. Fatigue (parasympathetic)
   s. Dry mouth (sympathetic)
   t. Weakness (sympathetic)
   u. Decreased pulse (parasympathetic)
   v. Facial flushing (sympathetic)
   w. Superficial vasoconstriction (sympathetic)
   x. Twitching (sympathetic)
   y. Decreased blood pressure (parasympathetic)

z. Nausea (parasympathetic)
aa. Urinary urgency (parasympathetic)
bb. Faintness (parasympathetic)
cc. Respiratory difficulties (sympathetic)
dd. Increased blood pressure (sympathetic)
ee. Trembling/hand tremors
ff. Shakiness

4. Cognitive
  a. Blocking of thought
  b. Confusion
  c. Preoccupation
  d. Forgetfulness
  e. Rumination
  f. Impaired attention
  g. Decreased perceptual field
  h. Fear of unspecified consequences
  i. Tendency to blame others
  j. Difficulty concentrating
  k. Diminished ability to problem solve and learn
  l. Awareness of physiologic symptoms

RELATED FACTORS[40]

1. Exposure to toxins
2. Unconscious conflict about essential values/goals of life/Familial Association/heredity
3. Unmet needs
4. Interpersonal transmission/contagion
5. Situational/Maturational crises
6. Threat of death
7. Threat to self-concept
8. Stress
9. Substance abuse
10. Threat or change in: role status, health status, interaction patterns, role function, environment, economic status.

RELATED CLINICAL CONCERNS

1. Any hospital admission
2. Failure to thrive
3. Cancer or other terminal illnesses
4. Crohn's disease
5. Impending surgery
6. Hyperthyroidism
7. Substance abuse
8. Mental health disorders
9. Actual, or threat of, significant life changing events
10. Perceptions of threat to self

 Have You Selected the Correct Diagnosis?

Fear
Fear is the response to an identified threat, whereas Anxiety is the response to threat that cannot be easily identified. Fear is probably the diagnosis that is most often confused with Anxiety. An example of a situation in which Fear would be an appropriate diagnosis is: After being released from jail, the prisoner threatened to kill the judge who placed him or her in jail. The judge, if experiencing psychological stress due to this threat and knowing the prisoner was out of jail, would receive the diagnosis of Fear.

Disturbed Personal Identity
This diagnosis is the most appropriate diagnosis if the individual's symptoms are related to a general disturbance in the perception of self. Anxiety would be used when the discomfort was related to other areas.

Dysfunctional Grieving
This would be considered an appropriate diagnosis if the loss was real, whereas the diagnosis of Anxiety would be used when the loss is a threat that is not necessarily real, such as a perceived loss of esteem from others.

Ineffective Individual Coping
This would be the appropriate diagnosis if the individual is not making the necessary adaptations to deal with daily life. This may or may not occur with Anxiety as a companion diagnosis.

Spiritual Distress
This diagnosis occurs if the individual experiences a threat to his or her value or belief systems. This threat may or may not produce Anxiety. If the primary expressed concerns are related to the individual's value or belief system, then the appropriate diagnosis would be Spiritual Distress.

EXPECTED OUTCOME

Will verbalize a decrease in concern about current life situation by _____ [date].

Will demonstrate _____ [number] alternative coping strategy(s) by _____ [date].

Will demonstrate absence of physiological signs and symptoms of anxiety (note those that have been most significant for this client) by _____ [date].[37]

TARGET DATES

A target date of 3 days would be realistic to start evaluating progress. The sooner anxiety is reduced, the sooner other problems can be dealt with.

ADDITIONAL INFORMATION

Anxiety is experienced at varying levels. The level of anxiety impacts the interventions selected. It is important for the nurse to assess anxiety level before selecting nursing interventions.[38]

Low: Adaptive and can motivate for normal activities of life

Mild: Prepares the person for action by sharpening the senses, increasing the perceptual field, alertness, and awareness. This level enhances learning and usually is not perceived as stressful.

Moderate: Reduction of perceptual field, reduced alertness to environment. Learning can occur at a reduced level with decreased attention span and ability to concentrate. Objective symptoms include increased restlessness, heart rate, respirations, perspiration, muscular tension, altered speech (rate, volume, pitch increased).

Severe: Perceptual field greatly diminished, focus on details or fixation on a single detail. Very limited attention span and great difficulty with concentration or problem-solving. Focus is on the self and desire to decrease anxiety. Objective symptoms include Headaches, dizziness, nausea, trembling, insomnia, palpitations, tachycardia, hyperventilation, urinary frequency, diarrhea.

Panic: Inability to focus on any details with misperceptions of the environment. Learning, concentration, and/or comprehension of simple directions cannot occur. Client experiences a sense of impending doom and/or terror. Objective symptoms include dilated pupils, labored breathing, severe trembling sleeplessness, palpitations, diaphoresis, pallor, muscular incoordination, immobility or purposeless hyperactivity, bizarre behavior, hallucinations, delusions.

NURSING ACTIONS/INTERVENTIONS WITH RATIONALES

Adult Health

ACTIONS/INTERVENTIONS	RATIONALES
Monitor anxiety behavior and relationship to activity, events, people, etc. every 2 hours on [odd/even] hour.	When anxiety increases, the ability to follow instructions or cooperate in the plan of care declines. Identification of the behavior and causative factors enhances intervention plans.
Give the patient an opportunity to verbalize perception of situation that is causing anxiety.	
Monitor vital signs at least every 4 hours while awake at [times].	Assists in determining the effects of anxiety. Helps determine the pathologic effects of anxiety.
Reassure the patient that anxiety may be a normal response. Assist the patient to learn to recognize and identify the signs and symptoms of anxiety (e.g., hyperventilation, rapid heartbeat, sweaty palms, inability to concentrate, and restlessness).	Helps identify the connection between the precipitating cause and the anxiety experience.
Provide a calm, nonthreatening environment: • Explain all procedures and rationales for the procedure in clear, concise, simple terms. • Decrease sensory input and distraction (e.g., lighting or noise). • If the presence of family is calming, encourage significant other(s) to stay with the patient	Conveys calm and helps the patient focus on conversation or activity.
Attend to primary physical needs promptly.	Conserves the patient's energy, and allows the patient to focus on coping with and reducing anxiety. Failure to attend to physical needs would increase anxiety.
Assist the patient to develop coping skills: • Review past coping behaviors and success or lack of success.	Determines what has helped, and whether these measures are still useful.
• Help identify and practice new coping strategies such as progressive relaxation, guided imagery, rhythmic breathing, balancing exercise and rest, appropriate food and fluid intake (e.g., reduced caffeine intake), and using distraction.	Methods that can be used successfully to decrease anxiety. Allows the patient to practice and become comfortable with skills in a supportive environment.
• Challenge unrealistic assumptions or goals.	Assists the patient to avoid placing extra stress on him- or herself.
• Place limits on maladaptive behavior (e.g., use of alcohol or fighting).	Promotes use of appropriate techniques for reducing anxiety while avoiding harm to self and others.

ACTIONS/INTERVENTIONS	RATIONALES
Provide at least 20 to 30 minutes every 4 hours while the patient is awake for focus on anxiety reduction. [List times here.] • Encourage the client to express feelings verbally and through activity. • Answer questions truthfully. • Offer realistic reassurance and positive feedback.	Provides an opportunity to practice the technique and express anxiety-provoking experiences.
Administer anti-anxiety medications as prescribed. Monitor and document effects of medication within 30 minutes of administration.	The effectiveness of medication is determined so modification can be provided if needed. Medication helps reduce anxiety to a manageable level.
Collaborate with the psychiatric nurse clinician regarding care (see Mental Health nursing actions).	Collaboration helps provide holistic care. The specialist may help discover underlying events for anxiety and assist in designing an alternate plan of care.
Refer the patient to, and collaborate with, appropriate community resources.	Support groups can provide ongoing assistance after discharge.

Child Health

ACTIONS/INTERVENTIONS	RATIONALES
Monitor for possible causes of anxiety to include situation, recent event, trauma, or medications.	Provides a realistic basis for plan of care.
Review, with the child and parents, coping measures used for daily changes and crises.	The identification of coping strategies provides essential information to deal with anxiety. Once they are identified, the nurse can begin to evaluate the strategies that are effective.
Identify ways the parents can assist the child to cope with anxiety (e.g., set realistic explanations or demands, and avoid bribing or not telling the truth).	A major starting point is to describe the feelings and attempt to create a sense of control, which is more likely in patients of a certain developmental capacity (e.g., those capable of abstract thinking). In younger infants, rocking can provide soothing repetitious notion when all other measures seem not to have calmed the infant.
Adapt the routine to best help the child regain control (e.g., use of speech according to situation, and simple but firm speech pattern).	Allowing the child to plan for meals or snacks with choices when possible or structuring the room to offer a sense of self is conducive to empowerment.
Modify procedures, as possible, to help reduce anxiety (e.g., do not use intramuscular injection when an oral route is possible).	Unnecessary pain or invasive procedures make overwhelming demands on the already stressed hospitalized child with anticipatory safety addressed.
*Exercise safe dosage administration of medications, especially amnesiacs and sedatives, with appropriate attention to back-up resuscitation equipment and staff.	
Use the child's developmental needs as a basis for care, especially for ventilation of anxiety (e.g., use of toys).	The developmental level of the patient serves to guide the nurse in care. A holistic approach is more likely to meet holistic health needs.
Allow the child and parents adequate time and opportunities to handle required care issues and thus reduce anxiety (e.g., when painful treatments must be done, prepare all involved according to an agreed-upon plan.	Appropriate time in preparation offers structure and allows focused attention, which empowers and helps reduce anxiety as efforts are directed to what is known.
*Use a child life specialist when available to assist in pre-procedural planning.	

(care plan continued on page 534)

NURSING ACTIONS/INTERVENTIONS WITH RATIONALES (continued from page 533)

Child Health

ACTIONS/INTERVENTIONS	RATIONALES
Facilitate family involvement with care as appropriate, including feeding, comfort measures, and stories.	Family involvement provides a sense of empowerment and growth in coping, thereby reducing anxiety and promoting a sense of security in the child.
Offer sufficient opportunities for rest according to age and sleep requirements.	Proper attention to rest for each individual child will foster coping capacities by conserving energy for coping.
Identify knowledge needs, and address these by having the family explain what they understand about treatments, procedures, needs, etc.	Provides a teaching opportunity that increases the patient's and family's knowledge about the situation, which assists in reducing anxiety.
Point out and reinforce successes in conquering anxiety.	Positive reinforcement that assists in learning.
Assist the patient and family to apply coping in future potential anxiety-producing situations by presenting possible scenarios that would call for utilization of the new skills (e.g., reviewing use of new coping behaviors before surgery).	Allows practice in a non-anxiety-producing environment. Increases skill in using coping strategy. Empowers the patient and family.
Discuss with the client and family alternative methods for coping with anxiety in the future.	Assists in an minimizing anxiety response to a more manageable degree.

Women's Health

ACTIONS/INTERVENTIONS	RATIONALES
Acute Anxiety Attack Provide a realistic, tranquil atmosphere (e.g., close door, sit with the patient, remind the patient you are there to help). • Do not leave the patient alone. • Speak softly using short, simple commands. • Be firm but kind. • Be prepared to make decisions for the patient. • Decrease external stimuli and provide a "safe" atmosphere.	Provides an atmosphere that assists in calming the patient and promotes the initiation of coping by the patient.
Administer anti-anxiety medication as ordered, and monitor effectiveness of medication within 30 minutes to 1 hour of administration.	Medication is best taken in moderation and only under the guidance of a physician. Today there are many natural and herbal remedies on the market. While some of these therapies can minimize the side effects of strong medications, they must be used with caution and guidance from those who understand and have utilized them in their practices. Practitioners of natural, alternative, or complementary heath care are becoming more well known in this country. Some of the terms used are alternative, complementary, natural, nonallopathic, and non-Western medicine.[41]
Mild or Moderate Anxiety Guide the patient through problem-solving related to the anxiety: • Assist the patient to verbalize and describe what she thinks is going to happen.	

ACTIONS/INTERVENTIONS	RATIONALES
• Describe to the patient what will happen (to the best of your ability), and compare with her expectations. • Assist the patient in describing ways she can more clearly express her needs. Assist the patient in changing unrealistic expectations by explaining procedures (e.g., labor process or sensations during a pelvic examination). Encourage the patient to participate in assertiveness training and/or to join an appropriate support group.[41]	By providing factual information, clarification of misconceptions, and emotional support, it is possible to enhance the patient's coping.[42,43]
Pregnancy and Childbirth Provide the patient and significant others with factual information about the physical and emotional changes experienced during pregnancy. Review the daily schedule with the patient and significant other. Assist them to identify lifestyle adjustments that may be needed for coping with pregnancy. • Practicing relaxation techniques when stress begins to build • Establishing a routine for relaxing after work • Developing a plan to provide frequent rest breaks throughout the day (particularly in the last trimester) Refer to a support group (e.g., childbirth education classes or maternal–child health (MCH) nurses in the community).	Helps reduce anxiety about financial concerns due to having to quit work. Good planning and working with the patient and partner to establish a realistic work schedule to present to the employer can assist the patient to reduce edema and fatigue and thus remain on the job longer.

Provide the patient and significant other with factual information about sexual changes during pregnancy:
• Answer questions promptly and factually.
• Introduce them to people who have had similar experiences.
• Discuss fears about sexual changes.
• Discuss aspects of sexuality and intercourse during pregnancy:
  • Positions for intercourse during different stages of pregnancy
  • Frequency of intercourse
  • Effect of intercourse on pregnancy or fetus
• Describe the healing process postpartum and timing of resumption of intercourse.
	Factual information provides the family with the essential knowledge needed in planning for the pregnancy, accomplishing the task of pregnancy, and adapting to a new infant.[44]

Provide the patient support during the birthing process (e.g., Montrice, doula, or other support person or coach).	Assists in reducing anxiety. Increases coping.
Provide support for significant others(s) during this process: • Encourage verbalization of fears. • Answer questions factually. • Demonstrate equipment. • Explain procedures.	Support of significant others leads to more support for the patient.
Postpartum Provide support for new parents during the first few days of the postpartum period. Provide new parents with telephone number to call with questions and concerns. Call new parents 36 to 48 hours after discharge:	Provides support and information from an "expert," helping to reduce the anxiety of being new parents.

(care plan continued on page 536)

NURSING ACTIONS/INTERVENTIONS WITH RATIONALES (continued from page 535)

Women's Health

ACTIONS/INTERVENTIONS	RATIONALES
• Formulate questions to receive simple one- or two-word answers.	
• Allow new parents time to ask questions and voice concerns.	
Before discharge from the hospital, give the new mother an appointment to return to follow-up clinic, or schedule home visit by nurse for herself and her infant.	Provides a continuity of services and support and education for the new family during time between discharge and follow-up visit to the primary health-care provider.
Assess the mother and baby for appropriate physical recovery from the birth:	
• Maternal: episiotomy, cesarean section incision, breasts (lactating and nonlactating), involution of uterus, lochia flow, fatigue level, etc.	
• Infant: Number of wet diapers in 24-hour period, number of stools in 24-hour period, color and consistency of stools, feeding patterns, bilirubin check, follow-up on newborn screening and hearing screening as mandated by most state law.	Check with your individual state as to the laws governing newborn screening (comprehensive blood testing) and newborn hearing screening.
Discuss with the mother and partner, or family, the psychosocial aspects of being new parents. Be alert to cues or signs and symptoms of depression in the mother. Pay special attention to any sleeping/eating disturbances, anxiety/insecurity, emotional lability, mental confusion, loss of self, guilt/shame or suicidal thoughts, ignoring the infant's cues, and actual neglect of the infant.[45]	Research has shown that postpartum depression can begin during pregnancy, in the postpartum period, or in the weeks and months after the delivery of the baby. A particularly vulnerable group are adolescents, with depression rates as high as 47 percent.[45–47]
Assist in developing and planning coping skills for new roles.	
Provide appropriate education. (May have to repeat all education done during stay in hospital on postpartum unit.)	Readiness for learning for new mothers does not always occur during the hospital stay and requires follow-up. Research has shown that the most important learning needs immediately postpartum were "stitches, episiotomy, and complications," followed by feeding and illness.[48,49]
Monitor the infant and parents for attachment behaviors.	
Refer the parents to appropriate resources for support and further follow-up:	
• Lactation consultants	
• Primary care provider (obstetrician, pediatrician, certified nurse midwife, family practitioner, or nurse practitioner)	
• Public health nurse	
• Visiting nursing services	
Provide documentation of follow-up to the patient's primary care provider.	

ACTIONS/INTERVENTIONS	RATIONALES
Midlife Women	
Provide information about hormone influences on sleep disorders, cardiac and mental functioning (forgetfulness), lack of energy, irritability, weight gain, and perceptions of anxiety.[50,51,53]	Research has shown that hormone influences create symptoms that many women report during the mid-life cycle, usually beginning with perimenopause. The health-care provider should address the concerns of these affective and cognitive disturbances in these women and refer them to appropriate resources.[50-54]
Refer the client to appropriate resources for support and further follow-up: • Physicians well versed in women's health • Women's health centers • Alternative health centers • Menopause and midlife centers	Some resources are: National Women's Health Network 514 10th Street NW, Suite 400 Washington, DC 20004 (202) 347-1140 http://www.Womenshealthnetwork.org The North American Menopause Society P.O. Box 94527 Cleveland, Ohio 44101 (440) 442-7550 http://www.menopause.org

Mental Health

ACTIONS/INTERVENTIONS	RATIONALES
Approach the client in a calm, reassuring manner, assessing the caregiver's level of anxiety and keeping this to a minimum.	Anxiety is contagious and can be communicated from the social network to the client.[33]
Provide a quiet, nonstimulating environment that the client perceives as safe. For the client experiencing severe or panic anxiety, this may be a quiet room setting. This may include providing objects that symbolize safety to the client. (Note here the special environmental adaptations necessary for this client.)	Inappropriate levels of sensory stimuli can contribute to the client's sense of disorganization and confusion.[38,55]
Provide frequent, brief interactions that assist the client with orientation. Verbal information should be provided at a level that the client can process based on his or her anxiety level. Note the client's anxiety level, frequency, and focus of interactions here. (See Additional Information for assistance in determining the client's anxiety level.)	Appropriate levels of sensory stimuli promote the client's sense of control.[28]
If the client is experiencing severe or panic anxiety, provide support in a non-demanding atmosphere. [Note client-specific adaptations here.]	Communicates acceptance of the client, which facilitates the development of trust and self-esteem.
If the client is experiencing severe or panic anxiety, provide a here-and-now focus. • Provide the client with a simple repetitive activity until anxiety decreases to the level at which learning can begin. Note client specific activity here.	High levels of anxiety decrease the client's ability to process information. High levels of anxiety decrease the client's ability to problem solve. Promotes the client's sense of control.
If the client is hyperventilating, guide in taking slow, deep breaths. If necessary, breathe along with the client, and provide ongoing, positive verbal reinforcement.	Re-establishes a normal breathing pattern, and promotes the client's sense of control.

(care plan continued on page 538)

NURSING ACTIONS/INTERVENTIONS WITH RATIONALES (continued from page 537)

Mental Health

ACTIONS/INTERVENTIONS	RATIONALES
Provide a constant, one-to-one interaction for the client experiencing severe or panic anxiety. This should preclude use of physical restraints, which tend to increase the client's anxiety.	Presence of a calm, trusted individual can promote a sense of control and calm in the client. Protects a client's right to the least restrictive environment.[38]
Provide the client with alternative outlets for physical tension. Note techniques to be used by client here. These could include walking, running, talking with a staff member, using a punching bag, listening to music, doing a deep muscle relaxation sequence [number] times per day at [state specific times]. The outlet should be selected with the client's input.	Promotes the client's sense of control, and begins the development of alternative, more adaptive coping behaviors.[56]
Discuss relaxation techniques with the client (visual imagery, deep muscle relaxation, massage, meditation, or music). Have the client select one activity he or she would like to incorporate into his or her coping behaviors. Schedule 30 minutes per day to practice this activity with the client. [Note here activity and practice time.]	These techniques promote physiologic relaxation and shift the client to a state of parasympathetic nervous system recuperation.[37] Repeated practice of a behavior internalizes and personalizes the behavior.[56]
Sit with the client [number] times per day at [times] for [number] minutes to discuss feelings and complaints. As the client expresses these openly, the nurse can then explore the onset of the anxiety with the purpose of identifying the sources of the anxiety.	Identification of precipitating factors is the first step in developing alternative coping behaviors and promoting the client's sense of control.[56,57]
• After the source of the anxiety has been identified, the time set aside can be utilized to assist the client in developing alternative coping styles.	Promotes the client's sense of control.
Provide [number] times per day to discuss interests in the external environment with the client (especially with clients who tend to focus strongly on nonspecific physical complaints).	Provides positive reinforcement through the nurse's attention for improved coping behaviors.[38]
Talk with the client about the advantages and disadvantages of the current condition. (Help the client to identify secondary gain from the symptoms.) This would be done in the individual discussion sessions or in group therapy when a trusting relationship has been developed.	Identification of contributing factors is the first step in developing alternative coping behaviors.[56]
• During the interaction point out dysfunctional thinking patterns. These could include overgeneralization, magnification, dichotomous thinking, catastrophic thinking, and minimization	Thoughts can influence feelings. Cognitive interventions have been demonstrated to have a positive impact on the long-term resolution of anxiety-related disorders.[38,56]
• When these thought patterns are identified (one of the following responses can be implemented): • Discuss alternative ways of viewing the situation • Make a statement or ask a question that challenges the perception • Examine the evidence for and against the thought	Alters distorted thought patterns.[58]

ACTIONS/INTERVENTIONS	RATIONALES
Provide the client with feedback on how his or her behavior affects others (this could be done in an individual or group situation). [The target behavior and goals should be listed here with appropriate informative positive reinforcers.]	Assists the client with consensual validation. Specific positive reinforcement encourages behavior and enhances self-esteem.[38]
Provide positive specific informative feedback as appropriate on changed behavior. (The target behavior and goals should be listed here.) [Note positive feedback to be used with this client here.]	Positive feedback encourages behavior and enhances self-esteem.[38,56]
Provide appropriate behavioral limits to control the expression of aggression or anger. These limits should be specific to the client and listed here on the care plan (e.g., the client will be asked to go to a private room for 15 minutes when he raises his voice to another client). The client should be informed of these limits, and the limits should not exceed the client's capability. The client should be informed of the time frame of the limits (e.g., the time limit for raising his voice is 15 minutes). No limit should be set for an indefinite time. All staff should be aware of the limits so they can be enforced consistently with consistent consequences.	Client and milieu safety is of primary importance.[38]
• Provide the client with an opportunity to discuss the situation after the consequences have been met.	Assists the client with an opportunity to review behavioral limits and provides the staff with an opportunity to communicate to the client that limit setting is not a punishment.
Interact with the client in social activities [number] times per day for [number] minutes. This will provide the client with staff time other than that which is used to set limits. The activities selected should be done with the client's input and stated here in the care plan.	Promotes the development of a trusting relationship. Provides social reinforcers for pro-social behaviors.
Provide medication as ordered, and observe for appropriate effects and side effects (these should be listed here).	Antidepressants are the most commonly prescribed and are supported as the primary pharmacological treatment for most anxiety disorders.[38,56,59]
Inform the client of community resources that provide assistance with crisis situations, and provide a telephone number before the client leaves the unit.	Promotes the client's sense of control and self-esteem.
Develop a list of alternative coping strategies that the client can use at home, and have the client practice them before leaving the unit. (Note strategies to be practiced and practice schedule here. This could include role playing those situations the client identifies as the most difficult to manage.)	Repeated practice of a behavior internalizes and personalizes the behavior.[55,59]
When signs of increasing anxiety are observed, talk the client through one of the coping strategies they have identified. [Note here the client's symptoms of anxiety that are to be addressed and the identified coping strategy.]	Repeated practice of a behavior internalizes and personalizes the behavior.
Provide the client with a written list of appointments that have been scheduled for outpatient follow-up.	Provides visible documentation of the importance of follow-up. Increases the likelihood that appointments will be kept.

(care plan continued on page 540)

Gerontic Health

In addition to the following interventions, the interventions for Adult Health can be applied to the aging client.

ACTIONS/INTERVENTIONS	RATIONALES
Monitor daily for side effects of anxiolytic medications agents if prescribed.	The potential for side effects and drug interactions is increased with older adults because of the decreased metabolism of drugs.
Assure consistent caregivers to the extent possible	Decreases anxiety and facilitates trust.
Identify environmental factors that may increase anxiety, such as noise level, harsh lighting, and high traffic flow.	The environmental factors mentioned, if not addressed, induce more stress in the older individual.
Provide direct, basic information on usual routines and procedures.	May help decrease autonomic nervous system activity and feelings of anxiety.

Home Health

In addition to the following interventions, the interventions for Adult Health can be applied to the home health client.

ACTIONS/INTERVENTIONS	RATIONALES
Teach the client and family appropriate monitoring of signs and symptoms of anxiety: • Increased pulse • Sleep disturbance • Fatigue • Restlessness • Increased respiratory rate • Inability to concentrate • Short attention span • Feeling of dread • Faintness • Forgetfulness	Provides baseline data for early recognition and intervention.
Involve the client and family in planning and implementing strategies to reduce and cope with anxiety: • Family conference: Identification of sources of anxiety and interventions designed to decrease anxiety • Mutual goal setting: Specific ways to decrease anxiety, and identification of role of each family member • Communication	Family and client involvement enhances effectiveness of intervention.
Assist the client and family in lifestyle adjustments that may be required: • Relaxation techniques (e.g., yoga, biofeedback, hypnosis, breathing techniques, or imagery) • Problem-solving techniques • Crisis intervention • Maintaining the treatment plan of health-care professionals who are guiding the therapy • Redirecting energy to meaningful or productive activities (e.g., active games and hobbies, walking, or sports) • Decreasing sensory stimulation	Lifestyle changes require changes in behavior. Self-evaluation and support facilitate these changes.

ACTIONS/INTERVENTIONS	RATIONALES
Assist the client and family to set criteria to help them determine when the intervention of a health-care professional is required (e.g., inability to perform activities of daily living or threat to self or others).	Early identification of issues requiring professional evaluation will increase the probability of successful interventions.
Teach the client and family purposes, side effects, and proper administration techniques of medications.	Provides necessary information for self-care.
Consult with or refer to assistive resources as indicated: • Caregiver support groups • Disease-specific support groups • Counseling services	Use of existing community services; provides for effective utilization of resources.

BODY IMAGE, DISTURBED

DEFINITION[40]

Confusion in mental picture of one's physical self.

DEFINING CHARACTERISTICS[40]

1. Nonverbal response to actual or perceived change in structure and/or function
2. Verbalization of feelings that reflect an altered view of one's body in appearance, structure, or function
3. Verbalization of perceptions that reflect an altered view of one's body in appearance, structure, or function
4. Behaviors of avoidance, monitoring, or acknowledgment of one's body
5. Objective
   a. Missing body part
   b. Trauma to nonfunctioning part
   c. Not touching body part
   d. Hiding or overexposing body part (intentional or unintentional)
   e. Actual change in structure and/or function
   f. Change in social involvement
   g. Change in ability to estimate spatial relationship of body to environment
   h. Not looking at body part
   i. Extension of body boundary to incorporate environmental objects
6. Subjective
   a. Refusal to verify actual change
   b. Preoccupation with change or loss
   c. Personalization of part or loss by name
   d. Depersonalization of part or loss by impersonal pronouns
   e. Extension of body boundaries to incorporate environmental objects
   f. Negative feelings about body (e.g., feelings of helplessness, hopelessness, or powerlessness)
   g. Verbalization of changes in lifestyle
   h. Focus on past strength, function, or appearance
   i. Fear of rejection or of reaction by others
   j. Emphasis on remaining strengths or heightened achievement
   k. Heightened achievement

RELATED FACTORS[40]

1. Psychosocial
2. Biophysical
3. Cognitive or perceptual
4. Cultural or spiritual
5. Developmental changes
6. Illness
7. Trauma or injury
8. Surgery
9. Illness treatment

RELATED CLINICAL CONCERNS

1. Amputation
2. Mastectomy
3. Acne or other visible skin disorders
4. Visible scarring from surgery or burns
5. Obesity
6. Anorexia nervosa

✔ Have You Selected the Correct Diagnosis?

Situational Low Self-Esteem
This diagnosis addresses the lack of confidence in one's self and is characterized by negative self-statements, lack of concern about personal appearance, and withdrawal from others not related to physical problems or attributes. Disturbed Body Image relates to alterations in the perceptions of self due to actual or perceived alterations in body structure or function. The research indicates that for clients with eating disorders the focus of care should be on the total collection of self-schemas or identities; therefore, the preferred diagnosis would be Self-esteem, Chronic or Situational Low.[60] The determination of which of the Self-esteem diagnoses to implement depends on the defining characteristics.

(box continued on page 542)

Have You Selected the Correct Diagnosis? *(box continued from page 541)*

Disturbed Personal Identity
Disturbed Personal Identity is defined as the inability to distinguish between self and nonself. This diagnosis is more involved in the mental health arena. Disturbed Body Image is a reaction to an actual or perceived change in the body structure or function and incorporates the adult health area as well as mental health.

EXPECTED OUTCOME

Will verbalize at least [number] positive body image statements by [date].

Demonstrates [number] of strategies to enhance body image or function by [date].

TARGET DATES

A target date of 3 to 5 days would be acceptable to use for initial evaluation of progress.

NURSING ACTIONS/INTERVENTIONS WITH RATIONALES

Adult Health

ACTIONS/INTERVENTIONS	RATIONALES
Monitor for pain every 2 hours on (odd/even) hour. Administer analgesics. Monitor effectiveness of analgesic within 30 minutes of administration and use noninvasive techniques to keep pain under control.	Uncontrolled pain contributes significantly to problems with body functioning, thus promoting the development and continuation of Disturbed Body Image.
Use anxiety-reducing techniques as often as needed.	Assists the patient in adapting to the changed body image.
Stay in frequent contact with the patient.	Promotes verbalization of feelings, and allows consistent intervention.
Be honest with the patient.	Any dishonesty in terms of recovery, return of function, or rehabilitation needs causes the patient to distrust caregivers and promotes maintenance of body image disturbance.
Point out and limit self-negation statements.	Self-negating statements prolong the problem and interfere with rehabilitation potential.
Do not support denial. Focus on reality and adaptation (not necessarily acceptance).	The patient does not have to accept the problem, but he or she does have to, and can, adapt to the problem.
• Set limits on maladaptive behavior.	Maladaptive behavior supports the continuation of Disturbed Body Image.
• Focus on realistic goals.	Supports continued progress. Allows positive feedback for achievement, and permits the patient to see progress.
• Be aware of own nonverbal communication and behavior.	Any avoidance behavior or nonverbal communication that indicates dismay would support the patient's idea of his or her unacceptability as a damaged person.
Assist and encourage the patient to look at and use affected body part during activities of daily living.	Helps the patient attend to altered body image constructively, and assists the patient to accept him- or herself.
Teach the patient and significant others self-care requirements.	Helps the patient adapt to body change, and improves self-care management. Provides support for self-care, and assists significant others to adapt also.
Refer the patient to available resources: • Prosthetic devices • Assistive devices • Reconstructive and corrective surgery • Occupational therapy	Facilitates adaptation and decreases isolation. Provides long-term support.

ACTIONS/INTERVENTIONS	RATIONALES
• Physical therapy • Rehabilitation services	
Collaborate with the psychiatric nurse clinician regarding care as needed. (See Mental Health nursing actions.)	Collaboration promotes a holistic care plan and hastens solving of the patient's problem.
Refer to and collaborate with community resources.	Provides long-term support. Cost-effective use of already available support.

Child Health

According to age/developmental status, some components of Adult, Women's, or Mental Health also apply, in addition to the following:

ACTIONS/INTERVENTIONS	RATIONALES
Monitor for contributory factors for Disturbed Body Image (e.g., disfigurement or perceived disfigurement) in addition to relationship issues. (The family may perceive such on behalf of the young infant or child.)	Provides database needed to plan interventions more accurately.
Utilize developmentally appropriate communication to assess and determine exact expression of Disturbed Body Image (e.g., use puppet play or constructive dialogue with the toddler).	Developmental capacity has to guide the interaction to gain accurate information.
Provide factual information to assist in dealing with Disturbed Body Image (e.g., availability of assistive devices or surgery).	Knowledge serves to reduce anxiety and assists the patient to cope. Provides options to assist in decision making.
Include other specialists, such as dietitian, occupational, physical, and speech therapist, and child life specialist as required.	Promotes a more accurate and developmentally appropriate holistic plan of care.
Monitor, on a daily basis, for attitude toward body.	Allows daily evaluation, which promotes changes in plan of care to best meet the patient's current status.
Refer patient and family to community support groups as appropriate. Note specific support group information here.	Offers support by peers.

● N O T E : *In some instances, such as an infant or child with an anomaly or a condition offering no hope of resolution, this alteration may accompany other disturbances such as self-esteem, parental coping, and loss.*

Women's Health

ACTIONS/INTERVENTIONS	RATIONALES
Body Image: Surgery Assist the patient to identify lifestyle adjustments that may be needed (e.g., recuperation time or prosthesis as necessary [mastectomy]).	Initiate discharge planning, and assist the health-care provider and patient identify needed resources before surgery, allowing resources to be available to the patient and family when needed.
Monitor the patient's anxiety level and discuss preoperatively: • Discuss routines related to surgery (e.g., anesthesia, pain, length of surgery, postoperative care, and resources available to patient after discharge home).	

(care plan continued on page 544)

NURSING ACTIONS/INTERVENTIONS WITH RATIONALES (continued from page 543)

Women's Health

ACTIONS/INTERVENTIONS	RATIONALES
• Physical changes (e.g., cessation of menstruation or menopausal symptoms related to surgical or natural menopause).	Regardless of how menopause occurs, it is the signal of life-cycle change and many women mourn the loss of the ability to bear children. Research has shown that while many women morn the loss of reproductive abilities, other women begin to feel both liberated and often begin to direct their energies toward the world outside of the home.[50,51,53]
Allow the patient to grieve loss of body image (e.g., no longer able to have children), and provide an empathetic atmosphere that will allow the patient to ventilate concerns about appearance or reaction of significant other.	
Dispel "old wives' tales" (usually connected to hysterectomy) such as: • You will no longer feel like a woman. (Reassure the patient that although there will be no more pregnancies or menstruation, hysterectomy does not affect sexual performance, enjoyment, or response.) • There will be masculinization. (There is no basis for this belief.) • There will be weight gain. (Weight gain will not occur if the patient participates in health living, including an exercise routine and proper diet.)	Provides factual information, allowing the patient to ask further questions and be realistic about her status and goals.
Involve significant others in discussion and problem-solving activities regarding life cycle changes that might affect self-esteem and interpersonal relationships (e.g., hot flashes, appearance, sexual relationships, or ability to have children).	Provides basic information, and allows early intervention for anxiety. Provides an opportunity for teaching and clarification of misinformation.[50,51,53]
In collaboration with other health-care providers, provide factual information on hormone replacement therapy.	Assists the patient in making decision regarding use or nonuse of estrogen therapy. Recent research has shown that some hormone replacement therapy does not support cardiac health and can lead to dementia in older women when not carefully watched. Many physicians and compounding pharmacists are working together to provide patients with individualized hormone replacement therapies, as well as natural sources of hormones.[41,50,51]
Body Image: Pregnancy Assist the patient in identifying lifestyle adjustments due to physiologic, physical, and emotional changes that will occur throughout pregnancy and postpartum.	Knowledge that body changes in pregnancy are normal and temporary encourages the patient to follow through on care. Assists the patient to cope with the pregnancy and adapt to the changing images.
Review with the patient the body changes that occur during pregnancy and the effect on body image (particularly for teenagers): • Weight gain • Breast tenderness and enlargement • Enlargement of abdomen	

ACTIONS/INTERVENTIONS	RATIONALES
• Change in gait • Chlosama (mask of pregnancy) • Striations (stretch marks) from pregnancy	
Consider the patient's age and preparation for pregnancy, including (particularly for teenagers):	Continued home care planning that encourages the patient to better apply good health practices and thus increase maternal and fetal well-being.
• Stress weight loss after delivery usually takes up to 4 to 6 weeks. • Discuss physical development. • Evaluate the patient's attitude toward health-care providers. • Discuss self-esteem. • Provide emotional support. • Prepare the patient for lifestyle interruptions. • Encourage the patient to bring an attractive, loose-fitting dress to wear home. • Caution breastfeeding women against purposeful weight loss while lactating. • Encourage non-breastfeeding mothers to follow low-calorie, high-protein diet for weight loss. • Encourage exercise (begin slowly and work up to desired plan). • Caution the patient to avoid fatigue.	It is important that the new mother not resort to fad diets to speed weight loss, especially if breastfeeding. She will lose the pregnancy weight by following a good diet and exercise program.

Mental Health

ACTIONS/INTERVENTIONS	RATIONALES
Spend [number] minutes with the client at [times] discussing their perception of the situation. After a therapeutic relationship has been established this discussion can be expanded to include: • Discuss with the client meaning of loss or change from a personal, religious and cultural perspective. This discussion should also consider the impact of race, gender, and age. • Discuss with the client the difference between the cultural ideal of physical appearance and the population norm based on the realities of physiology. This activity should be done by the primary care nurse who has developed a relationship with the client. • Discuss with the client his or her significant others' reaction to loss or change.	Promotes the client's sense of control, and provides information that can be utilized in developing a plan of care that will fit within the client's perception of self. Perceptions influence change.[61] Expression of feelings in an accepting environment can facilitate the client's problem solving. Cognitive maps influence the change process.[61] Helps promote reality orientation by contrasting real with ideal, and confronts irrational goals. Support system understanding and support can facilitate the client's adjustment.
Set an appointment to discuss with the client and significant others effects of the loss or change on their relationships. (Time and date of appointment and all follow-up appointments should be listed here.)	Expression of feelings and concerns in an accepting environment can facilitate problem solving. Social support enhances coping.[62,63]
Spend [number] minutes with the client each day to focus on values, thoughts, and feelings that perpetuate body image problems. During this discussion:	Cognitive maps influence behavior.[64]

(care plan continued on page 546)

NURSING ACTIONS/INTERVENTIONS WITH RATIONALES (continued from page 545)

Mental Health

ACTIONS/INTERVENTIONS	RATIONALES

• Point out dysfunctional thinking patterns. These could include overgeneralization, magnification, dichotomous thinking, catastrophic thinking, and minimization
• When these thought patterns are identified (one of the following responses can be implemented):
  • Discuss alternative ways of viewing the situation
  • Make a statement or ask a question that challenges the perception
  • Examine the evidence for and against the thought
	Thoughts can influence feelings. Cognitive interventions have been demonstrated to have a positive impact on the long-term resolution of anxiety-related disorders.[38,56] Alters distorted thought patterns.[58]

• Discrepancies between current behavior and client goals/values • Have client explore perspectives for and against acceptance of change • Utilize goals established by client and credit client with any progress toward their goals	Client-centered interaction facilitates change.[65]
Spend [number] minutes each day to discuss assertive communication skills and practice these with the client. [Note specific behaviors to be practiced here.]	Assists in developing appropriate interpersonal boundaries.[66]
Schedule time with the client's significant other to assess his or her perception of the client and provide him or her with the necessary information to support the client's change. [Note here the time and person responsible for this meeting.]	Support assists with the development of lifestyle changes. Positive support has a positive impact on body image.[63] The support system's response to change can impact the client's perception of self.[62]
Spend [number] minutes with the client at [times] to assist with efforts to enhance appearance.	Promotes the client's sense of control, and enhances self-esteem.
Discuss with the client role exercise plays in health, and develop an appropriate exercise plan. [Note here the plan for this client.]	Provides the client with the information necessary to make healthy lifestyle choices. Exercise has a positive impact on self-esteem and assists with the client developing comfort with changes.
Provide physical activities two times per day at [times] that provide the client opportunities to define boundaries of body. These activities should be ones the client identifies as enjoyable and that are easily accomplished by the client. Those activities that are selected should be listed here. If this diagnosis is in conjunction with an eating disorder, adjust exercise to appropriate levels for the client.	Assists the client in developing a new perception of his or her body.
Have the client draw a picture of self before and after body change, and discuss this with him or her. This activity can also be done with clay models constructed by the client. This activity should be done by the primary care nurse who has developed a relationship with the client.	Assists the client in contrasting and externalizing his or her perceptions of self to facilitate development of congruence between real and ideal.
When the client has begun to discuss issues related to body change with the primary care nurse, the client can then be asked to discuss reactions to image of self in a mirror. One hour should be allowed for this activity. This activity should be done by the primary care nurse who has developed a relationship with the client.	Facilitates the development of congruence between real and perceived self.

ACTIONS/INTERVENTIONS	RATIONALES
Discuss with the client the mental images held of what the altered body is like and what life will be like. One hour should be allowed for this activity, and it should be implemented by the primary care nurse after a relationship has been established. Note the schedule for this activity here.	Discussion of concerns in a safe environment facilitates the development of strategies of coping.
Collaborate with physical and occupational therapy to schedule a time for client to attend group with others experiencing similar loss or change and that fit with the client's comparison targets. This could include support groups, activity groups, or specialty sports teams (e.g., wheelchair basketball team). [Note group schedule here.]	Group membership provides role models for life skills necessary for adaptation and the opportunity for upward comparison.[60,63,67] In addition, groups instill hope, and enhance self-esteem.[38,55,63]
For clients with eating disorders evidence based practice supports using a more comprehensive self-esteem intervention. (See Have You Selected the Correct Diagnosis.) In addition, the following interventions related specifically to body image can be considered:	Disturbances related to perceptions of self are more comprehensive than those related to body image, and effective care addresses these broader concerns.[60]
• Monitor the client for suicidal thoughts or depression related to weight gain.	Change in body shape can negatively impact self-esteem and increase feelings of depression.[64]
• Have the eating disorder client draw a life-size picture of self on paper hung on the wall; then have the client stand against the picture and trace the real outline, and discuss the differences. This activity should be done by the primary care nurse who has developed a relationship with the client.	Assists the client in confronting the difference between his or her perception of his or her body and the real body size and shape.
Collaborate with social services to develop a discharge plan that includes building community support for the client and family.	

Gerontic Health

The interventions for Adult Health can be applied to the aging client.

Home Health

In addition to the following interventions, the interventions for Adult Health can be applied to the home health client.

ACTIONS/INTERVENTIONS	RATIONALES
Involve the client and family in planning and implementing strategies to reduce and cope with disturbance in body image:	Family involvement enhances effectiveness of interventions.
• Family conference: Discuss meaning of loss or change from family perspective and from the perspective of individual members. Discuss the effects of the loss on family relationship roles.	
• Mutual goal setting: Establish realistic goals, and identify specific activities for each family member (e.g., assisting with activities as required or attending support groups as needed).	

(care plan continued on page 548)

NURSING ACTIONS/INTERVENTIONS WITH RATIONALES (continued from page 547)	
Adult Health	
ACTIONS/INTERVENTIONS	RATIONALES
• Communication: Clarify responses to Disturbed Body Image. Assist the client and family in lifestyle adjustments that may be required: • Obtaining and providing accurate information regarding specific Disturbed Body Image and potential for rehabilitation. • Maintaining safe environment. • Encouraging appropriate self-care without encouraging dependence or expecting unrealistic independence. • Maintaining the treatment plan of the health-care professionals guiding therapy. • Altering family roles as required.	Rehabilitation is a long-term process. Permanent changes in behavior and family roles require evaluation and support.
Consult with, or refer to, assistive resources as indicated. • Support groups • Counseling services	Utilization of existing services is efficient use of resources. Rehabilitation therapists and support groups can enhance the treatment plan.

DEATH ANXIETY

DEFINITION[40]

The apprehension, worry, or fear related to death or dying.

DEFINING CHARACTERISTICS[40]

1. Worrying about the impact of one's own death on significant others
2. Powerlessness over issues related to dying
3. Fear of loss of physical and/or mental abilities when dying
4. Deep sadness
5. Fear of the process of dying
6. Concerns of overworking the caregiver as terminal illness incapacitates self
7. Concern about meeting one's creator or feeling doubtful about the existence of a God or higher being
8. Total loss of control over any aspect of one's own death
9. Negative death images or unpleasant thoughts about any event related to death or dying
10. Fear of delayed demise
11. Fear of premature death because it prevents the accomplishment of important life goals
12. Worrying about being the cause of others' grief or suffering
13. Fear of leaving family alone after death
14. Fear of developing a terminal illness

15. Denial of one's own mortality or impending death
16. Anticipated pain related to dying

RELATED FACTORS[40]

To be developed.

RELATED CLINICAL CONCERNS

1. Cancer
2. Any hospital admission
3. Impending surgery
4. Cardiovascular diseases
5. Serious symptoms related to unknown cause
6. Autoimmune diseases
7. Neurologic diseases
8. Progressive chronic diseases

 Have You Selected the Correct Diagnosis?

Anticipatory Grieving
This would be appropriate if the symptoms of grief are related to another's death. If the symptoms are related to one's own death, then the correct diagnosis would be Death Anxiety.

Anxiety
If the symptoms are nonspecific or unknown to the individual, then this would be the appropriate diagnosis. Symptoms of anxiety that relate to one's own death support the diagnosis Death Anxiety.

EXPECTED OUTCOME

Will verbally express concerns about death by [date].
   Will identify [number] of strategies to manage anxiety by [date].

TARGET DATES

Any type of anxiety requires a sufficient amount of time to deal with causes of the anxiety and to learn coping skills. A minimum of 7 days is appropriate before checking for progress.

NURSING ACTIONS/INTERVENTIONS WITH RATIONALES

Adult Health

ACTIONS/INTERVENTIONS	RATIONALES
Take time to create a trusting relationship and a safe place for the patient to talk about the things that make him or her feel anxious about death.	A trusting relationship in which the patient feels free to express his or her fears will assist the patient to open up.
Encourage patients to share their perception of the implications of the illness for their life.[68]	Promotes a trusting relationship, and encourages the patient to seek and acknowledge the value of his or her life.
Work with patient to identify potential sources of duress related to death (e.g., financial burdens, funeral arrangements, dysfunctional relationships etc.).	Identification of these sources can assist in aligning the patient with appropriate resources, thereby decreasing anxiety.
Respect the patient's spirituality. Allow the patient to express his or her own beliefs about what his or her life has meant, death, and after death.	Promotes a trusting relationship.
Invite questions; answer honestly the questions that are asked; give reassurance where reassurance is possible, and emotional support to grieve when reassurance is not possible.	
• **Listen** when the patient describes his or her pain, and help ease both the physical and emotional pain.[41]	Promotes a trusting relationship.
Give analgesics, anxiolytics, or antidepressant drugs as prescribed.	
Direct patient to appropriate resources for assistance to manage personal affairs if desired	
Consult with chaplain or other spiritual support if desired.	

Child Health

● N O T E : *Review developmental conceptual considerations with a keen appreciation of unique needs per each client plus, as applicable, those orders for Adult Health.*

ACTIONS/INTERVENTIONS	RATIONALES
Assess for all possible contributing factors to include, as applicable, the client's verbalization of feelings, family or caregiver perceptions, related family interactions or stressors, and risk indices, with attempt to identify anxiety to be mild, moderate, or acute.	A holistic assessment provides the most thorough database for individualized care.
Once determined, provide appropriate factual information to assist in how best to deal with anxiety.	There will be a difference in how mild, moderate, or acute anxiety is dealt with.
Determine previous effective coping strategies.	Successful coping strategies will assist in establishing possible ways to augment current needs with modification to offer a sense of empowerment.

(care plan continued on page 550)

NURSING ACTIONS/INTERVENTIONS WITH RATIONALES (continued from page 549)

Child Health

ACTIONS/INTERVENTIONS	RATIONALES
Identify ways to assist the child in coping with appropriate incorporation of these strategies in daily care, with identification of additional coping strategies.	Feelings of empowerment will result when attempts are made to adhere to a regimen that values previously successful coping strategies on which new strategies may then be more readily accepted.
Provide a calm atmosphere with limitation of excessive noise, interruptions, or numbers of caregivers.	Enhancement of coping is likely when the surrounding atmosphere does not add more stress.
Provide all health-care team members updates, and seek information as needed to coordinate care on a daily basis. *Ideally the same primary care nurses ought to care for this child and family during this time.	The nurse is in the best position to offer coordination of care while maintaining continuity and affording trust.
Facilitate appropriate involvement of all members of the health care team, especially the child life specialist, psychiatrist, or psychologist.	Child specialists are most appropriately suited to assist in anxiety reduction strategies.
Provide anti-anxiety medications as appropriate to provide adequate pain relief.	Provides augmentation of the therapeutic regimen and offers relief from disturbing symptoms related to anxiety and pain.
Provide opportunities for the child and family to share thoughts of death-related anxiety issues or related feelings on an ongoing basis, with a sensitivity to unexpected potential for same.	Creating a sense of safe haven for all fears and thoughts to be shared demonstrates a valuing of open communication and the worth of the individual, thereby reducing anxiety.
Provide developmentally appropriate tools to assist patient with expression of feelings such as puppets, video viewing, art, or story telling. Note the items that are most useful for this client here.	Age-appropriate expression of anxiety is fostered by preferences of the child per developmental capacity.
Provide opportunities for the utilization of family's cultural practices. [Note special family needs here.]	Individualized sensitivity to culture provides valuing of the person and the importance he or she places on food, beliefs, or specific ways to cope.
Identify with the child and family ways to cope with dying and meaning of death.	When anxieties are diminished, actual engagement with dying can be realistically approached.
Offer assistance in obtaining or notifying clergyman, counselors, or other supportive personnel as needed.	Anxiety may be further reduced with assistance from those who are experts in death and dying.
Provide reassurance according to personal family beliefs about an afterlife or beliefs of same according to age-appropriate concerns of the child.	Anxiety may be further reduced when the child's fears of being alone or separated can be alleviated, while also supporting valued family beliefs.

Women's Health

The interventions for this diagnosis in Women's Health are the same as those given in Adult Health and Gerontic Health.

Mental Health

ACTIONS/INTERVENTIONS	RATIONALES
Provide a quiet, nonstimulating environment. (Note specific adaptations to the environment that promote the client's relaxation, i.e., music, scents, lighting, etc.) [Note the behaviors that facilitate the development of a relationship with this client here.]	Inappropriate levels of sensory stimuli can contribute to the client's sense of anxiety.

ACTIONS/INTERVENTIONS	RATIONALES
Spend [number] minutes per shift talking with the client about concerns and feelings. Include perceptions of death and life.	Assists the client in establishing the link between the feelings of anxiety and thoughts, which facilitates development of coping behaviors.[70] An expression of feeling helps reduce intense emotion that can block problem solving.[71] Frank discussion of fears and concerns can decrease anxiety.[72]
Provide support necessary to meet identified client's spiritual needs. Note any special adaptations needed for this support here (e.g., time for special prayers, meditation, reading, or contact with members of the client's faith community).[58]	
After concerns are identified, validate and normalize the emotional response.	Validation of affect can decrease feelings of isolation and assist the client to connect with others, including the family.[71]
When concerns involve the family and/or support system, schedule [number] minutes each day to bring the family together and facilitate discussion of the issues and concerns. • Develop a list of issues that client/support system identify as important. • Explore beliefs/feelings that facilitate/hinder resolution of concerns. • Develop, with the client and support system, actions that are needed to resolve issues and concerns. This could include resolution of past misunderstandings and forgiveness. • During interactions with client and support system model positive communication skills and facilitate positive interactions between the client and support system.	Assists the support system in bringing forth their own resources and strengths to support one another and problem solve. Decreases the feeling of isolation in members of the support system who are coping with the impending death.[71]
Spend [number] minutes [number] times per day with the client identifying alternative ways of responding to concerns that decrease anxiety. • Once a relationship has been established these discussions can also include opportunities for life review and making appropriate future plans. Note those topics to be discussed with this client here.	Empowers the client and facilitates growth-promoting change.[71] Assists the client in identifying strengths and past coping mechanisms.[72]
Discuss with the support system their need to provide care, and provide them the necessary information and equipment to accomplish this at the level they feel comfortable. (Note the assistance needed to accomplish this care.)	Provides the support system with a sense of helpfulness and control.[71]
Monitor the support system's need for respite, and talk with them about taking breaks to increase their ability to support the client. (Note the family's need here.)	Assists the family in coping with guilt about their need to take a break to enhance their coping resources.[71]
Provide the client with information about his or her care.	Empowers the client and decreases concerns about the unknown.

(care plan continued on page 552)

NURSING ACTIONS/INTERVENTIONS WITH RATIONALES (continued from page 551)

Mental Health

ACTIONS/INTERVENTIONS	RATIONALES
Spend [number] minutes [number] times each day assisting the client with a relaxation sequence he or she has identified as helpful. This could be deep muscle relaxation, visual imagery, meditation, or deep breathing exercises. (Note the method identified by the client here.)	Shifts the physiologic state from sympathetic nervous system arousal to a state of parasympathetic recuperation.[73]
Provide massage for [number] minutes as needed to reduce anxiety. (Note the client's preference for massage here.)	Promotes physical and psychological relaxation.[74]
Identify support systems in the community, and provide the client with a connection to these systems before discharge. (Note those identified for this client here.)	Provides visual documentation of the importance of follow-up and community support, increasing the likelihood that these referrals will be utilized.

Gerontic Health

● NOTE: *Research on the presence of death anxiety in older adults is slowly evolving, with no clear predictors of which older adults are at risk for experiencing death anxiety. Generally, elders with increased physical and psychological problems, and decreased ego integrity, are more likely to have death anxiety. Which physical and/or psychological problems have an impact on death anxiety are not yet clearly identified. In addition to selecting interventions from the adult health and mental health section, nurses caring for older adults may find the following actions to be effective.[75–77]*

ACTIONS/INTERVENTIONS	RATIONALES
Consult as needed with social services, mental health professionals, and/or religious counselors as signs of death anxiety are noted.	Enables clients to discuss and address issues that may be contributing to distress.
Administer anxiolytics cautiously as needed.	Treatment of anxiety.
Assist the client in completing advanced directives.	Death anxiety decreases in clients who have advanced directives.[75]
When consistent with the nurse's personal values and beliefs, pray with the patient as requested by the patient.	Prayer is an important source of coping with death anxiety in older clients.[76]
Monitor older adults for signs of decreased ego integrity, such as statements of regret related to past life experiences, unresolved relational problems, and expressions of despair.	Decreased ego integrity is a contributor to death anxiety noted in older adults.
Assist and encourage the older adult in life review process.	Provides an opportunity to review prior successes, effective and ineffective coping strategies, personal strengths, sense of life satisfaction, and psychological well-being.
Refer the client to hospice services if the client meets admission criteria for hospice care.	The hospice care team is prepared to address needs surrounding death and dying.

Home Health

In addition to the following interventions, the interventions for Adult Health and Mental Health can be applied to the home health client.

ACTIONS/INTERVENTIONS	RATIONALES
Manage the client's pain and other troubling symptoms, such as nausea.	Physical symptoms often contribute to anxiety.
Encourage the family to become involved in the care of the client as much as they are able.	A sense of purpose and usefulness can replace anxiety.
Help the client to talk about his or her anxiety and its source.	Makes the client, the nurse, and the family more aware of issues that need discussing or problems that need to be addressed.
Listen to client and family concerns, and answer all questions truthfully. Tell the client and family as much as you can about the dying process and disease process to decrease the number of "surprises" they may experience with the dying process.[77]	Understanding helps promote a sense of control and order.
Acknowledge all fears, feelings, and perceived threats as valid to the client.	All client fears are valid to the client, whether they are realistic or not.
Reassure the client that even though the dying process cannot be stopped, someone will be with them and they will not be left alone. Then ensure that a family member or caregiver is with the patient at all times.	Fear of abandonment is an almost universal fear of dying persons.[77]
Administer anxiolytics as ordered, and educate the family or caregivers about prescribed medications, their effects, side effects, and scheduling.[77]	Promotes a sense of well-being.

FEAR

DEFINITION[40]

Response to perceived threat that is consciously recognized as danger.

DEFINING CHARACTERISTICS[40]

1. Report of:
   a. Apprehension
   b. Increased tension
   c. Decreased self-assurance
   d. Excitement
   e. Scared
   f. Jitteriness
   g. Dread
   h. Alarm
   i. Terror
   j. Panic
2. Cognitive
   a. Identifies object of fear
   b. Stimulus believed to be a threat
   c. Diminished productivity, problem solving ability, learning ability
3. Behaviors
   a. Increased alertness
   b. Avoidance or attack behaviors
   c. Impulsiveness
   d. Narrowed focus on "it" (i.e., the focus of the fear)
4. Physiologic
   a. Increased pulse
   b. Anorexia
   c. Nausea
   d. Vomiting
   e. Diarrhea
   f. Muscle tightness
   g. Fatigue
   h. Increased respiratory rate and shortness of breath
   i. Pallor
   j. Increased perspiration
   k. Increased systolic blood pressure
   l. Pupil dilation
   m. Dry mouth

RELATED FACTORS[40]

1. Natural or innate origin, for example, sudden noise, height, pain, or loss of physical support
2. Learned response, for example, conditioning or modeling from or identification with others
3. Separation from support system in a potentially threatening situation, for example, hospitalizations, or procedures
4. Unfamiliarity with environment experience(s)
5. Language barriers
6. Sensory impairment
7. Phobic stimulus
8. Innate releasers (neurotransmitters)

RELATED CLINICAL CONCERNS

1. Any hospitalization
2. Any threat to loss of a body part, loss of functioning, or loss of life
3. Perceived or Impending Death

 Have You Selected the Correct Diagnosis?

Anxiety

Anxiety is a vague uneasy feeling combined with an autonomic response to a source that is usually non-specific or unknown. Fear is the anxiety that is a response to recognized and realistic danger. The response to meeting a bear in the woods or the antici-pation of this would be fear. A threat that cannot be identified or linked to a specific situation would be anxiety.

Impaired Parenting

This diagnosis should be considered as the appropri-ate diagnosis when the child's fears result from the parent's modeling or reinforcing of a child's fear or when the parent is not providing the appropriate sup-port for the developmental fears. An example might be the child who becomes uncontrollable in the clinic each time an injection is indicated. During the assess-ment, the nurse discovers that, as a reinforcer to dis-cipline at home, the parent tells the child that if he or she does not behave, the nurse or doctor will give him or her a shot. In this situation, the parent's inappropri-ate use of the threat of the injection produced a fear in the child.

Deficient Knowledge

If the patient indicates that he or she is afraid of not being able to care for himself or herself, then the most appropriate diagnosis would be Deficient Knowledge. Providing the patient with information, teaching, and reinforcement of self-care ability will overcome this diagnosis.

EXPECTED OUTCOME

Will be able to identify specific source of fear by [date].

Will demonstrate normalization of physiological signs/symptoms [note specific signs to monitored for this client here] by [date].[37]

Will identify [number] of strategies for coping with fear by [date].

TARGET DATES

A target date of 2 to 3 days would be acceptable, because the sooner the fear can be reduced, the sooner other problems can be resolved.

NURSING ACTIONS/INTERVENTIONS WITH RATIONALES

Adult Health

ACTIONS/INTERVENTIONS	RATIONALES
Establish a therapeutic and trusting relationship with the patient and family by actively listening, being nonjudg-mental, sitting with the patient, etc.	Promotes an environment that encourages the patient and/or family to verbalize concerns. Promotes an empathetic environment.
Identify other primary nursing needs, and deal with these as needed.	Attention to basic needs may decrease feelings of hope-lessness and of being of no value.
Provide explanations and appropriate teaching for proce-dures, diagnosis, treatments, and prognosis.	
Involve the patient in developing attainable goals and plan of care.	
Assist the patient to identify positive aspects of the situa-tion	
Support the patent's efforts at objectively describing feel-ings of hopelessness	Allows the patient to validate reality.
Assist the patient to find alternatives to feelings of hope-lessness.	Validates reality and encourages use of alternate coping techniques.
Hopelessness may prompt unhealthy eating patterns. (See nursing care plans related to Imbalanced Nutrition and/or Fluid Balance.)	

ACTIONS/INTERVENTIONS	RATIONALES
Support active participation in activities of daily living. Allow for preferences in day-to-day decisions (e.g., establishing a bath time).	Helps restore sense of being in control.
Refer to psychiatric nurse clinician as needed. (See Mental Health nursing actions.)	Collaboration promotes a more holistic and complete plan of care.
Identify religious, cultural, or community support groups prior to discharge. Provide appointments for follow-up.	Support groups can provide advocacy for the patient and continued monitoring and support of the patient after discharge from the hospital.

Child Health

Depending on gender and age/developmental status, some content of Adult, Women's, and Mental Health may also apply.

ACTIONS/INTERVENTIONS	RATIONALES
Offer brief interactions that assist the patient and family with orientation (e.g., hospital unit, procedures, and aspects of care).	Brief explanations and factual information serve to empower the patient and family as the unknown is made known. The patient and family can then focus on dealing with the identified fear rather than with added fears.
In instances of severe fear: • Provide support in a nondemanding atmosphere. • Provide a here-and-now focus. • Provide one-to-one care. • Offer simple, direct, repetitive tasks.	Avoids overwhelming the patient. Promotes a sense of trust.
Provide the patient and family with ways to assist and alternative outlets for physical tension. These outlets should be stated specifically and could include walking, talking, etc., at least [number] times per day at [times]. These outlets should be designed with input from the patient.	Providing such outlets promotes release of tension.
Sit with the patient and parents [number] times per day at [times] for [number] minutes to discuss feelings and complaints. *The same primary care nurses would ideally participate in this process.	As the patient or parents express these factors openly, the nurse can explore the possible onset of fear with the purpose of individualizing the plan according to the patient's needs. The subjective verbalization of fears helps reduce the preoccupation of the patient with the fear in the trusting relationship of nurse–patient/family.
Monitor patient and parents to for changes in feelings about fears. Discuss these changes with the patient and parents.	Reflection on an ongoing basis demonstrates a sensitivity to need.
Provide appropriate behavioral limits to control the expression of aggression or anger. These limits should be specific in time, expected behavior, and consequences. Note the plan for this client here.	Structured rules regarding behavioral consequences create a sense of limits, which provides security for the child.
Provide the patient and parents with opportunities to discuss the behavior after consequences have been met.	Rediscussion and clarification of events serves to update needs and provides feedback for evaluation. Valuing of the patient is also shown.
Provide opportunities for socialization appropriate for the patient and family. Note patient and family preferences here.	Socialization is vital as the individual or family assumes coping behaviors and learns new coping skills.

(care plan continued on page 556)

NURSING ACTIONS/INTERVENTIONS WITH RATIONALES (continued from page 555)

Child Health

ACTIONS/INTERVENTIONS	RATIONALES
Develop a list of alternative coping strategies to be practiced by the patient and family before dismissal (e.g., communication or progressive relaxation). Note techniques to be used by patient here.	Allows practice in a nonthreatening environment. Increases skills.
Ensure follow-up appointments by scheduling them for the patient before dismissal.	Follow-up appointments help ensure follow-up care.
Assist the patient and family to view situation represented as something that can be managed. Model positive reinforcement of desired behavior patterns.	Validation of success in coping provides a sense of empowerment.
Consult with child mental health specialists for unresolved issues related to fear. Make necessary referrals as appropriate.	Provides appropriate anticipatory guidance and offers a greater likelihood of resolution or coping with fears.

Women's Health

● N O T E : *Phobias affect approximately 2 to 3 percent of the adult population, and 80 percent of the affected group are female. The most common phobias among women are agoraphobia, fear of animals, and fear of social situations.*[78,79]

ACTIONS/INTERVENTIONS	RATIONALES
Obtain a detailed history of the patient's fears: • Encourage the patient to discuss signs and symptoms or precipitating event. • Ascertain how often problem occurs. • Have the patient describe her reaction. • Identify coping mechanisms that have previously helped. • Identify those factors or coping mechanisms that do not help.	Provides an essential database for planning appropriate interventions.
Domestic Violence Provide a nonjudgmental, safe environment for all women patients to verbalize their fears. Obtain a good history that can identify high-risk families and high-risk situations. Be alert to subtle clues in the patient's history or physical examination that hint at physical abuse.	Domestic violence against women cuts across all socioeconomic, age, religious, and ethnic strata of the population. Physical abuse usually concerns control and power issues. Domestic violence is not necessarily physical; it refers to violence in any form, both physical and verbal.[51,80–84]
Patiently explain all procedures and their purpose to the patient before performing them. Be aware that procedures in labor and delivery can trigger unpleasant fears and anxieties in the patient, with possible flashbacks to an abusive situation or rape. Perform necessary procedures as quickly as possible and with empathy, allowing the patient to direct as much of the care as possible. Encourage the patient to verbalize her fears and verbally relive the birth experience in a nonjudgmental environment.	Be sensitive to cultural norms in dealing with pregnant women. It is important to be able to speak the patient's language if the health-care provider is to establish the needed rapport to care for the patient. Often immigrant women suffer more severe and repeated abuse before they are aware that they are being abused.[84] Women often delay care during pregnancy because of an abusive situation.[83]

ACTIONS/INTERVENTIONS	RATIONALES
Screen for abuse at every opportunity, during the hospital stay and on postpartum follow-up visits.[80–83]	
Educate women about resources available to them and how you, the health-care provider, can assist them.[80,83]	
Provide written educational material.	Although this material can be displayed in waiting rooms and public areas, it is best to duplicate the display in bathrooms where only the woman can go. Resources and "help lines" need to be on small cards that can be concealed easily by the woman.[80–83]
Inform patients of services and shelters for the battered woman. Post telephone numbers in conspicuous places. Post telephone numbers in the women's bathroom (unavailable to men, so they cannot see the partner getting the number). Tell women to memorize the number and never write it down.	It is important to provide information about resources to these women in an unobtrusive manner, so they can access the resources *when they are ready.*

Birthing Process

Provide a comfortable, nonjudging atmosphere to encourage the patient and her significant other to verbalize their fears of: • The unknown • Safety for herself and her baby • Pain during the birthing process • Mutilation during the birthing process • "Losing control" during the birthing process	Assists in decreasing fear through promotion of verbalization.
Refer the patient to appropriate support groups for information: • Childbirth education classes in the community • Special national organizations	Provides effective use of existing resources and long-range support.
Monitor the patient's level of confidence using prepared childbirth techniques during labor: • Encourage use of relaxation and prepared childbirth techniques during labor. • Provide ongoing and accurate information, during the labor and birth process, to both the patient and her significant other. • Assist the patient in using "imagery" to overcome fears during the birthing process.	Use of relaxation techniques and provision of information regarding progress facilitate the labor process by easing anxiety and promoting comfort.[44]
Provide continuity of care by remaining with and providing comfort for the laboring woman throughout the birthing process: • Provide clear answers to the patient's questions. • Keep the patient informed of her progress in the birthing process.	Encourages involvement in the process, which enhances coping.
Provide the patient and significant others with as many opportunities as possible to make decisions about her care during the birthing process.	

(care plan continued on page 558)

NURSING ACTIONS/INTERVENTIONS WITH RATIONALES (continued from page 557)

Mental Health

ACTIONS/INTERVENTIONS	RATIONALES
Provide a quiet, nonstimulating environment for the client. This would include removing persons and objects that the person perceives as threatening. If the person is experiencing a thought disorder with delusions and hallucinations, attention should be paid to the details of the environment that could be misinterpreted. At times a same-sex caregiver can increase fear in the client.	Inappropriate levels of environmental stimuli can increase disorientation and confusion. Manipulation of the environment can eliminate the fear response.[43]
Obtain the client's understanding of the threat. Use simple concrete questions to obtain information (e.g., "What do you need right now?")	Facilitates the development of interventions that directly address the client's concerns. High levels of anxiety decrease the client's ability to process complex information.[38]
Provide a one-to-one relationship for the client with a member of the nursing staff. This should be maintained until the symptoms return to normal levels. Remain with the client in unfamiliar situations.	Promotes a trusting relationship, and enhances the client's self-esteem. After the relationship is developed, provides a sense of security in unfamiliar situations
Provide clear answers to the client's questions.	Inappropriate amounts of sensory stimuli can increase the client's confusion and disorganization.
Carry on conversations in the client's presence or vision in a voice that the client can hear.	Meets safety needs of the client by eliminating stimuli that could be misinterpreted in a personalized manner.
Inform the client of plans related to care before the plans are implemented. If possible, discuss these with the client (e.g., if it is necessary to move the client to another room or institution, the client should be informed of this change before it takes place).	Promotes the client's sense of control and enhances self-esteem.
Orient the client to the environment.	Promotes safety needs by increasing the client's familiarity with the environment in the accompaniment of a trusted individual.
Maintain a consistent environment and routine. Record the client's daily routine here, along with notes about client's special reactions to visitors and staff members.	Promotes the client's sense of safety and trust by maintaining consistency in the environment.
Provide a primary care nurse for the client on each shift.	Promotes the development of a trusting relationship.
Sit with the client [number] minutes [number] times per shift. (Initially the times should reflect short, frequent contact. This can change with the client's needs.)	Promotes the development of a trusting relationship. Interaction with the nurse can provide positive reinforcement and enhance self-esteem.
Provide the client with objects in the environment that promote security. These may be symbolic items from home or religious objects. List significant items here.	Meets the need for affiliation by providing meaningful objects to which the client is attached.[43]
Note the client's desired personal space, and respect these limits (the general guidelines should be stated here).	Communicates respect for the client, while decreasing the client's anxiety by maintaining a comfortable personal space.
Assist the client with sorting out the fearful situation by: • Recognizing that the experience is real for the client even though it may not be your experience of the situation: "I can see that you are very upset. I can understand how those thoughts could make you fearful."	Communicates respect for the client, while encouraging reality testing.

ACTIONS/INTERVENTIONS	RATIONALES

- Providing feedback about distorted thoughts: "No, I am not going to punish you. I am here to talk with you about your concerns."
- Talking about client's perceptions specific terms and not vague generalizations: "When you say your family is out to get you, who and what do you mean?"
- Focusing conversations on the here and now; this includes information about the effects of the client's behavior on those around him or her, your experience of the client, and your perceptions of the environment.
- Not arguing about the client's perceptions; instead, provide feedback in the here and now with your perceptions of the situation. The client tells you that you must be angry with him or her because of the look you had on your face while reviewing the client's chart. Your response is, "I am not angry with you, when I was looking at your chart, I was thinking about the conversation we had this morning about your job."

Provide the client with as many opportunities as possible to make decisions about his or her care and the current situation.

Promotes the client's sense of control, and enhances self-esteem.

Develop, with the client, a list of potential solutions to the threatening situation.

Teaches the client problem-solving skills, while promoting the client's sense of control and strengths.

Review the developed list of solutions with the client, and assist him or her in evaluating the benefits and costs of each solution.

Facilitates the client's decision making process.

Rehearse with the client, if necessary, the solution selected, or have the client practice a new response to the threatening situation. Note times and frequency of this practice here.

Behavioral rehearsal helps facilitate the client's learning new skills through the use of feedback and modeling by the nurse.[43]

Provide positive informative verbal feedback to the client about efforts to resolve the threatening situation.

Positive feedback encourages behavior and enhances self-esteem.[43]

Spend [number] minutes [number] times each day with the client to develop alternative outlets for the feelings generated by the threatening situation, and provide the opportunity for the use of these outlets. These would be noted in the written care plan so other staff members would be aware of them and could talk the client through their use when they notice the client's discomfort increasing.

Planned coping strategies facilitate the enactment of new behaviors when the client is experiencing stress.

Provide the client feedback that identifies early behavioral cues indicating fear or that he or she is entering a fearful situation.

Early recognition and intervention enhances the opportunities for new coping behaviors to be effective.

Support the client in using alternative coping strategies developed by:
- Providing the necessary environment
- Providing the appropriate equipment
- Spending time with the client doing the activity
- Providing positive reinforcement for the use of the strategy (this could be verbal as well as with special privileges) [Note the special adaptations needed here.]

Promotes the client's perception of control. Positive reinforcement encourages behavior.

(care plan continued on page 560)

Mental Health

ACTIONS/INTERVENTIONS	RATIONALES
If fear is related to a specific object or situation, teach the client to use deep muscle relaxation, and then teach this along with progressively real mental images of the threatening situation. This is for those situations that will not cause the client harm if he or she is approached, such as riding in elevators. This could also include other methods of relaxation such as music, deep breathing, thought stopping, fantasy, assertiveness training, audiotapes with relaxation images or sequences, yoga, hypnosis, and meditation.	The relaxation response inhibits the activation of the autonomic nervous system's fight-or-flight response.
Note techniques to be taught with teaching schedule here.	
Explore with the client ways to increase the feeling of control in threatening situations; e.g., a fear of elevators could be altered by the client only riding in elevators with emergency telephones and only riding when he or she could stand near the telephone. The fear may also indicate that the client is feeling out of control in an unrelated area of his or her life. If this is suspected, this should be explored and ways of increasing control should be explored (e.g., a woman's fear of driving could indicate that she feels out of control in her marriage, and increased assertive behavior with her husband removes the fear). [Note schedule for this discussion here.]	
When the client shows signs and symptoms of fear (note those signs and symptoms unique to this client here), talk him or her through the coping and/or relaxation strategies that have been identified as useful to him or her. Note the client's specific coping strategies to be used here. This may include removing the client from the fear-producing context.	Shifts physiologic state from sympathetic nervous system arousal to a state of parasympathetic recuperation.[73] Behavioral rehearsal helps facilitate mastery of new behavior through the use of feedback and modeling by the nurse.[43] Promotes a sense of control.[70] Contextual stimuli can elicit the fear response.[43]
Provide positive reinforcement for the client's implementation of the new coping behaviors. Note those things that are to be used to reinforce this client here.	Positive reinforcement encourages behavior.
If the method to increase control involves interactions with the health-care team, these should be noted in specific terms on the client's chart.	Promotes the client's sense of control, and enhances self-esteem.
Assist the client in developing strategies to be used in the community after discharge, and role-play various situations with the client [number] times for [number] minutes.	Behavioral rehearsal provides opportunities for feedback and modeling from the nurse.
Collaborate with other members of the health-care team to provide clients with pharmacologic agents to be administered before exposure to a context that elicits fear. Monitor for side effects of these medications and provide appropriate client education.	Gamma-aminobutyric acid (GABA) agonists inhibit the amygdala, which is the location of the fear response.[43]

Gerontic Health

In addition to the following interventions, the interventions for Adult Health and Mental Health can be applied to the aging client.

ACTIONS/INTERVENTIONS	RATIONALES
Assist the patient in discussing the source of fear (e.g., pain, death, or loss of function) by scheduling at least 30 minutes twice a day at [times] to confer with the patient about the fear.	Addressing the source of fear enables the patient to develop a specific plan of action to reduce the fear.
During the interview, observe behaviors of the patient. Patients will not readily offer information of abuse. You may observe: • The patient is unable to provide information without the caregiver present.[87] • The caregiver demonstrates aggressive behavior toward patient.[87] • The patient seems to be controlled by the caregiver and the caregiver shows no affection or seems indifferent to situation.[87]	Elder abuse is not new, but it receives little attention as the elderly in this country seem to be "the invisible population."[87]
Identify which coping strategies that the client has previously used have been effective and which have not. Discuss ways that effective strategies can be used to cope with future fearful events.	This helps the client identify effective strategies while reinforcing that he or she can cope with his or her fear.
Assist the patient in determining what resources are available to enhance his or her coping skills.	Knowledge and use of appropriate resources aid in reducing fear-provoking experiences by increasing the patient's inventory of skills to deal with fear.

Home Health

In addition to the following interventions, the interventions for Adult Health and Mental Health can be applied to the home health client.

ACTIONS/INTERVENTIONS	RATIONALES
Ask the client to describe the precipitating event.	Assists the nurse in understanding the client's perception of the fear.
Determine the client's perception of the fear.	Assists the nurse in understanding the client's perception of the fear.
Assess sources of support, resources, and usual coping methods.	Assists the nurse in understanding the client's perception of the fear.
Identify which coping strategies that the client has previously used have been effective and which have not. Discuss ways that effective strategies can be used to cope with future fearful events.	This helps the client identify effective strategies while reinforcing that he or she can cope with his or her fear.
Help the client to talk about his or her fear and its source.	Makes the client, the nurse, and the family more aware of issues that need discussing or problems that need to be addressed.
Listen to the client's and family's concerns, and answer all questions truthfully. Tell the client and family as much as you can to decrease the number of "surprises" they may experience with the fear-producing event.	Understanding helps promote a sense of control and order.

(care plan continued on page 562)

NURSING ACTIONS/INTERVENTIONS WITH RATIONALES (continued from page 561)

Home Health

ACTIONS/INTERVENTIONS	RATIONALES
Acknowledge all fears, feelings, and perceived threats as valid to the client.	All client fears are valid to the client, whether they are realistic or not.
Administer anxiolytics as ordered, and educate the family or caregivers about prescribed medications, their side effects, and scheduling.	Promotes a sense of well-being.
Consult with and/or refer the patient to assistive resources as needed.	Utilization of existing services is an efficient use of resources.

HOPELESSNESS

DEFINITION[40]

A subjective state in which an individual sees limited or no alternatives or personal choices available and is unable to mobilize energy on own behalf.[33]

DEFINING CHARACTERISTICS[40]

1. Passivity, or decreased verbalization
2. Decreased affect
3. Verbal cues (despondent content, "I can't," sighing)
4. Closing eyes
5. Decreased appetite
6. Decreased response to stimuli
7. Increased or decreased sleep
8. Lack of initiative
9. Lack of involvement in care or passivity allowing care
10. Shrugging in response to speaker
11. Turning away from speaker

RELATED FACTORS[40]

1. Abandonment
2. Prolonged activity restriction creating isolation
3. Lost belief in transcendent values/God
4. Long-term stress
5. Failing or deteriorating physiologic condition

RELATED CLINICAL CONCERNS

1. Any disease of a chronic nature
2. Any disease with a terminal diagnosis
3. Any condition where a diagnosis cannot be definitely established

 Have You Selected the Correct Diagnosis?

Powerlessness
This diagnosis is present when the individual perceives that his or her actions will not change a situation regardless of the options that the person may see in a situation. Hopelessness occurs when the individual perceives that there are few or limited choices in a situation. Powerlessness may evolve out of Hopelessness. Powerlessness is the perception that one's actions will not make a difference, whereas Hopelessness is the perception that there are not options to act on. The decision about which is the most appropriate diagnosis is based on the clinical judgment of the nurse about which symptoms predominate.

Anxiety
Anxiety may have as a component a perception of Hopelessness. This could evolve out of the narrowed perception of the anxious client. Hopelessness may have Anxiety as a component. This situation could develop when the client is feeling overwhelmed with the perception that there are no alternatives in a difficult situation. The primary diagnosis evolves from the symptoms sequence. If Anxiety is the predominant symptom cluster, it should be the primary diagnosis because of the strong influence it has on the client's perceptions.

Disturbed Thought Process
If the individual cannot accurately assess the situation, then a sense of Hopelessness might occur. In this instance, Hopelessness would be a companion diagnosis.

Fear
If the client is fearful in a situation, perception can be narrowed and alternative options may be overlooked. When Fear and Hopelessness occur together, Fear should be the primary diagnosis.

EXPECTED OUTCOME

Expresses expectation of a positive future by [date].[37]
Develops [number] of personal goals by [date].[37]
Lists [number] reasons to live by [date].[37]

TARGET DATES

A target date ranging between 3 and 5 days would be appropriate for initial evaluation. A target date later than 5 days might lead to increased complications, such as potential for self-injury. A target date sooner than 3 days would not provide a sufficient length of time for realizing the effects of intervention.

NURSING ACTIONS/INTERVENTIONS WITH RATIONALES

Adult Health

ACTIONS/INTERVENTIONS	RATIONALES
Establish a therapeutic and trusting relationship with the patient and family by actively listening, being nonjudgmental, sitting with the patient, etc.	Promotes an environment that encourages the patient and/or family to verbalize concerns. Promotes an empathetic environment.
Identify other primary care nursing needs, and deal with these as needed.	Attention to basic needs may decrease feelings of hopelessness and of being of no value.
Provide explanations and appropriate teaching for procedures, diagnosis, treatments, and prognosis.	
Involve the patient in developing attainable goals and plan of care.	
Assist the patient to identify positive aspects of the situation	
Support the patent's efforts at objectively describing feelings of hopelessness	Allows the patient to validate reality.
Assist the patient to find alternatives to feelings of hopelessness.	Validates reality and encourages use of alternate coping techniques.
Hopelessness may prompt unhealthy eating patterns. (See nursing care plans related to Imbalanced Nutrition and/or Fluid Balance.)	
Support active participation in activities of daily living. Allow for preferences in day-to-day decisions (e.g., establishing a bath time).	Helps restore sense of being in control.
Refer to psychiatric nurse clinician as needed. (See Mental Health nursing actions.)	Collaboration promotes a more holistic and complete plan of care.
Identify religious, cultural, or community support groups prior to discharge. Provide appointments for follow-up.	Support groups can provide advocacy for the patient and continued monitoring and support of the patient after discharge from the hospital.

Child Health

Depending on the age and developmental status of the child, some components of Adult and Mental Health will also apply in addition to the following:

ACTIONS/INTERVENTIONS	RATIONALES
Monitor for the etiologic components contributing to hopelessness pattern.	Provides a database that results in a more accurate and complete plan of care.
Facilitate with patient and parents discussions of feelings about current status, with 30 minutes set aside each shift at [times] for this purpose.	Verbalization helps reduce anxiety and assigns value to the patient's concerns. Allows ongoing assessment.
Assist the patient and family to explore growth potential afforded by this specific experience.	Opportunity for growth may be overlooked in times of crisis.

(care plan continued on page 564)

NURSING ACTIONS/INTERVENTIONS WITH RATIONALES (continued from page 563)

Child Health

ACTIONS/INTERVENTIONS	RATIONALES
Allow opportunities for the child to "play out" feelings under appropriate supervision and guidance of child life specialist: • Play with dolls for toddler • Art and puppets for preschooler • Peer discussions for adolescents	Play and the acting out of feelings provide insight into coping and perceptions of the child in a noninvasive mode. Provides valuable data to monitor feelings, concerns, etc.
Refer, as appropriate, to child mental health specialist.	Provides actual and anticipatory guidance for resolution of the acute phase.

Women's Health

● N O T E : *The following nursing actions are for the couple (husband or wife) who has been unable to conceive a child, after testing and treatment. See Chapter 10 for detailed information on infertility. Provide a nonjudgmental atmosphere to allow the infertile couple to express their feelings such as anger, denial, inadequacy, guilt, depression, or grief.*

ACTIONS/INTERVENTIONS	RATIONALES
Infertility Support and allow the couple to work through the grieving process for loss of fertility, loss of children, loss of idealized lifestyle, and loss of feminine life experiences such as pregnancy, birth, and breastfeeding.	Provision of support for and encouragement of discussion regarding emotions allows the couple to begin to deal with emotions and lays the groundwork for future decision making.[44]
Encourage the couple to talk honestly with one another about feelings.	Most adults assume they will have children; finding they cannot conceive often leads to feelings of inferiority, doubts about their sexuality, and guilt or blame.[44]
Encourage the couple to seek professional help if necessary to deal with feelings related to sexual relationship, conflicts, anxieties, parenting, and coping mechanisms used for dealing with loss of fertility (their expectations, relatives' expectations, and society's expectations).	
Be alert for signs of depression, anger, frustration, and impending crisis.	Allows early intervention and avoidance of complications.[44]
Provide the infertile couple with accurate information on adoption and living without children.	Adoption choices in this country are limited because many single mothers are keeping their babies and because of the availability of birth control and abortion. Often couples in the United States look to foreign countries to adopt.[44]

Postpartum Depression

● N O T E : *The majority of patients who experience hopelessness that leads to postpartum depression have been found to have underlying psychiatric disorders, or life experiences other than pregnancy, that accounted for the depression.[80]*

ACTIONS/INTERVENTIONS	RATIONALES
Provide factual information to the patient and partner on postpartum depression. Describe the difference between "baby blues" and depression. Identify potential psychosocial triggers in the patient's environment that could lead to postpartum depression, such as: • Feelings of ambivalence • Feelings of inadequacy • Marital discord • Guilt and irritability	Give the patient and partner realistic guidelines for when they might need to seek professional help for depression beyond "baby blues."[80]

Domestic Violence[80–84,88]

ACTIONS/INTERVENTIONS	RATIONALES
Provide a nonjudgmental atmosphere that allows the patient to express anger, fears, and feelings of hopelessness. Refer the patient to an appropriate agency for assistance to find shelter and psychological counseling. Assist the patient in developing a plan of action in the event of a situation that could threaten her or her children's safety.	
Place telephone numbers for assistance in the women's bathroom and other places women can see and memorize it without fear of reprisal from their partner.	Provides resources and information to patients without putting them or their children in further danger.

Mental Health

ACTIONS/INTERVENTIONS	RATIONALES
Monitor the health-care team's interactions with the client for behavior (verbal and nonverbal) that would encourage the client not to be hopeful (e.g., using an example of a less that optimal outcome of a disease process such as "I am a diabetic and am currently waiting for my kidney transplant," or referring to adult incontinent underwear as diapers). If situations are identified, they should be noted here, and the team should discuss alternative ways of behaving in the situation. The actions needed to support the client's hope should be noted on the client's chart.	Negative attitudes from the staff can be communicated to the client.
Sit with the client [number] times per day at [times] for 30 minutes to discuss feelings and perceptions the client has about the identified situation. These times should also include discussions about the client's significant others, times the client has enjoyed with these persons, the projects or activities the client was planning with or for these persons that have not been accomplished, the client's values and beliefs about health and illness, and the attitudes about the current situation.	Promotes positive orientation by assisting the client in remembering past successes and important aspects of life that make it important that he or she succeed this time.[89,90]

(care plan continued on page 566)

Mental Health

ACTIONS/INTERVENTIONS	RATIONALES
Identify with the client's significant others times that they can talk with the staff about the current situation. Themes that should be explored during this interaction should be their thoughts and feelings about the current situation, ways in which they can support the client, the importance of their support for the client, questions they may have about the client's situation, and possible outcomes. (Note the time for this interaction here as well as the name of the person who will be talking with the significant others.)	Negative expectations from the support system can be communicated to the client.
Note the times when significant others will be visiting, and schedule this time so there will be a private time for them to interact with the client. (Note these times here, and designate those times that are scheduled as private visitation times.) Inform the client and significant others of places on the unit where they can have privacy to visit.	Assists the client in maintaining connections with the support systems, and increases the awareness of contributions the client has made in the past and can make in the future to this system.
Identify with the client preferences for the daily routine, and place this information on the chart to be implemented by the staff. It is vital to this client to have the information shared with all staff so that it will not appear that the time spent in providing information was wasted.	Promotes the client's sense of control.
Provide answers to questions in an open, direct manner.	Promotes the client's sense of control, while building a trusting relationship.
Provide information on all procedures at a time when the client can ask questions and think about the situation.	
Allow the client to participate in decision making at the level to which he or she is capable of doing so. A client who has never made an independent decision would be overwhelmed by the complexity of the decisions made daily by a corporation executive. If necessary, offer decision situations in portions that the client can master successfully (the amount of information that the client can handle should be noted here as well as a list of decisions that have been presented to the client).	Promotes the client's sense of control in a manner that increases the opportunities for success. This success serves as positive reinforcement.
Provide positive reinforcement for behavior changed and decisions made. The actions that are reinforcing for this client should be listed here along with the reward system that has been established with the client (e.g., play one game of cards with the client when a decision about ways to cope with a specific problem has been made).	Positive reinforcement encourages behavior while enhancing self-esteem.
Provide verbal informative social reinforcements along with behavioral reinforcements.	Promotes the development of a trusting relationship. Enhances self-esteem.[89]
Keep promises (specific promises should be listed on the chart so that all staff will be aware of this information).	
Accept the client's decision if the decision was given to the client to make. These decisions should be noted on the chart.	Promotes the client's sense of control, while enhancing self-esteem.

ACTIONS/INTERVENTIONS	RATIONALES
Provide ongoing, informative, positive feedback to the client on progress.	Provides positive reinforcement for accomplishments.[89]
Spend 30 minutes a day talking with the client about current coping strategies and exploring alternative coping methods. Note the time for this discussion here as well as the person responsible for this interaction. When alternative coping styles have been identified, this time should be used to assist the client with necessary practice. The alternative styles that the client has selected should be noted on the chart, and the staff should assist the client in implementing the strategy when appropriate. These could include deep muscle relaxation, visual imagery, prayer, or talking about alternative ways of coping with stressful events.	Interaction with the nurse can provide positive reinforcement. Behavioral rehearsal provides opportunities for feedback and modeling of new behaviors from the nurse.
Allow the client to express anger, and assist with discovering constructive ways of expressing this feeling (e.g., talking about this feeling, using a punching bag, playing Ping-Pong, or throwing or hitting a pillow). Talk with the client about signs of progress, and assist him or her in recognizing these as they occur with verbal reminders or by keeping a record of steps taken toward progress.	Promotes the development of a positive orientation.
Assist the client in establishing realistic goals and realistic expectations for situations. The goals should be short term and stated in measurable behavioral terms. Usually, dividing the goal set by the client in half provides an achievable goal. This could involve dividing one goal into several smaller goals. [Note goals and evaluation dates here.]	Goals that are achieved serve as positive reinforcement for behavior change and enhance self-esteem and a positive expectational set.
Determine times with the client to evaluate progress toward these goals and to discuss his or her observations about this progress. These specific times should be listed here with the name of the person responsible for this activity. Initially this may need to be done on a daily basis until the client develops competency in making realistic assessments.	Provides positive reinforcement for movement toward the goal, and provides an opportunity for the nurse to provide positive verbal reinforcement.
Assist the client in developing a list of contingencies for possible blocks to the goals. These would be "what-if" and "if-then" discussions. This would be done in the goal-setting session, and a record of the alternatives discussed would be made in the chart for future reference.	Provides direction for the client, with an opportunity to mentally rehearse situations that could require alteration of goals. This protects the client from all-or-none situations.
Discuss with the client values and beliefs about life, and assess the importance of formal religion in the client's life. If the client requires contact with a person of his or her belief system, arrange this, and note necessary information for contacting this person here. Provide the client with the time necessary to perform religious rituals that are important to him or her. Note the rituals here with the times scheduled and any assistance that is required from the nursing staff.	Spirituality can provide hope-giving experiences.

(care plan continued on page 568)

NURSING ACTIONS/INTERVENTIONS WITH RATIONALES (continued from page 567)

Mental Health

ACTIONS/INTERVENTIONS	RATIONALES
Provide the client with opportunities to enjoy aesthetic experiences that have been identified as important, such as listening to favorite music, having favorite pictures placed in the room, enjoying favorite foods, or having special flowers in the room. Spend 5 minutes three times a day discussing these experiences and assisting the client in becoming involved in the enjoyment of them. Note here activities that have been identified by the client as important and times when they will be discussed with the client.	Promotes the client's interest in the positive aspect of life, promoting a positive orientation.
Assist the client in developing an awareness and an appreciation for the here and now by helping him or her focus attention in the present by pointing out to him or her the beauty in the flowers in the room, the warmth of the sunshine as it comes through the window, the calmness or vitality of a piece of music, the taste and smell of a special food item, the odor of flowers, etc.	Provides the client with an opportunity to access past positive experiences in the present, thus promoting a positive orientation.
Establish a time to talk with the client about maximizing potential at his or her current level of functioning. Note date and time for this discussion here. This may need to be done in several stages during more than one time, depending on the client's level of denial. Note here the person responsible for these discussions.	Promotes the client's sense of control, enhancing self-esteem.

Gerontic Health

The nursing actions for the older adult with this diagnosis are the same as for the Adult Health and Mental Health patient.

Home Health

In addition to the following interventions, the interventions for Adult Health and Mental Health can be applied to the home health client.

ACTIONS/INTERVENTIONS	RATIONALES
Monitor for factors contributing to the hopelessness (e.g., psychological, social, economic, spiritual, or environmental factors).	Provides a database for early recognition and intervention.
Involve the client and family in planning, implementing, and promoting reduction or elimination of hopelessness: • Family conference: To identify and discuss factors contributing to hopelessness • Mutual goal setting: Setting goals with roles of each family member identified • Communication • Support for the caregiver	Clarifies roles. Personal involvement in planning, etc. Increases the likelihood of success in resolving the problem.

ACTIONS/INTERVENTIONS	RATIONALES
Assist the client and family in making lifestyle adjustments that may be required: • Use relaxation techniques: yoga, biofeedback, hypnosis, breathing techniques, or imagery. • Provide assertiveness training. • Provide opportunities for individual to exert control over the situation. Offer choice when possible; support and encourage self-care efforts. • Provide a sense of mastery; set accomplishable and meaningful goals in secure environment. • Look for meaning in the situation (e.g., what can be learned from the situation). • Provide treatment for the physiologic condition. • Provide grief counseling. • Provide spiritual counseling.	Lifestyle changes require significant behavior change. Self-evaluation and support can assist in ensuring that changes are not transient.
Consult with, or refer to, assistive resources as indicated.	Effective use of existing community resources.

LONELINESS, RISK FOR

DEFINITION[40]

At risk of experiencing vague dysphoria.

RISK FACTORS[40]

1. Affectional deprivation
2. Social isolation
3. Cathectic deprivation
4. Physical isolation

RELATED CLINICAL CONCERNS

1. Any chronic illness
2. AIDS
3. Mental health diagnoses
4. Cancer
5. Any condition causing impaired mobility
6. Anticipated loss of significant others or support systems

 Have You Selected the Correct Diagnosis?

Social Isolation
Social Isolation is an actual diagnosis and is given when the client is currently experiencing the isolation.

Loneliness is a risk diagnosis and is the client's perception of his or her situation. Social Isolation is a risk factor for the diagnosis of Loneliness.

Impaired Social Interaction
This diagnosis is also an actual diagnosis. In Impaired Social Interaction, the problem can be insufficient or excessive social activity. If a person is experiencing impaired social interaction, he or she could be at risk for loneliness.

EXPECTED OUTCOME

Will implement a plan to reduce risk for loneliness by [date].
Will verbalize a sense of belonging by [date].[37]
Will identify [number] of methods to increase interpersonal interactions by [date].[37]

TARGET DATES

This is a fairly long-term diagnosis and will require much support to offset. Therefore, an appropriate initial target date would be 10 to 14 days.

NURSING ACTIONS/INTERVENTIONS WITH RATIONALES

Adult Health

ACTIONS/INTERVENTIONS	RATIONALES
Include patient input in planning of activities. Determine patient preferences for visitation. Develop a schedule for appropriate times and lengths of time for visitation.	Assists in balancing social interaction with periods of rest.

(care plan continued on page 570)

NURSING ACTIONS/INTERVENTIONS WITH RATIONALES (continued from page 569)

Adult Health

ACTIONS/INTERVENTIONS	RATIONALES
Include and facilitate child visitation as appropriate.	
Initiate family involvement in care through providing explanations of patient status, teaching about procedures, and performing aspects of care.	
Facilitate family involvement by identifying accommodations for visitation (e.g., family house, local hotels, etc.)	
Evaluate whether strategies are meeting needs.	Enables monitoring of progress and allows for altering the plan of care.
Identify alternative social interactions including outreach groups or pet therapy.	
Assist the patient to find alternate support systems, even short, quality interactions with the nurse.	Patients perceive that nurses can offer psychological support with even short visits.[61]
If expected outcomes are not met, see interactions for Social Isolation and Impaired Social Interaction.	

Child Health

Same as for Adult Health, with attention to developmentally appropriate approach for all interventions. When other diagnoses (e.g., Grief or Loss, Parent–Infant Separation, Coping) also contribute to this pattern, seek follow-up with concurrent plan for loneliness as well.

ACTIONS/INTERVENTIONS	RATIONALES
If anaclitic depression is to be considered, stage appropriately for current/ongoing status (i.e., protest, despair, or withdrawal).	In separation anxiety, the infant or child may have different needs, but all will help direct caregivers to support client regain bonding with others.
Determine how to support the infant, child, or adolescent coping with loneliness as applicable [Note the methods most appropriate for this patient here.]: • Play therapy or counseling • Consideration of developmental capacity • Access to activities within the local community • Monitor physical or emotional readiness, for both the individual and the family • Allowance for regression due to illness • Support services, foster grandparents, volunteers, Child Protective Services (CPS), or college interest groups	Holistic planning according to realistic capacity of the infant, child, or adolescent will provide an appropriate chance to reestablish a sense of belonging.
Involve all who have input in establishing consistent long-term goals.	Often underlying dynamics may require long-range planning.
When necessary, advocate for the infant or child.	Loneliness may be related to abuse on the part of the parents and must be considered appropriately.
Schedule a time for counseling that provides appropriate valuing of family needs. Note schedule and special accommodations for this here.	Loneliness will undermine family dynamics if left unrecognized.
Offer 30 minutes each shift for the patient or parents to ventilate feelings about loneliness.	Frequent verbalization will offer cues to suggest insight into how loneliness is being perceived and provide the basis for the most appropriate treatment.
Determine the need for follow-up counseling or referral to child mental health specialist.	Provides actual or anticipatory guidance for resolution of related issues.

Women's Health

● **NOTE** : *The heath-care provider will see this diagnosis in many more females than in male clients as a result of women outliving men. This is one of the most frequent diagnoses in geriatric women.*

ACTIONS/INTERVENTIONS	RATIONALES
Postpartum Provide the patient with access to support by the providing telephone number and name of available support person she can call with questions.	Provides new parents support and guidance during the first days of the postpartum period, and assists in the transition to parenthood.
Encourage new parents to attend parenting support groups and participate in parent education programs in the acute care setting and in the community after discharge. Suggest to parents: • YWCA • Churches • Neighborhood groups • Friends who have had babies • State-funded follow-up programs	
Single Parents Assist the new mother to develop a plan for coordinating activities of daily living with the new infant.	
Assist the patient in identifying available resources: • Family • Significant others • Community agencies • Peer groups	
Assist the patient in identifying and developing intrapersonal skills.	
Encourage attendance at parenting classes or support groups. • Learn about baby cues and how to provide for psychological needs of new infant. • Identify others with similar concerns and needs. • Identify new sources of support and contact opportunities for developing new friendships.	
Encourage the patient to identify friends or acquaintances who have recently had new babies and to begin: • Discussing similar concerns and problems with caring for a new baby • Sharing babysitting activities to reduce costs and increase opportunities for the new mom to get away occasionally	Provides support and guidance during the transition to parenthood, as well as provides additional resources specific to assisting the single parent.
Divorce and Widowhood Provide a relaxed atmosphere that will encourage the patient to express feelings, identify concerns, and allow for grieving.	
Evaluate need for professional assistance and/or family support.	
Identify and clarify with the patient feelings of abandonment, anger, and loss of previous lifestyle.	

(care plan continued on page 572)

NURSING ACTIONS/INTERVENTIONS WITH RATIONALES (continued from page 571)

Women's Health

ACTIONS/INTERVENTIONS	RATIONALES
Assist the patient in identifying new opportunities for involvement with others, i.e., church groups, community volunteer groups, social groups (ski club, travel clubs, etc.) for people with similar interests, returning to college, cultural events, etc.	
Provide opportunities for new interactions in a supportive atmosphere (e.g., identify friend to accompany the patient to social events or identify friend she can talk to).	
Provide referrals to appropriate professional resources for assistance if necessary.	Provides support and guidance during a time of crisis for the patient. Assists the client to find and utilize available resources.

Mental Health

ACTIONS/INTERVENTIONS	RATIONALES
Spend [number] minutes [number] times a day discussing with the client his or her perception of the source of the loneliness and how they have tried to resolve the situation.	Assists in understanding the client's worldview, which facilitates the development of client-specific interventions. Increases the client's sense of involvement and empowerment.[90]
Have the client list the persons in the environment who are considered family, friends, and acquaintances. Then have the client note how many interactions per week occur with each person. Have the client identify what interferes with feeling connected with these persons. Note here the person responsible and schedule for this interaction.	Facilitates the client's reality testing of perception of being alone.
When contributing factors have been identified, develop a plan to alter them. This could include: • Assertiveness training • Role-playing difficult situations • Teaching the client relaxation techniques to reduce anxiety in social situations • Providing the client with aids to compensate for sensory deficits • Providing the client with special clothing or prosthetic devices to enhance physical appearance • Teaching the client personal hygiene necessary to maintain aesthetic appearance (ostomy care, incontinence care, or wound care)	Facilitates the development of alternative coping behaviors, and improves social skills, which improves role performance and social confidence.
Note here the specific interventions, and schedule necessary for this client with person responsible for the activity. For example, the primary care nurse will interact with the client 30 minutes 2 times a day to teach assertive skills, or the client will attend social skills group at [time].	

ACTIONS/INTERVENTIONS	RATIONALES
Develop a list of things the client finds rewarding, and provide these rewards as the client successfully completes progressive steps in the treatment plan. This schedule should be developed with the client. Note here the schedule for rewards and the kinds of behavior to be rewarded.	Positive reinforcement encourages behavior and enhances self-esteem. Increases the client's competence, and thus enhances role performance and self-esteem.
Consult with the occupational therapist if the client needs to learn specific skills to facilitate social interactions, such as cooking skills so friends can be invited to dinner, craft skills, or dancing so the client can join others in these social activities.	
Include the client in groups on the unit. Assign the client activities that can be accomplished easily and that will provide positive social reinforcement from other persons involved in the activities. Note here the group and activity schedule.	Successful accomplishment of a valued task can provide positive reinforcement, which encourages social behavior. Provides opportunities for the client to practice social interaction skills in a context where feedback can be obtained.[37,38]
If lack of activities contributes to the loneliness, refer to Deficient Diversional Activity in Chapter 5 for detailed interventions.	Decreased activities can increase the sense of time passing slowly, which perceptually increases the time spent alone, increasing the sense of loneliness.[90]
Consult with social services if transportation or financial resource problems contribute to social isolation.	Decreased mobility can decrease social interaction and sense of aloneness.
Discuss with clients those times it would be appropriate to be alone, and develop a plan for coping with these times in a positive manner. For example, the client will develop a list of books to read and music to listen to, or call a friend.[91]	Promotes the client's sense of control, while facilitating the development of alternative coping behaviors.
When the client is demonstrating socially inappropriate behavior, keep interactions to a minimum, inform the client that the behavior is inappropriate, and escort him or her to a place away from group activities. Note here the target behaviors for this client.	Lack of positive reinforcement decreases a behavior.
When inappropriate behaviors stop, discuss the behavior with the client, and develop a list of alternative kinds of behavior for the client to use in situations in which the inappropriate behavior is elicited. Note here the behaviors that are considered problematic, with the action to be taken if they are demonstrated. For example, the client will spend time out in seclusion or sleeping area.	Promotes the client's sense of control, while promoting the development of alternative coping behaviors.
The primary care nurse will spend 30 minutes once a day with the client at [time] discussing the client's reactions to social interactions and assisting the client with reality testing of social interactions, for example, what others might mean by silence, or various nonverbal and common verbal expressions. This time can also be used to discuss role relationships and the client's specific concerns about relationships.	Provides positive reinforcement for appropriate problem solving.
Assign the client a room near areas with high activity.	Facilitates the client's participation in unit activities.
Assign one staff person to the client each shift, and have this person interact with the client every 30 minutes while the client is awake.	Decreases the client's opportunities for socially isolating him- or herself.

(care plan continued on page 574)

NURSING ACTIONS/INTERVENTIONS WITH RATIONALES (continued from page 573)

Mental Health

ACTIONS/INTERVENTIONS	RATIONALES
Have the client identify activities in the community that are of interest and would provide opportunities for interactions with others. List the client's interests here.	
Develop with the client a plan for making contact with the identified community activities before discharge.	Promotes the client's sense of control, and begins the development of adaptive coping behaviors.
Arrange at least 1 hour a week for the client to interact with his or her support system in the presence of the primary care nurse. This will allow the nurse to assess and facilitate these interactions. [Note here the schedule and responsible person.]	Support system understanding facilitates the maintenance of new behaviors after discharge.
Discuss with the support system ways in which they can facilitate client interaction (e.g., frequent telephone calls, teaching the client to use public transportation, Meals-on-Wheels, or community telephone call check-in services).	
Model for the support system and for the client the kinds of behavior that facilitate communication.	Provides opportunities for the client to practice new role behaviors in a safe, supportive environment.
Limit the amount of time the client can spend alone in room. This should be a gradual alteration and should be done in steps that can easily be accomplished by the client. Note the specific schedule for the client here. For example, the client will spend 5 minutes per hour in the day area. Have the staff person remain with the client during these times until the client demonstrates an ability to interact with others.[90]	
Provide a guest book in the client's room for visitors to sign. This should include a space for visitor's name, date, and time of visit. A space for a summary of the discussion could also be included.	This intervention assists with situations in which the client's perception of visitation is not congruent with actual contact with support systems. Provides the client and staff with documentation of visits to aid with reality testing.
Refer the client to appropriate community agencies.	

Gerontic Health

See actions and interventions under Mental Health. The older adult who is experiencing losses associated with aging, such as loss of a spouse, decline in physical health, and changes in role, is especially vulnerable to loneliness.

Home Health

In addition to the following interventions, the interventions for Adult Health and Mental Health can be applied to the home health client.

ACTIONS/INTERVENTIONS	RATIONALES
Teach the client and family to identify and prevent risk factors of loneliness: • Physical and social isolation • Deprivation	Early recognition and intervention can interrupt development of loneliness.

ACTIONS/INTERVENTIONS	RATIONALES
A terminal diagnosis can result in less outside interaction. If friends stop visiting, assist the family and client to understand possible reasons: • It is difficult for others to face their own mortality. • Others may fear that the client is too sick for visitors. The client and family should speak frankly with friends and family about these issues and their wishes regarding visitors.	Reestablishes previous social contacts.
Assist the client and family in lifestyle adjustments that may be necessary: • Develop a plan for increased involvement (e.g., begin with social contacts that are least threatening). • Provide for personal hygiene. • Provide a supportive environment.	Home-based care requires involvement of the family. Loneliness can disrupt family schedules and role relationships. Adjustments in family activities and roles may be required.
Assist the family to set criteria to help them determine when additional intervention is required (e.g., inability of the client or family to care for the client).	Provides the family with background knowledge to seek appropriate assistance as the need arises.
Refer to appropriate assistive resources as indicated.	Additional assistance may be required for the family to care for the family member with loneliness.

PERSONAL IDENTITY, DISTURBED

DEFINITION[40]

Inability to distinguish between self and nonself.[40]

DEFINING CHARACTERISTICS[40]

To be developed.

This diagnosis is located in Domain 6 (Self-Perception) Class 1 (Self-concept) of the NANDA-I Taxonomy. Because the defining characteristics and related factors are not yet developed, it might be useful to consider this diagnosis integrated with additional diagnoses related to self-concept. These additional diagnoses may provide a more comprehensive approach to the client's response.

RELATED FACTORS[40]

None given.

RELATED CLINICAL CONCERNS

1. Autism
2. Mental retardation
3. Dissociative disorders (e.g., psychogenic amnesia, psychogenic fugue, multiple personality, depersonalization disorder)
4. Borderline personality disorder
5. Delirium (Disorientation to person is rare; the most common manifestations are disorientation to place and time.)[38,58]
6. Amnesic Disorders related to general medical conditions or substance use[38,58]

 Have You Selected the Correct Diagnosis?

Chronic Low or Situational Low Self-Esteem
This diagnosis addresses lack of confidence in one's self and is characterized by negative self-statements, lack of concern about personal appearance, and withdrawal from others not related to physical problems or attributes. The self is defined. If the client demonstrates an inability to differentiate self from the environment, then the most appropriate diagnosis is Disturbed Personal Identity. An example is the client who perceives a life-support machine as part of the self.

Disturbed Body Image
This diagnosis relates to alterations in perceptions of self in conjunction with actual or perceived alterations in body structure or function. Again, the self is known with this diagnosis.

EXPECTED OUTCOME[37]

Will list at least [number] characteristics of self versus nonself by [date].

Describes [number] aspects of self by [date].

Accurately describes appropriate personal role behaviors by [date].

TARGET DATES

A target date of 5 days would be acceptable for initial evaluation of progress toward expected outcomes.

NURSING ACTIONS/INTERVENTIONS WITH RATIONALES

Adult Health

● N O T E : *Should the patient develop this nursing diagnosis on an adult health care unit, referral should be made immediately to a mental health nurse clinician. See nursing actions under Mental Health*

Child Health

ACTIONS/INTERVENTIONS	RATIONALES
Monitor for contributing factors that might predispose the development of Disturbed Personal Identity: • Altered maternal–infant attachment (e.g., parents' over-protection or ignoring of the infant) • Altered development norms related to independent functioning (e.g., following commands; check for organic or sensory–perceptual deficits.) • Preference for solitary play • Display of self-stimulation and/or self-mutilation behaviors • History of altered identity problems in the family	Provides the database needed to more accurately and completely plan care.
Provide basic care for other needs with prioritization for safety needs. Close observation is mandatory.	In anticipatory safety planning, standards must be in accord with both the known and the unknown self-injury potential of the patient.
Administer medications as ordered, with attention to hydration and nutritional concerns.	The patient is prone to dehydration and malnutrition due to inability to rely on usual thirst or appetite regulators.
Provide appropriate follow-up and collaboration with the family. [Note special adaptations needed here.]	Appropriate use of specialists will offer a more individualized plan of care with greater likelihood of meeting needs.
Assist the family in decision making regarding long-term care (e.g., institutionalization versus day care).	Assistance and support in identification of options assists in decision making, reducing stress, and empowering the family.

Women's Health

The nursing actions for the woman with this nursing diagnosis are the same as those for the Mental Health client. Also see Risk for Loneliness and Anxiety.

Mental Health

ACTIONS/INTERVENTIONS	RATIONALES
Assign the primary care nurse to establish trusting nurse–client relationship.	Establishes boundaries so changes can be immediately processed.[90]
Monitor the client for mental status changes.	Alterations in mental status that result in identity confusion can be related to a delirium related to a general medical condition or substance withdrawal. These situations can be life threatening and need to be addressed with immediate consultation with client's primary care provider to determine contributing factors.[38,58]

ACTIONS/INTERVENTIONS	RATIONALES
Provide the client with information about unit structure, policies, expectations, and requirements.	Assists the client in establishing clear interpersonal boundaries.
Provide a quiet, nonstimulating environment.	Inappropriate levels of sensory stimuli can increase confusion and sense of disorganization.
Provide frequent interactions that assist the client with orientation.	Promotes the development of a trusting relationship within the client's attention span.
Provide environmental cues to enhance orientation. These could include calendar with day and date marked, schedule board, personal items of attachment, and the client's name or object that they connect with on door of room.	Clients who have experienced alterations in personal identity still respond to basic personality characteristics and familiar objects.[92,93]
Verbal information should be provided in simple, brief sentences.	Interactions with others also assist in reestablishing weak ego boundaries.
Sit with the client [number] minutes [number] times per day at [times] to provide the client with an opportunity to discuss feelings and thoughts.	Promotes the development of a trusting relationship. Provides positive reinforcement for the client, meeting needs in a more constructive way.
Provide the client with honest, direct feedback in all interactions.	Promotes the development of a trusting relationship.
Utilize constructive confrontation if necessary, to include: • "I" statements • Relationship statements that reflect the nurse's reaction to the interaction • Responses that will assist the client in understanding, such as paraphrasing and validation of perceptions	Assists the client in establishing ego boundaries, while supporting self-esteem.
Develop, with the health-care team, a clear set of boundaries and a list of expectations and the consequences for inappropriate behaviors. Schedule frequent team meetings to review the client's behavior and to make revisions in care. Note times of meetings here.	Firm limits facilitate the client's focusing on feelings rather than moving away from them.[93,94] Prevents staff splits, which are detrimental to clients who have identity and splitting problems.[93,94]
Discuss with the client the source of the threat.	Assists the client in developing more adaptive coping behaviors.
Develop with the client alternative coping strategies. Activities, items, or verbal responses that are rewarding for the client should be listed here.	Promotes the client's sense of control and positive expectational set by providing a concrete plan for responding to stressful situations.
When the client is presented with a threat, assist with progressing through one of the alternative coping methods, or practice with the client the alternative coping methods [number] minutes twice a day.	Behavioral rehearsal provides opportunities for feedback and modeling from the nurse.
Provide the client with anchors developed to assist him or her with reality orientation (stuffed animal, verbal phrase, article of clothing, etc.) when the client demonstrates signs of dissociation or impending dissociation. Note the anchor to be used here.	Grounding reconnects the client to the here and now and increases his or her sense of control over the traumatic situation.[95]
If there is not a predetermined anchor, use the five senses to connect person in the present. This is done in a calm and supportive manner.	
Develop achievable goals with the client. (The goals that are appropriate for this client should be listed here.)	Goal achievement enhances self-esteem and promotes a positive expectational set, which motivates the client to move on to more complex goals and behavior change.

(care plan continued on page 578)

Mental Health

ACTIONS/INTERVENTIONS	RATIONALES
As the client masters the first set of goals, develop increasingly complex goals and problems.	Moves the client toward health goals in a manner that promotes self-esteem.
Provide positive reinforcement for accomplishments at any level. (Activities, items, or verbal responses that are rewarding for the client should be listed here.)	Positive reinforcement encourages behavior while enhancing self-esteem.
Do not argue with a client who is experiencing an alteration in thought process. (See Chapter 7 for nursing actions related to Disturbed Thought Process.)	Arguing with the belief interferes with the development of a trusting relationship and does not serve to change the perceptions.
Monitor the client's mental status before attempting learning or confrontation. If the client is disoriented, orient to reality as needed.	Alterations in mental status can interfere with the client's ability to process information, and teaching at this point could increase stimuli to a level that would only increase the client's confusion and disorganization.
For clients with Dissociative Identity Disorder:	
• Do not ask for alter personalities.	Does not further dissociation.[73,94] Discourages dissociation and encourages integration.
• Remind alters they are part of the host personality.	Discourages dissociation, while encouraging integration.
• Discuss the feelings that have been dissociated, rather than asking for alters.	Encourages integration.
• Emphasize the normalcy of having a range of feelings. Point out that one day the host will be able to tolerate all feelings.	
• Do not assure calm alters that they will be protected from hostile alters.	Prevents the strengthening of angry alters and dissociation.
If disorientation is present related to organic brain dysfunction, distract the client from disorientations that are not correct with a brief, simple explanation.	Short-term memory loss will assist with changing the client's orientation without getting into a strong confrontation.

Gerontic Health

● N O T E : *In the event the patient is unable to distinguish between self and nonself, it is necessary to contact a mental health clinician to further assess and devise the plan of care. Please see Mental Health nursing actions.*

Home Health

● N O T E : *Should the patient develop this nursing diagnosis in a home health setting, referral should be made immediately to a mental health nurse clinician. (See nursing actions under Mental Health.) If the patient is in the home setting after stabilization of the condition, the interventions for Adult Health and Mental Health can be applied to the home health client. In addition, the following interventions may be used:*

ACTIONS/INTERVENTIONS	RATIONALES
Involve the client and family in planning and implementing strategies to reduce and cope with disturbance in personal identity:	Family involvement enhances effectiveness of interventions.

ACTIONS/INTERVENTIONS	RATIONALES
• Family conference: Discuss feelings related to disturbance in personal identity of the client. • Mutual goal setting: Establish realistic goals, and identify the roles of each family member (e.g., provide a quiet environment and provide the client with honest and direct feedback). • Communication: Clear and honest communication among family members is essential. If organic brain dysfunction is present, the nurse may need to use distraction techniques.	
Assist the client and family in lifestyle adjustments that may be required: • Maintaining a safe environment • Altering roles as necessary • Maintaining the treatment plan of the health-care professionals guiding therapy	Disturbed Personal Identity can be a chronic condition that alters family relationships. Permanent changes in behavior and family roles require evaluation and support.
Consult with or refer to assistive resources as indicated.	Utilization of existing services is efficient use of resources. Psychiatric nurse clinicians and support groups can enhance the treatment plan.

POWERLESSNESS, RISK FOR AND ACTUAL

DEFINITIONS[40]

Risk for Powerlessness   Risk for perceived lack of control over a situation and/or one's ability to significantly affect an outcome.

   Powerlessness   Perception that one's own action will not significantly affect an outcome; a perceived lack of control over a current situation or immediate happening.

DEFINING CHARACTERISTICS[40]

A. Risk for Powerlessness
  1. Physiologic
    a. Chronic or acute illness (hospitalization, intubation, ventilator, suctioning)
    b. Acute injury or progressive debilitating disease process (e.g., spinal cord injury or multiple sclerosis)
    c. Aging (e.g., decreased physical strength, decreased mobility)
    d. Dying
  2. Psychosocial
    a. Lack of knowledge of illness or health-care system

    b. Lifestyle of dependency with inadequate coping patterns
    c. Absence of integrality (e.g., essence of power)
    d. Decreased self-esteem
    e. Low or unstable body image
B. Powerlessness
  1. Low
    a. Expressions of uncertainty about fluctuation of energy levels
    b. Passivity
  2. Moderate
    a. Nonparticipation in care or decision making when opportunities are provided
    b. Expressions of dissatisfaction and frustration over inability to perform previous tasks and/or activities
    c. Does not monitor progress
    d. Expression of doubt regarding role performance
    e. Reluctance to express true feelings
    f. Fearing alienation from caregivers
    g. Passivity
    h. Inability to seek information regarding care
    i. Resentment, anger, and guilt
    j. Does not defend self-care practices when challenged
    k. Dependence on others that may result in irritability

3. Severe
   a. Verbal expressions of having no control or influ-
     ence over the situation, outcome, or self-care
   b. Depression over physical deterioration that occurs
     despite patient compliance with regimens
   c. Apathy

RELATED FACTORS[40]

A. Risk for Powerlessness
   The defining characteristics serve also as the risk factors.
B. Powerlessness
   1. Health-care environment
   2. Interpersonal interaction
   3. Illness-related regimen
   4. Lifestyle of helplessness

RELATED CLINICAL CONCERNS

1. Any diagnosis that is unexpected or new to the patient
2. Any diagnosis resulting from a sudden, traumatic event
3. Any diagnosis of a chronic nature
4. Any diagnosis with a terminal prognosis
5. Hospitalization
6. Enmeshed family pattern

 Have You Selected the Correct Diagnosis?

Anxiety
Anxiety may have as a component a perception of
Powerlessness, which would evolve into a situation in
which the anxious client does not attempt to resolve
the situation. Powerlessness can also have Anxiety as
a component. Deciding on the primary diagnosis is
based on the clinical judgment of the nurse about
which symptoms predominate.

Ineffective Individual Coping
A perception of Powerlessness can produce Ineffective Individual Coping because if one perceives that
one's own actions cannot influence a situation,
appropriate actions may not be taken. If Ineffective
Individual Coping is determined to result from a perceived lack of influence, then Powerlessness would
be the primary diagnosis.

Disturbed Thought Process
This diagnosis can produce a sense of Powerlessness
because of the individual's inability to assess the situation accurately. Thus, the most appropriate diagnosis
would be Disturbed Thought Process.

Fear
Fear can produce a sense of Powerlessness,
just as Powerlessness can produce Fear. Differ-

entiation is based on the predominant symptom
sequence.

Deficient Knowledge
If the client lacks sufficient knowledge about a situation, a perception of Powerlessness may result. Therefore, Deficient Knowledge would be the primary
diagnosis.

EXPECTED OUTCOME[37]

Will describe at least [number] areas of control over self by
[date].
   Verbalize plan to participate in health-care decisions
by [date].
   Initiates [number] of activities to obtain more information about current situation by [date].
   Verbalizes [number] of personal preferences related to
care by [date].

TARGET DATES

A target date of 3 days is realistic to check for progress
toward reduced feeling of powerlessness.

ADDITIONAL INFORMATION

The paradox of the metaphor of power has been presented in
the literature. Systems theorists and cyberneticians have presented the most useful information when one is planning
intervention strategies. Keeney presents a summary of the
debate over the power metaphor.[97] In sum, most cyberneticians find this to be an invalid metaphor when discussing
systems of interaction. The process of a system involves
mutual interactions, and within a system each member exerts
influence over the other members. Therefore, the individual
who acts as if he or she is powerless is exerting "power" over
the other parts of the system to act in a manner that would
increase this "lost" personal power. The "powerless" one is
then actually exercising power to motivate other parts of the
system to act in certain ways. Understanding this conceptual
model provides the client with an opportunity to know how
one's behavior affects the situation and provides nurses with
an opportunity to understand their reactions to and feelings
toward the client with the diagnosis of Powerlessness. If the
power metaphor is not accepted, this affects the concept of
internal versus external locus of control. The concepts of
internal and external loci of control become metaphors for
how a person perceives personal influence within an interac-
tional system. Persons with an external locus of control do
not understand their influence on the system, whereas persons with an internal locus of control have an understanding
of personal influence.

NURSING ACTIONS/INTERVENTIONS WITH RATIONALES

Adult Health

ACTIONS/INTERVENTIONS	RATIONALES
Provide a calm, safe environment throughout hospitalization: • Answer questions truthfully. • Explain all procedures and rationales for procedures. • Give positive reinforcement to the extent possible.	Allows for verbalization of feelings and acceptance of those feelings. Avoids overwhelming the patient and increasing sensation of powerlessness.
Assist the patient in identifying realistic, achievable goals and activities for managing care.	Provides an environment for goal attainment and thus an increase in control.
Plan daily care with an emphasis on patient preferences (e.g., routines, diet, activities).	Allows the patient to have control over the environment and care attributes. Imparts to the patient a sense of power.
Consider cultural and religious preferences when planning care.	
Determine the extent to which the patient can participate in care. Facilitate provision of as much of self-care as possible.	
Avoid reinforcing manipulative behavior and negative feedback	Sets limits on behavior. Facilitates a nonthreatening environment.
Involve significant others in care as needed.	Promotes involvement in care and advocacy for the patient, thus empowering both the patient and significant others.
Failure to meet expected outcome may signal a decline in the situation.	
Refer to appropriate community resources prior to discharge.	Support groups can encourage progress in building self-esteem, provide advocacy, and provide long-term support.

Child Health

ACTIONS/INTERVENTIONS	RATIONALES
Perform a thorough assessment appropriate for the patient's developmental needs to identify specific factors that are causing powerlessness. Collaborate with the child life specialist, especially for infants and young children. • Use of art • Use of puppetry • Use of group therapy	Developmentally appropriate assessment will provide cues and reveal data to generate a more accurate and complete plan of care.
Facilitate the family's participation in care as they are able and choose to. [Note adaptations needed to accomplish this process here.]	Family participation provides security to the child and empowerment for the parents, with increased growth in coping skills.
Include the child and family by providing opportunities for them to voice preferences whenever appropriate.	Valuing individual preferences is demonstrated by frequent encouragement to express choices. Promotes a sense of control.

(care plan continued on page 582)

NURSING ACTIONS/INTERVENTIONS WITH RATIONALES (continued from page 581)

Child Health

ACTIONS/INTERVENTIONS	RATIONALES
Identify and address educational needs that might be contributing to powerlessness. Note necessary adaptations here.	Misinformation and inadequate knowledge are contributing factors that can be easily overcome by teaching.
Refer to the patient by preferred name or nickname. List that name here.	Promotes personalized communication. Points out individuality, and serves to empower the patient.
Allow for privacy and need to withdraw to the family as a unit.	Demonstrates appropriate respect for the family. Attaches value to the family unit.
Keep the patient and family informed as changes occur.	Frequent updates and provision of information help clarify actions and reduce anxiety, which results in a greater sense of control.
Provide opportunities for the child and parents to demonstrate appropriate care before dismissal from the hospital.	Allows practice in a nonthreatening environment, which increases sense of control.
Consider referral to a child mental health specialist for unresolved issues.	Offers anticipatory guidance for prevention of secondary issues.

Women's Health

ACTIONS/INTERVENTIONS	RATIONALES
Provide the prospective parents with factual information about the type of choices available for birth, and assist them to identify their preference: • Traditional obstetric services • Family-centered maternity care units • Single-room maternity care • Mother–baby care • Birthing center	Provides basic information that assists the family in decision making, thus promoting empowerment of the family unit.[44,49]
Provide answers to questions in an open, direct manner.	
Provide information on all procedures so the patient can make informed choices: • Assist the patient and significant others in establishing realistic goals (list goals with evaluation dates here). • Allow the patient and significant others to participate in decision making.	
Allow the patient maximum control over the environment. This could include the husband's staying in the postpartum room to assist with infant care, keeping the newborn with the mother at all times, using different positions for birth (e.g., squatting or hand–knee position), having grandparents and siblings in the room with the mother and newborn.	Decreases perception of powerlessness and assists in transition to parenthood.
Provide positive reinforcement for parenting tasks.	
Assist the patient in identifying infant behavior patterns and understanding how they allow her infant to communicate with her.	

ACTIONS/INTERVENTIONS	RATIONALES
Support the patient's decisions (e.g., to breastfeed or not to breastfeed, or who she wants as significant others during the birthing process).	
Reassure the new mother that it takes time to become acquainted with her infant.	
Support and reassure the mother in learning infant care (e.g., breastfeeding, bathing, changing, holding a newborn, cord care, or bottle-feeding).	
Allow the parents to verbalize fears and insecure feelings about their new roles as parents.	Promotes decision making, and leaves decisions up to family by providing the guidance and support that is needed.
Assist the parents in identifying lifestyle adjustments that may be needed because of the incorporation of a newborn into the family structure.	
Involve significant others in discussion and problem-solving activities regarding role changes within the family.	Involvement enhances motivation to stay with plan, thus reinforcing decision-making capacity of new parents.[96]
Domestic Violence (See also Hopelessness)	
Provide the patient with support, and assist in identifying actions the patient can take to begin helping herself. Recognize that leaving the abuser is not necessarily the best option at all times and that leaving is a process that may take time for a client.	
Provide a safe atmosphere for identifying needs and making decisions.	
Provide information in an honest, clear manner to help with the decision-making process. Do not attempt to "convince" the client of the correct course of action. Tell the client that there are options, that no one deserves to be beaten, and that she can stop the cycle of violence with outside help.	
Assist the patient in identifying resources available to her and her children.	

Mental Health

ACTIONS/INTERVENTIONS	RATIONALES
Sit with the client [number] times per day at [times] for 30 minutes to discuss feelings and perceptions the client has about the identified situation.	Promotes the development of a trusting relationship, and assists the client in identifying factors contributing to the feelings of powerlessness.
Identify client preferences for daily routine, and place this information on the chart to be implemented by the staff.	It is vital to this client to have the information shared with all staff so that it will not appear that the time spent in providing information was wasted. Promotes the client's perception of control.
Provide information to questions in an open, direct manner.	Facilitates the development of a trusting relationship.
Provide information on all procedures at a time when the client can ask questions and think about the situation.	Facilitates the development of a trusting relationship, and promotes the client's sense of control.

(care plan continued on page 584)

NURSING ACTIONS/INTERVENTIONS WITH RATIONALES (continued from page 583)	

Mental Health

ACTIONS/INTERVENTIONS	RATIONALES
Allow the client to participate in decision making at the level to which he or she is capable. If necessary, offer decision situations in portions that the client can master successfully. (The amount of information that the client can handle should be noted here as well as a list of decisions the client has been presented with.)	The client who has never made an independent decision would be overwhelmed by the complexity of the decisions made daily by a corporation executive. Promotes the client's sense of control.
Identify the client's needs and how these are currently being met. If these involve indirect methods of influence, discuss alternative direct methods of meeting these needs. (The client who requests medication for headache every 15 minutes may be requesting attention and is encouraged to approach the nurse and ask to talk when the need for attention arises.)	Assertive direct communication increases the opportunity for the client's needs being met. When the client is successful in getting needs met in a direct manner, his or her sense of control and self-esteem will increase.
Provide positive reinforcement for behavior changed and decisions made. Things that are reinforcing for this client should be listed here along with the reward system that has been established with the client (e.g., play one game of cards with the client when a decision about what to eat for dinner is made, or walk with the client on hospital grounds when a decision in made about grooming).	Positive reinforcement encourages behavior while enhancing self-esteem.
Provide verbal social reinforcements along with behavioral reinforcements.	Promotes the development of a trusting relationship.
Keep promises (specific promises should be listed here so that all staff will be aware of this information).	
Assist the client in identifying current methods of influence and in understanding that influence is always there by providing feedback on how the influence is being used in the client's interactions with the nurse.	Promotes positive orientation by assisting the client in identifying ways in which he or she is already "powerful."[98]
Accept the client's decisions if the decisions were given to the client to be made (e.g., if the decision to take or not take medication was left with the client, the decision not to take the medication should be respected).	Promotes the client's sense of control and enhances self-esteem.
Allow the client maximum control over the environment. This could include where clothes are kept, how the room is arranged, and times for various activities. [Note preferences here.]	Promotes the client's sense of control.
Spend 30 minutes two times per day at [times] allowing the client to role-play interactions that are identified as problematic. (The specific situations as well as new behavior should be noted here.)	Promotes the client's sense of control in a manner that increases opportunities for success. This success serves as positive reinforcement.
Provide opportunities for significant others to be involved in care as appropriate. Careful assessment of the interactions between the client and significant others must be made to determine the best balance of influencing behavior between the client and support system. Specific situations should be listed here.	Provides opportunities for the support system and the client to practice new ways of interacting while in a situation where they can receive feedback from the health-care team.

ACTIONS/INTERVENTIONS	RATIONALES
Monitor the health-care team's interactions with the client for behavior patterns that would encourage the client to choose indirect methods of influence. This could include interactions that encourage the adult client to assume a childlike role. If situations are identified, they should be noted here.	The role of the nurse in the therapeutic milieu is to promote healthy interpersonal interactions.
Provide ongoing feedback to the client on progress.	Positive reinforcement encourages behavior.
Assist the client in establishing realistic goals. List goals with evaluation dates here. Usually dividing the goal set by the client in half provides an achievable goal; this could also involve dividing one goal into several smaller goals.	Realistic goals increase the client's opportunities for success, providing positive reinforcement and enhancing self-esteem.
Schedule meetings with the client's identified support system when the client verbalizes the need. Facilitate communication between the client and support system about decision making and communication of needs. Note schedule for this meeting here.	A change in one member of a system has impact on the whole system.[61]
Refer the client to outpatient support systems, and assist him or her with making arrangements to contact these before discharge. These could be systems that would assist the client in maintaining a perception of influencing ability and could include assertiveness training groups, battered persons' programs, and legal aid.	Provides the client with support for continuing new behaviors in the community after discharge.

Gerontic Health

In addition to the following interventions, the interventions for Adult Health and Mental Health can be applied to the aging client.

ACTIONS/INTERVENTIONS	RATIONALES
Ensure the client has easy access to call light, telephone, personal care items, and television control.[39]	Increases the patient's ability to take control of some aspects of care.
Advocate for the patient, ensuring that health care professionals are including client in decision making.	Decision-making capacity does not necessarily diminish with age.

Home Health

In addition to the following interventions, the interventions for Adult Health and Mental Health can be applied to the home health client.

ACTIONS/INTERVENTIONS	RATIONALES
Involve the client and family in planning and implementing strategies to reduce Powerlessness: • Family conference: Identify and discuss strategies. • Mutual goal setting: Agree on goals to reduce Powerlessness. Identify roles of all participants. • Discuss effective communication techniques.	Personal involvement and goal setting according to personal wishes enhance the likelihood of success in resolving problem.
Assist the client and family in lifestyle adjustments that may be required:	Lifestyle adjustments require permanent changes in behavior. Self-evaluation and support facilitate the success of these lifestyle changes.

(care plan continued on page 586)

NURSING ACTIONS/INTERVENTIONS WITH RATIONALES (continued from page 585)

Home Health

ACTIONS/INTERVENTIONS	RATIONALES
• Relaxation techniques: Yoga, biofeedback, hypnosis, breathing techniques, imagery • Providing opportunities for the individual to exert control over situation, giving choices when possible, supporting and encouraging self-care efforts • Problem solving and goal setting • Providing sense of mastery and accomplishable goals in secure environment • Maintaining the treatment plan of the health-care professionals guiding therapy • Obtaining and providing accurate information regarding condition	
Consult with or refer to assistive resources as indicated.	Use of existing community resources provides for effective use of resources.
Assist the client and family to set criteria to help them determine when the intervention of a health-care professional is required (e.g., inability to perform activities of daily living, or condition has declined rapidly).	Early identification of issues requiring professional evaluation will increase the probability of successful intervention.

SELF-CONCEPT, READINESS FOR ENHANCED

DEFINITION[40]

A pattern of perceptions of ideas about the self that is sufficient for well-being and can be strengthened.

DEFINING CHARACTERISTICS[40]

1. Expresses willingness to enhance self-concept.
2. Expresses satisfaction with thoughts about self, sense of worthiness, role performance, body image, and personal identity.
3. Actions are congruent with expressed feelings and thoughts.
4. Expresses confidence in abilities.
5. Accepts strengths and limitations.

RELATED FACTORS[40]

None listed

RELATED CLINICAL CONCERNS

1. History of abuse
2. Physical disability
3. Adolescence
4. Situations that require significant role changes
5. Amputations or surgeries that alter body image

☑ Have You Selected the Correct Diagnosis?

Self-Esteem: Chronic Low, Situational Low
Address situations in which the client is demonstrating alterations in self-perceptions and negative self-evaluation.

Self-Esteem: Risk for Situational Low
would be the appropriate diagnosis when the client is experiencing a situation that could have a negative impact on self-esteem.

Self-Concept: Readiness for Enhanced
is the appropriate diagnosis for situations where the client is expressing positive self-statements and expresses a desire to enhance this self-perception.

EXPECTED OUTCOME

Will identify [number] goals for self improvement by [date].
Will demonstrate achievement of personal goals by [date].
Will verbalize satisfaction with role performance by [date].

TARGET DATES

Self-improvement can be a life-long process. The enhancement of self-concept, as used here, should focus on specific goals that can be measured with in a reasonable time. This could include short-term goals with target dates measured in days and long-term goals that could be measured in weeks.

NURSING ACTIONS/INTERVENTIONS WITH RATIONALES

Adult Health

ACTIONS/INTERVENTIONS	RATIONALES
Use routine patient interactions to engage the patient in a discussion of self-perception.	
Collaborate with the patient in developing a plan to engage in activities that enhance self-concept.	
Assist the patient in identifying individuals and relationships that promote feelings of self-worth.	Promotes a positive support network.
Collaborate with the patient to develop a plan for appropriate coping and reconciliation of limitations.	
See psychiatric plan of care for additional actions.	

Child Health

ACTIONS/INTERVENTIONS	RATIONALES
Seek input from all members of the health-care team, including child life specialist, family or child counselor/psychologist, and clinical nurse specialist.	Engenders a collaborative effort to be of best support for facilitating goals for the individual child and family.
Assist the child and family in identifying strategies to foster desired plan, especially daily routine, personal diary, feedback, or goal setting sessions with follow-up progress sessions.	Specific identified goals offer structure with likelihood of marking aspired levels of manageable achievement.[106–108]
Offer basic and then incrementally more challenging daily routine management. Develop goals that are achievable by the child. [Note the specific plan for the client and family here.]	Scaffolding provides likelihood of learning and reinforcement for success as opposed to overwhelming the learner. When the child can successfully reach goals self-esteem is enhanced.[106–108]
Provide feedback in a timely manner according to developmental level and appropriate nature of plan. Note feedback to be used with this client here.	Offers reinforcement that is suitable and able to encourage greater goal achievement.
Determine barriers to plan for care, especially how to modify the desired plan in light of equipment, treatments, or necessary interruptions. If school issues are to be considered, relate with teachers and the school nurse as appropriate.	Anticipatory guidance alleviates crises and affords facilitative progress.
Assist the child and family to identify resources that will foster continued success in self-concept enhancement. [Note specific plan to facilitate this here.][106–108]	Provides support to value efforts.
Teach the family and client appropriate use of prostheses or equipment.	Anticipatory guidance alleviates secondary and tertiary events that are preventable.
Schedule a time for the client and family to be involved in support groups.	Facilitates the reception of positive feedback. Positive self reflection from others enhances self-esteem.
Teach parents how to develop behavioral reward systems and provide positive meaningful verbal feedback.[106–108]	Positive reflections of self from others enhance self-esteem.[106–108]

(care plan continued on page 588)

NURSING ACTIONS/INTERVENTIONS WITH RATIONALES (continued from page 587)

Women's Health

Note most of the interventions and rationales for women will be the same as for Adult Health and Mental Health, with the following additions.

ACTIONS/INTERVENTIONS	RATIONALES
Assist the client in making responsible choices to care for themselves within their various life-cycles.[99] Spend time discussing how to achieve selected goals for life-style choices such as nutritious diet, regular exercise, no smoking, and mind–spirit awareness.[99–101]	Enhanced self-concept comes with feeling good about yourself and choosing to do what is good for your physical, emotional, and spiritual health. The health-care provider must guide and offer information on many choices women can make, including natural/alternative/complementary health care (NAC) options.[101]
Offer information so that client can make informed choices. Provide the client with: • List of women's health tests from adolescence through elderly cycles of a woman's life.	Understanding which tests women should be participating in and at what age and frequency will assist women in monitoring and maintaining their health. Tests such as screening for Osteoporosis (Bone Density Test), Cholesterol, Blood Glucose, Blood Pressure, Colorectal Exams, Breast Cancer Screenings, Dental Checkup, Pap Test, and Pelvic Exam are just a few.[102]

Mental Health

ACTIONS/INTERVENTIONS	RATIONALES
Spend [number] minutes [number] times per day discussing the client's understanding of his or her concerns and personal goals. Establish a nurse–client relationship based on warm positive regard and empathy for the client.	Change depends on the client's perception of the problem.[61] Enhances the client's sense of control and self-esteem/self-efficacy.[89,98]
Develop with the client a list of goals that are specific and behavioral. Establish goals that will move client to their larger personal goals and that are going to be achievable by the client. [Note client specific goals here.] • Develop a list of positive reinforces for goal achievement. (Note reinforcers and schedule for reinforcement here.) • Spend [number] minutes [number] times each day reviewing client's progress towards goals. Provide specific informative praise for steps toward goal achievement.	Goal attainment increases the client's sense of self-efficacy. Positive reinforcement increases behavior.[38,65] Informative praise that is specific and provides clear direction about which behavior is being rewarded enhances self-esteem. (This is in contrast to bland praise such as using the word "good" without a behavioral reference.)[89]
Spend [number] minutes once a day exploring with client their interests and achievements. From this interaction develop a list of community or other groups that would promote client's interests.	Positive social support and the sense of belonging to a group enhance self-concept. Recognition of past achievements increases self-efficacy and therefore self-concept.[63,89]

ACTIONS/INTERVENTIONS	RATIONALES
Identify the steps client can take to establish a relationship with one or two of these groups or begin engagement with an activity. Note the groups selected and the steps to be taken here.	Specific, concrete, incremental steps increase the client's perceptions of the possibility of goal attainment.
Schedule client's attendance at [number] groups that provide the opportunity for positive social support per day that reflect client's goals. Note the group times here. Walk the client to the group and introduce him or her to other members. Note specific interventions needed to assist the client with group attendance here.	Positive social support and the sense of belonging to a group enhance self-concept.[63,89] Groups that provide a variety of role models and/or enhance social skills demonstrate positive effects on self-concept. It is important that the client be allowed to make his or her own comparisons.[62]
Collaborate with the client to establish an exercise routine. Note specific exercises and times here. If the client has not done regular exercises, establish moderate goals and activities.	Exercise and good health have a positive impact on self-concept.[104,105]
Provide the client with information on assertive skills training.	Positive social skills enhance self-concept.
• If the client identifies this as a need, schedule the client for assertiveness training group. Note the schedule for group here.	
• Role-play social interactions the client has identified as difficult.	
• Provide positive verbal reinforcement for achievements.	
Meet with the client and his or her social support system to discuss methods of continuing social support after discharge. Note the schedule for meetings here.	Positive social support and a sense of belonging enhance self-concept. Client involvement in goal setting enhances sense of self-efficacy and in turn self-concept is enhanced.
During the meeting:	
• Model assertive communication and other positive communication skills.	
• Model positive informative praise.	
Develop a specific plan for achieving the goals that evolved from this meeting. Note specific goals and plan for achieving goals here. Provide members of the social support system with written copies of this plan.	

Gerontic Health

ACTIONS/INTERVENTIONS	RATIONALES
Assist the patient in setting realistic goals for strengthening a sense of well-being and self concept.	Client will not become discouraged by unrealistic goals.
Provide an environment conducive to improved self-concept:	Maximizes the effectiveness of planning and maintaining a program for improvement.
• Client is not hungry, in pain, or sleepy.	
• Have a family member present if desired or needed.	
• Maximize the client's control of the environment.	
Provide referral as needed to include:	Use of the interdisciplinary team facilitates the client's ability to control his or her environment and determine strategies for maintaining a positive self-concept.
• Physical therapy	
• Occupational therapy	
• Pastoral care	
• Social work	

(care plan continued on page 590)

NURSING ACTIONS/INTERVENTIONS WITH RATIONALES (continued from page 589)

Home Health

ACTIONS/INTERVENTIONS	RATIONALES
Assist the patient in setting realistic goals for strengthening his or her sense of well-being and self-concept.	Client will not become discouraged by unrealistic goals.
Provide an environment conducive to improved self-concept: • Client is not hungry, in pain, or sleepy. • Have a family member present if desired or needed. • Maximize the client's control of the environment.	Maximizes the effectiveness of planning and maintaining a program for improvement.
Provide referral as needed to include: • Physical therapy • Occupational therapy • Pastoral care • Social work	Use of the interdisciplinary team facilitates the client's ability to control his or her environment and determine strategies for maintaining a positive self-concept.
Refer the client to community resources as appropriate: • Support groups for clients and families • Educational Web resources	Utilizing existing resources facilitates success and is time and cost efficient.

SELF-ESTEEM, CHRONIC LOW, SITUATIONAL LOW, AND RISK FOR SITUATIONAL LOW

DEFINITIONS[40]

Chronic Low Self-Esteem Long-standing negative self-evaluation or feelings about self or self-capabilities.

Situational Low Self-Esteem Development of a negative perception of self-worth in response to a current situation (specify).

Risk for Situational Low Self-Esteem Risk for developing a negative perception of self-worth in response to a current situation (specify).

DEFINING CHARACTERISTICS[40]

A. Chronic Low Self-Esteem
1. Rationalizes away, or rejects, positive feedback, and exaggerates negative feedback about self (long standing or chronic)
2. Self-negative verbalization (long standing or chronic)
3. Hesitant to try new things or situations (long standing or chronic)
4. Expressions of shame or guilt (long standing or chronic)
5. Evaluates self as unable to deal with events (long standing or chronic)
6. Lack of eye contact
7. Nonassertive or passive
8. Frequent lack of success in work or other life events
9. Excessively seeks reassurance
10. Overly conforming or dependent on others' opinions
11. Indecisive

B. Situational Low Self-Esteem
1. Verbally reports current situational challenges to self-worth
2. Self-negating verbalizations
3. Indecisive, nonassertive behavior
4. Evaluates self as unable to deal with situations or events
5. Expressions of helplessness and uselessness

C. Risk for Situational Low Self-Esteem
The risk factors also serve as the defining characteristics.

RELATED FACTORS[40]

A. Chronic Low Self-Esteem
To be developed.

B. Situational Low Self-Esteem
1. Developmental changes (specify)
2. Body image disturbance
3. Functional impairment (specify)
4. Loss (specify)
5. Social role changes (specify)
6. Lack of recognition or rewards
7. Behavior inconsistent with values
8. Failures or rejections

C. Risk for Situational Low Self-Esteem (Risk Factors)
1. Developmental changes (specify)
2. Body image disturbance
3. Functional impairment (specify)
4. Loss (specify)
5. Social role changes (specify)
6. History of learned helplessness
7. History of abuse, neglect, or abandonment
8. Unrealistic self-expectations
9. Behavior inconsistent with values
10. Lack of recognition or rewards
11. Failures or rejections
12. Decreased power or control over environment
13. Physical illness (specify)

RELATED CLINICAL CONCERNS[27]

1. Pervasive developmental disorders
2. Disruptive behavior disorders
3. Eating disorders
4. Organic mental disorders
5. Substance use or dependence or abuse disorders
6. Mood disorders
7. Adjustment disorders
8. Personality disorders
9. Trauma
10. Surgery
11. Medical problems that contribute to the loss of body functions
12. Pregnancy
13. Chronic diseases
14. Dysfunctional family processes

 Have You Selected the Correct Diagnosis?

Disturbed Body Image
This diagnosis relates to alterations in the perception of self when there is an actual or perceived change in body structure or function. If interviewing reveals the patient perceives a potential change in body structure or function, then Disturbed Body Image is the most appropriate diagnosis.

Disturbed Personal Identity
When the patient cannot differentiate self from non-self, some self-esteem problems probably exist; however, the primary diagnosis would be Disturbed Personal Identity. Working with the Disturbed Personal Identity will address the self-esteem problem.

Ineffective Individual Coping
This diagnosis results from the client's inability to cope with stress appropriately. If the client demonstrates a decreased ability to cope appropriately, he or she may also have some defining characteristics related to self-esteem disturbance. Teaching and supporting coping will also assist in correcting the self-esteem problem.

Self-Concept, Readiness for Enhanced
This diagnosis reflects a perception of self that is positive and supports well-being. If the client is expressing negative self perceptions then the diagnosis would be one of the compromised self-esteem diagnoses.

EXPECTED OUTCOME

Will list at least [number] positive aspects about self by [date].

Will verbalize [number] of situations where success was experienced by [date].

Will demonstrate assertive behavior in [describe situation] by [date].

TARGET DATES

A target date of 3 to 5 days is acceptable to begin monitoring progress.

NURSING ACTIONS/INTERVENTIONS WITH RATIONALES

● N O T E: *An attitude of genuine warmth, acceptance of clients, and respect for uniqueness are characteristics required for successful nursing interventions.*[109]

Adult Health

ACTIONS/INTERVENTIONS	RATIONALES
Promote a calm, safe environment by avoiding a judgmental attitude, actively listening, using reflection, being consistent in approach, and setting boundaries.	Decreases anxiety and promotes a trusting relationship.
Support the patient's self-care management activities. Teach the patient and significant others the patient's self-care requirements as needed.	Participation in own care increases confidence and self-esteem.

(care plan continued on page 592)

NURSING ACTIONS/INTERVENTIONS WITH RATIONALES (continued from page 591)

Adult Health

ACTIONS/INTERVENTIONS	RATIONALES
Reinforce assertive behavior in interacting with the patient. Assist the patient to review passive and aggressive behavior.	Helps the patient avoid vacillating from one behavior to another. Promotes self-control and a "win–win" situation, which increases self-esteem.
Allow the patient to progress at his or her own rate. Start with simple, concrete tasks. Reward success.	Helps the patient have a sense of mastering of tasks, and promotes self-esteem.
In interactions with the patient: • Be honest with the patient. • Point out and limit self-negating statements. • Do not support denial. • Focus on reality and adaptation (not necessarily acceptance). • Set limits on maladaptive behavior. • Focus on realistic goals. • Be aware of own nonverbal communication and behavior. • Avoid moral value judgments. • Encourage the patient to try to note differences in situations and events.	
Use routine interactions as an opportunity to have the patient verbalize feelings.	Assists in self-understanding and facilitates self-acceptance.
Help the patient to ascertain why he or she can maintain self-esteem in one situation and not in another.	
Build on coping mechanisms or interpretations that maintain or increase self-esteem. Assist to find alternative coping mechanisms.	Supports adaptive coping, and helps broaden the inventory of coping strategies.
Refer to and collaborate with community resources.	Provides ongoing and long-term support.
Collaborate with the psychiatric nurse clinician regarding care. (See Mental Health nursing actions.)	Collaboration promotes a more holistic and total plan of care.

Child Health

ACTIONS/INTERVENTIONS	RATIONALES
Monitor for contributory factors related to poor self-esteem, including: • Family crisis • Lack of adequate parenting • Lack of sensory stimulation • Physical scars, malformations, or disfigurement • Altered role performance • Social isolation • Developmental crisis	Generates the database needed to plan care more accurately and completely.
Identify ways the patient can formulate or reestablish a positive self-esteem according to developmental needs. Note the methods best for this patient here. • Coping skills • Communication skills	Developmental norms serve as the conceptual framework for assisting the child to increase self-esteem.

ACTIONS/INTERVENTIONS	RATIONALES
• Role expectations • Self-care • Activities of daily living • Basic physiologic needs; primary health care • Expression of self • Peer and social relationships • Feelings of self-worth • Decision making • Validation of self (e.g., setting developmentally appropriate expectations)	
Praise and reinforce positive behavior. [Note reinforcers that are most important for this patient here.]	Reinforcement of desired behavior serves to enhance the permanence of the behavior.
Explore value conflicts and their resolution.	Values must be clarified as one strives to find one's identity. A healthy sense of self contributes to a positive self-image.
Collaborate with other health-care team members as needed.	Collaboration promotes a more holistic plan of care.
Meet primary health needs in an expedient manner.	Conserves energy, minimizes stress, and enhances trust.
Provide appropriate attention to other alterations, especially those directly affecting this diagnosis such as Risk for Violence or Impaired Parenting.	Related issues must be considered as contributing factors to the diagnosis. Inattention to these factors means resolution of the problem will not occur.
Provide for follow-up before the child is dismissed from hospital.	Attaches value to follow-up, and promotes likelihood of compliance.
Use developmentally appropriate strategies in the care of these children: • Infant and toddlers: Play therapy or puppets • Preschoolers: Art • School-agers: Art or role-playing • Adolescents: Discussion or role-playing	Developmentally based strategies are most likely to not frighten the child or parent unnecessarily.
Teaching parents and child about appropriate health maintenance. This could include ways of dealing with crisis, or enhanced communication skills. [Note teaching plan here.]	Personal hygiene and self-care will enhance a positive self-esteem as the patient copes with daily living.

Women's Health

ACTIONS/INTERVENTIONS	RATIONALES
Postpartum and Parenting Roles	
Allow the patient to "relive" the birthing experience by listening quietly to her perception of the birthing experience.	Promotes ventilation of feelings, and provides a database for intervention.
Encourage the patient to express her concerns about her physical appearance.	
List here the activities in which the patient can engage to gain positive feelings about herself.	
Join friends or an exercise group with the same goals as the patient.	Provides a support system that demonstrates adaptive behaviors.

(care plan continued on page 594)

NURSING ACTIONS/INTERVENTIONS WITH RATIONALES (continued from page 593)

Women's Health

ACTIONS/INTERVENTIONS	RATIONALES
Encourage participation in activities outside of the home as appropriate (e.g., parenting support groups or women's groups).	Support and positive activities assist in adaptation to new parental role and increase sense of self-worth.
Encourage networking with other women with similar interests.	
Encourage the patient to "do something for herself": • Buy a new dress. • Fix her hair differently. • Find some time for herself during the day. • Take a walk. • Take a long bath. • Rest quietly. • Do a favorite activity (e.g., reading, sewing, or some other hobby) • Spend time with spouse, without the children	
Encourage the patient to engage in positive thinking.	
Encourage the patient to engage in assertiveness training.	
● N O T E : *Pregnant teenagers, single mothers, and battered women have similar needs in building or rebuilding their self-esteem.*	
Provide a safe, nonjudgmental atmosphere that will encourage the patient to verbalize her needs and concerns.	
Assist the patient in identifying support groups with similar concerns and available community resources.	
Encourage teen mothers to take advantage of opportunities provided by various school systems to finish their education.	

Mental Health

ACTIONS/INTERVENTIONS	RATIONALES
Sit with the client [number] minutes [number] times per shift to discuss the client's feelings about self.	Expression of feelings and concerns in an accepting environment can facilitate problem solving.
Answer questions honestly.	Promotes the development of a trusting relationship.
Provide feedback to the client about the nurse's perceptions of the client's abilities and appearance by: • Using "I" statements • Using references related to the nurse's relationship to the client • Describing the client's behavior in situations • Describing the nurse's feelings in relationship	Assists the client with reality testing in a safe, trusting relationship.
Provide positive informative reinforcement. List here the things that are reinforcing for the client and when they are to be used. Also list here the things that have been identified as nonreinforcers for this client, and include social rewards.	Positive reinforcement encourages behavior.

ACTIONS/INTERVENTIONS	RATIONALES
Provide group interaction with [number] persons [number] minutes three times a day at [times]. This activity should be gradual and within the client's ability (e.g., on admission the client may tolerate one person for 5 minutes). If the interactions are brief, the frequency should be high (i.e., 5-minute interactions should occur at 30-minute intervals).	Disconfirms the client's sense of aloneness, and assists the client to experience personal importance to others while enhancing interpersonal relationship skills. Increasing these competencies can enhance self-esteem and promote positive orientation. Group interaction provides opportunities for social comparison which can have a positive impact on self-esteem.[62]
Monitor the client during each interaction for thoughts of self-harm. If thoughts are present protect the client from harm by: (See Chapter 8, Self-Mutilation and Chapter 9, Violence, Self-Directed for comprehensive care plans on this behavior if present.)	Client safety is of primary concern. Low self-esteem can be related to thoughts of self-harm.
• Removing all sharp objects from the environment	
• Removing belts and strings from the environment	
• Providing a one-to-one constant interaction if risk for self-harm is high	
• Checking on the client's whereabouts every 15 minutes or providing constant visual supervision if the risk is high. Note the level of observation needed here.	
• Removing glass objects from the environment	
• Removing locks from the room and bathroom doors	
• Providing a shower curtain that will not support weight	
• Checking to see whether the client swallows medications	
• Removing any items in the environment that would facilitate the client implementing his or her plan for self-harm	
In a supportive attitude and manner, reflect back to the client negative self-statements he or she makes.	Increases the client's awareness of negative evaluations of self.
Set achievable goals for the client. [Note goals and support necessary to achieve goals here.]	Goals that can be accomplished increase the client's perceptions of power and enhance self-esteem.
Provide activities that the client can accomplish and that the client values.	Activities the client finds demeaning could reinforce the client's negative self-evaluation. Accomplishment of valued tasks provides positive reinforcement and enhances self-esteem.[38,58]
Provide positive informative verbal reinforcement for achievement of steps toward a goal.	Positive reinforcement encourages behavior while enhancing self-esteem.[89]
Have the client develop a list of strengths and potentials.	Promotes positive orientation and hope.[28]
Define the client's lack of goal achievement or failures as simple mistakes that are bound to occur when one attempts something new (e.g., learning comes with mistakes, or if one does not make mistakes one does not learn).	Promotes positive orientation.[28]

(care plan continued on page 596)

NURSING ACTIONS/INTERVENTIONS WITH RATIONALES (continued from page 595)

Mental Health

ACTIONS/INTERVENTIONS	RATIONALES
Make necessary items available for the client to groom self.	Physical grooming can facilitate positive self-esteem by encouraging positive feedback from others.
Spend [number] minutes at [time] assisting the client with grooming, providing necessary assistance, and providing positive informative reinforcement for accomplishments. Note special accommodations here.	Presence of the nurse can serve as a positive reinforcement. Positive reinforcement encourages behavior while enhancing self-esteem.
Reflect back to the client the statements that discount the positive evaluations of others.	Raises the client's awareness of this behavior, which facilitates change. Self-concept development is facilitated by reflections of others about the self.[32,98]
Focus the client's attention on the here and now.	Past happenings are difficult for the nurse to provide feedback on.
Present the client with opportunities to make decisions about care, and record these decisions in the chart.	Promotes the clent's sense of control which enhance self-esteem.
Develop with the client alternative coping strategies. Link these to client's past successes.	Promotes the client's sense of control, and enhances opportunities for positive outcome when stressful events are encountered. This supports client's competencies and provides a positive orientation of self.[28,61]
Practice new coping behaviors with the client [number] minutes at [times].	Behavioral rehearsal provides opportunities for feedback and modeling of new behaviors from the nurse.
Place the client in a therapy group for [number] minutes once a day where the focus is mutual sharing of feelings and support of each other.	Facilitates the client's awareness of others' thoughts about themselves and him or her.
Identify with the client the situations that are perceived as most threatening to self-esteem.	Facilitates developing alternative coping behavior.
Assist the client in identifying alternative methods of coping with the identified situations. These should be developed by the client and listed here.	Increases the client's opportunities for success, and each success enhances self-esteem.
Role-play with the client once per day for 45 minutes the high-risk situations that were identified and the alternative coping methods.	Behavioral rehearsal provides opportunities for feedback and modeling of new behaviors from the nurse.
Establish an appointment with the client and significant others to discuss their perceptions of the client's situation. (The time of this and follow-up appointments should be listed here.)	Support system understanding facilitates the maintenance of new behaviors after discharge.[110]
• During the sessions model positive communication and recognizing each other's accomplishments.	
• Teach the support system to provide positive informative verbal feedback.	
Discuss with the client current behavior and reactions of others to this behavior.	Provides opportunities for feedback on new behaviors in a safe, trusting environment.
Provide the client with [number] minutes of assertive skills training [number] times per week. This could be provided in a group or individual context.	Teaches clients they have a right to their feelings, beliefs, and opinions, and provides them with the skills to express themselves effectively.[73]
Practice with the client [number] minutes twice a day making positive "I" statements.	Promotes the development of a positive orientation.

Gerontic Health

In addition to the following interventions, the interventions for Adult Health and Mental Health can be applied to the aging client.

ACTIONS/INTERVENTIONS	RATIONALES
Assist the patient in developing self-care skills needed for managing the current illness.[111]	Enhances perception of control over the situation.
Assist the patient in identifying his or her unique abilities, and relate the benefits you as a nurse receive from your interactions.	Increases recognition of successes that come from the use of personal strengths with the patient.[111]
Review the patient's current abilities and how they may require role modification.[111]	Increases perception of functional ability in preferred life roles.
Assist with personal grooming needs, such as removal of excess facial hair and use of cosmetics, where applicable.[112]	Attention to personal appearance can have a positive influence on self-esteem and thus perception of the individual.

Home Health

In addition to the following interventions, the interventions for Adult Health and Mental Health can be applied to the home health client.

ACTIONS/INTERVENTIONS	RATIONALES
Involve the client and family in planning and implementing strategies to reduce and cope with disturbance in self-esteem: • Family conference: Discuss perceptions of the client's situations and identify realistic strategies. • Mutual goal setting: Establish goals and identify roles of each family member (e.g., provide safe environment, assist with grooming, or focus on here and now). • Communication.	Family involvement improves effectiveness of implementation.
Assist the client and family in lifestyle adjustments that may be required.[113] • Obtaining and providing accurate information • Clarifying misconceptions • Maintaining a safe environment • Encouraging appropriate self-care without encouraging dependence or expecting unrealistic independence • Providing an opportunity for expressing feelings • Realistic goal-setting • Providing a sense of mastery and accomplishable goals in a secure environment • Maintaining the treatment plan of the health-care professionals guiding therapy • Relaxation techniques: Yoga, biofeedback, hypnosis, breathing techniques, or imagery • Altering roles	Lifestyle changes require long-term changes in behavior. Such changes in behavior require support.
Consult with or refer to assistive resources as indicated.	Utilization of existing services is efficient use of resources. Psychiatric nurse clinician and support groups can enhance the treatment plan.

SELF-MUTILATION, RISK FOR AND ACTUAL

DEFINITIONS[40]

Risk for Self-Mutilation Risk for deliberate self-injurious behavior causing tissue damage with the intent of causing nonfatal injury to attain relief of tension.

Self-Mutilation Deliberate self-injurious behavior causing tissue damage with the intent of causing nonfatal injury to attain relief of tension.

DEFINING CHARACTERISTICS[40]

A. Risk for Self-Mutilation (Risk Factors)
   1. Psychotic state (command hallucination)
   2. Inability to express tension verbally
   3. Childhood sexual abuse
   4. Violence between parental figures
   5. Family divorce
   6. Family alcoholism
   7. Family history of self-destructive behavior
   8. Adolescence
   9. Peers who self-mutilate
   10. Isolation from peers
   11. Perfectionism
   12. Substance abuse
   13. Eating disorders
   14. Sexual identity crisis
   15. Low or unstable self-esteem
   16. Low or unstable body image
   17. History of inability to plan solutions or see long-term consequences
   18. Use of manipulation to obtain nurturing relationship with others
   19. Chaotic or disturbed interpersonal relationships
   20. Emotionally disturbed and/or battered children
   21. Feels threatened with actual or potential loss of a significant relationship
   22. Loss of a parent or parental relationship
   23. Experiences dissociation or depersonalization
   24. Experiences mounting tension that is intolerable
   25. Impulsivity
   26. Inadequate coping
   27. Experiences irresistible urge to cut or damage self
   28. Needs quick reduction of stress
   29. Childhood illness or surgery
   30. Foster, group, or institutional care
   31. Incarceration
   32. Character disorder
   33. Borderline personality disorders
   34. Loss of control over problem-solving situation
   35. Developmentally delayed and autistic persons
   36. History of self-injurious behavior
   37. Feeling of depression, rejection, self-hatred, separation anxiety, guilt, and depersonalization

B. Self-Mutilation
   1. Cuts or scratches on body
   2. Picking at wounds
   3. Self-inflicted burns (e.g., eraser or cigarette)
   4. Ingestion or inhalation of harmful substances or object
   5. Biting
   6. Abrading
   7. Severing
   8. Insertion of object(s) into body orifices
   9. Hitting
   10. Constricting a body part

RELATED FACTORS[40]

A. Risk for Self-Mutilation
   The risk factors also serve as the related factors.
B. Self-Mutilation
   1. Psychotic state (command hallucination)
   2. Inability to express tension verbally
   3. Childhood sexual abuse
   4. Violence between parental figures
   5. Family divorce
   6. Family alcoholism
   7. Family history of self-destructive behavior
   8. Adolescence
   9. Peers who self-mutilate
   10. Isolation from peers
   11. Perfectionism
   12. Substance abuse
   13. Eating disorders
   14. Sexual identity crisis
   15. Low or unstable self-esteem
   16. Low or unstable body image
   17. Labile behavior (mood swings)
   18. History of inability to plan solutions or see long-term consequences
   19. Use of manipulation to obtain nurturing relationship with others
   20. Chaotic or disturbed interpersonal relationships
   21. Emotionally disturbed and/or battered children
   22. Feels threatened with actual or potential loss of a significant relationship (e.g., loss of a parent or parental relationship)
   23. Experiences dissociation or depersonalization
   24. Experiences mounting tension that is intolerable
   25. Impulsivity
   26. Inadequate coping
   27. Experiences irresistible urge to cut or damage self
   28. Needs quick reduction of stress
   29. Childhood illness or surgery
   30. Foster, group, or institutional care
   31. Incarceration
   32. Character disorder

33. Borderline personality disorders
34. Developmentally delayed and autistic persons
35. History of self-injurious behavior
36. Feeling of depression, rejection, self-hatred, separation anxiety, guilt, and depersonalization
37. Poor parent–adolescent communication
38. Lack of family confidant

RELATED CLINICAL CONCERNS

1. Borderline personality disorder
2. Organic mental disorders
3. Autism
4. Schizophrenia
5. Major depression
6. Dissociative identity disorder (DID)
7. Sexual masochism
8. Affective disorder or mania
9. History of abuse

 Have You Selected the Correct Diagnosis?

Risk for Violence
This diagnosis is very similar to the Risk for Self-Mutilation. However, self-mutilation speaks only to the intent to injure oneself and specifically excludes suicide.

Ineffective Individual Coping
Certainly, self-mutilation would be indicative of ineffective coping. If self-mutilation is present then this would be the priority diagnosis to provide clients with strategies to cope with the precursors to the self-harm behaviors.

EXPECTED OUTCOME

Will demonstrate no self-mutilation attempts by [date].
Contracts to contact staff when feeling urge to injure self by [date].[37]
Contracts for no self harm by [date].
Demonstrates [number] alternative(s) to manage feelings/tension by [date].

TARGET DATES

Initially progress should be evaluated on a daily basis because of the danger involved for the patient. After stabilization has been demonstrated, the target date could be moved to 5- to 7-day intervals.

NURSING ACTIONS/INTERVENTIONS WITH RATIONALES

Adult Health

● NOTE: *Should this diagnosis be made on an adult health patient, immediately refer him or her to a mental health practitioner. (See Mental Health nursing actions.)*

Child Health

● NOTE: *Refer the patient to a mental health practitioner. (See Mental Health nursing actions related to this diagnosis.)*

Women's Health

The nursing actions for the woman with this diagnosis are the same as those given for Mental Health.

Mental Health

ACTIONS/INTERVENTIONS	RATIONALES
Sit with the client [number] minutes [number] times per shift at [times] to assess the client's mood, distress, needs, and feelings.	Promotes the development of a trusting relationship, and an opportunity to monitor risk for self harm, in a nonintrusive manner.[114] Also communicates to client that their emotional needs will be respected and attempts will be made to understand their behavior.[115]

(care plan continued on page 600)

NURSING ACTIONS/INTERVENTIONS WITH RATIONALES (continued from page 599)

Mental Health

ACTIONS/INTERVENTIONS	RATIONALES
Place the client on a frequent observation schedule. Note that schedule here. This observation should take place in a nonintrusive manner.	Client safety is of primary importance. Increased attention may inadvertently reinforce injury if it occurs in relation to self-injury episodes.[114]
Remove from the environment any object that the patient could use to harm him- or herself. Note the items most preferred by this client here.	Client safety is of primary importance.
Use one-to-one observation to protect the client during periods of risk for self-harming behavior.	Physical and chemical restraints have been demonstrated to escalate behavior. At times clients may escalate their behavior to be placed in restraints.[116]
Develop a baseline assessment of the self-injury patterns. This should include frequency of behavior, type of behavior, factors related to self-harm, and effects of self-harm on the client and other clients. Note this information here.	Provides baseline information on which to base criteria for behavioral change. Provides positive reinforcement.
Answer the client's questions honestly. Maintain an environment of reassurance and respect.	Promotes the development of a trusting relationship.[115]
Develop a no self-harm contract with the client.	Provides client with clear understanding of behavioral expectations.[58]
Reframe the client's self-harming behavior as a habitual behavior that can be changed, like any habit. While doing this, do not diminish the client's experience of emotional pain and discomfort.	Promotes a positive orientation, and supports the client's strengths.[117]
Identify, with the client, goals that are reasonable. Note the goals here (e.g., the client will contact staff when feeling need to harm self).	Assists the client in gaining internal control of problematic behaviors.[117] Achieving goals provides reinforcement of positive behavior and enhances self-esteem.
Provide positive verbal reinforcement for positive behavior change.	Positive reinforcement encourages behavior and enhances self-esteem.
Have the client develop a list of "feel-good" reinforcers. [Note those reinforcers here.][114]	Promotes the client's sense of control, while supporting a positive orientation.
Provide feel-good reinforcers according to the reinforcement plan developed. Note the plan here.	Provides consistency in behavioral rewards. Positive reinforcement encourages behavior and enhances self-esteem.
Identify with the client situations and feelings that trigger self-injury.[114]	Promotes the client's perception of control by pairing self-injurious behavior to specific situations and decreasing cognitive exaggerations.[118]
Identify with the client strategies that can be utilized to cope with these situations. [Note the identified strategies here.]	Promotes the client's sense of control, and assists the client with cognitive preparation for coping with these situations.[118]
	Assists with the development of emotional self-regulation.[115,119]
Select one identified strategy and spend 30 minutes a day at [times] practicing this with the client. This could be in the form of a role-play. Note here the person responsible for this practice.	Behavioral rehearsal provides opportunities for feedback and modeling from the nurse.
Meet with the client just prior to and after trigger situations to assist with planning coping strategies and processing outcome to revise plans for future situations.[116]	Promotes the client's sense of control, and provides an opportunity for the nurse to provide positive reinforcement for adaptive coping mechanisms.

ACTIONS/INTERVENTIONS	RATIONALES
Initiate the client's coping strategy or provide distraction, such as physical activity, when the client identifies that the urge to harm him- or herself is strong. Acknowledge that the distraction will not increase comfort as much as self-harm would at the present time, but the feelings of mastery will be satisfying.[117]	Provides opportunity for the client to practice new behaviors in a supportive environment where positive feedback can be provided. Promotes the client's sense of control, and enhances self-esteem. Promotes positive orientation.
Identify, with the client, areas of social skill deficits, and develop a plan for improving these areas. This could include assertiveness training, communication skills training, and/or relaxation training to reduce anxiety in trigger situations. Note plan and schedule for implementation here. This should be a progressive plan with rewards for accomplishment of each step.[116–118]	Enhances interpersonal skills by providing the client with more adaptive ways of achieving interpersonal goals.
Develop a schedule for the client to attend group therapies. Note this schedule here.	Provides an opportunity for the client to practice interpersonal skills in a supportive environment and to observe peers modeling interpersonal skills.
Administer medications as appropriate.	Assist with stabilizing mood and decreasing anxiety.[58]
Monitor for side effects of medication and desired outcomes.	
Meet with the client and the client's support system to plan coping strategies that can be used at home. Assist system in obtaining resources necessary to implement this plan.	Facilitates support system understanding of the behavior and facilitates appropriate response in the community.[115]
In the event that self-mutilation does occur, provide the necessary first aid in a matter-of-fact manner. If the injury does not require medical attention, provide the client with the tools to do self-care and instructions that can be used to provide this self-care in the future.	Prevents loss of function and further injury. Assists in developing self-responsibility for the consequences of behavior.[58]
• Avoid elaborate focusing on the injury.	Prevents the development of secondary gains from self-injury.[120]
• Sit with the client for [number] minutes to discuss the feelings that preceded the act.	Supports the development of appropriate methods of coping with feelings.

Gerontic Health

The nursing actions for the gerontic patient with this diagnosis are the same as those given for the Mental Health patient.

Home Health

Should the patient develop this nursing diagnosis on an adult health care unit, referral should be made immediately to a mental health nurse clinician. (See nursing actions under Mental Health.)

ACTIONS/INTERVENTIONS	RATIONALES
Monitor for factors contributing to risk for self-mutilation.	Provides database for early recognition and intervention.
Involve the client and family in planning, implementing, and promoting reduction or elimination of risk for self-mutilation:	Family involvement enhances effectiveness of interventions.
• Family conference: Discuss the perspective of each family member.	

(care plan continued on page 602)

NURSING ACTIONS/INTERVENTIONS WITH RATIONALES (continued from page 601)

Home Health

ACTIONS/INTERVENTIONS	RATIONALES
• Mutual goal setting: Develop short- and long-term goals with evaluative criteria. Tasks and roles of each family member should be specified. • Communication: Open, direct, reality-oriented communication.	
Assist the client and family in lifestyle adjustments that may be required: • Development and use of support networks • Provision of safe environment • Protection of client from harm • Necessity for long-term care	Adjustments in lifestyle require long-term behavioral changes. Such changes are enhanced by education and support.
Consult with or refer to assistive resources such as caregiver support groups as needed.	Utilization of existing services is efficient use of resources. A psychiatric nurse clinician, support group, and mental health–mental retardation expert can enhance the treatment plan.

REFERENCES

1. Gordon, M: Manual of Nursing Diagnosis. CV Mosby, St. Louis, 2002.
2. Le Mone, P: Analysis of a human phenomenon: Self-concept. Nurs Diagn 2:126, 1991.
3. Liberman, MD, and Disenberger, NI: Conflict and habit: A social cognitive neuroscience approach to the self. In Intesser, A, and Wood, JV, and Staple, DA (eds): On Building, Defending and Regulating the Self: A Psychobiological Perspective. Psychology Press, New York, 2004, pp.77-102
4. Zimmer C: The neurobiology of the self. Sci Am 293:92, 2005.
5. Turner, R: The self-conception in social interaction. In Gordon, C, and Gergen, KJ (eds): The Self in Social Interaction, Vol. 1. Classic and Contemporary Perspectives. John Wiley & Sons, New York, 1968.
6. Gordon, C, and Gergen, KJ (eds): The Self in Social Interaction, Vol 1. Classic and Contemporary Perspectives. John Wiley & Sons, New York, 1968.
7. James, W: The self. In Gordon, C, and Gergen, KJ (eds): The Self in Social Interaction, Vol 1. Classic and Contemporary Perspectives. John Wiley & Sons, New York, 1968.
8. Mead, GH: The genesis of self. In Gordon, C, and Gergen, KJ (eds): The Self in Social Interaction, Vol 1. Classic and Contemporary Perspectives. John Wiley & Sons, New York, 1968.
9. Sullivan, HS: Beginnings of the self-system. In Gordon, C, and Gergen, KJ (eds): The Self in Social Interaction, Vol 1. Classic and Contemporary Perspectives. John Wiley & Sons, New York, 1968.
10. Bruch, H: Interpersonal theory: Harry Stack Sullivan. In Burton, A (ed): Operational Theories of Personality. Brunner-Mazel, New York, 1968.
11. Perry, HS, and Gawel, ML: The Interpersonal Theory of Psychiatry. Norton & Co., New York, 1953.
12. Glasersfeld, EV: Cybernetics, experience and the concept of self. In Gergen, KJ, and Davis, RE (eds): The Social Construction of the Person. Springer-Verlag, New York, 1985.
13. Watts, A: The Book: On the Taboo Against Knowing Who You Are. Random House, New York, 1966, p. 12.
14. Stake, JE: Gender differences and similarities in self-concept within everyday life contexts. Psychol Women Q 16:349, 1992.
15. Stake, JE: Development and validation of the six-factor self-concept scale for adults. Educ Psychol Measure 54:56, 1994.
16. O'Dea, J, and Abraham, S: Association between self-concept and body weight, gender and pubertal development among male and female adolescents. Adolescence 34:69, 1999.
17. Harter, S: Manual of the Self-Perception Profile for Adolescents. University of Colorado, Denver, 1998.
18. Shina, A, Nakazato, M, Mitsumori, M, et al: An open trial of outpatient group therapy for bulimic disorders: Combination program of cognitive behavioral therapy with assertive training and self-esteem enhancement. Psychiatry Clin Neurosci 59:690, 2005.
19. McCay, E, and Seeman, M: A scale to measure the impact of a schizophrenic illness on an individual's self-concept. Arch Psychiatr Nurs 12:41, 1998.
20. Champion, J: Effects of abuse on self-perception of rural Mexican-American and non-Hispanic white adolescents. Arch Psychiatr Nurs 13:12, 1999.
21. Search Institute: The Asset Approach: Giving Kids What They Need to Succeed. Author, Minneapolis, MN, 1997.
22. Jourard, S: Healthy personality and self-disclosure. In Gordon, C, and Gergen, TJ (eds): The Self in Social Interaction, Vol 1. Classic and Contemporary Perspectives. John Wiley & Sons, New York, 1968, p. 427.
23. Dufault, K, and Martocchio, B: Hope: Its spheres and dimensions. Nurs Clin North Am 20:379, 1985.
24. Vaillot, M: Hope: The restoration of being. AJN 70:268, 1970.
25. McGee, R: Hope: A factor influencing crisis resolution. Adv Nurs Sci 7:34, 1968.
26. Miller, J: Inspiring hope. AJN 85:22, 1985.
27. Watson, J: Nursing: Applying the Arts and Sciences of Human Caring. NLN Press, New York, 1994.
28. Eirckson, H, Tomlin, E, and Swain, M: Modeling and Role-Modeling: A Theory and Paradigm for Nursing. Engelwood Cliffs, NJ, Prentice-Hall, 1983.
29. Lynch, WF: Image of Hope: Imagination as Healer of the Hopeless. University of Notre Dame Press, Notre Dame, IN, 1974.
30. Bateson, G: Steps to an Ecology of Mind. Ballantine, New York, 1972.
31. Search Institute: You Can Make a Difference for Kids. Author, Minneapolis, MN, 1997.
32. Poole, C, Miller, SA, and Church, EB: How children develop self-concept. Early Childh Today 10:31, 2004.
33. Erickson, H, and Kinney, C: Modeling and Role-Modeling: Theory, Research and Practice. Society for the Advancement of Modeling and Role-Modeling, Austin, TX, 1990.
34. St. Clevy, K: The contribution of self-concept in the etiology of adolescent delinquency. Adolescence 32:671, 1997.
35. Starkman, N, Scales, P, and Roberts, C: Great Places to Learn. Search Institute, Minneapolis, MN, 1999.

36. Santrock, JW: Life Span Development, ed 4. WC Brown, Dubuque, IA, 1992.
37. Moorhead, S, Johnson, M, and Maas, M: Nursing Outcomes Classification (NOC). CV Mosby, St. Louis, 2004.
38. Townsend, M: Psychiatric Mental Health Nursing. FA Davis, Philadelphia, 2006.
39. Eliopoulos, C: Manual of Gerontologic Nursing, ed 2. CV Mosby, St. Louis, 1999.
40. North American Nursing Diagnosis Association: Nursing Diagnosis: Definitions and Classification, 2005–2006. Author, Philadelphia, 2005.
41. Amaya, MA: Women's environmental health. In Breslin, ET, and Lucas, VA (eds): Women's Health Nursing: Toward Evidence-Based Practice. Saunders, St. Louis, 2003.
42. Bull, M, and Lawrence, D: Mother's use of knowledge during the first postpartum weeks. JOGNN J Obstet Gynecol Neonatal Nurs 14:315, 1985.
43. Bay, EJ, and Algase, DL: Fear and anxiety: A simultaneous concept analysis. Nurs Diagn 10:103, 1999.
44. Lowdermilk, DL, and Perry, SE: Maternity & Women's Care, ed 8. Mosby, St. Louis, 2004.
45. Beck, CT, and Indman, P: The many faces of postpartum depression. JOGNN J Obstet Gynecol Neonatal Nurs 34(5):569, 2005.
46. Goodman, JH: Postpartum depression beyond the early postpartum period. JOGNN J Obstet Gynecol Neonatal Nurs 33(4):410, 2004.
47. Logsdon, MC, Birkimer, JC, Simpson, T, and Looney, S: Postpartum depression and social support in adolescents. JOGNN J Obstet Gynecol Neonat Nurs 34(1):46, 2005.
48. Bowman, KG: Postpartum learning needs. JOGNN J Obstet Gynecol Neonat Nurs 34(4):438, 2005.
49. Weiss, ME, Ryan, P, and Lokken, L: Validity and reliability of the perceived readiness for discharge after birth scale. JOGNN J Obstet Gynecol Neonatal Nurs 35(1):34, 2006.
50. Vliet, EL: Screaming to be Heard: Hormonal Connections Women Suspect and Doctors Ignore. M. Evans and Co., New York, 1995.
51. Kanusky, C: Health concerns of women in midlife. In Breslin, ET, and Lucas, VA (eds): Women's Health Nursing: Toward Evidence-Based Practice. Saunders, St. Louis, 2003.
52. McVeigh, C: Perimenopause: More than hot flushes and night sweats for some Australian women. JOGNN J Obstet Gynecol Neonatal Nurs 34(1):21, 2005.
53. Northrup, C: The Wisdom of Menopause: Creating Physical and Emotional Health and Healing During the Change. Bantam Books, New York, 2001.
54. Rotem, M, Kushnir, T, Levine, R, and Ehrenfeld, M: A psychoeducational program for improving women's attitudes and coping with menopause symptoms. JOGNN J Obstet Gynecol Neonatal Nurs 34(2):233, 2005.
55. Kneisl, C, Wilson, H, and Trigoboff, E: Contemporary Psychiatric-Mental Health Nursing. Upper Saddle River, NJ, Pearson Education, 2004.
56. National Guideline Clearinghouse. Anxiety disorders. Agency for Healthcare Research and Quality (AHRQ). 1–8, 2005. Washington, DC, US Department of Health and Human Services.
57. Ossman, SS: Clinical consult. Motivational interviewing: A process to encourage behavioral change. Nephrol Nurs J 31:346, 2004.
58. McCloskey Dochterman J, and Bulechek, G: Nursing Interventions Classification. CV Mosby, St. Louis, 2004.
59. National Guideline Clearinghouse. Stress related conditions and other mental disorders. Agency for Health Care Research and Quality (AHRQ), 2006, Washington DC, US Department of Health and Human Services. http://www.guidelines.gov.
60. Stein, KF, and Corte, C: Reconceptualizing causative factors and intervention strategies in the eating disorders: A shift from body image to self-concept impairments. Arch Psychiatr Nurs 17:57, 2003.
61. Wright L, and Leahey, M: Nurses and Families: A Guide to Family Assessment and Intervention. FA Davis, Philadelphia, 2005.
62. Dewar, A: Boosting strategies: Enhancing the self-esteem of individuals with catastrophic illnesses and injuries. J Psychosoc Nurs Ment Health Serv 41:24, 2003.
63. McEvey, GL, and Davis, R: A program to promote positive body image: A 1-year follow-up evaluation. J Early Adolesc 22:96, 2002.
64. Conant, M: The client with an eating disorder. In Lego, S (ed): Psychiatric Nursing: A Comprehensive Reference. Lippincott, Philadelphia, 1996.
65. Lange, N, and Tigges, BB: Influence positive change with motivational interviewing. Nurse Pract 30:44, 2005.
66. White, J: The development and clinical testing of an outpatient program for women with bulimia nervosa. Arch Psychiatr Nurs 13:179, 1999.
67. Search Institute. You Can Make a Difference for Kids. 1999. Search Institute, Minneapolis.
68. Parkes, CM: The dying adult. BMJ 316:1313, 1998.
69. Maguire, P, and Parkes, CM: Loss and the reaction to physical disablement and surgery. BMJ 316:1086, 1998.
70. Smith-Ainimer, M: The client who is anxious. In Lego, S (ed): Psychiatric Nursing: A Comprehensive Reference. Lippincott, Philadelphia, 1996.
71. Wright, L, and Leahey, M: Nurses and Families, ed 4. FA Davis, Philadelphia, 2005.
72. Paice, JA: Managing Psychological Conditions in Palliative Care. Am J Nurs 102:36-42, 2002.
73. Haber, J, et al: Comprehensive Psychiatric Nursing, ed 5. Mosby–Year Book, St Louis, 1997.
74. Keegan, L: Touch: Connecting with the healing power. In Dossey, BM, et al (eds): Holistic Nursing: A Handbook for Practice. Aspen, Rockville, MD, 1988.
75. Palker, NB, and Nettles-Carson, B: The prevalence of advanced directives; Lessons from a nursing home. Nurse Pract 20(2):7, 1995.
76. Moberg, DO: Research in spirituality, religion, and aging. J Gerontol Social Work 45(1-2):11, 2005.
77. Kemp, C: Terminal Illness: A Guide to Nursing Care, ed 2. Lippincott, Williams & Wilkins, Philadelphia, 1999.
78. Fogel, CI, and Woods, NF: Health Care of Women: A Nursing Perspective. CV Mosby, St. Louis, 1981.
79. Griffith-Kenney, JW: Contemporary Women's Health: A Nursing Advocacy Approach. Addison-Wesley, Menlo Park, CA, 1986.
80. Teschendorf, M: Women during the reproductive years. In Breslin, ET, and Lucas, VA: Women's Health Nursing: Toward Evidence-Based Practice. Saunders, St. Louis, 2003.
81. Harner, HM: Domestic violence and trauma care in teenage pregnancy: Does Paternal age make a difference? JOGNN J Obstet Gynecol Neonat Nurs 33(3):312, 2004.
82. Haggerty, LA, Kelly, U, Hawkins, J, Pearce, C, and Kearney, MH: Pregnant women's perceptions of abuse, JOGNN J Obstet Gynecol Neonat Nurs 30(3):283, 2001.
83. Lutz, KF: Abused pregnant women's interactions with health care providers during the childbearing year. JOGNN J Obstet Gynecol Neonat Nurs 34(2):151, 2005.
84. Barcelona de Mendoza, V: Culturally appropriate care for pregnant Latina women who are victims of domestic violence. JOGNN J Obstet Gynecol Neonat Nurs 30(6):579, 2001.
85. Beck, C, Reynolds, M, and Rutowski, P: Maternity blues and postpartum depression. JOGNN J Obstet Gynecol Neonat Nurs 21(4):287, 1992.
86. National Guideline Clearinghouse. Anxiety disorders. Agency for Healthcare Research and Quality (AHRQ). 1–8, 2005. Washington, DC, US Department of Health and Human Services.
87. Sellers, JB: Health care for older women. In Breslin, ET, and Lucas, VA (eds): Women's Health Nursing: Toward Evidence-Based Practice. Saunders, St. Louis, 2003.
88. Gantt, L, and Bickford, A: Screening for domestic violence: How one hospital network started asking about abuse. Lifelines 3:36, 1999.
89. Colwell, J, and O'Connor, T: Understanding nurturing practices : A comparison of the use of strategies likely to enhance self-esteem in nurture groups and normal classrooms. Br J Spec Educ 30:119, 2003.
90. Drew, N: Combating the social isolation of chronic mental illness. J Psychosoc Nurs Ment Health Serv 29:14, 1991.
91. Hoeffer, B: A causal model of loneliness among older single women. Arch Psychiatr Nurs 1:366, 1987.
92. Liberman, MD, and Disenberger, NI: Conflict and habit: A social cognitive neuroscience approach to the self. In Tesser A, Wood JV, and Staple DA (eds): On Building, Defending and Regulating the Self: A Psychobiological Perspective. Psychology Press, New York, 2004, pp. 77–102.
93. Zimmer, C: The neurobiology of the self. Sci Am 293:92, 2005.
94. Lego, S: The client with dissociative identity disorder. In Lego, S (ed): Psychiatric Nursing: A Comprehensive Reference. Lippincott, Philadelphia, 1996.

95. McAllister, M, Higson, D, McIntosh, W, et al: Dissociative identity disorder and the nurse-patient relationship in the acute care setting: An action research study. Aust N Z J Ment Health Nurs 10:20, 2001.

96. Tulman, L, and Fawcett, J: Return of functional ability after childbirth. Nurs Res 37:77, 1988.

97. Keeney, BP: Aesthetics of Change. Guilford, New York, 1983.

98. Kahng, SK, and Mowbray, CT: What affects self-esteem of persons with psychiatric disabilities: the role of causal attributions of mental illnesses. Psychiatr Rehabil J 28:354, 2005.

99. Breslin, E: Women's health: Challenges and opportunities. In Breslin, ET, and Lucas, VA (eds): Women's Health Nursing: Toward Evidenced Based Practice. Saunders, St. Louis, 2003.

100. Upvall, MJ: Women and culture. In Breslin, ET, and Lucas, VA (eds): Women's Health Nursing: Toward Evidenced Based Practice. Saunders, St. Louis, 2003.

101. Huebscher, R: Natural, alternative and complementary health care. In Breslin, ET, and Lucas, VA (eds): Women's Health Nursing: Toward Evidenced Based Practice. Saunders, St. Louis, 2003.

102. Burns, M: Screening and diagnostic tests. In Breslin, ET, and Lucas, VA (eds): Women's Health Nursing: Toward Evidenced Based Practice. Saunders, St. Louis, 2003.

103. Bernhard, LA: Patriarchy, feminism, and women's health. In Breslin, ET, and Lucas, VA (eds): Women's Health Nursing: Toward Evidenced Based Practice.

104. Ekeland, E, Heian F, Hagen, KB, et al: Exercise to improve self-esteem in children and young people. Cochrane Library 2006.

105. Reitzes, DC, and Mutran, EJ: Self and health: Factors that encourage self-esteem and functional health. J Gerontol B Psychol Sci Soc Sci 61B:S44, 2006.

106. DeMoulin, DF: I like me! Enhancing self concept in kindergarten age children through active school/business partnerships. Natl Assoc School Psychol 27:8 (accessed March 20, 2006, http://www.likeme.org/article2.html).

107. DeMoulin, DF: Reconceptualizing the self-efficacy paradigm: Analysis of an eight-year study. Education 111:167, 1993.

108. DeMoulin, DF: Enhancing self-concept development of kindergartners through a personalized reading program. Natl Forum Appl Educ Res J 9(2):239, 1996.

109. Dossey, BM, Keegan, L, and Guzzetta, CE: Holistic Nursing: A Handbook for Practice, ed 3. Aspen, Gaithersburg, MD, 2000.

110. Gilliss, C, et al: Toward a Science of Family Nursing. Addison-Wesley, Menlo Park, CA, 1989.

111. Miller, JF: Coping with Chronic Illness: Overcoming Powerlessness. FA Davis, Philadelphia, 2000.

112. Burnside, IM: Nursing and the Aged: A Self-Care Approach, ed 3. McGraw-Hill, New York, 1988.

113. Norris, J: Nursing intervention for self-esteem disturbances. Nurs Diagn 3:48, 1992.

114. King, KS, Dimond, M, and McCance, KL: Coping with relocation. Geriatr Nurs 8:258, 1987.

115. Starr, D: Understanding those who self-mutilate. J Psychosoc Nurs Ment Health Serv 42:33, 2004.

116. Valente, S: Deliberate self-injury: Management in a psychiatric setting. J Psychosoc Nurs Ment Health Serv 29:19, 1991.

117. Gallop, R: Self-destructive and impulsive behavior in the patient with a borderline personality disorder: Rethinking hospital treatment and management. Arch Psychiatr Nurs 6:178, 1992.

118. Reeder, D: Cognitive therapy of anger management: Theoretical and practical considerations. Arch Psychiatr Nurs 5:147, 1991.

119. Swales, M, Heard, HL, and Williams, MG: Linehan's Dialectical Behavior Therapy (DBT) for borderline personality disorder: Overview and adaptation. J Ment Health 9:7, 2000.

120. Lego, S: The client with borderline personality disorder. In Lego, S (ed): Psychiatric Nursing: A Comprehensive Reference. Lippincott, Philadelphia, 1996.

9

ROLE-RELATIONSHIP PATTERN

PATTERN DESCRIPTION

The role-relationship pattern is concerned with how a person feels he or she is performing the expected behavior delineated by the self and others. Each of us has several roles in family, work, and social relationships during our daily lives, with the related responsibilities. Disruption in these roles, relationships, and responsibilities can lead a patient to seek assistance from the health-care system. Likewise, satisfaction with these is a patient strength that can be used in planning care for other health problem areas.

PATTERN ASSESSMENT

1. Is the client exhibiting distress over a potential loss?
   a. Yes (Anticipatory Grieving)
   b. No
2. Is the client denying a potential loss?
   a. Yes (Risk for Dysfunctional Grieving)
   b. No
3. Is the client exhibiting distress over an actual loss?
   a. Yes (Most people exhibit distress over an actual loss; that is not dysfunctional)
   b. No
4. Is the client displaying extended grief symptoms that are not improving?
   a. Yes (Dysfunctional Grieving)
   b. No
5. Does the client have risk factors for dysfunctional grief following a loss?
   a. Yes (Risk for Dysfunctional Grieving)
   b. No
6. Is the client denying an actual loss?
   a. Yes (Dysfunctional Grieving)
   b. No
7. Is the client making verbal threats against others?
   a. Yes (Risk for Violence)
   b. No
8. Is the client exhibiting increased motor activity?
   a. Yes (Risk for Violence)
   b. No
9. Can the patient speak English?
   a. Yes (Readiness for Enhanced Communication)
   b. No (Impaired Verbal Communication)
10. Does the patient demonstrate any difficulty in talking?
    a. Yes (Impaired Verbal Communication)
    b. No (Readiness for Enhanced Communication)
11. Does the client verbalize difficulty with social situations?
    a. Yes (Impaired Social Interaction)
    b. No
12. Does the client indicate strained relationships with his or her family or others?
    a. Yes (Impaired Social Interaction)
    b. No

13. Does the patient have family or significant others visiting or calling?
    a. Yes
    b. No (Social Isolation)
14. Is the patient uncommunicative, withdrawn, or not making eye contact?
    a. Yes (Social Isolation)
    b. No
15. Does the client indicate that admission might impact role (family, work, or leisure)?
    a. Yes (Ineffective Role Performance)
    b. No
16. Does the family or do significant others verbalize that admission might impact the patient's role (family, work, or leisure)?
    a. Yes (Ineffective Role Performance)
    b. No
17. Does the child show signs or symptoms of physical or emotional abuse?
    a. Yes (Impaired Parenting)
    b. No
18. Do the parents indicate difficulty in controlling the child?
    a. Yes (Impaired Parenting)
    b. No
19. Do the parents demonstrate attachment behaviors?
    a. Yes
    b. No (Risk for Impaired Parenting, Risk for Impaired Parent, Infant, and Child Attachment)
20. Do the parents make negative comments about the child?
    a. Yes (Risk for Impaired Parenting)
    b. No
21. Does the family demonstrate a capability to meet the child's physical needs?
    a. Yes
    b. No (Interrupted Family Processes)
22. Does the family demonstrate a capability to meet the child's emotional needs?
    a. Yes
    b. No (Interrupted Family Processes)
23. Does a family member exhibit signs and symptoms of alcoholism?
    a. Yes (Dysfunctional Family Processes: Alcoholism)
    b. No
24. Do the parents express concern about the ability to meet the child's physical or emotional needs?
    a. Yes (Parental Role Conflict)
    b. No
25. Are the parents frequently questioning decisions about the child's care?
    a. Yes (Parental Role Conflict)
    b. No
26. Was the infant premature?
    a. Yes (Risk for Impaired Parent, Infant, and Child Attachment)
    b. No

27. Do the parents express anxiety regarding the parental role?
    a. Yes (Risk for Impaired Parent, Infant, and Child Attachment)
    b. No
28. Has the patient recently received a diagnosis related to a chronic physical or mental condition?
    a. Yes (Chronic Sorrow)
    b. No
29. Is the patient verbally expressing prolonged sadness?
    a. Yes (Chronic Sorrow)
    b. No
30. Is the patient in the role of primary caregiver for another person?
    a. Yes (Risk for Caregiver Role Strain, Caregiver Role Strain)
    b. No
31. Does the patient verbally express difficulty in or concerns about caregiving role?
    a. Yes (Caregiver Role Stress)
    b. No
32. Has the patient recently moved from one living site to another?
    a. Yes (Risk for Relocation Stress Syndrome)
    b. No
33. Does the patient appear depressed following a change in living environments?
    a. Yes (Risk for Relocation Stress Syndrome)
    b. No
34. Does the patient facing a change in a living environment have a good support system?
    a. Yes
    b. No (Risk for Relocation Stress Syndrome)
35. Does the patient express concern over his or her recent move?
    a. Yes (Risk for Relocation Stress Syndrome)
    b. No

CONCEPTUAL INFORMATION

The social connotation for role performance and relationships is a major premise for the intended use of this pattern. A *role* is a comprehensive pattern of behavior that is socially recognized and that provides a means of identifying and placing an individual in a society. Role is the interaction point between the individual and society. It also serves as a means of coping with recurrent situations. The term "role" is a borrowed theatrical noun that emphasizes the distinction of the actor and the part. A role remains relatively stable even though different persons may be occupying the position or role; however, the expectations of the script, other players, and audience all influence role enaction.[1] The importance of each of these factors varies with the context of each interaction. In our personal roles, the script is equivalent to the societal "norms," and our audience can be real or imagined. Uniqueness of style may exist within the boundaries of the role as determined by society.

Because our roles are such an integral part of our lives, we seldom analyze them until they become a problem to our internal or external adaptation to life's demands. Roles that are often associated with stages of development serve as society's guides for meaningful and satisfying relationships in life by facilitating an orderly method for transferring knowledge, responsibility, and authority from one generation to the next.

During the childhood years, an individual will have numerous contacts with different individuals having different sets of values. The child learns to internalize the values of those significant in his or her life as personal goals are actualized. When the goals are realistic, consistent, and attainable, the individual is assisted in developing a sense of self-esteem as these various roles are mastered. Each new role carries with it the potential for gratification and increased ego identity if the role is acquired. If the role is not mastered, poor self-esteem and role confusion may ensue. The potential for successful role mastery is diminished with multiple role demands and the absence of suitable role models. In addition, role acquisition depends on adequate patterns of cognitive–perceptual ability and a healthy sense of self.[1]

Although all roles are learned within the context of one's culture, specific roles are delineated in two ways: acquired and achieved. *Acquired roles* have variables over which the individual has no choice, such as gender or race. *Role achievement* allows for some choice by the individual, with the result of purposefully earning a role, such as choosing to become a professional nurse.

Many roles are not clearly defined as being either acquired or achieved but rather are a combination of the two. Roles are not mutually exclusive, but interdependent. The roles an individual assumes usually blend well; however, those that a person achieves or acquires may not always make for a harmonious blend. Role conflicts can occur from the most internalized personal level to a generalized societal level.

Roles may be influenced by a multitude of factors, including economics, family dynamics, changing roles of institutions, and gender role expectations. Roles can be mediated through role-playing skills and self-conceptions. It is hoped that with the increased demands on the individual, society will continue to value human dignity with respect for life itself. Roles should allow for self-actualization.

One of the more recent eclectic theories of personality development encompassing role theory is that of *symbolic interaction*. In this orientation, social interaction has symbolic meaning to the participants in relation to the roles assigned by society. (For further related conceptual information, refer to Chapter 8.)

Symbolic interaction encompasses the roles assumed by humans in their constant interaction with other humans, communicating symbolically in almost all they do. This interaction has meaning to both the giver and the receiver of the action, thus requiring both persons to interact symbolically with themselves as they interact with each other.

Symbolic interaction involves *interpretation,* that is, ascertaining the meaning of the actions or remarks of the other person, and *definition,* that is, conveying indication to another person as to how he or she is to act. Human association consists of just such a process of interpretation and definition. It is through this process that participants fit their own acts to the ongoing acts of one another, and, in doing so, guide others.[2]

To explore further how relationships develop, a brief overview of kinship is offered. A *kinship system* is a structured system of relationships in which individuals are bound one to another by complex, interlocking relationships. These relationships are commonly referred to as *families.* It is not so much the family form in which one lives as how the family form functions that defines whether or not there is a cohesive family structure.[3] An ideal family environment consists of a family that has many routines and traditions, provides for quality time between adults and children, has regular contact with relatives and neighbors, lives in a supportive and safe neighborhood, has contact with the work world, and has adult members who model a harmonious and problem-solving relationship.[3]

The 1980s saw great change in family structures with an explosion of individualized living arrangements and lifestyles requiring new definitions of the "family."[3–6] Fewer nuclear families consisting of husband, wife, and children exist today. There are in today's society many different acceptable family forms that do not fit the definition of a nuclear family. The following are some of the different family forms identified in today's society.[3–6]

Nuclear family   Husband, wife, and children living in a common household, sanctioned by marriage

Nuclear dyad   Husband and wife alone; childless or children have left home

Single-parent family   One head of household, mother or father, as a result of divorce, abandonment, or separation

Single adult alone   Either by choice, divorce, or death of a spouse

Three-generation family   Three or more generations in a single household

Kin network   Nuclear households or unmarried members living in close geographic proximity

Institutional family   Children in orphanages or residential schools

Homosexual family   Homosexual couples with or without children

Despite the differences in family forms and cultural differences, primary relationships within various family structures reveal markedly similar characteristics in all societies. These relationships were described[7] in 1949, and still exist in the various family forms cited today:

Husband and wife   Economic specialization and cooperation, sexual cohabitation; joint responsibility for support, care, and upbringing of children; well-defined reciprocal rights with respect to property, divorce, and spheres of authority

Father and son   Economic cooperation in masculine activities under leadership of the father; obligation of material support vested in the father during childhood of the son and in the son during the old age of father; responsibility of father for instruction and discipline of son; duty of obedience and respect on the part of the son; tempered by some measure of comradeship

Mother and daughter   Relationship parallel to that between father and son, but with more emphasis on child care and economic cooperation, and less on authority and material support (However, strong relationships in the development of mothering skills and parenting techniques lead to obligations of emotional support and caretaking activities vested in the mother during the childhood of the daughter and in the daughter during old age of mother.)

Father and daughter   Responsibility of the father for protection and material support before marriage of the daughter; economic cooperation, instruction, and discipline appreciably less prominent than in father–son relationship; playfulness common in infancy of daughter, but normally yields to a measure of reserve with the development of a strong incest taboo

Mother and son   Relationship parallel to that of mother and daughter, but with more emphasis on financial and emotional support in later life of mother

Elder and younger brother   Relationship of playmates, developing into that of comrades; economic cooperation under leadership of elder; moderate responsibility of elder for instruction and discipline of younger

Elder and younger sister   Relationship parallel to that between elder and younger brother, but with more emphasis on physical care of the younger sister

Brother and sister   Early relationship of playmates, varying with relative age; gradual development of an incest taboo, commonly coupled with some measure of reserve; moderate economic cooperation; partial assumption of parental role, especially by the elder sibling

The nurse must exercise great caution in maintaining sensitivity to the individual meaning attached to various roles, and the way in which these roles are perceived and assumed. With the current societal and economic changes, the individual's roles are being impacted on a daily basis, even without the added stress of a health problem.

DEVELOPMENTAL CONSIDERATIONS
NEONATE AND INFANT

The newborn period is especially critical for the development of the first attachment that is so vital for all future human relationships. Attachment behavior includes crying, smiling, clinging, following, and cuddling. The infant is dependent on his or her mother and father for basic needs of survival. This is often demanding and requires parents to place self-needs secondary to the needs of the infant, making for a potential role-relationship alteration.

Although dependent on others, the infant is an active participant in role-relationship pattern development from conception on. The infant is capable of influencing the interactions of those caring for him or her. Reciprocal interactions also influence the maternal–paternal–infant relationship. Positive interactions will be greatly influenced by infant-initiated behavior, as well as maternal–paternal responses and the reciprocal interaction of all involved. The state of the infant as well as that of the parent interacting with the infant must be considered as critical.

It is important to note that any alteration in health status of the mother, the neonate, or both has the potential of interfering with the establishment of the maternal–infant relationship. This may not necessarily be the case, but it is often critical that the potential risk be acknowledged early so that residual, secondary problems can be prevented with appropriate nursing intervention. It is also important to keep in mind that the infant is taking in all situational experiences, and that as learning occurs through interaction with the environment, a gradual evolution of role-relationship patterns occurs.

By approximately 12 months of age, the infant shows fear of being left alone, and will search for the parents with his or her eyes. The infant will avoid and reject strangers. There is an obvious increasing interest in pleasing the parent. In protest, the infant cries, screams, and searches for the parent. In despair, the infant is listless, withdrawn, and disinterested with the environment. In detachment or resignation, a superficial "adjustment" occurs in which the infant appears happy, friendly, and interested in surroundings for short periods of time. The infant is emotionally changeable, from crying to laughing, with a beginning awareness of separation from the environment. Still, the infant uses the mother as a safe haven from which to explore the world. The infant will have a favorite toy, blanket, or other object that serves to comfort him or her in times of stress. (Sucking behavior may also serve to calm the infant, and eventually he or she will develop self-initiated ways of dealing with the stressors of life, such as thumb sucking versus the actual taking of formula or milk.)

The infant receives cues from significant others and primary caregivers regarding grief responses such as crying, with a preference for the mother. Depending on age and situational status, the infant may protest by crying for the mother. In a weakened state, the infant may make little response of preference for caregivers.[8]

According to family structure, the neonate or infant will adapt to usual socialization routines within reasonable limits. Actual isolation for the infant would perhaps occur if the primary caregiver could not exercise usual role-taking behavior for socialization. If this behavior is arrested for marked periods of time, there is a potential for developmental delays secondary to the lack of appropriate social stimulation.

The newborn period is especially critical for the development of the neonate's first attachment for future human relationships. During this period, the infant must depend on others for his or her care and basic needs. This is often a demanding situation for parents, who must sacrifice their own needs to best meet the needs of the infant.[8]

The infant is dependent on others for care, ranging from required food for physical growth to appropriate sensory and social stimulation. In the absence of the stability usually afforded by the family in its usual functioning pattern, the infant may be at risk for failure to thrive or developmental delay. Ultimately, rather than developing a sense of trust and a feeling that the world is a place in which one's needs are met, the infant will doubt and mistrust others. This in turn places the infant at risk for an abnormal pattern of development.

Crying serves as primitive verbal communication for the neonate and infant. As the infant begins to understand and respond to the spoken word, the world should be symbolized as comforting and safe. With time, basic attempts at verbalization are noted in imitation of what is heard. There is a correlation between parental speech stimulation and the actual development of speech in young children, suggesting a positive effect for early stimulation. *Echolalia* (the often pathologic repetition of what is said by other people as if echoing them) and attempts at making speech are most critical to note during this time.

The infant may be the recipient of violent behavior, and, all too often, it is because of crying. The attempt to quiet the infant can take the form of lashing out for those individuals unable to deal with the usual role-relationship patterns. The infant is unable to defend him- or herself, and therefore is to be protected by reporting of any suspected abusive or negligent behavior. At particular risk are infants with feeding or digestive disorders, premature or small-for-gestational-age infants who require feedings every 2 hours, or others perceived as "demanding" or "irritable." Also at risk are infants who are born with congenital anomalies or disfigurements.[8]

TODDLER AND PRESCHOOLER

The toddler has an increasing sense of identity and is aware of him- or herself as a separate person. The toddler treats other children as if they were objects and gradually becomes involved in parallel play, which then leads to more interactive play with peers. The sharing of possessions is not yet to be expected with toddlers. The toddler begins to formulate a sense of right and wrong, with the ability to conform to some social demand, as exemplified by the capacity for self-toileting. It is reasonable that a toddler would begin to work through problems of family relationships with other children while playing.

The preschool child talks and plays with an imaginary playmate as a projection. What is offered may be what the child views as bad in him- or herself. The preschooler may have some friends of the same sex, and opportunities for socialization serve critical functions. The preschool child lives in the "here and now" and is capable of internalizing more and more of society's norms. By this age, there is a sense or morality and conscience. A strong sense of family exists for the preschooler.

The toddler may be unusually dependent on the mother, objects of security, and routines.[8] He or she is capable of magical thinking and may believe in animation of inanimate objects, such as believing an X-ray machine is really a mean monster. Toddlers may be fearful of seeing blood. These fears may be unrelated to actual situations.

The preschooler may be critical of him- or herself and may blame him- or herself for a situation, with some attempt at viewing the current situation as punishment for previous behavior or thoughts. He or she will tolerate brief separation from parents in usual functioning. Play or puppet therapy, which is appropriate to the situation, will help the preschooler in expressing feelings.

The toddler must have room to explore safely, with a sense of autonomy evolving in the ideal situation. If social isolation limits these opportunities, the toddler will be limited in role-relationship exposure. This will often result in either social isolation or a form of forced precocious role-taking in which the toddler is perceived as being able to satisfy the companionship needs of adults. The toddler may misinterpret socialization opportunities as abandonment or punishment, so short intervals of parallel play with one peer, to begin with, would be appropriate. Toddlers who are denied opportunities for peer interaction are at risk for role-relationship problems.[8]

The child of the preschool age group may experience alteration in socialization attempts if overpowered by peers, if there are too many rigid or unrealistic rules, or if the situation places the child in a situation that presents values greatly different from those of the child and his or her family. If the child at this age experiences prolonged social isolation or rejection, there could be marked potential for difficulty in forming future relationships. If things do not go well in his or her socialization, the child at this age may blame him- or herself.

The toddler will seek out opportunities to explore and interact with the environment, provided there is a safe haven to return to as represented by the family.[8] When this facilitative factor is not present, the toddler may regress and become dependent on primary caregivers or others, or may manifest frustration via extremes in demanding behavior. The child's subsequent development may also be affected by family process alteration.

The preschool child is able to verbalize concerns regarding changes in family process but is unable to comprehend dynamics. It is critical to attempt to view the altered process through the eyes of the preschooler, who could blame him- or herself for the change or crisis, or who may think magically and have fears that may be unrelated to the situation. Subsequent development may be altered by family process dysfunction, with regression often occurring.

At this age, it is important to stress the need for ritualistic behavior as a means of mastering the environment with adequate anticipatory safety. This period allows for knowing "self" as a separate entity. The toddler is capable of attempting to conform to social demands but lacks the ability of self-control.

The importance of setting limits must be stressed with regard to safety and disciplinary management. At this age, the child begins to resist parental authority. Methods of dealing with differences or rules from one setting to another must be simple and appropriate to the situation.

For the toddler, this time can prove frustrating, with a need to be understood despite a limited vocabulary. Jargon and gestures may be misinterpreted, with resultant frustration for both the child and the parent. Patience and understanding go far with a child of this age. Pictures and the telling of stories serve as means of enhancing speech as well as instilling an appreciation for reading and speech. Feelings come to be expressed by the spoken word also. The child is able to refer to him- or herself as "I," "me," or by name.

By preschool age, the child is able to count to 10, define at least one word, and may name four or five colors. Speech now serves as a part of socialization in play with peers. Wants should be expressed freely as the child broadens his or her contact with persons other than primary family members. The preschooler enjoys stories and television programs and attempts to tell stories of his or her own creation.

If the toddler is unable to fulfill the expectations of parents or caregivers who demand unrealistic behavior, there is a risk of abuse. Especially noteworthy would be a desire for the young toddler to be capable of self-toileting behavior when in fact such is not possible. This places the toddler in a target population for abuse also. At this age, the toddler may be unable to express hostility or anger verbally, and so a common occurrence may be temper tantrums. At risk for violence would be the toddler who resists parental authority in discipline, and cannot meet demands of the parents.

SCHOOL-AGE CHILD

Learning social roles as male or female is a major task for the school-age child, with a preference for spending time with friends of the same sex rather than with the family. The school-ager is capable of role-taking and values cooperation and fair play. There may be a strict moralism that is "black and white," with no gray areas noted. The school-ager enjoys simple household chores, likes a reward system, and has the capacity for expressing feelings. Fear of disability and concern for missing school are typical concerns for this age group.

Illness may impose separation from the peer group. Although independent of parents in health, the school-ager may require close parental relationship in illness or crisis. Loss of control and fear of mutilation and death are real concerns. The school-age child may fear disgracing parents if loss of control, such as crying, occurs. He or she is aware of the severity of his or her prognosis and may even deal with reality better than parents or adults might. The school-age child may use art as a means of expressing his or her feelings.

This child is at risk of social isolation if a situation is different from previous socialization opportunities. He or she may experience value conflict and question the rules. He or she may also be afraid to express desires or concerns regarding socialization needs for fear of punishment. Peer involvement is a most vital component of assisting the school-ager to formulate views of acceptable social behavior.

The school-ager may try to assume the role of a parent if the dysfunction of the family relates to the parent of the same sex. This may be healthy with appropriate acknowledgment of limitations. At this age, the child is concerned with what other friends may think about the family, with some stigma attached in certain cultures to divorce, homosexuality, and alternate lifestyles. To best endure the altered family process, it is critical for the school-ager to have a close friend who might share the cultural views of his or her own family.

Allowance for increasing interests outside the home should be made with sensitivity to parental approval or disapproval. The child may rebel against parental authority in an attempt to be like peers.

Confidence in self and a general sense of well-being will promote adequacy in communication development. The child of this age continues to learn vocabulary and takes pride in his or her ability to demonstrate appropriate use of words. At this age, jokes and riddles serve as a means of encouraging peer interaction with speech. Reading is a leisure activity for the school-age child.

The child will usually enjoy school and consider peer interaction an enjoyable part of life. In instances in which the child feels inferior, there may be a risk for violence or abusive behavior as a cover-up for poor self-image or low self-esteem. Often there will be related role-relationship alterations as well. The family serves as a means of valuing the interaction, which should foster the appropriate enjoyment of friendships. At risk are children with learning disabilities or handicaps, parental conflicts, or related role-relationship alteration.

ADOLESCENT

Vacillation between dependence and independence is common for the adolescent who is attempting to establish a sense of identity. The adolescent questions traditional values, especially those of parents. There is a gradual trend to independent functioning that allows the adolescent to assume roles of adulthood, including the development of intensive relationships with members of the opposite gender.

The adolescent will be constantly weighing self-identity versus perceived identity expressed via peers. He or she may be fearful of expressing true feelings or concern for fear of rejection by peers, parents, or significant others. Isolation from peers places the adolescent at risk for altered self-identity as well as altered role-relationship patterns.

The adolescent is able to assist within the family during times of altered process. It is important to stress that in more and more dual-career or single-parent families, young adolescents spend more and more time alone. Nonetheless, adolescents should still have opportunities for peer interaction and socialization according to the family's needs.

There may be marked vacillations, as the adolescent strives to find self-identity, with dependence and independence issues. Even more marked rebellion against parental wishes may be manifest at this time as peer approval is sought.

Any factors that may interfere with usual speech patterns may prove especially difficult for the adolescent. Bracing of teeth may be common, with the potential for self-image alteration. Also, the eruption of 12-year molars could prove painful, as might the possible impaction of wisdom teeth later. Expressed wit is valued in this age group, as might be special colloquial expressions to qualify group or peer identity. Difficulty in expression of self may be a major problem for this individual. Respect for times of reflection and estrangement should be maintained.

The adolescent may be caught in the crossfire of strife for independence versus dependence. For this group, it is paramount that self-control be attained to develop the meaningful relationships so critical for appropriate role-relationship patterns. Often adolescents who have not acquired appropriate socialization skills resort to drugs or alcohol as a means of feeling better and escaping the reality of life. This may also foster loss of control, as reality is distorted. In many instances, there may be related juvenile delinquency, with resultant records of lawbreaking.

In addition, any adolescent who is assuming a role that stresses or negates the usual development of self-identity is at risk for violence as a means of coping. An example of this would be two young teenagers attempting to parent when they themselves still require parenting.

YOUNG ADULT

Although biophysical and cognitive skills reach their peak during the adult years, the young adult is still in a period of growth and development. Striving for achievement of an education, job security, meaningful intimate relationships with others, and establishment of a family are the primary focuses of the young adult. Although young adults usually have achieved independence, they find themselves learning socially relevant behavior and settling into specific acquired roles within a chosen profession or occupation. They begin to adopt some of the values of the group to which they belong, and to assume assured roles such as marriage and parenting.

Cognitively, young adults have reached their peak level of intellectual efficiency, and they are able to think abstractly and to synthesize and integrate their ideas, experiences, and knowledge. For the adult, thinking usually involves reasoning, taking into consideration past experiences, education, and the possible outcomes of a situation more realistically and less egocentrically than the adolescent.

Young adulthood is still a time of great adjustment. The individual is expected to look at the self in relation to society, learning how to deal with personal needs and desires as opposed to the needs and desires of others, and managing the economic and physical needs of life. Sexual activity focuses toward the development of a single intimate, meaningful relationship and the establishment of a family. In developing the role of parenting, the young adult often falls back on the parenting patterns and behavior of his or her own parents.

The young adult begins to assume the responsibility of providing for a family. Most young adults are members of dual-career families, and thus face the stresses of multiple roles. Many of these young adults become single parents, and the stresses of multiple responsibilities and roles are greater both at home and at work. Just as during adolescence, the negation of development of self-identity can lead to crises, role strain, conflict, and often failure in the young adult.

As the adult acquires full role responsibility, there may be difficulties related to role diffusion, role confusion, role strain, or related assumption of appropriate roles. Also, the ultimate developmental need for assumption of accountability for self may be unresolved. There may be a greater likelihood for the various demands of society on male and female roles to be experienced at this time as women assume the multiple roles of wife, mother, worker, housekeeper, and so on, just as men also have assumed more and more roles that were formerly assumed by females. This challenge also brings the potential for growth and fulfillment in self-actualizing individuals.

MIDDLE-AGE ADULT

Middle age, or middlescence, is often considered the most productive years of an individual. Persons in this age group are usually secure in a profession or career, are in the middle of raising a family, and often must assume responsibility for aging parents.

As biophysical changes occur, there is a concurrent adaptation of the cognitive and physical activities of the individual. The body ages in varying stages or degrees, and young middle-age adults usually retain the body structure and activity level they established as young adults. Middle-age adults with more sedentary lifestyles must establish exercise programs to retain their youthful figures. The greatest changes facing both men and women during this time are those associated with the climacteric and the loss of reproductive capabilities. These biologic and physical changes can affect sexual lifestyles either positively or negatively, depending on the perception and orientation of the individual.

Most middle-age adults function well and learn to gradually accept the changes of aging, and with proper nutrition, exercise, and a healthy lifestyle, they can experience excellent health and a productive middlescence. Middle-age people usually begin to face more accidents, illness, and death; they begin to deal with their own aging process and death, as well as that of their parents. There is often a role reversal, with the middle-age adult assuming the role of parent.

This is the time of life when individuals usually review their goals and aspirations, sometimes to find that they did not reach the potential they once dreamed. Most middle-age adults begin to feel that there is not enough time to accomplish all they want to accomplish, and they begin to adjust to the fact that they may not reach all the goals they set in their youth. This can result in a loss of self-esteem, or it can be a motivation to develop previously untapped reservoirs, which can lead to self-actualization and personal satisfaction.

OLDER ADULT

With aging, individuals may have fewer demands placed on them, thus leaving more time, and fewer potential opportunities, for role performance. This may also be a time when one is able to fulfill volunteer roles and roles of choice versus those of demand. A critical factor may be the freedom one feels as basic needs are met. If health is satisfactory and one has children or grandchildren to enjoy, financial stability, and the ability to pursue fulfillment via role engagement, this experience would be self-actualizing. On the other hand, if one's health fails, few meaningful family supports exist, and financial needs arise, self-actualizing role performance is potentially threatened.

The older adult must deal with decreasing function with resultant decreasing socialization potential. This is a time for retrospection and pondering the past, with sincere concerns regarding the future and death. In some instances, full functional level is possible, whereas for others life is lived vicariously. Elder role-modeling opportunities, with respect for those who have lived life, still exist in many cultures. For these individuals, the aging process is welcomed and enjoyed as the fullest potential is actualized for role-relationship patterning, namely the generation of values to the young in society. In instances in which aging is accompanied by loss in whatever form, the potential exists for the individual to become dependent. This dependency may range from a minor to a major form of total dependence on others. The onset of dependency may be gradual or sudden. In either instance, the nurse must recognize the impact of the loss for the patient according to the values of the patient and family.

TABLE 9.1 NANDA, NIC, and NOC Taxonomic Linkages

GORDON'S FUNCTIONAL HEALTH PATTERN	NANDA NURSING DIAGNOSIS	NIC PRIORITY INTERVENTIONS	NOC EVALUATIONS
Role-Relationship Pattern	Caregiver Role Strain, Risk For and Actual	**Actual** Caregiver Support Parenting Promotion	**Actual** Caregiver Emotional Health Caregiver Endurance Potential Caregiver Lifestyle Disruption Caregiver Performance: Direct Care; Indirect Care Caregiver Physical Health Caregiver Stressors Caregiver Well-Being Family Resiliency Family Support During Treatment Parenting Performance Role Performance
		Risk for Caregiver Support Parenting Promotion	**Risk for** Caregiver Emotional Health Caregiver Home Care Readiness Caregiver Lifestyle Disruption Caregiver-Patient Relationship Caregiver Performance: Direct Care; Indirect Care Caregiver Physical Health Caregiver Stressors Caregiving Endurance Potential Coping Family Coping Family Functioning Family Resiliency Family Support During Treatment Knowledge: Energy Conservation, Health Behaviors, Health Resources Rest Risk Control Risk Detection Role Performance Sleep Stress Level
	Communication, Impaired Verbal	Active Listening Communication Enhancement: Hearing Deficit; Speech Deficit	Communication: Expressive Communication: Receptive Information Processing
	Communication, Readiness for Enhanced	*Still in development	Communication Communication: Expressive Communication: Receptive
	Family Processes, Interrupted	Family Integrity Promotion Family Process Maintenance Normalization Promotion	Adaptation to Physical Disability Family Coping Family Functioning Family Normalization Family Resiliency Family Social Climate Parenting Performance

(table continued on page 614)

GORDON'S FUNCTIONAL HEALTH PATTERN	NANDA NURSING DIAGNOSIS	NIC PRIORITY INTERVENTIONS	NOC EVALUATIONS
	Family Processes, Dysfunctional: Alcoholism	Family Process Maintenance Substance Use Treatment	Family Coping Family Functioning Family Resiliency Family Social Climate Parenting Performance Role Performance Substance Addiction Consequences
	Family Processes, Readiness for Enhanced	*Still in development	Family Coping Family Functioning Family Resiliency Family Social Climate
	Grieving, Anticipatory	Family Integrity Promotion Grief Work Facilitation Grief Work Facilitation: Perinatal Death	Adaptation to Physical Disability Coping Family Coping Family Social Climate Grief Resolution Psychosocial Adjustment: Life Change
	Grieving, Dysfunctional	Family Integrity Promotion Grief Work Facilitation Grief Work Facilitation: Perinatal Death	Coping Family Coping Family Resiliency Grief Resolution Psychosocial Adjustment: Life Change Role Performance
	Grieving, Dysfunctional, Risk for	*Still in development	*Still in development
	Parent/Infant/Child Attachment, Risk for, Impaired	Attachment Promotion Environmental Management: Attachment Process Parent Education: Infant Parenting Promotion	Caregiver Adaptation to Patient Institutionalization Caregiver Performance: Direct Care Child Development: 1, 2, 4, 6, 12 Months Cognition Coping Depression Self-Control Family Functioning Family Social Climate Knowledge: Parenting Parent-Infant Attachment Parenting Performance Risk Control Risk Detection Role Performance Social Interaction Skills Stress Level Substance Addiction Consequences

GORDON'S FUNCTIONAL HEALTH PATTERN	NANDA NURSING DIAGNOSIS	NIC PRIORITY INTERVENTIONS	NOC EVALUATIONS
	Parenting, Impaired, Risk for and Actual, Readiness for Enhanced	**Actual** Abuse Protection Support: Child Attachment Promotion Family Integrity Promotion Parenting Promotion	**Actual** Child Development: 1, 2, 4, 6, 12 Months; 2, 3, 4 Years; Preschool; Middle Childhood; Adolescence Family Coping Family Functioning Family Social Climate Parent-Infant Attachment Parenting Performance Parenting: Psychosocial Safety Role Performance
		Risk for Abuse Protection Support: Child Attachment Promotion Family Integrity Promotion Normalization Promotion Parenting Promotion	**Risk for** Abuse Recovery Status Abuse Recovery: Emotional; Physical; Sexual Abusive Behavior Self-Restraint Aggression Self-Control Caregiver: Emotional Health; Physical Health; Stressors; Well-being Cognition Coping Decision Making Distorted Thought Self Control Family Coping Family Health Status Family Normalization Family Resiliency Family Social Climate Knowledge: Health Resources; Infant Care; Parenting Parent–Infant Attachment Parenting Performance Risk Control Risk Control: Alcohol Use; Drug Use; Tobacco Use Risk Detection Role Performance Social Interaction Skills Social Support
		Readiness for Enhanced *Still in development	**Readiness for Enhanced** Family Functioning Knowledge: Child Physical Safety; Infant Care; Parenting Parenting Performance Parenting: Psychosocial Safety
	Parental Role Conflict	Crisis Intervention Family Process Maintenance Parenting Promotion Role Enhancement	Caregiver Adaptation to Patient Institutionalization Caregiver Home Care Readiness Caregiver Lifestyle Disruption Coping Family Functioning Family Social Climate Parenting Performance

(table continued on page 616)

::: TABLE 9.1 NANDA, NIC, and NOC Taxonomic Linkages *(continued from page 615)*

GORDON'S FUNCTIONAL HEALTH PATTERN	NANDA NURSING DIAGNOSIS	NIC PRIORITY INTERVENTIONS	NOC EVALUATIONS
			Psychosocial Adjustment: Live Change Role Performance
	Relocation Stress Syndrome, Risk for and Actual	**Actual** Coping Enhancement Discharge Planning Relocation Stress Reduction	**Actual** Anxiety Level Child Adaptation to Hospitalization Coping Depression Level Loneliness Severity Psychosocial Adjustment: Life Change Quality of Life Stress Level
		Risk for Coping Enhancement Discharge Planning Relocation Stress Reduction	**Risk for** Acceptance: Health Status Adaptation to Physical Disability Anxiety Level Anxiety Self-Control Child Adaptation to Hospitalization Cognition Discharge Readiness: Supported Living Family Participation in Professional Care Information Processing Knowledge: Health Resources Leisure Participation Memory Mobility Participation in Health Care Decisions Personal Health Status Risk Control Risk Detection Role Performance Self-Care: ADLs, Instrumental Activities of Daily Living (IADLs) Self-Direction of Care Social Interaction Skills Social Involvement Stress Level
	Role Performance, Ineffective	Role Enhancement	Anxiety Level Caregiver Lifestyle Disruption Cognition Coping Depression Level Parenting Performance Psychosocial Adjustment: Life Change Role Performance Stress Level

GORDON'S FUNCTIONAL HEALTH PATTERN	NANDA NURSING DIAGNOSIS	NIC PRIORITY INTERVENTIONS	NOC EVALUATIONS
	Social Interaction, Impaired	Self-Esteem Enhancement	Child Development: Middle Childhood; Adolescence Family Social Climate Leisure Participation Play Participation Social Interaction Skills Social Involvement
	Social Isolation	Socialization Enhancement	Family Social Climate Leisure Participation Loneliness Severity Personal Well-Being Play Participation Social Interaction Skills Social Involvement Social Support
	Sorrow, Chronic	Grief Work Facilitation Hope Instillation	Acceptance: Health Status Depression Level Depression Self-Control Grief Resolution Hope Loneliness Severity Mood Equilibrium Psychosocial Adjustment: Life Change
	Violence: Self-Directed, Risk for and Other-Directed, Risk for	**Self-Directed, Risk for** Behavior Management: Self-Harm Mood Management Suicide Prevention	**Self-Directed, Risk for** Adaptation to Physical Disability Cognition Coping Depression Level Depression Self-Control Distorted Thought Self-Control Impulse Self-Control Loneliness Severity Mood Equilibrium Quality of Life Risk Control Risk Control: Alcohol Use; Drug Use Risk Detection Self-Mutilation Restraint Stress Level Suicide Self-Restraint Will to Live
		Other-Directed, Risk for Anger Control Assistance Environmental Management: Violence Prevention	**Other-Directed, Risk for** Abuse Cessation Abuse Protection Abusive Behavior Self-Restraint Aggression Self-Control Cognition Community Risk Control: Violence

(table continued on page 618)

::: TABLE 9.1 NANDA, NIC, and NOC Taxonomic Linkages *(continued from page 617)*

GORDON'S FUNCTIONAL HEALTH PATTERN	NANDA NURSING DIAGNOSIS	NIC PRIORITY INTERVENTIONS	NOC EVALUATIONS
			Community Violence Level
			Depression Self-Control
			Distorted Thought Self-Control
			Fear Level
			Fear Level: Child
			Hyperactivity Level
			Impulse Self-Control
			Risk Control
			Risk Control: Alcohol Use; Drug Use
			Risk Detection
			Stress Level

 APPLICABLE NURSING DIAGNOSES

CAREGIVER ROLE STRAIN, RISK FOR AND ACTUAL

DEFINITIONS[9]

Risk for Caregiver Role Strain The caregiver is vulnerable for felt difficulty in performing the family caregiver role.

Caregiver Role Strain Difficulty in performing the family caregiver role.

DEFINING CHARACTERISTICS[9]

A. Risk for Caregiver Role Strain
  The risk factors also serve as the defining characteristics.
B. Caregiver Role Strain
  1. Caregiving activities
    a. Difficulty in performing or completing required tasks
    b. Preoccupation with care routine
    c. Apprehension about the future regarding the care receiver's health and the caregiver's ability to provide care
    d. Apprehension about the care receiver's care if the caregiver were to become ill or die
    e. Apprehension about possible institutionalization of the care receiver
    f. Dysfunctional changes in the caregiver's activities
  2. Caregiver's health status
    a. Physical
      (1) Gastrointestinal upset (e.g., mild stomach cramps, vomiting, diarrhea, and recurrent gastric ulcer episodes)
      (2) Weight change
      (3) Rash
      (4) Hypertension
      (5) Cardiovascular disease
      (6) Diabetes
      (7) Fatigue
      (8) Headaches
    b. Emotional
      (1) Impaired individual coping
      (2) Feeling depressed
      (3) Anger
      (4) Somatization
      (5) Increased nervousness
      (6) Increased emotional lability
      (7) Impatience
      (8) Lack of time to meet personal needs
      (9) Frustration
      (10) Disturbed sleep
      (11) Stress
    c. Socioeconomic
      (1) Withdraws from social life
      (2) Changes in leisure activities
      (3) Low work productivity
      (4) Refuses career advancement
  3. Caregiver–care receiver relationship
    a. Difficulty watching the care receiver go through the illness
    b. Grief or uncertainty regarding changed relationship with the care receiver
  4. Family processes
    a. Family conflict
    b. Concerns about marriage

RELATED FACTORS[9]

A. Risk for Caregiver Role Strain (Risk Factors)
  1. Pathophysiologic
    a. Illness severity of the care receiver
    b. Addiction or codependency
    c. Premature birth or congenital defect

d. Discharge of family member with significant home care needs

e. Caregiver health impairment

f. Unpredictable illness course or instability in the care receiver's health

g. Caregiver is female

h. Psychological or cognitive problems in care receiver

2. Developmental
   a. Caregiver is not developmentally ready for caregiver role (e.g., a young adult needing to provide care for middle-age parent).
   b. Developmental delay or retardation of the care receiver or caregiver

3. Psychological
   a. Marginal family adaptation or dysfunction prior to the caregiving situation
   b. Marginal caregiver's coping patterns
   c. Past history of poor relationship between the caregiver and the care receiver
   d. The caregiver is the spouse.
   e. Care receiver exhibiting deviant or bizarre behavior

4. Situational
   a. Presence of abuse or violence
   b. Presence of situational stressors that normally affect families, such as significant loss, disaster or crisis, poverty or economic vulnerability, major life events
   c. Duration of caregiving required
   d. Inadequate physical environment for providing care (e.g., housing, transportation, community services, or equipment)
   e. Family or caregiver isolation
   f. Lack of respite and recreation for the caregiver
   g. Inexperience with caregiving
   h. Caregiver's competing role commitments
   i. Complexity or amount of caregiving tasks

B. Caregiver Role Strain

1. Care receiver health status
   a. Illness severity
   b. Illness chronicity
   c. Increasing care needs or dependency
   d. Unpredictability of illness course
   e. Instability of the care receiver's health
   f. Problem behaviors
   g. Psychological or cognitive problems
   h. Addiction or codependency

2. Caregiving activities
   a. Amount of activities
   b. Complexity of activities
   c. 24-hour care responsibilities
   d. Ongoing changes in activities
   e. Discharge of family members to home with significant care needs
   f. Years of caregiving
   g. Unpredictability of care situation

3. Caregiver health status
   a. Physical problems
   b. Psychological or cognitive problems
   c. Addiction or codependency
   d. Marginal coping patterns
   e. Unrealistic expectations of self
   f. Inability to fulfill one's own or other's expectations

4. Socioeconomic
   a. Isolation from others
   b. Competing role commitments
   c. Alienation from family, friends, and co-workers
   d. Insufficient recreation

5. Caregiver–care receiver relationship
   a. History of poor relationship
   b. Pressure of abuse or violence
   c. Unrealistic expectations of the caregiver by the care receiver
   d. Mental status of elder inhibiting conversation

6. Family processes
   a. History of marginal family coping
   b. History of family dysfunction

7. Resources
   a. Inadequate physical environment for providing care (e.g., housing, temperature, and safety)
   b. Inadequate equipment for providing care
   c. Inadequate transportation
   d. Inadequate community resources (e.g., respite services and recreational resources)
   e. Insufficient finances
   f. Lack of support
   g. Caregiver is not developmentally ready for caregiver role.
   h. Inexperience with caregiving
   i. Insufficient time
   j. Emotional strength
   k. Physical energy
   l. Assistance and support (formal and informal)
   m. Lack of caregiver privacy
   n. Lack of knowledge or difficulty in accessing community resources

RELATED CLINICAL CONCERNS

1. Any chronic, debilitating illness (e.g., Alzheimer's disease, cancer, or rheumatoid arthritis)
2. Severe mental retardation
3. Chemical abuse
4. Closed head injury
5. Schizophrenia
6. Personality disorders

 Have You Selected the Correct Diagnosis?

Ineffective Individual Coping
This diagnosis and Caregiver Role Strain are very close; however, the differentiating factor is whether or not the individual is involved in a caregiver role.

(box continued on page 620)

Have You Selected the Correct Diagnosis? *(box continued from page 619)*

If significant caregiving is a part of the individual's role, then initial interventions should be directed toward resolving the problems within the caregiving role.

Impaired Adjustment

Certainly needing to assume a caregiving role would require some adjustment. However, this diagnosis relates to an individual adjusting to his or her own illness or health problem, not adjustment to someone else's illness or health problem.

Compromised or Disabled Family Coping

These diagnoses could be companion diagnoses to Caregiver Role Strain. If the family cannot adapt to a change in a family member's condition and assigns the caregiver role to just one family member, then both Compromised or Disabled Family Coping and Caregiver Role Strain are likely to develop.

EXPECTED OUTCOME

The caregiver will identify [number] of services that will facilitate their care by [date].

The caregiver will identify [number] of strategies to facilitate their meeting their personal health needs by [date].

The caregiver will identify [number] of coping strategies to adapt to lifestyle disruption by [date].

TARGET DATES

A target date of 5 days would be the earliest date to begin evaluation of progress toward meeting the expected outcome.

NURSING ACTIONS/INTERVENTIONS WITH RATIONALES

Adult Health

ACTIONS/INTERVENTIONS	RATIONALES
Provide a forum for caregivers to freely express apprehensions regarding role expectations, role conflict, role strain, and role negotiation each day.	Opens communication and promotes cooperative problem solving.
Assist the caregiver in identifying necessary home modifications to facilitate patient care.	
Collaborate with case management to ensure any equipment required for patient care is available before discharge and that financial aspects are addressed.	
Set realistic expectations for care.	Prevents undue duress on the caregiver.
Collaborate with the caregiver in devising strategies that will facilitate resuming or maintaining personal schedule.	
Identify community support groups such as daycare centers, housekeeping services, home health aides, hospice, or respite care before discharge. Also, a cooperative arrangement could be made with friends and neighbors for release time from care activities.	Provides alternatives for resources to support in short-term and long-term problems.
Teach caregiver stress management techniques such as relaxation, meditation, or deep breathing. Note the caregiver's preferred technique and practice schedule here.	Relieves stress, identifies alternative coping strategies, and decreases depression.
Support use of respite care. Collaborate with social services to arrange this.	Allows the caregiver an opportunity to care for self.
Refer to the psychiatric nurse specialist as needed. (See Mental Health nursing actions.)	Collaboration promotes holistic health care. Interventions may require the expertise of a specialist.

Child Health

ACTIONS/INTERVENTIONS	RATIONALES
Monitor for contributing factors with a focus on high-risk populations: • Excessive demands exist secondary to a child requiring extensive care (e.g., several small children in family with one child requiring extensive assistance with physical or mental problems). This can be compounded when depression is a coexisting factor. • A patient who has a total self-care deficit • Caregiver indicates inability to carry out usual routines	Unrealistic demands of parenting or care provision increase the likelihood of role strain.
Schedule a daily conference with the caregiver of at least 30 minutes to focus on:	Allows identification of current perception of role strain by encouraging ventilation of feelings. Provides a teaching opportunity. Assists in identification of referrals that are needed.
• Exploring with the parent or caregiver options available to assist with the demands of the situation. • Encourage the caregiver to provide time for self on a daily basis through such means as seeking outside help (e.g., visiting nurse, housekeeping assistance, respite care, institutionalization such as temporary per day or, if appropriate and desired, permanent).	Support from others serves as a means of preventing further demise of desired role taking while also allowing for long-term needs. Time for self will enhance coping abilities and, ultimately, self-esteem.
• Identifying community resources that are available, especially parenting support groups.	Provides long-term support and information. Encourages sharing of concerns with others in the same situation.
• Assisting the caregiver and significant other(s) to explore inevitabilities and realities associated with the care	Expectations may be unrealistic. Clarification of expectations and reality assists in problem solving.
Schedule a family conference, as needed, to focus on the family's willingness to provide assistance in caregiving.	Assists in delineating roles for each family member. Assists in providing relief for the primary caregiver on a more regular basis.
Monitor for any unresolved guilt regarding role demands, "less-than-perfect child," or related aspects of situation (See Dysfunctional Grieving).	Unresolved conflict increases the likelihood of little change in behavior.
Preserve the effective functioning of the caregiver through teaching and support during all interactions. [Note specific ongoing support the caregivers might need here.]	The likelihood of secondary and tertiary alterations for the caregiver increases when primary needs of rest and own physical self are not met.

Women's Health

ACTIONS/INTERVENTIONS	RATIONALES
New Mother or Parent Role Assist the new mother in developing realistic plans for infant care at home. Have the mother review plans for self-care and plans for care of the infant in the home.	Provides time for assessment and planning for home care. Affords an opportunity to teach and give realistic feedback regarding the impact a newborn makes on the former lifestyle.
Include the significant other in plans for care of the new mother and infant after discharge from the hospital. Encourage discussion by the mother and significant other of various role changes in the family that will occur with the new infant's being incorporated into the household (e.g., sibling's, wife's, husband's, or grandparent's role).[10]	

(care plan continued on page 622)

Women's Health

ACTIONS/INTERVENTIONS	RATIONALES
Encourage discussion of the "new" role of being a mother and father, as well as being husband and wife.	
Assist with development of plan to save time, such as learning to sleep when the infant sleeps, turning telephone off when trying to rest, or putting sign on front door when sleeping.[11]	Assists in reducing fatigue, which is a significant contributor to the development of caregiver role strain.
Identify areas in which the significant other can assist the new mother and help reduce fatigue. For example, if breastfeeding, let dad get the infant, change the diaper, and bring the infant to the mother for feeding during the night.[11,12]	Provides long-term support and a source of information.[13]
Plan, cook, and freeze meals for the family before leaving for the hospital, so that they can be prepared easily during the first few weeks at home.[11]	

Teen Parenting

● NOTE: *The nursing actions for the teenage parent will be the same as those in the previous section with the following additions:*

Refer the young couple or teenager to young parents' groups in the community for social and personal support.	
Give the young couple telephone hot lines they can call for assistance and support (e.g., hospital nursery, young parent services, or the YWCA). Check with individual community agencies for what is available in your community.	
Assist the young parent to get into or stay in school by giving references for childcare.	Promotes long-range planning and reduces the likelihood of strain for the young parent.
Encourage the young couple to express their feelings about the new responsibilities they face.	

Parent to Your Parents

● NOTE: *Approximately 80 percent of women will become the primary care providers for their elderly parents. These interventions and rationales can also apply to spouse and/or other family members.[14]*

• Identify specific concerns and needs. • Explore the inevitabilities and realities of the situation. • Identify possible resources in the community (financial assistance, personal support, social work, or day care). • Identify methods by which the family members and siblings can share responsibilities. • Establish ties from the primary caretaker to other family members to provide relief for each other. • Identify methods of sharing expenses associated with housing (keeping parent[s] in own home, nursing home or extended care, or assisted living). • Assist with development of plan to provide supervision for parent while working (neighbors of parents, family members, day care, or home aide assistant).	Sharing responsibilities for elderly parents assists the entire family to lead better lives. Many women have the entire burden of caring for elderly parents while trying to maintain jobs and their own families. Often they will not speak of this; therefore, the nurse must patiently interview the women.[14]

ACTIONS/INTERVENTIONS	RATIONALES
Provide instructions to both the woman and spouse (significant other) about provision of needed care.	Ensures that both parties have the same instructions or information about care needed.
Provide telephone number where the caregiver can reach clinical, professional assistance, day or night.	Provides a resource to answer questions and give reassurance.
Discuss with the caregiver possible lifestyle changes that will occur: • Sleeplessness (worried about hearing if needed) • Arranging time needed for work and other family members' needs	Most caregivers are not professional health-care providers and have to understand the need to plan their daily schedules to incorporate the time required to provide needed care.[13,14]

● N O T E : *Abundant resources for caregivers exist in bookstores and on the Internet. In addition, most local hospitals and outpatient facilities host support group meetings for caregivers. Here's a short list of resources to help nurses, patients, and caregivers alike sharpen their skills:*

- **Alzheimer's Association,** (800) 677-1116, has a great World Wide Web site at http://www.alz.org, with a host of resources for caregivers.
- **Caregiver Network, Inc.,** is a Canadian resource dedicated to making caregivers' lives easier and hosts extensive caregiver links to other World Wide Web sites, including "Ask a Professional" link at http://www.caregiver.on.ca/.
- **Eldercare Locator** (800) 677-1116
- **Senior Net** has a library of caregiving resources at: http://www.seniornet.com/.
- **Today's Caregiver,** (800) 829-2734, a magazine written by and for caregivers, features a caregiver's bill of rights among other useful resources at http://www.caregiver.com/.

Mental Health

● N O T E : *For information related to the caregivers of clients with a medical diagnosis of dementia, refer to Gerontic Health. As used in this discussion, "caregiver" can mean one person or an extended family system.*

ACTIONS/INTERVENTIONS	RATIONALES
Spend [number] minutes [number] times per week interacting with the primary caregiver.	Promotes the development of a trusting relationship.
Provide a role model for effective communication by: • Seeking clarification • Demonstrating respect for individual family members and the family system • Listening to expression of thoughts and feelings • Setting clear limits • Being consistent	Family problem solving is improved when the family members can effectively communicate with one another and the health-care team.[15]
Include the caregiver in weekly treatment planning meetings with the client. [Note here the time for this meeting and persons responsible for providing the information.]	Assists in providing information to the caregiving system so they can better cope with the uncertainty of a psychiatric diagnosis.[15,16]
Provide the family with opportunities to provide the care and support they identify as important. [Note here the care the family is going to provide, with the assistance they need to complete these activities.]	Provides the family with a sense of helpfulness and control.[16]

(care plan continued on page 624)

NURSING ACTIONS/INTERVENTIONS WITH RATIONALES (continued from page 623)

Mental Health

ACTIONS/INTERVENTIONS	RATIONALES
Spend [number] minutes [number] times per week educating the primary caregiver about the client's diagnosis. Provide both written and verbal information.	Provides the caregiver with an increased understanding of the diagnosis, and assists in the development of a home care plan. When anxiety is high, caregivers may have difficulty remembering information provided only in verbal form. Increases the stability in the living environment by decreasing the caregiver's anxiety.
Communicate understanding of the difficulty of the caregiver role by: • Answering questions honestly • Providing time to interact with the caregiver when he or she visits • Inquiring about the caregiver's self-care activities • Encouraging the caregiver to use the time the client is in the hospital to rest and meet personal needs • Providing time for the caregiver to express feelings related to the client and the hospitalization • Commend the family on their competencies and strengths. For example, comment on what the caregiver has said or done that is effective and useful.	Promotes the development of a trusting relationship, and assists the caregiver in the process of working through feelings related to the client. Provides caregivers an opportunity to change their self-view, which opens them up to viewing the problem differently, and move toward solutions that are more effective.[17]
Normalize the caregiver's feelings of guilt and/or ambivalence by informing him or her that these are normal feelings for anyone who assumes the level of responsibility that he or she has assumed.	Promotes a positive orientation, and enhances self-esteem.
Have the caregiver identify areas where he or she feels a need for support on a daily basis, and assist him or her in networking community resources to meet these needs. This should be a process that allows the nurse to teach the caregiver the skills necessary to accomplish this networking on his or her own after discharge.	Promotes the caregiver's sense of control, and provides positive reinforcement when he or she can accomplish the task, which enhances self-esteem.
Spend [number] minutes [number] times per week discussing his or her self-care activities. This could include planning time away from the client, inviting friends to visit, going for a walk, or arranging to get uninterrupted sleep. Inform the caregiver that if he or she does not care for him- or herself, he or she will eventually not have the energy to care for the client. A specific plan should be developed and noted here.	Gives permission to the caregiver to care for self. Promotes the caregiver's strengths.
Before the client is discharged, meet with the client and caregiver to: • Review information about the diagnosis and hospital course. • Review special treatments the client is to receive. • Explain the client's medications. • Anticipate problems that may arise after discharge. A specific plan should be developed for coping with anticipated problems. This plan should be written down and given to both the client and the caregiver.	Anxiety can decrease an individual's ability to process information during hospitalization. A specific coping plan provides direction during times of crisis, and prevents reliance on ineffective patterns of coping. These actions increase the caregiver's repertoire of strategies to deal with the problems.[18]

Gerontic Health

● N O T E : *One of the twenty-first century trends in the United States is the increased number of multigenerational families, which is a direct result of the number of people who survive well into old age. The trend has increased the probability that older adults will ultimately be caregivers for an aging parent, an aging spouse, or perhaps younger family members with chronic illnesses. In come cases, these roles may exist concurrently, magnifying the stress of caregiving.[19] In addition to the following interventions, the interventions for Mental Health and Adult Health may also apply to the aging adult.*

ACTIONS/INTERVENTIONS	RATIONALES
Monitor for signs of increasing strain in the caregiver, such as an increase in episodes of illness.	The stresses of caregiving have a negative effect on the caregiver's immune system.[20]
Assess the quality and type of the prior relationship between the caregiver and patient.[19]	Dyads with previously tense or troubled relationships are at greater risk for caregiver role strain, violence, and illness.[19]
Assist the caregiver in discussing feelings about caregiving. For example, encourage sharing by use of statements such as "Often people in your situation say they feel angry, helpless, guilty, or depressed."	Provides an opportunity for ventilation of feelings about caregiving, which assists in reducing stress.
Determine the caregiver's knowledge of support services in the community, such as adult daycare, respite services, or family support groups.	Assists in identifying actual or potential resources based on the individual's current knowledge of services. Expands options available to the caregiver.
Discuss with the caregiver stress management techniques such as imagery, deep breathing, or exercise. What has been tried? How helpful was it?	
Encourage the caregiver to use a journal to evaluate stresses, prioritizing stresses and noting his or her usual response. Are there specific times, days, or circumstances when stress is especially high?	Provides a database to use in planning interventions to reduce stress.
If needed, consult with social services for increased support in home care.	Highlights attention to the caregiver. Realistic planning serves to reduce stress.
Discuss with the caregiver, before patient discharge, his or her plan for maintaining self-health and coping abilities.[21]	

Home Health

In addition to the following interventions, the interventions for Mental Health and Adult Health may also apply to the home health client.

ACTIONS/INTERVENTIONS	RATIONALES
Consult with and/or refer the patient to assistive resources as needed, to include: • Caregiver support groups • Assistance with client activities of daily living • Assistance with home maintenance (cleaning) • Financial assistance	Utilization of existing services is an efficient use of resources.
Provide respite care for the client to allow the caregiver rest as finances allow.	To allow the caregiver physical and emotional rest, which promotes the best possible care for the client.

(care plan continued on page 626)

NURSING ACTIONS/INTERVENTIONS WITH RATIONALES (continued from page 625)	

Home Health

ACTIONS/INTERVENTIONS	RATIONALES
Educate all family members about critical care issues for the client, and encourage the primary caregiver to delegate caregiving responsibilities as appropriate.	Knowledge helps promote a sense of control and order, as well as more appropriate delegation of tasks. Delegation promotes caregiver physical and emotional rest, which enhances client care.
Help the caregiver identify positive outcomes related to caregiving (e.g., increased relationship intimacy and feeling valued in the relationship) to balance negative feelings.	Positive feelings can balance negative feelings and provide a sense of purpose.
Provide written documentation of caregiving responsibilities as needed for the caregiver's employers.	To assist the caregiver in obtaining time away from work if needed to provide care.

COMMUNICATION, IMPAIRED VERBAL AND READINESS FOR ENHANCED

DEFINITIONS[9]

Impaired Verbal Communication Decreased, delayed, or absent ability to receive, process, transmit, and use a system of symbols.

    Readiness for Enhanced Communication A pattern of exchanging information and ideas with others that is sufficient for meeting one's needs and life's goals and can be strengthened.

DEFINING CHARACTERISTICS[9]

A. Impaired Verbal
1. Willful refusal to speak
2. Disorientation in the three spheres of time, space, and person
3. Inability to speak dominant language
4. Does not or cannot speak
5. Speaks or verbalizes with difficulty
6. Inappropriate verbalization
7. Difficulty forming words or sentences (e.g., aphonia, dyslalia, and dysarthria)
8. Difficulty forming words or sentences (e.g., aphasia, dysphasia, apraxia, and dyslexia)
9. Dyspnea
10. Absence of eye contact or difficulty in selective attending
11. Difficulty in comprehending and maintaining the usual communication pattern
12. Partial or total visual deficit
13. Inability or difficulty in use of facial or body expressions

14. Stuttering
15. Slurring

B. Readiness for Enhanced
1. Expresses willingness to enhance communication
2. Able to speak or write a language
3. Forms words, phrases, and language
4. Expresses thoughts and feelings
5. Uses and interprets nonverbal cues appropriately
6. Expresses satisfaction with ability to share information and ideas with others

RELATED FACTORS[9]

A. Impaired Verbal
1. Decrease in circulation to the brain
2. Cultural difference
3. Psychological barriers (e.g., psychosis or lack of stimuli)
4. Physical barrier (e.g., tracheostomy and intubation)
5. Anatomic defect (e.g., cleft palate or alteration of the neuromuscular visual system, auditory system, or phonatory apparatus)
6. Brain tumor
7. Differences related to developmental age
8. Side effects of medication
9. Environmental barriers
10. Absence of significant others
11. Altered perceptions
12. Lack of information
13. Stress
14. Alteration of self-esteem or self-concept
15. Physiologic conditions
16. Alteration of central nervous system
17. Weakening of the musculoskeletal system
18. Emotional conditions

B. Readiness for Enhanced
    There are no related factors for this wellness diagnosis.

RELATED CLINICAL CONCERNS

A. Impaired Verbal
1. Laryngeal cancer
2. Cleft lip or cleft palate
3. Cerebrovascular accident
4. Facial trauma
5. Respiratory distress
6. Late-stage Alzheimer's disease
7. Tourette's syndrome
8. Psychiatric disorders such as schizophrenic disorders, delusional disorders, psychotic disorders, or delirium
9. Autism

B. Readiness for Enhanced
There are no related clinical concerns for this wellness diagnosis.

 Have You Selected the Correct Diagnosis?

A. Impaired Verbal

Social Isolation
Social Isolation can occur because of the reduced ability or inability of an individual to use language as a means of communication. The primary diagnosis would be Impaired Verbal Communication, because resolution of the problem would assist in alleviating Social Isolation.

Disturbed Sensory Perception (Auditory)
If the individual has difficulty in hearing, then he or she would also reflect Impaired Verbal Communication. The primary problem would be the auditory difficulty, because correction of this deficit would help improve communication.

B. Readiness for Enhanced

Communication, Impaired Verbal
Communication, Impaired Verbal is the correct diagnosis when communication is not adequate to share information and can include processing, transmission, or reception abilities.

Readiness for Enhanced Communication
Readiness for Enhanced Communication applies to situations in which the client is effectively interacting with others and expresses a desire to improve these abilities.

EXPECTED OUTCOME

Impaired Verbal
Will communicate needs in a manner that is understood by caregivers via [state specific method (e.g., orally, esophageal speech, or computer)] by [date].

Readiness for Enhanced
Will verbalize increased satisfaction with communication by [date].

TARGET DATES

Impaired Verbal
The target date for resolution of this diagnosis will be long-range. However, 7 days would be appropriate for initial evaluation.

Readiness for Enhanced
This positive diagnosis is appropriate for both short- and long-term goals. An appropriate target date for initial evaluation of progress would be 1 to 3 days.

NURSING ACTIONS/INTERVENTIONS WITH RATIONALES

Adult Health

ACTIONS/INTERVENTIONS	RATIONALES
Impaired Verbal Maintain a patient, calm approach by: • Allowing adequate time for communication • Not interrupting the patient or attempting to finish sentences for him or her • Asking questions that require short answers or a nod of the head • Anticipating needs	Avoids interfering with the patient's communication attempts.
Provide materials that can be used to assist in communication (e.g., magic slate, flash cards, pad and pencil, "Speak and Spell" computer toy, pictures, or letter board).	Provides alternative methods of communication. Decreases anxiety and feelings of powerlessness and isolation.

(care plan continued on page 628)

NURSING ACTIONS/INTERVENTIONS WITH RATIONALES (continued from page 627)

Adult Health

ACTIONS/INTERVENTIONS	RATIONALES
Inform the family, significant others, and other health-care personnel of the effective ways the patient communicates.	Promotes effective communication. Avoids frustration for the patient.
Answer call bell promptly rather than using the intercom system.	Decreases stress for the patient by not straining communication resources.
Assure the patient that parenteral therapy does not interfere with the patient's ability to write.	Decreases anxiety.
Initiate referral to speech therapist if appropriate.	Initial teaching regarding speech may need interventions by specialist.
Initiate referrals to support agencies such as Lost Chord Club or New Voice Club as appropriate.	Groups that experienced the same problems can assist in rehabilitation and decrease social isolation. Promotes the patient's comfort.
Discuss use of electronic voice box and esophageal speech before discharge. Have the patient practice using device.	Reduces anxiety and increases self-confidence.
Encourage the patient to have recordings made for reaching police, fire department, doctor, or emergency medical service if impaired verbal communication is a long-term condition.	Promotes safety, increases comfort, and decreases anxiety.

Readiness for Enhanced

Assist the patient in identifying factors that enhance or inhibit open communication (e.g., environment, personal feelings, self-image) and address accordingly by:	Identifying limiting factors can enhance efforts for communication.
• Assisting patient in crafting message that clearly articulates needs, perceptions, or feelings.	Assists patient in clearly communicating these areas.
• Instructing patient in appropriate and acceptable methods for communication that do not alienate other parties.	
• Assisting patient in developing appropriate coping mechanisms to manage differences in opinion, such as using assertive communication techniques.	

Child Health

ACTIONS/INTERVENTIONS	RATIONALES
Impaired Verbal Monitor the patient's potential for speech according to subjective and objective components, to include: • Reported or documented previous speech capacity or potential • Health history for evidence of cognitive, sensory, perceptual, or neurologic dysfunction • Actual auditory documentation of speech potential • Assessment by a speech specialist • Patterns of speech of parents and significant others • Cultural meaning attached to speech or silence of children	Provides a database needed to plan more complete and accurate interventions.

ACTIONS/INTERVENTIONS	RATIONALES
• Any related trauma or pathophysiology • Parental perception of the child's status, especially in instances of congenital anomaly such as cleft lip or palate • Identification of dominant language and secondary languages heard or spoken in the family	
Assist the patient and parents to understand needed explanations for procedures, treatments, and equipment to be used in nursing care.	Provides a teaching opportunity. Decreases anxiety, which can interfere with communication.
Encourage feelings to be expressed by taking time to understand possible attempts at speech. For young children, use pictures if necessary.	Alternate methods of communication and sensitivity to attempts at communication attach value to the patient and serve to reinforce future attempts at communication.
Encourage family participation in the care of the patient as situation allows.	Family input provides an opportunity for communication and fosters the parent–child relationship.
Assist the family to identify community support groups.	Provides long-term support for coping.
Assist the patient and family in determining the impact Impaired Verbal Communication may have for family functioning.	Family functioning relies heavily on communication.
Provide information for long-term medical follow-up as indicated, especially for congenital anomalies.	Knowledge helps prepare the family for long-term needs and helps reduce anxiety about unknowns.
Assist in identification of appropriate financial support if the child is able to qualify for help according to state and federal legislation.	Funding by third-party payment may be available, depending on the patient's medical status.
Monitor for potential for related alterations in role-relationship patterns as a result of Impaired Verbal Communication.	Alterations in communication can affect the role-relationship pattern.
Monitor the potential for related alterations in self-concept or coping patterns as a result of Impaired Verbal Communication.	Alterations in communication may impact self-esteem and should be considered as a risk factor.
Provide appropriate patient and family teaching for care of the patient if permanent tracheostomy or related prosthetic is to be used, to include: • Appropriate number or size of tracheostomy tube • Appropriate duplication of size of tracheostomy tube in place in event of accidental dislodging or loss • Appropriate administration of oxygen via tracheostomy adapter • Appropriate suctioning technique, sterile and nonsterile • Appropriate list of supplies and how to procure them • Resources for actual care in emergency, with list of numbers including ambulance and nearest hospital • Appropriate indications for notification of physician.	Basic standards of care for the patient with a tracheostomy.

● N O T E : *These may vary slightly according to physician's plan or actual patient status.*

• Bleeding from tracheostomy
• Coughing out or dislodging of tracheostomy
• Difficulty in passing catheter to suction tracheostomy
• Fever higher than 101°F

(care plan continued on page 630)

NURSING ACTIONS/INTERVENTIONS WITH RATIONALES (continued from page 629)

Child Health

ACTIONS/INTERVENTIONS	RATIONALES
• Appropriate daily hygiene of tracheostomy • Caution regarding use of regular gauze or other substances that might be inhaled or ingested through tracheostomy • Need for humidification of tracheostomy	

Readiness for Enhanced

ACTIONS/INTERVENTIONS	RATIONALES
Determine need for aids or instruments to assist in communication (e.g., hearing aid or other augmentation).	Provides support for effective communication.
Facilitate child's expression of thoughts and feelings regarding desired issues related to communication with attention to: • Getting down to eye level of child. • Providing environment free of distractions. • Offering active listening. • Facilitating nonstressful and open engagement. • Avoiding interruptions. • Allowing the child to maintain control of the conversation as situations allows.	Fosters the likelihood of success in communication.
Offer positive reinforcement with encouraging feedback for efforts in communicating. [Note specific reinforcement plan here.]	Positive reinforcement encourages behavior.

Women's Health

This nursing diagnosis pertain to women the same as for all adults. The reader is referred to the other sections—Adult Health, Mental Health, and Home Health.

Mental Health

● N O T E : *If impaired communication is related to alterations in physiology or surgical alterations, refer to Adult Health nursing actions.*

ACTIONS/INTERVENTIONS	RATIONALES
Impaired Verbal Establish a calm, reassuring environment.	Inappropriate levels of sensory stimuli can increase confusion and disorganization.
If communication difficulties are related to disorientation to person, place, or time, provide appropriate environmental cues to support orientation. These can include: • Calendars • Orientation boards • Seasonal decorations and conversations • Clocks with large numbers • Name signs on doors • Current event groups	

ACTIONS/INTERVENTIONS	RATIONALES
Note items that are necessary for this client with the frequency of exposure needed to support the client's orientation. If disorientation is related to delusions, refer to Disturbed Thought Process in Chapter 7 for additional interventions.	
Provide the client with a private environment if experiencing high levels of anxiety, to assist him or her in focusing on relevant stimuli.	High levels of anxiety decrease the client's ability to process information.
Communicate with the client in clear, concise language. • Speak slowly to the client. • Do not shout. • Face the client when talking to him or her; make sure lips are visible by wearing lipstick or trimming beards. • Role-model agreement between verbal and nonverbal behavior. • Use "I" messages to request clarification from client when you do not understand what is being communicated (e.g., "I want to understand what you are saying, could you please repeat that?")	Inappropriate levels of sensory stimuli can increase confusion and disorganization. When verbal and nonverbal behavior is not in agreement, a double-bind or incongruent message may be sent. These incongruent messages place the receiver in a "darned if you do, darned if you don't" situation and promote interpersonal ineffectiveness.
Spend 30 minutes twice a day at [times] with the client discussing communication patterns. As the client progresses, this time could also include: • Constructive confrontation about the effects of the dysfunctional communication pattern on relationships • Role-playing appropriate communication patterns • Pointing out to the client the lack of agreement between verbal and nonverbal behavior and context • Helping the client understand purpose of dysfunctional communication patterns • Developing alternative ways for the client to have needs met	Promotes the development of a trusting relationship, while providing the client a safe environment in which to practice new behaviors. Behavioral rehearsal helps facilitate the client's learning new skills through the use of feedback and modeling by the nurse.
Develop, with the client's assistance, a reward program for appropriate communication patterns and for progress on goals. [Note here the kinds of behavior to be rewarded and schedule for reward.]	Reinforcement encourages positive behavior while enhancing self-esteem.
Instruct the client in assertive communication techniques, and practice these in daily interactions with the client. Note here those assertive skills the client is to practice and how these are to be practiced (e.g., each medication is to be requested by the client in an assertive manner).	Assertiveness improves the individual's ability to act appropriately and effectively in a manner that maximizes coping resources.[22]
Provide the client with positive verbal rewards for appropriate communication.	Reinforcement encourages positive behavior.
Sit with the client while another client is asked for feedback about an interaction.	The nurse's presence provides support while the client can receive feedback on interpersonal skills from a peer.
Keep interactions brief and goal directed when the client is communicating in dysfunctional manner.	Inappropriate levels of sensory stimuli can increase confusion and disorganization.
Spend an extra 5 minutes in interactions in which the client is communicating clearly, and inform the client of this reward of time.	Time with the nurse can provide positive reinforcement.

(care plan continued on page 632)

NURSING ACTIONS/INTERVENTIONS WITH RATIONALES (continued from page 631)

Mental Health

ACTIONS/INTERVENTIONS	RATIONALES
Reward improvement in the client's listening behavior. This can be evaluated by having the client repeat what has just been heard. Provide clarification for the differences between what was heard and what was said.	Improved attending skills improve the client's ability to understand communication from others and to clarify unclear portions of communication.
Have the support system participate in one interaction per week with the client in the presence of a staff member. The staff member will facilitate communication between the client and the support system. [Note time for these interactions here, with the name of the staff person responsible for this process.]	Behavioral rehearsal provides opportunities for feedback and modeling from the nurse. Support system understanding facilitates the maintenance of new behaviors after discharge.
Arrange for the client to participate in a therapeutic group. [Note schedule for these groups here.]	Provides an opportunity for the client to receive feedback on communication from peers and to observe the interactions of peers so that he or she may increase the requisite variety of responses in social situation.
Request that the client clarify unclear statements or communications in private language.	Models appropriate communication skills for the client.
Teach the client to request clarification on confusing communications. This may be practiced with role-play.	Repeated practice of a behavior internalizes and personalizes the behavior.
Include the client in unit activities, and assign appropriate tasks to the client. These should require a level of communication the client can easily achieve so that a positive learning experience can occur. [Note level of activity appropriate for the client here.]	Provides opportunities for the client to practice new behaviors in a supportive environment.
If communication problems evolve from a language difference, have someone who understands the language orient the client to the unit as soon as possible and answer any questions the client might have.	Decreases the client's sense of isolation and anxiety.
Use nonverbal communication to interact with the client when no one is available to translate.	Decreases the client's sense of social isolation, and promotes the development of a trusting relationship.
Obtain information about nonverbal communication in the client's culture and about appropriate psychosocial behavior. Alter interactions and expectations to fit these beliefs as they fit the client. [Note here information that is important in providing daily care for this client.]	Decreases the possibilities for misunderstanding to develop.
Determine whether the client understands any English and, if so, how it is best understood (i.e., written or spoken).	Promotes the development of a trusting relationship.
If the client does not understand English, determine whether a language other than the one from the culture of origin is spoken. Perhaps a common language for staff and the client can be found. For example, few people other than Navajos speak Navajo, but some older Navajos also speak Spanish.	Communication facilitates social interaction and increases the client's sense of control.
Do not shout when talking with someone who speaks another language. Speak slowly and concisely.	Inappropriate levels of sensory stimulation can increase confusion and disorganization.
Use pictures to enhance nonverbal communication.	Pictures facilitate communication when the caregiver and client do not share the same language.

ACTIONS/INTERVENTIONS	RATIONALES
If a staff member does not speak the client's language, arrange for a translator to visit with the client at least once a day to answer questions and provide information. Have a schedule for the next day available so this can be reviewed with the client and information can be provided about complex procedures. Have a staff member remain with the client during these interactions to serve as a resource person for the translator. Allow time for the client to ask questions and express feelings. Note schedule for these visits here, with the name of the translator.	Promotes the client's sense of control, and decreases social isolation.

Readiness for Enhanced

ACTIONS/INTERVENTIONS	RATIONALES
Spend [number] minutes with client [number] times per day to discuss what client understands about communication and clarifying what they want to learn. [Note client's goals here with education plan.]	Change is dependent on the client's perception of the problem.[23]
Introduce the client to assertive communication skills and provide opportunities to practice these skills in the areas clients find difficult. [Note client learning needs here and schedule for practice.]	Assertive communications enhance the ability to express one's needs.[24]
Provide positive verbal reinforcement for client goal achievement.	Positive reinforcement increases behavior.[24]
Refer the client to community resources that can assist him or her with continued communication skill enhancement. [Note those resources here and arrange contact with the client before discharge.]	

Gerontic Health

Impaired Verbal

The nursing actions for a gerontic patient with this diagnosis are the same as those given in Adult Health and Mental Health.

ACTIONS/INTERVENTIONS	RATIONALES
Readiness for Enhanced Collaborate with the client, family, and/or caregiver to determine appropriate goals for enhanced communication and preferred methods of communication. Collaborate with the client, family, and/or caregiver to determine previously effective modes or methods of communication and determine how those methods might be strengthened in the current situation. Assess client strengths in communication (written or verbal communication) and facilitate the use of the stronger modes of communication for the client: • Discuss ways to communicate in writing for the client with strong written communication skills to include e-mail, journaling, letters, poetry. • Discuss ways to strengthen the verbal communication of the person who prefers verbal communication to include brainstorming, reflecting, or telephone conferencing.	

(care plan continued on page 634)

NURSING ACTIONS/INTERVENTIONS WITH RATIONALES (continued from page 633)

Home Health

In addition to the interventions for Adult Health, Mental Health, and Gerontic Health, the following may be applied in the home setting.

ACTIONS/INTERVENTIONS	RATIONALES
Impaired Verbal	
Involve the client and family in planning and implementing strategies to decrease, prevent, or cope with Impaired Verbal Communication: • Family conference: Discuss each member's perspective of the situation. • Mutual goal setting: Set short-term accomplishable goals with evaluation criteria; specify tasks for each member. • Communication: Identify ways to communicate with the client.	Family involvement enhances effectiveness of interventions.
Teach the client and family appropriate information regarding the care of a person with Impaired Verbal Communication: • Use of pencil and paper, alphabet letters, hand signals, sign language, pictures, flash cards, or computer • Use of repetition • Facing the person when communicating • Using simple, one-step commands • Allowing time for the person to respond • Use of drawing, painting, coloring, singing, or exercising • Identifying tasks the person with Impaired Verbal Communication can do well • Decreasing external noise	Knowledge bases are required to interact with the family member who is verbally impaired.
Assist the patient and family in lifestyle adjustments that may be required: • Stress management • Changing role functions and relationships • Learning a foreign language • Acknowledging and coping with frustration with communication efforts • Obtaining necessary supportive equipment (e.g., hearing aid, special telephone, or artificial larynx)	Lifestyle changes require long-term behavioral changes. Support enhances permanent changes in behavior.
Consult with, or refer to, appropriate assistive resources as required.	Self-help groups and rehabilitation services can enhance the treatment plans.
Readiness for Enhanced	
Collaborate with the client, family, and/or caregiver to determine appropriate goals for enhanced communication and preferred methods of communication.	
Assist the client in obtaining resources to enhance communication to include telephones, e-mail, journals.	

FAMILY PROCESSES, INTERRUPTED, AND FAMILY PROCESSES, DYSFUNCTIONAL: ALCOHOLISM AND READINESS FOR ENHANCED

DEFINITIONS[9]

Interrupted Family Processes   Change in family relationships and/or functioning.

Dysfunctional Family Processes: Alcoholism   Psychosocial, spiritual, and physiologic functions of the family unit are chronically disorganized, which leads to conflict, denial of problems, resistance to change, ineffective problem solving, and a series of self-perpetuating crises.

Readiness for Enhanced Family Processes   A pattern of family functioning that is sufficient to support the well-being of family members and can be strengthened.

DEFINING CHARACTERISTICS[9]

A. Interrupted Family Processes

1. Changes in power alliances
2. Changes in assigned tasks
3. Changes in effectiveness in completing assigned tasks
4. Changes in mutual support
5. Changes in availability for effective responsiveness and intimacy
6. Changes in patterns and rituals
7. Changes in participation in problem solving
8. Changes in participation in decision making
9. Changes in communication patterns
10. Changes in availability for emotional support
11. Changes in satisfaction with family
12. Changes in stress-reduction behaviors
13. Changes in expression of conflict with and/or isolation from community resources
14. Changes in somatic complaints
15. Changes in expressions of conflict within family

B. Dysfunctional Family Processes: Alcoholism

1. Roles and relationships
   a. Inconsistent parenting or low perception of parental support
   b. Ineffective spouse communication or marital problems
   c. Intimacy dysfunction
   d. Deterioration in family relationships or disturbed family dynamics
   e. Altered role function or disruption of family roles
   f. Closed communication systems
   g. Chronic family problems
   h. Family denial
   i. Lack of cohesiveness
   j. Neglected obligations
   k. Lack of skills necessary for relationships
   l. Reduced ability of family members to relate to each other for mutual growth and maturation
   m. Family unable to meet security needs of its members
   n. Disrupted family rituals
   o. Economic problems
   p. Family does not demonstrate respect for individuality and autonomy of its members
   q. Triangulating family relationships
   r. Patterns of rejection
2. Behavioral
   a. Refusal to get help, or inability to accept and receive help appropriately
   b. Inadequate understanding or knowledge of alcoholism
   c. Ineffective problem-solving skills
   d. Loss of control of drinking
   e. Manipulation
   f. Rationalization or denial of problems
   g. Blaming
   h. Inability to meet emotional needs of its members
   i. Alcohol abuse
   j. Broken promises
   k. Criticizing
   l. Dependency
   m. Impaired communication
   n. Difficulty with intimate relationships
   o. Enabling to maintain alcoholic drinking pattern
   p. Inappropriate expression of anger
   q. Isolation
   r. Inability to meet spiritual needs of its members
   s. Inability to express or accept wide range of feelings
   t. Inability to deal constructively with traumatic experiences
   u. Inability to adapt to change
   v. Immaturity
   w. Harsh self-judgment
   x. Lying
   y. Lack of dealing with conflict
   z. Lack of reliability
   aa. Nicotine addiction
   bb. Orientation toward tension relief rather than achievement of goals
   cc. Seeking approval and affirmation
   dd. Difficulty having fun
   ee. Agitation
   ff. Chaos
   gg. Contradictory, paradoxical communication
   hh. Diminished physical contact
   ii. Disturbances in academic performance in children
   jj. Disturbances in concentration
   kk. Escalating conflict

ll. Failure to accomplish current or past developmental tasks, or difficulty with life cycle transitions

mm. Family special occasions are alcohol-centered

nn. Controlling communications or power struggles

oo. Self-blaming

pp. Stress-related physical illnesses

qq. Substance abuse other than alcohol

rr. Unresolved grief

ss. Verbal abuse of spouse or parent

3. Feelings

a. Insecurity

b. Lingering resentment

c. Mistrust

d. Rejection

e. Feelings of responsibility for the alcoholic's behavior

f. Shame or embarrassment

g. Unhappiness

h. Powerlessness

i. Anger or suppressed rage

j. Anxiety, tension, or distress

k. Emotional isolation or loneliness

l. Frustration

m. Guilt

n. Hopelessness

o. Hurt

p. Decreased self-esteem or feelings of worthlessness

q. Repressed emotions

r. Vulnerability

s. Hostility

t. Lack of identity

u. Fear

v. Loss

w. Emotional control by others

x. Misunderstood

y. Moodiness

z. Abandonment

aa. Being different from other people

bb. Being unloved

cc. Confused love and pity

dd. Confusion

ee. Failure

ff. Depression

gg. Dissatisfaction

C. Family Processes, Readiness for Enhanced

1. Expresses willingness to enhance family dynamics.

2. Family functioning meets physical, social, and psychological needs of family members.

3. Activities support the safety and growth of family members.

4. Communication is adequate.

5. Relationships are generally positive; interdependent with community; family tasks are accomplished.

6. Family roles are flexible and appropriate for developmental stages.

7. Respect for family members is evident.

8. Family adapts to change.

9. Boundaries of family members are maintained.

10. Energy level of family supports activities of daily living.

11. Family resilience is evident.

12. Balance exists between autonomy and cohesiveness.

RELATED FACTORS[9]

A. Interrupted Family Processes

1. Power shift of family members

2. Family role shifts

3. Shift in health status of a family member

4. Developmental transition and/or crisis

5. Situation transition and/or crisis

6. Informal or formal interaction with community

7. Modification in family social status

8. Modification in family finances

B. Dysfunctional Family Processes: Alcoholism

1. Abuse of alcohol

2. Genetic predisposition

3. Lack of problem-solving skills

4. Inadequate coping skills

5. Family history of alcoholism, resistance to treatment

6. Biochemical influences

7. Addictive personality

C. Family Processes, Readiness for Enhanced

Related factors are not provided for wellness diagnoses.

RELATED CLINICAL CONCERNS

1. Surgery

2. Trauma

3. Mental retardation

4. Chronic illness

5. Alcoholism

6. Chemical abuse

 Have You Selected the Correct Diagnosis?

Compromised or Disabled Family Coping
This diagnosis has a history of destructive patterns of behavior. For the diagnosis of Interrupted Family Processes to be applicable, there would be evidence that the usual adequacy in coping is altered in relation to a specific crisis.

EXPECTED OUTCOME

Will describe specific plan to cope with [specific stressor] by [date].

d satisfaction with family pro-

ce

native ways to manage

fa

use of [number] of family com-

m ...ate].

TARGET DATES

Five to 7 days would be the earliest acceptable target date. Even after the expected outcome has initially been met, there may be other precipitating events that will again alter family processes; therefore, a long-term date should be designated.

NURSING ACTIONS/INTERVENTIONS WITH RATIONALES

Adult Health

ACTIONS/INTERVENTIONS	RATIONALES
Discern interaction styles, communication patterns, and role behaviors in the family.[25]	Baseline information about family dynamics can assist the nurse with planning and developing family interventions.
Help the family to identify its strengths and weaknesses in dealing with the situation during family conference.	Identifies existing resources for crisis resolution and areas to strengthen. Provides positive feedback for strengths that already exist.
Help the family organize to continue usual family activities.	Decreases the sense of overwhelming loss of everything. Adds stability to activities.
Promote a trusting therapeutic relationship during interaction with the patient and family by being empathetic, actively listening, accepting feelings and attitudes, and being nonjudgmental.	Provides comfort and aids in crisis resolution.
Promote open, honest communications among the family members by facilitating group interaction. Encourage the patient and family to express feelings regarding current family processes by spending [specific time] each shift, while awake, for this purpose.	Promotes verbalization of feelings and shared understanding of problems. Assists the family to acknowledge and accept the problem. Promotes a common definition of the problem and assists in identifying ways to cope with the problem.
Family Processes, Dysfunctional: Alcoholism	
Determine the family's level of recognition of problems within the family unit associated with the patient's alcoholism.	Level of recognition may serve as an indicator of the family's acceptance or denial of problems.
Allow the family to grieve by providing time, giving permission, and referring them to clergy and/or bereavement group.	Assists in crisis intervention and provides extra coping mechanisms.
Support efforts of the family to deal with previously identified problems within the family unit associated with the patient's alcoholism.	Family may already be involved in therapy for previously identified family unit problems. Hospitalization can cause regression and/or intensification of problems.
Monitor readiness to learn; then teach the family about the precipitating situation, its implications, and the expected response to treatment.	Provides a knowledge base to assist in problem solving. Decreases anxiety.
Allow the family members to participate in patient care as possible.	
Refer the family to a health professional or organization specializing in substance abuse.	If the family is not already involved in therapy, it is essential to provide resources for treatment or rehabilitation after discharge from the hospital. Provides long-term support and effective use of already available resources.
See Mental Health nursing actions for more detailed interventions.	Collaboration promotes more holistic care; many need specific interventions by a specialist.

(care plan continued on page 638)

NURSING ACTIONS/INTERVENTIONS WITH RATIONALES (continued from page 637)

Adult Health

ACTIONS/INTERVENTIONS	RATIONALES
Family Process, Readiness for Enhanced	
Assist the patient in identifying appropriate adaptation to life changes. [Note specific assistance needed here.]	Maintains realistic expectations of the evolving role.
Help the patient in identifying areas of family dynamics that can be enhanced through discussions during the provision of care.	Strengthens interactions among family members.
Support the patient's efforts to organize family activities. [Note specific assistance needed here.]	Promotes cohesiveness.
Facilitate efforts toward enhanced communication by modeling appropriate communication and providing time for the family to interact.	

Child Health

● N O T E : *Depending on the age of the infant or child, a range of possible needs may be represented in the context of the family—all interventions should be developmentally appropriate. Include all children in family counseling as applicable. Refer to Mental Health for Readiness for Enhanced Family Processes.*

ACTIONS/INTERVENTIONS	RATIONALES
Promote sibling participation in the patient's hospitalization and plans for discharge (e.g., allowing visitation during game time).	Inclusion of sibling(s) fosters a sense of family concern, and the need for support is met for all involved. Undue prolonged separations increase stress for the sibling(s) and family relationships.
Provide for cultural preferences when possible, including diet, religious needs, and plans for health care.	Attention to preferences demonstrates valuing and sensitivity for the family.
Provide reinforcement to appropriately value caretaking behavior.	Reinforcement of desired behaviors serves to offer positive learning, with increased likelihood of compliance.
Advocate on the infant's or child's behalf to best offer management of alcohol or substance abuse impact on current or future development.	The infant, child, or adolescent may be unable to look after self-interests, and when this is so, it is legally and morally mandated that the client have an advocate.
Determine the child's or adolescent's feelings of the family per ventilation about same for 30 minutes each shift.	Assists in anxiety reduction, and values input of all individual family members. Also, data may be known for best treatment.

Women's Health

ACTIONS/INTERVENTIONS	RATIONALES
New Parents	
Assist the patient and significant others in establishing realistic goals related to changes in role due to newborn (e.g., sharing of tasks or parenting skills).	Assist the family with role changes during a normal, but often unexpected, amount of role change event. Provides basis for planning necessary changes.
Provide positive reinforcement for parenting tasks.	Provides motivation and enhances likelihood of effective parenting.
Assist the parents in identifying infant behavior patterns and understanding how they allow the infant to communicate with them (e.g., crying or fussing).	Assists in reducing stress and promotes positive parenting.

ACTIONS/INTERVENTIONS	RATIONALES
Assist the patient in verbalizing her perceptions of the infant's growth and development, individual and family needs, and the stresses of being a new parent.	Provides a database that allows more effective teaching and planning for effective parenting.
Identify support groups (e.g., formal groups, such as Mother's Day Out, and informal groups, such as parenting groups, family, or friends).	Promotes planning and allows early intervention for potential stress areas.
Encourage open communication between the mother and father about household tasks, discipline, fears, and anxieties (e.g., less-than-perfect baby).	
Help develop a plan for sharing household tasks and child caretaking activities: • Bathing • Feeding • Care of siblings • Quality time with older children	Reduces stress-provoking events.
Allow older children to assist with newborn care (even the smallest child can do this with parental supervision): • Bringing a diaper to the parent • Pushing the baby in the stroller • Holding the baby (while sitting on couch is best)	
Follow up with home visits after discharge from hospital to physically monitor the infant, monitor family interactions, provide support, and provide referrals to the proper agencies.	Provides long-term support.
Teach and reinforce methods of caring for, and coping with, the emotional and physiologic needs of the infant, siblings, parents, and other relatives, such as grandparents.	Provides measures and preplanning to cope with potential stressful events.

Parent to Your Parents

Assist the client and family to establish realistic goals related to increasing responsibilities in caring for elderly parents, e.g., sharing of tasks, time, and resources (financial and emotional).

Assist in identifying resources in the community:
• Daycare for the elderly
• Church groups
• YWCAs
• Professional help in the home, such as home health aides

Assist in exploring and identifying need for care of elderly parent outside of home (e.g., assisted living or skilled nursing care).

Alcoholism

● N O T E : *Interventions under Adult Health and Mental Health will apply here, in addition to the following:*

Perinatal

Check your state's laws. Because of the widespread drug use in this country, some states have mandatory screening for drug use during the perinatal period.[26,27]

(care plan continued on page 640)

NURSING ACTIONS/INTERVENTIONS WITH RATIONALES (continued from page 639)

Women's Health

ACTIONS/INTERVENTIONS	RATIONALES
Screen clients for chemical use during pregnancy by means of interview at first visit. Provide a relaxed, secure atmosphere for the client when trying to obtain a substance-abuse history. Include the following in your questions: • Use of nonprescription drugs • Use of coffee • Use of cigarettes • Use of alcohol • Use of prescription drugs • Use of recreational drugs, such as marijuana • Use of multiple drugs • Problems encountered in trying to abstain from drug use	
Assure the client of acceptance of her and her family, but not of self-destructive behaviors.[28]	
Support and praise the client for health-seeking behaviors.[28]	
Thoroughly assess the woman and the fetus who present with complications related to substance abuse in order to provide the best physiologic support for her and her fetal well-being.	
Obtain a sample for toxicology screening: • Maternal or neonatal urine toxicology screen • Meconium and maternal or neonatal hair samples	Because of slow growth of hair and meconium produced by the second trimester, these methods provide the best analysis of long-term data on drug use.[28]
Collaborate with the physician to provide appropriate pain control during labor.	Women with narcotic dependency problems have a high tolerance to analgesics and usually have a low pain threshold.[28]
Notify neonatal personnel of the patient's labor and history of substance abuse.	
Support and guide maternal–infant interactions in order to encourage maternal–infant attachment.	
● N O T E: *For the addicted infant, see Child Health.*	

Mental Health

ACTIONS/INTERVENTIONS	RATIONALES
Provide a role model for effective communication by: • Seeking clarification • Demonstrating respect for individual family members and the family system • Listening to expression of thoughts and feelings • Setting clear limits • Being consistent • Communicating with the individual being addressed in a clear manner • Encouraging sharing of information among appropriate system subgroups	Communication skills provide a framework for effective problem solving.

ACTIONS/INTERVENTIONS	RATIONALES
Demonstrate an understanding of the complexity of system problems by: • Not taking sides in family disagreements • Providing alternative explanations of behavior that recognize the contributions of all persons involved with the problem, including health-care providers, as appropriate • Requesting the perspective of multiple family members on a problem or stressor	Outcome improves when psychosocial problems are treated from a systems perspective.[17]
Include all family members in the first interview.	Provides an opportunity to assess all family members' perception of the problem, and in identification of problem-solving strategies that are acceptable to more family members.
Have each member provide his or her perspective to the current difficulties.	Assists the family in defining a problem that can be resolved. For example, rather than defining the problem as "We don't love each other any more," the problem can be defined as "We do not spend time together in family activities." This definition evolves from the family's description of what they mean by the more general problem description.
Assist the family in developing behavioral short-term goals by: • Asking what they would see happening in the family if the situation improved • Having them break the problem into several parts that combine to form the identified stressor • Asking them what they could do in a week to improve the situation (should include a response from each family member)	Setting achievable goals increases the opportunities for success, which increases the motivation to continue to work toward problem resolution.
Maintain the nurse's role of facilitator of family communication by: • Having family members discuss possible solutions among themselves • Having each family member talk about how he or she might contribute to both the problem and the problem's resolution	Maintains a context that enhances and supports the family's problem-solving skills.
Provide the family with the information necessary for appropriate problem solving.	
During each meeting with the family, provide positive comments about the family's strengths and competencies.	Promotes the family's positive opinions of themselves, which opens them up to viewing the problem differently and developing more effective problem solving.[17]
Answer all questions in an open, direct manner.	Promotes a trusting relationship.
Support the expression of affect by: • Having family members share feelings with one another • Normalizing the expression of emotion (e.g., "Most persons experience anger after they have experienced a loss.") • Providing a private environment for this expression	Promotes communication among family members, while developing a positive expectational set.
Maintain and support a functional family role For example, allow the parents private time alone, allow the children to visit parents, and encourage the presenting of problems to the "family leader."	Provides positive reinforcement for functional interactions, and serves to encourage this behavior while enhancing self-esteem.

(care plan continued on page 642)

Mental Health

ACTIONS/INTERVENTIONS	RATIONALES
Schedule a time with the family to discuss how the current situation affects family roles and possible changes that may be necessary.	
Have the family identify the systems in the community that could support them during this time, and assist the family in contacting these systems. Note here the systems to be contacted as well as how they will assist the family.	Promotes and develops the family's strengths.
Provide positive verbal reinforcement for the family's accomplishments.	Positive reinforcement encourages behavior and enhances self-esteem.
Assist the family in identifying patterns of interaction that interfere with successful problem resolution. For example, the husband frequently asks his wife closed-ended questions, which discourages her from sharing her ideas; the children interrupt the parents when their level of conflict increases to a certain level; or the wife walks out of the room when the husband brings up issues related to finances.	Facilitates the development of more appropriate coping behaviors.
Assist the family in planning fun activities together. This could include time to play or exercise together, or engage in a shared project.	Families in crisis often limit their emotional experience.
Teach the family methods of anxiety reduction; establish a practice schedule and a schedule for discussing how this method could be used on a daily basis in the family. The selected method, along with the schedule for discussion and practice, should be listed here.	Relaxation response inhibits the activation of the autonomic nervous system's fight-or-flight response. Repeated practice of a behavior internalizes and personalizes the behavior.
Include the family in discussions related to planning care and sharing information about the client's condition.	Support system involvement in problem solving increases the opportunities for a more positive outcome.
Assist the family in developing a specific plan when the client is scheduled for a pass or discharge. Note that plan here, with the assistance needed from the nursing staff for implementation.	Promotes the client's sense of control. Planned coping strategies facilitate the enactment of new behaviors when stress is experienced. This increases the opportunities for successful coping and enhances self-esteem.

Alcohol

Promote a trusting therapeutic relationship during interaction with the client and family by being empathetic, listening actively, accepting feelings and attitudes, and being nonjudgmental.	Provides comfort and aids in the development of a context that supports expressions of emotions and risking change.[29]
Spend time in the initial interactions with the family discussing the influence the problem or illness has on their lives and the influence they have on the problem.	Assists the family in viewing the problem as outside of themselves, objectifying the problem rather than the person, thus making it easier for the family to see the problem as something they can influence. Assists the family in developing a different perspective of the problem.[17]
Establish a therapeutic relationship with whatever part of the family system initiates treatment.	Working with the nonalcoholic spouse and family members can facilitate the entry of the alcoholic family member into treatment.[30]

ACTIONS/INTERVENTIONS	RATIONALES
Promote open, honest communications among family members by facilitating group interaction. Promote the expression of feelings regarding current family process by spending [specific time] each shift, while the patient is awake, for this purpose.	Promotes verbalization of feelings and shared understanding of problems. Assists the family to acknowledge and accept the problem. Promotes a common definition of the problem and assists in identifying ways to cope.
Schedule the family for psychoeducational groups that explore basic information, family responses to alcoholism, family roles in intervention, and codependence. Included topics should be: • Basic disease concepts • Family control behaviors • Anger • Threats • Covering up for or enabling the alcoholic • Personal responsibility • Self-care • Healthy communication	Family involvement in early treatment improves the outcome.[30]
Provide a role model for effective communication by: • Seeking clarification • Demonstrating respect for individual family members and the family system • Listening to expression of thoughts and feelings • Setting clear limits • Being consistent • Communicating clearly with the individual being addressed	Communication skills provide a framework for effective problem solving.
Demonstrate an understanding for the complexity of system problems by: • Not taking sides in family disagreements • Providing alternative explanations of behavior that recognize the contributions of all persons involved with the problem • Requesting the perspective of multiple family members on a problem or stressor	Outcome improves when family communication problems are addressed.[30]
Assist the family in defining a problem that can be resolved. For example, rather than defining the problem as "I want him to be more responsible around the house," try "I would like him to take responsibility for paying the bills by the first of the month."	
Assist the family in developing behavioral short-term goals by: • Asking what they would see happening in the family if the situation improved • Having them break the problem into several parts that can bring to fore the identified stressor • Asking them what they could do in a week to improve the situation	Setting achievable goals increases the opportunities for success, which increases the motivation to continue to work toward problem resolution.
Maintain the nurse's role of facilitator of family communication by: • Having family members discuss possible solutions among themselves • Having each family member take responsibility for his or her own actions and not accept responsibility for others	Maintains a context that enhances and supports the family's problem-solving skills.

(care plan continued on page 644)

NURSING ACTIONS/INTERVENTIONS WITH RATIONALES (continued from page 643)

Mental Health

ACTIONS/INTERVENTIONS	RATIONALES
Support the expression of affect: • Have family members share feelings with one another. • Normalize the expressions of emotion, for example, "Most families experience anger as part of the recovery process." • Provide a private environment for this expression.	Expression of affect is one of the most difficult areas for these families. Promotes learning positive ways of communicating among family members, while developing a positive expectational set.[31]
Schedule a time with the family to discuss how the current situation affects family roles, and possible changes that may be necessary. [Note that schedule here with responsible person.]	
Maintain and support functional family roles; for example, allow the parents private time alone, or allow the children to visit parents.	Provides positive reinforcement for functional interactions and serves to encourage this behavior while enhancing self-esteem.
Have the family identify those systems in the community that could support them in recovery, and assist them in contacting these systems (Alcoholics Anonymous, Al-Anon, Al-Ateen). [Note here the systems to be contacted and person responsible for this activity.]	Promotes and develops the family's strengths and provides support systems for behavior changes.
Provide positive verbal reinforcement for the family's accomplishments.	Positive reinforcement encourages behavior and enhances self-esteem.
Assist the family in planning fun activities together. This could include time to play together, exercise together, or engage in a shared project.	Families in crisis often limit emotional experiences.
Teach the family methods of anxiety reduction; establish a practice schedule and a schedule for discussing how this method could be used on a daily basis in the family. The selected method along with the schedule for discussion and practice should be listed here.	The relaxation response inhibits the activation of the autonomic nervous system's fight-or-flight response. Repeated practice of a behavior internalizes and personalizes the behavior.
Assist the family in developing a specific plan when the client is scheduled for a pass or discharge. [Note that plan here, including the assistance needed from the nursing staff for implementation.]	Promotes the client's sense of control. Planned coping strategies facilitate the enactment of new behaviors when stress is experienced. This increases the opportunities foe successful coping and enhances self-esteem.
Readiness for Enhanced	
Spend [number] minutes with family identifying their areas of concern and develop plan that will facilitate their meeting goals. [Note that plan here.]	Change is dependent on the client's perception of the problem.[23,24]
Refer the family to community programs that focus on positive skill building such as Couples Communication and Parent Effectiveness Training, Developmental Assets programs (Search Institute).	
Spend [number] minutes with family identifying positive family activities and establishing a schedule for participation.	Promotes positive family affect and enhances the focus on family strengths.[23]
Identify with family community organizations that share their values and can assist with their ongoing development (e.g., faith communities, youth groups, Developmental Assets Programs).	

Gerontic Health

● N O T E : *The nursing actions for the gerontic patient with these diagnoses would be the same as those given in Adult Health and Mental Health. The prevalence of alcoholism in older adults is reportedly lower than in the general population; however, this may be due to the lack of age-specific screening instruments.[32] In older adults, there may be late-onset alcoholism due to an increase in the stresses associated with aging, such as loss of a spouse, changes in health, and retirement.[33] Some researchers advocate programs that are connected to aging service programs, such as senior programs, to assist the older alcoholic and his or her family in dealing with aging issues as well as alcoholism.[34]*

Home Health

See Mental Health nursing actions for detailed psychosocial interventions.

ACTIONS/INTERVENTIONS	RATIONALES
Teach the client and family appropriate information regarding the care of family members: • Discipline strategies appropriate for developmental level • Normal growth and development • Expected family life cycles (e.g., childrearing or grandparenting) • Coping strategies for family growth • Care of health deviations • Developing and using support networks • Safe environment for family members • Anticipatory guidance regarding growth and development, discipline, family functioning, responses to illness, role changes, etc.	Basic knowledge that contributes to successful family functioning.
Involve the client and family in planning and implementing strategies to decrease or prevent alterations in family process: • Family conference to ascertain perspective of members on current situation and to identify strategies to improve situation • Mutual goal setting to identify realistic goals with evaluation criteria and specific activities for each family member • Encouragement of clear, consistent, and honest communication with positive feedback • Distribution of family tasks so that all members are involved in maintaining the family based on developmental capacity	Family involvement enhances effectiveness of the intervention.
Assist the client and family in lifestyle adjustments that may be required: • Separation or divorce • Temporary stay in community shelter • Family therapy • Communication of feelings • Stress reduction • Identification of potential for violence	Permanent changes in behavior and family roles require support.

(care plan continued on page 646)

NURSING ACTIONS/INTERVENTIONS WITH RATIONALES (continued from page 645)	

Home Health

ACTIONS/INTERVENTIONS	RATIONALES
• Providing safe environment • Therapeutic use of anger • Seeking and providing support for family members • Coping with catastrophic or chronic illness • Requirements for redistributing family tasks • Changing role functions and relationships • Financial concerns Consult with or refer to assistive resources as required.	Utilization of existing services is efficient use of resources. Support groups, psychiatric nurse clinicians, and teachers can enhance the treatment plan.

GRIEVING, ANTICIPATORY

DEFINITION[9]

Intellectual and emotional responses and behaviors by which individuals, families, or communities work through the process of modifying self-concept based on the perception of potential loss.

DEFINING CHARACTERISTICS[9]

1. Expression of distress at potential loss
2. Sorrow
3. Guilt
4. Denial of potential loss
5. Anger
6. Altered communication patterns
7. Potential loss of significant object (e.g., people, possessions, job, status, home, ideals, and parts and processes of the body)
8. Denial of the significance of the loss
9. Bargaining
10. Alterations in:
    a. Eating habits
    b. Sleep patterns
    c. Dream patterns
    d. Activity level
    e. Libido
11. Difficulty taking on new or different roles
12. Resolution of grief prior to the reality of loss

RELATED FACTORS[9]

To be developed.

RELATED CLINICAL CONCERNS

1. Cancer
2. Amputation
3. Spinal cord injury
4. Birth defects

5. Any diagnosis that the family has been told has a terminal prognosis

 Have You Selected the Correct Diagnosis?

Disturbed Sensory Perception
The diagnosis of Disturbed Sensory Perception is identified according to the patient's change in capacity to exercise judgment or think critically with appropriate sensory–perceptual functioning. This may well be related to Anticipatory Grieving.

Anxiety or Fear
Anxiety is the response the individual has to a threat that is for the most part unidentified. Fear is the response of an individual to an identified threat. When the patient is faced with the thought of death, loss of a limb, loss of functioning, loss of a loved one, and so on, Anxiety and Fear may arise as parallel diagnoses with Anticipatory Grieving.

Ineffective Individual Coping
Ineffective Individual Coping is the appropriate diagnosis if the individual is not making the necessary adaptations to deal with the threatened loss. This diagnosis can be a companion diagnosis to Anticipatory Grieving.

Spiritual Distress
When faced with a devastating loss, the client may well express Spiritual Distress. This quite often is a companion diagnosis to Anticipatory Grieving.

EXPECTED OUTCOME

Will identify at least two support systems by [date].

TARGET DATES

A target date ranging from 2 to 4 days would be appropriate in evaluating progress toward achievement of the expected outcome.

NURSING ACTIONS/INTERVENTIONS WITH RATIONALES

Adult Health

For this diagnosis, the Mental Health nursing actions serve as the generic actions. Please see those actions.

Child Health

ACTIONS/INTERVENTIONS	RATIONALES
Spend at least 30 minutes every 8 hours (or as the situation dictates) to address specific anticipated loss by: • Facilitating the patient's and family's expression of perceptions of current situation (may be facilitated by age and developmentally appropriate intervention such as drawing, play, or puppet therapy) • Providing active listening in a quiet, private environment • Offering clarification of procedures, treatment, or plans for the patient and family • Revising plan of care to honor preferences when possible • Discussing and identifying impact of anticipated loss	A structured discussion places value on the importance of grieving and provides critical data for the plan of care.
Collaborate with appropriate health-care professional members to meet needs of the patient and family in realistically anticipating loss.	Appropriate collaboration and coordination of efforts results in more holistic, versus fragmented, care at a time of special need. A sense of support remains long after the event itself.
Encourage the patient and family to realistically develop coping strategies to best prepare for anticipated loss through: • Engaging in diversional activities of choice • Reminiscing of times spent with loved one or associated with anticipated loss • Identification of support groups	Fostering coping strategies provides an opportunity for growth with minimal support from others, thereby increasing empowerment for the family.
Facilitate optimal functioning for as long as possible, with identification of need for proper attention to rest, diet, and health of all family members at this time of stress.	Participation in usual daily activities provides a sense of normalcy despite impending loss and provides validation of life.
Promote parental and sibling participation in care of the infant or child according to situation: • Feedings and selection of menu • Comfort measures such as holding the child or giving backrubs • Diversional activities, quiet games, or stories • Decisions regarding life-support measures and resuscitation	Maintenance of family input and participation in care offers continuation of the family unit at a time when unity can serve to positively influence daily coping for all.
Reassure the infant or child that he or she is loved and cared for, with ample opportunities to answer questions regarding specific anticipated loss, whether related to self or others. According to age and developmental status, provide reassurance that the cause of the situation is not the patient's own doing.	Reassurance lessens the likelihood of guilt, while demonstrating there is no need for assignment of blame to any member of the family.

(care plan continued on page 648)

NURSING ACTIONS/INTERVENTIONS WITH RATIONALES (continued from page 647)

Child Health

ACTIONS/INTERVENTIONS	RATIONALES
Remember that hearing is one of the last of the senses to remain functional. Exercise opportunities for loved ones and staff to continue to address the patient even though the patient may be unable to answer or respond.	Speaking can serve to reassure the child of worth; urge caution in conversations that indicate the child cannot hear.
Provide for appropriate safety and maintenance related to physiologic care of the patient.	Standard practice requires safety maintenance. Special attention is required when the infant or child is comatose or cannot respond regarding sensations, especially for pressure areas, heat, or cold.

Women's Health

ACTIONS/INTERVENTIONS	RATIONALES
Obtain a thorough obstetric history, including previous occurrences of fetal demise.	Provides an essential database needed to plan for effective interventions.
Ascertain whether there were any problems conceiving this pregnancy or any attempts to terminate this pregnancy.	
Assess and record the mother's perception of cessation of fetal movements.	
Monitor and record fetal activity or lack of activity.	
Inform the mother and significant others of antepartal testing and why it is being ordered, and explain results: • Nonstress testing • Oxytocin (Pitocin) challenge test • Ultrasound	
Be considerate and honest in keeping the patient and significant other(s) informed. Share information as soon as it becomes available.	Promotes a trusting relationship and provides support during a very difficult time.
Allow the mother and family to express feelings and begin the grieving process.	Provides support and care to the patient and family, who are unable to begin real grieving because death is not yet real to them while they are going through a "normal" birthing process.
With the collaboration of the physician, facilitate necessary laboratory tests and procedures (e.g., blood tests such as complete blood count, type, and crossmatch; disseminated intravascular coagulation [DIC] screening and coagulation studies; real-time or obstetric ultrasound; or amniotomy).	
Provide emotional support for the couple during labor and the birth process.	
Closely monitor the physiologic process of labor.	
Explain the procedure of induction of labor and the use of Pitocin, IVs, and the uterine contraction pattern.	In instances where fetal death has been ascertained, labor is induced to prevent further complications.
Watch for nausea, vomiting, and diarrhea.	
Provide comfort measures: analgesics, tranquilizers, and medications for side effects, or prostaglandins as ordered	

ACTIONS/INTERVENTIONS	RATIONALES
Change the patient's position at least every 2 hours on [odd/even] hour.	
Observe for full bladder. Record intake and output every 8 hours.	
Provide ice chips for dry mouth, and lip balm or petroleum jelly for dry lips.	
Monitor vital signs every 2 to 4 hours at [times].	
Utilize breathing and relaxation techniques with the patient for comfort.	
Inform the physician of the mother's wishes for use of anesthetic for birth (e.g., awake and aware, sedated, or asleep).	
Prepare the infant for viewing by the mother and significant others: • Clean the infant as much as possible. • Use clothing to hide gross defects, such as a hat for head defects and a T-shirt or diapers for trunk defects. • Wrap in a soft, clean baby blanket (allow the mother to unwrap the infant if she desires).	Initiates the grieving process in a supportive environment. Demonstrates respect for and understanding of the family's emotional state.
Provide a private, quiet place and time for the parents and family to: • See and hold the infant • Take pictures	Provides essential support for the family during time of grief. Provides reality by letting the parents hold the infant.
Provide a certificate with footprints, handprints, lock of hair, armbands, date and time of birth, weight of the infant, and name of the infant.	
Ask the client whether she has a faith community.	Asking about a faith community is less threatening than using the term religion. The client is more likely to respond.
Contact the religious or cultural leader as requested by the mother or significant other. Provide for religious practices such as baptism.	
Provide references to supportive groups within community, such as Resolve with Sharing or Parents of Miscarried Children.	
Explain the need for autopsy or genetic testing of the infant.	
In instances of infertility, assist in realistic planning for the future: • Possible extensive testing • Fear • Economics • Uncertainty • Embarrassment • Surgical procedures • Feelings of inadequacy • Life without children • Adoption	Provides a database that can be used in assisting the couple to cope with situation and initiate realistic planning for the future.

(care plan continued on page 650)

NURSING ACTIONS/INTERVENTIONS WITH RATIONALES (continued from page 649)

Mental Health

● N O T E : *It may take clients anywhere from 6 months to a year or more to grieve a loss. This should be taken into consideration when developing evaluation dates. In a short-stay hospitalization, a reasonable set of goals would be to assist the client system in beginning a healthy grieving process. It is also important to note the anniversary date because grief reaction can be experienced past the 1-year period noted here.*

ACTIONS/INTERVENTIONS	RATIONALES
Assign the client a primary care nurse, and inform client of this decision. This nurse must have a degree of comfort in discussing issues related to loss and grief.	Promotes the development of a trusting relationship.
The primary care nurse will spend 30 minutes once a shift with the client discussing his or her perceptions of the current situation. These discussions could include: • His or her perceptions of the loss • His or her values or beliefs about the lost "object" • Client's past experiences with loss and how these were resolved • The client's perceptions of the support system and possible support system responses to the loss	Promotes the development of a trusting relationship and provides a supportive environment for the expression of feelings, which facilitates a healthy resolution of the loss.
The primary care nurse will schedule 30-minute interactions with the client and support system to assist them in discussing issues related to the loss and answering any questions they might have. [Note time and date of this interaction here.]	
The primary care nurse will discuss with the client and family role adjustments and other anticipated changes related to the loss.	Anticipatory planning facilitates adaptation.
If necessary after the first interaction, the primary care nurse will schedule follow-up visits with the client and his or her support system. [Note schedule for these interactions here.]	
Spend [number] minutes (this should begin as 5-minute sessions, and can increase to 10 minutes as the client needs and unit staffing permit) with the client each hour. If the client does not desire to talk during this time, it can be used to give a massage (backrub) or sit with the client in silence. Inform the client of these times, and let him or her know if for some reason this schedule has to be altered, and develop a new time for the visit. Inform the client that the purpose of this time is for him or her to use as he or she sees fit. The nurse should be seated during this time if he or she is not providing a massage.	Promotes the development of a trusting relationship and the client's sense of control.
Provide positive verbal and nonverbal reinforcement to expressions of grief from both the client and the support system. This would include remaining with the client when he or she is expressing strong emotions.	Positive reinforcement encourages the behavior and enhances self-esteem.
Once the client and the support system are discussing the loss, assist them in scheduling a time when they can be alone with the client.	Facilitates healthy resolution of the loss.

ACTIONS/INTERVENTIONS	RATIONALES
Answer questions in an open, honest manner.	Promotes the development of a trusting relationship and the client's sense of control.
If the client expresses anger toward the staff, and this anger appears to be unrelated to the situation, accept it as part of the grieving process and support the client in its expression by: • Not responding in a defensive manner • Recognizing the feelings that are being expressed (e.g., "It sounds like you are very angry right now," or "It can be very frustrating to be in a situation where you feel you have little control.")	Expression of anger is a normal part of the grieving process, and it is "safer" to be angry with members of the health-care team than with the family.
Recognize that the stages of grief progress at individual rates and in various patterns. Do not "force" a client through stages or express expectations about what the "normal" next step should be.	Supports the client's perception of control and strengths.
If the client is in denial related to the loss, allow this to happen, and provide the client with information about the loss at the client's pace. If the client does not remember information given before, simply provide the information again.	Serves as a way for the client to protect him- or herself from information he or she is not ready to cope with. As coping behaviors are strengthened, the client will be able to accept and respond to this information.
Allow the client and the support system to participate in decisions related to nursing care. Areas in which client decision making is to be encouraged should be noted here along with the client's decisions.	Promotes the client's sense of control and enhances his or her strengths.
Normalize the client's and support system's experience of grief by telling the client that his or her experience is normal, and by discussing with him or her potential future responses to loss.	Promotes the client's sense of control and promotes a positive orientation, which enhances self-esteem.
Recognize that this is an emotionally painful time for the client and the support system, and share this understanding with the client system.	Encourages expression of feelings and facilitates progression through the grieving process.
Assist the client in obtaining the spiritual support needed.	
Monitor the use of sedatives and tranquilizers. Consult with the primary care provider if overuse is suspected.	Extensive use of these medications may delay the grieving process.
Monitor the client system's use of alcohol and nonprescription drugs as a coping method. (Refer to Ineffective Individual Coping in Chapter 11 if this is identified as a problem.)	These are symptoms of ineffective coping and interfere with the normal grieving process.
Have the client and the support system develop a list of concerns and problems, and assist them in determining those they have the ability to change and those they do not.	Promotes the client's strengths.
When they have a list of workable problems, have the client system list all of the solutions they can think of for a problem; encourage them to include those solutions they think are impossible or just fantasy solutions. Do this one problem at a time.	Facilitates creative problem solving by assisting the family to break the "more-of-the-same" problem-solving set.
After solutions have been generated, assist the client in evaluating solutions generated. Solutions can be combined, eliminated, or altered. From this list the best solution is selected. It is important that the solution selected is the client's solution.	Promotes the development of creative problem solutions.

(care plan continued on page 652)

NURSING ACTIONS/INTERVENTIONS WITH RATIONALES (continued from page 651)

Mental Health

ACTIONS/INTERVENTIONS	RATIONALES
Assist the client in developing a plan for implementing this solution. [Note here any assistance needed from the nursing staff.]	Planned coping strategies facilitate the enactment of new behaviors when the client is experiencing stress.
Monitor the client for signs and symptoms of dysfunctional grieving.	Early intervention promotes a positive outcome.
Monitor the client's nutritional pattern, and refer to appropriate nursing diagnoses if a problem is identified.	Nutritional status impacts the individual's ability to cope.
Develop an exercise plan for the client. Consult with the physical therapist as needed. Develop a reward schedule for the accomplishment of this plan. Note the schedule for the plan here. This can also include the support system.	Exercise increases the production of endorphins, which contribute to feelings of well-being.
Provide assistance for the support system by: • Having them develop a schedule for rest periods • Providing snacks for them and scheduling periods of high nursing involvement with the client at a time when support persons can obtain meals. (This can reassure the support person that the client will not be alone while he or she is gone.) • Assisting the support system in finding cafeteria and transportation • Suggesting that support persons rest or walk outside or around hospital while the client is napping • Helping support persons discuss their feelings with the client • Facilitating interaction with client's/significant other's faith community if they feel this will be supportive in coping with the loss.	Support system reactions can impact the client.

Gerontic Health

In addition to the interventions for Adult Health and Mental Health, the following may be utilized with the aging client:

ACTIONS/INTERVENTIONS	RATIONALES
Provide information to the patient regarding what is occurring, and expected or anticipated changes.	This intervention is viewed by survivors as especially helpful during the dying process.[35]
Discuss, with the individual, the grieving process, what can be anticipated, and how each person grieves in his or her own way.	Provides information on common responses to loss and what emotions are commonly experienced by grieving people. Promotes the grieving process and reassures the survivor that he or she is coping well.

Home Health

See Mental Health nursing actions for detailed interventions.

ACTIONS/INTERVENTIONS	RATIONALES
Teach the client and family appropriate monitoring of signs and symptoms of anticipatory grief: • Crying, sadness • Alterations in eating and sleeping patterns • Developmental regression • Alterations in concentration • Expressions of distress at loss • Denial of loss • Expressions of guilt • Labile affect • Grieving beyond expected time • Preoccupation with loss • Hallucinations • Violence toward self or others • Delusions • Prolonged isolation	Provides a database for early recognition and intervention.
Involve the client and family in planning and implementing strategies to reduce or cope with anticipatory grieving: • Family conference: Develop list of concerns and problems; identify those concerns that family can control. • Mutual goal setting: Set short-term realistic goals and evaluation criteria. Specify the role of each member. • Communication: Discuss the loss in a supportive environment.	Family involvement in planning enhances the effectiveness of the plan.
Assist the client and family in lifestyle adjustments that may be required: • Providing realistic hope • Identifying expected grief pattern in response to loss • Recognizing a variety of accepted expressions of grief • Developing and using support networks • Communicating feelings • Providing a safe environment • Therapeutic use of denial • Identifying suicidal potential or potential for violence • Therapeutic use of anger • Exploring meaning of situation • Stress reduction • Promoting expression of grief • Decision making for the future • Promoting family cohesiveness	Permanent changes in behavior and lifestyle are facilitated by knowledge and support.
Assist the client and family to set criteria to help them determine when intervention of a health-care professional is required (e.g., if the client is threat to self or others, or if the client is unable to perform activities of daily living).	Provides data for early intervention.
Consult and/or refer to assistive resources as indicated.	Utilization of existing services is efficient use of resources. Self-help groups, a religious counselor, or a psychiatric nurse clinician can enhance the treatment plan.

GRIEVING, DYSFUNCTIONAL, RISK FOR AND ACTUAL

DEFINITION[9]

Extended, unsuccessful use of intellectual and emotional responses by which individuals, families, or communities attempt to work through the process of modifying self-concept based on the perception of loss.

DEFINING CHARACTERISTICS[9]

1. Persistent anxiety
2. Depression
3. Altered activities of daily living
4. Prolonged difficulty coping
5. Loss-associated sense of despair
6. Intrusive images
7. Feelings of inadequacy
8. Decreased self-esteem
9. Diminished sense of control
10. Dependency
11. Death anxiety
12. Self-criticism

RELATED FACTORS[9]

1. General
   a. Preloss neuroticism
   b. Preloss psychological symptoms
   c. Frequency of major life events
   d. Predisposition for anxiety and feelings of inadequacy
   e. Past psychiatric or mental health treatment
2. Perinatal
   a. Later gestational age at time of loss
   b. Limited time since perinatal loss and subsequent conception
   c. Length of life of infant
   d. Absence of other living children
   e. Congenital anomaly
   f. Number of past perinatal losses
   g. Marital adjustment problems
   h. Viewing of ultrasound images of the fetus

RELATED CLINICAL CONCERNS

1. Cancer
2. Amputation
3. Spinal cord injury
4. Birth defects
5. Any diagnosis that the family has been told has a terminal prognosis
6. Sudden infant death syndrome (SIDS)
7. Stillbirth
8. Infertility
9. Loss of significant object (job, prestige, pet, relationship, etc.)

 Have You Selected the Correct Diagnosis?

Disturbed Sensory Perception
The diagnosis of Disturbed Sensory Perception is identified according to the patient's change in capacity to exercise judgment or think critically with appropriate sensory–perceptual functioning. This may well be related to Dysfunctional Grieving.

Anxiety or Fear
Anxiety is the response the individual has to a threat that is for the most part unidentified. Fear is the response made by an individual to an identified threat. When the patient has experienced a loss, it is not a threat but an actual event. Therefore, the diagnoses of Anxiety and Fear would not be appropriate.

Ineffective Individual Coping
Ineffective Individual Coping can be an appropriate diagnosis if the individual is not making the necessary adaptations to deal with crises in his or her life; however, if a real loss has occurred, the most appropriate diagnosis is Dysfunctional Grieving.

Spiritual Distress
When faced with a devastating loss, the client may well express Spiritual Distress. This quite often is a companion diagnosis to Dysfunctional Grieving.

EXPECTED OUTCOME

Will identify [number] ways to appropriately cope with grief by [date].

TARGET DATES

Grief work should begin within 1 to 2 days after the nurse has intervened; the complete process of grief may take several years.

NURSING ACTIONS/INTERVENTIONS WITH RATIONALES

Adult Health

For this diagnosis, the Mental Health nursing actions serve as the generic actions. Please see Mental Health nursing actions.

Child Health

● N O T E : *It is difficult to make general assumptions as to how each child views death, but according to previous patterns of behavior, including communication, it would be necessary to allow for developmental patterns previously attained. In young children, there may be manifestations of obsessive, ritualistic behavior related to the loss or activities surrounding the loss. For example, if a loved one died, young children may think that if they fall asleep they may also die. In the event of grieving, regardless of the precipitating event, the child must be allowed to respond in keeping with developmental capacity. At times when the child is in danger of self-injury or injuring others, the risk for violence must be considered.*

ACTIONS/INTERVENTIONS	RATIONALES
Provide opportunities for expression of feelings related to loss or grief according to developmental capacity (e.g., puppets or play therapy for toddlers).	Expression of feelings helps the client deal with the sense of loss and provides a database for intervention. Expression of grief reduces uncontrolled outbursts.
In the event of a family member's death, offer support in understanding the deceased family member's relationship to the patient, and status for the family, with special attention to siblings and their reactions. Identify the impact the grief has for family dynamics via monitoring of family dynamics.	Provides a database for more accurate intervention in dealing with the loss.
Allow for cultural and religious input in the plan of care, especially related to care of the dying patient and care of the patient at the time of death.	Demonstrates valuing of these beliefs to the family, and decreases stress for the family.
Collaborate with professionals and paraprofessionals to aid in resolution of grief according to family preferences.	Collaboration offers the most comprehensive plan of care and avoids fragmentation of care.
Identify support groups to assist in resolution of grief, such as Compassionate Friends Organization.	Support groups offer validation of feelings and a sense of hope as similar concerns are shared.
Assist the family members in identification of coping strategies needed for resultant role-relationship changes.	Provides for support during the adjustments that are required because of the loss of a loved one.
Assist the family members to resolve feelings of loss via reminiscing about loved one, positive aspects of situation, or personal growth potential presented. Remember that behavior often serves as the most effective communication for the child or young toddler.	Reminiscing and valuing past experiences will offer an opportunity to project the impact for the present and future.
Allow the family members time and space to face the reality of the situation and ponder the meaning of the loss for self and the family.	Time and readiness promote the willingness to discuss feelings after the major emotional shock has diminished.
Direct the family to appropriate resources regarding positive methods of acknowledging the loved one through memorials or related processes.	A sense of fulfillment may be derived from the sharing of time, talent, or money in honor of the loved one. This affords some sense of resolve of the guilt or emptiness associated with the loss.
Assist in referral to appropriate resources for funeral planning and arrangements if needed.	In times of emotional duress, objective decisions may be difficult. Providing assistance will offer empowerment and a sense of coping.
In the event of SIDS, provide an opportunity, through a scheduled conference, for verbalization of: • How the infant's death occurred • Police investigation • Sense of guilt	

(care plan continued on page 656)

NURSING ACTIONS/INTERVENTIONS WITH RATIONALES (continued from page 655)

Child Health

ACTIONS/INTERVENTIONS	RATIONALES
• Feelings of powerlessness • Questions • Anger • Disbelief • Fears for future pregnancies and birth	
Identify the impact the death or grief has on other family members, the relationship of the couple, and the couple's attitude toward having other children.	Provides the essential database that can assist in planning that will offset the development of dysfunctional grieving.
Make referrals, as appropriate, to psychiatrist, psychologist, mental health nurse clinician, or counselor.	Anticipatory guidance lessens likelihood of unresolved grief.

Dysfunctional Grieving, Risk for

Assess for contributory factors, especially precipitating loss of significant family member, friend, or situational move/catastrophic event.	Provides a relevant base for the plan.
Determine previous coping capacity with input from reliable informants (e.g., the caregiver).	Helps establish a realistic baseline.
Seek input from all primary paraprofessionals including child psychiatrist, psychologist, child life specialist, and nursing specialists during the time of greatest need.	Offers continuity with greater likelihood of trust in the team.
Institute the plan for assisting with those factors that are modifiable with truth and honesty as soon as possible: • Determine actual response versus usual expected response according to all factors surrounding the problem based on previous data, especially the meaning for the anticipated loss in the life of this child. • Set aside time for planning an approach to the problem. • Identify with the child, family, and team strategies for reduction of stress related to anticipated loss.	Provides anticipatory planning, thereby reducing stress with the likelihood of acceptance of the plan with a sense of control.
Honor cultural wishes, especially religious and cultural rituals that enhance positive coping capacity.	Demonstrates cultural sensitivity and increases the likelihood of reduction of sense of loss.
Provide information for the child and family about support groups in the community.	Offers realistic oneness for similar populations, thereby affording hope for acceptance of/dealing with anticipated loss.
Establish a plan for ongoing counseling or assistance after the current episode.	Offers anticipatory guidance to reduce secondary risk.
Reinforce plan of coping with realistic expectations for success using appropriate feedback. For example, for very young children use stickers or some other form of immediate reward.	Reinforces learning.

Women's Health

ACTIONS/INTERVENTIONS	RATIONALES
Schedule a 30-minute daily conference with the couple and focus on: • Expression of grief, anger, guilt, or frustration	Initiates expression of emotions that allows gradual transference through the grief process. Allows clarification of issues related to a pregnancy that has not resulted in a healthy infant.

ACTIONS/INTERVENTIONS	RATIONALES
• Exploring expectations regarding children (e.g., the couple's, relatives', and society's expectations) • Providing factual information (on whichever diagnosis is appropriate) regarding SIDS, stillbirth, or abortion • Encouraging the couple to honestly share feelings with each other During the conference, encourage the couple to ask questions through open-ended questions, reflection, etc.	
Monitor, during hospitalization, for signs and symptoms of depression, anger, frustration, and impending crisis.	Provides the database necessary to permit early intervention and prevention of more serious problems during this crisis.
Encourage the couple to seek professional help, as necessary, to deal with continued concerns, such as their sexual relationship, conflicts, anxieties, parenting, and coping mechanisms that can be used to deal with the loss of fertility.	Fetal demise, SIDS, the decision to have an abortion, and the like all have long-term effects; therefore, long-term support will be required.
Assist the couple, through teaching and provision of written information, to realize that grief may not be resolved for more than a year.	Avoids unrealistic expectations regarding grief resolution.

Mental Health

ACTIONS/INTERVENTIONS	RATIONALES
Monitor the source of the interference with the grieving process.	Early recognition and intervention can facilitate the grieving process.
Monitor the client's use of medications and the effects this may have on the grieving process. Consult with the physician regarding necessary alterations in this area.	Sedatives and tranquilizers may delay the grieving process.
Assign a primary care nurse to the client.	Facilitates the development of a trusting relationship.
Provide a calm, reassuring environment.	Excessive environmental stimuli can increase the client's confusion and disorganization.
When the client is demonstrating an emotional response to the grief, provide privacy and remain with the client during this time.	Encourages appropriate expression of feelings.
The primary care nurse will spend 15 minutes twice a day with the client at [times]. These interactions should begin as nonconfrontational interactions with the client. The goal is to develop a trusting relationship so the client can later discuss issues related to the grieving process. If the client and support system do not identify rituals that would facilitate the grieving process, assist them in developing rituals as appropriate. [Note here the rituals and any assistance needed in completing the ritual.]	Facilitates the development of a trusting relationship. Rituals are most helpful in situations where there is confusion because of incompatible demands.[16]
Monitor the level of dysfunction, and assist the client with activities of daily living as necessary. [Note type and amount of assistance here.]	Facilitates the development of a trusting relationship.
Monitor nutritional status, and refer to Imbalanced Nutrition in Chapter 3 for detailed care plan.	Alterations in nutrition can impact coping abilities, or diminished coping abilities can lead to alterations in nutrition.

(care plan continued on page 658)

NURSING ACTIONS/INTERVENTIONS WITH RATIONALES (continued from page 657)

Mental Health

ACTIONS/INTERVENTIONS	RATIONALES
Monitor significant others' response to the client, and have the primary care nurse set a schedule to meet with them and the client every other day to answer questions and facilitate discussion between the client and the support system. [Note schedule for these meetings here.]	Support system understanding facilitates the maintenance of new behaviors after discharge.
Provide the spiritual/cultural support that the client indicates is necessary. Note here the type of assistance needed from the nursing staff. (Refer to Chapter 12 for clients needing in depth spiritual support.)	Clients may find answers to their questions about life and loss through spiritual/cultural expression.
Allow the client to express anger, and assure him or her that you will not allow harm to come to anyone during this expression.	Violent behavior can evolve from unexpressed anger. Appropriate expression of anger promotes the client's sense of control and enhances self-esteem.
Provide the client with punching bags and other physical activity that assists with the expression of anger. [Note tools preferred by this client here. Note the specific activities that assist this client with this expression here.]	Assists the client in developing appropriate coping behaviors that enhance self-esteem.
Remind the staff and support system that the client's expressions of anger at this point should not be taken personally, even though they may be directed at these persons.	Support system understanding facilitates the maintenance of new behaviors after discharge.
Answer questions directly and honestly.	Promotes the development of a trusting relationship.
Provide the time and opportunity for the client to participate in appropriate religious rituals. [Note here assistance needed from nursing staff.]	Rituals provide clarity and direction for the grieving process.
Sit with the client and listen attentively while he or she is talking about the lost object.	The presence of the nurse provides positive reinforcement, which encourages the behavior.
When the client's verbal interactions increase with the primary care nurse to the level that group interactions are possible, schedule the client to participate in a group that allows expression of feelings and feedback from peers. [Note the schedule of the group here.]	Provides opportunities for peer feedback and peer assistance with problem solving.
Assign the client appropriate tasks in unit activities. Note type of tasks assigned here. These should be based on the client's level of functioning and should be at a level that the client can accomplish. [Note type of tasks to be assigned to the client here.]	Successful accomplishment of tasks enhances self-esteem.
If delusions, hallucinations, phobias, or depression are present, refer to Ineffective Individual Coping in Chapter 11, and Disturbed Thought Process in Chapter 7. Some persons in active functional grief may experience hallucinations of the lost person. Tell them that this is common and subsides as their grief is resolved.	
The primary care nurse will engage the client and the support system in planning for lifestyle changes that might result from the loss. [Note the schedule for these interactions here, along with the specific goals.]	Planned coping strategies facilitate the enactment of new behaviors when the client is experiencing stress, which enhances self-esteem.
Refer the client and family to community resources that support grieving individuals (e.g., hospice, faith communities, and grief centers).	These resources will provide ongoing support when the client is discharged.

Gerontic Health

ACTIONS/INTERVENTIONS	RATIONALES
Carefully assess the client for risk of self-harm. Should a risk for self harm be determined, please move directly to Violence: Risk for Self-Harm interventions.	Prevention of complications.
Listen to the client when they are ready to talk; avoid the temptation to offer advice or opinions and focus on listening.	Listening is an essential source of support.[36]
Access additional resources as appropriate to the client to include: • Chaplain • Psychiatrist • Physician • Social services • Palliative clinical nurse specialist	Collaboration with the interdisciplinary team provides the most comprehensive client care.[36]
Avoid artificial positivism. Accept the client's negative feelings.	Individualizes care and acknowledges the client's feelings.[37]

Home Health/Community Health

● NOTE: *The interventions listed here are geared toward a community experiencing complicated grief. This type of community grief is most likely to occur following a disaster (natural disaster, terrorist attack). The course of bereavement in a community often follows that of the bereaved individual. The nurse may observe an increase in suicide or suicidal ideation, drug and alcohol misuse or abuse, and worsening of preexisting health problems among members of the community.*

ACTIONS/INTERVENTIONS	RATIONALES
Assist community leaders in arranging grief support groups and grief counseling.	Prevention of complications.[38]
Provide information to the community about grief and its symptoms, course, and complications.	Allows the clients to know what to expect. Helps the client to identify complications.[38]
Educate community health-care providers about assessment and management of depression.	Depression is a common effect of grief and care providers should be equipped to identify and treat it.[38]
Educate community health-care providers about assessment and management of Post Traumatic Stress Syndrome (PTSD).	PTSD is a common effect of grief and care providers should be equipped to identify and treat it.[38]

PARENT, INFANT, AND CHILD ATTACHMENT, IMPAIRED, RISK FOR

DEFINITION[9]

Disruption of the interactive process between parent, or significant other, and infant that fosters the development of a protective and nurturing reciprocal relationship.

RISK FACTORS[9]

1. Physical barriers
2. Anxiety associated with the parent role
3. Substance abuse
4. Premature infant, ill infant, or child who is unable to effectively initiate parental contact as a result of altered behavioral organization
5. Lack of privacy
6. Inability of parents to meet personal needs
7. Separation

RELATED FACTORS[9]

The risk factors also serve as the related factors.

RELATED CLINICAL CONCERNS

1. Premature infant
2. Chronically ill child
3. Chronically ill parent

4. Mental retardation
5. Maternal complications and illness during pregnancy and birth

 Have You Selected the Correct Diagnosis?

Interrupted Family Processes
Interrupted Family Processes is an actual diagnosis and would be used if there were an actual problem with attachment.

Impaired Parenting
Again, this is an actual diagnosis. Risk for Impaired Parenting occurs beyond the attachment phase.

EXPECTED OUTCOME

Will make [number] positive statements about infant in 30-minute conversation by [date].
> Will smile and vocalize to infant by [date].
> Will respond appropriately to infant cues by [date].

TARGET DATES

This diagnosis will require time periods that are longer than those for other diagnoses to reduce the risk factors. An appropriate initial target date would be 5 to 7 days.

NURSING ACTIONS/INTERVENTIONS WITH RATIONALES

Adult Health

ACTIONS/INTERVENTIONS	RATIONALES
Make arrangement, when possible, for the patient to interact with the infant or child. Provide privacy, but remain nearby during parent–child interactions.	Provides an opportunity to practice parenting skills and obtain feedback in a supportive environment.
Facilitate referral for the patient with substance-abuse problem, including counseling, treatment, and support groups; initiate referrals as needed.	Provides long-term support and assistance.
Collaborate with the patient in developing a schedule that provides time for care of the infant or child, as well as time for self.	Helps the patient not to get overwhelmed with activities needed to care for the infant or child.
Allow the patient to talk about anxiety with parenting. Teach stress management and alternate coping strategies.	Provides alternate strategies for coping.
Have the child health clinical nurse specialist, or pediatric nurse practitioner, teach parenting skills and growth and development of premature infant.	Provides a knowledge base, and helps the patient know that some of the things he or she is experiencing are normal.

Child Health

ACTIONS/INTERVENTIONS	RATIONALES
Monitor for factors regarding the infant that contribute to or influence maternal or paternal or parent or infant reciprocity: • Inability to send cues for needs • Inability of the mother or father to attend to cues appropriately and in a timely manner. • Inability of the mother or father to comfort the infant • Mismatch of temperament of the infant to the mother or father • Parental verbalization of feelings about the infant less than ideal for appropriate bonding Explore actual parent–infant interactions and note strengths and deficits.	A thorough assessment of reciprocal behaviors will serve as a guide to specific needs of parent–infant dyad. Provides major concepts of maternal sensitivity that are antecedents to infant attachment.[39]

ACTIONS/INTERVENTIONS	RATIONALES
Identify behaviors so unsafe as to suggest the need for separation of the infant from the parent, that is, physical or emotional abuse. (Involve Child Protective Services according to protocols for location; a hotline is available nationally.)	Safety and legal needs will help protect the infant in an unsafe relationship.
Offer role modeling and parenting teaching modules at readiness of the parents and when deemed suitable to do so: • Normal growth and development • Special care for the infant	Often new parenting roles must be acquired as there may be no suitable role modeling in the parent's own childhood.[40]
When the parents must be absent, maintain communication that is consistent, ideally with the same few individuals, to maintain long-term relationship.	Trust and sincerity will support the parents in this demanding role.
Involve appropriate support services as indicated in a timely manner (e.g., Ronald McDonald House for lodging, and local social services agencies).	Support during the time of need will enable the parents to be near the infant as much as possible.
Ensure appropriate counseling and follow-up for all members as may be deemed essential.	Long-term goals are best established during the acute phase of the crisis.

Women's Health

ACTIONS/INTERVENTIONS	RATIONALES
Pregnancy Encourage the expectant parents to discuss their perceptions and expectations of the pregnancy.	Allows expectant parents to progress through pregnancy in a satisfactory and satisfying manner. Provides a knowledge base, and helps the parents know that what they are experiencing is normal.[39,40]
Provide a nonthreatening atmosphere to encourage the parents to discuss their fears and concerns.	
Assist the parents to dispel myths about birth, the postpartum period, and early parenthood.	
Assist the parents to plan for changes in financial requirements of pregnancy, birth, and early parenthood.	
Encourage the parents to talk to the fetus, spend time together feeling the fetus move, etc.	
Encourage attendance in various classes that can assist in the transition to parenthood.	
Assist the parents in identifying community resources available to expectant and new parents.	
Parenthood[39–42] Encourage the new parents to touch, talk to, and observe the newborn as soon as possible (immediately is best).	Allows time for new parents to become acquainted with their newborn, learn the infant's cues, and begin to respond to the needs of the infant.[40,41]
Encourage comparison of newborn characteristics to those of the fantasized newborn.	

Mental Health

Nursing actions for this diagnosis can be found in Child Health and Women's Health care plans.

(care plan continued on page 662)

NURSING ACTIONS/INTERVENTIONS WITH RATIONALES (continued from page 661)

Gerontic Health

This diagnosis is not appropriate to use with gerontic clients.

Home Health

ACTIONS/INTERVENTIONS	RATIONALES
Involve the client and family in planning and implementing strategies to decrease or prevent alterations in attachment: • Identify family strengths and weaknesses. • Design strategies to support strengths and correct weaknesses. • Provide a safe environment.	Family involvement enhances the effectiveness of the intervention.
Teach parenting strategies and techniques to enhance parent–child interactions. • Appropriate stimulation for the child • Consistent approach to parenting	Parenting is learned behavior.
Consult with or refer to community resources as required.	Provides efficient use of existing resources.

PARENTING, IMPAIRED, RISK FOR AND ACTUAL, READINESS FOR ENHANCED AND PARENTAL ROLE CONFLICT

DEFINITIONS[9]

Risk for Impaired Parenting   Risk for inability of the primary caretaker to create, maintain, or regain an environment that promotes the optimum growth and development of a child.*

   Impaired Parenting   Inability of the primary caretaker to create, maintain, or regain an environment that promotes the optimum growth and development of a child.*

   Parenting, Readiness for Enhanced   A pattern of providing and environment for children or other dependent person(s) that is sufficient to nurture growth and development and can be strengthened.

   Parental Role Conflict   Parent experience of role confusion and conflict in response to crisis.

DEFINING CHARACTERISTICS[9]

A. Risk for Impaired Parenting (Risk Factors)
   1. Social
      a. Marital conflict and/or declining satisfaction
      b. History of being abused

      c. Poor problem-solving skills
      d. Role strain or overload
      e. Social isolation
      f. Legal difficulties
      g. Lack of access to resources
      h. Lack of value of parenthood
      i. Relocation
      j. Poverty
      k. Poor home environment
      l. Lack of family cohesiveness
      m. Lack of or poor parental role model
      n. Father of child not involved
      o. History of being abusive
      p. Financial difficulties
      q. Low self-esteem
      r. Unplanned or unwanted pregnancy
      s. Inadequate child care arrangements
      t. Maladaptive coping strategies
      u. Lack of resources
      v. Low socioeconomic class
      w. Lack of transportation
      x. Change in family unit
      y. Unemployment or job problems
      z. Single parent
      aa. Lack of social support network
      bb. Inability to put child's needs before own
      cc. Stress
   2. Knowledge
      a. Low educational level or attainment

---

*It is important to state as a preface to this diagnosis that adjustment to parenting in general is a normal maturational process that elicits nursing behaviors of prevention of potential problems and health promotion.

b. Unrealistic expectations of child

c. Lack of knowledge about parenting skills

d. Poor communication skills

e. Preference for physical punishment

f. Inability to recognize and act on infant care

g. Low cognitive functioning

h. Lack of knowledge about child health maintenance

i. Lack of knowledge about child development

j. Lack of cognitive readiness for parenthood

3. Physiologic

a. Physical illness

4. Infant or Child

a. Multiple births

b. Handicapping condition or developmental delay

c. Illness

d. Altered perceptual abilities

e. Lack of goodness of fit (temperament) with parental expectations

f. Unplanned or unwanted child

g. Premature birth

h. Not gender desired

i. Difficult temperament

j. Attention deficit hyperactivity disorder

k. Prolonged separation from parent

l. Separation from parent at birth

5. Psychological

a. Separation from infant or child

b. High number of or closely spaced children

c. Disability

d. Sleep deprivation or disruption

e. Difficult labor and/or delivery

f. Young ages, especially adolescent

g. Depression

h. History of mental illness

i. Lack of or late, prenatal care

j. History of substance abuse or dependence

B. Impaired Parenting

1. Infant or child

a. Poor academic performance

b. Frequent illness

c. Runaway

d. Incidence of physical and psychological trauma or abuse

e. Frequent accidents

f. Lack of attachments

g. Failure to thrive

h. Behavioral disorders

i. Poor social competence

j. Lack of separation anxiety

k. Poor cognitive development

2. Parental

a. Inappropriate child care arrangements

b. Rejection or hostility to child

c. Statements of inability to meet child's needs

d. Inflexibility to meet needs of child or situation

e. Poor or inappropriate caretaking skills

f. Frequently punitive

g. Inconsistent care

h. Child abuse

i. Inadequate child health maintenance

j. Unsafe home environment

k. Verbalization of inability to control child

l. Negative statements about child

m. Verbalization of role inadequacy frustration

n. Abandonment

o. Insecure or lack of attachment to infant

p. Inconsistent behavior management

q. Child neglect

r. Little cuddling

s. Maternal–child interaction deficit

t. Poor parent–child interaction

u. Inappropriate visual, tactile, or auditory stimulation

C. Parenting, Readiness for Enhanced

1. Expresses willingness to enhance parenting

2. Children or other dependent person(s) express satisfaction with home environment

3. Emotional and tacit support of children or dependent person(s) is evident; bonding or attachment evident

4. Physical and emotional needs of children/dependent person(s) are met

5. Realistic expectations of children/dependent person(s) exhibited

D. Parental Role Conflict

1. Parent(s) express concerns about changes in parental role, family functioning, family communication, or family health

2. Parent(s) express concerns or feelings of inadequacy to provide for child's physical and emotional needs during hospitalization or in the home

3. Demonstrated disruption in caretaking routines

4. Expresses concern about perceived loss of control over decisions relating to his or her child

5. Reluctant to participate in usual caretaking activities even with encouragement and support

6. Verbalizes and/or demonstrates feelings of guilt, anger, fear, anxiety, and/or frustration about the effect of the child's illness on family process

RELATED FACTORS[9]

A. Risk for Impaired Parenting

The defining characteristics (risk factors) also serve as the related factors.

B. Impaired Parenting

1. Social

a. Lack of access to resources

b. Social isolation

c. Lack of resources

d. Poor home environment

   e. Lack of family cohesiveness
   f. Inadequate child care arrangements
   g. Lack of transportation
   h. Unemployment or job problems
   i. Role strain or overload
   j. Marital conflict, declining satisfaction
   k. Lack of value of parenthood
   l. Change in the family unit
  m. Low socioeconomic class
   n. Unplanned or unwanted pregnancy
   o. Presence of stress (e.g., financial, legal, recent crisis, and cultural move)
   p. Lack of, or poor, role model
   q. Single parents
   r. Lack of social support network
   s. Father of child not involved
   t. History of being abusive
   u. Financial difficulties
   v. Maladaptive coping strategies
   w. Poverty
   x. Poor problem-solving skills
   y. Inability to put child's needs before own
   z. Low self-esteem
  aa. Relocation
  bb. Legal difficulties
  cc. History of being abused

2. Knowledge
   a. Lack of knowledge about child health maintenance
   b. Lack of knowledge about parenting skills
   c. Unrealistic expectations for self, infant, and partner
   d. Limited cognitive functioning
   e. Lack of knowledge about child development
   f. Inability to recognize and act on infant cues
   g. Low educational level or attainment
   h. Poor communication skills
   i. Lack of cognitive readiness for parenthood
   j. Preference for physical punishment

3. Physiologic
   a. Physical illness

4. Infant or child
   a. Premature birth
   b. Illness
   c. Prolonged separation from parent
   d. Not gender desired
   e. Attention deficit hyperactivity disorder
   f. Difficult temperament
   g. Separation from parent at birth
   h. Lack of goodness of fit (temperament) with parental expectations
   i. Unplanned or unwanted child
   j. Handicapping condition or developmental delay
   k. Multiple births
   l. Altered perceptual abilities

5. Psychological
   a. History of substance abuse or dependencies

   b. Disability
   c. Depression
   d. Difficult labor and/or delivery
   e. Young age, especially adolescent
   f. History of mental illness
   g. High number of or closely spaced pregnancies
   h. Sleep deprivation or disruption
   i. Lack of, or late, prenatal care
   j. Separation from infant or child
   k. Multiple births

C. Parenting, Readiness for Enhanced
  Not provided for wellness diagnoses.

D. Parental Role Conflict
1. Change in marital status
2. Home care of a child with special needs (e.g., apnea monitoring, postural drainage, or hyperalimentation)
3. Interruptions of family life as a result of home care regimen (treatments, caregivers, or lack of respite)
4. Specialized care centers policies
5. Separation from child as a result of chronic illness
6. Intimidation with invasive or restrictive modalities (e.g., isolation or intubation)

RELATED CLINICAL CONCERNS

1. Birth defect
2. Multiple births
3. Chronically ill child
4. Substance abuse
5. Parental chronic illness
6. Major depressive episode
7. Manic episode
8. Phobic disorders
9. Dissociative disorders
10. Organic mental disorders
11. Schizophrenic disorders

☑ Have You Selected the Correct Diagnosis?

Interrupted Family Processes
The diagnosis of Interrupted Family Processes indicates dysfunctioning on part of the entire family, not just the parents. If the entire family is indicating difficulties dealing with current problems or crises, then Interrupted Family Processes is a more correct diagnosis than one of the Parenting diagnoses, which is related to the parents only.

Compromised or Disabled Family Coping
The diagnosis of Compromised Disabled Family Coping usually arises from the client's perspective that his or her primary support is no longer fulfilling this role. If the problem relates to parents and their child(ren), then one of the Parenting diagnoses is the most appropriate diagnosis.

EXPECTED OUTCOME

Will demonstrate appropriate parental role of [specify exactly what, e.g., feeding or medication administration] behavior by [date].

Will verbalize satisfaction with parental role by [date].

Parent verbalizes appropriate developmental expectations of child by [date].

Parent develops developmentally appropriate plan to meet child's needs by [date].

TARGET DATES

The diagnosis will require a lengthy amount of time to be totally resolved. However, progress toward resolutions could be evaluated within 7 days.

NURSING ACTIONS/INTERVENTIONS WITH RATIONALES

Adult Health

ACTIONS/INTERVENTIONS	RATIONALES
Assist the patient in assessing the home environment.	Identifies areas that require strengthening to meet primary needs.
Assist the patient in identifying areas that will strengthen the parenting role.	Will facilitate aligning the patient with appropriate resources.
Initiate a dialogue with the patient to discern the perception of expectations of role. Discuss the patient's perception of the impact of change in life role. Provide anticipatory guidance for the patient in regard to life changes.	Lends insight into potential areas of role strain.
Refer the patient to community resources that supplement finances, assist nutrition, or provide social support.	Can assist in reducing common stressors that can cause strain.
Provide information relative to normal growth and development of self and the child by sitting and talking with the patient for 30 minutes twice a day at [times].	Provides a knowledge base, and assists the patient to know that some of the things he or she is experiencing are normal.
Assist the parent to recognize when stress is becoming distress (e.g., irritability turns to rage and/or verbal or physical abuse, sleeplessness, disturbed thought process, or tunnel perception of situation).	Prevents a crisis situation. Promotes self-knowledge.
Teach stress management and parenting techniques (e.g., relaxation, deep breathing, Mother's Day Out, safety precautions, or toileting process).	Provides strategies for coping and information integral to parenting.
Provide opportunities for the parent to gradually assume the caregiver role with adequate support.	Provides an opportunity to practice parenting skills and obtain feedback in a supportive environment.
Discuss disciplinary methods other than physical (e.g., grounding, time out, positive reinforcement, and verbal praise for "good" behavior).	Physical discipline can lead to abuse; sends wrong message to the child.
Convey the necessity for the patient to meet his or her own needs.	Own needs must be met to decrease stress and facilitate meeting the needs of others.
Develop an emergency contact system.	
Refer the patient to support groups. Initiate referrals as needed.	Provides an outlet for the parents with other parents in similar situations. Provides long-term support and assistance.

Parenting, Readiness for Enhanced

Assist the patient in ongoing efforts to provide an environment suitable for dependents and maintaining safety. [Note assistance needed from the health-care team here, e.g., contacting social services, referring to community resources.]

(care plan continued on page 666)

NURSING ACTIONS/INTERVENTIONS WITH RATIONALES (continued from page 665)

Adult Health

ACTIONS/INTERVENTIONS	RATIONALES
Discuss with the patient strategies to meet Their emotional needs. [Note that plan here with the assistance needed from the health care team to implement.]	Self-care is an essential foundation for being supportive to others.
Explore the patient's feelings regarding the parenting role. Address any areas of concern. [Note plan for addressing these concerns here.]	

Child Health

ACTIONS/INTERVENTIONS	RATIONALES
Review current level of knowledge regarding parenting of the infant or child to include: • Parental perception of the infant or child • Parental views of expected development of the infant or child • Health status of the infant or child • Current needs of the infant or child • Infant or child communication (remember, behaviors reveal much about feelings) • Infant's or child's usual responsiveness • Family dynamics (e.g., who offers support for emotional needs or the child's view of mother and father)	Provides a database needed to accurately plan care.
Determine needs for specific health or developmental intervention from other health-care providers as needed.	Needs may be identified with assistance from experts in multidisciplinary domains. Collaboration is essential to avoid fragmentation of care.
Observe parental readiness, and encourage caretaking in a supportive atmosphere in the following ways, as applicable: • Feeding • Bathing • Anticipatory safety measures • Clarification of medical or health maintenance regimen • Play and developmental stimulations for age and capacity • Handling and carriage of the infant or child • Diapering and dressing of the infant or child • Social interaction appropriate for age and capacity • Other specific measures according to the patient's status and needs	Provides data needed to plan teaching and to provide individualization of the plan of care.
Schedule a daily conference of at least 1 hour with the parents, and encourage the parents to verbalize perceived parenting role, both current and desired.	Provides a teaching opportunity. Verbalization reveals thoughts and data needed to more accurately plan care.
Allow the parents to gradually assume total care of the infant within the hospital setting at least 48 hours before dismissal. If more time is required to validate appropriate parenting success, collaborate with the pediatrician regarding extending the child's stay for 24 hours.	Provides an opportunity for practice of needed skills or roles; fosters growth and confidence in parenting.

ACTIONS/INTERVENTIONS	RATIONALES
Readiness for Enhanced	This is a wellness concept and, as such, the health-care provider should be a resource and support for the parents, providing them with correct information and helping them sort out the appropriate information about parenting.
Provide parents with resources for information and support in the early days of parenting. • Parenting classes • Parenting support groups • Being available to help translate and sort out information if needed.	

Women's Health

ACTIONS/INTERVENTIONS	RATIONALES

Assist the patient, through monthly conferences, in completing the tasks of pregnancy by encouraging verbalization of:
• Fears
• The mother's perception of marriage
• The mother's perception of the "child within" her
• The mother's perception of the changes in her life as a result of this birth:
  • Relationship with the partner
  • Relationship with other children
  • Effects on career
  • Effects on family
Allow the mother to question the pregnancy: "Now" and "Who, me?"[42]
	Acceptance of pregnancy and working through the tasks of pregnancy provide a strong basis for positive parenthood and appropriate attachment and bonding.[39–42]

Assist the mother in realizing the existence of the child by encouraging the mother to: • Note when the infant moves. • Listen to fetal heart tones during the visit to the clinic. • Discuss body changes and their relationship to the infant. • Verbalize any questions she may have. Assist in preparation for birth by: • Encouraging attendance at childbirth education classes • Providing factual information regarding the birthing experience • Involving significant others in preparation for birthing process Assist the patient in preparing for role transition to parenthood by encouraging: • Economic planning (e.g., physician, hospital, or prenatal testing fees) • Social planning (e.g., changes in lifestyle)	Provides a basis for appropriate attachment behaviors and coping skills for transition to the maternal role.
Assist the patient in identifying needs related to the family's acceptance of the newborn: • Mother's perceived level of support from family members	Assists in identifying patients at high risk for the development of this diagnosis.

(care plan continued on page 668)

NURSING ACTIONS/INTERVENTIONS WITH RATIONALES (continued from page 667)

Women's Health

ACTIONS/INTERVENTIONS	RATIONALES
• Stressors present in the family (e.g., economics, housing, or level of knowledge regarding parenting)	
Monitor for the following behaviors:	
• Refuses to plan for the infant	
• No interest in pregnancy or fetal progress	
• Overly concerned with own weight and appearance	
• Refuses to gain weight (diets during pregnancy)	
• Negative comments about "What this baby is doing to me!"	
Postpartum	
Assist the patient and significant others in establishing realistic goals for integration of the baby into the family.	
Provide positive reinforcement for parenting tasks:	Promotes realistic planning for the new baby as well as bonding and attachment.[39–42]
• Encourage use of birthing room: labor, delivery, and recovery (LDR) room and labor, delivery, recovery, and postpartum (LDRP) rooms—for birth to allow active participation in birth process by both parents.	
• Allow the mother and partner time with the infant (do not remove to nursery if stable) after delivery.	
• Provide mother–baby care to allow maximum continuity of mother–infant contact and nursing care.	
Assist the parents in identifying different kinds of infant behavior and understanding how they allow the infant to communicate with them:	Provides the parents with essential information they need to care for the infant.
• Perform gestational age assessment with the parents, and explain the significance of the findings.	
• Perform Brazelton neonatal assessment with the parents, and explain the significance of the findings.	Teaches parents to recognize their infant's cues and how to respond to them. This interaction between parent and infant is a major factor in the brain development of the infant.
• Demonstrate how to hold the infant for maximum communication.	
• Explain infant reflexes (e.g., rooting or Moro) and the importance of understanding them.	
Assist the parents in identifying support systems:	
• Friends from childbirth classes	
• Parents and parents-in-law	
• Siblings	
• Nurse specialists	
Encourage the parents to reminisce about the birthing experience.	
Assist the patient in identifying needs related to family functioning:	Provides the database needed for planning to offset factors that would result in ineffective parenting.[39–42]
Identify negative maternal behavior:	
• No interest in the new baby	
• Talks *excessively* to friends on the telephone	
• Is more interested in TV than in feeding the infant	
• Refuses to listen to infant teaching	

ACTIONS/INTERVENTIONS	RATIONALES

• Asks no questions
• *Extraordinary* interest in self-appearance:
  • *Severe dieting* to gain pre-pregnancy figure
  • *Overutilization* of exercise to gain pre-pregnancy figure
• Crying, moodiness
• Lack of interest in the family and other children
• Failure to perform physical care for the infant
• Noncompliance: Breaks appointments with health-care providers for self and the infant
Identify negative paternal behavior:
• Refusal to support wife by:
  • Not assisting in child care
  • Not sharing household tasks
  • Keeping "his" social contacts and going out while the wife remains at home with the child
• Not providing financial support
• Abandonment	

Assist the patient in identifying methods of coping with stress of the newborn in the family: • Seek professional help from the nurse specialist, physician (obstetrician or pediatrician), or psychiatrist • Identify the support system in the family or among friends • Refer to appropriate community or private agencies	Provides long-term support.
Readiness for Enhanced	This is a wellness concept and as such the health-care provider should be a resource and support for the parents, providing them with correct information and helping them sort out the appropriate information about parenting.
Provide parents with resources for information and support in the early days of parenting. • Parenting classes • Parenting support groups • Being available to help translate and sort out information if needed.	

Mental Health

ACTIONS/INTERVENTIONS	RATIONALES
Monitor the degree to which drugs and alcohol interfere with the parenting process. If this is a factor, discuss a treatment program with the client.	Early intervention and treatment increase the likelihood of a positive outcome.
Ask the client who is caring for the children while he or she is hospitalized, and assess his or her level of comfort with this arrangement. If a satisfactory arrangement is not present, refer to social services so arrangements can be made.	Early intervention and treatment increase the likelihood of a positive outcome.
Discuss with the client expectations and problem perception.	Promotes the client's sense of control.

(care plan continued on page 670)

NURSING ACTIONS/INTERVENTIONS WITH RATIONALES (continued from page 669)

Mental Health

ACTIONS/INTERVENTIONS	RATIONALES
Have the client identify support systems, and gain permission to include these persons in the treatment plan as necessary. This could include spouse, parents, close friends, etc.	Support system understanding facilitates the maintenance of behaviors after discharge.
If the client desires to maintain parenting role, arrange to have the children visit during hospitalization. Assign a staff member to remain with the client during these visits. The staff person can serve as a role model for the client and facilitate communication between the child and the client. [Note schedule for these visits here and the staff person responsible for the supervision of these interactions.]	A continuous relationship between the parent and the child is necessary for the normal development of the child.[43]
Answer the client's questions in a clear, direct manner.	Promotes the development of a trusting relationship.
Spend 15 minutes twice a day at [times] with the client discussing his or her perception of the parenting role and his or her expectations for self and the children.	Promotes the development of a trusting relationship, and provides information abut the client's worldview that can be utilized in constructing interventions.
Arrange 30 minutes a day for interaction between the client and one member of the support system. A staff member is to be present during these interactions to facilitate communication and focus the discussion on parenting issues.	Supports the maintenance of these relationships, and provides opportunities for the nurse to do positive role modeling.
Provide the client with information on normal growth and development and normal feelings of the parents. Provide the client with concrete information about building age-appropriate developmental assets. This could include setting appropriate boundaries, providing appropriate support, and constructive use of time.[44]	Provides information that will assist the client in making appropriate parenting decisions, enhancing self-esteem. Provides parents with specific strategies for affirmation of parent and child interactions that support positive child development.
Assist the client in developing a plan for disciplining the children. This plan should be based on behavioral interventions, and the primary focus should be on positive social rewards.[44]	Facilitates the development of positive coping behaviors and promotes a positive expectational set.
Teach the client ways of interacting with the child that reduce levels of conflict (e.g., providing the child with limited choices, spending scheduled time with the child, and listening carefully to the child).	Promotes positive orientation and enhances self-esteem.
Encourage the client to maintain telephone contact with the children by providing a telephone and establishing a regular time for the client to call home, or have the children call the hospital.	Assists in maintaining these important relationships to make the transition home easier.
Encourage the support system to continue to include the client in decisions related to the children by having them bring up these issues in daily visits, and by assisting the client and the support system to engage in collaborative decision making regarding these issues.	Assists in maintaining the client's role functioning, thus enhancing self-esteem.
Have the client identify parenting models, and discuss the effect these persons had on their current parenting style.	

ACTIONS/INTERVENTIONS	RATIONALES
Observe the interaction between the parents to assess for problems in the husband–wife relationship that may be expressed in the parenting relationship. If this appears to be happening, refer the parents to family therapy.	Children can be triangled into parental conflicts in an unconscious effort to preserve the marital relationship.[22,45]
Have the client develop a list of problem behavior patterns, and then assist him or her in developing a list of alternative behavior patterns. For example, Current: When I get frustrated with my child, I spank him with a belt. New: When I get frustrated with my child, I arrange to send him to the neighbors for 30 minutes while I take a walk around the block to calm down.	Promotes the client's sense of control and begins the development of alternative, more adaptive coping behaviors.
Role-play with the client situations that are identified as being most difficult, and provide opportunities to practice more appropriate behavior. This should be done daily in 30-minute time periods. Note the schedule for this activity here, list time periods, and list situations that are to be practiced. It would be useful to include the spouse.	Behavioral rehearsal provides opportunities for feedback and modeling of new behaviors by the nurse.
Have the client attend group sessions where feelings and thoughts can be expressed to peers and the thoughts and feelings of peers can be heard. [Note the schedule for the group here.]	Assists the client to experience personal importance to others, while enhancing interpersonal relationship skills. Increasing these competencies can enhance self-esteem and promote positive orientation.
Assist the client in identifying personal needs and in developing a plan for meeting these needs at home. For example, the parents will exchange babysitting time with neighbors so they can have an evening out once a month. [Note this plan here.]	Assists the parents to develop strategies for coping with role strain.
Monitor staff attitudes toward the client, and allow them to express feelings, especially if child abuse is an issue with this client.	Negative attitudes of staff can be communicated to the client, decreasing the client's self-esteem and increasing the client's defensiveness.
Assist the client with grieving separation from the child, and refer to Anticipatory Grieving for detailed nursing actions.	
Provide the client with positive verbal support for positive parenting behavior and for progress on behavior change goal. For example, "You demonstrate a great deal of concern for your child's welfare," or "You have taught your child to be very sensitive." Make sure these comments are honest and fit the client's awareness of the situation.	Positive reinforcement encourages behavior and enhances self-esteem.
Assist the client in developing stress reduction skills by: • Teaching deep muscle relaxation and practicing this with the client 30 minutes a day at [time]. • Discussing with the client the role physical exercise plays in stress reduction and developing a plan for exercise. [Note plan and type of exercise here.] Have the staff member remain with the client during these exercise periods. [Note time for these periods here.]	
When the client's level of tension or anxiety is rising on the unit, remind him or her of the exercise or relaxation technique, and work through one of these with him or her.	

(care plan continued on page 672)

NURSING ACTIONS/INTERVENTIONS WITH RATIONALES (continued from page 671)

Mental Health

ACTIONS/INTERVENTIONS	RATIONALES
Observe the interaction between the parents to monitor for problems in the parental dyad that may be expressed in the parenting relationship with the children. If this appears to be happening, refer the patient to family therapy.	Conflict in one part of the family system can impact interactions in other parts of the system.

Readiness for Enhanced

ACTIONS/INTERVENTIONS	RATIONALES
Spend time with the client identifying areas they want to enhance and develop a plan to meet these needs. [Note that plan here.]	Change is dependent on client's perception of the problem.
Refer to community programs that focus on positive skill building such as Couples Communication and Parent Effectiveness Training, Developmental Assets programs (Search Institute).	
Spend [number] minutes with parents identifying positive family activities and establishing a schedule for participation.	Promotes positive family affect and enhances focus on family strengths.[23]
Identify with parents community organizations that share their values and can assist with their ongoing development (e.g., faith communities, youth groups, Developmental Assets Programs)	
Refer to community programs that focus on positive skill building such as Couples Communication and Parent Effectiveness Training, and Developmental Assets programs (Search Institute).	

Gerontic Health

● N O T E : *This would be an unusual diagnosis for the gerontic patient, but might develop if the grandparents had to take grandchildren into their home as a result of a family crisis. In that instance, the nursing actions would be the same as those given in Adult Health and Child Health.*

Home Health

ACTIONS/INTERVENTIONS	RATIONALES
Act as role model through use of positive behaviors when interacting with the child and parents.	Role modeling provides an example for parenting skills.
Report child abuse and neglect to the appropriate authorities.	Meets legal requirements and provides for intervention.
Teach the client and family appropriate information regarding the care and discipline of children: • Cultural norms • Normal growth and development • Anticipatory guidance regarding psychosocial, cognitive, and physical needs for children and parents • Expected family life cycles	Knowledge is necessary to provide appropriate child care.

ACTIONS/INTERVENTIONS	RATIONALES
• Development and use of support networks • Safe environment for family members • Nurturing environment for family members • Special needs of the child requiring invasive or restrictive treatments	
Involve the client and family in planning and implementing strategies to decrease or prevent alterations (risk for or actual) in parenting: • Family conference: Identify each member's perspective of the situation. • Mutual goal setting: Develop short-term, realistic goals with evaluation criteria. • Communication: Use open, honest communication with positive feedback. • Distribution of family tasks: Tasks are performed by all family members as developmentally and physically appropriate. • Promoting the parent's self-esteem: Provide positive support of existing positive parenting skills.	Involvement of the family in planning enhances the effectiveness of the interventions.
Assist the client and family in lifestyle adjustments that may be required: • Development of parenting skills • Use of support network • Establishment of realistic expectations of the children and spouse	Long-term behavioral changes require support.
Refer to appropriate assistive resources.	Support groups, family therapist, school nurse, and teachers can enhance the treatment plan.

RELOCATION STRESS SYNDROME, RISK FOR AND ACTUAL

DEFINITIONS[9]

Risk for Relocation Stress Syndrome Risk for physiologic and/or psychosocial disturbances pending a transfer from one environment to another.

Relocation Stress Syndrome Physiologic and/or psychosocial disturbances following a transfer from one environment to another.

DEFINING CHARACTERISTICS[9]

A. Risk for Relocation Stress Syndrome (Risk Factors)
1. Decreased psychosocial or physical health status
2. Feelings of powerlessness
3. Lack of adequate support system or group
4. Moderate competence (e.g., alert enough to experience changes)
5. Lack of predeparture counseling
6. Moderate to high degree of environmental change (e.g., physical, ethnic, or cultural)
7. Passive coping
8. Past, current, or recent losses
9. Temporary and/or permanent moves
10. Unpredictability of experience
11. Voluntary or involuntary move

B. Relocation Stress Syndrome
1. Aloneness, alienation, or loneliness
2. Depression
3. Anxiety (e.g., separation)
4. Sleep disturbance
5. Withdrawal
6. Anger
7. Loss of identity, self-worth, or self-esteem
8. Increased verbalization of needs, unwillingness to move, or concern over relocation
9. Increased physical symptoms or illness (e.g., gastrointestinal disturbance or weight change)
10. Dependency
11. Insecurity
12. Pessimism
13. Frustration
14. Worry
15. Fear

RELATED FACTORS[9]

A. **Risk for Relocation Stress Syndrome (Risk Factors)**
   The risk factors also serve as the related factors.
B. **Relocation Stress Syndrome**
   1. Unpredictability of experiences
   2. Temporary or permanent move
   3. Voluntary or involuntary move
   4. Past, concurrent, or recent losses
   5. Feelings of powerlessness
   6. Lack of adequate support system or group
   7. Lack of predeparture counseling
   8. Passive coping
   9. Impaired psychosocial health
   10. Decreased health status
   11. Isolation from family and/or friends
   12. Language barrier

RELATED CLINICAL CONCERNS

1. Any diagnosis that would require transfer of the patient to a long-term care facility
2. A chronic disease that would require the older adult to move in with his or her children
3. Placement in foster care
4. Crisis that results in a forced change in living situation (e.g., fires, floods and other natural disasters, war, divorce)

 Have You Selected the Correct Diagnosis?

Ineffective Individual Coping
Ineffective Individual Coping and Relocation Stress Syndrome do sound similar in some ways; however, the differentiating factor is whether or not the individual is being or recently has been involved in a transfer from one care setting to another. If such a transfer is being considered or has occurred, initial interventions should be directed toward resolving the problems associated with relocation of the patient.

Impaired Adjustment
Certainly any move, whether for an ill or healthy individual, would require some adjustment. However, this diagnosis relates to an individual's adjusting to his or her own illness or health problem, not adjustment to a change in the health-care setting.

EXPECTED OUTCOME

The patient will verbalize increased satisfaction with the new environment by [date].

TARGET DATES

An initial target date of 7 days would be reasonable to assess for progress toward meeting the expected outcome.

NURSING ACTIONS/INTERVENTIONS WITH RATIONALES

Adult Health

ACTIONS/INTERVENTIONS	RATIONALES
Explain all rationales for transfer before implementation.	Prepares the patient for a new environment and decreases anxiety.
Allow the patient to verbalize feelings that interfere with becoming acclimated to the new environment.	Brings feelings out into the open, and clarifies emotions and makes them easier to cope with.
Identify coping strategies that will facilitate adjustment.	Provides an understanding of problem and information to further develop interventions. Determines previously used coping strategies, which ones were successful or unsuccessful, and what alternative strategies may be tried.
Gradually transfer control regarding daily routines to the patient.	Increases self-confidence and decreases feeling of powerlessness.
Provide consistency in daily care, such as the same primary care nurse, same daily routines, and the same environment.	Provides security, thus facilitating adjustment.
Involve the patient in groups with similar interests.	Decreases anxiety.
Teach stress management techniques such as relaxation, meditation, deep breathing, exercise, or diversional activities. Have the patient return-demonstrate the technique for 15 minutes twice a day at [times].	Decreases anxiety so that energy can be used to implement effective coping strategies.

ACTIONS/INTERVENTIONS	RATIONALES
Consult with other health-care professionals as necessary.	Collaboration promotes care that incorporates physiologic and psychosocial interventions that may be needed as a result of relocation stress.
Help the patient maintain former relationships by providing letter-writing materials or a telephone.	Decreases feelings of isolation and depression.
Provide the patient with a list of organizations and community services available for newcomers (e.g., Welcome Wagon, senior citizens' groups, churches, or singles' groups).	Assists the patient to develop new relationship and may hasten adjustment.

Child Health

ACTIONS/INTERVENTIONS	RATIONALES
Assess, to the degree possible, the emotional stability of the patient and family. (Can use Chess-Thomas Temperament Scale.)[46]	Adaptability to change is determined to a large degree by temperament and previous coping.
Schedule a family conference of at least 1 hour daily and focus on: • Feelings of the patient and family regarding move • Aspects of relocation that are problematic (e.g., school or friends) • Identification of potential benefits and growth the relocation might offer	Provides support to cope with changes caused by relocation.
Facilitate plans for maintaining desired relationships despite physical move (e.g., letter, telephone calls, or visits).	
Facilitate expression of feelings with referral to mental health nurse clinician, psychiatrist, psychologist, or counselor.	Provides anticipatory or actual guidance for control of risk for unresolved issues.

Women's Health

The nursing actions for a woman with this nursing diagnosis are the same as those found in Adult Health, Mental Health, and Gerontic Health.

Mental Health

In addition to those interventions identified under Adult Health and Gerontic Health, the following interventions apply:

ACTIONS/INTERVENTIONS	RATIONALES
Monitor the client's cognitive resources.	Nursing interventions should be adapted to the client's cognitive abilities.[47]
Arrange to have objects familiar to the client in the environment. This could include photographs, clothing, furniture, or other significant personal items.	Familiar objects decrease anxiety and increase the sense of control while helping to reestablish personal space.
Provide the client with a sense of personal space by labeling the room, having him or her seated at the same place at mealtimes, and assisting him or her in the protection of this space and his or her belongings. [Note those adaptations here.]	Facilitates the reestablishment of a personal space.

(care plan continued on page 676)

NURSING ACTIONS/INTERVENTIONS WITH RATIONALES (continued from page 675)

Mental Health

ACTIONS/INTERVENTIONS	RATIONALES
Involve the client in the decision to change location. This is adjusted to fit the client's cognitive abilities, and the degree to which the client is involved should be noted here.	Promotes a sense of personal control and facilitates the psychological and emotional preparation for the move.
Sit with the client [number] minutes each day to discuss the move and memories of the former home. Having a picture of the former residence may facilitate this. [Note the person responsible for this discussion here.]	Facilitates adjustment to the new milieu.[22]
Provide sensory adaptive devices such as hearing aids and eyeglasses. [Note the devices needed by this client here.]	Facilitates orientation to the environment and promotes a sense of control. Promotes safety in the new environment.

Gerontic Health

● N O T E : *This diagnosis is appropriate for clients who have already experienced relocation. The reader is encouraged to view the Web site http://www.guidelines.gov before relocation to facilitate effective planning of relocation Post-relocation, all interventions should be tailored to meet the individual values, culture, and needs of the elder.[48]*

ACTIONS/INTERVENTIONS	RATIONALES
Offer choices such as where and when to move, room choice, where to locate items in the room, a daily schedule, and activities.	Involvement in decision making increases control.[48]
Assist the client with unpacking his or her own belongings.	Promotes personal sense of control and mastery.[48]
Provide opportunities to see old friends, make new friends, volunteer, or continue meaningful roles and activities.[48]	Provides social support and activities.[48]
Facilitate support from, and interaction with, family, friends, and new neighbors by introducing neighbors, extending invitations to social gatherings, and scheduling visits.[48]	Provides social support and activities.[48]
Facilitate the development of relationships with others (peers and staff), especially if there are no former friends in the new environment.[48]	Provides social support and activities.[48]
Establish a buddy system between the new resident and a person living in the new environment.	Provides social support and activities.[48]
Make available animal visits and visits with children if desired.[48]	Provides social support and activities.[48]
Assess preferences and opportunities for being alone in addition to meeting the need for social support.[48]	Individualizes care.[48]
Promote coping with the relocation: • Assist with grieving processes, providing more intense support in the first month. • Listen and allow the client to talk about feelings regarding the move.	Addresses the feelings of loss.[48]

ACTIONS/INTERVENTIONS	RATIONALES
• Encourage activities/rituals to say goodbye to the old residence and welcome the new space. • Discuss usual coping strategies with the client. • Assist the client in identifying positive aspects of the move (increased physical safety, fewer household responsibilities).[79]	
Orient the client to the new environment: • Welcome the client. • Promote communication among residents, family, and staff. • Establish a trusting relationship with the client. • Orient the client to the physical environment and routines. • Provide adequate lighting and mark the room so it is easy to find.[48]	A planned approach to relocation promotes adjustment.[48]
Maintain stability or continuity of care: • Develop and adhere to a plan of care. • Assist the client as needed to ensure continuity in taking medications, keeping physician appointments. • Maintain continuity in daily patterns of living • Maintain consistency in the physical environment by keeping favorite items readily available (i.e., chair, afghan, photos).[48]	Promotes coping with relocation.[48]
Ensure meeting of physical and psychosocial needs: • Support the client's highest level and functioning, thus his or her autonomy. • Refer to social support services as needed. • Ensure adequate assistance with personal care. • Maintain appropriate use of assistive devices (glasses, hearing aids, walkers).[48]	Promotes coping with relocation.[48]
Identify whether the patient is at risk for relocation syndrome. In older adults, this may include those with no confidant (social support), those who perceive themselves as worriers, those in poor health, and those with low self-esteem.[49]	Early identification of patients at risk can mean earlier intervention and a possible decrease in the negative consequences of relocation.
Assist the patient in realistic perception of event: what has occurred, reasons for transfer based on physical needs, changed health status.	May assist in accepting the need for relocation.
Discuss possible occurrence of the syndrome with significant others.	Provides anticipatory information that avoids undue stress on the family.
If not returning to prehospitalization location, discuss with the patient his or her proposed plans, reasons for transfer, and the patient's response to the proposal.	Allows time for ventilation of feelings related to the relocation.

Home Health

See Gerontic and Mental Health for additional interventions.

ACTIONS/INTERVENTIONS	RATIONALES
Assist the client or caregiver to make the new environment as much like the previous environment as possible:	Enhances the client's sense of security and comfort.

(care plan continued on page 678)

NURSING ACTIONS/INTERVENTIONS WITH RATIONALES (continued from page 677)

Home Health

ACTIONS/INTERVENTIONS	RATIONALES
• Similar schedules and routines • Decorations from previous environment • Significant items such as blankets, artwork, and music • Foods served should be as familiar as possible.	
Educate the client or caregiver as far in advance as possible of necessary changes in location, and tell them what to expect.	Promotes a sense of control and avoids unpleasant surprises.
When the change in location involves separation from significant others, help the client or caregiver to obtain items that may increase the client's comfort: • Photographs of loved ones • Letters and cards from loved ones • Videotapes and/or audiotapes of loved ones	Enhances the client's sense of security and comfort.

ROLE PERFORMANCE, INEFFECTIVE

DEFINITION[9]

Patterns of behavior and self-expression that do not match the environmental context, norms, and expectations.*

DEFINING CHARACTERISTICS[9]

1. Change in self-perception of role
2. Role denial
3. Inadequate external support for role enactment
4. Inadequate adaptation to change or transition
5. System conflict
6. Change in usual patterns of responsibility
7. Discrimination
8. Domestic violence
9. Harassment
10. Uncertainty
11. Altered role perception
12. Role strain
13. Inadequate self-management
14. Role ambivalence
15. Pessimistic attitude
16. Inadequate motivation
17. Inadequate confidence
18. Inadequate role competency and skills
19. Inadequate knowledge
20. Inappropriate developmental expectations
21. Role conflict
22. Role confusion
23. Powerlessness
24. Inadequate coping
25. Anxiety or depression
26. Role overload
27. Change in other's perceptions of role
28. Change in capacity to resume role
29. Role dissatisfaction
30. Inadequate opportunities for role enactment

RELATED FACTORS[9]

1. Social
   a. Inadequate or inappropriate linkage with the health-care system
   b. Job schedule demands
   c. Young age or developmental level
   d. Lack of rewards
   e. Poverty
   f. Family conflict
   g. Inadequate support system
   h. Inadequate role socialization (e.g., role model, expectations, and responsibilities)
   i. Low socioeconomic status
   j. Stress and conflict
   k. Domestic violence
   l. Lack of resources
2. Knowledge
   a. Inadequate role preparation (e.g., role transition, skill rehearsal, and validation)
   b. Lack of knowledge about role, role skills
   c. Role transition
   d. Lack of opportunity for role rehearsal
   e. Developmental transitions
   f. Unrealistic role expectations
   g. Education attainment level
   h. Lack of or inadequate role model

---

*There is a typology of roles: socio-personal (friendship, family, marital, parenting, community); home management; intimacy (sexuality, relationship building); leisure, exercise, or recreation; self-management; socialization (developmental transitions); community contributor; and religious.

3. Physiologic
   a. Inadequate or inappropriate linkage with the health-care system
   b. Substance abuse
   c. Mental illness
   d. Body image alteration
   e. Physical illness
   f. Cognitive defects
   g. Health alterations (e.g., physical health, body image, self-esteem, mental health, psychosocial health, cognition, learning style, or neurologic health)
   h. Depression
   i. Low self-esteem
   j. Pain
   k. Fatigue

RELATED CLINICAL CONCERNS

1. Any major surgery
2. Any chronic disease
3. Any condition resulting in hemiplegia, paraplegia, or quadriplegia
4. Chemical abuse
5. Cancer

 Have You Selected the Correct Diagnosis?

Social Isolation
The diagnosis of Social Isolation relates to the patient who, because of physical, communicative, or social problems, chooses to be alone or perceives that he or she is alone and therefore isolated from society. This diagnosis deals mainly with the individual who cannot or will not perform any role.

Interrupted Family Processes
Interrupted Family Processes refers to an entire family that must in one way or another alter the processes that go on within the family. Many times this will involve altered role performances of the individual family members; however, the overall focus is on the alteration within the family and not with the individual members of the family.

EXPECTED OUTCOME

Will describe role changes necessitated by life change [note specific change here] by [date].

Will describe plan to adapt to role changes by [date].

Will demonstrate [number] new role behavior by [date].

Will verbalize satisfaction with new role performance by [date].

TARGET DATES

Target dates for this diagnosis will have to be highly individualized according to each situation. A minimum target date would be 5 days to allow time to identify impinging factors and methods to cope with those factors.

NURSING ACTIONS/INTERVENTIONS WITH RATIONALES

Adult Health

ACTIONS/INTERVENTIONS	RATIONALES
Encourage the patient to express his or her perception of role responsibilities. Facilitate the development of a plan for client to address perceived inadequacies. Note that plan here. Reinforce the client's strengths.	Relieves stress and helps the patient clarify feelings in a safe environment.
Help the patient and significant others realistically negotiate role responsibilities by assisting in the problem-solving process.	Facilitates problem solving. Promotes cooperation among involved persons.
Teach the patient regarding the role (e.g., parent, caregiver, or breadwinner). Allow time for discussion and questioning before discharge.	Clarifies misconceptions and provides realistic role expectations.
Help the patient identify community resources to assist in role responsibilities before discharge.	Provides support for short-term and long-term problem solving.
Refer to the psychiatric nurse clinician as needed. (See Mental Health nursing actions for more detailed interventions.)	Collaboration promotes a holistic plan of care, and the problem may need specialized interventions.

(care plan continued on page 680)

NURSING ACTIONS/INTERVENTIONS WITH RATIONALES (continued from page 679)

Child Health

ACTIONS/INTERVENTIONS	RATIONALES
Determine how the child and parent perceive the expected role for the child.	Provides the essential database necessary to plan care.
Identify confusion or diffusion of role according to the child's and parent's expectations versus the actual role.	Problem identification serves to establish common areas to be further explored in role performance.
Determine the value the child has in the family.	The value a child has for each family is critical to expectations for all involved.
Determine the child's self-perception.	One's self-perception provides insight into how one evaluates his or her own performance.
Identify ways to alleviate role performance alteration according to the actual cause. If the child is temporarily unable to participate in certain physical activities, explore other nonphysical ways the child can participate.	Alleviation of one or more role performance alterations may prevent further deterioration in role functioning, with a greater appreciation for the value of all roles.
Allow for ventilation of feelings by the child via puppetry, art, or other age-appropriate methods. Schedule at least 30 minutes during each 8-hour shift, while the patient is awake, for this activity. [Note times here.]	Feelings are most critical in exploring one's role performance. Appropriate aids in communication serve to foster focused play or behaviors to reveal thoughts of the child who is unable to express him- or herself.
Provide the patient and parents with options to best facilitate needs for future implications of compromised role performance (e.g., shared experiences with peers who have temporarily had to forsake physical activities because of illness. How did they keep up with the team?)	Vicarious involvement allows for shared activities and the sense of maintaining closeness with the desired groups or person.
Allow for family time and support for choices to uphold role needs (e.g., visitation by peers).	Shared time of family and friends is important, especially in times of role stress, to maintain the value of self.
Provide for safety needs of the child and family.	Standard care includes safety. The tendency is to relax concerns in times of less stressful activity.
Assist in follow-up plans with appropriate appointments for psychiatric or pediatric care.	Arrangements for follow-up promote valuing of follow-up and increase the likelihood for compliance.
Provide support in identification of risk to normal actualization of potential of the child. Refer to the child or family mental health practitioner as appropriate.	Early identification of primary or secondary risks may prevent or minimize tertiary risks for the child and family.

Women's Health

ACTIONS/INTERVENTIONS	RATIONALES
Allow the patient to describe her perception of her role as a mother, wife, and working woman.	Provides a database to initiate care planning.
Identify sources of role stress and strain that contribute to role conflict and fatigue.	
Assist in developing a schedule that manages time well, both at home and at work.	
Involve significant others in planning methods of reducing role stress and strain at home by: • Assisting with child care • Assisting with household duties • Sharing carpooling and children's activities	Encourages the patient to identify various roles she is currently fulfilling, and provides support that allows planning of coping strategies and techniques.

ACTIONS/INTERVENTIONS	RATIONALES
Encourage the patient to use time at work for "work activities" and time at home for "home activities," i.e., do not take work home.	
Look at possibility of job sharing or part-time employment while the children are at home.	
Plan home activities in advance, such as shopping for and cooking meals in advance, and freezing them for later use.	
Encourage division of workload by exchanging childcare activities with friends or other families in the neighborhood.	

Mental Health

ACTIONS/INTERVENTIONS	RATIONALES
Sit with the client [number] minutes [number] times per day to discuss the client's feelings about self and role performance.	Provides information about the client's perceptions and expectations that can be utilized in developing specific interventions.
Answer questions honestly.	Promotes the development of a trusting relationship.
Provide feedback to the client about nurse's perceptions of the client's abilities and appearance by: • Using "I" statements • Using references related to the nurse's relationship to the client • Describing the nurse's feelings in relationship	Assists the client in realistically evaluating his or her perceptions.
Provide positive reinforcement. List here those things, including social rewards, that are reinforcing for the client and when they are to be used. Also list those things that have been identified as nonreinforcers for this client.	Reinforcement encourages positive behavior and enhances self-esteem.
Provide group interaction with [number] persons [number] minutes three times a day at [times]. This activity should be gradual within the client's ability. For example, on admission the client may tolerate one person for 5 minutes. If the interactions are brief, the frequency should be high, e.g., 5-minute interactions should occur at 30-minute intervals.	Assists the client to experience personal importance to others, while enhancing interpersonal relationship skills. Increasing these role competences can enhance self-esteem and promote a positive orientation.
Reflect back to the client negative self-statements. This should be done with a supportive attitude in a manner that will increase the client's awareness of these negative evaluations of self.	This will increase the client's awareness of these statements and facilitate the development of alternative cognitive patterns.
Set achievable goals for the client.	Achievement of goals provides positive reinforcement that encourages the behavior and enhances self-esteem.
Provide activities that the client can accomplish and that the client values. Care should be taken not to provide tasks that the client finds demeaning, which could reinforce the client's negative self-evaluation.	Accomplishment of valued tasks provides positive reinforcement that encourages behavior and enhances self-esteem.
Provide verbal reinforcement for the achievement of steps toward a goal.	Promotes a positive orientation.
Have the client develop a list of his or her strengths and potentials.	

(care plan continued on page 682)

NURSING ACTIONS/INTERVENTIONS WITH RATIONALES (continued from page 681)

Mental Health

ACTIONS/INTERVENTIONS	RATIONALES
Define the client's lack of goal achievement or failures as simple mistakes that are bound to occur when one attempts something new. For example, learning comes with mistakes; if one does not make mistakes, one does not learn.	Promotes a positive orientation.
Define past failures as the client's best attempts to solve a problem; for example, if the client had known a better solution, he or she would have used it; one does not set out to fail.	
Make necessary items available for the client to groom self.	Appropriate grooming improves the client's self-evaluation.
Spend [number] minutes at [time] assisting the client with grooming, providing necessary assistance and positive reinforcement for accomplishments.	The nurse's presence can provide positive reinforcement, and reinforcement encourages positive behavior.
Focus the client's attention on the here and now.	It is difficult for the nurse to provide feedback on past happenings.
Present the client with opportunities to make decisions about care, and record these decisions on the chart.	Promotes the client's sense of control, and enhances self-esteem.
Develop with the client alternative coping strategies.	Promotes the development of more adaptive coping behaviors and increases the client's role competence.
Practice new coping behavior with the client [number] minutes at [time].	Repeated practice of a behavior internalizes and personalizes the behavior.
Discuss with the client ideal versus current perceptions of role performance.	Assists the client in a cognitive appraisal of perceptions to eliminate unrealistic or irrational beliefs.
Discuss with the client the factors that are perceived to be interfering with role performance.	Assists the client in cognitive evaluation of perception of role performance.
Have the client develop a list of alternatives for resolving interfering factors. [This list should be noted here.]	Facilitates the development of alternative coping behaviors.
Establish an appointment with significant others to discuss their perceptions of the client's role performance and their perceptions of the various roles involved in the identified situations. [Date and time of this meeting should be written here.]	Assists in establishing agreement on the performance of role pairs to decrease role conflict and strain. This is of primary importance because roles occur in interactions.
Discuss with the client and significant others alterations in role that will facilitate successful performance. [Date and time of this meeting should be written here.]	
Develop a specific list of necessary changes, and provide the client system with a written copy.	
Role-play altered role situations with the client system for 1 hour once a day at [time]. This would include opportunities for clients to practice the areas of role performance that may be new or unique.	Repeated practice of a behavior internalizes and personalizes the behavior.
If the client and client system cannot achieve agreement on the problematic role, refer to: • Psychiatric mental health clinical nurse specialist • Family therapist • Social worker	Interactions with the health-care system involve role pairs with the role expectations that are present in any social situation. As in any interaction, there can be differing expectations about role performance, which can lead to role conflict and strain.

ACTIONS/INTERVENTIONS	RATIONALES
If problematic roles involve interactions between the client and members of the health-care team (nurses, physicians, etc.), request consultation with psychiatric mental health clinical nurse specialist or mental health specialist with experience in the area of resolving system problems (i.e., family therapists or social workers).	
Refer the client and significant others to community resources that will continue to support role development (e.g., family therapist, occupational therapist, rehabilitation counseling).	

Gerontic Health

In addition to the interventions for Adult Health and Mental Health, the following may be utilized with the aging client:

ACTIONS/INTERVENTIONS	RATIONALES
Discuss with the patient how he or she perceives his or her role performance has altered.	Provides an opportunity to gain the patient's exact perspective on the situation. Provides database needed for most effective planning.
Discuss with the patient potential role modifications or substitutions, such as foster grandparenting, friendly visitor at a long-term-care facility, participant in intergenerational programs, or telephone reassurance visitor or caller.	Depending on the patient's interests and abilities, these measures would provide an alternate method to achieve role satisfaction.

Home Health

ACTIONS/INTERVENTIONS	RATIONALES
Monitor for factors contributing to disturbed role performance.	Provides a database for early recognition and intervention.
Involve the client and family in planning, implementing, and promoting reduction or elimination of disturbance in role function: • Family conference: Clarify expected role performance of all family members. • Mutual goal setting: Set realistic goals and evaluation criteria. Identify tasks for each family member. • Communication: Use open, direct communication and provide positive feedback.	Family involvement in planning increases the likelihood of effective intervention.
Assist the client and family in lifestyle adjustments that may be required: • Treatment of physical or emotional disability • Stress management • Adjustment to changing role functions and relationships • Development and use of support networks • Requirements for redistribution of family tasks	Long-term behavioral changes require support.
Consult with assistive resources as indicated.	Utilization of existing services is efficient use of resources. Psychiatric nurse clinician, occupational and physical therapists, and support groups can enhance the treatment plan.

SOCIAL INTERACTION, IMPAIRED

DEFINITION[9]

Insufficient or excessive quantity or ineffective quality of social exchange.

DEFINING CHARACTERISTICS[9]

1. Verbalized or observed inability to receive or communicate a satisfying sense of belonging, caring, interest, or shared history
2. Verbalized or observed discomfort in social situations
3. Observed use of unsuccessful social interaction behaviors
4. Dysfunctional interaction with peers, family, and/or others
5. Family report of change of style or pattern of interaction

RELATED FACTORS[9]

1. Knowledge or skill deficit about ways to enhance mutuality
2. Therapeutic isolation
3. Sociocultural dissonance
4. Limited physical mobility
5. Environmental barriers
6. Communication barriers
7. Altered thought process
8. Absence of available significant others or peers
9. Self-concept disturbance

RELATED CLINICAL CONCERNS

1. Any condition causing paraplegia, hemiplegia, or quadriplegia
2. AIDS
3. Alzheimer's disease
4. Cancer of the larynx
5. Mental retardation
6. Substance abuse
7. Communicable disease
8. Altered physical appearance secondary to disease or trauma

9. Psychiatric disorders (e.g., major depression, borderline personality disorder, schizoid personality disorder)

 Have You Selected the Correct Diagnosis?

Deficient Knowledge
Deficient knowledge, particularly as related to mutuality, would be the most appropriate alternate diagnosis if the individual verbalized or demonstrated an inability to attend to significant others' social actions in the context of independent and dependent aspects of their role.

Impaired Verbal Communication
Impaired Verbal Communication would be the most appropriate diagnosis if the individual is unable to receive or send communication. Certainly Impaired Verbal Communication could relate to Impaired Social Interaction and would be the primary problem that has to be resolved.

Social Isolation
Social Isolation would be the more appropriate diagnosis when the individual is placed in or chooses isolation because of physiologic, sociologic, or emotional concerns. Further assessment is required to completely delineate the exact problem when self-isolation is chosen as the diagnosis.

EXPECTED OUTCOME

Will describe [number] behaviors that will improve social exchanges by [date].

Will demonstrate [number] of behaviors that will improve social interactions by [date].

Will participate in [number] social interaction(s) by [date].

TARGET DATES

Assisting the patient to modify social interactions will require a significant amount of time. A target date ranging between 7 and 10 days would be appropriate for evaluating progress.

NURSING ACTIONS/INTERVENTIONS WITH RATIONALES

Adult Health

ACTIONS/INTERVENTIONS	RATIONALES
Explore the patient's feelings regarding fears in a social situation. Assist the client to put the fears in perspective and work through the fears.	Assists the patient to examine social experience and verbalize feelings. Encourages the therapeutic relationship.
Evaluate the patient's communication skills, identify areas for development.	Improves communication skills.
Help the patient obtain a realistic perception of self by focusing on and enhancing strengths.	Helps the patient see that no one is perfect, and improves self-concept.

ACTIONS/INTERVENTIONS	RATIONALES
Help the patient participate in group interactions. [Note assistance the patient needs to accomplish this here.]	Increases social skills by providing social contact.
Involve the patient in daily care. Help the patient make decisions about own care.	Improves self-concepts. Increases motivation. Decreases feeling of powerlessness.
If the patient is in isolation, spend at least 10 minutes for each routine patient interaction.	Avoids feeling of total isolation for the patient.
Initiate referrals to support groups before discharge.	Puts the patient in contact with community groups to interact with the patient to decrease social isolation.

Child Health

ACTIONS/INTERVENTIONS	RATIONALES
Monitor for contributory factors to altered social interaction pattern (e.g., role-play with puppets).	Provides a database needed to plan appropriate care.
Determine the effect the altered social interaction has on the child, parent, family, and school.	Provides a database needed to accurately plan intervention.
Develop a plan of care to best meet the child's potential for succeeding with appropriate social interaction—this will be impacted by social class and values.	Individual family values will dictate the way in which they deal with social interaction.
Determine whether conflict exists between the parent's and the child's desired social interaction.	Conflict may prevent appropriate attention to actual social interaction, but must be dealt with as it will remain a critical component. This may be true particularly at times of authority issues (e.g., adolescence).
If conflict exists regarding social interaction, deal with this as needed in values or beliefs pattern.	Values and beliefs may be in conflict, and some resolution of the problem is essential to prevent further long-term effects.
Assist the child, parents, and family in ventilation of feelings regarding social interaction impairment, including actual consequences of the impairment. *Best facilitated with same primary care nurse.	Ventilation of feelings and the opportunity to do so serve to value the importance for the patient to help reduce anxiety and initiate problem resolution.
Make referrals as appropriate to professionals best able to assist in dealing with problem (e.g., psychiatric nurse clinical specialist, play therapist, or family therapist).	Referral serves to best deal with problems according to a match of needs and resources.
Identify local support groups to appropriately match needs (e.g., parent–child support groups for the handicapped, United Cerebral Palsy Association, or Spina Bifida Association).	Resource groups provide vital support through provision of a common, shared sense of concern, coping, and empowerment.
If impaired social interaction also relates to the school, include the teacher and essential school personnel in plans for resolving the impairment and for best follow-up.	Valuing the importance of school and the need to provide the best for the child and family in the development of positive social interaction is showing respect for the patient and family.
Identify follow-up appointment needs and ways to monitor progress for the child and family (e.g., stickers as incentives to reinforce desired behavior).	Provides reinforcement and attaches value to follow-up.
Anticipate discrepant or unrealistic parental expectations of the child. Monitor for potential abuse of the child according to pattern for this.	Unrealistic demands or expectations are risk indicators for abuse.

(care plan continued on page 686)

NURSING ACTIONS/INTERVENTIONS WITH RATIONALES (continued from page 685)

Women's Health

This nursing diagnosis pertains to women the same as to any other adult. The reader is referred to the other sections—Adult Health, Child Health, Mental Health, Gerontic Health, and Home Health—for specific nursing actions.

Mental Health

ACTIONS/INTERVENTIONS	RATIONALES
If delusions or hallucinations are present, refer to Disturbed Sensory Perception for detailed interventions.	
Assign a primary care nurse to the client.	Promotes the development of a trusting relationship.
The primary care nurse will spend [number] minutes twice a day at [times] with the client. The focus of this interaction will change as a relationship is developed. Initially, the nurse should model for the client how to develop a relationship through his or her behavior in developing a relationship with the client. This modeling should include demonstrating respect for the client; consistency in interaction; congruence between thoughts, feelings, and actions; and empathy.	Promotes the development of a trusting relationship and provides opportunities for the client to observe the nurse in appropriate interpersonal interactions.
Have the client identify the persons who are considered family, friends, and acquaintances. Then have the client note how many interactions per week occur with each person. Have the client identify his or her thoughts, feelings, and behavior about these interactions.	Assists the client in reality testing of the belief that he or she is having difficulty with interpersonal relationships.
Provide appropriate confrontation with the client about his or her behavior patterns that inhibit interaction in relationships with the nurse.[16]	Assists the client in developing alternative coping behaviors that are adaptive.
Observe the client in interactions with others on the unit, and identify patterns of behavior that inhibit social interaction.	Facilitates the provision of feedback to the client on methods he or she could use to improve interpersonal effectiveness.
Develop a list of things the client finds rewarding, and provide these rewards as the client successfully completes progressive steps in treatment plan.	Positive reinforcement encourages behavior.
When the client is demonstrating socially inappropriate behavior, keep interactions to a minimum and escort the client to a place away from activities.	Continuing the interaction could provide positive reinforcement and encourage inappropriate behavior.
When the inappropriate behavior stops, discuss the behavior with the client and develop a list of alternative kinds of behavior for the client to use in situations where the inappropriate behavior is elicited. [Note here the kinds of behavior that are identified as problematic, with the action to be taken if they are demonstrated; e.g., the client will spend time out in seclusion and away from group activity.]	Promotes the client's sense of control and begins the development of alternative, more adaptive coping behaviors. Social isolation assists in decreasing behaviors.
Develop a schedule for gradually increasing time of the client in group activities. For example, the client will spend [number] minutes in the group dining hall during mealtimes, or will spend [number] minutes in a group game. [Note the client's specific activities here.]	Social interaction can provide positive reinforcement and opportunities for the client to practice new behaviors in a supportive environment.

ACTIONS/INTERVENTIONS	RATIONALES
Primary nurse will spend 30 minutes a day with the client exploring thoughts and feelings about social interactions and assisting with reality testing of social interaction (e.g., what others might mean by silence and other nonverbal responses).	
Identify with the client areas of social skill deficit, and develop a plan for improving these areas. This could include: • Assertiveness training • Role-playing difficult situations • Teaching the client relaxation techniques to reduce anxiety in social situations. [Note here the plan and schedule for implementation. This should be a progressive plan with rewards for accomplishment of each step.]	Promotes the client's sense of control and begins the development of alternative, more adaptive coping behaviors by increasing role competence.
Consult with the occupational therapist if the client needs to learn specific skills to facilitate social interactions (e.g., cooking skills so friends can be invited to dinner, or craft skills so the client can join others in social interactions around these activities).	Increasing behavioral repertoire increases role competence, which enhances self-esteem.[1]
Include the client in group activities on the unit, and assign the client activities that can be easily accomplished, and that will provide positive social reinforcement from other persons involved in the activities.	Reinforcement encourages positive behavior and enhances self-esteem.
When the client demonstrates tolerance for group interactions, schedule a time for the client to participate in a group therapy that provides opportunities for feedback about relationship behavior from peers, and for listening to the thoughts and feelings of peers.	Disconfirms the client's sense of aloneness, and assists the client to experience personal importance to others, while enhancing interpersonal relationship skills. Increasing these competencies can enhance self-esteem and promote positive orientation.
Discuss with the support system ways in which they can facilitate client interaction.	Support system understanding facilitates the maintenance of new behaviors after discharge.
Have the client identify the activities in the community that are of interest and would provide opportunities for interaction. List the activities here, and develop a plan for the client to develop necessary skills to ensure opportunities for interactional success during these activities (e.g., practice a card game or tennis while in the hospital).	Increases the client's ability to perform these roles successfully, which provides positive reinforcement, thereby encouraging the behavior and enhancing self-esteem.
When the client reports problems in an interaction, review his or her perceptions of the interaction and an evaluation of when the problems began.	Assists the client with reality testing of his or her perceptions.
Limit the amount of time the client can spend alone in room. This should be a gradual alteration and done in steps that can easily be accomplished by the client. Note specific schedule for the client here. Have a staff person remain with the client during these times until client demonstrates an ability to interact with others.	Successful accomplishment of a task provides positive reinforcement and promotes a positive orientation.
Have the referral source make contact with the client before discharge and schedule a post-discharge meeting.	Promotes the development of a trusting relationship while the client is in a safe environment.

(care plan continued on page 688)

NURSING ACTIONS/INTERVENTIONS WITH RATIONALES (continued from page 687)

Gerontic Health

The nursing actions for the gerontic patient with this diagnosis are the same as those given in Adult Health and Mental Health.

Home Health

ACTIONS/INTERVENTIONS	RATIONALES
Monitor for factors contributing to the impaired social interaction (e.g., psychological, physical, economic, or spiritual).	Provides database for early recognition and intervention.
Involve the client and family in planning, implementing, and promoting reduction or elimination of Impaired Social Interaction: • Family conference: Identify the perspective of each member. Establish consistent rules for behaviors. • Mutual goal setting: Set consistent rules for behavior and provide support for care providers. Identify tasks for each member.	Family involvement enhances the effectiveness of the interventions.
Assist the patient and family in lifestyle adjustments that may be required: • Providing a safe environment • Development and use of support networks • Change in role functions • Prescribed treatments (e.g., medications or behavioral interventions) • Assistance with self-care activities • Possible hospitalization or placement in halfway house • Treatment of drug or alcohol abuse • Development and practice of social skills • Independent living skills • Finances • Stress management • Suicide prevention	Permanent changes in behavior and family roles require support.
Assist the client and family to develop criteria to determine when a crisis exists and professional intervention is necessary: • Violence • Sudden change in ability to care for self • Hallucinations or delusions	Provides a database for early recognition and intervention.
Consult with or refer to assistive resources as indicated.	Utilization of existing services is efficient use of resources. Respite care and support groups can enhance the treatment plan.

SOCIAL ISOLATION

DEFINITION[9]

Aloneness experienced by the individual and perceived as imposed by others and as a negative or threatened state.

DEFINING CHARACTERISTICS[9]

1. Objective
   a. Absence of supportive significant other(s) (family, friends, group)

b. Projects hostility in voice or behavior
c. Withdrawn
d. Uncommunicative
e. Shows behavior unaccepted by dominant cultural group
f. Seeks to be alone, or exists in a subculture
g. Repetitive, meaningless actions
h. Preoccupation with own thoughts
i. No eye contact
j. Evidence of physical or mental handicap or altered state of wellness
k. Sad, dull affect
l. Inappropriate or immature interests or activities for developmental age or stage

2. Subjective
   a. Expresses feelings of aloneness imposed by others
   b. Expresses feelings of rejection
   c. Inadequacy in or absence of significant purpose in life
   d. Inability to meet expectations of others
   e. Expresses values acceptable to the subculture but unacceptable to the dominant cultural group
   f. Expresses interests inappropriate to the developmental age or stage
   g. Experiences feelings of difference from others
   h. Insecurity in public

RELATED FACTORS[9]

1. Alterations in mental status
2. Inability to engage in satisfying personal relationships
3. Unaccepted social values
4. Unaccepted social behavior
5. Inadequate personal resources
6. Immature interests
7. Factors contributing to the absence of personal relationships (e.g., delay in accomplishing developmental tasks)
8. Alterations in physical appearance
9. Altered state of wellness

RELATED CLINICAL CONCERNS

1. Any condition that has resulted in scarring
2. Alzheimer's disease

3. AIDS
4. Tuberculosis
5. Any condition causing impaired mobility
6. Psychiatric disorders such as major depression, schizophrenic disorders, paranoid disorders, or conduct disorders

 Have You Selected the Correct Diagnosis?

Deficient Knowledge
Deficient knowledge, particularly as related to mutuality, would be the most appropriate alternate diagnosis if the individual verbalized or demonstrated an inability to attend to significant others' social actions in the context of independent and dependent aspects of their role.

Impaired Verbal Communication
Impaired Verbal Communication would be the most appropriate diagnosis if the individual is unable to receive or send communication. Certainly Impaired Verbal Communication could be related to Impaired Social Interaction and would be the primary problem that has to be resolved.

Impaired Social Interaction
Impaired Social Interaction can be either too much or too little in terms of social activity and is more focused on the individual's choice. In Social Isolation, the patient sees this problem as being caused by others.

EXPECTED OUTCOME

Will identify [number] of behaviors that will increase social interactions by [date].

Will participate in [number] of social activities by [date].

TARGET DATES

A target date range of 2 to 7 days would be acceptable depending on the exact social interaction chosen.

NURSING ACTIONS/INTERVENTIONS WITH RATIONALES

Adult Health

ACTIONS/INTERVENTIONS	RATIONALES
Explore feelings of isolation and aloneness during routine patient encounters.	Promotes a therapeutic relationship in which the patient can verbalize feelings in a nonthreatening environment.
Support the patient in maintaining personal appearance.	Increases self-confidence.
Provide positive feedback and support for social interactional skills as appropriate.	Increases self-confidence. Decreases anxiety in social situations.

(care plan continued on page 690)

Adult Health

ACTIONS/INTERVENTIONS	RATIONALES
Facilitate visits from the family, friends, and significant others daily. If appropriate, arrange for family to room-in. Involve in patient care to the extent feasible.	Increases social contacts and interactional skills.
Facilitate the patient's involvement in diversional activities.	Increases social contacts and interactional skills, especially those involving groups, daily.
Encourage the patient to identify and use community support systems and groups before discharge.	Increases social contacts. Promotes assistance with short-term and long-term goals.

Child Health

ACTIONS/INTERVENTIONS	RATIONALES
Provide opportunities for expression of feelings about desired social activity by spending 15 to 20 minutes per shift, during waking hours, at [times] with the patient and family.	Ventilation of feelings allows for insight into the patient's thinking and assists in reducing anxiety.
Determine what obstacles are perceived by the patient and family in pursuit of desired social activities by asking both direct and open-ended questions; for example, "What do you think prevents you from doing what you want to?"	Directed inquiry into obstacles that prevent the patient from engaging in desired social interaction increases the likelihood of a more complete database that will allow more individualized planning.
Identify what realistic patterns for socialization are applicable for the patient and family in collaboration with the patient and family.	Realistic goals are more likely to bring about the desired changes for more effective social interaction.
Collaborate with other health-care professionals to meet realistic goals for patient and family socialization.	Appropriate use of resource personnel ensures optimal likelihood for goal attainment.
Monitor for contributory related factors to best consider the social activity pattern.	All factors must be considered to provide a holistic plan of care.
Identify support groups to assist in realization of desired social activities.	Support groups provide a sense of sharing and empowerment.
Monitor the patient's and family's perceptions of the effect desired social activities might have on the current role-relationship pattern.	Roles are closely impacted by patterns of social interaction.
Provide appropriate opportunities for assessment of the young child's perceptions of situational needs and how he or she views self.	The child's view of him- or herself in relationship to social patterns is vital to planning the most effective interventions.
Assist the patient to develop a schedule for consideration of desired social activities at least 2 days before dismissal from hospital.	Appropriate planning serves to increase success with desired activities.
Provide for appropriate follow-up appointment as needed before dismissal from the hospital.	Follow-up plans attach value to long-term care for the patient.

Women's Health

● N O T E : *When women experience social isolation, it is especially important to assess for the presence of domestic violence. Social isolation may be one of the methods by which an abuser controls his or her partner. The following nursing actions apply to the social isolation experienced by the patient who has sexually transmitted diseases such as herpes genitalis, syphilis, chlamydia, gonorrhea, and AIDS.*

ACTIONS/INTERVENTIONS	RATIONALES
Assure the patient of confidentiality.	Promotes sharing of information by the patient.
Refer for counseling and/or treatment to: • Support groups • Professionals (e.g., public health clinic, nurse specialists, or physician)	Provides long-term support and care for the patient.
Provide a nonjudgmental atmosphere[50] to encourage verbalization of concerns: • Recurrent nature of disease, especially herpes and Chlamydia • Lack of cure for disease (AIDS) • Economics in treating the disease • Social stigma associated with the disease • Opportunity for entrance into the health-care system	Provides the database needed to provide appropriate care and teaching.
Encourage honesty in answers to such question as: • Multiple sexual partners (identify contacts) • Describing sexual behavior	
Encourage honest communication with sexual partners.	Sexual partners will also need to seek health care.

Mental Health

ACTIONS/INTERVENTIONS	RATIONALES
If delusions and/or hallucinations are present, refer to Disturbed Sensory Perception for detailed interventions.	Assists in understanding the client's worldview, which facilitates the development of client-specific interventions.
If social isolation is related to the client's feelings of powerlessness, refer to Powerlessness in Chapter 8 for detailed interventions.	
Discuss with the client his or her perception of the source of the social isolation, and have him or her list those things he or she has tried to resolve the situation.	Change is dependent on the client's perception of the problem.[23]
Have the client list the persons who are considered family, friends, and acquaintances. Then have the client note how many interactions per week occur with each person. Have the client identify what interferes with feeling connected with these persons. This activity should be implemented by the primary care nurse. [Note schedule for this interaction here.]	Facilitates the client's reality testing of his or her perception of being socially isolated.
When contributing factors have been identified, develop a plan to alter these factors. This could include: • Assertiveness training • Role-playing difficult situations • Teaching the client relaxation techniques to reduce anxiety in social situations [Note plan and schedule for implementation here.]	Facilitates the development of alternative coping behaviors that enhance role performance.

(care plan continued on page 692)

NURSING ACTIONS/INTERVENTIONS WITH RATIONALES (continued from page 691)

Mental Health

ACTIONS/INTERVENTIONS	RATIONALES
Develop a list of things the client finds rewarding, and provide the rewards as the client successfully completes progressive steps in the treatment plan. This schedule should be developed with the client. [Note here the schedule for rewards and the kinds of behavior to be rewarded.]	Reinforcement encourages positive behavior and enhances self-esteem.
Consult with the occupational therapist if the client needs to learn specific skills to facilitate social interactions (e.g., cooking skills so friends can be invited to dinner, craft skills so the client can join others in social interactions around these activities, or dancing).	Increases the client's competencies, which enhances role performance and self-esteem.
Provide the client with the prostheses necessary to facilitate social interactions, (e.g., hearing aids or eyeglasses). [Note here the assistance needed from nursing staff in providing these to the client. Also note where they are to be stored while not in use.]	
Include the client in group activities on the unit. Assign the client activities that can be easily accomplished and that will provide positive social reinforcement from other persons involved in the activities. This could include things like having the client assume responsibility for preparing a part of a group meal, or for serving a portion of a meal.	Successful accomplishment of a valued task can provide positive reinforcement, which encourages behavior.
Role-play with the client the social interactions identified as most difficult. This will be done by primary nurse. [Note schedule for this activity here.]	Repeated practice of a behavior internalizes and personalizes the behavior.
Discuss with the client the times it would be appropriate to be alone, and develop a plan for coping with these times in a positive manner (e.g., the client will develop a list of books to read, music to listen to, or community activities to attend).	Promotes the client's sense of control, while facilitating the development of alternative coping behaviors.
When the client is demonstrating socially inappropriate behavior, keep interactions to a minimum, and escort to a place way from group activities.	Lack of positive reinforcement decreases a behavior.
When inappropriate behavior stops, discuss the behavior with the client, and develop a list of alternative kinds of behavior for the client to use in situations where the inappropriate behavior is elicited. [Note here the kinds of behavior that are identified as problematic, with the action to be taken if they are demonstrated, e.g., the client will spend a time-out in seclusion or a sleeping area.]	Promotes the client's sense of control, while facilitating the development of alternative coping behaviors.
Develop a schedule of gradually increasing time for the client in group activities. For example, the client will spend [number] minutes in the group dining hall during mealtimes or will spend [number] minutes in a group game twice a day. [Note specific goals for the client here.]	Provides the client with opportunities to practice new behaviors in a safe, supportive environment.

ACTIONS/INTERVENTIONS	RATIONALES
The primary care nurse will spend 30 minutes once a day with the client at [time] discussing the client's reactions to social interactions and assisting the client with reality testing social interactions (e.g., what others might mean by silence or various nonverbal and common verbal expressions). This time can also be used to discuss relationship roles and the client's specific concerns about relationships.	
Assign the client a room near areas with high activity.	Facilitates the client's participation in unit activities.
Assign one staff person to the client each shift, and have this person interact with the client every 30 minutes while the client is awake.	Decreases the client's opportunities for socially isolating self.
Be open and direct with the client in interactions, and avoid verbal and nonverbal behavior that requires interpretation from the client.	Promotes a trusting relationship.
Have the client tell staff his or her interpretation of interactions.	Assists the client in reality testing his or her perceptions that might inhibit social interactions.
Have the client identify the activities in the community that are of interest and would provide opportunities for interactions with others. List the client's interests here.	Promotes the client's sense of control.
Develop, with the client, a plan for making contact with the identified community activities before discharge.	Promotes the client's sense of control and begins the development of adaptive coping behaviors.
When the client demonstrates tolerance for group interactions, schedule a time for the client to participate in a therapy group that provides opportunities for feedback about relationship behavior from peers and for listening to the thoughts and feelings of peers.	Disconfirms the client's sense of aloneness and assists the client to experience personal importance to others, while enhancing interpersonal relationship skills. Increasing these competencies can enhance self-esteem and promote positive orientation.
Arrange at least 1 hour a week for the client to interact with his or her support system in the presence of the primary nurse. This will allow the nurse to assess and facilitate these interactions.	Support system understanding facilitates the maintenance of new behaviors after discharge.
Discuss with the support system ways in which they can facilitate client interaction.	
Model for the support system and for the client those kinds of behavior that facilitate communication.[40]	
Limit the amount of time the client can spend alone in the room. This should be a gradual alteration and should be done in steps that can easily be accomplished by the client. Note specific schedule for the client here; for example, the client will spend 5 minutes per hour in day area. Have staff person remain with the client during these times until the client demonstrates an ability to interact with others.	Provides opportunities for the client to practice new role behaviors in a safe, supportive environment.
Refer the client to appropriate community agencies.	

(care plan continued on page 694)

NURSING ACTIONS/INTERVENTIONS WITH RATIONALES (continued from page 693)

Gerontic Health

In addition to the interventions for Adult Health and Mental Health, the following may be utilized with the aging client:

ACTIONS/INTERVENTIONS	RATIONALES
Discuss with the patient what efforts he or she has made to increase social contacts and what results have been obtained.	Assists in determining what interventions may result in positive outcomes.
Ask the patient to identify hobbies and activities that have been a part of his or her adult life.	Provides information on preferred activities and guides the nurse in seeking resources that match the patient's interests.
Ask the patient to identify barriers to continuing with the hobbies and activities he or she enjoyed.	Barriers may be indicators of need for use of specific resources such as adaptive equipment or transportation.
Assist the patient in identifying and contacting community support services.	In many areas, initial contact with support services can entail numerous telephone calls to reach the appropriate resource.

Home Health

See Mental Health nursing actions for detailed interventions.

ACTIONS/INTERVENTIONS	RATIONALES
Involve the client and family in planning and implementing strategies to reduce social isolation: • Family conference: Discuss perceptions of source of social isolation, and list possible solutions. • Mutual goal setting: Set realistic goals with evaluation criteria. List specific tasks for each family member. • Communication: Provide positive feedback.	Family involvement in planning enhances the effectiveness of interventions.
Assist the family and patient with lifestyle adjustments that may be required: • Promote social interaction. • Provide transportation. • Provide activities to keep busy during lonely times. • Provide communication alternatives for those with sensory deficits. • Assist with disfiguring illness (e.g., refer the patient to enterostomal therapist or prosthesis manufacturer). • Control incontinence, or provide absorbent undergarments when socializing. • Promote self-worth. • Promote self-care. • Develop and utilize support groups. • Use pets. • Establish regular telephone contact. • Inform of volunteer programs in the community that person could work for.	Permanent changes in behavior and family roles require support.
Consult with or refer to assistive resources as indicated.	Utilization of existing services is efficient use of resources. Self-help groups, occupational therapists, or home-bound programs can enhance the treatment plan.

SORROW, CHRONIC

DEFINITION[9]

Cyclical, recurring, and potentially progressive pattern of pervasive sadness that is experienced (by a parent, caregiver, or individual with chronic illness or disability) in response to continual loss, throughout the trajectory of an illness or disability.

DEFINING CHARACTERISTICS[9]

1. Feelings that vary in intensity, are periodic, may progress and intensify over time, and may interfere with the client's inability to reach his or her highest level of personal and social well-being
2. Expresses periodic, recurrent feelings of sadness
3. Expresses one or more of the following feelings:
    a. Anger
    b. Being misunderstood
    c. Confusion
    d. Depression
    e. Disappointment
    f. Emptiness
    g. Fear
    h. Frustration
    i. Guilt or self-blame
    j. Helplessness
    k. Hopelessness
    l. Loneliness
    m. Low self-esteem
    n. Recurring loss
    o. Overwhelmed

RELATED FACTORS[9]

1. Death of a loved one
2. Experiences chronic physical or mental illness or disability, such as mental retardation, multiple sclerosis, prematurity, spina bifida or other birth defects, chronic mental illness, infertility, cancer, or Parkinson's disease
3. Experiences one or more triggering events (e.g., crises in management of the illness or crises related to developmental stages and missed opportunities or milestones that bring comparisons with developmental, social, or personal norms)
4. Unending caregiving as a constant reminder of loss

RELATED CLINICAL CONCERNS

1. Any chronic physical or mental illness
2. Any terminal diagnosis
3. Less-than-perfect newborn

 Have You Selected the Correct Diagnosis?

Ineffective Individual Coping
Chronic Sorrow has different and more specific related factors. Chronic Sorrow could lead to Ineffective Individual Coping as the individual loses physical and mental energy. The primary differentiation will be in the related factors.

Anticipatory Grieving
Chronic Sorrow relates to a continual loss, whereas Anticipatory Grieving relates to a specific potential loss. These could well be companion diagnoses, and the nursing interventions designed to assist the client with either diagnosis would be beneficial in assisting with resolution of the other diagnosis.

EXPECTED OUTCOME

Will verbalize less sadness by [date].

Will describe [number] of strategies of coping with loss by [date].

Will demonstrate [number] of coping behaviors by [date].

TARGET DATES

Resolving this diagnosis will require long-term intervention; however, the development of a plan to address client's concerns can be evaluated on a short-term basis. An appropriate target date for initial evaluation of long-term goals would be 10 to 14 days. A target date to evaluate the short term goals would be 2 to 3 days.

NURSING ACTIONS/INTERVENTIONS WITH RATIONALES

Adult Health

ACTIONS/INTERVENTIONS	RATIONALES
Assess the events that precipitate chronic sorrow and make the patient feel disparity between self and others.	Provides information for anticipatory guidance.
Assess the patient's coping methods. Support the coping strategies that work. Teach other strategies that may help if these are insufficient for meeting needs.	Supports the patient and helps the patient learn effective coping methods.

(care plan continued on page 696)

NURSING ACTIONS/INTERVENTIONS WITH RATIONALES (continued from page 695)

Adult Health

ACTIONS/INTERVENTIONS	RATIONALES
Take time to listen, empathize, and support the patient.	Listening conveys respect, compassion, and a nonjudgmental position.
Have the patient participate in his or her own care and maintain involvement in personal interests and activities.[41]	Helps the patient feel control over own life.
Provide opportunities for the patient to interact with others who have experienced the same type of loss.	Helps the patient to see that he or she is not alone in the grief process.
Refer to the Mental Health nursing actions for additional information.	

Child Health

● N O T E : *Identify developmentally appropriate approach, with incorporation of appropriate nursing interventions.*

ACTIONS/INTERVENTIONS	RATIONALES
Monitor for all possible contributing factors to chronic sorrow, including history, family, child, or others as feasible.	Provides the most holistic database to offer appropriate individualization.
Facilitate the child's and family members' verbalization of feelings about sorrow.	Expression of feelings helps reduce anxiety and offers clues to related issues.
Identify preferences of the child to further express feelings per age-appropriate play, art, discussion, or, when appropriate, support groups.	Free and creative expression provides a noninvasive insight to monitor feelings on an ongoing basis.
Help the child and family to identify the meaning the chronic sorrow provides.	Significance of sorrow is often the key to acceptance and reducing negative effects of sorrow.
Identify ways to cope with factors that contributed or contribute to chronic sorrow by determining previously successful coping patterns.	Growth is enhanced when coping strategies familiar to the client are valued.
Introduce additional coping strategies according to the child's and family's readiness.	Reinforcement is best timed when the client is successfully dealing with demands and is more likely to accept additional modes.
Determine the effect chronic sorrow has on basic daily functioning.	Sorrow may be interfering with basic daily activities.
Support the child's and family's daily progress in expression of feelings and ways to cope with sorrow.	Ongoing assessment and expression foster trust and open communication.
Identify the need for other pediatric specialists as needed (e.g., play therapist, child psychologist, and psychiatrist).	Experts will best be able to deal with the child's and family's long-range needs.
Determine a support group for long-term follow-up.	Peer support is valued, with the likelihood of bonding and reduction of feelings of isolated sorrow.
Provide sensitive inquiry as related to anniversaries or events that may hold significance for the child or family.	Valuing of the importance of events for the child and family provides respect and facilitates sharing to foster trust.
Identify, with the child's and family's input, ways to cope effectively with chronic sorrow.	Actual resolution of chronic sorrow is possible with an individualized plan known to be effective and familiar to the client, thereby lessening the likelihood of recurrence.

Women's Health

For this diagnosis, the Women's Health nursing actions are similar to Adult Health, Child Health, Gerontic Health, and Mental Health, except for the following:

ACTIONS/INTERVENTIONS	RATIONALES
Fetal Demise or Stillborn The following are important *first* steps to help the parents cope with chronic sorrow: • Allow the parents to express feelings and participate in needed decision making. • Prepare the infant for viewing by the parents and significant others. • Provide a private, quiet place and time for the parents and family to see and hold the infant. • Take pictures, and complete a "memory box" for the parents. • Contact faith-based or cultural leader as requested by the parents for desired ceremonies for the infant. • Provide references to supportive groups within community, such as Resolve with Sharing or other parents who have lost infants.	Initiates the grieving process in a supportive environment, as well as providing a database that can be used by the family and therapist when dealing with chronic sorrow.
Obtain from the client or other family members information about the cause of sorrow that could help with understanding and therefore planning actions to support the client. • Determine, if possible, the cause of death and the gestational age of fetus and/or infant at the time of death. • Determine the nature of attachment of the parents to the infant. • Discuss past unresolved grief. • Determine social support of parents. (Beware of a "conspiracy of silence.")[51,52]	Some deaths of babies are a relief to the parents, such as in the case of congenital abnormalities or a long, difficult illness of a child. This does not mean they do not love their babies, and could result in experiencing feelings of guilt because of the feeling of relief. Many family members and relatives do not know what to say or do, and therefore ignore the subject, believing this is better for the parents so they can forget sooner.
Discuss with the parents the aspect of anniversaries, birthdays, or holidays. Give suggestions of how to observe the child's memory, such as: • Have a small ceremony with the family and friends at gravesite, home, or place of worship. • Plant a tree or flowers in the child's memory. • Encourage the family and friends to acknowledge awareness of special day to the parent.	Such dates often become an anticlimax; they have dreaded the date and find it either easy or very difficult. Acknowledgment tells the parents that you share their pain without becoming intrusive. Holidays are very difficult, particularly when other children are celebrating. It often becomes a reminder that they will never be able to do these things with their child.

Mental Health

● N O T E : *Because this is a normal response, clients most likely to have this diagnosis will be seen as outpatients. Inpatient clients may experience this response if a trigger event occurs during hospitalization.*

ACTIONS/INTERVENTIONS	RATIONALES
Provide the client with the information he or she requests related to illness and the disease process.	Assists with decision making and promotes a sense of control.[53,54]
Sit with the client [number] minutes [number] times a day to explore and provide specific information he or she may need to cope with the identified situation.	Assists with coping, and promotes a sense of control.[53]

(care plan continued on page 698)

NURSING ACTIONS/INTERVENTIONS WITH RATIONALES (continued from page 697)

Mental Health

ACTIONS/INTERVENTIONS	RATIONALES
Provide information that indicates to the client that his or her reaction is normal. This information should be provided in a manner that does not diminish the individual's personal experience.	Alleviates feelings of "difference" or isolation, and increases sense of control. Assists the client in making room for grief, as a normal process, in his or her life.[16,54]
Discuss with the client the situations that might contribute to the increase or recurrence of grief feelings. These situations could include comparisons with norms, management crises, anniversaries, unending caregiving, and awareness of role changes. [Note here the person responsible for this discussion.]	Promotes client understanding of the experience, and assists with the normalizing of the experience, while providing anticipatory guidance.[55] Facilitates the development of the belief that grief is a life process and not something that is "dealt with" or ended.[54]
Sit with the client [number] minutes [number] times per day to provide an opportunity for him or her to tell his or her story with the effect of the experience.	Validates the client's experience, and legitimizes the emotions.[16,56]
Discuss with the client his or her beliefs about grief and how it affects his or her life.	Understanding the client's perceptions provides the foundation for necessary change.[54]
Discuss with the client previous strategies utilized to cope with loss, and the extent to which these were successful. [Note here the person responsible for this discussion and ongoing follow-up.]	Supports strengths and assists with the development of client-specific coping strategies.[16,52]
Provide the client with necessary supports to utilize identified coping strategies. Note here the supports, specific for this client, needed from staff. This could include referrals to community support groups, arrangements for respite care, supporting the use of humor and play as a coping strategy, arrangements to interact with spiritual leader, and providing opportunities for physical activity.	Facilitates the use of coping strategies.[53]
Schedule a meeting with the support system to explore their beliefs and experiences related to loss. [Note here the time for this meeting and the person responsible.]	Something that affects one member of the support system affects other members.[54]
Meetings with support systems should also include:	
• Normalization of the support system emotions. • Provide stories of the successes of other support systems. • Sit with them as they express their thoughts and feelings related to the situation. • Support strengths of this system. • Modeling of good communication.	Normalizes the experience and increases the sense of control, while providing a context that supports positive coping.[54]
• Include open, honest communication about the issues the system finds most difficult to discuss.	Addressing both the perceived positive and negative aspects of a situation opens communication and decreases guilt.[54]
• Provide information the system needs about the situation and disease process.	Promotes a sense of control, and facilitates decision making.
• Refer the support system to community support groups.	Normalizes the experience and provides a source for information on coping.
• Discuss opportunities for respite from caregiving responsibilities.	Decreases guilt related to the need to withdraw from the caregiving role.[16]

Gerontic Health

In addition to the nursing actions provided here, the nurse is referred to the Mental Health section for this diagnosis.

ACTIONS/INTERVENTIONS	RATIONALES
Provide the client and/or caregiver with information that is understandable and focused on the specific information needed for the situation, and practical.	Assists the client and/or caregiver to have a sense of control in meeting care needs.
Encourage use of community, facility, or Web site support services dealing with the specific disability or chronic illness involved.[57]	Gives the client or caregiver access to information and resources that may help meet the challenges of their condition.
Promote use of available respite services as needed.	Provides a means of positive coping for the individual.
Advise the older adult to maintain personal interests and activities as much as possible.	Identified in research as a means of coping and maintaining control.[57,58]
Use empathetic presence (listening, offering support and encouragement and validation of feelings).	Helps the client or caregiver feel supported by professionals involved in care needs.
Discuss with the client or caregiver milestones and events that may trigger episodes of feeling sorrow, such as anniversaries, birthdays, or celebrations that contrast what could have been with what is.[55]	Presents opportunities for anticipatory guidance.

Home Health

ACTIONS/INTERVENTIONS	RATIONALES
Actively listen to the client's story, helping him or her to put events in sequence, increasing his or her recall of details, and separating what is real from what is not.[59]	There is an almost universal need to describe the feelings and events of a death or major diagnosis.
Teach the client and significant others the importance of expressing and accepting sadness[59]: • Avoid platitudes. • Avoid quiet suffering and suppression of grief. • Change settings as necessary to allow expressions of grief.	Removes impediments to healthy expression of sadness.
Assist the client to acknowledge and express feelings of guilt.	This is the first step in resolution of feelings of guilt.
If the chronic sorrow is related to death, assist the client in reviewing his or her relationship with the deceased[59]: • Exploring the early days of the relationship, covering negative aspects as well as positive aspects • Exploring what might have been had the death not occurred	Talking about the relationship is an important element of healing.
Consult with and/or refer the patient to assistive resources as needed.	Utilization of existing services is an efficient use of resources.

VIOLENCE, SELF-DIRECTED AND OTHER-DIRECTED, RISK FOR

DEFINITIONS[9]

Risk for Self-Directed Violence Behaviors in which an individual demonstrates that he or she can be physically, emotionally, and/or sexually harmful to self.

    Risk for Other-Directed Violence Behaviors in which an individual demonstrates that he or she can be physically, emotionally, and/or sexually harmful to others.

DEFINING CHARACTERISTICS[9]

A. Risk for Other-Directed Violence (Risk Factors)

1. Body language: Rigid posture, clenching of fists and jaw, hyperactivity, pacing, breathlessness, threatening stances
2. History of violence against others (e.g., hitting, kicking, spitting at, scratching, throwing objects at, or biting someone; attempted rape; rape; sexual molestation; urinating or defecating on a person)
3. History of threats of violence (e.g., verbal threats against property, verbal threats against person, social threats, cursing, threatening notes/letters, threatening gestures, sexual threats)
4. History of violent antisocial behavior (e.g., stealing, insistent borrowing, insistent demands for privileges, insistent interruption of meetings, refusal to eat, refusal to take medication, ignoring instructions)
5. History of violence, indirect (e.g., tearing off clothes, ripping objects off walls, writing on walls, urinating on floor, defecating on floor, stamping feet, temper tantrum, running in corridors, yelling, throwing objects, breaking a window, slamming doors, sexual advances)
6. Neurological impairment (e.g., positive EEG, CAT, MRI, neurological findings; head trauma; seizure disorders)
7. Cognitive impairment (e.g., learning disabilities, attention deficit disorder, decreased intellectual function)
8. History of childhood abuse
9. History of witnessing family violence
10. Cruelty to animals
11. Firesetting
12. Pre-/perinatal complications/abnormalities
13. History of drug/alcohol abuse
14. Pathological intoxication
15. Psychotic symptomatology (e.g., auditory, visual, or command hallucinations; paranoid delusions; loose, rambling, or illogical thought processes)
16. Motor vehicle offenses (e.g., frequent traffic violations, use of a motor vehicle to release anger)
17. Suicidal behavior
18. Impulsivity
19. Availability/possession of weapon(s)

B. Risk for Self-Directed Violence (Risk Factors)

1. Suicidal ideation (frequent, intense prolonged)
2. Suicidal plan (clear and specific lethality; method and availability of destructive means)
3. History of multiple suicide attempts
4. Behavioral clues (e.g., writing forlorn love notes, directing angry messages at a significant other who has rejected the person, giving away personal items, taking out a large life insurance policy)
5. Verbal clues (e.g., talking about death, "better off without me," asking questions about lethal dosages of drugs)
6. Emotional status (hopelessness, despair, increased anxiety, panic, anger, hostility)
7. Mental health (severe depression, psychosis, severe personality disorder, alcoholism or drug abuse)
8. Physical health (hypochondriasis, chronic or terminal illness)
9. Employment (unemployed, recent job loss/failure)
10. Age 15 to 19
11. Age over 45
12. Marital status (single, widowed, divorced)
13. Occupation (executive, administrator/owner of business, professional, semiskilled worker)
14. Conflictual interpersonal relationships
15. Family background (chaotic or conflictual history of suicide)
16. Sexual orientation (bisexual [active], homosexual [inactive])
17. Personal resources (poor achievement, poor insight, affect unavailable and poorly controlled)
18. Social resources (poor rapport, socially isolated, unresponsive family)
19. People who engage in autoerotic sexual acts

RELATED FACTORS[9]

None listed.

RELATED CLINICAL CONCERNS

1. Physical abuse
2. Organic brain syndrome; Alzheimer's disease
3. Attempted suicide
4. Epilepsy, temporal lobe
5. Panic episode
6. Depression
7. Command hallucinations

 Have You Selected the Correct Diagnosis?

Compromised or Disabled Family Coping
The diagnosis of Compromised or Disabled Family Coping relates to the inability of the primary caregiver or caretaker to meet the needs of the patient. No violence is included in this diagnosis. If such abuse has been assessed, then the diagnosis should be changed.

Impaired Parenting
Impaired Parenting relates to the relationship between the nurturing figure and the child. Child abuse is included within this diagnosis, but as an actual fact, not as a risk for. If a risk for abuse exists, then Risk for Violence is the most appropriate diagnosis.

Suicide, Risk for
Suicide, Risk for would be the appropriate diagnosis for a client who demonstrates behaviors or thoughts that indicate an intention is to end his or her life. This diagnosis would initiate interventions to directly address the suicidal ideation/behavior.

Self-Directed Violence, Risk for
Self-Directed Violence, Risk for would be appropriate for the client who is at risk of harming themselves physically, emotionally or sexually without the intent to die.

Self-Mutilation
Self-Mutilation is the appropriate diagnosis for the client who is actively involved in self-injurious behavior that results in tissue damage and would not be fatal. The goal of the behavior is to attain relief from tension.

EXPECTED OUTCOME

A. Self-Directed Violence, Risk for
Will sign a no self-harm contract by [date].
  Will identify feelings that precede thoughts of self-injury by [date].
  Will identify [number] of methods to cope with feelings by [date].
B. Other-Directed Violence, Risk for
Will identify [number] of methods that will facilitate self-restraint of abusive behavior
  Will demonstrate and or identify the use of [number] of coping behaviors by [date].
  Will verbalize empathy for the victim by [date].

TARGET DATES

For the sake of all concerned, the patient should begin to demonstrate progress within 3 to 5 days. However, the patient must be monitored on a daily basis. To control violent behavior completely may take months.

NURSING ACTIONS/INTERVENTIONS WITH RATIONALES

Adult Health

ACTIONS/INTERVENTIONS	RATIONALES
Provide a safe environment by removing clutter, breakables, or potential weapons. Restrain or seclude the patient as needed.	Promotes safety and reduces the risk of harm to patients or others.
Observe, at least once an hour, for indications of suicidal behavior (e.g., withdrawal, depression, or planning for and organizing an attempt).	Prevents self-inflicted violence.
Monitor for signs of anger or distress such as restlessness, pacing, wringing of hands, or verbally abusive behavior.	Monitors for deterioration of condition and promotes early intervention.
Accept the anger of the patient, but do not participate in it when interacting with the patient.	Anger is an acceptable behavior if appropriately handled, but escalation of anger is to be avoided.
Remain calm. Set limits on the patient's behavior, and reduce environmental stimuli.	Decreases sensory stimuli. Decreases anxiety and violence-provoking situations.
Encourage the patient to verbalize angry feelings rather than physically demonstrating them or to physically demonstrate them in constructive ways (e.g., working out on a punching bag, banging a trash can, or taking a walk). Schedule 30 minutes twice a day at [times] to confer with the patient regarding this topic.	Promotes an acceptable alternative strategy for dealing with anger.
Let the patient know that he or she has control of, and is responsible for, own actions. Help the patient identify situations that interfere with his or her control during conferences with the patient.	Reinforces reality and maintains limits on behavior.
Give medications as ordered (tranquilizer, sedative, etc.), and monitor effects of medication.	Determines the effectiveness of medication as well as monitoring for unwanted side effects.
Refer to a psychiatric nurse clinician. (See Mental Health nursing actions.)	Violence or risk for violence requires specific interventions by a specialist in the area of mental health.

(care plan continued on page 702)

NURSING ACTIONS/INTERVENTIONS WITH RATIONALES (continued from page 701)

Child Health

ACTIONS/INTERVENTIONS	RATIONALES
Assist the patient and family to describe usual patterns of role-relationship activities.	Insight into role-relationships is basic in determining the risk for violence.
Monitor for precipitating or triggering events that seem to recur as the pattern for violence is explored.	Risk indicators can be identified as assessment for repeated violence is considered.
Assist the patient and family to describe their perception of the actual or potential violence pattern.	Insight of the patient or parents reveals basic data about the violence pattern, which assists in accurate intervention.
Provide opportunities for expression of emotions related to the violence appropriate for age and developmental capacity (e.g., a toddler could use dolls, puppets, or other noninvasive methods).	Expression of thoughts and feelings in a directive age-appropriate manner helps the child understand the impact of the violence and assists in reducing his or her anxiety.
Provide appropriate collaboration for long-term follow-up regarding appropriate intervention.	Valuing long-term follow-up fosters compliance and shows sensitivity to the patient's needs for long-term support. Safety is also at risk. In many instances, legal mandates dictate the exact protocols to be enforced.
Provide for role-taking by parents in a supportive manner when possible.	Supportive role-modeling provides a safe and nonjudgmental milieu for the parents to practice parenting and appropriate behaviors with the child. It also allows for observation of behaviors to follow reciprocity of parent–infant dyad or triad.
Provide consistency in caregivers to best develop a trust for the nursing staff during hospitalization.	Consistency increases trust in caregivers.
Provide for confidentiality and privacy.	These standards are too often overlooked.
Ensure that discussions regarding the child and family are carried out with objectivity.	Objective dialogues are less threatening for all involved.
Address appropriate authorities as needed for protection of the child and family members, to include security or police members according to institutional policy.	Appropriate child protective measures must be taken.
Provide support in determining usual coping patterns and how these may be enhanced to deal with altered role-relationship pattern of violence.	Support in coping and dealing with violence will help reduce the likelihood of increasing violence and assist in reducing anxiety.
Assist in plans for placement, transitional placement, or dismissal to return home for the family.	Appropriate planning for changes in care and the environment lessens the emotional trauma of these changes.
Assist in identification of specific resources for long-term planning as appropriate.	Follow-up ensures attention to long-term needs and attaches value to follow-up care.
Maintain objectivity in documentation of parent–child interactions.	

Women's Health

● N O T E : *These actions relate specifically to the abused, battered woman.*[60–63]

ACTIONS/INTERVENTIONS	RATIONALES
All female clients should be screened for the presence of violence on entry into the health-care system: • Have you ever been intentionally hurt by someone?	

ACTIONS/INTERVENTIONS	RATIONALES
• Are you afraid of your partner or significant other? • Has your partner or significant other ever made you feel afraid, inadequate, or worthless? Be alert for cues that might indicate battering, such as: • Hesitancy in providing detailed information about injury and how it occurred • Explanation for injuries that are inconsistent with the injury (e.g., trunk injury not consistent with a fall) • Inappropriate affect for the situation • Delayed reporting of symptoms • Types and sites of injuries, such as bruises to head, throat, chest, breast, or genitals • Inappropriate explanations • Increased anxiety in the presence of the batterer • Injuries that are proximal, rather than distal, may indicate a battering injury. • Injuries that are in various stages of healing (e.g., old bruises along with new bruises) • Vague somatic symptoms with no visible cause	Provides the database necessary to accurately assess the true causative factor.
Provide a quiet, secure atmosphere to facilitate verbalization of fears, anger, rage, guilt, and shame. All discussions about violence should be initiated and conducted with the patient isolated away from the partner.	Provides emotional support to the patient. Fosters security for the patient so that she will realize that she is not alone, or not the only person to have had this experience.
Provide information on options available to the patient (e.g., women's shelters and legal aid societies).	Provides basic information needed by the patient for future planning.
Assist the patient in raising her self-esteem by: • Asking permission to do nursing tasks • Involving the patient in decision making • Providing the patient with choices • Encouraging the patient to ask questions • Assuring the patient of confidentiality • Listening to her concerns and choices without judging	
Assist the patient in reviewing and understanding family dynamics.	
Facilitate the patient's planning for economic and financial needs, such as housing, job, child care, food, clothing, schooling for the children, and legal assistance.	Provides the information, long-range support, and essentials for resolving the problem.
Refer the patient to social services or battered women's support programs for immediate financial assistance for shelter, food, clothing, and child care.	
Assist the patient in identifying lifestyle adjustments that each decision could entail.	
Encourage development of community and social network systems.	
The nurse should monitor his or her own biases about victims of domestic violence: • Belief that they deserve the abuse because they choose to stay with the abuser • Belief that the patient is powerless to change the situation	Biases negatively impact appropriate nursing interventions. (Refer to Rape Trauma Syndrome in Chapter 10.)

(care plan continued on page 704)

NURSING ACTIONS/INTERVENTIONS WITH RATIONALES (continued from page 703)	

Mental Health

ACTIONS/INTERVENTIONS	RATIONALES
Introduce self to the client, and call the client by name.	Conditions that make people feel anonymous facilitate aggressive behavior.[64]
If aggressive behavior is resulting from toxic substances, consult with the primary care provider for medication and detoxification procedure.	Staff and client safety is of primary concern.
Observe the client every 15 minutes during detoxification, assessing vital signs and mental status, until the condition is stable.	Client safety is of primary concern.
Place the client in a quiet environment for detoxification.	Inappropriate levels of sensory stimuli can increase confusion and disorganization.
Eliminate environmental stimuli that affect the client in a negative manner. This could include staff, family, and other clients. Establish a balance between being in control and being controlling.	Inappropriate levels of sensory stimuli can increase confusion and disorganization, increasing the risk for violent behavior.
Provide a calm, reassuring environment. Respect the client's requests for quiet, alone time.	
Protect the client from harm by: • Removing sharp objects from environment • Removing belts and strings from the environment • Providing a one-to-one constant interaction if risk for self-harm is high • Checking on the client's whereabouts every 15 minutes • Removing glass objects from environment • Removing locks from room and bathroom doors • Providing a shower curtain that will not support weight • Checking to see whether the client swallows medication	Provides basic client safety.
Observe the client's use of physical space, and do not invade client's personal space.	Encroachment of the client's personal space may be perceived as a threat.[65]
If it is necessary to have physical contact with the client, explain this need to the client in brief, simple terms before approaching.	Clarifies the role of the staff to the client so that the intent of these interactions is framed in a positive manner.
Remove unnecessary clutter and excess stimuli from the environment.	Inappropriate levels of sensory stimuli can increase the client's confusion and disorganization, thus increasing the risk for violent behavior.
Talk with the client in a calm, reassuring voice.	
Do not make sudden moves.	
Remove persons who irritate the client from the environment. Observe the client carefully for signs of increasing anxiety and tension.	The best intervention for violent behavior is prevention.
Do not assume physical postures that are perceived as threatening to the client.	
If an increase in tension is noted, talk with the client about his or her feelings.	Assists the client in developing coping behaviors.
Help the client attach feelings to appropriate persons and situations; for example, "Your boss really made you angry this time."	Assists the client in developing coping behaviors that are appropriate to the situation. Promotes the client's sense of control.[65]

ACTIONS/INTERVENTIONS	RATIONALES
Suggest to the client alternative behavior for releasing tension, for example, "You really seem tense right now. Let's go to the gym so you can use the punching bag." Or, "Let's go for a walk."	Assists the client in releasing physical tension associated with high levels of anger.
Provide medication as ordered, and observe the client for signs of side effects, especially orthostatic hypotension.	Provides the least restrictive way of assisting the client to control behavior.
Answer questions in an open, direct manner.	Promotes the development of a trusting relationship, and promotes consistency in interventions.[65]
Orient the client to reality in interactions. Use methods of indirect confrontation that do not pose a personal threat to the client. Do not agree with delusions, for example, "I do not hear voices other than yours or mine," or "This is the mental health unit at [name] Hospital."	Direct confrontations could be perceived as a threat to the client and precipitate violent behavior.[66]
Refer to Disturbed Thought Process in Chapter 7 for detailed interventions for delusions and hallucinations.	Promotes the development of a trusting relationship. In crisis, clients are more likely to respond positively to someone with whom they have a trusting relationship. Increases consistency in interventions.[65]
Assign one staff member to be primary caregiver to the client to facilitate the development of a therapeutic relationship.	
Inform the client before any attempts to make physical contact are made in the process of normal provision of care. For example, explain to the client you would like to assist him or her with dressing, and would this be all right?	Clients who are prone to violence need increased personal space. Intrusions could provoke violent behavior.[65]
Assist the client in identifying potential problem behavior with feedback about his or her behavior.	Promotes the client's sense of control, which decreases the risk for violent behavior.[65]
Have the client talk about angry feelings toward self and others.	Assists the client to understand the reasons for the anger, which can defuse the situation.[65]
Contract with the client to talk with staff member when he or she feels an increase in internal tension or anger.	Promotes the client's sense of control by assuring the client that if he or she can no longer maintain control, the staff has a specific plan to assist him or her.[65]
Set limits on inappropriate behavior, and discuss these limits with the client. Note these limits here, as well as the consequences for these kinds of behaviors. This information should be very specific so that the intervention is consistent from shift to shift. Present these limits as choices.	
If conflict occurs between the client and someone else, sit with them as they resolve the conflict in an appropriate manner. The nurse will serve as a facilitator during this interaction.	Staff presence can reinforce using appropriate problem-solving skills as the client practices these new behaviors.
Discuss tension-reduction techniques with the client, and develop a plan for the client to learn these techniques and apply them in difficult situations. [Note the plan here.]	Promotes the client's sense of control. Repeated practice of a behavior internalizes and personalizes the behavior.
Develop with the client a reward system for appropriate behavior. [Note reward system here.]	Positive reinforcement encourages behavior.
Talk with the client about the differences between feelings and behavior. Role-play with the client, attaching different kinds of behavior to feelings of anger.	Promotes the client's sense of control by establishing limits around feelings in the cognitive realm. Repeated practice of a behavior internalizes and personalizes the behavior.

(care plan continued on page 706)

NURSING ACTIONS/INTERVENTIONS WITH RATIONALES (continued from page 705)

Mental Health

ACTIONS/INTERVENTIONS	RATIONALES
Help the client in determining whether the feeling being experienced is really anger. Explain that at times of high stress we can misinterpret feelings and must be very careful not to express the wrong feeling. What we are expressing as anger may actually be, for example, anxiety or frustration.	Placing other names on the feeling may open new behavior possibilities to the client, while promoting a positive orientation. For example, if this were anger, lashing out would be appropriate, but because it is anxiety, it is more appropriate to relax.
When the client is capable, assign him or her to group in which feelings can be expressed and feedback can be obtained from peers. [Note the schedule for group activity here.]	Promotes the client's sense of control by providing role models for alternative ways of coping with feelings.
Review with the client consequences of inappropriate behavior, and assess the gains of this behavior over the costs.	Assesses the possibility for secondary gain for inappropriate behavior.
Accept all threats of aggressive behavior as serious.	Client and staff safety are of primary importance.
Remind the staff to not take aggressive acts personally, even if they appear to be directed at one staff member.	As the nurse's level of arousal increases, judgment decreases, making the nurse less effective when working with the client who is experiencing difficulty.[65]
Provide the client with positive verbal feedback about positive behavior changes.	Positive feedback encourages behavior.
Do not place the client in frustrating experiences without a staff member to support the client during the experience.	Frustration can increase the risk for aggression.[64]
If the client is suicidal, place him or her in a room with another client.	Decreases the amount of time the client is alone.
Provide the client with opportunities to regain self-control without aggressive interventions by giving the client choices that will facilitate control; for example, "Would you like to take some medication now or spend some time with a staff member in your room?" Or "We can help you into seclusion, or you can walk there on your own."	Promotes the client's perception of control while supporting self-esteem.
Provide the client with opportunities to maintain his or her dignity.	
Assure the client that you will not allow him or her to harm self or someone else.	
Reinforce this by having more staff in attendance than necessary to physically control the client if necessary. Persons from other areas of the institution may be needed in these situations. If others are used, they should be trained in proper procedures.	Client and staff safety are of primary concern.
If potential for physical aggression is high[65,66]:	
• Place one staff member in charge of the situation.	Promotes consistency in intervention and decreases inappropriate levels of sensory stimulation.
• As the primary care person attempts to "talk the client down," other staff member should remove other clients and visitors from the situation.	Client and staff safety are of primary concern.

ACTIONS/INTERVENTIONS	RATIONALES
• Other staff members should remove potential weapons from the environment in an unobtrusive manner. This could include pool cues and balls, chairs, flower vases, or books.	Assists in reducing levels of emotion.
• Avoid sudden movements.	
• Never turn your back on the client.	
• Maintain eye contact (this should not be direct, for this can be perceived as threatening to the client), and watch the client's eyes for cues about potential targets of attack.	Assists in assessing the client's intentions without appearing threatening.
• **Do not** attempt to subdue the client without adequate assistance.	Client and staff safety are of primary concern.
• Put an increased distance between the client and self.	Clients who have a potential for violent behavior need more personal space.
• Tell the client of the concern in brief, concise terms.	Maintains appropriate levels of sensory stimuli.
• Suggest alternative behavior.	Promotes the client's sense of control.
• Help the client focus aggression away from the staff.	May prevent the need for more restrictive interventions.
• Encourage the client to discuss concerns.	Assists in reducing levels of emotion and de-escalation of behavior.
If talking does not resolve the situation:	
• Have additional assistance prepared for action (at least four persons should be present).	Client and staff safety are of primary concern.
• Have those who are going to be involved in the intervention remove any personal items that could harm client or self (e.g., eyeglasses, guns, long earrings, necklaces, or bracelets).	
• Have seclusion/restraints ready for the client, remove glass objects and sharp objects, and open doors for easy entry.	Prevents sensory overload while providing reassurance to the client.
• Briefly explain to client what is going to happen and why.	
• Use method practiced by intervention team to place the client in seclusion or restraints.	Client and staff safety and coordination are of primary concern.
• Protect self with blankets, arms bent in front of the body to protect the head and neck.	Contains the client's body and blocks the client's vision if it is necessary to disarm the client.[66]
• Be prepared to leave the situation, and be aware of location of exits.	Client and staff safety is of primary concern.
See Impaired Physical Mobility, Chapter 5, for care of the client in seclusion or restraints.	
Discuss the violent episode with the client when control has been regained. Answer questions the client has about the situation, and provide the client with opportunities to express thoughts and feelings about the episode.	Debriefing diminishes the emotional impact of the intervention, and provides an opportunity to clarify the circumstances for the intervention, offer mutual feedback, and promote the client's self-esteem.[67]
Inform the client of the behavior that is necessary to be released from seclusion or restraints.	Promotes the client's sense of control and enhances self-esteem.
Process the situation with the client after incident and explore alternative coping strategies for future situations.	
Assess the milieu for "organizational provocation."	
If the client has a history of violent acts:	Provides offenders with the opportunity to rebuild their relationship style.[68]

(care plan continued on page 708)

NURSING ACTIONS/INTERVENTIONS WITH RATIONALES (continued from page 707)

Mental Health

ACTIONS/INTERVENTIONS	RATIONALES

• Provide the client with individual or group opportunities to:
  • Take responsibility for the violent act.
  • Develop empathy for the victim.
  • In some way, develop an apology to the victim. (This method may be indirect if it would not be in the best interest of the victim to receive a direct apology.)
  • Explore the interactions of thoughts, feelings, and behaviors in their violent acts.
  • Develop a plan for alternative ways of responding to the identified thoughts and feelings.
• Note persons responsible for facilitating this process here, along with the meeting schedule.
• If partner or family violence is an issue, arrange conjoint, solution-oriented treatment. This should include a no-violence contract between the partners.
	Provides partners with an opportunity to develop alternative ways of communicating and problem solving.[69,70]

Educate the client about personal behaviors that could result in self-harm or are high risk (e.g., autoerotic asphyxia, failure to use personal protective sports equipment).	Client's may not be aware of the risks involved in these behaviors.

Gerontic Health

● **NOTE:** *Suicide or attempted suicide is a serious functional consequence of depression in elders. Particularly at risk are elderly clients who are: males; Protestant with rare church attendance; Caucasian; widowed or divorced; living alone or living in an urban environment; recently relocated; retired or unemployed; depressed; alcoholic or dependent on other substances; experiencing low self-esteem, decreased life satisfaction, or hopelessness; or has a family history of suicide or mental illness. Elders who attempt suicide are typically successful on the first attempt. If there is a failed attempt, the elder should be considered high risk for further attempts.[71] Remember that for the client who has intent to end their life the correct nursing diagnosis would be Suicide, Risk for.*

Psychoses and agitation are common in clients with dementia. In cases of agitation, it is critical to consider the safety of the patient and that of those around him or her. The health-care team should carefully evaluate the medical, psychiatric, or psychosocial problems that underlie the disturbance and tend to those in an effort to resolve the problem.[72]

ACTIONS/INTERVENTIONS	RATIONALES
Risk for Self-Directed Violence Carefully conduct an assessment of verbal, behavioral, situational, or syndromatic warning signs that may signal suicidal ideology: • Stockpiling medications • Purchasing a gun • Making or changing a will • Putting personal affairs in order • Giving money or possessions away	These are warning signs that may signal suicidal ideology.[71]

ACTIONS/INTERVENTIONS	RATIONALES
• Donating one's body to science • Sudden interest or disinterest in religion • Self-neglect • Difficulty in performing household or social tasks • Deterioration of relationship behaviors • A general downturn in health status • Failure to thrive • Scheduling an appointment with a physician for vague symptoms • Recent move • Death of a spouse, child, or friend • Diagnosis of a terminal illness • Depression accompanied by anxiety • Tension, agitation, guilt, and dependency • Rigidity, impulsiveness, and isolation • Changes in sleeping and eating habits • Sudden recovery from a deep depression	
Carefully assess the client for the presence of protective factors and draw upon these when working with the client: • The potential for understanding, relating, benefiting from experience, benefiting from knowledge, acceptance of help • The capacity for loving, wisdom, sense of humor, social interest • Possession of a sense of purpose or meaning in life • A history of successful transitions, coping independently, acquisition of life skills, the ability to reminisce (especially about life successes) • The presence of a caring and available family and supportive community network • The presence of a caring, available, and knowledgeable nurse or health-care provider and health network • Membership in a religious community, particularly Catholic or Jewish • Commitment to personal values and ideals, people, groups, creative work, and/or social, political, or intellectual causes	These are important resources that the nurse can draw upon when working with a suicidal elder.[71]
Determine the agency's suicide policy/protocol and adhere to it.[71]	

Risk for Other-Directed Violence
When bathing the client with a tendency toward violence[73]:
• Keep the bathing area warm.
• If the sound of running water agitates the client, run the water before the client enters the bathing area.
• Avoid rushing; task-oriented behavior by the caregiver is associated with agitated behavior.
• Use "rescuing" if necessary to reduce agitation; a negative response to one caregiver can be "solved" by the second caregiver.

(care plan continued on page 710)

| NURSING ACTIONS/INTERVENTIONS WITH RATIONALES (continued from page 709) | |

Gerontic Health

ACTIONS/INTERVENTIONS	RATIONALES
• Assess early signs of agitation; back off for a few minutes until the client calms. • Remove dentures in clients who tend to bite. • Offer gum or other foods or engage the client in singing if he or she tends to bite. For clients who "grab," offer distraction or something for them to hold. Ensure that an adequate number of caregivers are present for lifting and transferring so the client feels safe.[74]	
In cases of dementia, discuss with the caregiver whether there is a usual pattern of violence. For example, does startling or speaking in loud tones, or having several people speaking at once, usually result in a violent outburst by the patient?	Awareness of violence triggers provides guidelines to adjust environment and staff behaviors.

Home Health

ACTIONS/INTERVENTIONS	RATIONALES
Teach the client and family appropriate monitoring of signs and symptoms of the risk for violence: • Substance abuse • Increased stress • Social isolation • Hostility • Increased motor activity • Disorientation to person, place, and time • Disconnected thoughts • Clenched fists • Throwing objects • Verbalizations of threats to self or others	Provides a database for early recognition and intervention.
Assist the client and family in lifestyle adjustments that may be required: • Recognition of feelings of anger or hostility • Developing coping strategies to express anger and hostility in acceptable manner, such as exercise, sports, art, music, etc. • Prevention of harm to self and others • Treatment of substance abuse • Management of debilitating disease • Coping with loss • Stress management • Decreasing sensory stimulation • Provision of a safe environment • Removal of weapons, toxic drugs, etc. • Development and use of a support network • Restriction of access to weapons, especially handguns[75,76]	Permanent changes in behavior require support.

ACTIONS/INTERVENTIONS	RATIONALES
Discuss workplace issues related to violence.[77]	Homicide is a leading cause of occupational death. Prevention is needed.
Develop anticipatory guidance materials for violence prevention.[77,78]	Age-appropriate prevention strategies provide support for change.
Involve the patient and family in planning and implementing strategies to reduce the risk for violence: • Family conference • Mutual goal setting • Communication	Provides for early intervention.
Assist the client and family to set criteria to help them determine when intervention of law enforcement officials or health professionals is required (e.g., if the patient becomes threat to self or others).	
Consult with or refer to assistive resources as appropriate.	Utilization of existing services is efficient use of resources. The psychiatric nurse clinician and support groups can enhance the treatment plan.

REFERENCES

1. Turner, J: The Structure of Sociological Theory, ed 6. Dorsey Press, Homewood, IL, 1998.
2. Shibutani, R: Human Nature and Collective Behavior: Papers in Honor of Herbert Blumer. Prentice-Hall, Englewood Cliffs, NJ, 1970.
3. Johnson, GB: American families: Changes and challenges. Fam Sociol 72:502, 1991.
4. Clemen-Stone, S, Eigsti, DG, and McGuire, SL: Comprehensive Community Health Nursing: Family, Aggregate and Community Practice, ed 5. CV Mosby, St. Louis, 1998.
5. Mallinger, KM: The American family: History and development. In Bomar, PJ (ed): Nurses and Family Health Promotion: Concepts, Assessment, and Interventions. WB Saunders, Philadelphia, 1996.
6. Stanhope, M, and Lancaster, J: Community & Public Health Nursing, ed 6. Mosby–Year Book, St. Louis, 2003.
7. Murdock, G: Social Structure. Macmillan, New York, 1949.
8. Ainsworth, M, Blehar, M, Walter, E, and Wall, S: Patterns of Attachment: A Psychological Study of the Strange Situation. Lawrence Erlbaum, Hillsdale, NJ, 1978.
9. North American Nursing Diagnosis Association: Nursing Diagnosis: Definitions and Classification, 2005–2006. North American Nursing Diagnosis Association, Philadelphia, 2005.
10. Gennaro, S: Postpartal anxiety and depression of mothers of term and preterm infants. Nurs Res 37:82, 1988.
11. Weiss, ME, and Armstrong, M: Postpartum mothers' preferences for nighttime care of the neonate. JOGNN J Obstet Gynecol Neonatal Nurs 20:290, 1991.
12. Nichols, FH, and Zwelling, E: Maternal-Newborn Nursing: Theory and Practice. WB Saunders, Philadelphia, 1997.
13. Gregory, CM: Caring for caregivers: Proactive planning eases burden on caregivers. Lifelines 1:51, 1997.
14. Kanusky, C: Health concerns of women in midlife. In Breslin, ET, and Lucas, VA (eds): Women's Health Nursing: Toward Evidence Based Practice. WB Saunders, St. Louis, 2003.
15. Chafetz, L, and Barnes, L: Issues in psychiatric caregiving. Arch Psychiatr Nurs 3:61, 1989.
16. Kneisl, CR, Wilson, HS, and Trigoboff, E: Contemporary Psychiatric-Mental Health Nursing. Pearson Education, Upper Saddle River, NJ, 2004.
17. Wright, L, and Leahey, M: Nurses and Families: A Guide to Family Assessment and Intervention, ed 4. FA Davis, Philadelphia, 2005.
18. Anderson, CM, Hogarty, GE, and Reiss, DJ: The psychoeducational family treatment of schizophrenia. In Goldstein, M (ed): New Directions for Mental Health Services. Jossey-Bass, San Francisco, 1981.

19. Thompson, C, and Spilsbury, K: Support for carers of people with Alzheimer's type dementia, Chochrane Database of Systematic Reviews 1, 2006.
20. Baldwin, BA: Family caregiving: Trends and forecasts. Geriatr Nurs 11:172, 1990.
21. Gaynor, S: When the caregiver becomes the patient. Geriatr Nurs 10:120, 1989.
22. Haber, J, et al: Comprehensive Psychiatric Nursing, ed 5. Mosby–Year Book, St. Louis, 1997.
23. Wright, L, and Leahey, M: Nurses and Families: A Guide to Family Assessment and Intervention, ed 4. FA Davis, Philadelphia, 2005.
24. Kneisl, C, Wilson, H, and Trigoboff, E: Contemporary Psychiatric-Mental Health Nursing. Pearson Education, Upper Saddle River, NJ, 2004.
25. Krupnick, SLW, and Wade, AJ: Psychiatric Care Planning, ed 2. Springhouse, Springhouse, PA, 1999.
26. ACOG Committee on Ethics: Patient Choice: Maternal-Fetal Conflict. Committee Opinion, Washington, DC, 1990.
27. Mercer, R, and Ferketich, S: Maternal-infant attachment of experienced and inexperienced mothers during infancy. Nurs Res 43:344, 1994.
28. May, KA, and Mahlmeister, LR: Maternal and Neonatal Nursing: Family-Centered Care, ed 3. JB Lippincott, Philadelphia, 1994.
29. Lindeman, M, Hawks, J, and Bartek, J: The alcoholic family: A nursing diagnosis validation study. Nurs Diagn 5:65, 1991.
30. Edwards, M, and Steinglass, P: Family therapy treatment outcomes for alcoholism. J Marital Fam Ther 21:475, 1995.
31. Stanton, D, and Todd, T: The Family Therapy of Drug Abuse and Addiction. Guilford Press, New York, 1982.
32. Mudd, SA, et al: Alcohol withdrawal and related nursing care in older adults. J Gerontol Nurs 20:17, 1994.
33. Atkinson, RM: Alcohol and substance use disorders in the elderly. In Birren, J, et al (eds): Handbook of Mental Health and Aging. Academic Press, New York, 1992.
34. Stone, JT, Wyman, JF, and Salisbury, SA: Clinical Gerontological Nursing: A Guide to Advanced Practice. WB Saunders, Philadelphia, 1999.
35. Richter, JM: Support: A resource during crisis of role loss. J Gerontol Nurs 13:18, 1991.
36. National Guide Clearinghouse: Family bereavement support before and after the death of a nursing home resident. http://www.guideline.gov, 2006.
37. Prigerson, HG, and Jacobs, SC: Caring for bereaved patients: All the doctors just suddenly go. JAMA 286:1373, 2001.
38. National Center for Post Traumatic Stress Disorder: Managing grief after disaster. http://www.NCPTSD.VA,gov, 2006.

39. Lowdermilk, DL, and Perry, SE: Maternity & Women's Health Care, ed 8. CV Mosby, St. Louis, 2004.
40. Teschendorf, M: Women during the reproductive years. In Breslin, ET, and Lucas, VA (eds): Women's Health Nursing: Toward Evidenced-Based Practice. WB Saunders, St. Louis, 2003.
41. Pridham, KF, et al: Early postpartum transition: Progress in maternal identity and role attainment. Res Nurs Health 14:21, 1991.
42. Condon, J, and Corkindale, C: The correlates of antenatal attachment in pregnant women. Br J Med Psychol 70:359, 1997.
43. Gilliss, C, et al: Toward a Science of Family Nursing. Addison-Wesley, Menlo Park, CA, 1989.
44. Roehlkepartain, E: You Can Make a Difference for Kids. Search Institute, Minneapolis, MN, 1999.
45. Patterson, G: Families. Research Press, Champaign, IL, 1971.
46. Wong, DL: Whaley and Wong's Nursing Care of Infants and Children, ed 6. CV Mosby, St. Louis, 1999.
47. Abraham, IL, and Reel, S: Cognitive nursing interventions with long-term care residents: Effects on neurocognitive dimensions. Arch Psychiatr Nurs VI:356, 1992.
48. National Guide Clearinghouse: National guidelines for management of relocation in cognitively intact older adults. http://www.guideline.gov, 2006.
49. King, KS, Dimond, M, and McCance, KL: Coping with relocation. Geriatr Nurs 8:258, 1987.
50. Flake, KJ: HIV testing during pregnancy: Building the case for voluntary testing. Lifelines 4:13, 2000.
51. Stewart, A, and Dent, A: At a Loss: Bereavement Care When a Baby Dies. Bailliere Tindall, London, 1994.
52. Cote-Arsenault, C, and Mahlangu, N: Impact of perinatal loss on the subsequent pregnancy and self: Women's experiences. JOGNN J Obstet Gynecol Neonatal Nurs 28:274, 1999.
53. Hainsworth, M: Helping spouses with chronic sorrow related to multiple sclerosis. J Psychosoc Nurs 34:36, 1996.
54. Moules, N: Legitimizing grief: Challenging beliefs that constrain. J Fam Nurs 4:142, 1998.
55. Burke, M, Eakes, G, and Hainsworth, M: Milestone of chronic sorrow: Perspectives of chronically ill and bereaved persons and family caregivers. J Fam Nurs 5:374, 1999.
56. Eakes, G: Chronic sorrow: The lived experience of parents of chronically mentally ill individuals. Arch Psychiatr Nurs 9:77, 1995.
57. Lindgre, CL, and Connely, CT: Grief in spouse and children caregivers of dementia patients. West J Nurs Res 21:521, 1999.
58. Lindgren, CL: Chronic sorrow in persons with Parkinson's and their spouses. Scholast Inquiry Nurse Pract 10:351, 1996.
59. Kemp, C: Terminal Illness: A Guide to Nursing Care, ed 2. Lippincott, Williams & Wilkins, Philadelphia, 1999.
60. Phillips, DSH: Culture and systems of oppression in abused women's lives. JOGNN J Obstet Gynecol Neonatal Nurs 27:678, 1998.
61. Parker, B, and McFarlane, J: Identifying and helping battered pregnant women. MCN Am J Matern Child Nurs 16:161, 1991.
62. Sampselle, CM: The role in preventing violence against women. JOGNN J Obstet Gynecol Neonatal Nurs 20:481, 1991.
63. Farley, M, and Keaney, JC: Physical symptoms, somatization, and dissociation in women survivors of childhood sexual assault. Women's Health 25:33, 1997.
64. Zimbardo, P: In review. In Evans, R: The Making of Psychology. Alfred Knopf, New York, 1976.
65. Stevenson, S: Heading off violence with verbal de-escalation. J Psychosoc Nurs Ment Health Serv 29:6, 1991.
66. Morton, P: Staff roles and responsibilities in incidents of patient violence. Arch Psychiatr Nurs 1:280, 1987.
67. Norris, M, and Kennedy, C: The view from within: How patients perceive the seclusion process. J Psychosoc Nurs Ment Health Serv 30:7, 1992.
68. Sheela, RA: A nurse's experiences working with sex offenders. J Psychosoc Nurs 37:25, 1999.
69. Stith, S: Domestic violence. Clin Update 2000 1:1, 2000.
70. Robinson, C, Wright, L, and Watson, WA: A nontraditional approach to family violence. Arch Psychiatr Nurs 8:30, 1994.
71. National Guideline Clearinghouse: Evidenced-based protocol: Elderly suicide, secondary prevention. http://www.guideline.gov, 2006.
72. National Guideline Clearinghouse: Guideline for the treatment of patients with Alzheimer's disease and other dementias of late life. http://www.guideline.gov, 2006.
73. National Guideline Clearinghouse: Prevention of violence. http://www.guideline.gov, 2006.
74. National Guideline Clearinghouse: Bathing persons with dementia. http://www.guideline.gov, 2006.
75. Loftin, C, et al: Effects of restrictive licensing of handguns and homicide and suicide in the District of Columbia. N Engl J Med 325:1615, 1991.
76. Kellerman, A, et al: Suicide in the home in relation to gun ownership. N Engl J Med 327:467, 1992.
77. Centers for Disease Control/National Institute of Occupational Safety and Health: Homicide in US Workplaces: A Strategy for Prevention and Research. US Department of Health and Human Services, Morgantown, WV, 1992.
78. Roberts, C, and Quillian, J: Preventing violence through primary care intervention. Nurse Pract 17:62, 1992.
79. National Guidelines for Management of Relocation in Cognitively Intact Older Adults, http://www.guidelines.gov (accessed February 8, 2006).

10

SEXUALITY– REPRODUCTIVE PATTERN

PATTERN DESCRIPTION

This pattern focuses on the sexual–reproductive aspects of individuals over the entire life span. Sexuality patterns involve sex role behavior, gender identification, physiologic and biologic functioning, as well as the cultural and societal expectations of sexual behavior. An individual's anatomic structure identifies sexual status, which determines the social and cultural responses of others toward the individual and, in turn, the individual's responsive behavior toward others.

Reproductive patterns involve the capability to procreate, actual procreation, and the ability to express sexual feelings. The success or failure of psychologically and physically expressing sexual feelings and procreating can affect an individual's lifestyle, health, and self-concept.

The nurse may care for clients who, because of illness, violence, or lifestyles, experience alterations or disturbances in their sexual health that affect their sexuality and reproductive patterns.

PATTERN ASSESSMENT

1. Following a rape, is the patient experiencing multiple physical symptoms?
   a. Yes (Rape-Trauma Syndrome: Compound Reaction)
   b. No
2. Following a rape, is the patient indicating severe emotional reactions?
   a. Yes (Rape-Trauma Syndrome: Compound Reaction)
   b. No
3. Is the client using alcohol or drugs to cope following a rape?
   a. Yes (Rape-Trauma Syndrome: Compound Reaction)
   b. No
4. Has the client changed her relationship with men?
   a. Yes (Rape-Trauma Syndrome: Silent Reaction)
   b. No
5. Does the client indicate increased anxiety in follow-up counseling?
   a. Yes (Rape-Trauma Syndrome: Silent Reaction)
   b. No
6. Does the client verbalize any problems related to sexual functioning?
   a. Yes (Sexual Dysfunction)
   b. No
7. Does the client exhibit any indications of physical or psychosocial abuse?
   a. Yes (Sexual Dysfunction)
   b. No
8. Does the client relate any changes in sexual behavior?
   a. Yes (Ineffective Sexuality Patterns)
   b. No
9. Does the client report any difficulties or limitations in sexual behavior?
   a. Yes (Ineffective Sexuality Patterns)
   b. No

CONCEPTUAL INFORMATION

Gender development and sexuality are closely entwined with biologic, psychological, sociologic, spiritual, and cultural aspects of human life. The biologic sex of an individual is decided at the time of conception, but sexual patterning is influenced from the moment of birth by the actions of those surrounding the individual. From that moment, males and females receive messages about who they are and what it means to be masculine or feminine.[1]

The sexuality of an individual is composed of biologic sex, gender identity, and gender role. The biologic and psychological perspectives of culture and society determine how an individual develops sexually, particularly in the sense one has of being male or female (gender identity). Biologic identity begins at the moment of fertilization, when chromosomal sex is determined, and becomes even more defined at 5 to 6 weeks of fetal life. At this time, the undifferentiated fetal gonads become ovaries (XX, female chromosomal sex) or testes (XY, male chromosomal sex), and hormones finalize the genital appearance between the 7th and 12th weeks. Fetal androgens (testicular hormones) must be present for male reproductive structures to develop from the wolffian ducts. If fetal androgens are not present, the fetus will develop female reproductive structures. By the 12th week of fetal life, biologic sex is well established.[1,2]

Reactions by others begin the moment the biologic sex of the fetus or infant is known. Whether the sex of the infant is known before birth or not until the time of birth, the parents and those about them prepare for either a boy or a girl by buying clothes and toys for a boy (color blue, pants, shirts, football) or a girl (color pink, frilly dresses, dolls), as well as speaking to the infant differently according to sex. Girls are usually spoken to in a high, singsong voice: "Oh, isn't she cute!" whereas boys are spoken to in a low-pitched, matter-of-fact voice: "Look at that big boy. He will really make a good football player one of these days!" These actions contribute to the infant's gender identity and perception of self. Behavioral responses from the infant are elicited by the parents, based on their views of what roles a boy or girl should fulfill.

Gender role is determined by the kinds of sex behavior that are performed by individuals to symbolize to themselves and others that they are masculine or feminine.[3] Early civilizations assigned roles according to who performed what tasks for survival. Women were relegated to specific roles because of the biologic nature of bearing and rearing children and gathering food. The men were the hunters and soldiers. Advanced technologies, changing mores, birth control, and alternative methods of securing food and rearing children have led to changes in roles based on gender in Western society. Gender roles are influenced by cultural, religious, and social pressures. "Gender role stereotypes are culturally assigned clusters of behaviors or attributes covering everything from play activities and personal traits to physical appearance, dress and vocational activities."[4]

As in gender identity, researchers have noticed gender role-play in children as young as 13 months. Schoolchildren are particularly exposed and pressured into gender role stereotyping by parents, teachers, and peers, who demand expected, rigid behavior patterns according to the sex of the child. Molding into gender roles is often accomplished by handling girls and boys differently. Little girls are usually handled gently as infants, and adults fuss with their baby's hair and tell her how pretty she is; little boys are usually roughhoused and are told "What a big boy you are." Sex directional training is also accomplished by such verbalizations as "Where's Daddy's girl?" and "Big boys don't cry; be a man."[5]

North American society is moving toward a blending of male and female roles; however, stereotyping still exists. According to Schuster and Ashburn,[4] stereotyping is not all bad, as it can help "reduce anxiety arising from gender differences and may aid in the process of psychic separation from one's parents." Therefore, they conclude that stereotypes can provide structure and facilitate development as well as restrict development and become too rigid, thus interfering with a child's potential.

One's sexuality is a continuing lifetime evolution, changing as one matures and progresses through the life cycle. It is impossible to separate an individual's sexuality from his or her development, as sexuality combines the interaction of the biophysical and psychosocial elements of the individual.

According to a national research study,[8] "Rape in America," rape occurs far more often than previously recognized. This study found that 683,000 American women were raped in 1990, which is a far higher number than had been estimated. Almost 62 percent of these women stated they were minors when they were raped, and about 29 percent stated they were younger than 11 when the rape occurred. This indicates rape is most definitely a traumatic event for our young in America. Of the rapists, 75 percent were known by the victim, and included such persons as neighbors, friends, relatives, boyfriends, ex-boyfriends, husbands, or ex-husbands. Only 22 percent of the rapists were strangers to the victim. In 28 percent of the cases, injuries to the victim, beyond the rape itself, occurred. Sadly, only 16 percent of the victims told police about the attack, with the victims being concerned about the family finding out, being blamed by others for the attack, and others knowing about the attack. These concerns have decreased in victims raped in the past 5 years. Nonetheless, in this group there were increased concerns about having their name become public, getting AIDS and other sexually transmitted diseases, and becoming pregnant. Confidentiality of identity is a high priority for these victims.

DEVELOPMENTAL CONSIDERATIONS

INFANT

Erickson defines the major task of infancy as the development of trust versus mistrust.[4] The act of the parents' nur-turing and providing care-taking activities allows the infant to begin experiencing various pleasures and physical sensations, such as warmth, pleasure, security, and trust,[1] and it is through these acts of nurturing that the infant begins to develop a sense of masculinity or femininity (gender identity). The infant is further molded by the parents' perceptions of sex-appropriate behavior through reward and punishment. Female infants tend to be less aggressive and develop more sensitivity because girls are usually rewarded for "being good," and male infants develop more aggressively and learn to be independent because boys are told that "big boys don't cry" and they learn to comfort themselves. By the age of 13 months, sexual behavior patterns and differences are in place,[1,4] and core gender identity is theorized to be formed by 18 months.[7] "These early behaviors are so critical to one's core gender-identity that children who experience gender reassignment after the age of 2 years are high-risk candidates for psychotic disorders."[4]

The infant who is sexually abused is usually physically traumatized and, many times, dies. Developmental delays can be recognized in these children by failure to thrive, low weight or no weight gain, lethargy, and flat affect.

TODDLER AND PRESCHOOLER

Neuromuscular control allows toddlers to explore their environment, interact with their peers,[1,4] and develop autonomy and independence.[7] Genital organs continue to increase in size but not in function. The toddler's vocabulary increases; he or she distinguishes between male and female by recognizing clothing and body parts; and he or she develops pride in his or her own body, especially the genital area, as he or she becomes aware of elimination or excretory functions. They need guidance and require parents to set limits as they learn to "hold on" or "let go" in order to achieve a sense of autonomy.[4] By the age of 3, they have perfected verbal terms for the sexes, understand the meaning of gender terms and the roles associated with those terms (e.g., girl is sister or mother, and boy is brother or father),[1] and receive pleasure from kissing and hugging.[7]

The preschooler is busy developing a sense of socialization and purpose. Learning suitable behavior for girls and boys or sex role behavior is the major task during the preschool years. Preschoolers will often identify with the parent of the same sex while forming an attachment to the parent of the opposite sex. They are inquisitive about sex and are often occupied in exploration of their own bodies and friends' bodies, which will often be exhibited in group games such as "doctor–nurse," urinating "outside," or masturbating.[7] The toddlers' concept of their bodies, not as a whole but as individual parts, changes when as preschoolers they begin to develop "an awareness of themselves as individuals, and become more concerned about body integrity and intactness."[4]

It is important to note that 6-year-olds are the age group most subjected to sexual abuse.[8] How a child handles this experience, and his or her future developmental and psychological growth, depend largely on the reactions and actions of the significant adult in the child's life.[7] Rape that occurs during early childhood may simply be acknowledged by the child as part of the experience of growing up and may have no long-term effects if not repeated. Usually counseling during this developmental age has great effect. All claims of abuse by a child should be investigated and should be handled through someone who has the experience and knowledge to deal with the child and his or her parents in a professional and understanding manner.

SCHOOL-AGE CHILD

Play is the most important work of children—it allows them to be curious and investigate social, sexual, and adult behavior. "Through play children learn how to get their needs met and how to meet the needs of others."[4] Different socialization of boys and girls tends to become apparent in play during the school years, with boys engaging in aggressive team play and girls in milder play and forming individual friendships. These activities can lead to stereotyping and exaggeration of gender difference.

Going to school allows children to begin to be more independent and form peer groups of the same sex. Although the peer group becomes very important to them, they need adult direction in learning socially acceptable forms of sexual behavior and when they may engage in them. If they do not receive the information they are seeking, negative feelings and apprehension about sexuality may develop.[1]

Great trauma can occur when rape occurs during these years. It is very damaging to the value systems that are being formed. Sexual identity can be disturbed, and sexual confusion can occur.

ADOLESCENT

Puberty, "the period of maturation of the reproductive system,"[4] causes profound changes in the individual's sexual anatomy and physiology and is a major developmental crisis for the adolescent. Secondary sex characteristics appear—breasts, pubic hair, and menstruation in girls; testicular enlargement, penile enlargement, pubic hair, ejaculation, and growth of muscle mass in boys. The configuration, contour, and function of the body changes rapidly and dramatically point out sexual differences and the onset of adulthood. These changes bring new feelings that create role confusion and increase awareness of sexual feelings. "The major task of adolescence is the establishment of identity in the fact of role confusion."[1]

Peer groups have an important influence on the young adolescent (12 to 15 years), but during late adolescence (16 to 19 years) the peer group influence lessens and more intimate relationships with the opposite sex develop.[7] These relationships can involve a wide range of sexual behavior from exploring behavior to intercourse, sometimes with the result of teenage pregnancy. Exploring behavior can be either with the opposite sex (foreplay and intercourse), the same sex (homosexuality), or self (masturbation). How the teenager views him- or herself sexually will depend on the reassurance and guidance he or she receives from a significant adult in his or her life. The greatest misunderstandings of teenagers involve homosexuality, masturbation, and conception and contraception. How these subjects are approached, taught, and supported can influence their adult sexuality.[1,7]

It is during adolescence, when new experiences of sexual maturity begin, that questions about maleness or femaleness are asked by the individual and concerns arise about "who one is within the peer group."[1] Adolescents must evaluate their masculinity and femininity and question and then decide on their gender identity, gender orientation, and gender preference. The adolescent not only deals with physical changes, but also integrates past experiences and role models with new experiences and new role models into his or her own gender identity.

Violent sexual occurrences during this period of life can devastate a person for the rest of his or her life. Adolescents are dealing with sexual confusion and identification; rape can stop or slow or change this process. Fear and loss of self-esteem can dictate actions and influence the sexual identity and gender expression.

YOUNG ADULT

This period of an individual's life (usually 20s and early 30s) is concerned with selecting a vocation, obtaining an education, military service, choosing a partner, building a career, and establishing an intimate relationship. This is a period of maximal sexual self-consciousness, commitment to a relationship, and social legitimization of sexual experiences.[1,4,7] There is a concern with parenting and establishment of the marital relationship.

Rape can slow or stop normal sexual relationships during the adult years. Fear can become the greater part of life for the victim. These years are ones for forming lasting relations with a sexual partner, marrying, and beginning families. Rape can cause withdrawal from any interaction with a sexual partner; relationships can break up, not only because of the reaction of the victim of rape, but also because of the reactions of the family and partner of the victim.

ADULT

Demands placed on adults by their careers and raising children may interfere with their sexual interest and activity.[1] The major task of this period of life is to accent one's own lifestyle and decisions rather than feeling frustrated and disappointed. "Social pressures and expectations, feedback from significant others and, finally, self-perception all influence how one evaluates the success of one's life."[1]

Although the adult is at the peak of his or her career or profession, physiologic changes begin to influence the adult's lifestyle. The aging process, illnesses, and menopause (male and female) cause changes in lifestyles and everyday activities. Changes in sexual activities can occur because of these physical and physiologic changes; however, the adult who lives a healthy lifestyle, has good nutrition, exercises, and has an optimistic outlook usually feels good and functions well sexually. Often middle-age adults, just as they have finished raising their children, are faced with the task of caring for their elderly parents.

OLDER ADULT

As in adolescence, dramatic body changes begin in late adulthood and continue into old age. There is no reason that healthy men and women cannot continue to enjoy their sexuality into old age. Women must deal with menopause and postmenopause, and men must often deal with impotence; however, with an interested sexual partner, good healthy sexuality can continue.

Older women are viewed by rapists as easy victims. Slowing of physical reactions and disabilities of old age (impaired seeing or hearing, or slow gait) keep them from being alert to danger and from reacting quickly. More important, the older woman often views herself as inferior, and this contributes to her own victimization.[9] Because most women outlive men and face changes in lifestyles and economic status, they are reluctant, and often cannot afford, to leave familiar older parts of cities that often change and deteriorate. This may expose them to the accompanying increase in crime rate.[9]

 APPLICABLE NURSING DIAGNOSES

RAPE-TRAUMA SYNDROME: COMPOUND REACTION AND SILENT REACTION

DEFINITIONS[10]

Rape-Trauma Syndrome Sustained maladaptive response to a forced, violent sexual penetration against the victim's will and consent.

Rape-Trauma Syndrome: Compound Reaction Forced, violent sexual penetration against the victim's will and consent. The trauma syndrome that develops from this attack or attempted attack includes an acute phase of disorganization of the victim's lifestyle, and a long-term process of reorganization of lifestyle.

Rape-Trauma Syndrome: Silent Reaction Forced, violent sexual penetration against the victim's will and con-

sent. The trauma syndrome that develops from this attack, or attempted attack, includes an acute phase of disorganization of the victim's lifestyle and a long-term process of reorganization of lifestyle.

DEFINING CHARACTERISTICS[10]

A. **Rape-Trauma Syndrome**
  1. Disorganization
  2. Change in relationships
  3. Physical trauma (e.g., bruising and tissue irritation)
  4. Suicide attempts
  5. Denial
  6. Guilt
  7. Paranoia
  8. Humiliation
  9. Embarrassment
  10. Aggression
  11. Muscle tension and/or spasms
  12. Mood swings
  13. Dependence
  14. Powerlessness
  15. Nightmares and sleep disturbance
  16. Sexual dysfunction
  17. Revenge
  18. Phobias
  19. Loss of self-esteem
  20. Inability to make decisions
  21. Dissociative disorders
  22. Self-blame
  23. Hyperalertness
  24. Vulnerability
  25. Substance abuse
  26. Depression
  27. Helplessness
  28. Anger
  29. Anxiety
  30. Agitation
  31. Shame
  32. Shock
  33. Fear

B. **Rape-Trauma Syndrome: Compound Reaction**
  1. Change in lifestyle, for example, changes in residence, dealing with repetitive nightmares and phobias, seeking family support, or seeking social network support in long-term phase
  2. Emotional reaction, for example, anger, embarrassment, fear of physical violence and death, humiliation, revenge, or self-blame in acute phase
  3. Multiple physical symptoms (e.g., gastrointestinal irritability, genitourinary discomfort, muscle tension, or sleep pattern disturbance in acute phase)
  4. Reactivated symptoms of previous conditions, that is, physical illness or psychiatric illness in acute phase
  5. Reliance on alcohol and/or drugs (acute phase)

C. Rape-Trauma Syndrome: Silent Reaction
1. Increased anxiety during interview, that is, blocking of associations, long periods of silence, minor stuttering, or physical distress
2. Sudden onset of phobic reactions
3. No verbalization of the occurrence of rape
4. Abrupt changes in relationships with men
5. Increase in nightmares
6. Pronounced changes in sexual behavior

RELATED FACTORS[10]

A. Rape-Trauma Syndrome
1. Rape
B. Rape-Trauma Syndrome: Compound Reaction
To be developed.
C. Rape-Trauma Syndrome: Silent Reaction
To be developed.

RELATED CLINICAL CONCERNS

Not applicable.

 Have You Selected the Correct Diagnosis?

Sexual Dysfunction
Rape can be the cause of Sexual Dysfunction in a patient who cannot learn to put into perspective, or deal with, the rape experience. Rape-Trauma is always the result of a violent act, and must be dealt with according to the individual situation. Although Sexual Dysfunction can occur as the result of rape, the nurse must assist the patient to deal with the trauma of the rape in order to assist with the sexual dysfunction.

EXPECTED OUTCOME

Will verbalize [number] positive self-statements related to personal response to the incident by [date].

TARGET DATES

Because of the varied physical and emotional impact of rape, a target date of 3 days would not be too soon to evaluate for progress.

NURSING ACTIONS/INTERVENTIONS WITH RATIONALES

Adult Health

ACTIONS/INTERVENTIONS	RATIONALES
Explore your own feelings about rape before initiating patient care. Maintain a nonjudgmental attitude. Actively listen when the survivor wants to talk about the event. Encourage verbalization of thoughts, feelings, and perceptions of the event. Explore the basis for and reality of thoughts, feelings, and perceptions.	The nurse's feelings can be sensed by the survivor and can influence the survivor's coping and sense of self.
Attend to physical and health priorities such as lacerations or infection with appropriate explanations and preparation.	Prompt attention to physical needs provides comfort and facilitates a trusting relationship.
Promote a trusting, therapeutic relationship by spending at least 30 minutes every 4 hours (while the survivor is awake) at [times] with the survivor.	Promotes expression of feelings and validates reality.
Use a calm, consistent approach when interacting with the survivor. Respect the survivor's rights.	Assists in reducing anxiety.
Be supportive of the survivor's values and beliefs.	The survivor's sexuality is intimately linked to his or her value-belief system.
Explain the need for medicolegal procedures, procedures to assess for sexually transmitted diseases, prophylactic medications, and medications to avoid postcoital contraception before performing procedures. Refer to Women's Health nursing actions for specifics about procedures.	Enlists the survivor's cooperation, and prepares her for events in case charges are filed against the alleged rapist.

ACTIONS/INTERVENTIONS	RATIONALES
Provide for appropriate privacy and health teaching as care is administered. Allow the survivor to see her own anatomy if this seems appropriate as part of health teaching.	Avoids perpetuating the survivor's fear as a result of necessity of examination and treatment in the same body area involved in the rape. Could promote a sensation of rape recurrence.
Assist the survivor in activities of daily living (ADLs) after examination.	Promotes a slight sense of return to normalcy. Emotional shock may render the survivor temporarily unable to perform basic ADLs.
Determine to what degree or extent symptoms of physical reactions exist, such as: • Pain or body soreness • Disturbances in sleep • Altered eating patterns • Anger • Self-blame • Mood swings • Feelings of helplessness	Basic database needed to plan for long-term effects of rape.
Administer medications as ordered to alleviate pain, anxiety, or inability to sleep, and teach the survivor how to safely take such medications.	Allows time for the survivor to process event in a way that maintains self-integrity and self-esteem.
When interacting with the survivor, recognize that she will proceed at her own rate in resolving rape trauma. Do not rush or force the survivor.	
Identify available support systems (e.g., rape crisis center, and involve the significant other as appropriate).	Support systems that know signs and symptoms of rape-trauma syndrome can provide help for both short-term and long-term interventions. Promotes effective coping for the survivor.
Monitor coping in the survivor and significant other until discharge from the hospital.	Monitors for adaptive and maladaptive coping strategies. Provides an opportunity to assist the survivor and significant other to practice alternative coping strategies.
Assist the survivor to identify own strengths in dealing with the rape.	Helps build the survivor's self-esteem and overcome self-blame.
Provide anticipatory guidance about the long-term effects of rape. Promote self-confidence and self-esteem through positive feedback regarding strengths, plans, and reality.	Helps prepare for expected and unexpected reactions in self, friends, and significant others.
Provide for appropriate epidemiologic follow-up in cases of venereal disease.	Required by law.
Collaborate with other health-care professionals as needed.	Promotes a holistic approach and more complete plan of care.
Arrange for appropriate long-term follow-up before discharge from the hospital (e.g., counseling).	Provides for long-term support.

Male Rape Victim

Provide the same considerations as with a female survivor. (Usually these are the result of homosexual relationships. Most reported cases are children and early adolescents.)	The act of rape is an act of violence regardless of the gender of the patient, and requires the same type of care and concern.
Refer the patient to a trained male counselor (rape crisis center).	

(care plan continued on page 720)

NURSING ACTIONS/INTERVENTIONS WITH RATIONALES (continued from page 719)

Child Health

ACTIONS/INTERVENTIONS	RATIONALES
Encourage collaboration among health-care professionals to best address the patient's needs.	A specialist will be required to deal with the unique needs of the young child enduring rape. The likelihood exists for incest or a closely related individual's being identified as the one who committed the act.
Try to establish trust as dictated by age and circumstances related to rape trauma (with nurse being same sex as the patient). **Do not** leave the child alone. Be gentle and patient. • *Infants and toddlers:* Ensure continuity of caregivers. Explain procedures with dolls and puppets. • *Preschoolers:* Ensure continuity of caregivers. Allow the patient to perform self-care behavior as ability allows. Use art and methods that deal with the general view of what happened, singling out the child as not being the "cause" of this incident. • *School-agers:* Maintain continuity of caregivers. Assist the patient to express concerns related to incident. Use appropriate techniques in interviewing to determine the extent of sexual dysfunction or potential threat to future functioning. • *Adolescents:* Maintain continuity of caregivers. Encourage the patient to express how this experience affects own self-identity and future sexual activities. Encourage psychiatric assistance in resolving this crisis for any patients of this age group. Look for signs of growth of secondary sex characteristics.	
Follow up with appropriate documentation and coordination of child protective service needs. Assist the parents or guardians in signing proper release forms. Determine whether the situation involves incest.	Appropriate protocols for documentation and reporting of rape or incest must be followed according to state and federal guidelines.
Assist the patient to deal with residual feelings such as guilt for revealing or identifying assailant (in young children this often must be dealt with within the family or extended-family situations) by allowing at least 30 minutes per shift (while the patient is awake) at [times]. Use simple language when dealing with the child.	Resolution of unresolved guilt or feelings about the event must be dealt with as soon as the client's condition permits.
Encourage the family members to assist in care and follow-up of the patient's reorganization plans: • Be alert for signs of distress such as refusing to go to school, dreams, nightmares, or verbalized concerns. • Identify ways to gradually resume normal daily schedule. • Assist the family to identify how best to resolve and express feelings about the incident.	Risk behaviors serve as cues to alert the family or caregiver to monitor the child's progress in resolving the crisis.
Carry out appropriate health teaching regarding normal sexual physiology and functioning according to age and developmental capacity.	Normalcy is afforded as attempts are realistically made to resolve any aspects of rape trauma.

ACTIONS/INTERVENTIONS	RATIONALES
Incest	
Monitor for inappropriate sexual behavior among family members.	Provides a database needed to accurately assess for incest.
Monitor for children who know more about the actual mechanics of sexual intercourse than their developmental age indicates they would.	
Monitor for girls who seem to have taken over the mother's role in the home.	
Monitor for mothers who have withdrawn from the home, either emotionally or physically.	

Women's Health

ACTIONS/INTERVENTIONS	RATIONALES
Assist the survivor through the procedures for provision of necessary health care treatment. Explain each phase of examination to the survivor. Remain with the survivor at all times.	Provides a database necessary for intervention. Secures chain-of-evidence procedure, and assists in reducing anxiety for the client.
Obtain history: • List of previous venereal diseases • List of previous pelvic infections • Any injuries that were present before attack • Obstetric and menstrual history	
Assist in gathering information to provide proper health and legal care.	
Secure the survivor's description of any objects used in the attack and how these objects were used in the attack.	

Maintain sequencing and collection of evidence (chain of evidence):
• Label each specimen with:
  • Survivor's name and hospital number
  • Date and time of collection
  • Area from which specimen was collected
  • Collector's name
• Ensure proper storage and packaging of specimens:
  • Clothing and items that are wet (e.g., with blood or semen) should be put in paper bags, not plastic.
	Plastic bags will cause molding of wet items.

• Specimens obtained on microscopic slides or swabs need to be air dried before packaging.	

• Comb pubic hair for traces of the attacker's pubic hair or other evidence:
  • Submit paper towel placed under the victim to catch combings, as well as the comb used, along with pubic hair.
  • Pluck (do not cut) two or three pubic hairs from the patient, and label properly. These are used for comparison.	

(care plan continued on page 722)

NURSING ACTIONS/INTERVENTIONS WITH RATIONALES (continued from page 721)

Women's Health

ACTIONS/INTERVENTIONS	RATIONALES
• When custody of evidence is transferred to police, be certain written evidence of transfer is properly recorded: 　• Signatures of individuals involved in transfer 　• Name of person to whom the evidence is being transferred 　• Date and time • Take photographs of injuries or torn clothing. • Have the survivor sign forms for release of information to authorities. • Provide medical treatment and follow-up for: 　• Injuries 　• Sexually transmitted disease: AIDS, gonorrhea, or syphilis 　• Pregnancy	
Report to proper authorities any suspicion of family violence.	Initiates long-range support for the patient.
Evaluate for increased rate of changing residences, repeated nightmares, and sleep pattern disturbance.	Provides a database that allows accurate interpretation of the long-range impact. Provides information needed to plan long-term care.
Encourage the patient to discuss phobias, frustrations, and fears.	
Be available and allow the patient to express difficulties in establishing normal ADLs and redescribe the attack as needed.	Provides long-term essential support.
Assist the patient in developing a plan of reorganization of ADLs.	Promotes realistic planning for problem while avoiding continued denial of problem.

Mental Health

ACTIONS/INTERVENTIONS	RATIONALES
Assign a primary care nurse to the client. This nurse should be of the sex the client demonstrates most comfort with at the current time.	Promotes the development of a trusting relationship.
The primary care nurse will remain with the client during the orientation to the unit.	Promotes the development of a trusting relationship.
Limit visitors, as the client feels necessary.	Promotes the client's sense of control, while meeting security needs.
Answer the client's questions openly and honestly.	Promotes the development of a trusting relationship.
The primary care nurse will be present to provide support for the client during medical or legal examinations if the client has not identified another person.	Promotes the development of a trusting relationship, while meeting the client's security needs.
Assist the client in identifying a support person, and arrange for this person to remain with the client as much as necessary. [Note the name of this person here.]	Promotes the client's sense of control, while meeting security needs.

ACTIONS/INTERVENTIONS	RATIONALES
Provide information to the client's support system as the client indicates is needed.	Support system understanding enhances their ability to support the client in a constructive manner.
Allow the client to talk about the incident as much as is desired. Sit with client during these times, and encourage expression of feelings.	Facilitates the confrontation of the memories of the event and attachment of meaning to the situation, which will promote a sense of control.[11]
Communicate to the client that his or her response is normal. This could include expressions of anger, fear, and discomfort with persons of the opposite sex, discomfort with sexuality, or personal blame.	Normalization of the client's feelings, without diminishing his or her experience, enhances self-esteem and helps him or her move from a position of victim to that of a survivor.[12]
Inform the client that rape is a physical assault rather than a sexual act and that rapists choose victims without regard for age, physical appearance, or manner of dress.	Promotes the client's resolution of guilt and feelings of responsibility.
Assist the client in developing a plan to return to ADLs. The plan should begin with steps that are easily accomplished so that the client can regain a sense of personal control and power. [Note the steps of the plan here.]	Promotes the client's sense of control, and inhibits the tendency toward social isolation.[12]
Provide positive social rewards for the client's accomplishment of established goals. [Note here the kinds of behavior that are to be rewarded and the rewards to be used.]	Positive reinforcement encourages behavior while enhancing self-esteem.
Provide the client with opportunities to express anger at the assailant in a constructive manner, e.g., talking about fantasies of revenge, use of punching bag or pillow, or physical activity.	Assists the client in moving from the powerless position of victim to a position of survivor.
When the client can interact with small groups, arrange for the client's involvement in a therapeutic group that provides interaction with peers. [Note time of group meetings here.]	Provides the client opportunities to resolve his or her feelings of being different, while decreasing social isolation. Promotes consensual validation of the experience with others from similar situations, which enhances self-esteem and emotional resources available for coping.[12]
Involve the client in unit activities. Assign the client activities that can be easily accomplished. [Note the client's level of functioning here along with those tasks that are to be assigned to the client.]	Prevents social isolation. Accomplished tasks enhance self-esteem with positive reinforcement. Also provides opportunities to reality test self-perceptions against those of peers on the unit.
Primary nurse will spend [number] minutes with the client twice a day at [times] to focus on expression of feelings related to the rape. Encourage the client not to close these feelings off too quickly. Assist the client in reducing stress in other life situations while healing emotionally from the rape experience. Begin to facilitate the client's use of cognitive coping resources by logically assessing various aspects of the situation.	Promotes reality testing of feelings related to the rape, and inhibits the development of self-blame and guilt, which often occur in survivors.
Assist the client in developing a plan to reduce life stressors so emotional healing can continue. [Note this plan here, with the support needed from the nursing staff in implementing this plan.]	Promotes the client's sense of control and provides a positive orientation.
The primary care nurse will meet with the client andprimary support person once per day to facilitate their discussion of the rape. If the client is involved in an ongoing relationship, such as a marriage, this interaction is very important. The support person should be encouraged to express his or her thoughts and feelings in a constructive manner. If it is assessed that the rape has resulted in potential long-term relationship difficulties such as rejection or sexual problems, refer to couple therapy.	Support system understanding and acceptance facilitate the client's coping and the maintenance of these relationships.

(care plan continued on page 724)

NURSING ACTIONS/INTERVENTIONS WITH RATIONALES (continued from page 723)

Mental Health

ACTIONS/INTERVENTIONS	RATIONALES
Refer the client to appropriate community support groups, and assist him or her with contacting these before discharge.	Promotes the client's reintegration into the community, and inhibits the isolating behavior often exhibited by these clients.[12]

Gerontic Health

ACTIONS/INTERVENTIONS	RATIONALES
In the event of the rape being secondary to elder abuse, refer the patient to adult protective services.	Provides a resource for the older adult to explore options and prevent recurrence of problem.

Home Health

ACTIONS/INTERVENTIONS	RATIONALES
During the acute phase, be sure that appropriate assessment, law enforcement involvement, and treatment of physical injuries or sexually transmitted diseases are provided.	Early and accurate intervention decreases sequelae and provides documentation for any legal action.
Assist the client and family in lifestyle changes that may be needed: • Treatment for physical injuries or sexually transmitted disease • Testimony in court • Protection • Coping with terror, nightmares, or fear • Coping with alterations in sexual response to significant others • Development and use of support networks • Stress management • Changing telephone number or moving • Traveling with companion • Strategies for prevention of rape	Provides support and enhances recovery.
Assist the client and family in planning and implementing strategies for resolution of Rape-Trauma Syndrome: • Communication (e.g., discussion of feelings among family members) • Mutual sharing and trust • Problem solving (e.g., providing support for the family members and client; strategies to reduce possibility of future attacks)	Crimes of violence upset the family equilibrium and require support to correct. Involvement of the client and significant others is important to ensure successful resolution.
Consult with, or refer the patient to, assistive resources as appropriate.	Use of existing resources and expertise provides high-quality care and is effective use of already available resources.

SEXUAL DYSFUNCTION

DEFINITION[10]

Change in sexual function that is viewed as unsatisfying, unrewarding, or inadequate.

DEFINING CHARACTERISTICS[10]

1. Change of interest in self and others
2. Conflicts involving values
3. Inability to achieve desired satisfaction
4. Verbalization of problem
5. Alteration in relationship with significant other
6. Alteration in achieving sexual satisfaction
7. Actual or perceived limitation imposed by disease and/or therapy
8. Seeking confirmation of desirability
9. Alterations in achieving perceived sex role

RELATED FACTORS[10]

1. Misinformation or lack of knowledge
2. Vulnerability
3. Values conflict
4. Psychosocial abuse, for example, harmful relationships
5. Physical abuse
6. Lack of privacy
7. Ineffectual or absent role models
8. Altered body structure or function (pregnancy, recent childbirth, drugs, surgery, anomalies, disease process, trauma, or radiation)
9. Lack of significant others
10. Biopsychosocial alteration of sexuality

RELATED CLINICAL CONCERNS

1. Endocrine, urologic, neuromuscular, and skeletal disorders
2. Genital trauma

3. Agoraphobia
4. Pelvic surgery
5. Malignancies of the reproductive tract
6. Female circumcision[13]
7. Psychiatric disorders such as mania, major depression, dementia, borderline personality disorder, substance abuse or use, anxiety disorder, and schizophrenia

 Have You Selected the Correct Diagnosis?

Ineffective Sexuality Patterns
In this diagnosis, the individual is expressing concern about his or her sexuality. This diagnosis could be a result of Sexual Dysfunction, but it is not necessarily a problem to the patient. Ineffective Sexuality Patterns can be compatible with the patient's lifestyle for whatever reason, and create no overwhelming problems for the patient.

Rape-Trauma Syndrome
The diagnosis of Rape-Trauma Syndrome could result in Sexual Dysfunction because of the patient's inability to deal with the violence, trauma, and lifestyle changes as a result of rape. It is absolutely essential for the nurse to ascertain the cause of the Sexual Dysfunction, and to determine whether it is the result of the patient's perception of sexuality in general, pathophysiology, or trauma.

EXPECTED OUTCOME

Will report return, as near as possible, to previous levels of sexual functioning by [date].

TARGET DATES

Depending on the patient's perception of the sexual dysfunction, target dates may range from 1 week to several months.

NURSING ACTIONS/INTERVENTIONS WITH RATIONALES

Adult Health

ACTIONS/INTERVENTIONS	RATIONALES
Facilitate communication between the patient and partner by providing at least [number] minutes per day for privacy to communicate.	Promotes identification of issues involved in sexual dysfunction.
Encourage the patient and partner to talk about concerns and problems during conference.	Sexual behavior includes verbal, nonverbal, genital, and nongenital activities.
Talk with the patient and partner about alternative ways to attain sexual satisfaction and express sexuality (e.g., hugging, touching, kissing, masturbation, hand holding, or sexual aids). Provide factual informational material.	
Clarify misconceptions as needed (e.g., sexual activity after a heart attack, older people don't engage in sexual activity, or hysterectomy decreases sexual drive).	Misinformation and myths contribute to sexual dysfunction.

(care plan continued on page 726)

NURSING ACTIONS/INTERVENTIONS WITH RATIONALES (continued from page 725)

Adult Health

ACTIONS/INTERVENTIONS	RATIONALES
Be nonjudgmental in your attitudes.	Sexuality is a highly personal experience. Nonjudgmental attitudes reduce anxiety and open the way for therapeutic communication.
Respect the patient's values and attitudes about sexuality and sexual functioning.	Sexual behavior is intimately linked to the value-belief system. Demeaning these values and beliefs will cause anxiety in the patient.
Provide accurate information on effects of medical diagnosis or treatment on sexual functioning.	Clarifies misconceptions. Provide information on changes or modifications in sexual activities that may need to occur as a result of disease process.
Implement measures to improve self-concept (e.g., positive self-talk, assertiveness, new hairdo, new clothes, or new social surroundings).	How one feels about self is important in self-perception of sexuality.
Provide privacy for expressing sexuality (e.g., masturbation, sexual intercourse), particularly when the patient has been hospitalized for a significant length of time, or has been separated from his or her significant other for a significant length of time.	Sexuality expression may be inhibited by hospitalization, but the need still exists.
Teach the patient the importance of adequate rest before and after sexual activity.	Sexual activity increases basal metabolic rate and initiates the sympathetic nervous system, creating a high level of stress.
If dyspareunia is a problem, teach the patient and significant other to: • Use adequate amounts of water-soluble lubricant. • Use vaginal steroid cream. • Take sitz baths.	Increases comfort and reduces trauma. Eases dryness and avoids irritation.
If impotence is a problem, advise the patient to: • Consult with a physician regarding a complete physical examination. • Consult with a sex therapist. • Consider a penile prosthesis.	Discover the underlying causes of impotence. Provides an alternative method of penile erection to find satisfaction in intercourse.

Child Health

This diagnosis is not appropriate for a child.

Women's Health

● N O T E : *Very little information is found in the literature on Sexual Dysfunction of lesbian women, as they often conceal their sexual orientation when they receive health care and some choose not to receive health care if there is a danger of exposure.[14] The following actions refer to those who have a heterosexual relationship.*

ACTIONS/INTERVENTIONS	RATIONALES
Obtain a detailed sexual history. Determine who the patient is: • Female • Male • Couple or partners	Provides a database needed to plan accurate intervention.

ACTIONS/INTERVENTIONS	RATIONALES
Review communication skills between partners.	
Ascertain the couple's knowledge of:	
• Sexual performance	
• Female and male anatomy and physiology	
• Female and male orgasm	
• Anticipatory performance anxiety	
• Unrealistic romantic ideas	
• Rigid religious conformity	
• Negative conditioning in formative years	
• Erection and ejaculation	
• Stimulation	
• Arousal	
• Sexual anxiety	
• Fear of failure	
• Demand for performance	
• Fear of rejection	
Dispel sexual myths and fallacies or misinformation about sexuality by:	Provides basic information and support that can assist the patient in long-term care.
• Allowing the patient to talk about beliefs and practices in a nonthreatening atmosphere	
• Providing correct information	
• Answering questions in an honest manner	
• Referring to the appropriate agencies or health-care providers	
Obtain description of current problem:	Provides an essential database to permit narrowing of focus for intervention.
• Psychological	
• Physical	
• Social	
Determine the type of sexual dysfunction:	
• General	
• Lack of erotic feeling	
• Lack of sexual responses	
• No pleasure in the sexual act	
• Consider it an ordeal	
• Avoidance	
• Frustration	
• Disappointment	
• Fear	
• Disgust	
• Orgasmic difficulties	
If the client is sexually responsive but cannot complete the sexual response cycle, determine whether this is:	
• *Situational:* Client is inhibited, disappointed, or disinterested.	
• *Physiologic:* Interruption results from lack of lubrication, impotence, or interference with the sexual response cycle.	
• *Psychological:* Ambivalence, guilt, or fear is present.	
• If vaginismus (tight closing of vaginal muscle with any attempt at penetration) is present, determine whether this results from:	
• Fear of vaginal penetration	
• Spasm of vaginal muscle	

(care plan continued on page 728)

NURSING ACTIONS/INTERVENTIONS WITH RATIONALES (continued from page 727)

Women's Health

ACTIONS/INTERVENTIONS	RATIONALES
• Frustration • Fear of inadequacy • Guilt • Pain • Prior sexual trauma • Strict religious code • Rape • Dyspareunia	
Discuss consequences of sexual acts and situations in an honest and nonthreatening manner.	Initiates intervention in a supportive environment.
Collaborate with appropriate therapists.	Provides the long-term care and support that is needed to resolve the basic problem

Mental Health

● N O T E : *If sexual dysfunction is related to physiologic limitations, loss of body part, or impotence, refer to Adult Health care plan. If dysfunction is related to ineffective coping or poor social skills, initiate the following actions:*

ACTIONS/INTERVENTIONS	RATIONALES
Set limits on the inappropriate expression of sexual needs. Note the kinds of behavior to be limited and the consequences for inappropriate behavior here; for example, when the client approaches staff member with sexually provocative remarks, the staff member will use constructive confrontation and discontinue the interaction).[15] Inform the client of these limits.	Promotes the client's sense of control, while maintaining the safety of the milieu.
Assign a primary care nurse to the client on each shift. The primary care nurse will spend 15 minutes with the client twice per shift at [times] to develop a relationship, and then begin to explore with the client the effects this behavior has on others and the needs that are being met by the behavior.	Promotes the development of a trusting relationship.
Assist the client in identifying environmental stimuli that provoke sexual behavior and in developing alternative responses to these stimuli in inappropriate situations.	
Develop with the client a list of alternative kinds of behavior to meet the need currently being met by the sexual behavior. [Note alternative behavior patterns here with plan for implementing them.]	Promotes the client's sense of control.
Provide the client with information about appropriate sexual behavior—for example, what are "normal" sexual expressions, what are appropriate ways to meet sexual needs (intercourse with appropriate person or masturbation at suitable time in an appropriate place).	Facilitates the development of appropriate coping behaviors.
Role-play with the client social situations that have been identified as problematic. These could include setting limits on other's inappropriate behavior toward the client, or situations in which the client needs to practice appropriate social responses.	Behavioral rehearsal provides opportunities for feedback and modeling of new behaviors by the nurse.

ACTIONS/INTERVENTIONS	RATIONALES
Assist the client in appropriate labeling of feelings and needs. For example, anxiety may be inappropriately labeled as "sexual tension."	Promotes the client's sense of control, and facilitates the development of adaptive coping behaviors.
Plan a private time and place for the client. Inform the client that this can be used for appropriate sexual expression. [Note this plan here.]	
If the client begins inappropriate sexual behavior while involved in group activities, remove the client from group to a private place and explain to the client purpose of this. Inform the client that he or she may return to the group when (the limit set by the care team will be noted here).	Social isolation inhibits inappropriate behavior by removing social rewards.
If sexual behavior results from anxiety, refer to Anxiety (Chapter 8) for detailed care plan.	
Assign the client tasks in unit activities that are appropriate for the client's level of comfort with group interaction. For example, if the client is uncomfortable with persons of opposite sex, assign a task that requires involvement with a same-sex group, or involvement with an opposite-sex staff member who can begin a relationship.	Promotes the development of adaptive interpersonal skills in an environment that provides supportive feedback from peers.
Recognize and support the client's feelings; for example, "You sound confused."	Promotes the development of a trusting relationship. Models for the client appropriate expressions of feelings in a supportive environment. Helps the client learn to talk about feelings rather than act on them.
Engage the client in a socialization group once a day at [time]. This should provide the client with an opportunity to interact with peers in an environment that provides feedback to the client in a supportive manner.	Decreases social isolation, and provides the client with an opportunity to practice interpersonal skills in a supportive environment.
Arrange a consultation with occupational therapist to assist the client in developing needed social skills (e.g., cooking skills or skills at games that require socialization).	Increases the client's interpersonal competence and enhances self-esteem.
Provide an environment that does not stimulate inappropriate sexual behavior; for example, a staff member indirectly encourages the client's behavior with dress or verbal comments, or other clients interact with the client in a sexual manner.	Promotes an environment that increases the opportunities for the client to succeed with new behaviors. This success serves as reinforcement that encourages positive behavior and enhances self-esteem.
Sit with the client [number] minutes once a shift at [time] to discuss non-sexual-related information.	Nurses' interactions can provide social reinforcement for the client's appropriate interactions. Provides an opportunity for the client to practice new behaviors in a supportive environment. Success in this situation provides reinforcement that encourages positive behavior and enhances self-esteem.
Provide positive social rewards for appropriate behavior (the rewards, as well as the kinds of behavior to be rewarded, should be noted here).	Reinforcement encourages positive behavior and enhances self-esteem.
Evaluate the effects of the client's current medication on sexual behavior, and consult with the physician as needed for necessary alterations.	Basic monitoring of medication efficiency.

(care plan continued on page 730)

NURSING ACTIONS/INTERVENTIONS WITH RATIONALES (continued from page 729)

Mental Health

ACTIONS/INTERVENTIONS	RATIONALES
Develop a structured daily activity schedule for the client, and provide the client with this information.	Assists the client in focusing away from issues of sexuality and engage in socially appropriate activity.
Schedule a time for the client to engage in physical activity. This activity should be developed with the client's assistance and could include walking, jogging, basketball, cycling, dancing, "soft" aerobics, etc. A staff member should participate with the client in these activities to provide positive social reinforcement. [Note schedule and type of activity here.]	Physical activity decreases anxiety and increases the production of endorphins, which increase the client's feelings of well-being.[16] Provides opportunities for the client to learn alternative ways of coping with anxiety in a supportive environment.
If the client's concerns are related to his or her relationship with his or her significant other, initiate the following actions:	
• Assess the role current medications and nonprescription drug use may have on sexual functioning. Note here the person responsible for this assessment. If the medications could have a negative impact on sexual functioning, assist the client in discussing a medication change with the primary care provider. For example, an antidepressant with fewer sexual side effects, such as bupropion, could be prescribed.	Medications and nonprescription drugs can have a negative impact on sexual functioning. These can include antidepressants, antihypertensives, and alcohol.[17]
• Explore with the client, and his or her significant other, their understanding of normal sexual functioning. Provide information as appropriate. This could include referring clients to appropriate references. [Note here information and follow-up needed.]	Poor understanding of the normal sexual response cycle can have a negative impact on sexual functioning.[18,19]
• Provide the client system with opportunities to discuss concerns while modeling communication skills. Note here the person responsible for this interaction.	Assists clients with developing skills to communicate about their sexual relationship.
• If providing basic information does not resolve client concerns, arrange a referral to a health-care provider with expertise in addressing issues related to sexual functioning. [Note here the name of referral source and appointment time.]	Sex therapy requires advanced preparation.

Gerontic Health

ACTIONS/INTERVENTIONS	RATIONALES
Monitor for use of medications that may induce sexual dysfunction. Male impotency may be related to antihypertensive medications.	Identifies correctable source of impotency.
Determine the individual patient's knowledge of facts and myths regarding sexual changes in aging.	Knowledge of expected aging changes may encourage the individual to discuss changes experienced and seek treatment for dysfunction.
Identify resources for assistance with sexual dysfunction, such as Impotents Anonymous groups.[20]	Provides an information source and support for individuals with a common problem. Impotence, regardless of etiology, shows marked increase beyond age 65.

ACTIONS/INTERVENTIONS	RATIONALES
Provide resources for patients with chronic illnesses, such as chronic obstructive pulmonary disease (COPD) or arthritis, that address and assist in problem solving regarding disease-related sexual difficulties.[21]	
Provide uninterrupted time for couples, particularly in long-term-care settings, where it may be difficult to maintain or attain privacy.	Assists patients in maintaining sexuality as long as possible.

Home Health

ACTIONS/INTERVENTIONS	RATIONALES
Involve the client and significant other in planning and implementing strategies for reducing sexual dysfunction and enhancing sexual relationship: • Communication (e.g., discussion of concerns and ideas for intervention) • Mutual sharing and trust • Problem solving (e.g., identification of specific strategies with roles defined, such as second honeymoon or specific sexual arousal exercises)	Sexual dysfunction affects and is affected by relationships. Involvement of significant people in strategies is vital to enhance the potential for success.
Assist the patient and significant other with lifestyle adjustments that may be required by: • Providing accurate and appropriate information regarding contraception • Teaching stress management • Providing information regarding sexuality and clarifying myths regarding sexuality • Exploring strategies for coping with disabling injury or disease • Using massage • Using touch • Treating substance abuse • Exercising regularly • Coping with changes in role functions and role relationships • Using water-soluble lubricants • Obtaining treatment for physical problems (e.g., vaginal infections or penile discharge) • Teaching changes accompanying pregnancy • Teaching side effects of medication	Lifestyle changes require permanent behavior changes. Support and self-evaluation can improve the probability of successful change.
Consult with, or refer to, assistive resources as indicated.	Use of existing resources provides for high-quality care and effective use of services.

SEXUALITY PATTERNS, INEFFECTIVE

DEFINITION[10]

Expressions of concern regarding own sexuality.

DEFINING CHARACTERISTICS[10]

1. Reported difficulties, limitations, or changes in sexual behaviors or activities

RELATED FACTORS[10]

1. Lack of significant others
2. Conflicts with sexual orientation or variant preferences
3. Fear of pregnancy or of acquiring a sexually transmitted disease
4. Impaired relationship with a significant other
5. Ineffective or absent role models

6. Knowledge or skills deficit about alternative responses to health-related transitions, altered body function or structure, illness or medical treatment
7. Lack of privacy

RELATED CLINICAL CONCERNS

1. Mastectomy
2. Hysterectomy
3. Cancer of the reproductive tract
4. Any condition resulting in paralysis
5. Sexually transmitted disease (e.g., syphilis, gonorrhea, or AIDS)

 Have You Selected the Correct Diagnosis?

Sexual Dysfunction
Sexual Dysfunction indicates there are problems in sexual functioning. Ineffective Sexuality Patterns refers to concerns about sexuality but does not necessarily mean an overwhelming problem. In some instances, this diagnosis may involve a lifestyle different from heterosexual norms.

Rape-Trauma Syndrome
Certainly a traumatic event such as a rape could result in an Ineffective Sexuality Patterns. The nurse would focus, however, on assisting the patient to deal with the rape trauma first. Resolving this problem would assist in resolving the Ineffective Sexuality Patterns.

Many of the other nursing diagnoses can impact sexual feelings and functioning in both men and women. Examples are Disturbed Body Image, Pain, Chronic Pain, Fear, Anxiety, Dysfunctional Grieving, and Ineffective Role Performance.

EXPECTED OUTCOME

Will identify at least [number] factors contributing to ineffective sexual pattern by [date].

TARGET DATES

Because of the extremely personal nature of sexuality, the patient may be reluctant to express needs or problems in this area. For this reason, a target date of 5 to 7 days would be acceptable.

NURSING ACTIONS/INTERVENTIONS WITH RATIONALES

Adult Health

ACTIONS/INTERVENTIONS	RATIONALES
Establish a therapeutic and trusting relationship with the patient and significant other.	Promotes therapeutic and open communication.
Address other primary nursing needs, especially physiologically related and self-image related.	Meeting these needs promotes solving of the ineffective sexuality pattern.
Actively listen to the patient's and significant other's efforts to talk about fears or changes in body image affecting sexuality or altered sexual preferences. Assist the patient and family to identify how the desired sexual function may be attained.	Promotes open and therapeutic communications.
Help the patient and significant other to understand that sexuality does not necessarily mean intercourse.	Misinformation and myths may create unrealistic expectations about sexuality and the sexual experience.
Discuss alternative methods for expressing sexuality, including masturbation.	Sexuality includes verbal, nonverbal, genital, and nongenital sexual activities.
Do not be judgmental with the patient or significant other.	Sexuality is a highly personal behavior. The nurse's attitude can create guilt feelings and stress in the patient.
Provide privacy and time for the patient and significant other to be alone if so desired.	Allows for sexual expressions.
Administer medications as ordered, with monitoring of potential side effects.	
Monitor for contributory causative components, and provide appropriate education and follow-up.	Permits a more fully developed and accurate plan of care. Provides for long-term support.

Child Health

ACTIONS/INTERVENTIONS	RATIONALES
Encourage the child and family to verbalize perception of altered sexual functioning (e.g., undescended testicle).	Provides the database necessary to accurately plan intervention.
Assist the patient and family to identify how the desired sexual function may be attained.	Specific plans for goals of sexual function desired will assist in how the client will be treated (e.g., surgeries for future procreation).
Include appropriate collaboration with other health-care team members as needed.	Specialist may best meet the unique needs represented with ineffective sexual functioning.
Provide attention to developmentally appropriate role modeling for age and situation.	Opportunities appropriate for age with role models serve as valuable learning modes.
Encourage peer support during hospitalization as appropriate.	Peer support fosters sense of self, which is also a composite of sexuality.
Plan for potential long-term nursing follow-up.	The chronic nature of many physiologic components will necessitate serial rechecks and treatment over time as the child grows and matures.

Women's Health

ACTIONS/INTERVENTIONS	RATIONALES
Assist the patient to describe her sexuality and understanding of sexual functioning as it relates to her lifestyle and lifestyle decisions.	Provides database needed to plan for successful interventions.
Allow the patient time to discuss sexuality and sex-related problems in a nonthreatening atmosphere. Obtain a complete sexual history, including current emotional state.	
Assist the patient in listing lifestyle adjustments that need to be made, e.g., different methods of achieving sexual satisfaction in the presence of mutilating surgery.	
Identify significant others in the patient's life and involve them, if so desired by the patient, in discussion and problem-solving activities regarding sexual adjustments.	
Provide an atmosphere that allows the patient to discuss freely: • Partner choice • Sexual orientation • Sexual roles	Assists the patient in planning coping strategies to various life situations, and provides information the patient needs to achieve the planning.
Assist the patient in identifying lifestyle adjustments to each different cycle of reproductive life: • Puberty • Pregnancy • Menopause • Postmenopause	
Discuss pregnancy and the changes that will occur during pregnancy and the postpartum period: • Sexuality • Mood swing	Provides essential information needed by the patient to offset concerns regarding maintaining sexuality during and after pregnancy.

(care plan continued on page 734)

NURSING ACTIONS/INTERVENTIONS WITH RATIONALES (continued from page 733)

Women's Health

ACTIONS/INTERVENTIONS	RATIONALES
Discuss aspects of sexuality and intercourse during pregnancy. Answer questions promptly and factually: • Positions • Frequency • Effects on fetus • Effects on pregnancy • Fears about sexual changes	
Discuss the postpartum healing process, and timing of resumption of intercourse.	
Assist the patient facing surgery or body structure changes in identifying lifestyle adjustments that may be needed (e.g., ileostomy, colostomy, mastectomy, or hysterectomy).	
Allow the patient to grieve loss of body image.	
Reassure the patient that she can still participate in sexual activities.	Provides support to the patient who is questioning continuance of sexuality.
Ensure confidentiality for the patient with sexually transmitted diseases.	Promotes sharing of information necessary to plan care.
Encourage verbalization of concerns with sexually transmitted diseases: • Recurrent nature of disease, especially herpes and *Chlamydia* • Lack of cure for the disease (AIDS) • Economics of treating the disease • Social stigma associated with disease	Provides the database needed to most accurately plan care.
Encourage honesty in answers to such questions as: • Multiple sex partners • Describing sexual behavior	

Encourage honest communication with sexual partners(s).
• Discuss the impact of the male partner's prostate surgery and possible impotence.
• Discuss the impact on either partner of medication that may affect libido.
• Discuss means of satisfying sexual desires other than intercourse:
  • Cuddling
  • Massaging, stroking, or touching partner
  • Masturbation
	Sexual partner will require health care.

Mental Health

● NOTE: *If alteration is related to altered body function or structure or illness, refer to Adult Health nursing actions.*

ACTIONS/INTERVENTIONS	RATIONALES
Assign a primary care nurse who is comfortable discussing related material with the client.	Promotes the development of a trusting relationship.

ACTIONS/INTERVENTIONS	RATIONALES
The primary care nurse will spend [number] minutes [number] times a day with the client discussing issues related to diagnosis. These discussions will include:	
• Client's use of prescription and nonprescription medications. If current medications could have a negative impact on sexual functioning, assist the client in discussing possible medication changes with the primary health-care provider.	Prescription and nonprescription medications can have a negative impact on sexual functioning.
• Client's current physiologic health	Disease states can have a negative impact on sexual functioning. This can include cardiovascular disease and diabetes.
• Client's thoughts and feelings about alteration	Expression of feelings and perceptions in a supportive environment facilitates the development of alternative coping behaviors.
• Other stressors and concerns in the client's life that could affect sexual patterns • Client's perceptions of partner's responses • Client's perceptions of self as a sexual person without a partner • Client's perceptions of social or cultural expectations • Client's thoughts and feelings about sexuality	
If alteration is related to lack of information, develop a teaching plan. [Note teaching plan here.]	Provides a guide to ensure that the client gets accurate and consistent information.
When the client identifies specific difficulties that contribute to the concern, develop a specific action plan to cope with these and note the plan here.	Promotes the client's sense of control and enhances self-esteem.
If the alteration is related to problems with the significant other, arrange a meeting with the client and significant other to discuss the perceptions each has about the problem. If these difficulties are related to a lack of information, develop a teaching plan and note it here. If alteration is related to a long-term relationship or if alteration is only one of several problems, refer to a marriage and family therapist or clinical nurse specialist.	Provides an opportunity for the nurse to facilitate communication between the partners and for the partners to communicate their relationship needs as well as personal needs in a nonthreatening environment.
Arrange a private time for the client and partner to discuss relationship issues, including sexuality. [Note time and place arranged for this discussion here.]	Provides recognition and support for this relationship.
During interactions with the client and significant other, have them express feelings about their relationship. These should be both positive and negative feelings.	Promotes the development of a positive expectational set. Positive feelings enhance self-esteem and enhance personal psychological resources for coping with the difficult aspects of the relationship.

Gerontic Health

The nursing actions for the older adult with this diagnosis are the same as for the Adult Health patient.

(care plan continued on page 736)

NURSING ACTIONS/INTERVENTIONS WITH RATIONALES (continued from page 735)

Home Health

ACTIONS/INTERVENTIONS	RATIONALES
Monitor for factors contributing to Ineffective Sexuality Patterns by [date].	Provides a database for early identification and intervention.
Involve appropriate family members (e.g., significant others or parents of child) in planning, implementing, and promoting reduction or elimination of Ineffective Sexuality Patterns: • Communication (e.g., discussion of values and sexual mores) • Mutual sharing and trust • Problem solving (e.g., identification of strategies acceptable to all involved with the role of each person identified) • Sex education (e.g., clarify any misconceptions regarding sexual behavior and sexuality)	Sexual behavior can affect the entire family. Involvement of the family in problem identification and intervention enhances the probability of successful intervention.
Assist the client and family with lifestyle adjustments that may be required:	Provides knowledge and support necessary for permanent behavioral change.
Providing accurate and appropriate information regarding sexuality and contraception.	
Providing time and privacy for development and improvement of sexual relationship: • Teaching stress management • Coping with loss of sexual partner • Providing accurate and appropriate information regarding sexually transmitted diseases • Providing accurate and appropriate information regarding sexual orientation (e.g., homosexuality, heterosexuality, or transsexuality) • Coping with physical disability • Explaining side effects of medical treatment	
Consult with assistive resources as indicated.	Specialized counseling may be indicated. Effective use of existing resources provides continuity.

REFERENCES

1. Gordon, M: Manual of Nursing Diagnosis. McGraw-Hill, New York, 2002.
2. Fogel, CI: Female sexuality. In Breslin, ET, and Lucas, VA (eds): Women's Health: Toward-Based Practice. WB Saunders, St. Louis 2003.
3. Youngkin, EQ, and Davis, MS: Woman's Health: A Primary Care Clinical Guide. Appleton & Lange, Norwalk, CT, 1994.
4. Speroff, L, Glass, RH, and Kase, NG: Clinical Gynecologic Endocrinology and Infertility, ed 6. Lippincott, Williams & Wilkins, Philadelphia, 1999, p 321.
5. Fogel, CI, and Woods, NF: Health Care of Women: A Nursing Perspective. CV Mosby, St. Louis, 1981.
6. Schuster, CS, and Ashburn, SS: The Process of Human Development: A Holistic Life-Span Approach, ed 3. JB Lippincott, Philadelphia, 1992.
7. Biddle, BJ, and Thomas, EJ: Role Theory: Concepts and Research. Robert E. Drieger, Huntington, NY, 1979.
8. Associated Press: Study finds greater number of rape victims than supposed. Lubbock Avalanche J 70:A-11, April 24, 1992.
9. Molcan, KL, and Fickley, BS: Sexuality and the Life Cycle. In Poorman, SG (ed): Human Sexuality and the Nursing Process. Appleton & Lange, Norwalk, CT, 1988.
10. Ames, LB, and Ilg, FL: Child Behavior. Dell, New York, 1976.
11. Warner, CG: Rape and Sexual Assault: Management and Intervention. Aspen Systems, Germantown, MD, 1980.
12. NANDA: Nursing Diagnosis: Definitions and Classification, 2005–2006. North American Nursing Diagnosis Association, Philadelphia, 2005.
13. Ben-David, S, and Schneider, O: Rape perceptions, gender role attitudes and victim-perpetrator acquaintance. Sex Roles J Res 53(5-6):385, 2005.
14. Associated Press: Shock Rape Survey: Asking for It. The Mirror, London, November 21, 2005.
15. Erickson, EH: Childhood and Society. Triad/Paladin, St. Albans, England, 1978.
16. Scott, LD: Sexuality & older women: Exploring issues while promoting health. Lifelines 6(6):520, 2003.
17. American Academy of Pediatrics: The evaluation of sexual abuse in children. Kellogg and the Committee on Child Abuse and Neglect 116(2):506 American Academy of Pediatrics Policy, 2005.

18. American Academy of Pediatrics: Guidelines for the Evaluation of Sexual Abuse of children: Subject Review—Committee on Child Abuse and Neglect 103:1, 186, American Academy of Pediatrics Policy, 1999.

19. Hockenberry, MJ: Wong's Essentials of Pediatric Nursing, ed 7. CV Mosby, St. Louis, 2006.

20. Muram, D: Child sexual abuse: Relationship between sexual acts and genital findings. Child. (http://aappolicy.aappublications.org).

21. Dienemann, J, Campbell, J, Wiederhorn, N, Laughon, K, and Jordan, E: A critical pathway for intimate partner violence across the continuum of care. JOGNN J Obstet Gynecol Neonatal Nurs 32(5):594, 2003.

22. Anderson, C: Battered & pregnant: A nursing challenge. Lifelines 6(2):95, 2002.

23. Hartman, SJ: Battered woman in a small town: Encountering violence through the story of one woman. Lifelines 4(4):35, 2000.

24. Lutz, KF: Abused pregnant women's interactions with health care providers during the childbearing year, JOGNN J Obstet Gynecol Neonatal Nurs 34(2):151, 2005.

25. Haggerty, LA, Kelly, R, Hawkins, J, Pearce, C, and Kearney, MH: Pregnant women's perceptions of abuse. JOGNN J Obstet Gynecol Neonatal Nurs 30(3):283, 2001.

26. McCloskey Dochterman, J, and Bulecheck, G: Nursing Interventions Classification. CV Mosby, St. Louis, 2004.

27. Haber, J, et al: Comprehensive Psychiatric Nursing, ed 5. CV Mosby, St. Louis, 1997.

28. McArthur, M: Reality therapy with rape victims. Arch Psychiatr Nurs 4:360, 1990.

29. Townsend, M: Psychiatric Mental Health Nursing: Concepts of Care in Evidence-Based Practice, ed 5. FA Davis, 2006.

30. Brown, K, Streubert, G, and Burgess, A: Effectively detect and manage elder abuse. Nurse Pract Am J Primary Health Care 29(8):22, 2005.

31. Teschendorf, M: Women during the reproductive years. In Breslin, ET, and Lucas, VA (eds): Women's Health Nursing: Toward Evidence-Based Practice. WB Saunders, St. Louis, 2003.

32. Sellers, JB: Health care for older women. In Breslin, ET, and Lucas, VA (eds): Women's Health Nursing: Toward Evidence-Based Practice. WB Saunders, St. Louis, 2003.

33. Maxmen, J, and Ward, N: Psychotropic Drugs Fact Facts. WW Norton, New York, 2002.

34. Dossey, B, Keegan, L, and Guzzetta, CE: Holistic Nursing: A Handbook for Practice, ed 3. Aspen, Gaithersburg, MD, 2000.

35. Love, P: What is this thing called love? Family Therapy Network 23:34, 2000.

36. Butler, K: The evolution of modern sex therapy. Family Therapy Network 23:28, 1999.

37. Wright, L, and Leahey, M: Nurses and Families: A Guide to Family Assessment and Intervention. F.A. Davis, Philadelphia, 2005.

38. Buczny, B: Impotence in older men: A newly recognized problem. J Gerontol Nurs 18:25, 1992.

39. Eliopoulos, C: Manual of Gerontological Nursing, ed 2. CV Mosby, St. Louis, 1999.

40. Lightfoot-Klain, H, and Shaw, E: Special needs of ritually circumcised women patients. JOGNN J Obstet Gynecol Neonatal Nurs 20:102, 1991.

41. Northrup, C: The Wisdom of Menopause: Creating Physical and Emotional Health and Healing During the Change. Random House, New York, 2003.

42. Berg, JA: Dimensions of sexuality in the perimenopausal transition: A model for practice, JOGNN J Obstet Gynecol Neonatal Nurs 30(4):421, 2001.

43. Katz, A: Sexuality after hysterectomy. JOGNN J Obstet Gynecol Neonatal Nurs 31:256, 2001.

11

COPING–STRESS TOLERANCE PATTERN

PATTERN DESCRIPTION

Stress has been defined as the response of the body or the system to any demand made on it.[1] This response can be both physiologic and psychosocial. Because demands are synonymous with living, stress has been defined as "life itself."[1] The system's (individual, family, or community) ability to respond to the demands has an effect on the well-being of the system. Also considered is the system's reserve to respond to the demands. *Stress tolerance pattern* refers to the system's usual manner of responding to stress, or to the amount of stress, previously experienced and includes the stress response history of the individual, family, or community.[2] *Coping* has been defined as "efforts to master condition of harm, threat, or challenge when a routine or automatic response is not readily available."[3] Thus, the coping pattern is the system's pattern of responding to nonroutine threats. The client's ability to respond to stress is affected by a complex interaction of physical, social, and emotional reactions. Assessment of this pattern focuses on gaining an understanding of the interaction of these factors within the system. Interventions are related to maximizing the system's well-being.[1–3]

PATTERN ASSESSMENT

1. Does the client verbalize an inability to cope?
   a. Yes (Ineffective Individual Coping)
   b. No (Readiness for Enhanced Coping)
2. Does the client demonstrate inability to problem solve?
   a. Yes (Ineffective Individual Coping)
   b. No
3. Does the client deny problems or weaknesses in spite of evidence to the contrary?
   a. Yes (Defensive Coping)
   b. No
4. Is the client projecting blame for the current situation on other persons or events?
   a. Yes (Defensive Coping)
   b. No
5. Did the patient delay seeking health care assistance to the detriment of his or her health?
   a. Yes (Ineffective Denial)
   b. No
6. Does the patient downplay his or her condition?
   a. Yes (Ineffective Denial)
   b. No
7. Does the patient verbalize nonacceptance of health status change?
   a. Yes (Impaired Adjustment)
   b. No
8. Is the patient moving toward independence?
   a. Yes (Readiness for Enhanced Coping)
   b. No (Impaired Adjustment)
9. Is the client's primary caregiver denying the severity of the client's problem?
   a. Yes (Disabled Family Coping)
   b. No (Readiness for Enhanced Family Coping)
10. Does the client demonstrate indications of neglect?
    a. Yes (Disabled Family Coping)
    b. No
11. Does the client state concerns about care being received from the primary caregiver?
    a. Yes (Compromised Family Coping)
    b. No
12. Can the primary caregiver verbalize understanding of care requirements?
    a. Yes (Readiness for Enhanced Family Coping)
    b. No (Compromised Family Coping)
13. Does the family indicate physical and emotional support for the client?
    a. Yes (Readiness for Enhanced Family Coping)
    b. No
14. Does the family or primary caregiver indicate an interest in a support group?
    a. Yes (Readiness for Enhanced Family Coping)
    b. No
15. Does the patient exhibit re-experience of traumatic events (flashbacks or nightmares)?
    a. Yes (Post-Trauma Syndrome)
    b. No
16. Does the patient exhibit vagueness about traumatic event?
    a. Yes (Post-Trauma Syndrome)
    b. No
17. Is there evidence of positive communication and community participation in planning for predicted community stressors?
    a. Yes (Readiness for Enhanced Community Coping)
    b. No
18. Is there evidence of community conflict and deficits in community participation?
    a. Yes (Ineffective Community Coping)
    b. No
19. Has the patient threatened to kill him- or herself?
    a. Yes (Risk for Suicide)
    b. No
20. Has the patient demonstrated marked changes in behavior, attitude, or school performance?
    a. Yes (Risk for Suicide)
    b. No

CONCEPTUAL INFORMATION

To understand coping, one must first understand the concept of stress, because coping is the system's attempt to adapt to stress. An understanding of these concepts and their relationship is crucial for the promotion of well-being. Research has clearly demonstrated that undue stress can be related to major health problems if inappropriate coping is present.[1,4]

Stress has been defined as the body's nonspecific response to any demand placed on it.[1] These demands can be any situation that would require the system to adapt. For the individual, this could include anything from getting out of bed in the morning to experiencing the loss resulting from a major environmental disaster. Stress is life.

The body's physiologic response to stress involves activation of the autonomic nervous system. The symptoms of this activation can include sweating, tachycardia, tachypnea, nausea, and tremors. This process has been labeled the *general-adaptation syndrome (GAS)*[5] and occurs in three stages: alarm reaction, resistance, and exhaustion. The alarm stage mobilizes the system's defense forces by initiating the autonomic nervous system response. The system is prepared for "fight or flight." In the resistance stage, the system fights back and adapts, and normal functioning returns. If the stress continues and all attempts of the system to adapt fail, exhaustion occurs, and the system is at risk for experiencing major disorganization.

Four levels of psychophysiologic stress responses have been described.[5] The first level comprises the day-to-day stressors that all systems experience as a part of living. This stress calls on the self-regulating processes of the system for adaptation. Intersystem coping mechanisms are used, and the system does not require assistance from outside sources to adapt. Level 2 responds to less routine or new experiences encountered by the system. The system experiences a mild alarm reaction that is not prolonged. The individual system might experience a mild increase in heart rate, sensations of bladder fullness and increased frequency of urination, temporary insomnia, tachypnea, anxiety, fear, guilt, shame, or frustration. Some outside assistance may be necessary to facilitate adaptation. This assistance could be in the form of identifying stressors and strengths or encouraging the individual to solve problems. Level 3 consists of the moderate amount of stress that occurs when a persistent stress is encountered or when a new situation is perceived as threatening. Emergency adaptation processes are activated. The individual experiences tachycardia, palpitations, tremors, weakness, cool pale skin, headache, oliguria, vomiting, constipation, and increased susceptibility to infections. This level of stress usually requires assistance from a professional helper and can include identifying problems and coping strengths, teaching, performing tasks for the client, or altering the environment to facilitate coping. When the system cannot adapt to a stressful situation with assistance, a severe degree of stress is experienced, which is labeled Level 4. This occurs when all coping strategies are exhausted. Intervention at this level requires the assistance of professionals who have the skills to assist with the development of unique coping strategies.

Because stress is life itself, adaptation to reduce the effects of stress on the system is imperative. To begin this process, it is important to understand those factors that can influence the system's ability to respond to stress. Stress can arise from biophysical, chemical, psychosocial, and cultural sources. The basic health of the affected system improves the ability to respond to these stressors. Response to the biophysical–chemical stressors can be improved by improving the condition of the biologic system, including proper nutrition, appropriate amounts of rest, appropriate levels of exercise, and reduced exposure of the system to toxic chemicals.[1]

The literature[1] indicates that a great deal of psychosocial–cultural stress evolves from a philosophy of life that is impossible to fulfill. This would indicate that a great deal of stress arises from the perception of events, not from the events themselves. This is compounded by the social and cultural influences on the system. The sociocultural influences could include the cultural attitudes about age, body appearance, and family roles and the social approaches to assistance for working mothers, advancement in employment status, and so on. The system's beliefs about these sociocultural stressors can affect the degree to which the stressors affect the system. If the stressor is perceived as unnatural or impossible to adapt to, the system's stress level will be increased. Response to the psychosocial–cultural stressors can be improved with attitude assessment and interventions that reduce the physiologic response to psychosocial stressors.

Coping has been defined as behavior (conscious and unconscious) that a system uses to change a situation for the better or to manage the stress-resultant emotions.[6] These kinds of behavior can occur on the biologic, psychological, and social levels. Effective coping uses biologic, psychological, and social resources in attempts to manage the situation.

A coping model has been developed[3] that addresses the biologic, psychological, and sociocultural aspects of this process. The model indicates that systems have *generalized resistance resources (GRRs)* to facilitate coping. GRRs are those characteristics of the system that can facilitate effective tension management. Genetic characteristics that provide increased resistance to the effects of stressors are considered physical and biochemical GRRs. These GRRs can include levels of immunity, nutritional status, and the adaptability of the neurologic system. Valuative and attitudinal GRRs describe consistent features of the system's coping behavior, which could include personality characteristics and the system's perception of the stressor. The more flexible, rational, and long term these are, the more effective they are as GRRs. Interpersonal–relational GRRs include social support systems and can provide an important resource in managing stress. Finally, those cultural supports that facilitate coping are referred to a macrosociocultural GRRs. *Macrosociocultural GRRs* could include religions, rites of passage, and governmental structures.

In 1979, Kobasa introduced the concept of hardiness to the literature on coping.[7,8] She described the hardy individual as having three characteristics that provide him or her with the ability to cope effectively with stress. The first characteristic is commitment, or a purpose and involvement in life. Challenge is the second characteristic of the hardy individual. Challenge is the belief that the changes in life can be meaningful opportunities for personal growth. The third characteristic is control. Control has three components: cognitive control, decisional control, and a repertoire of coping skills. Kobasa and other authors proposed that the hardy individual would remain healthier and experience less disabling psychological stress.

An understanding of the concept of hardiness can facilitate the nurse's assessment of the client's potential ability to cope with life's stresses. Based on this assessment, the nurse can then develop interventions that support or develop commitment, challenge, and control for the client. These interventions might include providing the client with as much control as possible in the situation, facilitating his or her positive orientation with reframes, and assisting in the development of a variety of coping strategies.[8]

Wagnild and Young[9] have questioned the validity of hardiness as a concept. The concern of these authors evolves from their observation that the tools utilized to measure the various components of hardiness do not provide clear distinctions between the identified concepts and other influencing variables. Wagnild and Young conclude that it is important to continue the research related to a hardiness concept, and, until a more precise understanding of what constitutes this concept is developed, it will be difficult to apply it to therapeutic interventions.[9] From a clinical perspective, hardiness is a useful concept to consider when interacting with the client system, for it both provides a model for understanding client response and presents fertile content for clinical nursing research related to psychosocial aspects of coping.

Effective coping can occur when the system has a strong physiologic base combined with adequate psychosociocultural support. This implies that any intervention that addresses coping behavior should address each of these areas. Interventions that have been applied to this process include therapeutic touch, kinesiology, meditation, relaxation training, hypnosis, family therapy, nutritional counseling, massage, and physical exercise.

DEVELOPMENTAL CONSIDERATIONS

The number of resources available to the system greatly affects its ability to cope with stressors. Thus, there is a need to maximize physical, cognitive, and psychosocial development. Cross-cultural research has identified the characteristics that are common to individuals who are perceived as mature and capable of coping effectively. These characteristics include an ability to anticipate consequences; calm, clear thinking; potential fulfillment; problem solving that is orderly and organized; predictability; purposefulness; realisticness; reflectiveness; strong convictions; and implacability.[9] The development of these characteristics is maximized

in environments that provide children with a loving, warm environment; respect and acceptance for personal interests, ideas, needs, and talents; stable role models; challenges that foster development of competence and responsibility; opportunities to explore all of their feelings; a variety of experiences; opportunities for age-appropriate problem solving and the knowledge that they must live with the consequences of their decisions; opportunities to develop commitments to others; and encouragement in the development of their own standards, values, and goals.[10]

According to developmental stages, there are some specific etiologies and symptom clusters.

INFANT

Interactions with significant others are the primary source of the infant's response to trauma or stress. If the significant other is supportive and consistent, the effects of the event on the infant are minimized. Events that separate infants from their significant others also pose a threat to this age group. Primary symptoms are disruptions in physiologic responses.

Chronic diseases place this age group at special risk. Because the development of coping behavior is limited at this age, the primary caregivers (usually the parents) provide the child with the support to cope. If the caregivers cannot provide the proper supports, then the child is affected. Chronic illness in a child places an extreme stress on the family and can result in divorce. Support for the parents is crucial in supporting the child's coping.

TODDLER AND PRESCHOOLER

Responses of significant others are still the primary supports for the child in this age group. Thus, as for the infant, the response of significant others or separation from these persons can have an effect on the toddler and preschooler. In addition, threats to body integrity pose a special threat to this age group. Traumatic events that inflict physical damage on these children place the child at greatest risk. Regression is the primary symptom and coping behavior. This can be frustrating to caregivers who expect the child to assist in a time of crisis with age-appropriate developmental behavior when the child may regress to a very dependent stage. Other methods used by young children in coping include denial, repression, and projection. Coping may be more difficult because adults may not recognize that young children can experience crisis and will, therefore, not provide assistance with the coping process.[11]

SCHOOL-AGE CHILD

Symptoms include problems with school performance, withdrawal from family and peers, behavioral regression, physical problems related to anxiety, and aggressive behavior to self or others. Coping behavior includes that used by the younger child, only in a more effective manner. This age group may find a great deal of support from siblings during a crisis. Situations that can precipitate crisis in this age group include school entry, threats to body image, peer problems, and family stress such as divorce or death of a loved one.[11]

Chronic disease or disability also affects the adjustment of this age group. Again, the primary support for adaptation comes from the primary caregivers, usually the parents.

ADOLESCENT

The adolescent demonstrates more adult-like coping behavior. Symptoms of stress include anxiety; increased physical activity, daydreaming, and apathy; change in mood cycles; alteration in sleeping patterns; aggressive behavior directed at self or others; and physical symptoms associated with anxiety. Crisis-producing situations can include role changes, peer difficulties, threats to body integrity, rapidly changing body functioning, conflict with parents, personal failures, sexual awareness, and school demands.[11]

Response to traumatic events is similar to that of adults. Etiologies of crisis-producing events, for this age group, are also similar to those for adults. Specific events that place this age group at greater risk are those that affect the peer group and could have effects on body image or sexual functioning. Coping behavior is adult-like. This age group may find support from peers especially useful in facilitating coping. Coping may also be affected by limited life experience and impulsive behavior.

Illnesses that threaten body image could result in difficulties in adjustment. Peers again provide a primary support system and can have a great impact on the adolescent's acceptance. Educating significant peers about the client's situation could facilitate their acceptance of the client, and in turn facilitate the client's adjustment to the change in health status. Adjustment could also be facilitated by involving the client in a support group composed of peers with similar alterations.

YOUNG ADULT

Symptoms of problems with coping include changes in performance of roles at home and at work, aggressive behavior directed at self or others, and physical symptoms associated with anxiety and denial. Changes in role performance might include loss of interest in sexual relationships or withdrawal from the community. Situations that might tax the coping abilities of the young adult include balancing increasing role responsibilities, dealing with threats to the self or to body integrity, leaving home, and making career choices.[11]

Alterations in health status that affect the ability of role performance place this age group at risk for impaired adjustment. This could include loss of ability to function in job responsibilities. Behavior can include regression, but this does not necessarily indicate that the client is experiencing impaired adjustment.

ADULT

Coping resources have broadened for this age group as a result of past successful coping experiences and the possible addition of adult children as supports during crisis. Symptoms of difficulties with coping are similar to those of the young adult. Age-related stressors include loss, such as significant others and physical functioning; role changes, such as job loss and the leaving of adult children; aging parents; career pressures; and cultural role expectations.[11]

OLDER ADULT

Older adults face many psychosocial challenges; loss of autonomy, ageist stereotypes, retirement, chronic illness, relocation, and death of friends and spouses. Symptoms of extreme stress in this age group may be overlooked and attributed to senility. These symptoms include withdrawal, decreased functioning, increased physical complaints, and aggressive behavior. Decreased function of hearing, vision, and mobility, as well as loss of support systems and other resources, affects coping behavior. These problems can be balanced by life experience that has provided the individual with many situations of successful coping to fall back on during stressful times.

The effects of multiple losses related to alteration in health status and the loss of support systems place the older adult at risk for impaired adjustment. In the absence of illness affecting cognitive functioning, the older adult can assume responsibility for making decisions related to alterations in health status. This ability, combined with life experience, can facilitate creative problem solving with the support of health-care personnel.[12]

FAMILY LIFE CYCLE

The following is a presentation of the developmental framework of the family life cycle as described by Carter and McGoldrick.[13]

Between Families. The unattached young adult: The process of this level is accepting parent–child separation. The individual must separate from his or her family of origin and develop intimate peer relationships and a career.

Joining of Families Through Marriage. The newly married couple: The process of this level involves commitment to a new system. The individuals form a marital system and realign relationships with extended families and friends to include spouse.

Family with Young Children. The task faced is to accept a new generation of members into the system. The marital system adjusts to make space for the child(ren) and assumes parental roles. Additional realignment takes place to include parenting and grandparenting roles.

Family with Adolescents. The family task is to increase flexibility of family boundaries to include children's independence. The parent–child relationships shift to allow the adolescents to move in and out of the system. The parents refocus on midlife marital and career issues, and there is a beginning shift toward concerns for the older generation.

Family in Later Life. Accepting the shifting of generational roles is the task of this stage. The system maintains individual and couple functioning and interests in conjunction with physiologic decline. There is an exploration of new role options with more support for a more central role for the middle generation. The system also makes room for the wisdom and experience of the elderly and to support the older generation without overprotecting them. This stage will also include coping with the deaths of significant others and preparation for death.

Specific problems can arise in family coping when the family developmental cycle or expectations do not correspond with the developmental tasks of individual family members. There are three stages that are nodal points in family development.

The joining of families through marriage requires a commitment to a new system. If the separation from the parents is not successful, then the new family does not have an opportunity to form its own identity by combining the experiences both bring into this new relationship. Symptoms of unsuccessful resolution of this stage could result in the marital partners returning home to their parents when conflict arises or an ongoing struggle over loyalties to families of origin.

The second major shift occurs when children enter the system. The new role of parent is assumed, and the couple boundaries must be opened to accept the child. Unsuccessful resolution of this stage could result in physical or emotional abuse of the child. If there is a developmental delay in the parents and they are not ready to assume the responsibilities that accompany parenthood, family dysfunction can occur.

A family with adolescents is faced with the task of increasing flexibility to include children's independence. This may require a major shift in family rules. This is also influenced by the parents' perception of the adolescent and the environment. If the adolescent is seen as being competent, and the environment that the adolescent interacts in is seen as safe, then it will be much easier for the family to provide the necessary shifts in relationships. When this stage is not resolved successfully, the adolescent may enhance behavior that highlights his or her differences with the family to force separation, or the frequency and intensity of family conflict may increase. Unsuccessful resolution of this stage may indicate that the family has overly rigid boundaries to the external world and individual boundaries that are overly permeable.

Application of the concept of coping at the aggregate or community level is in the process of development. Additional research is needed to identify and validate community-based diagnoses. Successful communities are healthy communities.[13–15]

● N O T E : *For the individual diagnoses in this chapter, the psychiatric health nursing actions serve as the generic nursing actions, because the nature of the diagnoses in this chapter calls for the skills, knowledge, and expertise of a psychiatric–mental health nursing specialist.*

⣿ TABLE 11.1 NANDA, NIC, and NOC Taxonomic Linkages

GORDON'S FUNCTIONAL HEALTH PATTERN	NANDA NURSING DIAGNOSIS	NIC PRIORITY INTERVENTIONS	NOC EVALUATIONS
Coping-Stress Tolerance Pattern	Adjustment, Impaired	Coping Enhancement Mutual Goal Setting	Acceptance: Health Status Adaptation to Physical Disability Compliance Behavior Coping Health-Seeking Behavior Motivation Psychosocial Adjustment: Life Change Treatment Behavior: Illness or Injury
	Community Coping, Ineffective and Readiness for Enhanced	**Ineffective** Communicable Disease Management Community Disaster Preparedness Community Health Development Environmental Management: Community	**Ineffective** Community Competence Community Disaster Readiness Community Risk Control: Chronic Disease; Communicable Disease; Lead Exposure; Violence

GORDON'S FUNCTIONAL HEALTH PATTERN	NANDA NURSING DIAGNOSIS	NIC PRIORITY INTERVENTIONS	NOC EVALUATIONS
		Readiness for Enhanced Bioterrorism Preparedness Health Policy Monitoring Program Development	**Readiness for Enhanced** Community Competence Community Disaster Readiness
	Family Coping, Compromised and Disabled	**Compromised** Family Involvement Promotion Family Mobilization Family Support	**Compromised** Caregiver Emotional Health Caregiver–Patient Relationship Caregiver Performance: Direct Care; Indirect Care Caregiving Endurance Potential Family Coping Family Normalization
		Disabled Family Support Family Therapy	**Disabled** Caregiver–Patient Relationship Caregiver Performance: Direct Care; Indirect Care Caregiver Well-Being Caregiving Endurance Potential Family Coping Family Normalization
	Family Coping, Readiness For Enhanced	Family Involvement Promotion Family Support Normalization Promotion	Caregiver–Patient Relationship Caregiver Well-Being Family Coping Family Normalization Health-Promoting Behavior Health-Seeking Behavior Participation in Health Care Decisions
	Coping, a. Defensive b. Ineffective c. Readiness for Enhanced	**Defensive** Self-Awareness Enhancement	**Defensive** Acceptance: Health Status Adaptation to Physical Disability Child Development: Adolescence Coping Self-Esteem Social Interaction Skills
		Ineffective Coping Enhancement Decision-Making Support	**Ineffective** Acceptance: Health Status Adaptation to Physical Disability Child Adaptation to Hospitalization Coping Decision Making Impulse Self-Control Knowledge: Health Resources Psychosocial Adjustment: Life Change Role Performance Stress Level
		Readiness for Enhanced *Still in development*	**Readiness for Enhanced** Acceptance: Health Status Adaptation to Physical Disability Coping Personal Well-Being Role Performance Stress Level

(table continued on page 746)

⣿ TABLE 11.1 NANDA, NIC, and NOC Taxonomic Linkages (continued from page 745)

GORDON'S FUNCTIONAL HEALTH PATTERN	NANDA NURSING DIAGNOSIS	NIC PRIORITY INTERVENTIONS	NOC EVALUATIONS
	Post-Trauma Syndrome, Risk for and Actual	**Actual** Counseling Support System Enhancement	**Actual** Abuse Recovery: Emotional; Financial; Physical; Sexual Anxiety Level Coping Depression Level Fear Level Fear Level: Child Impulse Self-Control Self-Mutilation Restraint Stress Level Suicide Self-Restraint
		Risk for Crisis Intervention Support System Enhancement	**Risk for** Abuse Cessation Abuse Protection Abuse Recovery Status Abuse Recovery: Emotional; Sexual Adaptation to Physical Disability Aggression Self-Control Anxiety Level Anxiety Self-Control Body Image Cognition Concentration Coping Depression Level Depression Self-Control Distorted Thought Self-Control Grief Resolution Impulse Self-Control Information Processing Mood Equilibrium Psychosocial Adjustment: Life Change Quality of Life Risk Control Risk Control: Drug Use Risk Detection Self-Esteem Self-Mutilation Restraint Sleep Social Support Spiritual Health Stress Level Suicide Self-Restraint
	Suicide, Risk for	Mood Management Suicide Prevention	Abuse Recovery: Status; Emotional; Financial; Physical; Sexual Client Satisfaction: Psychological Care Depression Level Impulse Self-Control Loneliness Severity Mood Equilibrium Pain: Adverse Psychological Response

GORDON'S FUNCTIONAL HEALTH PATTERN	NANDA NURSING DIAGNOSIS	NIC PRIORITY INTERVENTIONS	NOC EVALUATIONS
			Pain Control
			Personal Well-Being
			Psychomotor Energy
			Risk Control
			Risk Control: Alcohol Use; Drug Use
			Risk Detection
			Social Interaction Skills
			Social Support
			Stress Level
			Substance Addiction Consequences
			Suicide Self-Restraint
			Will to Live

 APPLICABLE NURSING DIAGNOSES

ADJUSTMENT, IMPAIRED

DEFINITION[16]

Inability to modify lifestyle or behavior in a manner consistent with a change in health status.

DEFINING CHARACTERISTICS[16]

1. Denial of health status change
2. Failure to achieve optimal sense of control
3. Failure to take actions that would prevent further health problems
4. Demonstration of nonacceptance of health status change

RELATED FACTORS[16]

1. Low state of optimism
2. Intense emotional state
3. Negative attitudes toward health behavior
4. Absence of intent to change behavior
5. Multiple stressors
6. Absence of social support for changed beliefs and practices
7. Disability or health status change requiring change in lifestyle
8. Lack of motivation to change behaviors

RELATED CLINICAL CONCERNS

1. Alzheimer's disease
2. Head injury sequelae
3. Any new diagnosis for the patient
4. Couvade syndrome
5. Postpartum depression or puerperal psychosis
6. Personality disorders
7. Substance use or abuse disorders
8. Psychotic disorders

 Have You Selected the Correct Diagnosis?

Ineffective Individual Coping
Ineffective Individual Coping results from the client's inability to cope appropriately with stress. Impaired Adjustment is the client's inability to adjust to a specific disease process. If the client's behavior were related to the adjustment to a specific disease process, the diagnosis would be Impaired Adjustment; however, if the behavior were related to coping with general life stressors, the diagnosis would be Ineffective Individual Coping.

Powerlessness
Powerlessness is appropriate as a primary or co-diagnosis if the client demonstrates the belief that personal action cannot affect or alter the situation. Impaired Adjustment may result from Powerlessness. If this is the situation, then the appropriate primary diagnosis would be Powerlessness.

Disturbed Sensory Perception
Disturbed Sensory Perception can affect the individual's ability to adjust to an alteration in health status. If it is determined that perceptual alterations are affecting the client's ability to adapt, then the appropriate primary diagnosis would be Disturbed Sensory Perception.

Disturbed Thought Process
This diagnosis can inhibit the client's ability to adapt effectively to an alteration in health status. If the inability to adapt to the alteration is related to an alteration in thought processes, then the appropriate primary diagnosis would be Disturbed Thought Process.

Dysfunctional Grieving
Grieving can have a strong effect on the client's ability to adjust to an alteration in health status. The differentiation is complicated by the fact that

(box continued on page 748)

Have You Selected the Correct Diagnosis? *(box continued from page 747)*

a normal response to an alteration in health status can be grief. If, however, the client is not reporting a sense of loss, then the appropriate diagnosis would be Impaired Adjustment. If the client reports a sense of loss with the appropriate defining characteristics, then the appropriate diagnosis would be Grieving. If the grieving is prolonged or exceptionally severe, then an appropriate co-diagnosis with Impaired Adjustment would be Dysfunctional Grieving.

EXPECTED OUTCOME

Will return-demonstrate measures necessary to increase independence by [date].

Performs self-care tasks by [date].

Requests information about health status by [date].

TARGET DATES

Adjustment to a change in health status will require time; therefore, an acceptable initial target date would be no sooner than 7 to 10 days following the date of diagnosis.

NURSING ACTIONS/INTERVENTIONS WITH RATIONALES

Adult Health

ACTIONS/INTERVENTIONS	RATIONALES
Establish a therapeutic relationship with the patient and significant others by showing empathy and concern for the patient, calling the patient by name, answering questions honestly, involving the patient in decision making, etc.	A therapeutic relationship promotes cooperation in the plan of care and gives the patient a person to talk with.
Explain the disease process and prognosis to the patient.	Knowledge of disease process and limitations is necessary for adjustment.
Encourage the patient to ask questions about health status by allowing opportunity and asking the patient to share his or her understanding of the situation.	Increasing knowledge and understanding leads to improved coping and adjustment.
Encourage the patient to express feelings about disease process and prognosis by sitting with the patient for 30 minutes once a shift at [times]. Use techniques such as active listening, reflection, and asking open-ended questions.	Verbalization of feelings leads to understanding and adjustment.
Identify previous coping mechanisms, and assist the patient to find new ones.	Determines what coping strategies have been successful, and provides an opportunity to try new strategies.
Help the patient find alternatives or modification in previous lifestyle behavior by using assistive devices, changing level of participation in activities, learning new behaviors, etc.	Helps the patient continue to have satisfaction in activities, and provides a sense of control in lifestyle.
Encourage independence in self-care activities by focusing on the patient's strengths, rewarding small successes, etc.	Provides a sense of control, and increases self-esteem and adjustment.
Refer to the psychiatric nurse practitioner. (See Mental Health nursing actions.)	Collaboration promotes a holistic approach to care, and problems may need intervention by a specialist.

Child Health

ACTIONS/INTERVENTIONS	RATIONALES
Monitor for all possible etiologic factors via active listening by asking questions that are appropriate for the child (who, what, where, and when) regarding first feeling of not being able to adjust.	Provides the database needed to most accurately plan care.

ACTIONS/INTERVENTIONS	RATIONALES
Help the child realize it is normal to need some time and assistance in adjusting to changes (e.g., the child needing assistance with ambulating following surgery).	Realistic planning increases the likelihood of compliance and increases the sense of success.
Explore the child's and family's previous coping strategies.	Previous coping strategies serve as critical information in developing interventions for the current status.
Identify ways the child can feel better about coping with the needed adjustment, including reinforcement of desired behavior.	Effective coping can empower the child and family and thereby afford a positive adjustment.
Assist the child and family in creating realistic goals for coping.	Realistic goals enhance success.
Collaborate with related health-care team members as needed.	Collaborations with specialists serve to meet the unique needs of the patient and family.
Provide clear and simple explanations for procedures.	Simple and clear instructions promote the child's functioning while he or she is in a stressful situation.
Address educational needs related to health care.	Knowledge serves to empower and provide guidelines for compliance with the expected behavior.
Deal with other primary care needs promptly.	Basic primary needs require prompt attention to offer the best likelihood of minimizing adjustment difficulty.
Provide for posthospitalization follow-up with home care as needed.	Follow-up affords long-term resolution of adjustment.
Assist the patient and family in identification of community resources that can offer support.	Identification of resources before discharge will encourage the patient and family to use the resources as needed and will help them cope with the changes in their lifestyle.

Women's Health

ACTIONS/INTERVENTIONS	RATIONALES
Couvade Syndrome	
When counseling with expectant fathers, be alert for characteristics for Couvade Syndrome.[17]	Provides a database that allows early intervention.
• The syndrome affects males only.	
• Wives are pregnant and usually in the third or ninth month of gestation.	
• Symptoms are confined to the gastrointestinal (GI) or genitourinary (GU) system; notable exceptions are toothache and skin growths.	
• Anxiety and affective disturbances are common (e.g., constant worrying about labor events, "I can't do this" or "I just know I will faint,") and/or over-managing arrangements for the new baby (e.g., painting the nursery three times).	
• Physical findings are minimal.	
• Laboratory and X-ray testing yields normal results.	
• Patient makes no connection between his symptoms and his wife's pregnancy.	
Provide a nonjudgmental atmosphere to allow the patient (in this instance, a man with the medical diagnosis of Couvade Syndrome)[17] to express concerns of:	Encourages the patient to talk about feelings, and allows planning of how to channel feelings into activities that will assist in preparing for fatherhood.
• Self-image as a father	
• Relationship with his father	

(care plan continued on page 750)

NURSING ACTIONS/INTERVENTIONS WITH RATIONALES (continued from page 749)

Women's Health

ACTIONS/INTERVENTIONS	RATIONALES
• Self-responsibility • Feelings about the wife's or partner's pregnancy • Concerns about the safety of the wife or partner	
Accurately record physical symptoms described by the expectant father: • Fatigue • Weight gain • Nausea or vomiting • Headaches • Backaches • Food cravings	Allows more effective interventions and planning.
Support and guide the expectant father through the changes being experienced.	
Assure the expectant couple that: • Expectant fathers can suffer physical symptoms during partner's pregnancy. • Pregnancy affects both partners. • Fathers also have emotional needs during pregnancy.	Emphasizes that this is not necessarily unusual behavior. Assists with positive actions that support both partners, and allows the man to view the pregnancy realistically.[17]

Postpartum Affective Disorders

Postpartum Blues
This affects approximately 50 to 85 percent of all delivering women, is viewed as part of the adaptation process to childbirth, and usually resolves with normal support of the family. Therefore, it is not considered an impairment and is not discussed here.

Postpartum Depression

ACTIONS/INTERVENTIONS	RATIONALES
Described as postpartum major affective disorder in psychiatric literature (usually occurs 2 weeks to 3 months postpartum).	The following tools assist health-care personnel in checking for postpartum depression: **PDPI**—Postpartum Depression Prediction Inventory **PDSS**—Postpartum Depression Screening Scale **EPDS**—Edinburgh Postnatal Depression Scale[19,20]
Encourage the client to express fears about a less-than-perfect infant. This can include: • Low-birth-weight infant • Different sex than desired by parents • Fussy infant • Premature infant • Unwanted infant (the infant could be the result of an unwanted pregnancy or of rape).	Research has shown that not one factor alone creates an environment that makes the woman vulnerable to postpartum depression.[19–22]
Continually assess the new mother's mood, observing for signs of: • Continuous crying • Insomnia not related to care of the infant • Mood swings • Loss of appetite • Withdrawal • Irritability	Nursing observations can be critical in getting these patients the professional help they need. Too often women feel this is just part of being a new mother and that they have no one who will listen. Often these signs and symptoms go unreported and unrecognized by family members.[18–20]

ACTIONS/INTERVENTIONS	RATIONALES
• Guilt feelings • Feeling of inability to care for self or the infant or function in roles of wife and mother • Impaired memory • Lowered self-image Provide nonjudgmental atmosphere for the patient to discuss problematic situations. Issues may include: • Partner's lack of sexual interest • Any illness or problems with older children • Marital status • Disappointment in experience (Unwanted cesarean section, medications administered during labor, or any unexpected occurrences.) • Isolation during the postpartum period (Unable to return to work immediately, no adults available to talk to during day, unable to complete daily activities owing to fatigue, demands of infant, uncooperative partner, lack of support system, and so on.)	Encourages the patient to discuss feelings and verbalize disappointments or problems, so that plans for coping with reality of birth experience can be initiated.[21,22]

Postpartum Psychosis

The incidence of postpartum psychosis is approximately 1 in 1000 deliveries. Onset is acute and abrupt.[18]

Obtain a complete patient and family history, particularly regarding previous depressive or psychotic episodes. (Usually has familial and/or genetic basis.)

Collaborate with family members to never leave the patient alone, particularly with the infant.

Arrange for the family to take and care for the infant.

If needed, arrange for community resources for care of the infant.

ACTIONS/INTERVENTIONS	RATIONALES
Obtain immediate assistance from mental health colleagues for the mother.	This diagnosis needs professional assistance immediately and is beyond the scope of practice for perinatal nursing. The main duty of the perinatal nurse is to see that no harm comes to the mother or infant until mental health colleagues can assume care of the mother.
Explain to family the likelihood of repetition of psychosis with subsequent pregnancies.	

Mental Health

ACTIONS/INTERVENTIONS	RATIONALES
Call the client by the name he or she has identified as the preferred name with each interaction. [Note this name on the chart.]	Promotes a positive orientation, while enhancing self-esteem.
Discuss with the client his or her perception of the current alteration in health status. This should include information about the coping strategies that have been attempted and his or her assessment of what has made them ineffective in promoting adaptation.	Communicates respect for the client and his or her experience of the stressor, which promotes the development of a trusting relationship. Provides information about the client's strengths that can be utilized to promote coping, and provides the nurse with an opportunity to support these strengths in a manner that promotes a positive orientation.

(care plan continued on page 752)

NURSING ACTIONS/INTERVENTIONS WITH RATIONALES (continued from page 751)	

Mental Health

ACTIONS/INTERVENTIONS	RATIONALES
Provide the client with clocks and calendars to promote orientation and involvement in the environment.	Maintains the client's cognitive strengths in a manner that will facilitate the development of coping strategies.[7]
Give the client information about the care that is to be provided, including times for treatments, medicines, group, and other therapy.	Promotes the client's sense of control.
Assign the client appropriate tasks during unit activities. These should be at a level that can easily be accomplished. Provide the client with positive verbal support for completing the task. Gradually increase the difficulty of the tasks as the client's abilities increase.	Accomplishment of tasks provides the positive reinforcement that enhances self-esteem and motivates behavior. Also assists the client to develop a positive expectational set.
Sit with the client [number] minutes [number] times per day at [times] to discuss current concerns and feelings.	Communicates concern for the client, and facilitates the development of a trusting relationship. Promotes the client's sense of control by communicating that his or her ideas and concerns are important.
Provide the client with familiar needed objects. These should be noted here. These should assist the client in identifying a personal space over which he or she feels some control. This space is to be respected by the staff, and the client's permission should be obtained before altering this environment.	Promotes the client's sense of control, while meeting safety and security needs.
Provide the client with an environment that will optimize sensory input. This could include hearing aids, eyeglasses, pencil and paper, decreased noise in conversation areas, and appropriate lighting. (These actions should indicate an awareness of sensory deficit as well as sensory overload, and the specific interventions for this client should be noted here—e.g., place hearing aid in when client awakens and remove before bedtime (9:00 P.M.)	Appropriate levels of sensory input decrease confusion and disorganization, maximizing the client's coping abilities.
Communicate to the client an understanding that all coping behavior to this point has been his or her best effort and asking for assistance at this time is not failure—a complex problem often requires some outside assistance to resolve.	
Have the client dress in "street clothing." This should be items of clothing that have been brought from home and in which the client feels comfortable.	Promotes positive orientation and the client's sense of control by supporting normal daily routine and activities.
Provide the client with opportunities to make appropriate decisions related to care at his or her level of ability. This may begin as a choice between two options and then evolve into more complex decision making. It is important that this be at the client's level of functioning so that confidence can be built with successful decision-making experiences. [Note here those decisions that the client has made.]	Promotes the client's sense of control, and enhances self-esteem when appropriate decisions are made.

ACTIONS/INTERVENTIONS	RATIONALES
Provide the client with a primary care nurse on each shift. Nurse will spend 30 minutes once per shift at [time] developing a relationship with the client. This time could be spent answering the client's questions about the hospital, daily routines, etc., or providing the client with a backrub.	Promotes the development of a trusting relationship, while promoting the client's sense of control with knowledge about the environment.
Identify with the client methods of anxiety reduction. The specific method selected by the client should be noted here. For the first 3 days, the staff should remain with the client during a 30-minute practice of the selected method. The method should be practiced 30 minutes, three times a day at [times]. (See Anxiety in Chapter 8 for specific instructions about anxiety reduction methods.)	High levels of anxiety interfere with decision making. Increased control over anxiety promotes the client's sense of control. The presence of the nurse can provide positive reinforcement, which encourages behavior. Behavioral rehearsal internalizes and personalizes the behavior.
Provide positive social reinforcement and other behavioral rewards for demonstration of adaptation. The things that the client finds rewarding should be listed here with a schedule for use. The kinds of behavior that the team is to be rewarding should also be listed with the appropriate reward.	Reinforcement encourages positive behavior and enhances self-esteem.
Assist the client in identifying support systems and in developing a plan for their use. The support systems identified should be noted along with the plan for their use.	Support systems can facilitate the client's coping strategies.[23]
Schedule a meeting with members of the identified support system to assist them in understanding alterations in the client's health. Provide time to answer any questions they may have. [Note the time for this meeting here and the person responsible for this meeting.]	Promotes the development of a trusting relationship, and provides the support system with the information they can utilize to provide more effective support.
Provide the client with group interaction with [number] persons, [number] minutes, [number] times per day at [times]. This activity should be graded with the client's ability. For example, on admission, the client may tolerate one person for 5 minutes. If the interactions are brief, the frequency should be high; for example, 5-minute interactions should occur at 30-minute intervals. If the client is meeting with a large client group, this may occur only once a day. The larger groups should include persons who are more advanced in adapting to their alterations and persons who may be less advanced.	Disconfirms the client's sense of aloneness, and assists the client to experience personal importance to others while enhancing interpersonal relationship skills. Increasing these competencies can enhance self-esteem and promote a positive orientation.[24]
Make available items necessary for the client to groom him- or herself. Have these items adapted as necessary to facilitate client use. List the items that are necessary here, along with any assistance that is needed from the nursing staff. Assign one person per day to be responsible for this assistance. Provide positive social reinforcement for the client's accomplishments in this area.	Appropriate grooming enhances self-esteem. Reinforcement encourages positive behavior while enhancing self-esteem.[24]
Set an appointment to discuss with the client and significant others effects of the loss or change on their relationship (time and date of appointment and all follow-up appointments should be listed here). [Note the person responsible for these meetings.]	Promotes communication in the system that can serve as the basis for developing coping strategies.[25,26]

(care plan continued on page 754)

NURSING ACTIONS/INTERVENTIONS WITH RATIONALES (continued from page 753)

Mental Health

ACTIONS/INTERVENTIONS	RATIONALES
Monitor the nurse's nonverbal reactions to loss or change, and provide the client with verbal information when necessary to establish the nurse's acceptance of the change.	Promotes the development of a trusting relationship and the development of a positive orientation.
If the nursing staff is having difficulty coping with the client's alterations, schedule a staff meeting where these issues can be discussed. An outside clinical nurse specialist may be useful in facilitating these meetings. Schedule ongoing support meetings as necessary.	Staff thoughts and feelings can be indirectly communicated to the client, which could have a negative effect on the client's developing a positive orientation.
Utilize constructive confrontation if necessary to include "I" statements, relationship statements that reflect nurse's reaction to the interaction, and responses that will assist the client in understanding, such as paraphrasing and validation of perceptions.	Models appropriate communication skills, while providing the client with information that facilitates consensual validation.
When a relationship has been developed, the primary care nurse will spend 30 minutes twice a day at [time] with the client discussing thoughts and feelings related to the alteration in health status. These discussions could include memories that have been activated by this alteration, the client's fears and concerns for the future, the client's plans for the future before the alteration in health status, the client's perceptions of how this alteration will affect daily life, and the client's perceptions of how this alteration will affect the lives of significant others.	Promotes the development of adaptive coping strategies.
Provide the client with information about care and treatment. Give information in concise terms appropriate to the client's level of understanding. Note here those areas for which the client needs the most information, and include a plan for providing this information.	Promotes the client's sense of control. Inappropriate levels of sensory input can increase the client's confusion and disorganization.
Do not argue with the client while he or she is experiencing an alteration in thought process. (Refer to Disturbed Thought Process in Chapter 7 for related nursing actions.)	Arguing with these perceptions decreases the client's self-esteem and increases his or her needs to enlist dysfunctional coping behavior.
Develop with the client a very specific behavioral plan for adapting to the alteration in health status. Note that plan here. It should include achievable goals so the client will not become frustrated.	Achievement of a specific plan provides positive reinforcement and enhances self-esteem, which motivates positive behavior.
Refer the client to occupational therapy to develop the necessary adaptations to the occupational role. [Note times for these meetings here.]	Successful adaptation to the occupational role enhances self-esteem.[27]
Schedule a time for the client and his or her support system to be together without interruptions. The times for these interactions should be noted here.	Provides opportunities for the support system to maintain normal relationships while the client is hospitalized.
If the client is disoriented, orient to reality as needed and before attempting any teaching activity. Provide the client with clocks and calendars, and refer to day, date, and time in each interaction with this client.	Enhances the client's cognitive functioning, improving his or her ability to problem solve and to cope.
Refer the client to appropriate assistive resources as indicated. [Note here those referrals made and the name of the contact person.]	Establishes the client's support system in the community. Social support enhances coping.

Gerontic Health

In addition to the following, the nursing actions for the Adult Health and Mental Health patient may also be used.

ACTIONS/INTERVENTIONS	RATIONALES
Communicate your own positive views about aging, and the client's ability to cope, to the client and caregivers.	Promotes positive anticipatory coping.
Avoid ageist remarks such as "You look so good for someone who is 90 years old."	Promotes positive self-esteem.
Assist the client to maintain functional abilities or make referrals for Occupational Therapy or Physical Therapy to assist the client to improve his or her functional abilities.	Self-esteem and coping are closely related with physical health and functional ability.
Discuss the client's roles in life (grandparent, parent, roommate) and the associated responsibilities with the roles.	Persons with greater numbers of role identities have improved perceptions of self worth.
Utilize reminiscence therapy, either in a group or individually, with the client.	Reminiscence therapy assists the client in identifying unresolved conflicts and focusing on their achievements.
Promote a sense of control for the client: • Include the client in the decision-making process. • Speak to the client rather than about him or her. • Show respect for the client's privacy (knock before entering his or her room, keep the curtains drawn, be careful with personal possessions). • Promote physical fitness in clients able to participate in activities.	Older clients who feel a sense of control are better able to cope.

Home Health

In addition to the interventions for Adult Health and Mental Health, the following may be used for the home health client.

ACTIONS/INTERVENTIONS	RATIONALES
Monitor for factors contributing to impaired adjustment (e.g., psychological, social, economic, spiritual, or environmental factors).	Provides a database for intervention.
Involve the client and family in planning, implementing, and promoting reduction or elimination of impaired adjustment: • Family conference: Discuss feelings and altered roles, and identify coping strategies that have worked in the past. • Mutual goal sharing: Establish realistic goals and specify role of each family member; for example, provide a safe environment and support self-care. • Communication: Clear and honest communication should be promoted among family members. If sensory impairments exist, corrective interventions are needed (e.g., eyeglasses or a hearing aid).	Family involvement enhances the effectiveness of interventions.
Assist the client and family in lifestyle adjustments that may be required: • Stress management • Development and use of support networks • Treatment for disability	Family relationships can be altered by impaired adjustment. Permanent changes in behavior and family roles require evaluation and support.

(care plan continued on page 756)

NURSING ACTIONS/INTERVENTIONS WITH RATIONALES (continued from page 755)	

Home Health

ACTIONS/INTERVENTIONS	RATIONALES
• Appropriate balance of dependence and independence • Grief counseling • Change in role functions • Treatment for cognitive impairment • Provision of comfortable and safe environment • Activities to increase self-esteem	
Consult with or refer to appropriate assistive resources as indicated.	Utilization of existing services is efficient use of resources. Resources such as an occupational therapist, a psychiatric nurse clinician, and support groups can enhance the treatment plan.

COMMUNITY COPING, INEFFECTIVE AND READINESS FOR ENHANCED

DEFINITIONS[16]

Ineffective Community Coping Pattern of community activities for adaptation and problem solving that is unsatisfactory for meeting the demands or needs of life in the community.

Readiness for Enhanced Community Coping Pattern of community activities for adaptation and problem solving that is satisfactory for meeting the demands or needs of life in the community but can be improved for management of current and future problems or stressors.

DEFINING CHARACTERISTICS[16]

A. Ineffective Community Coping
1. Expressed community powerlessness
2. Deficits of community participation
3. Excessive community conflicts
4. Expressed vulnerability
5. High illness rate
6. Stressors perceived as excessive
7. Community does not meet its own expectations
8. Increased social problems, for example, homicides, vandalism, arson, terrorism, robbery, infanticide, abuse, divorce, or unemployment

B. Readiness for Enhanced Community Coping
One or more characteristics that indicate effective coping:
1. Positive communication between community or aggregates and larger community
2. Programs available for recreation and relaxation
3. Resources sufficient for managing stressors
4. Agreement that the community is responsible for stress management

5. Active planning by the community for predicted stressors
6. Active problem solving by the community when faced with issues
7. Positive communication among community members

RELATED FACTORS[16]

A. Ineffective Community Coping
1. Natural or man-made disasters
2. Ineffective or nonexistent community systems (e.g., lack of emergency medical system, transportation system, or disaster planning systems)
3. Deficits in community social support services and resources
4. Inadequate resources for problem solving

B. Readiness for Enhanced Community Coping
1. Community has a sense of power to manage stressors.
2. Social supports are available.
3. Resources are available for problem solving.

RELATED CLINICAL CONCERNS

1. High incidence of violence
2. High illness rates
3. Few opportunities or locations for community connectedness.

 Have You Selected the Correct Diagnosis?

Effective Management of Therapeutic Regimen, Community
This is an actual diagnosis that indicates a community has resolved its problems. Ineffective Community Coping and Readiness for Enhanced Community Coping indicate the community is either still in the throes of its problem or has just started problem solving.

EXPECTED OUTCOME

Community problem solving forums have representation by all stake holders by [date].

There will be a [number] percent increase in member attendance at community forums by [date].

There will be a [number] percent decrease in community violence by [date].

TARGET DATES

These diagnoses are very long term. Appropriate target dates would be expressed in terms of months or years.

NURSING ACTIONS/INTERVENTIONS WITH RATIONALES

Adult Health

Nursing actions specific for this diagnoses will require implementation in the home and community environment; therefore, the reader is referred to the Home Health nursing actions for this diagnosis.

Child Health

Same as for Adult Health, with acknowledgement of parents and caregivers assuming the advocacy role. Use developmentally appropriate approach. May be dependent on funding or interest of local potential supporters.

Women's Health

ACTIONS/INTERVENTIONS	RATIONALES
Ineffective Community Coping	
● N O T E : *It has been noted that with early discharge of the new mother and baby, many communities are ineffective in having in place follow-up programs to assist these new mothers and their infants in the first critical postpartum days. Even with states' mandating "48-hour stays," there still exists a great need to support new mothers and their newborns after discharge from the hospital.*	
Investigate what programs are available to the new mother and her infant in the community. Different communities have different programs, such as: • Well-baby clinics[30,31] • Public health department programs • Nursing centers (usually at schools of nursing in university settings) • State and federal programs such as First Steps, First Start, and maternity support programs Network with nursing colleagues in the community to assess how you can assist one another in providing continuity of care for these mothers and their newborns.	Provides a coordinated flow of care for the patient. Allows for more equal distribution of scarce resources, which can eliminate duplication of services to some while others have none.[28-31]
Readiness for Enhanced Community Coping	
● N O T E : *Many private nursing agencies and acute care hospitals have or are putting into place follow-up programs to deal with the issue of early discharge of the new mother and her infant. These programs include telephone follow-up, postpartum after-care centers, and home visits.[28-31]*	
Telephone Follow-up	
Call the discharged mother within 36 to 48 hours after discharge. Allow the mother time to answer questions and expand on her answers if necessary. (Sometimes this takes some leading and directed questioning by the nurse.)	Provides follow-up contact with the new mother and her family. This contact can provide important information and monitoring, reinforcement of previous education, emotional and professional support to new parents, and referral to appropriate professional services, if needed.

(care plan continued on page 758)

NURSING ACTIONS/INTERVENTIONS WITH RATIONALES (continued from page 757)

Women's Health

ACTIONS/INTERVENTIONS	RATIONALES
Provide a nonjudgmental atmosphere that allows the new mother and/or father to verbalize concerns and needs.	
Ask for descriptions of the infant's color, cord, circumcision (if appropriate), feeding patterns, stool patterns, and number of wet diapers.	
Ask the mother to describe feeding sessions. If breastfeeding: • How often and how long does the infant nurse? • Does the infant nurse on both sides? • How do her breasts look (cracks, bleeding, or sore)? • Does the infant latch on correctly? • What does the infant's stool look like, and how many wet diapers are there in a 24-hour period?	
If formula feeding: • How often does the infant feed? • How many ounces does the infant take? • Is the infant tolerating formula (not spitting excessively or having projectile vomiting)? • What is the color of the stool and pattern? How many wet diapers?	
Discuss potential for injury to the infant, covering the following topics: • Use of approved car seat • Smoking in the presence of the infant or in home where the infant is • Use of proper bedding and proper positioning of the infant in bed (on back or side) • Environmental safety ("childproofing" the house)	
Ask the mother how she is feeling (tired, overwhelmed, out of sorts, etc.). Inquire about her physical well-being: • Episiotomy • Incision (if cesarean section) • Any alterations in involution (lochia—rubra, serosa, or alba) • Breasts • Stools (diarrhea or constipation) • Any signs and symptoms of infection (increased temperature, increased tenderness of uterus [abdomen], foul-smelling lochia)	
Instruct the mother and/or father to call primary health-care provider if any signs or symptoms of infection are noted.	
If concerns are noted, make arrangements for the mother, father, and infant to return to postpartum follow-up center or clinic, and/or schedule a home visit by a nurse. If concerns are urgent, recommend that the mother, father, and infant go to emergency room and/or their primary health care provider immediately.	Provides a creative solution to the early discharge of new mothers and their infants from the acute care system after birth. Allows for continuation of quality nursing care and monitoring of the postpartum progress of the mother and her infant.[28–31]

ACTIONS/INTERVENTIONS	RATIONALES
Follow-up Clinic and/or Home Visit	
Assess interaction between the parents and the parents with the newborn. If siblings are present, assess interaction with the parents and the new baby.	
Assess the mother for physical and psychological well-being. (See previous interventions for physical well-being. See also Impaired Adjustment for psychological well-being.)	
Assess the home for social economic needs and referrals, such as: • Enough to eat • Cleanliness • Whether the new mother have help in home • Transportation	
Assess the infant for physical well-being. (See previous interventions.)	
Document findings, and place them in the mother's and infant's charts when returning to hospital. Send a copy of the documentation to primary health-care provider for both the mother and infant.	

Mental Health

Refer to Home Health actions and interventions for these care plans.

Gerontic Health

● N O T E : *This diagnosis covers community as a whole, and affects all areas of health care.*

ACTIONS/INTERVENTIONS	RATIONALES
Ineffective Community Coping	
Discuss examples of ineffective coping in order to begin problem solving.	Increases awareness of problems in the community and stimulates interest.
Clarify questions related to coping that arise from problem-solving sessions.	Helps identify strategies that may increase coping skills.
Identify fiscal resources available to the community for problem solving.	Local, regional, state, or federal programs may have funds dedicated to addressing problems related to aging.
Identify local leaders (formal as well as informal) who have power within the community, and gain their perspective.	
Facilitate use of community services to network for problem solving, such as radio or television stations that offer to air public service announcements, newspapers to publish letters to the editor, or libraries to make available access to community internets.	Conserves money. Also increases likelihood of reaching the target audience in the community.

(care plan continued on page 760)

NURSING ACTIONS/INTERVENTIONS WITH RATIONALES (continued from page 759)

Gerontic Health

ACTIONS/INTERVENTIONS	RATIONALES
Readiness for Enhanced Community Coping Facilitate participation in community activities.	Older adults are more likely to be involved in organized activities, such as senior citizens' groups. They are also more likely to vote and actively support or campaign for governmental candidates.
Enlist older adults in community setting in problem-solving meetings.	Can provide historical perspective on the community and its growth pattern and needs.
Consult with organized community resources such as RSVP or American Association of Retired Persons (AARP) groups for problem solving and future planning.	Provides a wealth of life experiences for problem solving within the community.
Consider use of telephone trees, computer connections, or letter writing for older adults with decreased mobility who can still add to community life and growth.	Time is an important factor in community growth and planning, and older adults may have more time to assist the community. Activities such as those mentioned may be possible even for those with limited mobility.

Home Health

ACTIONS/INTERVENTIONS	RATIONALES
Involve community groups in problem identification and program development: • Identify local needs for addressing problems or stressors. • Facilitate participation in the community process.	Involvement at the local level enhances community development and communication.
Identify community strengths and weaknesses. • Develop strategies to enhance strengths and correct weaknesses. • Identify resources needed and resources available.	Community recognition of strengths, weaknesses, and resources enhances the potential.
Develop collaborative relationships within the community to promote development of the community.	Supportive relationships enhance the success of the plan.
Utilize strategies identified for enhanced community coping to identify factors leading to Ineffective Community Coping: • Develop strategies to correct the deficits. • Develop a plan with community involvement to correct deficits.	

FAMILY COPING, COMPROMISED AND DISABLED

DEFINITIONS[16]

Compromised Family Coping Usually supportive primary person (family member or close friend) provides insufficient, ineffective, or compromised support, comfort, assistance, or encouragement that may be needed by the client to manage or master adaptive tasks related to his or her health challenge.

Disabled Family Coping Behavior of significant person (family or other primary person) that disables his or her own capacities and the client's capacities to effectively address tasks essential to either person's adaptation to the health challenge.

DEFINING CHARACTERISTICS[16]

A. Compromised Family Coping
1. Subjective
   a. The client expresses or confirms a concern or complaint about significant other's response to his or her health problems.
   b. A significant person describes or confirms an inadequate understanding or knowledge base that interferes with effective assistive or supportive behaviors.
   c. A significant person describes preoccupation with personal reaction (e.g., fear, anticipatory grief, guilt, or anxiety) to client's illness, disability, or other situational or developmental crises.
2. Objective
   a. A significant person attempts assistive or supportive behaviors with less than satisfactory results.
   b. A significant person displays protective behavior disproportionate (too little or too much) to the client's abilities or need for autonomy.
   c. A significant person withdraws or enters into limited or temporary personal communication with the client at the time of need.

B. Disabled Family Coping
1. Intolerance
2. Agitation, depression, aggression, or hostility
3. Taking on illness signs of client
4. Rejection
5. Psychosomaticism
6. Neglectful relationships with other family members
7. Neglectful care of the client in regard to basic human needs and/or illness treatment
8. Impaired restructuring of a meaningful life for self
9. Impaired individualization or prolonged over concern for client
10. Distortion of reality regarding the client's health problem, including extreme denial about its existence or severity
11. Desertion
12. Decisions and actions of the family that are detrimental to economic or social well-being
13. Carrying on usual routines, disregarding client's needs
14. Abandonment
15. Client's development of helpless, inactive dependence
16. Disregarding needs

RELATED FACTORS[16]

A. Compromised Family Coping
1. Temporary preoccupation by a significant person who is trying to manage emotional conflicts and personal suffering and is unable to perceive or act effectively in regard to the client's needs
2. Temporary family disorganization and role changes
3. Prolonged disease or disability progression that exhausts supportive capacity of significant people
4. Other situational or developmental crises or situations the significant person may be facing
5. Inadequate or incorrect information or understanding by a primary person
6. Little support provided by the client, in turn, for primary person

B. Disabled Family Coping
1. Significant person with chronically unexpressed feelings of guilt, anxiety, hostility, despair, etc.
2. Arbitrary handling of the family's resistance to treatment, which tends to solidify defensiveness, as it fails to deal adequately with underlying anxiety
3. Dissonant discrepancy of coping styles for dealing with adaptive tasks by the significant person and the client or among significant people
4. Highly ambivalent family relationships

RELATED CLINICAL CONCERNS

1. Alzheimer's disease
2. AIDS
3. Any disorder resulting in permanent paralysis
4. Cancer
5. Any disorder of a chronic nature (e.g., rheumatoid arthritis)
6. Substance abuse or use
7. Somatoform disorders
8. Multiple co-occurring family crises
9. Unresolved family conflicts

☑ Have You Selected the Correct Diagnosis?

Compromised versus Disabled Coping
Compromised dysfunction reflects the family that cannot provide appropriate support to the identified patient. This problem removes a possible support system from the client. If the family dysfunction results in further dysfunction for the identified patient, then the diagnosis is Disabled. Because this diagnosis is used to describe family processes, it may be difficult at times to differentiate between compromised and disabled because there is not an identified patient or the effects of the family patterns on the client cannot be determined. When this is the situation, the diagnosis can be made as Ineffective Family Coping with no attached label.

Family Coping, Readiness for Enhanced
Family Coping, Readiness for Enhanced is an appropriate diagnosis for families that are coping well with current stressors and are in a position to enhance their coping abilities. Ineffective Family Coping describes a family that has a deficit in coping abilities that threatens the family's existence.

(box continued on page 762)

Have You Selected the Correct Diagnosis? *(box continued from page 761)*

Impaired Parenting
Impaired Parenting refers to an inability to fulfill the parenting role. This dysfunction is circumscribed to the parent–child relationship and is time limited, in contrast with Ineffective Family Coping.

EXPECTED OUTCOME

Family Coping, Compromised
Caregiver will identify [number] social connections by [date].
Caregiver will identify [number] of positive self statements per interaction by [date].
Caregiver will problem solve with client by [date].

Family Coping, Disabled
Caregiver will problem solve with client by [date].
Caregiver will verbalize understanding of disease process by [date].
Caregiver will verbalize [number] of positive statements per interaction about client by [date].
Will identify the effects current coping strategies have on the family by [date].

TARGET DATES

The target dates should reflect the complexity and power of the system. Four-week intervals would be appropriate to assess for progress. It may be necessary to refer family to community agency for ongoing follow-up in acute care settings.

NURSING ACTIONS/INTERVENTIONS WITH RATIONALES

Adult Health

ACTIONS/INTERVENTIONS	RATIONALES
Encourage and assist the family and significant others to verbalize their needs, fears, feelings, and concerns by sitting with the patient for 30 minutes per shift at [times] or planning a family conference. Actively listen and facilitate discussion.	Allows for identification of specific stressors, and promotes creative problem solving.
Provide accurate information about the situation.	Clarifies misconceptions and misunderstanding.
Include the family and significant others in decision making and plan of care when planning care and intervening.	Promotes active participation, motivation, and compliance.
Assist the family and significant others to identify and explore alternatives to dealing with the situation (e.g., respite care, Mom's day out, or daycare centers).	Promotes creative problem solving.
Assist the family and significant others to identify before discharge sources of community support that could assist them to cope with their feelings and to supply relief when needed.	Community resources can help strengthen family coping process and prevent isolation of the family.
Encourage the family to provide time for themselves on a regular basis.	Reduces stresses and strengthens coping skills.
Initiate referral to a psychiatric clinical nurse specialist as needed.	Problems may need intervention by a specialist.

Child Health

Obvious concern is for safety of child; when necessary, child protective services will be involved. Many nursing actions are related to those of women's health and psychiatric nursing. A developmentally appropriate basis for care is paramount.

ACTIONS/INTERVENTIONS	RATIONALES
Encourage the child and family to express feelings and fears by allotting 30 minutes per shift, while the client is awake, for this purpose.	Expression of concerns provides insight into views about problem and the values of the patient and family.

ACTIONS/INTERVENTIONS	RATIONALES
Review family dynamics in place before the crisis.	Family dynamics in usual times is paramount in understanding coping dynamics during times of stress.
Facilitate family member participation in the child's care, as appropriate, including bathing, feeding, comfort, and diversional activity.	Family and patient input ensures individualized plan of care. Provides a teaching opportunity and increases the child's security.
Provide education to all family members regarding the child's illness, prognosis, and special needs as appropriate.	Reduces anxiety, increases likelihood of compliance, and empowers the family.
Involve health-care team members in collaboration for care with focus on role modeling desired behaviors.	Increases the likelihood of a holistic plan of care for both short-term and long-term goals.
Provide referral to appropriate community resources for support purposes.	Provides for long-term follow-up and support.
Provide for home discharge planning at least 5 days before discharge.	Allows time for teaching, practice, and return-demonstration.
Make referral for home health care and other community resources as needed (e.g., parenting support groups).	Provides for long-term follow-up and support.[32]

Women's Health

● N O T E : *This diagnosis would be most likely to relate to the single mother in the area of Women's Health.*

ACTIONS/INTERVENTIONS	RATIONALES
Review the physical, mental, social, and economic status of the single mother, taking into account whether she is widowed; divorced; single, and a parent by choice; or single, and a parent not by choice. (See Impaired Adjustment.)	Provides a database that can be used to plan appropriate interventions and locate support systems for the patient.
Identify support system available to the single mother (e.g., family, friends, co-workers, or formal support groups such as church or community organizations).	
Review the patient's perception of employment status (e.g., educational level and skills, job opportunities, and opportunity for improvement of employment status).	Assists the patient to realistically plan for fiscal needs of herself and her infant. Allows identification of resources that could assist in improving income status.
Identify child care requirements considering the age of children, who has legal custody of children, and child support (financial and emotional).	
Suggest strategies for exposing the children to male role models.[32] • Assign to classes with male teachers. • Ask for assistance from brothers or grandparents. • Involve the children in sports. (Coaches are usually male.)	Provides for male role modeling in the absence of a father figure.

Mental Health

ACTIONS/INTERVENTIONS	RATIONALES
Role-model effective communication by: • Seeking clarification	Models for the family effective communication that can enhance their problem-solving abilities.

(care plan continued on page 764)

Mental Health

ACTIONS/INTERVENTIONS	RATIONALES
• Demonstrating respect for individual family members and the family system • Listening to expression of thoughts and feelings • Setting clear limits • Being consistent • Communicating with the individual being addressed in a clear manner • Encouraging sharing of information among appropriate system subgroups	
At each meeting with the family, provide positive verbal reinforcement related to the observed strengths.	Promotes hope, and helps the family develop a positive view of themselves and their abilities, promoting an environment for change. Supports the development of a positive therapeutic relationship.[32]
Demonstrate an understanding of the complexity of system problems by: • Not taking sides in family disagreements • Providing alternative explanations of behavior patterns that recognize the contributions of all persons involved in the problem, including health care providers, if appropriate • Requesting the perspective of multiple family members on a problem or stressor	Promotes the development of a trusting relationship, while developing a positive orientation.
Determine the risk for physical harm, and refer to appropriate authorities if the risk is high (child protective services, battered women's centers, or police).	Client safety is of primary concern.
Assist the family in developing behavioral short-term goals by: • Asking what changes they would expect to see when the problem is improved • Having them break the problem into several parts that combine to form the identified stressor or crisis • Setting a time limit of 1 week to accomplish a taskl for example, "What could you do this week to improve the current situation?"	Accomplishments of goals provide reinforcement, which motivates continued positive behavior and enhances self-esteem.
Develop a priority list with the family.	Promotes the family's sense of control and promotes the development of a trusting relationship by communicating respect for the client system.
Begin work with the presenting problem, and enlist the system's assistance in resolving concerns.	Promotes the development of a trusting relationship, while enhancing the client system's sense of control.
Include assessment data in determining how to work on the presenting problem. For example, if behavioral controls for a child are requested, the nurse can develop a plan for teaching and implementing them in the home that includes both parents.	
Support communication between family members by: • Having the family members discuss alternatives to the problem in the presence of the nurse • Having each family member indicate how he or she might help resolve the problem	Assists the family in developing problem-solving skills that will serve them in future situations.

ACTIONS/INTERVENTIONS	RATIONALES
• Having each family member indicate how he or she contributes to the maintenance of the problem, or how he or she does not help the identified patient change behavior • Spending time having the family members give each other positive feedback	
Discuss with the family the need for taking breaks from the focus on the health challenge. Options to accomplish this might include: • Arranging for respite care • Planning a family vacation • Planning a family play day Note here the family plan and support needed from the staff.	Provides the family with balance between illness demands and the need for self-care activities.[32] Assists the family in discovering positive aspects of their relationships.
Support the development of appropriate subgroups by: • Presenting problems to the appropriate subsystems for discussion—for example, if the problem involves a discussion of how the sexual functioning of the marital couple will change as a result of illness, this issue should be discussed with the husband and wife • Providing an opportunity for the children to discuss their concerns with their parents • Supporting appropriate generational boundaries—for example, parent's attempts to exclude children from parental roles	Promotes healthy family functioning.
Develop direct interventions that instruct a family to do something different or not to do something. If direct interventions are not successful and reassessment indicates they were presented appropriately, this may indicate the family system is having unusual problems with the change process and should be referred to an advanced practitioner for further care.	Provides information on the family's ability to change at this point in time, while promoting a positive orientation.
Provide experiences for the family to learn how they can think differently about the problem, for example, a job loss can be seen as an opportunity to reevaluate family goals, focus on interpersonal closeness, and enhance family problem-solving skills.	Promotes a positive orientation, while assisting the family in developing problem-solving skills.
Provide opportunities for the expression of a range of affect; this can mean laughing and crying together. This may require that the nurse "push" the family to express feelings with the skills of confrontation or providing feedback.[32,33]	Validates the family members' emotions, and helps identify the appropriateness of their affective responses.
Develop a teaching plan to provide the family with information that will enhance their problem solving. (This could include information about the disease process and skills necessary for self-care.) [Note that teaching plan here.]	
Assist the family with interactions with other systems by: • Providing information about the system • Maintaining open communication between nurse and other agencies or systems	Facilitates the development of support networks in the community that can be called on in future situations.

(care plan continued on page 766)

NURSING ACTIONS/INTERVENTIONS WITH RATIONALES (continued from page 765)

Mental Health

ACTIONS/INTERVENTIONS	RATIONALES
• Having the family identify what their relationship is with the system, and how they could best achieve the goals they have for their interactions with this system	
Provide constructive confrontation to the family about problematic coping behavior.[33] Those kinds of behavior identified by the treatment team as problematic should be listed here.	Facilitates the development of functional coping behaviors in a warm, supportive environment.
Teach the family methods to reduce anxiety, and practice and discuss the use of these methods with the family [number] times per week. This should be done at least once a week until family members are using this as a coping method. This could include deep muscle relaxation, physical exercise, family games that require physical activity, or cycling. Those methods selected by the family should be listed here, with the time schedule for implementation. The family should be given "homework" related to the practice of these techniques at home on a daily basis.	High levels of anxiety can interfere with adaptive coping behaviors. Repeated practice of a behavior internalizes and personalizes the behavior.
Provide the family with the information about proper nutrition that was indicated as missing on the assessment. This should include time spent on discussing how proper nutrition can fit the family lifestyle. This teaching plan should be listed here. A "homework" assignment related to the necessary pattern change should be given. This should involve all the family members. Make an assignment that has high potential for successful completion by the family.	Proper nutrition promotes physical well-being, which facilitates adaptive coping. Successful accomplishment of goals provides positive reinforcement and motivates behavior, while enhancing self-esteem.
If a homework assignment is not completed, **do not** chastise the family. Indicate that the nurse misjudged the complexity of the task, and assess what made it difficult for the family to complete the task. Develop a new, less complex task based on this information. If a family continues not to complete tasks, they may need to be referred to an advanced practitioner for continued care.	Promotes positive orientation.
Monitor the family's desire for spiritual counseling, and refer to appropriate resources. The name of the resource person should be listed here.	
Assist the family in identifying support systems and in developing a plan for their use. This plan should be recorded here.	
Refer the family to community resources as necessary for continued support.	Provides resources that can provide support in the community.

Gerontic Health

In addition to the interventions for Adult Health and Mental Health, the following may be used for the older client:

ACTIONS/INTERVENTIONS	RATIONALES
Refer to adult protective services if risk of physical harm is high.	Provides means for monitoring the patient and family. Effective use of resources to reduce risk of harm for the patient.

Home Health

In addition to the interventions for Adult Health and Mental Health, the following may be used for the home health client.

ACTIONS/INTERVENTIONS	RATIONALES
Involve the client and family in planning and implementing strategies to improve family coping: • Crisis management: Identify actions to identify crisis and intervene (e.g., removing individuals from situation). • Mutual goal setting: Identify realistic goals and specify activities for each family member. • Communication: Provide realistic feedback in positive manner. • Family conference: Each member identifies how he or she is involved, and possible interventions are considered. • Support for the caregiver.	Family involvement and clarification of roles are necessary to enhance interventions.
Assist the family and client in lifestyle adjustments that may be required: • Stress management • Altering past ineffective coping strategies • Treatment for substance abuse • Treatment for physical illness • Appropriate use of denial • Avoiding scapegoating • Activities of daily family living • Financial concerns • Change in geographic or sociocultural location • Potential for violence • Identify family strengths • Obtain temporary assistance (e.g., housekeeper, sitter, or temporary placement outside the home)	Changes in family roles and behaviors require long-term behavioral changes. Support is required to facilitate these lifestyle changes.
Consult with and refer to assistive resources as appropriate.	Utilization of existing services is efficient use of resources. Such resources as a family therapist, protective services, a psychiatric nurse clinician, and community support groups can enhance the treatment plan.

FAMILY COPING, READINESS FOR ENHANCED

DEFINITION[16]

Effective managing of adaptive tasks by family member involved with the client's health challenge, who now is exhibiting desire and readiness for enhanced health and growth in regard to self and in relation to the client.

DEFINING CHARACTERISTICS[16]

1. Individual expressing interest in making contact on a one-to-one basis or on a mutual-aid group basis with another person who has experienced a similar situation
2. Family member moving in direction of health-promoting and enriching lifestyle, which supports and monitors maturational processes, audits and negotiates treatment

programs, and generally chooses experiences that optimize wellness

3. Family member attempting to describe the growth impact of crisis on his or her own values, priorities, goals, or relationships

RELATED FACTORS[16]

Needs sufficiently gratified and adaptive tasks effectively addressed to enable goals of self-actualization to surface.

RELATED CLINICAL CONCERNS

1. Alzheimer's disease
2. AIDS
3. Any disorder resulting in permanent paralysis
4. Cancer
5. Any disorder of a chronic nature (e.g., rheumatoid arthritis)

 Have You Selected the Correct Diagnosis?

Ineffective Family Coping and Interrupted Family Processes
Readiness for Enhanced Family Coping addresses the family that is currently handling stresses well

and that is in a position to enhance their coping abilities. The other nursing diagnoses related to family functioning address various aspects of family dysfunction. If any dysfunction is present, Readiness for Enhanced Family Coping would not be the diagnosis of choice.

EXPECTED OUTCOME

Will verbalize satisfaction with current progress toward family goals by [date].

Participates in mutual aide group with others in similar situation by [date].

Identifies [number] of activities that can be initiated to improve personal/family health by [date].

TARGET DATES

Depending on the family size and the commitment of each member toward growth, the target date could range from weeks to months. A reasonable initial target date would be 2 weeks.

NURSING ACTIONS/INTERVENTIONS WITH RATIONALES

Adult Health

ACTIONS/INTERVENTIONS	RATIONALES
Provide opportunities for the family and significant others to discuss the patient's condition and treatment modalities by scheduling at least one family session every other day.	Promotes understanding, open communication, creative problem solving, and growth.
Include the family and significant others in planning and providing care as care is planned and implemented.	Promotes active participation, motivation, and compliance. Provides a teaching opportunity and an opportunity for the family to practice in a supportive environment.
Provide instruction as needed in supportive and assistive behavior for the patient.	Understanding and knowledge base are needed to adapt to situations. Reduces anxiety.
Answer questions clearly and honestly.	Promotes a trusting relationship.
Refer the family and significant others to support groups and resources as indicated.	Coordination and collaboration organize resources and decrease duplication of services. Provides a broader range of networked resources.

Child Health

ACTIONS/INTERVENTIONS	RATIONALES
Identify how the child views the current crisis by using play, puppetry, etc.	The impact of the crisis on the child is basic data needed for planning care.
Identify the family's and the child's previous and current coping patterns.	Family coping behaviors serve as reference data to understand the child's response and behavior. Will also provide needs assessment data for planning of teaching.
Assist the child in identifying ways the current crisis or situation can enhance his or her coping for future needs.	Viewing current situation for beneficial outcomes can assist in a positive outcome.
Identify appropriate health members who can assist in providing support for growth potential.	Specialists may best assist the patient in positive resolution of crisis.
Offer educational instruction to meet the patient's and family's needs related to health care.	Knowledge serves to empower the patient and family and reduces anxiety.
Allow for sufficient time while in hospital to reinforce necessary skills for care (e.g., range of motion (ROM) exercises).	Learning in a supportive environment provides reinforcement of desired content.

Women's Health

ACTIONS/INTERVENTIONS	RATIONALES
Encourage participation of significant others in preparation for birth (e.g., spouse, boyfriend, partner, children, in-laws, grandparents, and others who are important to the individual).	Enhances the support system for the patient, and promotes positive anticipation of birth.
Discuss childbirth and the changes that will occur in the family unit.	
Encourage the patient to list family lifestyle adjustments that need to be made. Involve significant others in discussion and problem-solving activities regarding family adjustments to the newborn (e.g., child care, working, household responsibilities, social network, or support groups).	Provides directions for anticipation of birth, and allows more long-range planning that can prevent crises.
Encourage the woman and partner (significant other) to attend childbirth education or parenting classes in preparation for the birthing experience.	Provides basic information that assists in easing labor experience. Promotes a more positive birth experience and reduces anxiety.

Mental Health

ACTIONS/INTERVENTIONS	RATIONALES
Talk with the family to identify their goals and concerns.	Promotes development of a trusting relationship by communicating respect and concern for the family.
Assist the family in identifying strengths.	Promotes a positive orientation.
Commend family strengths at each meeting with the family.	Promotes hope and helps the family develop a positive view of themselves and their abilities, promoting an environment for change. Supports the development of a positive therapeutic relationship.[32]
Refer the family to appropriate community support groups.	Parents and families with social supports demonstrate enhanced relationships and coping.[23]

(care plan continued on page 770)

NURSING ACTIONS/INTERVENTIONS WITH RATIONALES (continued from page 769)

Mental Health

ACTIONS/INTERVENTIONS	RATIONALES
Teach the family the skills necessary to provide care to an ill member.	Provides the family with an increased repertoire of behavior that they can use to effectively cope with the situation.
Talk with the family about the role flexibility necessary to cope with an ill member and how this may be affecting their family.	Assists the family in anticipatory planning for the necessary adjustments that could evolve from the present situation. Anticipatory planning increases their opportunities for successful coping, which enhances self-esteem.
Provide the family with information about normal developmental stages and anticipatory guidance related to these stages.	Promotes a sense of control and increases opportunities for successful coping.
Discuss with the family normal adaptive responses to an ill family member, and relate this to their current functioning.	Promotes the family's strengths.
Support appropriate family boundaries by providing information to the appropriate family subgroup.	Promotes healthy family functioning.
Model effective communication skills for the family by using active listening skills, "I" messages, problem-solving skills, and open communication without secrets.	Effective communication improves problem-solving abilities.
Spend [number] minutes with the family per [day or week] providing them with the opportunity to practice communication skills and to share feelings (if this is an identified goal). [Note the schedule for these meetings here.]	Behavioral rehearsal provides opportunities for feedback and modeling of new behaviors by the nurse.
Arrange [number] minute appointments with the family [weekly or daily] for [number] times to assess progress on the established goals. The need for continued follow-up can be decided at the end of the last scheduled visit.	Provides opportunities for the nurse to give positive reinforcement and promotes positive orientation.
Accept the family's decisions about goals for care.	Promotes the family's sense of control.
Discuss with the family the role nutrition has in health maintenance, and develop a family nutritional plan. Consult with nutritionist as necessary.	Nutrition impacts coping abilities.
Discuss with the family the role exercise has in improving ability to cope with stress, and assist in the development of a family exercise plan. Consult with physical therapist as necessary.	Exercise improves physical stamina and increases the production of endorphins.

Gerontic Health

In addition to the interventions for Adult Health and Mental Health, the following may be used for the older client.

ACTIONS/INTERVENTIONS	RATIONALES
Communicate your own positive views about aging and the client's ability to cope to the client and caregivers.	Promotes positive anticipatory coping.
Avoid ageist remarks. For example, "You look so good for someone who is 90 years old."	Promotes positive self-esteem.

ACTIONS/INTERVENTIONS	RATIONALES
Assist the client to maintain functional abilities or make referrals for Occupational Therapy or Physical Therapy to assist the client to improve their functional abilities.	Self-esteem and coping are closely related with physical health and functional ability.
Discuss the client's roles in life (grandparent, parent, room mate) and the associated responsibilities with the roles.	Persons with greater numbers of role identities have improved perceptions of self-worth.
Utilize reminiscence therapy, either in a group or individually, with the client.	Reminiscence therapy assists the client in identifying unresolved conflicts and focusing on their achievements.
Promote a sense of control for the client: • Include the client in the decision making process. • Speak to the client rather than about him or her. • Show respect for the client's privacy (knock before entering their room, keep the curtains drawn, be careful with personal possessions). • Promote physical fitness in clients able to participate in activities.	Older clients who feel a sense of control are better able to cope.

Home Health

In addition to interventions for Adult Health and Mental Health, the following may be used for the home health client.

ACTIONS/INTERVENTIONS	RATIONALES
Involve the client and family in planning and implementing strategies to enhance health and growth: • Family conference: Identify family strengths. • Mutual goal setting: Establish family goals, and identify specific activities for each family member. • Communication: Enhance family discussions and support.	Family involvement in planning enhances growth and implementation of the plan.
Assist the family and client in lifestyle adjustments that may be required: • Provide information related to health promotion. • Provide information related to expected growth and development milestones, both individual and family. • Assist in development and use of support networks.	Support enhances permanent behavioral changes.
Consult with and refer to assistive resources as appropriate.	Community services provide a wealth of resources to enhance growth (e.g., service organizations such as Lion's Club, Altrusa, etc., colleges and universities, or recreational facilities).

COPING, INEFFECTIVE AND READINESS FOR ENHANCED

DEFINITIONS[16]

Ineffective Coping   Inability to form a valid appraisal of the stressors, inadequate choices of practiced responses, and/or inability to use available resources.

Readiness for Enhanced   A pattern of cognitive and behavioral efforts to manage demands that is sufficient for well-being and can be strengthened.

Defensive Coping   Repeated projection of falsely positive self-evaluation based on a self-protective pattern that defends against underlying perceived threats to positive self-regard.

Ineffective Denial   Conscious or unconscious attempt to disavow the knowledge or meaning of an event to reduce anxiety or fear to the detriment of health.

DEFINING CHARACTERISTICS[16]

A. Ineffective Coping
1. Lack of goal-directed behavior or resolution of problem, including inability to attend to and difficulty with organizing information
2. Sleep disturbance
3. Abuse of chemical agents
4. Decreased use of social supports
5. Use of forms of coping that impede adaptive behavior

6. Poor concentration
7. Inadequate problem solving
8. Verbalization of inability to cope or inability to ask for help
9. Inability to meet basic needs
10. Destructive behavior toward self or others
11. Inability to meet role expectations
12. High illness rate
13. Change in usual communication pattern
14. Fatigue
15. Risk taking

B. Readiness for Enhanced
1. Defines stressors ad manageable.
2. Seeks social support.
3. Uses a broad range of problem-oriented and emotion-oriented strategies.
4. Uses spiritual resources.
5. Acknowledges power.
6. Seeks knowledge of new strategies.
7. Is aware of possible environmental changes.

C. Defensive Coping
1. Grandiosity
2. Rationalization of failures
3. Hypersensitive to slight or criticism
4. Denial of obvious problems or weaknesses
5. Projection of blame or responsibility
6. Lack of follow-through or participation in treatment or therapy
7. Superior attitude toward others
8. Hostile laughter or ridicule of others
9. Difficulty in perception of reality or reality testing
10. Difficulty establishing or maintaining relationships

D. Ineffective Denial
1. Delays seeking or refuses health care attention to the detriment of health.
2. Does not perceive personal relevance of symptoms or danger.
3. Displaces source of symptoms to other organs.
4. Displays inappropriate affect.
5. Does not admit fear of death or invalidism.
6. Makes dismissive gestures or comments when speaking of distressing events.
7. Minimizes symptoms.
8. Unable to admit impact of disease on life pattern.
9. Uses home remedies (self-treatment) to relieve symptoms.
10. Displaces fear of impact of the condition.

RELATED FACTORS[16]

A. Ineffective Coping
1. Gender differences in coping strategies
2. Inadequate level of confidence in ability to cope
3. Uncertainty

4. Inadequate social support created by characteristics of relationship
5. Inadequate level of perception of control
6. Inadequate resources available
7. High degree of threat
8. Situational or maturational crises
9. Disturbance in pattern of tension release
10. Inadequate opportunity to prepare for stressor
11. Inability to conserve adaptive energies
12. Disturbance in pattern of appraisal of threat

B. Coping, Readiness for Enhanced
To be developed.

C. Defensive Coping
To be developed.

D. Ineffective Denial
To be developed.

RELATED CLINICAL CONCERNS

1. Eating disorders
2. Substance abuse or use disorders
3. Psychotic disorder
4. Somatoform disorders
5. Dissociative disorders
6. Adjustment disorders
7. A diagnosis with a terminal prognosis
8. Chronic illnesses or disabilities
9. Any condition that can cause alterations in body image or function
10. New diagnosis

 Have You Selected the Correct Diagnosis?

Anxiety
Ineffective Individual Coping would be used if the client demonstrates both an inability to cope appropriately and anxiety. If the client is demonstrating anxiety with appropriate coping, then the diagnosis would be Anxiety. Ineffective Individual Coping would be used only if the client could not adapt to the anxiety.

Risk for Violence
If the aggressive behavior of the client poses a threat of physical or psychological harm, the most appropriate diagnosis would be Risk for Violence. If the client's risk for violence is assessed to be very low, then this would be the secondary diagnosis, with Ineffective Individual Coping being the primary diagnosis. In this situation, the diagnosis of Risk for Violence would serve as a reminder to care providers to remain alert to the potential for this behavior.

Disturbed Sensory Perception
If coping abilities are affected by alterations in sensory input, then Disturbed Sensory Perception would be the most appropriate primary diagnosis.

Disturbed Thought Process

The diagnosis of Disturbed Thought Process can affect the individual's ability to cope. If these alterations are present with Ineffective Individual Coping, then the primary diagnosis should be Disturbed Thought Process. Effective problem solving is inhibited as long as this disruption in thinking is present.

Dysfunctional Grieving

If the client's behavior can be related to resolving a loss or change, then the appropriate diagnosis is Dysfunctional Grieving. The loss can be actual or perceived. If the client demonstrates an inability to manage this process, then the appropriate diagnosis would be Ineffective Individual Coping.

Powerlessness

This diagnosis can produce a personal perception that would result in Ineffective Individual Coping. If one perceives that one's own actions cannot influence the situation, then Powerlessness would be the primary diagnosis.

Impaired Adjustment

This diagnosis is appropriate when the client is having difficulty adapting to a change in health status that is specific and recent. Ineffective coping would be the correct diagnosis when multiple stressors require adaptation or the inability to cope is more pervasive and not time limited.

EXPECTED OUTCOME

Ineffective Coping

Will return-demonstrate at least [number] new coping strategies by [date].

Identifies [number] of support systems by [date].

Coping, Readiness for Enhanced

Goals for ineffective coping can be adapted for use with this diagnosis.

Defensive Coping

In addition to the goals foe ineffective coping you may consider:

Requests assistance with coping by [date].

Identifies [number] of alternative coping strategies by [date].

Ineffective Denial

In addition to the goals for ineffective coping and defensive coping you may consider:

Requests information about [describe client's personal areas of concern] by [date].

TARGET DATES

A realistic target date, considering assessment and teaching time, would be 7 days fromthe date of the diagnosis.

NURSING ACTIONS/INTERVENTIONS WITH RATIONALES

Adult Health

ACTIONS/INTERVENTIONS	RATIONALES
Assist the patient to identify and explore specific situations that are creating stress and possible alternatives for dealing with the situation by allowing at least 1 hour per shift for interviewing and teaching.	Identification of problem area is the first step in problem solving and promotes creative problem solving.
Help the patient evaluate which methods he or she has used that have not been successful or have been only partially successful.	Allows for strengthening of effective coping methods and elimination of ineffective ones.
Monitor for and reinforce behavior suggesting effective coping continuously.	Strengthens and enhances coping skills. Increases confidence to risk new coping strategies.
Maintain consistency in approach and teaching whenever interacting with the patient.	Reduces stress. Promotes a trusting relationship.
Encourage participation in care by assisting the patient to maintain activities of daily living to degree possible.	Promotes self-care, enhances coping, builds self-esteem, and increases motivation and compliance.
Encourage support from the family and significant others by allowing participation in care, encouraging questions, and allowing expression of feelings.	Broadens support network. Builds self-esteem in support systems.
Teach relaxation techniques such as meditation, exercise, yoga, deep breathing, or imagery. Have the patient practice for 10 minutes twice a shift at [times].	Reduces stress and provides alternative coping strategies.

(care plan continued on page 774)

NURSING ACTIONS/INTERVENTIONS WITH RATIONALES (continued from page 773)

Adult Health

ACTIONS/INTERVENTIONS	RATIONALES
Assist the patient to identify and use available support systems before discharge from hospital.	Broadens the support network to reach short-term and long-term goals.
Initiate referral to psychiatric clinical nurse specialist as needed.	Specialized skills may be needed to intervene in significant problem areas.

Child Health

ACTIONS/INTERVENTIONS	RATIONALES
Ineffective Coping	
Establish a trusting relationship with the child and respective family by allowing time (30 minutes) per shift, while the patient is awake, for verbalization of concerns and their perception of the situation.	Promotes communication and allows gathering of data that enhance care planning.
Identify the need for collaboration with related health team members.	Specialist (e.g., mental health, may best be able to deal with the problem).
Reinforce appropriate behavior of choosing or coping by verbal praise.	Positive reinforcement will enhance learning of coping mechanisms.
Assist the patient and family in setting realistic goals.	Realistic goals enhance success, which increases coping ability.
Provide appropriate attention to primary nursing needs.	Meeting of primary care needs allows the patient to focus energy on coping.
Offer education to provide clarification of information as needed, regarding any health-related needs.	Provides basic knowledge needed to avoid future crises. Increases options for coping choices.
Determine appropriate developmental baseline behavior versus actual coping behavior.	Baseline data will provide valuable information for comparative follow-up.
Administer medications as ordered, including sedatives.	Relaxation assists in decreasing anxiety. Conserves energy to deal with crisis.
Set aside time each shift [specify] to deal with how the child and parents feel about the defensive behavior. This may require art, puppetry, or related expressive dynamics.	Acting out or expression of feelings provides valuable data that increase the likelihood of a successful plan of care.
Provide feedback with support for progress. When progress is not occurring, provide reflective referral back to the child and parent as applicable.	Feedback serves to clarify and allows for reviewing the specific coping activity with reteaching as needed.
Provide ongoing information regarding the child's health status, which could affect defensive behavior by the child or parents.	Factors related to coping may well be influenced by residual effects from illness. Misinformation or lack of information can also be detrimental to positive coping.
Throughout defensive coping period, monitor and ensure the child's safety.	Basic standard of care.
Determine disciplinary plans for all to abide by with safety in mind.	Structured limit setting will provide security and safety.
Provide appropriate reality confrontation according to readiness of the child and parents.	Reality confrontation helps keep perspective on here and now and is a useful approach to initiate coping with current situation.

ACTIONS/INTERVENTIONS	RATIONALES
Provide for discharge planning with reinforcement of importance of follow-up appointments as needed.	Attaching value to follow-up increases the likelihood of satisfactory attendance for appointments and other follow-up activities.
Identify, along with the patient and family, resources to assist in coping, including support groups.	Support groups provide empowerment and a sense of shared concern.
Readiness for Enhanced[34]	
Monitor for defining characteristic for enhanced coping readiness plan.	Provides a relevant base.
Facilitate health-care team paraprofessionals, especially child life specialist, provision of developmentally appropriate coping strategies.	Provides the likelihood of addressing child and family's needs within a realistic scope.
Assist the child and family to generate ways to incorporate the plan into daily routine with allowance for alterations of role, time, activity, or related aspects, including school and extracurricular activities.	Offers a realistic approach.
Offer opportunities for discussion in group or with child alone regarding the desired level of change the coping offers.	Offers a sense of input for each member.
Promote ongoing evaluation and reinforcement of small changes related to application of enhanced coping.	Enhances and empowers the child to see effects of behavior changes.
Refer, as appropriate, for counseling to promote enhanced coping.	Provides anticipatory guidance with likelihood of continued success.
Assist the child and family to communicate to relevant persons how to best assist in maintenance of plan, especially school teacher and nurse, as applicable.	Offers continuity of plan for daily routine.

Women's Health

● **N O T E** : *Women's health will be the same as Adult Health, Mental Health, and Gerontic Health for these diagnoses, in addition to the following:*

ACTIONS/INTERVENTIONS	RATIONALES
Ineffective Coping	
Identify groups at risk for ineffective individual coping (e.g., single parents, minority women, women with "superwoman" syndrome, and lesbians).	Provides a database that allows for early recognition, planning, and action.[35–37]
Identify situations that place patients at risk for ineffective individual coping, e.g., unwanted or unplanned pregnancy, unhappy home situation (marriage), demands at work, or demands of children or spouse. (See Impaired Adjustment for Postpartum Depression.)	
Assist the patient in identifying typical stressful times (e.g., at home, at work, in social situations, or during an average day).	
Assist the patient in identifying lifestyle adjustments that may be made to lower stress levels (e.g., planning for divorce or planning for job change, either part-time or unemployment for a period of time).	Supports the patient in identification and planning of strategies to reduce stress.[35–37]

(care plan continued on page 776)

NURSING ACTIONS/INTERVENTIONS WITH RATIONALES (continued from page 775)

Women's Health

ACTIONS/INTERVENTIONS	RATIONALES
Assist the patient in identifying factors that contribute to ineffective coping, for example, depression, guilt (blaming self), assuming helplessness, passive acceptance of traditional feminine role, anger toward self and others (aggressive behavior, suicide threats, or substance abuse), and failure to make time for self (relaxation, pleasure, or self-care).	Identification of factors that contribute to the situation is the first step in learning positive rather than negative skills.
Assist the patient in developing problem-solving skills to modify stressors, for example, using 12-step plan (as developed by Alcoholics Anonymous), or planning time for self-rewarding activities such as exercise or long quiet baths.	Assists the patient in planning positive actions and in communicating her needs to others.
Assist the patient in identifying negative and positive responses to stressors (e.g., pressures at work such as being constantly interrupted or become defensive when challenged).	
Assist the patient in developing an individual plan of stress management (e.g., relaxation techniques or assertiveness training).	
Involve significant others in discussion and problem-solving activities.	
Provide a nonjudgmental atmosphere that allows the patient to discuss her feelings about the pregnancy, including such areas as lifestyle, children, or support systems.	
Explore the patient's use of what she perceives are contraceptives[38] (e.g., pills, intrauterine devices, diaphragm, withdrawal, feminine hygiene products, douching, spermicide foams, or rhythm).	Provides a basis for planning lifestyle options.[35–37]
Explore the patient's lack of contraceptive use[39] due to ignorance ("It won't happen to me" syndrome), guilt ("If I use the pill, then I am not good"), spontaneity, excitement due to risk, loneliness, crisis or pressure, or uncertainty in sex role relationships or self-image.	Provides health-care personnel information to plan care that enhances likelihood of successful compliance.

Readiness for Enhanced Coping

Refer clients to natural resources and activities to enhance their coping skills, such as the following: • Bibliotherapy—readings that help clients through difficult times • Journaling, writing, storytelling, creativity, arts—writings of personal thoughts, memories, and/or experiences kindles introspection and meaning • Affirmations—positive personal statements in present tense that express a desirable outcome • Presence, deep breathing, centering—presence with all senses focused • Relaxation, imagery, visualization • Prayer, religion, spirituality, meditation	Self-care practices are practices an individual can pursue on their own to assist in coping, comforting, and healing activities.[66]

ACTIONS/INTERVENTIONS	RATIONALES
• Music therapy—application of pleasant sounds to produce desired changes • Color therapy—display of colors for healing • Light therapy—for those with seasonal affective disorder. • Hydrotherapy—water used in healing process • Nutrition/herbs, etc. • Health-care provider assistance.[66]	

Mental Health

ACTIONS/INTERVENTIONS	RATIONALES
Ineffective Coping Determine the client's functional abilities and developmental level for the adaptation of all future interventions. The results of this assessment should be noted here.	Cognitive abilities can impact the client's ability to develop appropriate coping behaviors.
Discuss with the client his or her perception of the current crisis and stressors. This should include information about the coping strategies that the client has attempted and his or her assessment of what has made them ineffective in resolving this stressor or crisis.	Promotes the development of a trusting relationship by communicating respect for the client.
Assist the client in developing an appropriate time frame for the resolution of the situation. (Often when experiencing a crisis, the individual has the perception that resolution must take place immediately.) This could include, as appropriate to the client's situation: • Informing the client that any difficulty that has taxed his or her resources as much as this one has will take an extended time to resolve because it must be complex. • Informing the client that a situation that is as important as this one is to the individual's future deserves a well-thought-out answer and that a decision should not be made hastily. • Assisting the client in determining the source of the time pressure and the appropriateness of this time frame. • Assisting the client in developing an appropriate perspective on the time frame. (One question that could be useful is "What would be the worst that could happen if this problem is not resolved by [put client's stated time frame here]?")	"De-catastrophizes" the client's perceptions of the situation.[44]
• Assist the client in understanding that goals should be modest. Complex change should be taken slowly.	Provides an opportunity for client success in achieving change while enhancing self-esteem.
Provide a quiet, nonstimulating environment or an environment that does not add additional stress to an already overwhelmed coping ability. (Potential environmental stressors for this client should be listed here with the plan for reducing them in this environment.)	Inappropriate levels of sensory stimuli can increase confusion and disorganization.
Sit with the client [number] minutes [number] times per day at [specify times here] to discuss current concerns and feelings.	Communication of concerns in a supportive environment can facilitate the development of adaptive coping behaviors. Continues the development of a trusting relationship.

(care plan continued on page 778)

NURSING ACTIONS/INTERVENTIONS WITH RATIONALES (continued from page 777)

Mental Health

ACTIONS/INTERVENTIONS	RATIONALES
Assist the client with setting appropriate limits on aggressive behavior. (See Risk for Violence in Chapter 9 for more detailed nursing actions if this diagnosis develops.)	Inappropriate levels of environmental stimuli can increase disorganization and confusion, increasing the risk for acting-out behavior.
Decrease environmental stimulation as appropriate. (This might include a secluded environment.)	
Provide the client with appropriate alternative outlets for physical tension. (This should be stated specifically and could include walking, running, talking with a staff member, using a punching bag, listening to music, or doing a deep muscle relaxation sequence.) Strategies should be used [number] times per day at [times] or when increased tension is observed. These outlets should be selected with the client's input.	Physical activity decreases the tension that is related to anxiety. Appropriate control of behavior promotes the client's sense of control and enhances self-esteem.
Orient the client to date, time, and place. Provide clocks, calendars, and bulletin boards. Make references to this information in daily interactions with the client. The frequency needed for this client should be noted here (e.g., every 2 hours, every day, or three times a day).	Orientation enhances the client's coping abilities.
Provide the client with familiar or needed objects. These should be noted here.	Promotes the client's sense of control, while meeting security needs.
Provide the client with an environment that will optimize sensory input. This could include hearing aids, eyeglasses, pencil and paper, decreased noise in conversation areas, or appropriate lighting. (These interventions should indicate an awareness of sensory deficit as well as sensory overload.) The specific interventions for this client should be noted here, for example, place hearing aid in when client awakens and remove before bedtime (9:00 P.M.).	Inappropriate levels of sensory stimuli can increase confusion and disorganization.
Provide the client with achievable tasks, activities, and goals (these should be listed here). These activities should be provided with increasing complexity to give the client an increasing sense of accomplishment and mastery.	Accomplishment of these goals provides reinforcement and encourages positive behavior, while enhancing self-esteem.
Communicate to the client an understanding that all coping behavior to this point has been his or her best effort and that asking for assistance at this time is not failure. A complex problem often requires some outside assistance to resolve.	Assists the client to maintain self-esteem, diminishes feelings of failure, and promotes a positive orientation.
Provide the client with opportunities to make appropriate decisions related to care at his or her level of ability. This may begin as a choice between two options and then evolve into more complex decision making.	
It is important that decision making be at the client's level of functioning so that confidence can be built with successful decision-making experience.	Promotes the client's sense of control.
Provide the client with a primary care nurse on each shift.	Promotes the development of a trusting relationship.

ACTIONS/INTERVENTIONS	RATIONALES
When a relationship has been developed with primary care nurse, this person will sit with the client [number] minutes per shift to discuss concerns about sexual issues, fears, and anxieties (begin with 30 minutes and increase as the client's ability to concentrate improves).	Promotes development of a trusting relationship. Discussion of concerns in a supportive environment promotes the development of alternative coping behaviors.
Provide constructive confrontation for the client about problematic coping behavior.[33] Those kinds of behavior identified by the treatment team should be listed here.	Assists the client in reality testing of coping behaviors.
Provide the client with information about care and treatment. Give information in concise terms appropriate to the client's level of understanding.	Promotes the client's sense of control. Inappropriate levels of sensory stimuli increase confusion and disorganization.
Identify with the client methods for anxiety reduction. Those specific methods selected should be listed here.	High levels of anxiety decrease the client's coping abilities and interfere with the learning of new behaviors.
Assist the client with practice of anxiety reduction techniques, and remind him or her to implement these techniques when level of anxiety is increasing.	Repeated practice of a behavior internalizes and personalizes the behavior.
Provide the client with opportunities to test problem solutions either by role-playing or by applying them to graded real-life experiences.	Behavioral rehearsal helps facilitate the client's learning new skills through the use of feedback and modeling by the nurse.
Assist the client to revise problem solutions if they are not effective. (This will assist the patient to learn that no solution is perfect or final and that problem solving is a process of applying various alternatives and revising them as necessary.)	Promotes positive orientation and enhances the client's self-esteem by turning disadvantages into advantages.[44]
Allow the client to discover and develop solutions that best fit his or her concerns. The nurse's role is to provide assistance and feedback and to encourage creative approaches to problem behavior.	Promotes the client's sense of control, and development of new behaviors enhances the client's problem-solving behaviors and improves self-esteem.
Teach the client skills that facilitate problem solving, such as assertive behavior, goal setting, relaxation, evaluation, information gathering, requesting assistance, and early identification of problem behavior. Those skills that are identified by the treatment team as being necessary should be listed here with the teaching plan. This should include a schedule of the information to be provided and identification of the person responsible for providing the information.	Increases repertoire of coping behaviors, decreasing all-or-none thinking.[44]
Spend [number] minutes two times per day at [times] with the client role-playing and practicing problem solving and implementation of developed solutions. This will be the responsibility of the primary care nurse.	Repeated practice of a behavior internalizes and personalizes the behavior.
Assist the client in identifying those problems he or she cannot control or resolve and in developing coping strategies for these situations. This may involve alteration of the client's perception of the problem.	Increases the client's opportunities for success in early problem-solving attempts. This success provides reinforcement, which motivates positive behavior and enhances self-esteem.
Monitor the client's desire for spiritual counseling, and refer to appropriate resources.	Increases the resources available to the client.
Provide positive social reinforcement and other behavioral rewards for demonstration of adaptive problem solving. (Those things that the client finds rewarding should be listed here with a schedule for use. The kinds of behavior that are to be rewarded should also be listed).	Reinforcement encourages positive behavior and enhances self-esteem.

(care plan continued on page 780)

NURSING ACTIONS/INTERVENTIONS WITH RATIONALES (continued from page 779)

Mental Health

ACTIONS/INTERVENTIONS	RATIONALES
Assist the client in identifying support systems and in developing a plan for their use.	Decreases the client's sense of social isolation.
The following interventions relate to the client who is experiencing problems related to organic brain dysfunction:	
• Maintain a consistent environment; do not move furniture or personal belongings.	Inappropriate levels of sensory stimuli increase confusion and disorganization.
• Remove hazardous objects from the environment, such as loose rugs or small items on the floor.	Client safety is of primary concern.
• Provide environmental cues to assist the client in locating important places such as the bathroom, own room, or the dining room.	
• Do not argue with the client about details of the recent past.	The client cannot remember this information, and arguing increases the client's levels of frustration, which can precipitate aggressive behavior.
• Avoid situations that result in aggressive behavior by redirecting the client's attention.	Prevention provides the safest approach to aggression.
• Provide a constant daily routine and a homelike atmosphere, to include personal belongings, music, and social mealtimes with assistance with meal preparation. This can often provide appetite cues to the client and stimulate memories.	Appropriate levels of sensory stimuli can increase orientation and organization.
• Provide group experiences that explore current events, seasonal changes, reminiscence, and organizing life experiences.	Promotes the client's orientation, and maximizes cognitive abilities.
The following interventions related to the client who is experiencing Defensive Coping:	
• Approach the client in a positive, nonjudgmental manner.	Promotes the development of a trusting relationship.
• Focus any feedback on the client's behavior.	Communicates acceptance of the client, while providing information on coping behaviors that create problems.
• Provide an opportunity for the client to share his or her perspectives and feelings.	Promotes the development of a trusting relationship by communicating acceptance of the individual. This relationship will decrease the need for defensive coping.
• Use "I" statements, e.g., "I feel angry when I see you breaking the window."	Provides modeling of more effective coping behaviors.
• Develop a trusting relationship with the client before using confrontation or requesting major changes in behavior.[45,46]	Trusting relationship decreases need for defensive coping and increases the client's ability to respond to this information constructively.
• Provide positive reinforcement for the client when issues are addressed. (Things that are reinforcing for this client should be noted here.)	Reinforcement encourages positive behavior while enhancing self-esteem.
• When the client's defenses increase, reduce anxiety in situation. (See Anxiety in Chapter 8 for precise information on anxiety control.)	Anxiety increases the client's use of familiar coping behaviors and makes it difficult to practice new behaviors.
• Determine the kinds of behavior by staff members that increase the client's defensive coping, and note them here with a plan to decrease them.	Provides an environment that is supportive of the client's learning new coping behaviors.
• Be clear and direct with the client.	Inappropriate levels of sensory stimuli can increase confusion and disorganization.

ACTIONS/INTERVENTIONS	RATIONALES
• If defensive coping is related to alteration in self-concept, refer to the appropriate nursing diagnosis for interventions.	
• Reduce or eliminate environmental stressors or threats.	
• Arrange a time for the client to be involved in activity that he or she enjoys, and that provides him or her with positive emotional experiences. [Note activity and time for this activity here.]	Promotes positive orientation.
The following interventions are for the client experiencing Denial:	High levels of anxiety increase the client's use of familiar coping behaviors and make it difficult to practice new behaviors.
• Determine whether current use of denial is appropriate in the current situations. (Facilitates coping with situation in a manner that does not compromise normal functioning)	
• If denial is determined to be non-health promotive, initiate the following interventions:	Communicates acceptance of the client, promoting the development of a trusting relationship.
• Provide a safe, secure environment.	
• Allow the client time to express feelings.	
• Provide a positive, nonjudgmental environment.	Promotes positive orientation.
• Develop a trusting relationship with the client before presenting threatening information.	A trusting relationship decreases the client's need to enlist dysfunctional coping behaviors.
• Present information in a clear, concise manner.	Inappropriate levels of sensory stimuli can increase the client's confusion and disorganization.
• Determine which kinds of staff behavior reinforce denial, and note them here with alternative behavior.	Models appropriate coping behavior, while decreasing direct threats to the client's self-system.
• Utilize "I" messages, and reflect on the client's behavior.[32]	
• Present the client with information that demonstrates inconsistencies between thoughts and feelings, between thoughts and behavior, and between thoughts about others and their perceptions of the situation.	Places in question the client's current coping behaviors, and facilitates the examining of options and alternatives.[44]
• Arrange for the client to participate in a group that will provide feedback from peers regarding the stressful situation.	Assists the client to experience personal importance to others, while enhancing interpersonal relationship skills. Increasing the client's competencies can enhance self-esteem and promote positive orientation.
• Present the client with differences between his or her perceptions and the nurse's perceptions with "I" messages.	Assists the client in questioning the evidence that he or she has been using to support ineffective coping behaviors without directly challenging them. This decreases the need for the client to use ineffective coping behaviors.[44]
• Do not agree with the client's perceptions that are related to denial.	Would support and reinforce ineffective coping behaviors.
• Schedule a time for the client and support system to discuss issues related to the current problem. [Note this time here with the name of the staff person responsible for this session.]	Support system understanding promotes the continuation of new coping behaviors after discharge.
• Assist the support system in learning constructive ways of coping with the client's denial.	
• Schedule time for the client to be involved in positive esteem-building activity. (This activity should be selected with client input.) [Note activity and times here.]	

(care plan continued on page 782)

NURSING ACTIONS/INTERVENTIONS WITH RATIONALES (continued from page 781)

Mental Health

ACTIONS/INTERVENTIONS	RATIONALES
• Provide positive feedback for the client, addressing concerns in a direct manner. [Note here those things that are rewarding for the client.] • Determine needs that are being met with denial. Establish and present the client with alternative kinds of behavior for meeting these needs. [Note alternatives here.]	Feedback encourages positive behavior and enhances self-esteem.

Readiness for Enhanced Coping

Talk with the client to identify their goals and concerns. [Note client's goals here.]

Assist the client in identifying strengths and purpose in life.

Commend client's strengths at each meeting.

Identify, with the client, the support needed from staff to strengthen coping behaviors and build on strengths. Note the support needed here (e.g., music, quiet time, training in a specific relaxation technique).

• Collaborate with other health-care providers to provide assistance needed in developing additional coping strategies (e.g., physical therapy, music therapist, occupational therapists, and leaders of the client's faith community). Note those providers involved here with those supports needed to facilitate their work with the client (meeting schedules, group times).

Spend [number] minutes [number] time(s) per day discussing client's progress toward goals. Provide informative positive verbal reinforcement for goal attainment.

Provide client with the information necessary to facilitate enhanced wellness. [Note the information needed here.]

Before discharge, meet with the client's support system and client to develop a plan for addressing stressors. [Note the time for this meeting here.]

Refer the client to appropriate community support groups. [Note groups here with supports needed from staff to facilitate the client's connecting with these groups.]

Gerontic Health

In addition to the interventions for Adult Health and Mental Health, the following may be used for the older client:

ACTIONS/INTERVENTIONS	RATIONALES
Ineffective Coping Discuss with the patient any recent life changes that may have affected his or her coping, such as loss of a loved one, relocation, loss of best friend, or loss of a pet.[47]	Recent or multiple losses may significantly impact usual coping skills.

ACTIONS/INTERVENTIONS	RATIONALES
Assess the client for physical factors that may contribute to impaired coping: • hearing impairment • communication barriers • chronic illness • fatigue • social isolation • mobility limitations	Identifies factors that can be changed or addressed to facilitate coping.

Readiness for Enhanced

ACTIONS/INTERVENTIONS	RATIONALES
Communicate your own positive views about aging and the client's ability to cope to the client and caregivers.	Promotes positive anticipatory coping.
Avoid ageist remarks such as, "You look so good for someone who is 90 years old."	Promotes positive self-esteem.
Facilitate the client's maintenance of functional abilities or make referrals for Occupational Therapy or Physical Therapy to assist the client to improve his or her functional abilities.	Self-esteem and coping are closely related with physical health and functional ability.
Discuss the client's roles in life (grandparent, parent, roommate) and the associated responsibilities with the roles.	Persons with greater numbers of role identities have improved perceptions of self worth.
Utilize reminiscence therapy, either in a group or individually, with the client.	Reminiscence therapy assists the client in identifying unresolved conflicts and focusing on their achievements.
Promote a sense of control for the client. • Include the client in the decision-making process. Speak to the client rather than about him or her. • Show respect for the client's privacy (knock before entering their room, keep the curtains drawn, be careful with personal possessions). • Promote physical fitness in clients able to participate in activities.	

Home Health

In addition to the interventions for Adult Health and Mental Health, the following may be used for the home health client.

ACTIONS/INTERVENTIONS	RATIONALES
Ineffective Coping Involve the client and family in planning and implementing strategies to improve individual coping: • Family conference: Identification of problem and role each family member plays. • Mutual goal setting: Set realistic goals. Specify activities for each family member. Establish evaluation criteria. • Communication: Use accurate and honest feedback in a positive manner.	Family involvement enhances effectiveness of interventions.
Assist the family and client in lifestyle adjustments that may be required: • Stress management • Development and use of support networks • Alteration of past ineffective coping strategies	

(care plan continued on page 784)

NURSING ACTIONS/INTERVENTIONS WITH RATIONALES (continued from page 783)

Home Health

ACTIONS/INTERVENTIONS	RATIONALES
• Treatment for substance abuse • Treatment for physical illness • Activities to increase self-esteem: Exercise or stress management • Temporary assistance: Babysitter, housekeeper, or secretarial support	
Identify signs and symptoms of illness.	Permanent changes in behavior and family roles require support and accurate information.
Point out hazards and benefits of home remedies, self-diagnosis, and self-prescribing.	
Consult with and refer the patient to assistive resources as appropriate.	Utilization of existing services is efficient use of resources. Resources such as a psychiatric nurse clinician, a family therapist, and support groups can enhance the treatment plan.
Readiness for Enhanced	
Monitor for factors contributing to adaptive coping (psychological, social, economic, spiritual, or environmental factors).	Provides a basis for continued improvement.
Involve the client and family in planning, implementing, and promoting continued adaptive coping. • Family conference: Discuss feelings, roles, and identify coping strategies that have worked in the past. • Mutual goal sharing: Establish realistic goals and specify role of each family member (e.g., provide safe environment and support self-care). • Communication: Clear and honest communication should be promoted among family members. If sensory impairments exist, corrective interventions are needed (e.g., eyeglasses or a hearing aid).	Family involvement enhances effectiveness of interventions.
Assist the client and family in lifestyle adjustments that may be required: • Stress management • Development and use of support networks • Treatment for disability • Appropriate balance of dependence and independence • Grief counseling • Change in role functions • Treatment for cognitive impairment • Provision of comfortable and safe environment • Activities to increase self-esteem	Family relationships can be altered by impaired adjustment. Permanent changes in behavior and family roles require evaluation and support.
Consult with or refer to appropriate assistive resources as indicated.	Utilization of existing services is efficient use of resources. Resources such as an occupational therapist, a psychiatric nurse clinician, and support groups can enhance the treatment plan.

POST-TRAUMA SYNDROME, RISK FOR AND ACTUAL

DEFINITIONS[16]

Risk for Post-Trauma Syndrome At risk for sustained maladaptive response to a traumatic, overwhelming event.

Post-Trauma Syndrome Sustained maladaptive response to a traumatic, overwhelming event.

DEFINING CHARACTERISTICS[16]

A. Risk for Post-Trauma Syndrome (Risk Factors)
1. Occupation (e.g., police, fire, rescue, corrections, emergency room staff, and mental health)
2. Exaggerated sense of responsibility
3. Perception of event
4. Survivor's role in event
5. Displacement from home
6. Inadequate social support
7. Nonsupportive environment
8. Diminished ego strength
9. Duration of the event

B. Post-Trauma Syndrome
1. Avoidance
2. Repression
3. Difficulty in concentrating
4. Grief
5. Intrusive thoughts
6. Neurosensory irritability
7. Palpitations
8. Enuresis (in children)
9. Anger and/or rage
10. Intrusive dreams
11. Nightmares
12. Aggression
13. Hypervigilance
14. Exaggerated startle response
15. Hopelessness
16. Altered mood states
17. Shame
18. Panic attacks
19. Alienation
20. Denial
21. Horror
22. Substance abuse
23. Depression
24. Anxiety
25. Guilt
26. Fear
27. Gastric irritability
28. Detachment
29. Psychogenic attachment
30. Irritability
31. Numbing
32. Compulsive behavior
33. Flashbacks
34. Headaches

RELATED FACTORS[16]

A. Risk for Post-Trauma Syndrome
The risk factors also serve as the related factors.

B. Post-Trauma Syndrome
1. Events outside the range of usual human experience
2. Physical and psychosocial abuse
3. Tragic occurrence involving multiple deaths
4. Sudden destruction involving one's home or community
5. Epidemic
6. Being held prisoner of war or criminal victimization (torture)
7. Wars
8. Rape
9. Natural disasters and/or man-made disasters
10. Serious accidents
11. Witnessing mutilation, violent death, or other horrors
12. Serious threat or injury to self or loved ones
13. Industrial and motor vehicle accidents
14. Military combat

RELATED CLINICAL CONCERNS

1. Rape victim
2. Multiple injuries (motor vehicle accident)
3. Victims of assault and torture[31]
4. Post-traumatic stress disorder
5. Multiple personality disorder
6. Victims of natural disasters
7. First responders (e.g., emergency medical personnel, law enforcement personnel, and volunteers).
8. Victims of child physical or sexual abuse
9. Experience combat in a war zone
10. Sudden life-threatening physical illness

 Have You Selected the Correct Diagnosis?

Anxiety
Anxiety may be the initial diagnosis given to the individual. As the relationship with the client progresses, it may become evident that the source of the anxiety is a traumatic event. If this is the case, then the diagnosis of Post-Trauma Syndrome would be added. As long as the symptoms of Anxiety are predominant, this would be the primary diagnosis.

Disturbed Thought Process
Some of the symptoms of Post-Trauma Syndrome are similar to those of Disturbed Thought Process. If these alterations are present in the client who has experienced a traumatic event, then the primary diagnosis would be Post-Trauma Syndrome. If the disruption in thinking persists after intervention has begun for Post-Trauma Syndrome, then Disturbed Thought Process should be reconsidered as a diagnosis.

(box continued on page 786)

Have You Selected the Correct Diagnosis? *(box continued from page 785)*

Dysfunctional Grieving

Dysfunctional Grieving is the appropriate diagnosis if the client's behavior is related to resolving a loss or change and this loss or change is not the result of an overwhelming traumatic event. If it is the result of a traumatic event, then Post-Trauma Syndrome is the most appropriate diagnosis for the behavior the client is demonstrating.

Rape-Trauma Syndrome

Rape-Trauma Syndrome is the correct diagnosis if the individual's symptoms are related to a rape. If the symptoms are related to another overwhelming traumatic event, or if the rape occurred in conjunction with another overwhelming traumatic event, then the appropriate diagnosis would be Post-Trauma Syndrome.

EXPECTED OUTCOME

Post-Trauma Syndrome, Risk for

Identifies [number] of strategies to increase personal safety by [date].

Identifies [number] of support systems and methods for using them by [date].

Demonstrates use of [number] of positive coping strategies by [date].

Describes signs and symptoms of Post-Trauma Syndrome and a realistic plan for obtaining assistance if these are identified by [date].

Post-Trauma Syndrome

Demonstrates use of [number] of positive coping strategies by [date].

Participates in [number] of support group meeting (s) per [day or week] by [date].

Demonstrates ability to maintain social roles by [date].

TARGET DATES

Because of the highly individualized and personalized response to trauma, target dates will need to be highly individualized and based on initial assessment. A reasonable initial target date would be 7 days.

NURSING ACTIONS/INTERVENTIONS WITH RATIONALES

Adult Health

ACTIONS/INTERVENTIONS	RATIONALES
Establish a therapeutic relationship by actively listening, calling the person by name, showing empathy and concern, not belittling feelings, etc.	Promotes trust and open expression of feelings.
Avoid prolonged waiting periods for the patient for routine procedures.	This tactic may have been one used by the torturer, and standard care procedures, e.g., drawing blood or electrocardiography, may be perceived as torture because of the memories they evoke.[48]
Encourage the patient to express feelings about the event by actively listening, asking open-ended questions, reflection, etc.	Provides database for planning interventions.
Help the patient see the event realistically by clarifying misconceptions and looking at both sides of the situation.	Provides objective view. Promotes problem solving.
Before discharge, help the patient identify support groups who have previously experienced the same or similar traumatic events.	Enhances coping methods. Promotes use of community resource networks to help meet short- and long-term goals and advocate for the patient.
Initiate a psychiatric nursing consultation as needed.	Situation may require specialized skills to intervene.
Help the patient identify diversional activities to activate when he or she feels he or she is going to reexperience the event.	Provides alternative coping strategy.
Orient the patient to reality as needed.	Helps the patient focus on here and now rather than on past events.
Engage the patient in social interactions with nurses or with other support groups as appropriate.	Decreases isolation. Encourages communication. Provides diversional activity.
Teach the patient relaxation and stress management techniques before discharge.	Reduces stress. Promotes alternative coping methods.

Child Health

ACTIONS/INTERVENTIONS	RATIONALES
Monitor for details surrounding the incident causing Post-Trauma Syndrome.	Circumstances surrounding the event may provide clues as to how the child may be internalizing people, places, and objects as symbols or reminders.
Allow for developmental needs in encouraging the child to express feelings about trauma: • Play for infants • Puppets or dolls for toddlers • Stories or play for preschoolers	Appropriate methods should help resolve the emotions surrounding the incident and avoid further traumatization.
Deal appropriately with other primary nursing needs (e.g., nutrition or rest).	Allows focusing of energy on dealing with the crisis.
Provide for one-to-one care and continuity of staff.	Enhances trust.
Encourage the patient and family to note positive outcomes of experience (e.g., being able to deal with crisis).	Potential for growth exists in crisis management.
Review previous coping skills.	Coping may be enhanced by consideration of previous skills within framework of current situation.
Address educational needs according to situation (e.g., rights of the individual or related follow-up).	Knowledge provides empowerment and enhances decision making.
Allow for visitation by the family and significant others.	Family visitation offers opportunity for reassurance and promotes resuming daily routines and relationships.
Refer the patient appropriately for continuity and follow-up after discharge from hospital.	Continuity and follow-up will foster likelihood of resolution of major conflicts.
Provide for diversional activity of the child's choice.	Promotes relaxation.
Allow for potential sleep disturbances. Provide favorite toy or security object. Offer adequate comforting, such as holding the infant on waking.	Recurrent nightmares may occur as a result of the trauma.
Provide for follow-up for delayed Post-Trauma Syndrome up to 2 years after the trauma.	Delayed response can be noted long after the initial event, and must be included in the planning of care.[49]
Reassure the child that he or she is not being punished and is not responsible for trauma.	Depending on the cognitive level and coping ability, the child may associate the event as being caused by something "wrong" he or she did or said.

Women's Health

This nursing diagnosis will pertain to the woman the same as to any other adult. The reader is referred to Rape-Trauma Syndrome (see Chapter 10) and to the other nursing actions in this section (Adult Health, Mental Health).

Mental Health

ACTIONS/INTERVENTIONS	RATIONALES
Risk for Inform persons exposed to trauma of the signs and symptoms of PTSD and indicate that this response is normal. • Emphasize strength of natural resilience (persons before us have survived similar situations).	Normalizes the response and provides them with the knowledge to seek early assistance.[50]
Discuss with client methods for coping with situation and have them identify those coping strategies that would be most useful.	

(care plan continued on page 788)

NURSING ACTIONS/INTERVENTIONS WITH RATIONALES (continued from page 787)

Mental Health

ACTIONS/INTERVENTIONS	RATIONALES
Facilitate client's connections with their support systems. [Note type of assistance needed here.]	
Develop, with client, plan for providing adequate nutrition, sleep, and exercise. [Note client's plan here.]	Physiological well-being facilitates emotional well-being.[50]
Facilitate client's maintenance of daily routine. Note client's routines and type of assistance needed here.	Stability assists in reducing stress.[50]
Actual	
Assign a primary care nurse to the client, and assign the same staff member to the client each day on each shift and establish a daily routine. [Note the client's specific routine there.]	Promotes the development of a trusting relationship and sense of safety.[50]
Monitor for sleep disturbance and refer to Sleep pattern, Disturbed for appropriate interventions.	
Begin appropriate anxiety-reducing interventions if this is a significant problem for the client. (See Anxiety in Chapter 8 for detailed intervention strategies and assessment criteria.)	Provides the client with increased repertoire of coping behaviors to cope with intense emotional experiences.
Discuss with the client his or her perception of the current situation and stressors. This should include information about the coping strategies that the client has attempted, and his or her assessment of what has made them ineffective in resolving this situation, and information about PTSD symptoms.	Promotes the client's sense of control, while communicating respect for the client's experience.[50]
If the client describes or demonstrates high levels of guilt, assess for suicide risk or risk for self-harm, and implement appropriate precautions. Note here the actions to be taken. (See Suicide, Risk for, or Self-Mutilation, Risk for, for detailed interventions.)	Clients with guilt related to the experience may view suicide as a way to end this guilt.[33] Clients experiencing high stress reactions can't be at greater risk for self-harm.[50]
Monitor the client for risk for harming others. Refer to Other Directed Violence, Risk for, for appropriate interventions if defining characteristics are present.	Clients experiencing stress reactions can be at increased risk for harming others.[50]
Monitor the client for signs and symptoms of substance intoxication or withdrawal.	Clients with acute stress reactions may utilized substances as a coping strategy.[50]
Provide a quiet, nonstimulating environment, or an environment that does not add additional stress, to an already overwhelmed coping ability. [Potential environmental stressors for this client should be listed here, with the plan for reducing them in this environment.]	Inappropriate levels of sensory stimuli can increase confusion and disorganization and decrease sense of safety.[50]
Provide the client with basic needs such as food, hygiene, sleep, fluids.	Physiological stability facilitates recovery.[50]
Sit with the client [number] minutes [number] times a day at [times] to discuss the traumatic event. This should be directed by the client's need to discuss various aspects of their experience and not forced. Person responsible for this activity should be listed here. This should be the nurse who has established a relationship with the client.	Promotes the development of a trusting relationship, while providing the client with an opportunity to review and attach meaning to the client's experience.[45,50]

ACTIONS/INTERVENTIONS	RATIONALES
Assist the client with setting appropriate limits on aggressive behavior (see Risk for Violence in Chapter 9 for nursing actions if this is an appropriate diagnosis) by:	
• Decreasing environmental stimulation as appropriate. (This might include a secluded environment or a time-out.)	Inappropriate levels of sensory stimuli can increase confusion and disorganization, which increases the risk for aggressive behavior.
• Providing the client with appropriate alternative outlets for physical tension. (This should be stated specifically, and could include walking, running, talking with staff member, using a punching bag, listening to music, journaling, or doing a deep muscle relaxation sequence [number] times per day at [times] or when increased tension is observed.) These outlets should be selected with the client's input. Those outlets that the client selects should be listed here.	Physical activity decreases physical tension and increases the production of endorphins, which can increase the feeling of well-being. This also provides the client with opportunities to practice new coping behaviors in a supportive environment.
• Talking with the client about past situations that resulted in loss of control, and discussing alternative ways of coping with these situations. (Persons responsible for this discussion should be noted here. This will not be accomplished in one discussion; the time and date for the initial discussion should be noted, with the times and dates for follow-up discussions.)	Increases the client's coping options, and assists with cognitive appraisal of past coping behaviors.[44]
Once the symptoms have been identified and linked to the traumatic event, the primary nurse will sit with the client [number] minutes (begin with 30 and increase as the client's ability to concentrate improves) per shift to discuss the traumatic event These discussions should include:	Promotes the client's positive orientation.
• The uniqueness of the situation, noting that one could not plan for the behavior that might be needed to endure the situation.	
• Ways of evaluating behavior, noting that the usual moral and ethical standards may be inappropriate for the unique situation of a traumatic event.	Assists the client to evaluate and gain perspective on behavior, while moving away from all-or-none thinking.[44]
• Details of the event as the individual remembers them, and the thoughts and feelings that occur with these memories.	Assists the client in attaching meaning to the experience.
• Meaning of life since the event, and the implications this has for the future.	Promotes positive orientation, while assisting the client to review cognitive distortions.[27]
• Client's perceptions of the current actions of those around them and information about the care provider's perceptions. This should include normalization of the client's responses. (Person is experiencing a normal response to an abnormal situation).	Assists the client with reality testing his or her perceptions of current situations and motivations of others.[50,51]
Talk with client about thoughts rather than feelings about the event if feelings become extreme, such as with rage or despondency.	Inhibits automatic behavioral responses.[44]
Provide constructive confrontation for the client about problematic coping behavior.[32] Those kinds of behavior identified by the treatment team as problematic should be listed here with the selected method of confrontation.	Assists the client to gain a perspective on the experience and to label cognitive distortions that inhibit effective coping.[44]
Provide the client with information about care and treatment.	Promotes the client's sense of control.

(care plan continued on page 790)

NURSING ACTIONS/INTERVENTIONS WITH RATIONALES (continued from page 789)

Mental Health

ACTIONS/INTERVENTIONS	RATIONALES
Provide the client with opportunities to make appropriate decisions related to care at his or her level of ability. This may begin as a choice between two options and then evolve into more complex decision making. It is important that this decision making be at the client's level of functioning so confidence can be built with successful decision-making experiences. Those decisions that the client has made should be noted.	Success in this activity provides positive reinforcement and promotes the client's utilizing alternative coping behaviors, while enhancing self-esteem.
Provide positive social reinforcement and other behavioral rewards for demonstration of adaptive problem solving and coping. Those things that the client finds rewarding should be listed here, with a schedule for use. Those kinds of behavior that are to be rewarded should also be listed.	Reinforcement encourages positive behavior and enhances self-esteem.
Assist the client in identifying support systems and in developing a plan for their use. This plan should be noted here.	Support system understanding promotes their appropriate support of the client.
Inform significant others of the relationship between the client's behavior and the traumatic event. Discuss with them their thoughts and feelings about the client's behavior. The person responsible for these discussions should be noted here, along with the schedule for the discussion times. This should also include information about the importance of supporting the client in discussing the event and how this might be facilitated. The concerns the significant others have about their response to this sharing should be discussed as well as planning for the types of information they might be exposed to.	Support system understanding promotes their appropriate support of the client.[50]
When the client develops a degree of comfort discussing the traumatic event, meetings between the client and significant others should be scheduled. Content of these meetings should include: • Opportunities for the client to share thoughts and feelings about the event • Opportunities for the significant others to share their thoughts and feelings about the client's behavior • Sharing of thoughts and feelings related to other events in the relationship as they surface as important topics of discussion during the meetings • Sharing of caring thoughts and feelings with each other	Promotes the development of adaptive coping within the support system.
Arrange for the client to attend support group meetings with others who have experienced similar traumas. The times and days for these meetings should be noted here with any special arrangements that are needed to facilitate the client's attendance (e.g., transportation to group meeting place). This could include veterans groups, groups for survivors of natural disasters, and victims' groups.	Decreases the sense of social isolation, and decreases feelings of deviance. Consensual validation from other group members enhances self-esteem, providing increased emotional resources for coping.[50]

ACTIONS/INTERVENTIONS	RATIONALES
Schedule client involvement in unit activities. [Note here the client's responsibilities in these activities, with times the client will be involved in the activity.]	Decreases social isolation, and provides opportunity to practice new coping skills in a supportive environment.
Provide medications as ordered and monitor for therapeutics response and side effects.	Medication may be utilized for clients who do not respond to non-pharmacological treatment. These are targeted to specific symptoms such as sleep disturbance or excessive anxiety/panic attacks.[50]

Gerontic Health

The nursing actions for a gerontic patient with this diagnosis are the same as those given for the Adult Health and Mental Health patient.

Home Health

See Mental Health nursing actions for detailed interventions. If family violence is involved, refer to Chapter 9.

ACTIONS/INTERVENTIONS	RATIONALES
Ask the client to describe the precipitating event.	Assists the nurse in understanding the client's perception of the crisis and its impact.
Determine the client's perception of the stress.	
Assess sources of support, resources, and usual coping methods.	
Identify which coping strategies that the client has previously used have been effective and which have not. Discuss ways that effective strategies can be used to cope with future crises.[29]	Crisis can produce growth if effective skills are applied in future situations.
Assist the client in implementing adaptive coping mechanisms.	
Reinforce and encourage the use of healthy coping responses.	Assists the nurse in mobilizing resources and reinforcing adaptive actions.
Refer the client to existing community resources such as support groups.	Utilizes existing resources to promote adaptive coping.

SUICIDE, RISK FOR

DEFINITION[16]

At risk for self-inflicted, life-threatening injury.

DEFINING CHARACTERISTICS[16]

1. Behavioral factors
   a. History of prior suicide attempt
   b. Impulsiveness
   c. Buying a gun
   d. Stockpiling medicines
   e. Making or changing a will
   f. Giving away possessions
   g. Sudden emphatic recovery from a major depression
   h. Marked changes in behavior, attitude, or school performance

2. Verbal factors
   a. Threats of killing oneself
   b. States a desire to die or "end it all"
3. Situational factors
   a. Living alone
   b. Retired
   c. Relocation or institutionalization
   d. Economic instability
   e. Loss of autonomy or independence
   f. Presence of gun in home
   g. Adolescents living in nontraditional settings: juvenile detention center, prison, halfway house, or group home
4. Psychological factors
   a. Family history of suicides
   b. Alcohol and substance use or abuse

c. Psychiatric illness or disorder, for example, depression, schizophrenia, and bipolar disorder
d. Abuse in childhood
e. Guilt
f. Gay or lesbian youth

5. Demographic factors
   a. Age: elderly, young adult males, or adolescents
   b. Race: Caucasian or Native American
   c. Gender: male
   d. Divorced or widowed

6. Physical factors
   a. Physical illness
   b. Terminal illness
   c. Chronic pain

7. Social factors
   a. Loss of important relationships
   b. Disrupted family life
   c. Grief or bereavement
   d. Poor support systems
   e. Loneliness
   f. Hopelessness
   g. Helplessness
   h. Social isolation
   i. Legal or disciplinary problem
   j. Cluster suicides

RELATED FACTORS[16]

The risk factors also serve as the related factors.

RELATED CLINICAL CONCERNS

1. Any chronic or terminal disorder (e.g., rheumatoid arthritis, multiple sclerosis, cancer, or chronic pain)
2. Psychiatric illness or disorder
3. Chemical use or abuse

4. Recent, multiple losses
5. Post-Traumatic Stress Disorder

 Have You Selected the Correct Diagnosis?

Risk for Self-Mutilation
This diagnosis refers to the patient causing self-injury; however, there is no intent to kill oneself.

Risk for Violence Self-Directed
This diagnosis can be labeled as a combination of Risk for Self-Mutilation and Risk for Suicide. Using this diagnosis rather than Risk for Suicide would not be a problem because the interventions for both diagnoses are essentially the same. Risk for Suicide, when the intention was to end one's life, is the more accurate diagnosis, and incorporates actions that were not necessarily violent.

EXPECTED OUTCOME

Contracts to contact staff member when suicidal thoughts are present by [date].

Demonstrates use of [number] of positive coping strategies by [date].

Describes plans for future by [date].

TARGET DATES

Because of the life-threatening consequences of this diagnosis, progress should be monitored as frequently as the client's condition warrants. If the client is highly suicidal this could be on a constant basis even in a secure inpatient setting. Other common times for evaluation include every 15 minutes and every 30 minutes.

NURSING ACTIONS/INTERVENTIONS WITH RATIONALES

Adult Health

The Mental Health nursing actions also serve as the Adult Health nursing actions.

Child Health

ACTIONS/INTERVENTIONS	RATIONALES
Monitor for all contributing factors, including the child's or parental subjective data, objective data, primary and secondary references. If a child is taking antidepressants, monitor for side effects.	A holistic and complete assessment will provide the most thorough database for individualized care. Antidepressants have been associated with an increased risk of suicide in youth.[52,53]
Identify any threats or expression of related high-risk factors suggesting low self-esteem or lack of self-worth.	Verbalization of ideation must be taken seriously.
Identify history of any past suicidal ideation.	Tendency for recurrence is often noted with one suicide ideation providing risk index.
Identify ways to enhance communication for the child and family to best express feelings on an ongoing basis.	Communication will provide cues to how the client is feeling, with an avenue for dialogue.

ACTIONS/INTERVENTIONS	RATIONALES
Explore value conflicts and meaning these have for the client and family.	Freedom to explore thoughts about values will assist in noting uniqueness of each individual, while attempting to also respect the family's views.[53–55]
Identify ways to assist the child and family to identify cues suggestive of suicidal risk.	Knowledge is enhanced with recognition of patterns per individual and family.[53–55]
Provide appropriate attention to role of medications if these are ordered, with focus on desired effect, appropriate dosing and timing, importance of parent's securing supply in a safe place, expected side effects, possible toxicity, and ways to reduce toxicity vs. importance of maintenance of blood levels.	Knowledge about drugs will assist in safe, effective compliance with regimen.[52,55]
Ensure environmental safety as noted per adult plus frequent surveillance every 10 minutes, or constant, as may be required.	Client safety is paramount.
Identify appropriate peer support group activities, and encourage group activities.	The sense of isolation is reduced with peers who may be able to relate to similar feelings.
Collaborate with other members of health team, such as child life specialist, child psychologist, or psychiatrist.	Expertise will best provide for needs of the child and family.
Utilize developmentally appropriate strategies to encourage ongoing expression of feelings and/or ways to cope with suicidal tendency.	Expression of feelings may be facilitated through means other than verbalization and must be considered paramount in the child with suicidal risk.
Identify with the child and family a plan to deal with the risk for suicide.	Input from the child and family will best reflect and demonstrate the need for anticipatory planning in event of possible recurrence.
Identify a plan for gradual resumption of daily activities, such as school and extracurricular activities, well before actual dismissal.	Prior planning lessens anxiety and affords time to resume activities per individual coping strategies.
Identify a plan for follow-up in advance of dismissal.	Appropriate follow-up planning lessens likelihood of crisis or recurrence before situational or precipitating factors can be controlled.

Women's Health

The nursing interventions for a woman with this diagnosis are the same as those actions in Adult Health and Mental Health.

Mental Health

ACTIONS/INTERVENTIONS	RATIONALES
Introduce self and call the client by name.	Conditions that encourage feelings of anonymity facilitate aggressive behavior.[34]
Frame suicide as one option or solution to the problem.	Promotes a problem-solving approach without prompting a power struggle between the staff and the client around this option.
Inform the client about the limits of confidentiality. Plans to harm himself or herself or someone else must be shared with the treatment team and necessary authorities.	Honesty promotes the development of a trusting relationship.

(care plan continued on page 794)

NURSING ACTIONS/INTERVENTIONS WITH RATIONALES (continued from page 793)

Mental Health

ACTIONS/INTERVENTIONS	RATIONALES
Protect the client from harm by: • Asking the client what in the environment could pose harm for them • Removing sharp objects from environment • Removing belts and strings from environment • Providing a one-to-one constant interaction if risk for self-harm is high • Checking on the client's whereabouts every 15 minutes if not on one-to-one observation • Removing glass objects from environment • Removing locks from room and bathroom doors • Providing a shower curtain that will not support weight • Providing staff to supervise client areas at times when clients would normally expect less supervision, such as change of shift • Checking to see whether the client swallows medication	Provides an environment that promotes client safety.
Sit with the client [number] minutes [number] times each day. (Note person responsible for this here.) Use this time to: • Have the client tell his or her perspective of the situation, including feelings.	Facilitates the development of a trusting environment for open expression of concerns.[32] Communicates to the client that his or her welfare is important to the staff.[56]
• Commend the client's strengths.	Increases the client's awareness of strengths, which promotes a context of change and alternative problem solutions, while providing hope.[32,39]
• Explore the client's past attempts to cope with concerns.	Facilitates understanding of the client's perception of the problem. Change is dependent on problem perception.[32]
If suicidal behavior is influenced by intoxication, consult with the primary care provider for detoxification procedure.	Intoxication with drugs and alcohol can have a negative impact on the client's ability to make decisions.[56]
If suicidal behavior is influenced by command hallucinations, provide one-to-one observation until the client no longer describes these thoughts. Refer to Disturbed Thought Process (see Chapter 7) for detailed interventions for hallucinations.	Command hallucinations place clients at high risk for self-harm.[56]
Contract with the client to talk with staff member when he or she feels or thinks the risk for suicide is high.	Promotes the client's sense of control by assuring the client that if he or she needs help controlling his or her behavior, the staff has a specific plan to help. Assures the client of staff availability.[56,57]
When the client is capable of group interactions, assign him or her to a support group. [Note schedule for group interactions here.]	Facilitates the client's development of social skills and social contacts.[58]
Schedule regular times with primary nurse for the client to [Note times and person responsible for these interactions here.]: • Explore the need to carry out this problem solution at this time.	Removing the immediacy of this solution set can provide the client with time to develop alternative solutions.
• Explore past solutions.	Assists in facilitating understanding of the client's perception of the problem.

ACTIONS/INTERVENTIONS	RATIONALES
• Explore solution sets that enlist creative problem solving. These might include what the client would tell a friend to do, three wishes, generating a long list of solutions that are not assessed for their practicality in the initial problem-solving stages. • When solutions are generated, note the support the client needs from staff to implement these solutions here. • Develop with the client a plan to initiate new problem-solving strategies when problems arise after discharge. Provide the client with a written copy of this plan.	Facilitates the client's learning new problem-solving strategies. Promotes the client's sense of control.
Develop with the client a system to reward the use of new problem-solving strategies. Note the behavior that is to be rewarded and the reward system here.	Positive reinforcement encourages behavior.
Attend recreational activities with the client. Choose activities that have a high potential for client success. [Note activities here and person responsible for attending with the client.]	Provides the client with alternative outlets for anger or aggression, while promoting a sense of belonging and self-worth.[59]
Develop with the client a list of support groups in the community that will be utilized after discharge. [Note the support groups here with names of contact persons.]	Social isolation increases the risk for suicide.[58,59]
Arrange meeting with the client's support system to provide information about alternative coping strategies and develop positive communication patterns. [Note times and frequency of these meetings here.]	Promotes connection with support system, and facilitates problem solving.[58]

Gerontic Health

● N O T E : *In the United States, the highest suicide rate is seen in the older, white male population. Older adults rarely threaten to commit suicide. Usually they successfully take action rather than discuss the possibility. With the "graying" of America comes a need for health-care professionals to increase their own, and public, awareness of this problem. The Mental Health section for this diagnosis provides information on nursing actions that can be used in conjunction with the following interventions.*

ACTIONS/INTERVENTIONS	RATIONALES
Obtain information regarding risk factors associated with suicide in the elderly, such as loss of spouse in the past year, history of depression, social isolation, physical decline, loss of independence, and terminal diagnosis.[60]	A combination of these risk factors is frequently present in older adults who commit suicide.
Refer to social support services for assistance in meeting changing care needs.[61]	Introduces means of dealing with changing life circumstances.
Refer for hospice support if the older adult has been diagnosed with a terminal illness and meets hospice admission criteria.[61,62]	Provides interdisciplinary resources and support for the older client.
Question older adults about possible suicidal thoughts or plans.[63–65]	Encourages the client to discuss feelings of possible suicidal intent.
Refer the client for psychiatric assessment and treatment if risk for suicide is determined to be present.[62,65]	Places the client in contact with necessary resources for treatment.

(care plan continued on page 796)

NURSING ACTIONS/INTERVENTIONS WITH RATIONALES (continued from page 795)

Home Health

ACTIONS/INTERVENTIONS	RATIONALES
Consult with and/or refer the patient to assistive resources such as caregiver support groups as needed.	Utilization of existing services is an efficient use of resources.
Monitor the client and family closely for warning signs or risks for suicide.	Understanding helps promote a sense of control and order.
Consider all threats seriously.	
When a threat is made, do not leave the client alone for any period of time.	Minimizes risk of a suicide attempt.
Ask direct questions about intent:	Helps determine the seriousness and lethality of the suicide plan.
• Have you thought about killing yourself? • Have you thought about how and when you might do this? • What can I or we do to help you through this time?	Indicates to the client that you take him or her seriously and are willing to help.
Assist the family or caregivers in removing the most lethal means of suicide, such as weapons and medications.	Although it is not possible to remove all potentially destructive items, removal of the most lethal items reduces the likelihood of an attempt or successful effort.
Develop a written "no-suicide contract" with the client; that is, the client agrees that he or she will not hurt or kill himself or herself during a specific time period; that if such thoughts occur he or she will contact the nurse or other involved person; and if the contact person is not immediately available, the client will continue trying to reach him or her.	Allows time for intervention should the client decide to attempt suicide. Provides the client with a sense of responsibility to another and a sense that he or she is important to others.

REFERENCES

1. Sutterly, D: Stress in health: A survey of self regulation modalities. Top Clin Nurs 1:1, 1979.
2. Gordon, M: Manual of Nursing Diagnosis. McGraw-Hill, New York, 2002.
3. Ziemer, M: Coping behavior: A response to stress. Top Clin Nurs 4:4, 1982.
4. Kneisl, C, Wilson, H, and Trigoboff, E: Contemporary Psychiatric-Mental Health Nursing. Pearson Education, Upper Saddle River, NJ, 2004.
5. Frain, M, and Valiga, T: The multiple dimensions of stress. Top Clin Nurs 1:43, 1979.
6. Mengel, A: Coping. Top Clin Nurs 4:80, 1982.
7. Davis, L: Hardiness. In Creasia, J, and Parker, B (eds): Conceptual Foundations of Professional Nursing Practice, ed 2. CV Mosby, St. Louis, 1996.
8. Simoni, P: Hardiness and coping approach in the workplace of the nurse [Unpublished manuscript]. West Virginia University School of Nursing, Morgantown, WV, 1991.
9. Wagnild, G, and Young, H: Another look at hardiness, Image 23:257, 1991.
10. Schuster, CS, and Ashburn, SS: The Process of Human Development: A Holistic Life-Span Approach, ed 3. JB Lippincott, Philadelphia, 1992.
11. Smitherman, C: Nursing Actions for Health Promotion, FA Davis, Philadelphia, 1981.
12. Dixon, J, and Dixon, JP: An evolutionary-based model of health and viability. Adv Nurs Sci 6:1, 1984.
13. Carter, E, and McGoldrick, M (eds): The Changing Family Life Cycle: A Framework for Family Therapy, ed 2. Gardner Press, New York, 1988.
14. Ridenour, N: Aggregate nursing diagnoses for community health. In Carroll-Johnson, RM, and Paqvette, M (eds): Classification of Nursing Diagnoses: Proceedings of the Tenth Conference. JB Lippincott, Philadelphia, 1994.
15. Lunney, M, et al: Community Diagnosis: Analysis and Synthesis of the Literature. Association of Community Health Nursing Educators, Chicago, 1994.
16. NANDA International: Nursing Diagnoses: Definitions and Classification, NANDA International, 2005–2006, Philadelphia, 2005.
17. Viken, RM: The modern couvade syndrome. Female Patient 7:40, 1982.
18. Wong, DL and Perry, SE: Maternal Child Nursing Care. CV Mosby, St Louis, 1998.
19. Hanna, B, Jarman, H, Savage, S, and Layton, K: The early detection of postpartum depression: Midwives and nurses trial a check list. JOGNN J Obstet Gynecol Neonatal Nurs 33(2):191, 2004.
20. Beck, CT: Revision of the postpartum depression predictors inventory. JOGNN J Obstet Gynecol Neonatal Nurs 31(4):394, 2002.
21. Beck, CT, and Indman, P: The many faces of postpartum depression. JOGNN J Obstet Gynecol Neonatal Nurs 34(5):569, 2005.
22. Goodman, JH: Postpartum depression beyond the early postpartum period. JOGNN J Obstet Gynecol Neonatal Nurs 33(4):410, 2004.
23. Letvak, S: The importance of social support for rural mental health. Issues Ment Health Nurs 23:249, 2002.
24. Townsend, M: Psychiatric Mental Health Nursing, ed 5. FA Davis, Philadelphia, 2006.
25. Upton, N, and Reed, V: The influence of social support on caregiver coping, Int J Psychiatr Nurs Res 11:1256, 2006.
26. Sachs, B, Hall, L, Lutenbacher, M, and Rayens, K: Potential for abusive parenting by rural mothers with low-birth-weight children. Image J Nurs Scholar 31:21, 1999.

27. Sang, KK, and Mowbray, CT: What affects self-esteem of persons with psychiatric disabilities: The role of causal attributions of mental illnesses. Psychiatr Rehab J 28:354, 2005.

28. Evans, C: Personal interview. Swedish Medical Center, Seattle, WA, November, 1995.

29. Evans, C: Postpartum home care in the U.S. JOGNN J Obstet Gynecol Neonatal Nurs 24:181, 1995.

30. Keppler, AB: Personal interview. Evergreen Hospital, Kirkland, WA, December, 1995.

31. Keppler, AB: Postpartum care center: Follow-up care in a hospital-based clinic. JOGNN J Obstet Gynecol Neonatal Nurs 24:17, 1995.

32. Wright, LM, and Leahey, M: Nurses and Families: A Guide to Family Assessment and Intervention, ed 4. FA Davis, Philadelphia, 2005.

33. Wilson, H, Kneisl, C, and Trigoboff, E: Contemporary Psychiatric-Mental Health Nursing. Pearson Education, Upper Saddle River, NJ, 2004.

34. Hockenberry, MJ: Wong's Essentials of Pediatric Nursing, ed 7. CV Mosby, St. Louis, 2005.

35. Blankenship, V: Psychosocial development of women. In Breslin, ET, and Lucas, VA (eds): Women's Health Nursing: Toward Evidence-Based Practice. WB Saunders, St. Louis, 2003.

36. Upvall, MJ: Women and culture. In Breslin, ET, and Lucas, VA (eds): Women's Health Nursing: Toward Evidence-Based Practice. WB Saunders, St. Louis, 2003.

37. Bernhard, LA: Patriarchy, feminism, and women's health. In Breslin, ET, and Lucas, VA (eds): Women's Health Nursing: Toward Evidence-Based Practice. WB Saunders, St. Louis, 2003.

38. King, J: Helping patients choose an appropriate method of birth control. MCN Am J Matern Child Nurs 17:91, 1992.

39. Lightfoot-Klain, H, and Shaw, E: Special needs of ritually circumcised women patients. JOGNN J Obstet Gynecol Neonatal Nurs 20:102, 1992.

40. Miller, JF: Coping with Chronic Illness, ed 3. FA Davis, Philadelphia, 2000.

41. Sarason, I, and Sarason, B: Abnormal Psychology: The Problem of Maladaptive Behavior, ed. 11. Prentice-Hall, Upper Saddle River, NJ, 2004.

42. Ossman, SS: Clinical consult. Motivational interviewing: A process to encourage behavioral change. Nephrol Nurs J 31:346, 2004.

43. McCloskey Dochterman, J, and Bulechek, G: Nursing Interventions Classification, ed 4. CV Mosby, St. Louis, 2004.

44. Reeder, C: Cognitive therapy of anger management: Theoretical and practical considerations. Arch Psychiatr Nurs 5:147, 1991.

45. Haber, J, et al (eds): Comprehensive Psychiatric Nursing, ed 5. Mosby–Year Book, St. Louis, 1997.

46. Stuart, GW, and Laraia, MT: Principles and Practice of Psychiatric Nursing, ed 7. CV Mosby, St. Louis, 2001.

47. Matteson, MA, and McConnell, ES: Gerontological Nursing: Concepts and Practices, ed 2. WB Saunders, Philadelphia, 1997.

48. Laborde, JM: Torture: A nursing concern. Image 21:31, 1989.

49. Wong, DL: Whaley and Wong's Nursing Care of Infants and Children, ed 6. CV Mosby, St. Louis, 1999.

50. US Department of Defense: Clinical Practice Guideline for the Management of Post-Traumatic Stress. (Rep No Version 1.0). Washington, DC: Veterans Health Administration, Department of Defense, 2004.

51. Symes, L: Post traumatic stress disorder: An evolving concept. Arch Psychiatr Nurs 9:195, 1995.

52. Maxmen, J, and Ward, N: Psychotropic Drugs Fast Facts, ed. 3. WW Norton, New York, 2002.

53. American Academy of Pediatrics: Preventing youth suicide. Available at http://www.keepkidshealthy.com, 2006.

54. American Academy of Pediatrics: About teen suicide. Available at http://www.kidshealth.org, 2006.

55. Pharmaceutical Drugs: Risk of suicide from children prescriptions. Available at http://www.hpakids.org, 2006.

56. Egan, M, et al: The "No Suicide Contract": Helpful or harmful? J Psychosoc Nurs 35:31, 1997.

57. Stevenson, S: Heading off violence with verbal de-escalation. J Psychosoc Nurs 29:6, 1991.

58. Editors News: Eight factors critical in evaluating suicide risk. J Psychosoc Nurs 38:7, 2000.

59. Townsend, M: Psychiatric-Mental Health Nursing: Concepts of Care, ed 5. FA Davis, Philadelphia, 2006.

60. Lambert, MT, and Fowler, DR: Suicide risk factors among veterans: Risk management in the changing culture of the Department of Veterans Affairs. J Ment Health Admin 24:350, 1997.

61. Morrow-Howell, N, et al: Evaluating an intervention for the elderly at increased risk of suicide. Res Social Work Pract 8:29, 1998.

62. Stanley, M, and Beare, PG: Gerontological Nursing: A Health Promotion-Protection Approach, ed 2. FA Davis, Philadelphia, 1999.

63. Wattis, J, and Burns, E: What an old age psychiatrist does. BMJ 313:101, 1996.

64. Tyson, SR: Gerontological Nursing Care. WB Saunders, Philadelphia, 1999.

65. Butler, RN, and Lewis, MI: Late-life depression: When and how to intervene. Geriatrics 50:44, 1995.

66. Huebscher, R: Natural, alternative and complementary health care. In Breslin, ET, and Lucas, VA (eds): Women's Health Nursing: Toward Evidence-Based Practice. WB Saunders, St. Louis, 2003.

12

VALUE–BELIEF PATTERN

PATTERN DESCRIPTION

The nurse may care for patients who, because of health alterations, experience disturbances in their individual value-belief systems. A person's value-belief system is the core of his or her existence, his or her interconnectedness with his or her spiritual side as well as his or her interconnectedness with the environment. This value-belief system gives meaning and purpose to life. Some call this faith "Faith carries us forward when there is no longer reason to carry on. It enables us to exist during the in-between times: between meanings, amid dangers or radical discontinuity, even in the face of death. Faith is a sine qua non of life, a primal force we cannot do without" Faith can be in many things–a superior being, the environment, self, family, or community. The nurse may care for patients who, because of their faith or value-belief system, cope and even increase their spiritual well-being when faced with health alterations. Other patients the nurse cares for may experience disturbances in their individual value-belief system or faith because of health alterations. These alterations may take a form ranging from being disturbed to being demolished. These disturbances can be manifested by the inability to practice formal religious directions, such as attending church or following a specific diet, to being totally unable to manage their own spiritual needs and live within a certain spiritual structure. Conversely, religion can affect physical or emotional well-being if the practice of the religion results in spiritual distress. An individual's value-belief system can contribute to alterations in health, just as alterations in health can contribute to disturbances in the individual's values and beliefs.

On the other hand alterations in health can strengthen a person's faith, values and beliefs.These patients are experiencing "enhanced spirituality" and often search for the greater meaning in their health alteration experience. Many times the nurse may encounter the patient who will refuse treatment and/or seek alternative methods of dealing with illness. The nurse must individualize care to help enhance and support faith while minimizing spiritual distress when meeting the specific needs of the individual patient within his or her value-belief system.

The value-belief pattern looks not only at how the individual retains faith and enhances his or her value-belief system in times of stress but at how physical illness can interfere with the individual's ability to practice religion and maintain beliefs, values, and spiritual life, as well as how a person's judgment and interpretation of the meaning of life (faith) for himself or herself can affect or interfere with health care practices.

PATTERN ASSESSMENT

1. Does the patient express anger toward a supreme being regarding his or her current condition?
   a. Yes (Spiritual Distress)
   b. No (Readiness for Enhanced Spiritual Well-Being)

2. Does the patient verbalize conflict about personal spiritual beliefs?
   a. Yes (Risk for Spiritual Distress)
   b. No (Readiness for Enhanced Spiritual Well-Being)
3. Does the patient indicate positive thoughts about spirituality?
   a. Yes (Readiness for Enhanced Spiritual Well-Being)
   b. No (Risk for Spiritual Distress)
4. Does the patient indicate comfort with self and his or her purpose in life and life stage?
   a. Yes (Readiness for Enhanced Spiritual Well-Being)
   b. No (Risk for Spiritual Distress)
5. Is the patient unable to participate in rites and/or religious activities and services because of illness or life circumstance?
   a. Yes (Impaired Religiosity)
   b. No (Risk for Impaired Religiosity)
6. Does the practice of religious rites bring the patient and family comfort and stronger feelings of well-being and strength?
   a. Yes (Readiness for Enhanced Religiosity)
   b. No (Risk for impaired religiosity)

CONCEPTUAL INFORMATION

According to several authors, spirituality and religiousness are two very different concepts that are often used interchangeably.[1] The nurse may care for patients who, because of health alterations, experience disturbances in their individual value–belief systems, as well as interruptions in their involvement in their religious community.[1,2] A person's value–belief system is the core of his or her existence. This belief system facilitates a connection with the spiritual self by providing interconnectedness with the environment. This system gives meaning and purpose to life. Some call this faith, and some call this spirituality. "Faith carries us forward when there is no longer reason to carry on. It enables us to exist during the in-between times: between meanings, amid dangers of radical discontinuity, even in the face of death. Faith is a sine qua non of life, a primal force we cannot do without."[3] An individual can have faith in many things—a Superior Being, the environment, self, family, or community. The nurse may care for patients who, because of their faith or value–belief system, cope and even increase their spiritual well-being when faced with health alterations. Other patients may experience disturbances in their individual value–belief system or faith because of health alterations to themselves, their family, or friends. These alterations may range from being disturbed to being demolished and can be manifested by the inability to exercise formal religious practices such as attending church or following a specific diet (religiosity), to being totally unable to manage their own spiritual needs and live within a certain spiritual structure (spiritual distress). Conversely, religion can enhance physical or emotional well-being if the practice of the religion results in stronger feelings of well-being and strength (readiness for enhanced religiosity). An individual's value–belief system can contribute to alterations in health, just as alterations in health can contribute to disturbances in the individual's values and beliefs. Nursing must individualize care to help enhance and support faith, while minimizing spiritual distress when meeting the specific needs of the individual patient within his or her value–belief system.

The value–belief pattern looks not only at how the individual retains faith and enhances his or her value–belief system in times of stress, but also at how physical illness can interfere with the individual's ability to practice religion and maintain beliefs. It also looks at how, when faced with stress and/or alterations in health, an individual or family can either maintain or lose the ability to discern meaning and purpose (faith) in life. How this is accomplished by the individual and/or family can affect or interfere with health-care practices.

It is important for the practitioner to be able to distinguish between spirituality and religiousness. Spirituality is defined by many authors as the manner in which people find meaning and purpose in life. This can be accomplished through relationships with others, art, music, literature, nature, and the ability to connect to a higher power through prayer, meditation, or thought.[1,4]

Religiousness is how individuals or groups express their spirituality, and is more closely linked to culture and social subgroups. Religion is expressed and/or practiced by individuals in many different ways, and usually consists of a set of beliefs, rites, and rituals.[1]

The faith, belief, or value system of a person can be described as the predominating force (spirituality) that provides the vital direction to that person's existence. This predominating force can be a faith in a supreme being or God, a belief in one's self, or a belief in others.[5] It is conceptualized that each person must find his or her place in the world, nature, and in relationships with other beings. This faith, belief, or value system is expressed by the individual in the form of organized religion, attitudes, and actions related to the individual's sense of what is right, cultural beliefs, and the individual's internal motivations.

All persons have some philosophical orientation to life that assists in constructing their reality, regardless of whether or not they practice a formal religion. Spirituality is interwoven into a person's cultural background, beliefs, and individual value system. This spirituality is what gives life meaning and allows the person to function in a more total manner. These beliefs and values influence a person's behavior and attitudes toward what is right and what is wrong with the lifestyle he or she practices. Many authors[1,6,7] stress that the nurse must not only take into consideration the patient's beliefs and value system, but also must recognize his or her own beliefs and values. The nurse must know about, or develop resources to assist with understanding, the different beliefs and religious practices of individuals and groups encountered in practice settings. Further understanding and assessment of a patient's beliefs can be ascertained by asking questions such as "Do you have a faith community?" or "Which beliefs and practices are important to you?"[7]

Studies have shown that the value of specific rituals such as prayer to the individuals who practice them is not affected by the fact that they can or cannot be proved scientifically. Longitudinal studies have found a protective link between religious participation and increased chances for living longer.[7–10] The impact of values and beliefs is best described by the following quote, "When as much emphasis is placed on the symbolic and intuitive as is placed on the analytical, consciousness develops more fully."[11] The expansion of consciousness is what life, and therefore health, is all about; health can coexist with illness and even encompass it as a meaningful aspect. This can be seen in those individuals who consider suffering, illness, and even death as having "meaning in life" or as "God's will."[7,11]

Many individuals believe that the only value of life, and the source of strength and power, is the will of the individual and that there is no need for assistance from the outside. This focus has been described as "a person's authority within himself."[12] This focus may actually revolve around work, physical activity, or self—"I can do anything I want to when I want to."[11,12] Three predominant indicators have been listed that must be considered when judging the value of continued life: mental capacity, physical capacity, and pain.[9] This would indicate that, in and of itself, life is not intrinsically valuable to the possessor of it. Rather, it is the quality of conscious life that is important.

In one phenomenological study[13] of spirituality, the constituents of spirituality, as reported by the study subjects, were described and included (1) realization of humanity of self or valued other; (2) event of nonhuman intervention; (3) receiving divine intervention; (4) visceral knowing; (5) willingness to sacrifice; (6) physical sensations; (7) a personal experience; (8) a reality experience; (9) not easily explained; and (10) different from or more than daily experience.

In 1981, Fowler[3] described his faith development theory, which was influenced by the work of Piaget and Kohlberg. Fowler describes faith as not always religious in its content or context, but "a person's or group's way of moving into the force field of life. It is our way of finding coherence in and giving meaning to the multiple forces and relations that make up our lives."[3] Fowler described the experience of spirituality in different stages of the life cycle. He states that one transitions from one stage to another, some fast and some slow, and that it is not a simple change of mind or even a conscious movement from one phase to another. He also states that it can be a long and painful process. Six states of faith are recognized by Fowler:

1. **Intuitive–Projective.** This stage is characterized by experiencing the world as a child, fluid and full of novelty, with a rudimentary awareness of self as the center of the universe. Preoperational reasoning and judgment are employed by people in this stage. There is no reasoning or logic to thought; therefore, the capacity for taking the role or perspective of others is extremely limited.
2. **Mythic–Literal.** People in this stage can separate real from unreal on the basis of experience, and therefore the

world becomes more linear and orderly than in stage one. This is accompanied by a private world of speculation, fantasy, and wonder. Bounds of the social world widen, and the questioning of "good and evil" is begun. Often these thoughts, which can be reassuring, hopeful, or full of terror and fear, are symbolized in dreams and daydreams.[3,14]

3. **Synthetic–Conventional.** One begins to structure the world and the environment in interpersonal terms. The individual constructs an image of self as seen by others and becomes aware that others are performing the same operations in their relationships. This is a conformist stage, in which peers and their values become most important. Influences from earlier stages are carried "within" as reference points by which beliefs and values are valued, and actions are valued, validated, and sanctioned.

4. **Individuative–Reflexive.** The individual begins to construct and maintain his or her own identity, autonomy, and faith, without relying on others. The sense of self is now reciprocal with a faith outlook or worldview that negotiates between self and significant others. One knows he or she is different from others, and his or her views and faith are vulnerable to challenge and change.

5. **Paradoxical–Consolidative.** Many previous dimensions that were formally suppressed or ignored are integrated. One becomes open to the voices of one's innermost self. There is a coming to terms with one's social unconsciousness: the myths, norms, ideal images, and prejudices that have, until now, formed one's life. One can see injustice because of an expanded awareness of the demands of justice, and the implications of those demands.

6. **Universalizing.** The individual at this stage becomes a disciplined activist. He or she exhibits qualities that shake the usual criteria of normalcy. He or she leads and embraces strategies of nonviolent suffering and of ultimate respect for life. "They often become martyrs to the visions they incarnate."[7,16]

Other studies[1,6,13,16] provide insights regarding the interactive process of caring as it relates to spiritual needs. Trust, meaningful support systems, and a respect for personal beliefs were identified by participants as central to care.

Because of the conscious, subconscious, and unconscious components of the value–belief system, nurses must be continually alert for disruptions in the system. There is a need to be aware that every individual expresses disruptions in spirituality differently.[7,16] Some withdraw, some become more religious, and some become angry and defiant. Nurses need to be cognizant of not only the patient's spiritual beliefs but also the stage of spiritual development in which both the patient and nurse are.[1,6,13,16] This will affect and determine not only the needs and concerns of the patients but how the nurse will approach the patient to care for those needs and concerns. This awareness of and respect for the impact and influence values and beliefs have on the patient

cannot be overemphasized in planning and providing high-quality care for the patient.

DEVELOPMENTAL CONSIDERATIONS

The geographic, social, political, and home environment in which one lives has a major effect on how a person develops, how he or she will view health, and how spirituality, values, and beliefs are formulated. The values a person holds influence all facets of life. How one perceives the world about him or her, as well as his or her basic philosophy, guides all interactions with others and ultimately reflects a person's individuality.[17]

Fowler, in describing his developmental stages of faith, states he has found adults in all stages, regardless of their chronological age. Adolescents have been found in stages two and three. However, persons are usually found in the various stages as shown in the parentheses at the end of each developmental stage in the text that follows.[3]

INFANT

The infant is totally dependent on the parents and those about him or her and is busy building trust or mistrust.[18] Unable at this age to form values or distinguish spirituality, the infant is a mirror image of those about him or her. The parent's method of interaction, communication, and fulfillment of the emotional and physiologic needs of the infant forms the basis for value development. (Fowler's Stage One)

TODDLER AND PRESCHOOLER

The toddler imitates those about him or her, such as parents, siblings, and other adults. The toddler develops by mimicking observed behavior and receiving either positive or negative reinforcement. Values begin to form as the toddler starts to become aware of others and to interact with those around him or her. Values become known to individuals through the process of social cognition, which begins in early childhood. This arises neither from objects, nor the subject, but from the interaction between the subject and those objects.[16] (Fowler's Stage One)

SCHOOL-AGE CHILD

The school-age child begins to be influenced by peers outside the family structure, and also begins to question and make choices. The school-age child actively participates in his or her own moral development. Individual reasoning develops through various stages, beginning in the school-age years.[18,19] Play is the major mechanism of learning throughout the school-age years. (Fowler's Stage Two)

ADOLESCENT

The adolescent searches for his or her own identity and begins to practice values that are separate, and yet congruent with, his or her family unit. The adolescent is constantly questioning, trying, and searching for the "truth of life". This search is the adolescent's method of understanding his or her identity in the scheme of things. They see values as being either "black or white," and there can be no overlapping. The adolescent is still struggling with his or her own independence, while trying to formulate his or her own values, beliefs, and spirituality.[3,10] (Fowler's Stages Two and Three)

YOUNG ADULT

Young adults are constantly examining, reformulating, and changing their values, beliefs, and spirituality. Often they change completely the values and beliefs they developed during adolescence, although it is important to note that they often keep the basic values and beliefs they learned during their young years with their families. (Fowler's Stages Three and Four)

ADULT

Adults usually strengthen the values and beliefs they have formed according to their life experiences. Adult are continually exploring and trying to see whether their value system fits within his or her lifestyle.[3,10] They are busy teaching children the values and beliefs they hope their children will adopt for their lives. (Fowler's Stages Four and Five)

OLDER ADULT

Older adults find great solace in their spirituality and the values and beliefs they have formed through a lifetime. In general, the older adult continues to use the values, beliefs, and spiritual patterns adopted in adulthood.[3,8,10] (Fowler's Stages Five and Six)

TABLE 12.1 NANDA, NIC, and NOC Taxonomic Linkages

GORDON'S FUNCTIONAL HEALTH PATTERN	NANDA NURSING DIAGNOSIS	NIC PRIORITY INTERVENTIONS	NOC EVALUATIONS
Value–Belief Pattern	Spiritual Distress, Actual and Risk for	**Actual** Spiritual Growth Facilitation Spiritual Support	**Actual** Dignified Life Closure Hope Spiritual Health
		Risk for Spiritual Growth Facilitation Spiritual Support	**Risk for** Anxiety Level Client Satisfaction: Cultural Needs Fulfillment Comfortable Death Coping Dignified Life Closure Grief Resolution Hope Loneliness Severity Mood Equilibrium Personal Autonomy Personal Well-Being Psychosocial Adjustment: Life Change Quality of Life Risk Control Risk Detection Social Interaction Skills Spiritual Health
	Spiritual Well-Being, Readiness for Enhanced	Spiritual Growth Facilitation	Hope Personal Well-Being Quality of Life Spiritual Health
	Religiosity, Impaired	*Still in development*	* Still in development
	Religiosity, Impaired, Risk for	* Still in development	* Still in development

APPLICABLE NURSING DIAGNOSES

RELIGIOSITY, IMPAIRED

DEFINITION[4]

Impaired ability to exercise reliance on beliefs and/or participate in rituals of a particular faith.

DEFINING CHARACTERISTICS[4]

1. Demonstrates or explains difficulty adhering to prescribed religious beliefs and rituals, such as the following:
   a. Religious ceremonies
   b. Dietary regulations
   c. Clothing
   d. Prayer
   e. Worship/religious services
   f. Private religious behaviors/reading religious materials/media
   g. Holiday observances
   h. Meetings with religious leaders
2. Expresses emotional distress because of separation form faith community
3. Expresses emotional distress regarding religious beliefs and/or religious social network
4. Expresses a need to reconnect with previous belief patterns and customs
5. Questions religious belief patterns and customs

RELATED FACTORS[4]

A. Physical
   1. Sickness/illness
   2. Pain
B. Psychological Factors
   1. Ineffective support/coping
   2. Personal disaster/crisis
   3. Lack of security
   4. Fear of death
   5. Ineffective coping with disease
   6. Use of religion to manipulate
C. Sociocultural
   1. Barriers to practicing religion (cultural and environmental)
   2. Lack of social integration
   3. Lack of social/cultural interaction

D. Spiritual
   1. Spiritual crises
   2. Suffering
E. Developmental and Situational
   1. End-stage life crises
   2. Life transitions
   3. Aging

RELATED CLINICAL CONCERNS

1. Victims of disasters
2. Pain
3. Physical or mental ability to function independently
4. Restrictive medical regimens
5. Immobility
6. Loss or lessening of senses (e.g., hearing loss)
7. Isolation from usual spiritual/faith community that impedes religious practice (i.e., can not obtain special foods or paraphernalia).

EXPECTED OUTCOME

The patient and/or family will be able to express needs related to religious practices by [date].

Patient and family will be able to describe an alternative plan for certain religious practices by [date].

TARGET DATES

A target date of 1 to 2 days is appropriate. The sooner this can be accomplished, the sooner an individual can practice religious rites that are meaningful to them. This will allow them to achieve enhanced religiosity and maintain enhanced spiritually in a timely manner.

 Have You Selected the Correct Diagnosis?

Spiritual Distress
Spiritual Distress is the correct diagnosis when an individual and/or family has given up all belief and hope in the meaning and purpose of life. If the patient and family express concern only about inability to practice certain rites that strengthen their spirituality, but are not concerned with meaning and purpose in life, then impaired religiosity is the correct diagnosis.

NURSING ACTIONS/INTERVENTIONS WITH RATIONALES

Adult Health

ACTIONS/INTERVENTIONS	RATIONALES
Engage in active listening with the patient and significant others, providing opportunities for them to express areas of concern related to religious practice.	
Assist the patient in determining current factors perceived to interfere with religious practice and develop a plan to meet identified needs. [Note that plan here with information about the assistance needed from nursing for implementation.]	
Arrange accommodations for religious practice when possible (e.g., special foods, treatments about times of prayer, recognition of special days of religious observance, religious texts, religious healing practices).	
Confer with community resources such as a parish nurse and leaders in the client's faith community.	Allows for development of plan aimed to minimize barriers to practice.

Child Health

This pattern is primarily related to Adult Health, Women's Health, and Mental Health aspects according to developmental stage and capacity, in addition to those noted for the school-aged child or older.

ACTIONS/INTERVENTIONS	RATIONALES
Assess for all factors contributing to the alteration, especially those verbalized by the child. Be alert to potential circumstantial school related activities or perceived barriers	Provides a realistic base for plan.
Identify the effect the problem is having in the child's world and how to intervene with assistance of family, child life specialist, religious clergy, or other identified support persons. Involve the child and encourage their engagement in the plan.	Provides likelihood of fullest exploration of problem within child's realm.
Assist the child, family, and relevant paraprofessionals in developing a plan that will satisfy the altered religiosity issue. Especially note ways to feel freedom of self-expression of desired worship, while also remaining in compliance with societal constraints.	Allows for child's regaining a sense of the right to express religiosity in appropriate manner and setting.
*Issues may require legal or school-related input if conflicts are of these domains.	
Provide a plan for follow-up to re-explore progress in near future.	Offers anticipatory guidance.
Refer to community resources with similar valued religiosity, as faith-based centers.	Empowers and provides shared experiences for child and family.

(care plan continued on page 806)

NURSING ACTIONS/INTERVENTIONS WITH RATIONALES (continued from page 805)

Women's Health

Women's health will be the same as for Adult Health or Mental Health with the following additions:

ACTIONS/INTERVENTIONS	RATIONALES
Discuss a situation that is producing anxiety and strategize activities to reduce stress and increase religiosity.	Research conducted at Arizona State University pinpointed specific traits associated with religion and spirituality that positively affect health. One aspect of religion and spirituality was linked to a specific physiological response, and people who communicated with a "higher-power" (prayer) throughout the day were less reactive when exposed to an anxiety-causing situation.[20]
Allow women to discuss fears related to role loss, declining health, poor economic status, and widowhood.	Older women cope and thrive in a variety of creative, productive ways many of which involve participating in their religion.[21]
Discuss the connection between spirituality, religion, and productive activities.	Religious practices and values are one way older women become involved.[21]
Facilitate bible reading, mediating, praying, and participation in religious activities. [Note client's preferred practice here with support needed from nursing staff.]	Research shows these activities increase with age and engagement in these activities related to strong personal spirituality.[21]

Mental Health

ACTIONS/INTERVENTIONS	RATIONALES
Spend [number] minutes per [day/shift] with the client and/or significant others identifying needs for religious practice, and the influence it has on the client's well-being.	Communicates concern and acceptance. Clients report wanting increased support for religious beliefs by health-care providers. Religious practice that is predicated on restrictive and punitive dogma may impede the experience and healing potential of **spirituality**.[22]
Develop, with the client and/or significant others, plan for meeting needs of religious practice in a manner that facilitates emotional well-being. [Note the client's plan here with assistance needed from nursing staff for implementation.]	Familiar practices enhance emotional sense of well being and religious practice can facilitate healing and wholeness in times of stress.[22]
Arrange religious accommodations that enhance client's sense of emotional well-being, for example, special foods, schedule treatments around times for prayer, meetings with religious leaders or members of their faith community, recognition of special days of religious observance, religious texts, and religious healing practices.	
Demonstrate respect for client's religious practices by: • Providing special space to keep religious objects • Maintaining safety of these objects (e.g., checking gowns for medals before sending them to laundry).	
Educate staff about religious practices and the support needed from staff to facilitate client's plan. [Note plan for this here.]	Enhances staff cultural competence and increases their ability to facilitate plan of care.

ACTIONS/INTERVENTIONS	RATIONALES
Collaborate with other health-care providers that have an understanding of mental health issues and religious practice (chaplain, parish nurse, dietary, etc.) to meet the client's needs.	The client's well-being is enhanced when health-care providers recognize the complex relationship between mental health issues and religious beliefs "Perceptions of mental illness as divine will or punishment may cause increased distress when there is fear of displeasing a punitive God or a sense of being unheard or abandoned by a God of comfort."[22]

Gerontic Health

ACTIONS/INTERVENTIONS	RATIONALES
Engage in active listening with the client by: • Presence (creating a relationship with sincere communication) • Using therapeutic/caring touch as tolerated by client • Facilitating the client's search for meaning • Facilitating reminiscence	This assists the nurse in collecting data about client status and establishing a trusting relationship with the client. Caring touch can improve a client's self-esteem, sense of well being, and faith.[23]
Assess which needs can be met in the client's current circumstance, and which needs are most important to the client. Assist the client in meeting those needs (pastoral consult, visitors from church) as health status allows.	Assists the nurse in determining the client's priorities and preferences.
Encourage the client to seek forgiveness or to forgive others.	Through forgiveness, older adults can discover new meaning and continue the development of the spiritual self.[23]
Offer to pray, meditate, or read spiritual text with the client, or arrange for another member of the health-care team to do so while respecting the client's time for quietness and prayer.	Supports the client's existing spirituality.[23]

Home Health

ACTIONS/INTERVENTIONS	RATIONALES
Engage in active listening with the client by: • Presence (creating a relationship with sincere communication) • Using therapeutic/caring touch as tolerated by client • Facilitating the client's search for meaning	This assists the nurse in collecting data about client status and establishing a trusting relationship with the client. Caring touch can improve a client's self-esteem, sense of well-being, and faith.[23]
Assess which needs can be met in the client's current circumstance, and which needs are most important to the client. Assist the client in meeting those needs (pastoral consult, visitors from church) as health status allows.	Assists the nurse in determining the client's priorities and preferences.
Encourage the client to seek forgiveness or forgive others.	Through forgiveness, older adults can discover new meaning and continue the development of the spiritual self.[23]
Offer to pray, meditate, or read spiritual text with the client, or arrange for another member of the health-care team to do so while respecting the client's time for quietness and prayer.	Supports the client's existing spirituality.[23]

RELIGIOSITY, READINESS FOR ENHANCED

DEFINITION[4]

Ability to increase reliance on religious beliefs and/or participate in rituals of a particular faith tradition

DEFINING CHARACTERISTICS[4]

1. Expresses desire to strengthen religious belief patterns and customs that had provided comfort/religion in the past
2. Request for assistance to increase participation in prescribed religious beliefs through:
   a. Religious ceremonies
   b. Dietary regulations/rituals
   c. Clothing
   d. Prayer
   e. Worship/religious services
   f. Private religious behaviors/reading religious materials/media
   g. Holiday observances
   h. Requests assistance expanding religious options
   i. Requests meeting with religious leaders/facilitators
   j. Requests forgiveness, reconciliation
   k. Requests religious material and/or experiences
   l. Questions or rejects belief patterns and customs that are harmful

RELATED FACTORS[4]

None listed.

RELATED CLINICAL CONCERNS

1. Victims of abuse
2. Change in lifestyle
3. Chronic illness
4. Pain
5. Terminal illness
6. Immobility

EXPECTED OUTCOME

The patient and/or family will be able to express needs related to religious practices by [date].

The patient and family will be able to describe an alternative plan for certain religious practices by [date].

TARGET DATES

A target date of 1 to 2 days is appropriate. The sooner this can be accomplished, the sooner an individual can practice religious rites that are meaningful to him or her. This will allow him or her to achieve enhanced religiosity and maintain enhanced spiritually in a timely manner.

 Have You Selected the Correct Diagnosis?

Readiness for Enhanced Spiritual Well-Being
Readiness for Enhanced Spiritual Well-Being is the correct diagnosis when the client is requesting assistance with integrating meaning and purpose into life through connectedness. If the client is concerned with increasing his or her reliance on current religious beliefs or participation in the rituals of a faith tradition, then the correct diagnosis would be Readiness for Enhanced Religiosity.

NURSING ACTIONS/INTERVENTIONS WITH RATIONALES

Adult Health

ACTIONS/INTERVENTIONS	RATIONALES
Collaborate with the patient, family, and staff to determine how faith needs can best be met and accommodate to the extent feasible. [Note accommodations needed here.]	Determines how staff can facilitate meeting practice needs.
Contact and arrange for visits from members and leaders of the patient's faith community.	Provides support for patient
Provide time and privacy to allow the patient to practice his or her faith. Be considerate to any rituals associated with days of special concern and healing. Plan nursing interventions around rituals. [Note this schedule here.]	Allows for time and privacy.
Align the patient with community resources (e.g., classes or discussion groups that will facilitate religious practice).	

Child Health

This pattern incorporates the applicable components of the adult and women's components in a developmentally appropriate manner in addition to the following:

ACTIONS/INTERVENTIONS	RATIONALES
Monitor for cues to confirm readiness to engage in enhanced spirituality from child and/or parents: • The child or family may verbalize willingness and acceptance of current status.	Offers a base for considering plan.
Honor the practice of the desired plan within daily routine. • Allow for music, reading, or play as appropriate with spiritual focus. • Allow quiet time without undue interruptions. • Respect privacy during times of spiritual expression or participate according to the nurse's and family's mutual comfort.	Continually practicing the plan models for the caregivers, so that they begin to value the plan.
Determine the need for visitation or referral to clergy persons or other support persons.	Provides anticipatory guidance.
Assist the child and/or family in developing plan for continued practice of plan.[24]	

Women's Health

ACTIONS/INTERVENTIONS	RATIONALES
When requested, describe for the client such therapies as: • Alternative medical systems • Mind–body interventions • Biologically based therapies • Manipulative and body-based methods • Energy therapies	Support the client in exploring alternative practices if he or she desires. Many practices of self-care and alternative health care reflect an inner focus, for instance, physical, mental, and spiritual, that sustains and supports when needed to enhance beliefs and values.[25] To some individuals, religiosity and spirituality has to do with a "mystical feeling" or "a flowing dynamic quality of unity" rather than a formal religious practice.[25]
Discuss the situation that is producing anxiety and strategize activities to reduce stress and increase religiosity.	Research conducted at Arizona State University pinpointed specific traits associated with religion and spirituality that positively affect health. One aspect identified was a specific physiological response, and people who communicated with a "higher-power" (prayer) throughout the day were less reactive when exposed to an anxiety-causing situation.[20]
Allow women to discuss fears related to role loss, declining health, poor economic status, and widowhood.	Older women cope and thrive in a variety of creative, productive ways many of which involve participating in their religion.[21]
Discuss the connection between spirituality, religion, and productive activities.	Religious practices and values are one way older women become involved.[21]
Facilitate bible reading, mediating, praying and participation in religious activities. [Note the client's preferred practice here with support needed from nursing staff.]	Research shows these activities increase with age, and engagement in these activities is related to strong personal spirituality.[21]

(care plan continued on page 810)

NURSING ACTIONS/INTERVENTIONS WITH RATIONALES (continued from page 809)

Mental Health

Refer to Mental Health nursing actions for Impaired Religiosity.

Gerontic Health

ACTIONS/INTERVENTIONS	RATIONALES
Engage in active listening with the client by: • Presence (creating a relationship with sincere communication) • Using therapeutic/caring touch as tolerated by client • Facilitating the client's search for meaning • Facilitating reminiscence	This assists the nurse in collecting data about client status and establishing a trusting relationship with the client. Caring touch can improve a client's self-esteem, sense of well-being, and faith.[23]
Assess which needs can be met in the client's current circumstance, and which needs are most important to the client. Assist the client in meeting those needs (pastoral consult, visitors from faith community) as health status allows.	Assists the nurse in determining the client's priorities and preferences.
Encourage the client to seek forgiveness or forgive others.	Through forgiveness, older adults can discover new meaning and continue the development of the spiritual self.[23]
Offer to pray, meditate, or read spiritual text with the client, or arrange for another member of the health-care team to do so while respecting the client's time for quietness and prayer.	Supports the client's existing spirituality.[23]

Home Health/Community Health

ACTIONS/INTERVENTIONS	RATIONALES
Engage in active listening with the client by: • Presence (creating a relationship with sincere communication) • Using therapeutic/caring touch as tolerated by client • Facilitating the client's search for meaning • Facilitating reminiscence	This assists the nurse in collecting data about client status and establishing a trusting relationship with the client. Caring touch can improve a client's self-esteem, sense of well-being, and faith.[23]
Assess which needs can be met in the client's current circumstance, and which needs are most important to the client. Assist the client in meeting those needs (pastoral consult, visitors from faith community) as health status allows.	Assists the nurse in determining the client's priorities and preferences.
Encourage the client to seek forgiveness or forgive others.	Through forgiveness, older adults can discover new meaning and continue the development of the spiritual self.[23]
Offer to pray, meditate, or read spiritual text with the client, or arrange for another member of the health-care team to do so while respecting the client's time for quietness and prayer.	Supports the client's existing spirituality.[23]

RELIGIOSITY, RISK FOR IMPAIRED

DEFINITION[4]

At risk for an impaired ability to exercise reliance on religious beliefs and/or participate in rituals of a particular faith tradition

RELATED FACTORS[4]

A. Physical
1. Illness/hospitalization
2. Pain

B. Psychological
1. Ineffective support/coping/caregiving
2. Depression
3. Lack of security

C. Sociocultural
1. Lack of social interaction
2. Cultural barrier to practicing religion
3. Social isolation

D. Spiritual
Suffering

E. Environmental
1. Lack of transportation
2. Environmental barriers to practicing religion

F. Developmental
Life transitions

RELATED CLINICAL CONCERNS

1. Victims of disasters
2. Pain

3. Physical or mental ability to function independently
4. Restrictive medical regime
5. Immobility
6. Loss of senses, such as a hearing loss

EXPECTED OUTCOME

The patient and/or family will be able to express needs concerning religious practices by [date].

The patient and/or family will be able to accept an alternative plan for certain religious practices by [date].

TARGET DATES

A target date of 1 to 2 days is appropriate. The sooner the risk is addressed the sooner the patient and or family can move on to enhanced religiosity.

 Have You Selected the Correct Diagnosis?

Impaired Religiosity
Impaired Religiosity would be the correct diagnosis if the patient and family has no interest in or is angry, and refuses to discuss or practice any religious rites.

Risk for Impaired Religiosity
Risk for Impaired Religiosity would be correct when a patient or family comes into "harms way" and wishes to still practice their religious rites. However, they cannot achieve this without assistance or finding alternative methods for practicing, because of the mental, physical, or social situation they find themselves in.

NURSING ACTIONS/INTERVENTIONS WITH RATIONALES

Adult Health

Nursing actions for Adult Health are similar to those for Impaired Religiosity, but require the nurse to recognize the occurrence of factors that would potentially lead to the diagnosis of Impaired Religiosity.

Child Health

ACTIONS/INTERVENTIONS	RATIONALES
Ensure quiet and time for worship as child or family desire to degree possible.	
Maintain the child's room in a manner that permits presence of religious articles available in periphery vision of the child.	

(care plan continued on page 812)

NURSING ACTIONS/INTERVENTIONS WITH RATIONALES (continued from page 811)

Women's Health

ACTIONS/INTERVENTIONS	RATIONALES
Arrange for religious practices if requested and desired (e.g., baptism or other rituals).	
Contact a religious or cultural leader as requested by the mother or family.	
Provide support for the woman facing an unwanted pregnancy:	Let the client express his or her anger; sometimes he or she will refuse to practice religious rites or talk about "faith issues."[26–29]
Encourage questions and verbalization of the patient's life expectations by providing at least 15 minutes of one-to-one time at least twice a day at [times].	Provides information about choices and consequences of each choice, which can assist with decision making. Gives long-term support by providing referrals.
Provide information on options available to the patient (e.g., adoption, abortion, or keeping the baby).	Not making judgments, but providing factual information can provide support for the client and help him or her retain his or her faith and progress to enhanced religiosity and enhanced spiritual well-being.[28,30]
Assist the patient in identifying lifestyle adjustments that each decision could entail (e.g., dealing with guilt or finances).	
Involve significant others and include the patient's religious or cultural leader, if so desired by the patient, in discussion and problem-solving activities regarding lifestyle adjustments.	

Mental Health

Refer to Mental Health nursing actions for Impaired Religiosity.

Gerontic Health

Refer to Gerontic Health nursing actions for Impaired Religiosity.

Home Health/Community Health

Refer to Home Health nursing actins for Impaired Religiosity.

SPIRITUAL DISTRESS

DEFINITION[4]

Impaired ability to experience and integrate meaning and purpose in life through a person's connectedness with self, other, art, music, literature, nature, or a power greater than oneself

DEFINING CHARACTERISTICS[4]

A. Connections to Self
   1. Express lack of:
      a. Hope
      b. Meaning and purpose in life
      c. Peace/serenity

d. Acceptance
e. Love
f. Forgiveness of self
g. Courage
2. Anger
3. Guilt
4. Poor Coping

B. Connections with Others
1. Refuses interactions with spiritual leaders
2. Refuses interactions with friends, family
3. Verbalizes being separated from their support system
4. Expresses alienation

C. Connections with Art, Music, Literature, Nature
1. Inability to express previous state of creativity (singing/listening to music/writing)
2. No interest in nature
3. No interest in reading spiritual literature

D. Connections with a Power Greater than Self
1. Inability to pray
2. Inability to participate in religious activities
3. Expresses being abandoned by or having anger toward God
4. Inability to experience the transcendent
5. Requests to see a religious leader
6. Sudden changes in spiritual practices
7. Inability to be introspective/inward turning
8. Expresses being without hope, suffering

RELATED FACTORS[4]

1. Self-alienation
2. Loneliness/social alienation
3. Anxiety
4. Sociocultural deprivation
5. Death and dying of self or others
6. Pain
7. Life change
8. Chronic illness of self or others

RELATED CLINICAL CONCERNS

1. Chronic illnesses, for example, rheumatoid arthritis or multiple sclerosis
2. Terminal illness, such as cancer
3. Mental retardation
4. Burns or scaring of body
5. Loss of limbs

6. Sudden infant death syndrome (SIDS)
7. Stillbirth, fetal demise, or miscarriage
8. Infertility

EXPECTED OUTCOME

Will verbalize concerns and feelings by [date].

Will describe at least [number] persons they feel comfortable in confiding and speaking with by [date].

TARGET DATES

Because of the largely subconscious nature of spiritual beliefs and values, it is recommended the target date be at least 5 days from the date of diagnosis.

 Have You Selected the Correct Diagnosis?

Ineffective Individual Coping
Many individuals use religion or beliefs as a means of bargaining in unwanted life situations, or denying their role in the situation by blaming it on a superior being. Others will find their source of strength and hope in their beliefs in a superior being or God, and are able to live fully functional lives despite physical handicaps. If the patient mentions any of the defining characteristics of this diagnosis then the primary diagnosis is Spiritual Distress, which must be attended to before trying to intervene for Ineffective Individual Coping.

Risk for Spiritual Distress
Life events often place individuals in situations where they begin to question their beliefs, values, and the meaning and purpose of life. These events can affect individuals or groups of people. For instance, during the blitzkreig over England before America's entry into World War II, Winston Churchill stated; "These are times which try men's souls." Many groups of people were at risk for spiritual distress just as in more modern times, when many groups of people were at risk for spiritual distress after 9/11. Some people fought back, kept going, and actually enhanced their spiritually, even though they were at risk for a while. Some who gave up, were totally overwhelmed, became chronically depressed, or totally denied their faith and the existence of a Superior Being reverted to Spiritual Distress. *But until that point in time when they made the decision of which way to react,* they were only at risk for Spiritual Distress.

NURSING ACTIONS/INTERVENTIONS WITH RATIONALES

Adult Health

ACTIONS/INTERVENTIONS	RATIONALES
Demonstrate respect for and acceptance of the patient's values, beliefs, and doubts about spiritual system by not judging, moralizing, or arguing.	Spiritual values and beliefs are highly personal. When faced with life altering events it is natural to question and blame. Asking "Why me" and feeling they have been deserted by a Higher Being can be temporary or permanent. A nurse's attitude can positively or negatively influence the therapeutic relationship and support the patient in time of need.[1,6,7]
Encourage conversation that assists patient in sorting out spiritual, mental, and physical concerns.	Such conversation without judgment on the part of the health-care provider can assist the patient and family begin to learn how to deal with life events and to decide what sort of, if any, spiritual or religious intervention he or she would wish to have.[6]
Arrange visits from support persons (e.g., chaplain, pastor, rabbi, priest, or prayer group), if requested by the patient.	Each offers good listening skills that promote comfort and reduce anxiety and could engage patient in conversation that assists the patient in sorting out spiritual, mental, and physical concerns.
Plan to spend at least 15 minutes twice a day at [times] with the patient to allow verbalization, questioning, counseling, and support on a one-to-one basis.	Promotes mutual sharing, and builds a trusting relationship.
Assist the patient to develop problem-solving behavior through practice of problem-solving techniques at least twice daily at [times] during hospitalization.	Involves the patient in self-management activities. Increases motivation.

Child Health

In addition to the following, this pattern is basically related to the Adult Health or Women's Health pattern as noted, with appropriate allowance for developmental capacity.

ACTIONS/INTERVENTIONS	RATIONALES
Assess for situational related factors including: actual onset of life-limiting situation, barriers to usual spiritual enjoyment, or inability to express how the problem is perceived.	Offers a base for planning that allows support of the child or the parents (caregivers) of the child as needed.
Seek input from appropriate paraprofessionals including child life specialist, psychiatric nurse, clergy person, ethicist and counselor, as well as the primary care nurse.	Provides a developmental approach to satisfy child's need.
Provide input with child, family, and team for best ways to incorporate the plan into child's daily routine in light of current health status.	Assists the family unit to value and learn how to make the plan a part of the child's daily routine.
Respect and honor the child's wishes within realm of what is possible.	Offers respect for choice of expressed spirituality, with cues for availability of articles and environment suited to enhanced potential for spirituality.
Establish ways to acknowledge the ways the plan can assist in acceptance of current situation.	
Provide clear and honest communication to answer child's questions, while also honoring family's values.	Promotes a trusting relationship.
*It is ideal to have the same primary care nurses involved in times of need for close communication and times of distress.	

Women's Health

ACTIONS/INTERVENTIONS	RATIONALES
Allow the mother and family to express feelings about the less-than-perfect pregnancy outcomes.[26,27]	Allows the family to express their feelings and the health-care provider to support and facilitate patient and family coping with unexpected outcomes of pregnancy. Guilt, loneliness, lack of emotions and an inability to take interest in life, family and former values or beliefs can be signs of spiritual distress and Postpartum Depression.[27]
Stillborn or infant death: • Provide time for the mother and family to see, hold, and take pictures of the infant if so desired. • Provide quiet, private place where the mother and family can be with the infant. • Refer to appropriate support groups within the community. • Do legacy building, for example, cap, bracelets, certificate of life (acknowledgement of baby), and footprints.[26]	Contact religious or cultural leader as requested by the mother or family. Positive spiritual perspectives has been shown to be related to satisfaction with social support from others during pregnancy.[28]
Less-than-perfect baby, for example, sick baby or infant with anomaly[26,27]: • Provide a quiet, private place for the mother and family to visit with the infant. • Encourage verbalization of fears and asking of any question by providing time for one-to-one interactions at least twice a day at [times]. • Encourage touching and holding of the infant by the mother and family. • Teach methods of caring for the infant (e.g., special feeding techniques). • Teach methods of coping with the stress connected with caring for the infant (e.g., planned alone time for relaxation techniques). • Assign one staff member to care for both the mother and infant. • Provide the patient with information and referrals to appropriate support groups and community agencies. If requested, contact religious or cultural leader.	Provides consistency and encourages the mother and family to build trust with provider of care. Provides support and information and assists with coping.
Assist the patient facing gynecologic surgery to express her perceptions of lifestyle adjustments: • Provide an explanation of the surgical procedure and perioperative nursing care. • Provide factual information as to physiologic and psychological reactions she may experience. • Allow the patient to grieve the loss of body image (e.g., inability to have a child). • Involve significant others in discussion and problem-solving activities regarding life cycle changes that could affect self-concept and interpersonal relationships (e.g., hot flashes, sexual relationships, or ability to have children).	Provides support and give preoperative information, which assists with postoperative recovery. Although sexuality is not changed due to hysterectomy or mastectomy, some women have problems that cannot be accounted for physically. Depression, fear of rejection, and changed body image may occur and can result in loss of sexual drive and spiritual distress.[30]

(care plan continued on page 816)

NURSING ACTIONS/INTERVENTIONS WITH RATIONALES (continued from page 815)

Mental Health

ACTIONS/INTERVENTIONS	RATIONALES
Remove items from the environment that increase problem behavior (list specific items for each client, e.g., Bible or religious pictures).	The environment will assist the client in demonstrating appropriate coping behaviors, which increases opportunities for succeeding with new coping behaviors. Success provides reinforcement, which encourages positive behavior and enhances self-esteem. Faith and involvement in spiritual activities when practices are not dogmatic and involvement is seen as a source of solace and support.[22]
Restrict visitors who increase problem behavior for the client. Discuss with the family and other frequent visitors the necessity of not discussing the problem ideas with the client.	Promotes the client's sense of control.
Request consultation from leader of client's faith community who has had education and experience in assisting clients to cope with this type of spiritual distress.	Meets the client's spiritual needs in a constructive manner. Spiritual messages that indicate mental illness is a punishment or that one is being abandoned by a source of spiritual power can increase spiritual distress.[22]
Do not discuss with the client belief systems that are related to problem behavior. (Specifically state what that content is here.)	These discussions only serve to reinforce the client's misconceptions and decrease their spiritual well-being.
Do not argue with the client about spiritual belief system or behaviors that evolve from this system.	This would reinforce the dysfunctional belief system that promotes the client's distress.
Do not joke with the client about belief system or behavior that evolves from this system.	Protects the client's self-esteem at a time when it is most vulnerable.
Spend time with the client when themes of conversation are not related to the problem behavior.	Presence of the nurse, at this time, provides reinforcement for this behavior, which encourages the positive behavior and enhances self-esteem.
Limit topics of conversation to daily activities or situations that do not include problematic spiritual beliefs.	Environmental structure helps turn the client focus away from problem areas, which supports his or her efforts to enlist more appropriate coping behaviors.
Provide activities that decrease client time alone to reflect on the problem beliefs. Suggested activities include: • Physical exercise such as walks, bicycle riding, swimming, or exercise classes. • Group activities such as board games, meal preparation, sports, or arts and crafts.	Provides the client with opportunities to practice alternative coping behaviors in a supportive environment.
Facilitate positive spiritual connections by:	Spirituality can support emotional healing when it is expressed in the discovery of the true self, through caring relationships, giving thanks, and embracing grace. Higher levels of spirituality have been associated with lower anxiety and lower risk of suicide.[22]
• Spending [number] minutes per [shift/day] discussing client's previously used strengths for solace and hope. Elicit the client's perceptions of what is needed, do not suggest activities, beliefs.	Being with the client can being the process of spiritual connection and can mediate interventions at the spiritual level. It is important for nurse to remain self-aware and neutral to diminish coercion and countertransference. These interactions must be guided by the client's values and understandings, and not used as an opportunity to share the nurse's belief system. Seek supervision if having difficulty determining appropriate boundaries for the therapeutic relationship.[22]

ACTIONS/INTERVENTIONS	RATIONALES
• Facilitating the client's connections with faith communities he or she has found supportive in the past.	Can facilitate client's movement from existential loneliness when the connection is client focused. When spiritual experiences are viewed as a source of solace and strength they can have a positive effect on mental health.[22]
• Facilitating the client's involvement in supportive rituals that bring solace and hope.	Positive spiritual involvement can contribute to emotional well-being.[22]
• Facilitating client-initiated and -led expressions of spirituality by sitting with them during this process. This could include prayer, meditation, guided imagery, and other activities that connect persons to inner sources of solace and hope.	Before expression of spirituality is initiated, assess meaning this has to client to validate that this will be a source of solace and hope. Client-initiated and led prayer diminishes the risk of inadvertent provider coercion.[22] Use meditation and guided imagery cautiously with clients who are experiencing sensory-perceptual alternations, especially when this has negative content. It may be difficult for the client to control the negative content during these activities.
• Referring to health-care providers, or a member of the client's spiritual network who specialize in spirituality and have an understanding of mental health and spirituality, for in-depth spiritual counseling and community support.	Provides ongoing support for client upon discharge.[22]

Gerontic Health

ACTIONS/INTERVENTIONS	RATIONALES
Establish a therapeutic relationship with the client through active listening, nonjudgmental behaviors, and offering as much time as is needed.	A therapeutic relationship must be established for the client to continue to share concerns.
Discuss with the client the factors or events that are contributing to spiritual distress and can be addressed (anxiety, loneliness, pain, life changes).	Assessment of the client's concerns and priorities is the first step toward resolution.
Involve the client in addressing the factors contributing to the distress than can be addressed.	Personal involvement in the process increases the likelihood of successful resolution.
Tend to the client's basic needs, particularly pain.	Addresses one of the risk factors for the problem.
Offer social activities as appropriate for the client's health status.	Addresses one of the risk factors for the problem.

Home Health/Community Health

ACTIONS/INTERVENTIONS	RATIONALES
Establish a therapeutic relationship with the client and family through active listening, nonjudgmental behaviors, and offering as much time as is needed.	A therapeutic relationship must be established for the client and family to continue to share concerns.
Discuss with the client and family the factors or events that are contributing to spiritual distress and can be addressed (anxiety, loneliness, pain, life changes).	Assessment of the client and family's concerns and priorities is the first step toward resolution.
Involve the client and family in addressing the factors contributing to the distress that can be addressed.	Personal involvement in the process increases the likelihood of successful resolution.
Personal involvement in the process increases the likelihood of successful resolution.	Assist the client and family in making lifestyle and home adjustments that are needed to facilitate resolution of the distress:

(care plan continued on page 818)

NURSING ACTIONS/INTERVENTIONS WITH RATIONALES (continued from page 817)	
Mental Health	
ACTIONS/INTERVENTIONS	RATIONALES
• Support groups • Visits from spiritual leaders • scheduled time for the client to be outside • Scheduled times for visitors Consult with, or refer to, assistive services as indicated.	Effective use of existing community resources.

SPIRITUAL DISTRESS, RISK FOR

DEFINITION[4]

At risk for an impaired ability to experience and integrate meaning and purpose in life through a person's connectedness with self, other persons, art, music, literature, nature, and/or a power greater than oneself

DEFINING CHARACTERISTICS[4]

None given.

RELATED RISK FACTORS[4]

A. Physical
1. Physical illness
2. Substance abuse/excessive drinking
3. Chronic illness

B. Psychosocial
1. Low self-esteem
2. Depression
3. Anxiety
4. Stress
5. Poor relationships
6. Separate from support systems
7. Blocks to experiencing love
8. Inability to forgive
9. Loss
10. Racial/cultural conflict
11. Change in religious rituals
12. Change in spiritual practices

C. Developmental
1. Life change
2. Developmental life changes

D. Environmental
1. Environmental changes
2. Natural disasters

RELATED CLINICAL CONCERNS

1. Potential diagnosis of terminal illness such as cancer
2. Potential diagnosis of chronic illnesses
3. Accident or injury that could potentially lead to change in physical or mental status
4. Accident or injury that could potentially lead to change in body image
5. Potential for less than perfect outcome for pregnancy
6. Divorce, loss of spouse or other life changing event(s)

EXPECTED OUTCOMES

Will describe at least [number] support systems to use when spiritual conflict arises by [date].

TARGET DATES

Because of the largely subconscious nature of spiritual beliefs and values, it is recommended the target date be at least 5 days from the date of diagnosis.

 Have You Selected the Correct Diagnosis?

Ineffective Individual Coping
Many individuals use religion or beliefs as a means of bargaining in unwanted life situations or denying their role in the situation by blaming it on a superior being. Others will find their source of strength and hope from their beliefs in a superior being or God and are able to live fully functional lives despite physical handicaps. If the patient mentions any of the defining characteristics of this diagnosis, then the primary diagnosis is Spiritual Distress, which must be attended to before trying to intervene for Ineffective Individual Coping.

Impaired Religiosity
If patients and families are unable because of the situation, disease, and/or treatment to practice religious rites, such as participate in communion or follow a special diet (Kosher), and they seek help or verbalize frustration with the situation. If they do not view this situation as a crisis or concern about finding meaning or purpose in life then risk for impaired religiosity is the correct diagnosis.

Spiritual Distress
When a person or family learn about a terminal diagnosis or a permanent life change, question their faith and beliefs and lose their purpose in life. The health care provider often hears questions such as , "What did I do wrong?" or "Why me?" If the patient and/or family refuse to be consoled or change their attitude, then spiritual distress is the correct diagnosis.

NURSING ACTIONS/INTERVENTIONS WITH RATIONALES

Adult Health

ACTIONS/INTERVENTIONS	RATIONALES
Assist the patient to articulate his or her values, particularly in relation to health and illness, through the use of value clarification techniques such as sentence completion, rank-ordering exercises, and completion of health-value scales.	Clarifies values and beliefs and helps the patient understand impact of values and beliefs on health and illness.
Demonstrate respect for and acceptance of the patient's values and spiritual system.	Spiritual values and beliefs are highly personal. A nurse's attitude can positively or negatively influence the therapeutic relationship.[1,6]
Adapt nursing therapeutics as necessary to incorporate values and religious beliefs, e.g., in regard to diet, administration of blood or blood products, or religious rites.	Maintains and respects the patient's preferences during hospitalization.
Arrange for religious rites and practices as needed (e.g., baptism, confession, or communion).	Provides comfort for the patient and allows for expression of religious practices. Shows respect for the patient's spiritual values and needs.[31]
Coordinate visits from support persons (e.g., chaplain, pastor, rabbi, priest, or prayer group, as needed).	Each offers good listening skills that promote comfort and reduce anxiety. Spiritual leader can assure patient. They are okay to consult, even when the patient is unable to practice certain rites.[1]
Encourage the family to bring significant symbols to the patient (e.g., Bible, rosary, or icons, as needed).	Promotes comfort.
Spend at least 15 minutes twice a day at [times] with the patient to allow verbalization, questioning, counseling, and support on a one-to-one basis.	Promotes mutual sharing and builds a trusting relationship.

Child Health

In addition to the following, this pattern is basically related to the Adult Health or Women's Health pattern as noted with appropriate allowance for developmental capacity.

ACTIONS/INTERVENTIONS	RATIONALES
Assess for situational related factors including: actual onset of life limiting situation, barriers to usual spiritual enjoyment, or inability to express how the problem is perceived.	Offers a base for planning.
Seek input from appropriate paraprofessionals including child life specialist, psychiatric nurse, clergy person, counselor, and primary care nurse; if possible, ethicist also advisable.	Provides developmental approach to satisfy child's need.
Provide input with the child, family, and health-care team for best ways to incorporate the plan into the child's daily routine in light of current health status.	Values how to make the plan a part of the child's daily routine.
Respect and honor the child's wishes within realm of what is possible. • Ensure quiet and time for worship as child or family desire to the degree possible. • Establish ways to acknowledge the ways the plan can assist in acceptance of the current situation.	Offers respect for choice of expressed spirituality with cues for availability of articles and environment suited to enhanced potential for spirituality.[24]

(care plan continued on page 820)

NURSING ACTIONS/INTERVENTIONS WITH RATIONALES (continued from page 819)	

Mental Health

ACTIONS/INTERVENTIONS	RATIONALES
• Maintain the child's room in a manner that permits presence of religious articles available in periphery of the child.	
Provide clear and honest communication to answer the child's questions while also honoring family's values.	Promotes a trusting relationship.[24]
*It is ideal to have the same primary care nurses involved in times of need for close communication and times of distress.	

Women's Health

ACTIONS/INTERVENTIONS	RATIONALES
Allow the mother and family to express feelings at the less-than-perfect pregnancy outcome[26,29]:	Allows the family to receive religious and social support as a means of coping.
• Stillborn or infant death:	
• Provide time for the mother and family to see, hold, and take pictures of the infant if so desired.	
• Provide quiet, private place where the mother and family can be with the infant.	
• Arrange for religious practices requested (e.g., baptism or other rituals).	
• Contact religious or cultural leader as requested by the mother or family.	
• Refer to appropriate support groups within the community.	
• Do legacy building (e.g., cap, bracelets, certificate of life, and footprints).[26]	
• Spontaneous abortion:	
• Provide the patient with factual information regarding the etiology of spontaneous abortion.	Assists in reducing guilt, blame, etc.
• Encourage verbal expressions of grief.	
• Allow expression of feelings such as anger.	
• Do legacy building (e.g., cap, bracelets, certificate of life, and footprints).[26]	
• Provide information on miscarriage and grief.	
• Contact a religious or cultural leader as requested by the patient.	
• Provide referrals to appropriate support groups within the community.	Provides information and support for the family.
• Less-than-perfect baby (e.g., sick baby or infant with anomaly)[29]:	
• Provide a quiet, private place for the mother and family to visit with the infant.	
• Encourage verbalization of fears and asking of any question by providing time for one-to-one interactions at least twice a day at [times].	
• Encourage touching and holding of the infant by the mother and family.	
• Teach methods of caring for the infant (e.g., special feeding techniques).	

ACTIONS/INTERVENTIONS	RATIONALES
• Teach methods of coping with the stress connected with caring for the infant (e.g., planned alone time for relaxation techniques).	
• Assign one staff member to care for both the mother and infant.	
• Contact religious or cultural leader as requested by the mother or family.	Encourage religious rites if requested and appropriate. For example, pin religious medal on baby's clothing.
• Provide the patient with information and referrals to appropriate support groups and community agencies.	Provides support and information, and assists with coping.
Provide support for the woman facing an unwanted pregnancy:	
• Encourage questions and verbalization of the patient's life expectations by providing at least 15 minutes of one-to-one time at least twice a day at [times].	Provides information about choices and consequences of each choice, which can assist with decision making. Gives long-term support by providing referrals.
• Provide information on options available to the patient (e.g., adoption, abortion, or keeping the baby).	
• Assist the patient in identifying lifestyle adjustments that each decision could entail (e.g., dealing with guilt or finances).	
• Involve significant others and include the patient's religious or cultural leader, if so desired by the patient, in discussion and problem-solving activities regarding lifestyle adjustments.	
Assist the patient facing gynecologic surgery to express her perceptions of lifestyle adjustments:	Provides support and gives preoperative information, which assist with postoperative recovery.
• Provide explanation of surgical procedure and perioperative nursing care.	
• Provide factual information as to physiologic and psychological reactions she may experience.	
• Allow the patient to grieve loss of body image (e.g., inability to have a child).	
• Involve significant others in discussion and problem-solving activities regarding life cycle changes that could affect self-concept and interpersonal relationships (e.g., hot flashes, sexual relationships, or ability to have children).	
Participate with the patient in religious support activities (e.g., praying or reading religious literature aloud).	Demonstrates visible support for the role these activities play in the patient's life.

Mental Health

ACTIONS/INTERVENTIONS	RATIONALES
Remove items from the environment that increase problem behavior (list specific items for each client, e.g., Bible or religious pictures).	Environment will assist the client in demonstrating appropriate coping behaviors, which increases opportunities for succeeding with new coping behaviors. Success provides reinforcement, which encourages positive behavior and enhances self-esteem.
Restrict visitors who increase problem behavior for the client. Discuss with the family and other frequent visitors the necessity of not discussing the problem ideas with the client.	Promotes the client's sense of control.

(care plan continued on page 822)

NURSING ACTIONS/INTERVENTIONS WITH RATIONALES (continued from page 821)

Mental Health

ACTIONS/INTERVENTIONS	RATIONALES
Request consultation from religious leader who has had education and experience in assisting clients to cope with this type of spiritual distress.	
Do not discuss with the client belief systems that are related to problem behavior. [Specifically state what that content is here.]	Meets the client's spiritual needs in a constructive manner.
Do not argue with the client about religious belief system or behaviors that evolve from this system.	These discussions only serve to reinforce the client's misconceptions.
Do not joke with the client about belief system or behavior that evolves from this system.	This would reinforce the dysfunctional belief system.
Spend time with the client when themes of conversation are not related to the problem behavior.	Protects the client's self-esteem at a time when it is most vulnerable.
Limit topics of conversation to daily activities or situations that do not include religious beliefs.	Presence of the nurse, at this time, provides reinforcement for this behavior, which encourages the positive behavior and enhances self-esteem.
Provide activities that decrease client time alone to reflect on the problem beliefs. Suggested activities include:	Environmental structure helps the client focus away from problem areas, which supports his or her efforts to enlist more appropriate coping behaviors.
• Physical exercise such as walks, bicycle riding, swimming, or exercise classes	Provides the client with opportunities to practice alternative coping behaviors in a supportive environment.
• Group activities such as board games, meal preparation, sports, or arts and crafts	
Facilitate positive spiritual connections by:	Spirituality can support emotional healing when it is expressed in the discovery of the true self, through caring relationships, giving thanks, and embracing grace. Higher levels of spirituality have been associated with lower anxiety and lower risk of suicide.[22]
• Spending [number] minutes per [shift/day] discussing client's previously used strengths for solace and hope. Elicit the client's perceptions of what is needed; do not suggest activities, beliefs. Note support from nursing needed to facilitate the client's meeting spiritual needs.	Being with the client can being the process of spiritual connection and can mediate interventions at the spiritual level. It is important for nurse to remain self-aware and neutral to diminish coercion and countertransference. These interactions must be guided by client's values and understandings and not used as an opportunity to share the nurse's belief system. Seek supervision if having difficulty determining appropriate boundaries for the therapeutic relationship.[22]
• Facilitate the client's connections with faith communities he or she has found supportive in the past.	Can facilitate client's movement from existential loneliness when the connection is client focused. When spiritual experiences are viewed as a source of solace and strength they can have a positive effect on mental health.[22]
• Facilitate the client's involvement in supportive rituals that bring solace and hope	Positive spiritual involvement can contribute to emotional well-being.[22]

ACTIONS/INTERVENTIONS	RATIONALES
• Facilitate client-initiated and -led expressions of spirituality by sitting with them during this process. This could include prayer, meditation, guided imagery, listening to music and other activities that connect persons to inner sources of solace and hope.	Before expression of spirituality is initiated assess meaning this has to client to validate that this will be a source of solace and hope. Client initiated and led prayer diminishes the risk of inadvertent provider coercion.[39] Use meditation and guided imagery cautiously with clients who are experiencing sensory-perceptual alternations, especially when this has negative content. It may be difficult for the client to control the negative content during these activities.
• Refer to health-care providers or a member of the client's spiritual network who specialize in spirituality and have an understanding of mental health and spirituality for in-depth spiritual counseling and community support.	Provides ongoing support for the client upon discharge.[22]

Gerontic Health

ACTIONS/INTERVENTIONS	RATIONALES
Engage in active listening with the client by: • Presence (creating a relationship with sincere communication) • Use of therapeutic/caring touch as tolerated by client • Facilitating the client's search for meaning • Facilitating reminiscence	This assists the nurse in collecting data about client status and establishing a trusting relationship with the client. Caring touch can improve a client's self-esteem, sense of well-being, and faith.[23]
Assess which needs can be met in the client's current circumstance, and which needs are most important to the client. Assist the client in meeting those needs (pastoral consult, visitors from church) as health status allows.	Assists the nurse in determining the client's priorities and preferences.
Encourage the client to seek forgiveness or to forgive others.	Through forgiveness, older adults can discover new meaning and continue the development of the spiritual self.[23]
Offer to pray, meditate, or read spiritual text with the client or arrange for another member of the health-care team to do so while respecting the client's time for quietness and prayer.	Supports the client's existing spirituality.[23]

Home Health/Community Health

ACTIONS/INTERVENTIONS	RATIONALES
Engage in active listening with the client by: • Presence (creating a relationship with sincere communication) • Use of therapeutic/caring touch as tolerated by client • Facilitating the client's search for meaning • Facilitating reminiscence	This assists the nurse in collecting data about client status and establishing a trusting relationship with the client. Caring touch can improve a client's self-esteem, sense of well-being, and faith.[23]
Assess which needs can be met in the client's current circumstance, and which needs are most important to the client. Assist the client in meeting those needs (pastoral consult, visitors from church) as health status allows.	Assists the nurse in determining the client's priorities and preferences.

(care plan continued on page 824)

NURSING ACTIONS/INTERVENTIONS WITH RATIONALES (continued from page 823)

Mental Health

ACTIONS/INTERVENTIONS	RATIONALES
Encourage the client to seek forgiveness or to forgive others.	Through forgiveness, older adults can discover new meaning and continue the development of the spiritual self.[23]
Offer to pray, meditate, or read spiritual text with the client or arrange for another member of the health care team to do so while respecting the client's time for quietness and prayer.	Supports the client's existing spirituality.[23]

SPIRITUAL WELL-BEING, READINESS FOR ENHANCED

DEFINITION[4]

Ability to experience and integrate meaning and purpose in life through connectedness with self, others, art, music, literature, nature, or a power greater than oneself.

DEFINING CHARACTERISTICS[4]

A. Connections to Self
  1. Desire for enhanced:
     a. Hope
     b. Meaning and purpose in life
     c. Peace/serenity
     d. Acceptance
     e. Surrender
     f. Love
     g. Forgiveness of self
     h. Satisfying philosophy of life
     i. Joy
     j. Courage
  2. Heightened coping
  3. Meditation
B. Connections with Others
  1. Provides service to others.
  2. Requests interactions with spiritual leaders.
  3. Requests forgiveness of others.
  4. Requests interactions with friends, family.
C. Connections with Art, Music, Literature, Nature
  1. Displays creative energy (e.g., writing, poetry).
  2. Sings/listens to music.
  3. Reads spiritual literature.
  4. Spends time outdoors.
D. Connections with Power Greater than Self
  1. Prays.
  2. Reports mystical experiences.
  3. Participates in religious activities.
  4. Expresses reverence, awe.
1. **Inner Strengths**: A sense of awareness, self-consciousness, sacred source, unifying force, inner core, and transcendence

2. **Unfolding Mystery**: One's experience about life's purpose and meaning, mystery, uncertainty, and struggles
3. **Harmonious Interconnectedness**: Harmony, relatedness, and connectedness with self, others, Higher Power or God, and the environment

RELATED FACTORS[4]

None given.

RELATED CLINICAL CONCERNS

1. Any terminal diagnosis
2. Any chronic disease diagnosis
3. Any life change
4. Moving from one life stage to another

EXPECTED OUTCOME

Will identify practices that bring strength and hope by [date].
  Will participate to extent possible, in religious rites that provide comfort and meaning by [date].

TARGET DATES

Because of the subconscious and individual nature of spiritual beliefs and practices, it is recommended the target date be at least 5 to 7 days from the date of diagnosis.

 Have You Selected the Correct Diagnosis?

Readiness for Enhanced Coping
Individuals under stress use different patterns of cognitive and behavioral efforts to manage disruptions in their lives. They can even use spiritual resources to allow themselves to achieve enhanced coping. However, it is only when they embrace their sense of spiritual identity that they move beyond coping to promote resiliency and enhance their spiritual well-being.[10]

Readiness for Enhanced Religiosity
Is the correct diagnosis in the case of the patient who because of mental or physical illness cannot participate in religious rites or practices; but does not express spiritual concern or crisis and only wants assistance to be able to participate in religious rituals. Often the practice of or the ability to participate in religious rituals must be dealt with first as they some-

times have great meaning to the individual and their ultimate connectiveness to the meaning and purpose of life. If the patient or family express any of the characteristics of spirituality as central to their beliefs and faith and that they use religiosity to achieve peace, harmony, and a sense of balance in life, then the diagnosis is enhanced spiritual well-being.

NURSING ACTIONS/INTERVENTIONS WITH RATIONALES

Adult Health

ACTIONS/INTERVENTIONS	RATIONALES
Establish a trusting relationship. Inquire about religion, values, relationships, transcendence, affective feeling, communication, and spiritual practices.	A trusting relationship assists the patient to express his or her feelings to the nurse. Spirituality is expressed in all these areas.[32]
Demonstrate compassion and acceptance. Be sensitive to the patient's spiritual needs.	Spiritual nursing care needs to be based on a more universal concept of inspiring rather than focusing around religious concepts.[33] However, depending on the patient's beliefs, religious concepts may be integral to care.
Show respect and support of the patient's beliefs and values.[24]	Shows respect and support of the patient's beliefs and values.[29]
Listen and talk to the patient. Facilitate reflection on hopes, dreams, God, faith, religious beliefs, social support, acceptance, health, forgiveness, hopelessness; provide privacy and personal time for reflection; assure presence of a Higher Being.	Solitude may liberate the spirit and lead to true knowledge of self, peace and joy, and an appreciation of life on a more profound level.[31]
Have the patient express his or her health and well-being through connectedness—intrapersonally, interpersonally, and transpersonally.	Expressions of self-transcendence may differ across individuals and life phases in general.[26] Interactions, both within the person and with the environment, generate conflicts that can provide the impetus for development through self-transcendence. Finding meaning in life is integral to human development and enhancement of health.[34]
Be present: touch, make eye contact, and use appropriate facial expressions.	
Assist the patient to meet own spiritual needs. Assist the patient to use spiritual resources to meet personal situation.	
Support and enhance the patient's spirituality by convening family, clergy, and other support persons.	
Refer to chaplain, clergy, or spiritual advisor. Participate in spiritual practices initiated by the patient as appropriate	
If appropriate, allow the patient to provide spiritual support for and with other patients.	Provides an expansion of personal boundaries through connectedness. Provides a sense of wholeness and well-being. Person may be "ill," yet still be "healthy" in terms of spirituality, as spirituality provides the patient with the capacity for health through transcendence of ordinary boundaries and various modes of connectedness.[35]

(care plan continued on page 826)

NURSING ACTIONS/INTERVENTIONS WITH RATIONALES (continued from page 825)

Adult Health

ACTIONS/INTERVENTIONS	RATIONALES
Support family and friends' expression of love and support for the patient	Shows respect and support of the patient's beliefs and values.[33]
Advocate for the patient's spiritual beliefs with the health team.	Significant symbols can be a source of consolation and spiritual support.[36]
Consider the patient's spiritual beliefs and values. When developing plan of care with the health-care team.[29]	A patient's spiritual needs are complex and individual.[33]
Allow and support the patient's to keeping significant symbols nearby.	Awareness of the nurse's own feelings is helpful in guiding and/or controlling his or her actions.[33]
Inform the patient and family where chapel or prayer room is located.	
Determine own values and spirituality.	

Child Health

This pattern would incorporate the applicable components of the adult and women's components in a developmentally appropriate manner in addition to the following:

ACTIONS/INTERVENTIONS	RATIONALES
Assess for cues to confirm readiness to engage in enhanced spirituality from child and/or parents:	Offers a base for considering a plan.
• Child or family may verbalize willingness and acceptance of status.	
• Honor the practice of desired plan within daily routine.	Values the plan.
• Allow for music, reading, or play as appropriate with spiritual focus.	
• Allow quiet time without undue interruptions.	
• Respect privacy during times of spiritual expression or participate according to nurse's and family's mutual comfort.	
Determine need for visitation or referral to clergypersons or other support persons.	Provides anticipatory guidance.[24]
Help the child and/or family to determine how to continue to practice the plan.	

Women's Health

ACTIONS/INTERVENTIONS	RATIONALES
Allow the woman and her family to direct the spiritual care needed when possible.	By allowing the patient to express her own beliefs and values, strengths, and relationships, great insight into how health-care providers can provide high-quality care to the whole person can emerge. This can form the basis of care or support to patients.
Be available and willing to call whatever spiritual advisor the woman and family wish.	
Provide quiet, noninterruptive space for discussion, prayer, or communication with spiritual advisor.	
Allow the patient and family to participate in rituals as requested when possible.	

ACTIONS/INTERVENTIONS	RATIONALES
Be open to spiritual awareness in both the patient's life and in the nurse's own life. This could be accomplished through being a participant in a dream-telling group.[6,8,14]	
Assess how the patient views her "sense of fit" in her world.[7,9,37]	
Assess the patient's sources of strength and relationships that are important to her.[7,8,38]	Life satisfaction in older women is related to their engagement in social activities.[21,32]
Encourage the woman to give voice to her story.[7,8,38]	
Encourage time for self-reflection and making connections.	
	Older women cope and thrive in a variety of creative and productive ways. Research shows older women's lives are enhanced by volunteer activities and do-it-yourself tasks.[21,32]

Mental Health

Refer to Mental Health interventions for Spiritual Distress, Risk for.

Gerontic Health

ACTIONS/INTERVENTIONS	RATIONALES
Engage in active listening with the client by: • Presence (creating a relationship with sincere communication) • Use of therapeutic/caring touch as tolerated by client • Facilitating the client's search for meaning • Facilitating reminiscence	This assists the nurse in collecting data about client status and establishing a trusting relationship with the client. Caring touch can improve a client's self-esteem, sense of well-being, and faith.[23,39]
Assess which needs can be met in the client's current circumstance, and which needs are most important to the client. Assist the client in meeting those needs (pastoral consult, visitors from church) as health status allows.	Assists the nurse in determining the client's priorities and preferences.
Encourage the client to seek forgiveness or to forgive others.	Through forgiveness, older adults can discover new meaning and continue the development of the spiritual self.[23,40]
Offer to pray, meditate, or read spiritual text with the client or arrange for another member of the health-care team to do so while respecting the client's time for quietness and prayer.	Supports the client's existing spirituality.[23]

Home Health

ACTIONS/INTERVENTIONS	RATIONALES
Engage in active listening with the client by: • Presence (creating a relationship with sincere communication) • Use of therapeutic/caring touch as tolerated by client • Facilitating the client's search for meaning • Facilitating reminiscence	This assists the nurse in collecting data about client status and establishing a trusting relationship with the client. Caring touch can improve a client's self-esteem, sense of well-being, and faith.[23,39]

(care plan continued on page 828)

NURSING ACTIONS/INTERVENTIONS WITH RATIONALES (continued from page 827)

Home Health

ACTIONS/INTERVENTIONS	RATIONALES
Assess which needs can be met in the client's current circumstance, and which needs are most important to the client. Assist the client in meeting those needs (pastoral consult, visitors from church) as health status allows.	Assists the nurse in determining the client's priorities and preferences.
Encourage the client to seek forgiveness or to forgive others.	Through forgiveness, older adults can discover new meaning and continue the development of the spiritual self.[26]
Offer to pray, meditate, or read spiritual text with the client or arrange for another member of the health-care team to do so while respecting the client's time for quietness and prayer.	Supports the client's existing spirituality[23,39]

REFERENCES

1. Burkhart, L, and Solari-Twadell, A: Spirituality and religiousness: Differentiating the diagnoses through a review of the nursing literature, Nurs Diagn 12(2):45, 2001.
2. Gordon, M: Manual of Nursing Diagnosis. McGraw-Hill, New York, 2002.
3. Fowler, J: Stages of Faith: The Psychology of Human Development and the Quest for Meaning. Harper & Row, San Francisco, 1981.
4. North American Nursing Diagnosis Association: Nursing Diagnoses: Definitions and Classification, 2005–2006, North American Nursing Diagnosis Association, Philadelphia, 2005.
5. Fowler, J, and Keen, S: Life Maps: Conversations on the Journey of Faith. Word, Waco, Texas, 1978.
6. Cavendish, R, Konecny, L, Mitzeliotis, C, Russo, D, Luise, BK, Lanza, M, Medefindt, J, and McPartlan-Bajo, MA: Spiritual care activities of nurses using nursing interventions classification (NIC) labels. Int J Nurs Terminol Classif 14(4):113, 2003.
7. Larson, DB, and Larson, SB: Spirituality's potential relevance to physical and emotional health: A brief review of quantitative research. J Psychol Theol 31(1):37, 2003.
8. Corrine, BV, et al: The unheard voices of women: Spiritual interventions in maternal–child health. MCN Am J Matern Child Nurs 17:141, 1992.
9. Bayles, MD: The value of life - By what standard? Am J Nurs 80: 2226, 1980.
10. Poll, JB, and Smith, TB: The spiritual self: Toward a conceptualization of spiritual identity development. J Psychol Theol 31:68, 2003.
11. Potter, PA, and Perry, AG: Fundamentals of Nursing: Concepts, Process and Practice, ed 3. Mosby-Year Book, St. Louis, 1993.
12. Stoll, RI: Guidelines for spiritual assessment. Am J Nurs 79:1574, 1979.
13. Burns, PB: Elements of spirituality and Watson's theory of transpersonal caring: Expansion of focus. In Chinn, P (ed): Anthology on Caring: National League for Nursing, New York, 1991.
14. Dombeck, MG: Dream telling: A means of spiritual awareness. Holis Nurs Pract 9:37, 1995.
15. Clark, CC, et al: Spirituality: Integral to quality care. Holis Nurs Pract 5:67, 1991.
16. Nagi-Jackson, MG, and Buckhardt, MA: Spirituality: Cornerstone of holistic nursing practice. Holist Nurs Pract 3:18, 1990.
17. Chandler, JJ: Social Cognition A selective review of current research. In Overton, WF, and Gallagher, JM (eds): Knowledge and Development, Vol. 1: Research and Theory. Plenum Press,New York, 1977.
18. Erickson, EH: Childhood and Society. Triad/Paladin, St. Albans, England, 1978.
19. Kohlberg, L: The Philosophy of Moral Development. Harper & Row, San Francisco, 1981.
20. Norstrom-Ojeda, O, Ross, B, and Michonski, L: Mind-body breakthrough. FIRST 18(11):28, 2006.
21. Neill, CM, and Kahn, AS: The role of personal spirituality and religious social activity on the life satisfaction of older widowed women. Sex Roles J Res 40(3-4):319, 1999..
22. O'Reilly, M: Spirituality and mental health clients. J Psychosoc Nurs Ment Health Serv 42:44, 2004.
23. Gaskamp CD, Sutter R, Meraviglia M:Promoting spirituality in the older adult. University of Iowa Gerontological Nursing Interventions Research Center, Research Dissemination Core, Iowa City, IA, 2004, p50.
24. Hockenberry, MJ: Wong's Essentials of Pediatric Nursing, ed 7. CV Mosby, St. Louis, 2006.
25. Huebscher, R: Natural, alternative, and complementary health care. In Breslin, ET, and Lucas, VA (eds): Women's Health Nursing: Toward Evidence-Based Practice. WB Saunders, St. Louis, 2003.
26. Lanham, CC: Pregnancy After a Loss: A Guide to Pregnancy After a Miscarriage, Stillbirth, or Infant Death. Penguin Putnam, New York, 1997.
27. Vieria, T: When joy becomes grief. Lifelines 6(6):506, 2003.
28. Jesse, DE, and Reed, PG: Effects of spirituality and psychosocial well-being on health risk behaviors in Appalachian pregnant women. JOGNN J Obstet Gynecol Neonatal Nurs 33(6):739, 2004.
29. Cox, BE: What if? Coping with unexpected outcomes. Childbirth Instructor 1:24, 1991.
30. Sellers, JB: Health care for older women. In Breslin, ET, and Lucas, VA (eds): Women's Health Nursing: Toward Evidence-Based Practice, Saunders, St. Louis, 2003.
31. Taylor, EF, Amenta, M, and Highfield, M: Spiritual care practices of oncology nurses. Oncol Nurs Forum 22:31, 1995.
32. Maas, M, Buckwalter, K and Hardy, M: Nursing Diagnosis and Interventions for the Elderly. Addison-Wesley, Redwood City, CA, 1991.
33. Carson, VB: Spiritual Dimensions of Nursing Practice. WB Saunders, Philadelphia, 1989.
34. Broten, PS: Spiritual care given by nurses and spiritual well being of terminally ill cancer patients (Dissertation). Western Michigan University, 1991.
35. Reed, PG: An emerging paradigm for the investigation of spirituality in nursing. Res Nurs Health 15:349, 1992.
36. Potter, PA, and Perry AG: Basic Nursing: Theory and Practice, ed 3. CV Mosby, St. Louis, 1995.
37. Fitzpatrick, JJ, and Whall, AL: Conceptual models of nursing: Analysis and application. Appleton & Lange, Stamford, CT, 1996.
38. Burkhardt, MA: Spirituality: An analysis of the concept. Holist Nurs Pract 3:69, 1989.
39. Emblen, JD, and Halstead, L: Spiritual needs and interventions. Comparing the views of patients, nurses and chaplains. Clin Nurse Specialist 7:175, 1993.
40. Burkhardt, MA: Becoming and connecting: Elements of spirituality for women. Holist Nurs Pract 8:12, 1994.

NANDA'S AXES DEFINITIONS*

AXIS 1

The diagnostic concept is the root of the diagnostic statement. This statement may contain one or more nouns, each contributing a unique meaning (e.g., Infant Feeding Pattern). This list contains the foundation for each diagnosis and is not repeated here. Refer to *NANDA Nursing Diagnosis: Definitions and Classification, 2005–2006* for a complete list.

AXIS 2: TIME

Acute: Lasting less than 6 months
Chronic: Lasting more than 6 months
Intermittent: Stopping or starting again at intervals, periodic, cyclic
Continuous: Uninterrupted, going on without stop

AXIS 3: SUBJECT OF DIAGNOSIS

This axis refers to the person for whom the diagnosis is determined.

Individual: A single human being distinct from others, a person
Family: Two or more people having continuous or sustained relationships, perceiving reciprocal obligations, sensing common meaning, and sharing certain obligations toward others; related by blood and/or choice
Group: A number of people with shared characteristics
Community: A group of people living in the same locale under the same governance. Examples include neighborhoods and cities.
When the subject of the diagnosis is not stated, the default subject is individual.

AXIS 4: AGE

This axis refers to the length of time the individual has been living.

Fetus   Adolescent
Neonate   Young adult
Infant   Middle-age adult
Toddler   Young old adult
Pre-school child   Middle old adult
School-age child   Old-old adult

AXIS 5: HEALTH STATUS

This axis refers to the position or rank on the health continuum of wellness to illness (or death).

Wellness: The quality or state of being healthy, especially as a result of deliberate effort
Risk: Vulnerability, especially as a result of exposure to factors that increase the chance of injury or loss
Actual: Existing in fact or reality, existing at the present time

*From North American Nursing Diagnosis *Association*: NANDA Nursing Diagnosis: Definitions and Classification, 2005–2006. NANDA, Philadelphia, 2005, pp 233–239, with permission.

AXIS 6: DESCRIPTORS

Ability: Capacity to do or act

Anticipatory: To realize beforehand, foresee

Balance: State of equilibrium

Compromised: To make vulnerable to threat

Decreased: Lessened; lesser in size, amount, or degree

Deficient: Inadequate in amount, quality, or degree; not sufficient; incomplete

Defensive: Used or intended to protect from a perceived threat

Delayed: To postpone, impede, and retard

Depleted: Emptied wholly or in part; exhausted of

Disproportionate: Not consistent with a standard

Disabling: To make unable or unfit; to incapacitate

Disorganized: To destroy the systematic arrangement

Disturbed: Agitated or interrupted; interfered with

Dysfunctional: Abnormal, incomplete functioning

Effective: Producing the intended or expected effect

Excessive: Characterized by an amount or quantity that is greater than is necessary, desirable, or useful

Functional: Normal complete functioning

Imbalanced: State of disequilibrium

Impaired: Made worse, weakened, damaged, reduced, deteriorated

Inability: Incapacity to do or act

Increased: Greater in size, amount, or degree

Ineffective: Not producing the desired effect

Interrupted: To break the continuity or uniformity

Low: Containing less than the norm

Organized: To form as into a systematic arrangement

Perceived: To become aware of by means of the senses; assignment of meaning

Readiness for enhanced (for use with wellness diagnoses): To make greater; to increase in quality; to attain the more desired

Situational: Related to particular circumstances

Total: Complete, to the greatest extent or degree

AXIS 7: TOPOLOGY

This axis refers to parts/regions of the body and/or other related functions.

Auditory

Bladder

Cardiopulmonary

Cerebral

Gastrointestinal

Gustatory

Intracranial

Mucous membranes

Oral

Olfactory

Peripheral neurovascular

Peripheral vascular

Renal

Skin

Tactile

Visual

ADMISSION ASSESSMENT FORM AND SAMPLE

ADMISSION ASSESSMENT FORM

DEMOGRAPHIC DATA

Date: _____ Time: _____

Name: _____

Date of Birth: _____ Age: _____ Sex: _____

Primary Significant Other: _____ Telephone # _____

Name of Primary Information

Source: _____

Admitting Medical Diagnosis: _____

VITAL SIGNS

Temperature: _____ F _____ C _____ ; Oral _____ Rectal _____ Axillary _____ Tympanic _____

Pulse Rate: Radial _____ Apical _____ ; Regular _____ Irregular _____

Respiratory Rate: _____ Abdominal _____ Diaphragmatic _____

Blood Pressure: Left arm _____ ; Right arm _____ ; Sitting _____ Standing _____ Lying down _____

Weight: _____ pounds, _____ kilograms; Height: _____ feet _____ inches, _____ meters

Do you have any allergies? No _____ Yes _____ What? _____

(Check reactions to medications, foods, cosmetics, insect bites, etc.)

Review admission CBC, urinalyses, and chest x-ray. Note any abnormalities here: _____

HEALTH PERCEPTION–HEALTH MANAGEMENT PATTERN

Subjective

1. How would you describe your usual health status? Good _____ Fair _____ Poor _____
2. Are you satisfied with your usual health status? Yes _____ No _____
   Source of dissatisfaction _____
3. Tobacco use? No _____ Yes _____ Number of packs per day_____
4. Alcohol use? No _____ Yes _____ How much and what kind? _____

5. Street drug use? No _____ Yes _____ What and how much?_____
6. Any history of chronic diseases? No _____ Yes _____ Describe. _____
_____
7. Immunization History: Tetanus _____; Pneumonia _____; Influenza _____; MMR _____;
Polio _____; Hepatitis B _____ ; Hib _____
8. Have you sought any health care assistance in the past year? No _____ Yes _____
If yes, why? _____
9. Are you currently working? Yes _____ No _____ How would you rate your working conditions
(e.g., safety, noise, space, heating, cooling, water, ventilation)?
Excellent _____ Good _____ Fair _____ Poor _____
Describe any problem areas _____
_____
10. How would you rate living conditions at home? Excellent _____ Good _____ Fair _____ Poor _____
Describe any problem areas _____
11. Do you have any difficulty securing any of the following services?
Grocery store? Yes _____ No _____ ; Pharmacy? Yes _____ No _____;
Health care facility? Yes _____ No _____ ; Transportation? Yes _____ No _____;
Telephone (for police, fire, ambulance, etc.)? Yes _____ No _____
If any difficulties, note referral here _____
12. Medications (over-the-counter and prescriptive)

NAME/DOSAGE AMT.	TIMES/DAY	REASON	TAKING AS ORDERED
_____			Yes _____ No _____
_____			Yes _____ No _____
_____			Yes _____ No _____
_____			Yes _____ No _____
_____			Yes _____ No _____
_____			Yes _____ No _____
_____			Yes _____ No _____
_____			Yes _____ No _____

13. Have you followed the routine prescribed for you? Yes _____ No _____
Why not? _____
14. Did you think this prescribed routine was the best for you? Yes _____ No _____
What would be better? _____
15. Have you had any accidents/injuries/falls in the past year? No _____ Yes _____
Describe. _____
16. Have you had any problems with cuts healing? No _____ Yes _____
Describe. _____
17. Do you exercise on a regular basis? No _____ Yes _____ Type and Frequency _____
_____
18. Have you experienced any ringing in the ears? Right ear: Yes _____ No _____
Left ear: Yes _____ No _____
19. Have you experienced any vertigo? Yes _____ No _____ How often and when? _____
_____
20. Do you regularly use seat belts? Yes _____ No _____
21. For infants and children, are car seats used regularly? Yes _____ No _____
22. Do you have any suggestions or assistance requests for improving your health?
No _____ Yes _____
23. Do you do (breast/testicular) self-examination? No _____ Yes _____
How often? _____
24. Were you or your family able to meet all your therapeutic needs? Yes _____ No _____
25. Are you scheduled for surgery? Yes _____ No _____
26. Have you recently had surgery? No _____ Yes _____ Date _____

Objective
1. Mental Status (Indicate assessment with an X)
   a. Oriented _____ Disoriented _____ Length of time _____
   Time: Yes _____ No _____ Length of time _____

Place: Yes _____ No _____ Length of time _____

Person: Yes _____ No _____ Length of time _____

b. Sensorium

Alert _____ ; Drowsy _____ ; Lethargic _____ ;

Stuporous _____ ; Comatose _____ ; Cooperative _____ ;

Combative _____ ; Delusions _____ ; Fluctuating levels of consciousness?

Yes _____ No _____

Appropriate response to stimuli? Yes _____ No _____

c. Memory

Recent: Yes _____ No _____ ; Remote: Yes _____ No _____ ;

Past 4 hours: Yes _____ No _____

d. Is there a disruption of the flow of energy surrounding the person? Yes _____ No _____

Change in color? Yes _____ No _____; Change in temperature? Yes _____ No _____ ;

Field? Yes _____ No _____ ; Movement? Yes _____ No _____ ;

Sound? Yes _____ No _____

e. Responds to simple directions? Yes _____ No _____

2. **Vision**

   a. Visual Acuity: Both eyes 20/_____ Right 20/_____ Left 20/_____ Not assessed _____

   b. Pupil Size: Right: Normal _____ Abnormal _____ ; Left: Normal _____

   Abnormal _____ Description of abnormalities _____

   c. Pupil Reaction: Right: Normal _____ Abnormal _____ ; Left: Normal _____

   Abnormal _____ Description of abnormalities _____

   d. Wears glasses? Yes _____ No _____ ; Contact lenses? Yes _____ No _____

3. **Hearing:** Not assessed _____

   a. Right ear: WNL _____ Impaired _____ Deaf _____ ;

   Left ear: WNL _____ Impaired _____ Deaf _____

   b. Hearing aid? Yes _____ No _____

4. **Taste**

   a. Sweet: Normal _____ Abnormal _____ Describe. _____

   b. Sour: Normal _____ Abnormal _____ Describe. _____

   c. Tongue Movement: Normal _____ Abnormal _____ Describe. _____

   d. Tongue Appearance: Normal _____ Abnormal _____ Describe. _____

5. **Touch**

   a. Blunt: Normal _____ Abnormal _____ Describe. _____

   b. Sharp: Normal _____ Abnormal _____ Describe. _____

   c. Light Touch Sensation: Normal _____ Abnormal _____ Describe. _____

   d. Proprioception: Normal _____ Abnormal _____ Describe. _____

   e. Heat: Normal _____ Abnormal _____ Describe. _____

   f. Cold: Normal _____ Abnormal _____ Describe._____

   g. Any numbness? No _____ Yes _____ Describe. _____

   h. Any tingling? No _____ Yes _____ Describe. _____

6. **Smell**

   a. Right Nostril: Normal _____ Abnormal _____ Describe. _____

   b. Left Nostril: Normal _____ Abnormal _____ Describe._____

7. Assess Cranial Nerves: Normal _____ Abnormal _____

   Describe deviations _____

8. Cerebellar Exam (Romberg, balance, gait, coordination, etc.): Normal _____ Abnormal _____

   Describe. _____

9. Assess Reflexes: Normal _____ Abnormal _____ Describe. _____

10. Throat: Enlarged tonsils? No _____ Yes _____ Location_____

    Tenderness? No _____ Yes _____ Exudate on tonsils? No _____ Yes _____ Color_____

    Uvula midline? No _____ Yes _____

11. Neck: Any enlarged lymph nodes? No _____ Yes _____ Location and size_____

    _____

12. General Appearance
   a. Hair_____
   b. Skin_____
   Does the patient exhibit any eczema? No _____ Yes _____ Where? _____
   c. Nails_____
   d. Body Odor_____
13. Does the patient have a history of multiple surgeries or a history of reaction to latex?
   No _____Yes _____ Which one? _____ Multiple surgeries _____ Reaction to latex
14. Is the patient's surgical incision healing properly? N/A _____ Yes _____ No _____
   Describe. _____

NUTRITIONAL–METABOLIC PATTERN

Subjective
1. Any weight gain in last 6 months? No _____ Yes _____ Amount _____
2. Any weight loss in last 6 months? No _____ Yes _____ Amount _____
3. Would you describe your appetite as: Good _____ Fair _____ Poor _____
4. Do you have any food intolerances? No _____ Yes _____ Describe. _____
   _____
5. Do you have any dietary restrictions? (Check for those that are a part of a prescribed regimen as well as those that patient restricts voluntarily; for example, to prevent flatus.)
   No _____ Yes _____ What _____
6. Describe an average day's food intake for you (meals and snacks).
   _____
   _____
   _____
   _____
7. Describe an average day's fluid intake for you._____
   _____
8. Describe food likes and dislikes. _____
   _____
9. Would you like to: Gain weight? _____ Lose weight? _____ Neither _____
10. Any problems with:
   a. Nausea? No _____ Yes _____ Describe. _____
   b. Vomiting? No _____ Yes _____ Describe. _____
   c. Swallowing? No _____ Yes _____ Describe. _____
   d. Chewing? No _____ Yes _____ Describe. _____
   e. Indigestion? No ___ Yes ___ Describe. _____
11. Would you describe your usual lifestyle as: Active _____ Sedate _____
12. Do you have any chronic health problems? No _____ Yes _____ Describe. _____
   _____

For breastfeeding mothers only:
13. Do you have any concerns about breastfeeding? No _____ Yes _____
   Describe. _____
14. Are you having any problems with breastfeeding? No _____ Yes _____
   Describe._____

Objective
1. Skin Examination
   a. Warm _____ Cool _____ Moist _____ Dry _____
   b. Lesions? No _____ Yes _____ Describe. _____
   c. Rash? No _____ Yes _____ Describe. _____
   d. Turgor: Firm _____ Supple _____ Dehydrated _____ Fragile _____
   e. Color: Pale _____ Pink _____ Dusky _____ Cyanotic _____ Jaundiced _____ Mottled _____
   Other_____
2. Mucous Membranes
   a. Mouth

(1) Moist _____ Dry _____

(2) Lesions? No _____ Yes _____ Describe. _____

(3) Color: Pale _____ Pink _____

(4) Teeth: Normal ___ Abnormal _____ Describe. _____

(5) Dentures? No _____ Yes _____ Upper _____ Lower _____ Partial _____

(6) Gums: Normal _____ Abnormal _____ Describe. _____

(7) Tongue: Normal _____ Abnormal _____ Describe. _____

b. Eyes

(1) Moist _____ Dry _____

(2) Color of conjunctivae: Pale _____ Pink _____ Jaundiced _____

(3) Lesions? No _____ Yes _____ Describe. _____

3. Edema

a. General? No _____ Yes _____ Describe. _____

_____

Abdominal Girth: _____inches; Not measured _____

b. Periorbital? No _____ Yes _____ Describe. _____

c. Dependent? No _____ Yes _____ Describe. _____

Ankle Girth: Right _____ inches; Left _____ inches; Not measured _____

4. Thyroid: Normal _____ Abnormal _____ Describe. _____

5. Jugular vein distention? No _____ Yes _____

6. Gag Reflex: Present _____ Absent _____

7. Can the patient move self easily (turning, walking)? Yes _____ No _____ Describe limitations. _____

_____

8. Upon admission was the patient dressed appropriately for the weather? Yes _____ No _____

Describe. _____

For breastfeeding mothers only:

9. Breast Exam: Normal _____ Abnormal _____ Describe. _____

_____

10. Weigh the infant. Is the infant's weight within normal limits? Yes _____ No _____

ELIMINATION PATTERN

Subjective

1. What is your usual frequency of bowel movements?

a. Have to strain to have bowel movement? No _____ Yes _____

b. Same time each day? No _____ Yes _____

2. Has the number of bowel movements changed in the past week? No _____ Yes _____

Increased _____ Decreased _____

3. Character of stool:

a. Consistency: Hard _____ Soft _____ Liquid _____

b. Color: Brown _____ Black _____ Yellow _____ Clay colored_____

c. Bleeding with bowel movements? No _____ Yes _____

4. History of constipation? No _____ Yes _____ How often?_____

Use bowel movement aids (laxatives, suppositories, diet)? No _____ Yes _____ Describe. _____

_____

5. History of diarrhea? No _____ Yes _____ When_____

6. History of incontinence? No _____ Yes _____

Related to increased abdominal pressure (coughing, laughing, sneezing)? No _____ Yes_____

7. History of recent travel? No _____ Yes _____ Where?_____

8. Usual voiding pattern:

a. Frequency (times/day) _____ Decreased _____ Increased _____

b. Change in awareness of need to void? No _____ Yes _____ Increased _____ Decreased _____

c. Change in urge to void? No _____ Yes _____ Increased _____ Decreased _____

d. Any change in amount? No _____ Yes _____ Decreased _____ Increased _____

e. Color: Yellow _____ Smoky _____ Dark _____

f. Incontinence? No _____Yes _____ When_____

Difficulty holding voiding when urge to void develops? No _____ Yes _____

Have time to get to bathroom? Yes _____ No _____

How often does problem of reaching the bathroom occur?

g. Retention? No _____ Yes _____ Describe. _____

h. Pain/burning? No _____ Yes _____ Describe. _____

i. Sensation of bladder spasms? No _____ Yes _____ When _____

Objective

1. Auscultate abdomen.
   a. Bowel Sounds: Normal _____ Increased _____ Decreased _____ Absent _____
2. Palpate abdomen.
   a. Tender? No _____ Yes _____ Where? _____
   b. Soft? Yes _____ No _____ ; Firm? Yes _____ No _____
   c. Masses? No _____ Yes _____ Describe. _____
   d. Distention (include distended bladder)? No _____ Yes _____ Describe. _____
   e. Overflow urine when bladder palpated? Yes _____ No _____
3. Rectal Exam
   a. Sphincter tone: Describe. _____
   b. Hemorrhoids? No _____ Yes _____ Describe. _____
   c. Stool in rectum? No _____ Yes _____ Describe. _____
   d. Impaction? No _____ Yes _____ Describe. _____
   e. Occult blood? No _____ Yes _____
4. Ostomy present? No ___ Yes ___ Location _____

ACTIVITY–EXERCISE PATTERN

Subjective

1. Using the following Functional Level Classification, have the patient rate each area of self-care.*
   0 = Completely independent
   1 = Requires use of equipment or device
   2 = Requires help from another person for assistance, supervision, or teaching
   3 = Requires help from another person and equipment or device
   4 = Dependent, does not participate in activity

   Feeding _____; Bathing/hygiene _____; Dressing/grooming _____;
   Toileting _____; Ambulation _____; Care of home _____; Shopping _____;
   Meal preparation _____; Laundry _____; Transportation _____
2. Oxygen use at home? No _____ Yes _____ Describe. _____
3. How many pillows do you use to sleep on? _____
4. Do you frequently experience fatigue? No _____ Yes _____ Describe. _____
   _____
5. How many stairs can you climb without experiencing any difficulty (can be individual number or number of flights)?
   _____
6. How far can you walk without experiencing any difficulty? _____
7. Any history of falls? No _____ Yes _____ How often? _____
8. Has assistance at home for care of self and maintenance of home? No _____ Yes _____
   Who _____
   If no, would like to have or believes needs to have assistance? No _____ Yes _____
   With what activities? _____
9. Occupation (if retired, former occupation) _____
10. Describe your usual leisure time activities/hobbies. _____
    _____
11. Any complaints of weakness or lack of energy? No _____ Yes _____
    Describe. _____
12. Any difficulties in maintaining activities of daily living? No _____ Yes _____
    Describe. _____

---

*(Code adapted by NANDA from Jones, E, et al: Patient Classification for Long-Term Care: Users' Manual, HEW Publication No. HRA-74-3107. November, 1974.)

13. Any problems with concentration? No _____ Yes _____
Describe. _____

14. If in wheelchair, do you have any problems manipulating the wheelchair? No _____ Yes _____
Describe. _____

15. Can you move yourself from site to site with no problems? Yes _____ No _____
Describe. _____

Objective

1. Cardiovascular
  a. Cyanosis? No _____ Yes _____ Where? _____
  b. Pulses: Easily palpable?
    Carotid: Yes _____ No _____; Jugular: Yes _____ No _____; Temporal: Yes _____ No _____;
    Radial: Yes _____ No _____; Femoral: Yes _____ No _____; Popliteal: Yes _____ No _____;
    Post-tibial: Yes _____ No _____; Dorsalis pedis: Yes _____ No _____
  c. Extremities
    (1) Temperature: Cold _____ Cool _____ Warm _____ Hot _____
    (2) Capillary Refill: Normal _____ Delayed _____
    (3) Color: Pink _____ Pale _____ Cyanotic _____ Other _____
    Describe. _____
    (4) Homans' sign? No _____ Yes _____
    (5) Nails: Normal _____ Abnormal _____ Describe. _____
    _____
    (6) Hair Distribution: Normal _____ Abnormal _____ Describe. _____
    _____
    (7) Claudication? No _____ Yes _____ Describe. _____
  d. Heart: PMI Location
    (1) Abnormal rhythm? No _____ Yes _____ Describe. _____
    _____
    (2) Abnormal sounds? No _____ Yes _____ Describe. _____
    _____

2. Respiratory
  a. Rate _____ ; Depth: Shallow _____ Deep _____ Abdominal _____ Diaphragmatic _____
  b. Have the patient cough. Any sputum? No _____ Yes _____ Describe. _____
    _____
  c. Fremitus? No _____ Yes _____
  d. Any chest excursion? No _____ Yes _____ Equal _____ Unequal _____
  e. Auscultate chest.
    Any abnormal sounds (rales, rhonchi)? No _____ Yes _____ Describe. _____
    _____
  f. Have the patient walk in place for 3 minutes (if permissible):
    (1) Any shortness of breath after activity? No _____ Yes _____
    (2) Any dyspnea? No _____ Yes _____
    (3) BP after activity _____ in (right/left) arm
    (4) Respiratory rate after activity _____
    (5) Pulse rate after activity _____

3. Musculoskeletal
  a. Range of motion: Normal _____ Limited _____ Describe. _____
  b. Gait: Normal _____ Abnormal _____ Describe. _____
  c. Balance: Normal _____ Abnormal _____ Describe. _____
  d. Muscle Mass/Strength: Normal _____ Increased _____ Decreased _____
    Describe. _____
  e. Hand Grasp: Right: Normal _____ Decreased _____
                       Left: Normal _____ Decreased _____
  f. Toe Wiggle: Right: Normal _____ Decreased _____
                       Left: Normal _____ Decreased _____
  g. Posture: Normal _____ Kyphosis _____ Lordosis _____

    h. Deformities? No _____ Yes _____ Describe. _____

    i. Missing limbs? No _____ Yes _____ Where_____

    j. Uses mobility assistive devices (walker, crutches, etc.)? No _____ Yes _____
    Describe. _____

    k. Tremors? No _____ Yes _____ Describe. _____

    l. Traction or casts present? No _____ Yes _____ Describe._____

    m. Easily turns in bed? Yes _____ No _____ Describe. _____

4. Spinal cord injury? No _____ Yes _____ Level_____

5. Paralysis present? No _____ Yes _____ Where _____

6. Conduct developmental assessment. Normal _____ Abnormal _____ Describe. _____
_____

7. Responds appropriately to stimuli? Yes _____ No _____ Describe. _____
_____

8. Are there any abnormal movements? No _____ Yes _____ Describe. _____
_____

9. Frequent walking in hall? No _____ Yes _____

10. Episodes of trespassing or getting lost? No _____ Yes _____

SLEEP–REST PATTERN

Subjective

1. Usual sleep habits: Hours/night _____ ; Naps? No _____ Yes _____ A.M. _____ P.M. _____
Feel rested? Yes _____ No _____ Describe. _____

2. Any problems:

    a. Difficulty going to sleep? No _____ Yes _____

    b. Awakening during night? No _____ Yes _____

    c. Early awakening? No _____ Yes _____

    d. Insomnia? No _____ Yes _____ Describe. _____

3. Methods used to promote sleep: Medication? No _____ Yes _____ Name_____
Warm fluids? No _____ Yes _____ What_____
Relaxation techniques? No _____ Yes _____

Objective
None

COGNITIVE–PERCEPTUAL PATTERN

Subjective

1. Pain

    a. Location (have the patient point to area) _____

    b. Intensity (have the patient rank on scale of 0–10) _____

    c. Radiation? No _____ Yes _____ To where? _____

    d. Timing (how often; related to any specific events) _____
_____

    e. Duration _____

    f. What do you do to relieve pain at home? _____

    g. When did pain begin? _____

2. Decision Making

    a. Find decision making: Easy _____ Moderately easy _____ Moderately difficult _____ Difficult_____

    b. Inclined to make decisions: Rapidly _____ Slowly _____ Delay _____

    c. Difficulty choosing between options? Yes _____ No _____ Describe. _____
_____

3. Knowledge Level

    a. Can define what current problem is? Yes _____ No _____

    b. Can restate current therapeutic regimen? Yes _____ No _____

Objective

1. Review sensory and mental status completed in Health Perception–Health Management Pattern.

2. Any overt signs of pain? No _____ Yes _____ Describe. _____

3. Any fluctuations in intracranial pressure? Yes _____ No _____

SELF-PERCEPTION AND SELF-CONCEPT PATTERN

Subjective

1. What is your major concern at the current time? _____
   _____

2. Do you think this admission will cause any lifestyle changes for you? No _____ Yes _____
   What? _____

3. Do you think this admission will result in any body changes for you? No _____ Yes _____
   What? _____

4. My usual view of myself is: Positive _____ Neutral _____ Somewhat negative _____

5. Do you believe you will have any problems dealing with your current health situation?
   No _____ Yes _____ Describe. _____

6. On a scale of 0–5, rank your perception of your level of control in this situation_____

7. On a scale of 0–5, rank your usual assertiveness level _____

8. Have you recently experienced a loss? No _____ Yes _____ Describe. _____

Objective

1. During assessment, the patient appears: Calm _____ Anxious _____ Irritable _____ Withdrawn _____ Restless _____

2. Did any physiologic parameters change: Face reddened? No _____ Yes _____
   Voice volume changed? No _____ Yes _____ Louder _____ Softer _____
   Voice quality changed? No_____ Yes_____ Quavering _____ Hesitation _____
   Other_____

3. Body language observed_____

4. Is current admission going to result in a body structure or function change for the patient?
   No _____ Yes _____ Unsure at this time _____

5. Is the patient expressing any fears about dying? No _____ Yes _____

6. Is the patient expressing worries about the impact of his or her death on his or her family and/or friends?
   No _____ Yes _____ N/A _____

ROLE-RELATIONSHIP PATTERN

Subjective

1. Does the patient live alone? Yes _____ No _____With whom_____

2. Is the patient married? Yes _____ No _____ ; Children? No _____ Yes _____ ; # of children _____
   Age(s) of children _____
   Were any of the children premature? No _____ Yes _____ Describe. _____

3. How would you rate your parenting skills: Not applicable _____
   No difficulty with _____ Average _____ Some difficulty with _____ Describe. _____

4. Any losses (physical, psychological, social) in past year? No _____ Yes _____ Describe. _____

5. How is the patient handling this loss at this time? _____

6. Do you believe this admission will result in any type of loss? No _____ Yes _____ Describe. _____

7. Has the patient recently received a diagnosis related to a chronic physical or mental illness? No _____ Yes _____

8. Is the patient verbally expressing sadness? No _____ Yes _____

9. Ask both the patient and family: Do you think this admission will cause any significant changes in (the patient's)
   usual family role? No _____ Yes _____ Describe._____

10. How would you rate your usual social activities? Very active _____ Active _____ Limited _____ None _____

11. How would you rate your comfort in social situations? Comfortable _____ Uncomfortable _____

12. What activities/jobs, etc., do you like to do? _____

13. What activities/jobs, etc., do you dislike doing? _____

14. Does the person use alcohol or drugs? No _____ Yes _____ Kind_____
    Amount _____

15. Is the patient in the role of primary caregiver for another person? No _____ Yes _____

Objective

1. Speech Pattern
   a. Is English the patient's native language? Yes _____ No _____
      Native language is _____ ; Interpreter needed? No _____ Yes _____
   b. During interview have you noted any speech problems? No _____ Yes _____ Describe. _____
2. Family Interaction
   a. During interview have you observed any dysfunctional family interactions? No _____ Yes _____ Describe. _____
   b. If the patient is a child, is there any physical or emotional evidence of physical or psychosocial abuse?
      No _____ Yes _____ Describe. _____
   c. If the patient is a child, is there evidence of attachment behaviors between the parents and child?
      Yes _____ No _____ Describe. _____
   d. Any signs or symptoms of alcoholism? No _____ Yes _____ Describe. _____

SEXUALITY–REPRODUCTIVE PATTERN

Subjective
Female

1. Date of LMP _____ ; Any pregnancies? Para _____ Gravida _____
   Menopause? No _____ Yes _____ Year _____
2. Use birth control measures? No _____ N/A _____ Yes _____ Type _____
3. Any history of vaginal discharge, bleeding, lesions? No _____ Yes _____ Description _____
4. Pap smear annually? Yes _____ No _____ Date of last Pap smear _____
5. Date of last mammogram _____
6. History of STD (sexually transmitted disease)? No _____ Yes _____ Describe. _____

If admission secondary to rape:

7. Is the patient describing numerous physical symptoms? No _____ Yes _____ Describe. _____
8. Is the patient exhibiting numerous emotional reactions? No _____ Yes _____ Describe. _____
9. What has been your primary coping mechanism to handle this rape episode? _____
10. Have you talked to persons from the rape crisis center? Yes _____ No _____
    If no, does the patient want you to contact them for her? No _____ Yes _____
    If yes, was this contact of assistance? No _____ Yes _____

Male

1. Any history of prostate problems? No _____ Yes _____ Describe. _____
2. Any history of penile discharge, bleeding, lesions? No _____ Yes _____ Describe. _____
3. Date of last prostate exam _____
4. History of STD (sexually transmitted disease)? No _____ Yes _____ Describe. _____

Both

1. Are you experiencing any problems in sexual functioning? No _____ Yes _____ Describe. _____
2. Are you satisfied with your sexual relationship? Yes _____ No _____ Describe. _____
3. Do you believe this admission will have any impact on sexual functioning? No _____ Yes _____ Describe. _____

Objective

Review admission physical exam for results of pelvic and rectal exams. If results not documented, nurse should perform exams. Check history to see whether admission resulted from a rape.

COPING–STRESS TOLERANCE PATTERN

Subjective

1. Have you experienced any stressful or traumatic events in the past year in addition to this admission?
   No _____ Yes _____ Describe. _____
2. How would you rate your usual handling of stress? Good _____ Average _____ Poor _____
3. What is the primary way you deal with stress or problems? _____
4. Have you or your family used any support or counseling groups in the past year?
   No _____ Yes _____ Group Name _____
   Was support group helpful? Yes _____ No _____ Additional comments: _____
5. What do you believe is the primary reason behind the need for this admission? _____
6. How soon, after first noting symptoms, did you seek health care assistance? _____

7. Are you satisfied with the care you have been receiving at home? Yes _____ No _____ Comments: _____

8. Ask primary caregiver: What is your understanding of the care that will be needed when the patient goes home?
_____

Objective

1. Observe behavior. Are there any overt signs of stress (e.g., crying, wringing of hands, clenched fists, etc.)? Describe. _____

2. Ask the family or primary caregiver if the patient has threatened to kill himself or herself. No _____ Yes _____

3. Ask the family or primary caregiver if they have noticed any marked changes in the patient's behavior, attitude, or school performance? No _____ Yes _____

VALUE–BELIEF PATTERN

Subjective

1. Satisfied with the way your life has been developing? Yes _____ No _____ Comments: _____

2. Will this admission interfere with your plans for the future? No _____ Yes _____ How? _____

3. Religion: Protestant _____ Catholic _____ Jewish _____ Islam _____ Buddhist _____ Other _____

4. Will this admission interfere with your spiritual or religious practices? No _____ Yes _____ How? _____

5. Any religious restrictions to care (diet, blood transfusions)? No _____ Yes _____ Describe. _____

6. Would you like to have your (pastor, priest, rabbi, hospital chaplain) contacted to visit you? No _____ Yes _____ Who? _____

7. Have your religious beliefs helped you deal with problems in the past? No _____ Yes _____ Comments: _____

Objective

1. Observe behavior. Is the patient exhibiting any signs of alterations in mood (e.g., anger, crying, withdrawal, etc.)? No _____ Yes _____ Describe. _____

GENERAL

1. Is there any information we need to have that I have not covered in this interview? No _____ Yes _____ Comments: _____

2. Do you have any questions you need to ask me concerning your health, plan of care, or this agency? No _____ Yes _____ Questions: _____
_____

3. What is the first problem you would like to have assistance with? _____

CASE STUDY: MR. FRED CARSON

Mr. Fred Carson is a 63-year-old man who has been admitted with a medical diagnosis of hyperglycemia secondary to diabetes mellitus. He was first diagnosed as having adult onset diabetes 2 years ago.

On admission Mr. Carson's vital signs are temperature 101.4° F orally, pulse 98, respiration 20, blood pressure 98/70. Mr. Carson is 5 feet 9 inches tall and weighs 230 pounds. He states he has gained 20 pounds over the past 6 weeks. His fasting glucose is 200 mg/dL. His hemoglobin level is 20 g/dL, with a hematocrit of 56 vol/dL. Mr. Carson tells you he regulates his insulin according to what he eats and eats whatever he is hungry for. You find, in interviewing Mr. Carson, that he has been drinking three or four "iced tea glasses" of water every hour stating, "I'm always thirsty." He has been voiding at least once an hour. His urine specimen is dilute and a very pale yellow. Mr. Carson's urine glucose, as measured by a Clinitest, is 4+. In the past 2 hours Mr. Carson voided 1500 mL in addition to the urine specimen, and his intake has been 500 mL.

Mr. Carson says he doesn't pay any attention to his urine tests—"They're just a waste of time"—but, he adds, "I've been peeing a lot more the past few days. Does this mean I'm not behaving?" Mr. Carson states he was taught about his diabetes but thinks "They were just trying to scare me. I don't think I really have diabetes. Kids develop that—not old codgers like me. I only check in with the doctor when I feel like it. He wants me to come in every other month, but I think he's just trying to get more money." When asked to discuss what he was taught regarding his diabetes, Mr. Carson relates a high level of understanding of his prescribed regimen.

You find out this is Mr. Carson's fourth admission over the last 8 months. All of the admissions have been due to complications secondary to the diabetes. He exhibits anger on each admission and refuses to have home health nurses visit him.

In examining Mr. Carson's skin you find that his toenails and fingernails are dry, thick, and brittle. Both his skin and mucous membranes are dry in spite of the amount of fluid Mr. Carson indicates he was drinking prior to admission. His extremities are shiny and cool to the touch, and his legs become cyanotic when they are kept in a dependent position. When elevated, his legs become pale, and color is very slow to return when his legs are returned to a neutral position. His pedal pulses are difficult to locate and diminished in volume. He has a 10 cm+ size lesion on his left shin, and you can see that the lesion has begun to impact the muscle tissue. Mr. Carson tells you he hit his leg on a table 3 weeks ago. You note three round scars with atrophied skin on his right leg and 1 similar scar on his left leg. Mr. Carson describes a sensation of "pins and needles when walking, but if I stop it goes away."

SAMPLE ADMISSION ASSESSMENT

DEMOGRAPHIC DATA

Date: <u>10/25/92</u>   Time: <u>9:25</u> A.M.

Name: <u>CARSON, FRED</u>

Date of Birth: <u>6/10/29</u>   Age: <u>63</u>   Sex: <u>MALE</u>

Primary Significant Other: <u>WIFE—RUTH CARSON</u>   Telephone #: <u>806-745-5689</u>

Name of Primary Information Source: <u>PATIENT</u>

Admitting Medical Diagnosis: <u>HYPERGLYCEMIA SECONDARY TO INSULIN-DEPENDENT DIABETES</u>

VITAL SIGNS

Temperature <u>101.4</u> F <u>X</u>   C   Oral <u>X</u>   Rectal   Axillary   Tympanic

Pulse Rate: Radial <u>98</u>   Apical   ; Regular <u>X</u>   Irregular

Respiratory Rate: <u>20</u>   Abdominal   Diaphragmatic <u>X</u>

Blood Pressure: Left arm <u>98/60</u>   ; Right arm <u>100/64</u>   ; Sitting <u>X</u>   Standing   Lying down

Weight: 230 pounds,   kilograms; Height: <u>5</u> feet <u>9</u> inches,   meters

Do you have any allergies? No <u>X</u>   Yes   What?

(Check reactions to medications, foods, cosmetics, insect bites, etc.)

Review admission CBC, urinalyses, and chest x-ray. Note any abnormalities here:

<u>FASTING GLUCOSE 200 MG/DL; HGB 20 G/DL; HCT 56 VOL/DL</u>

HEALTH PERCEPTION–HEALTH MANAGEMENT PATTERN

Subjective
1. How would you describe your usual health status? Good   Fair <u>X</u>   Poor
2. Are you satisfied with your usual health status? Yes   No <u>X</u>
   Source of dissatisfaction <u>"I'M ALWAYS THIRSTY."</u>
3. Tobacco use? No <u>X</u>   Yes   Number of packs per day
4. Alcohol use? No <u>X</u>   Yes   How much and what kind
5. Street drug use? No <u>X</u>   Yes   What
6. Any history of chronic diseases? No   Yes <u>X</u>   What <u>"THE DOCTOR SAYS I HAVE DIABETES, BUT I DON'T BELIEVE IT. KIDS DEVELOP THAT, NOT OLD CODGERS LIKE ME."</u>
7. Immunization History: Tetanus <u>1960</u>   ; Pneumonia <u>NO</u>   ; Influenza <u>NO</u> ; MMR <u>HAD DISEASES AS CHILD</u> ; Polio <u>NO</u> ; Hepatitis B <u>NO</u> ; Hib <u>NO</u>
8. Have you sought any health care assistance in the past year? No   Yes <u>X</u>
   If yes, why? <u>"I'M THIRSTY ALL THE TIME." "SORES ON MY LEGS." FOUR ADMISSIONS IN PAST MONTHS FOR COMPLICATIONS OF DIABETES</u>
9. Are you currently working? Yes   No <u>RETIRED</u>   How would you rate your working conditions (e.g., safety, noise, space, heating, cooling, water, ventilation)?
   Excellent   Good   Fair   Poor   Describe any problem areas
10. How would you rate living conditions at home? Excellent <u>X</u>   Good   Fair
    Poor   Describe any problem areas <u>"NEED ANOTHER BATHROOM. WE HAVE ONLY ONE AND I NEED TO PEE ALL THE TIME."</u>

11. Do you have any difficulty securing any of the following services?
Grocery store? Yes _____ No X_____ ; Pharmacy? Yes _____ No X_____ ;
Health care facility? Yes _____ No X_____ ; Transportation? Yes _____ No X_____ ;
Telephone (for police, fire, ambulance, etc.)? Yes _____ No X_____
If any difficulties, note referral here _____

12. Medications (over-the-counter and prescriptive)

NAME	DOSAGE AMT.	TIMES/DAY	REASON	TAKING AS ORDERED
INSULIN	REGULATES ACCORD. TO GLUCOSE METER READING	1–3 TIMES	DIABETES	Yes _____ No ___X__
				Yes _____ No _____
				Yes _____ No _____
				Yes _____ No _____
				Yes _____ No _____
				Yes _____ No _____

13. Have you followed the routine prescribed for you? Yes _____ No X_____
Why not? "I TAKE THE INSULIN, BUT I DON'T LIKE THE DIET."

14. Did you think this prescribed routine was the best for you? Yes _____ No X_____
What would be better? "I EAT WHAT I WANT."

15. Have you had any accidents/injuries/falls in the past year? No _____ Yes X_____
Describe. "I HIT MY LEG ON THE TABLE A FEW WEEKS AGO."

16. Have you had any problems with cuts healing? No _____ Yes X_____ Describe. "THIS SORE HAS BEEN HERE SINCE I HIT IT 3 WEEKS AGO (POINTS TO LT SHIN). THESE SCARS ARE FROM SORES THAT TOOK AGES TO HEAL (POINTS TO RT LEG)."

17. Do you exercise on a regular basis? No X_____ Yes _____ Type and Frequency "I USED TO WALK EVERY AFTERNOON, BUT SINCE I HAVE TO PEE SO MUCH I CAN'T LEAVE THE HOUSE."

18. Have you experienced any ringing in the ears?   Right: Yes _____ No X_____
Left: Yes _____ No X_____

19. Have you experienced any vertigo? Yes _____ No X_____ How often and when?_____

20. Do you regularly use seat belts? Yes _____ No X_____

21. For infants and children, are car seats used regularly? Yes _____ No _____

22. Do you have any suggestions or assistance requests for improving your health? No _____ Yes X_____ What?
"I WANT TO STOP PEEING SO MUCH."

23. Do you do (breast/testicular) self-examination? No X_____ Yes _____
How often? _____

24. Were you or your family able to meet all your therapeutic needs? Yes X_____ No _____

25. Are you scheduled for surgery? Yes _____ No X_____

26. Have you recently had surgery? No X_____ Yes _____ Date_____

Objective

1. Mental Status (Indicate assessment with an X)
   a. Oriented X_____ Disoriented _____ Length of time_____
      Time: Yes X_____ No _____ Length of time_____
      Place: Yes X_____ No _____ Length of time_____
      Person: Yes X_____ No _____ Length of time_____
   b. Sensorium
      Alert _____ ; Drowsy X_____ ; Lethargic _____ ; Stuporous _____; Comatose _____ ; Cooperative X___;
      Combative _____ ; Delusions _____ ; Fluctuating levels of consciousness? Yes _____ No X_____
      Appropriate response to stimuli? Yes X_____ No _____
   c. Memory
      Recent? Yes X_____ No _____ ; Remote? Yes X_____ No _____ ; Past 4 hours? Yes _____ No _____
   d. Is there a disruption of the flow of energy surrounding the person? Yes X_____ No _____
      Change in color? Yes _____ No X_____ ; Change in temperature? Yes _____ No X_____ ;
      Field? Yes _____ No X_____ ; Movement? Yes _____ No X_____; Sound? Yes _____ No X_____
   e. Responds to simple directions? Yes X_____ No _____
2. Vision
   a. Visual Acuity: Both eyes 20/_____ Right 20/_____ Left 20/_____ Not assessed X_____
   b. Pupil Size: Right: Normal X_____ Abnormal _____ ; Left: Normal X_____ Abnormal _____

Description of abnormalities_____

   c. Pupil Reaction: Right: Normal <u>X</u>_____ Abnormal _____ ; Left: Normal <u>X</u>_____ Abnormal _____
Description of abnormalities <u>NONE</u>_____

   d. Wears glasses? Yes <u>X</u>_____ No _____ ; Contact lenses? Yes _____ No <u>X</u>_____

3. Hearing: Not assessed _____

   a. Right: WNL <u>X</u>_____ Impaired _____ Deaf _____ ;
Left: WNL <u>X</u>_____ Impaired _____ Deaf _____

   b. Hearing aid? Yes _____ No <u>X</u>_____

4. Taste

   a. Sweet: Normal _____ Abnormal _____ Describe. <u>NOT EXAMINED</u>_____

   b. Sour: Normal _____ Abnormal _____ Describe. <u>NOT EXAMINED</u>_____

   c. Tongue Movement: Normal <u>X</u>_____ Abnormal _____ Describe. <u>MIDLINE</u>_____

   d. Tongue Appearance: Normal <u>X</u>___ Abnormal _____ Describe. <u>PINK, NO LESIONS OR EXUDATE</u>

5. Touch

   a. Blunt: Normal <u>X</u>_____ Abnormal _____ Describe. <u>RESPONDS TO TOUCH ON ALL EXTREMITIES</u>
<u>WITH FLAT TONGUE DEPRESSOR</u>_____

   b. Sharp: Normal _____ Abnormal <u>X</u>_____ Describe. <u>DIMINISHED RESPONSE ON LT FOOT</u>_____

   c. Light Touch Sensation: Normal _____ Abnormal <u>X</u>___ Describe. <u>HYPERESTHESIA LT ANKLE AND RT LEG</u>

   d. Proprioception: Normal <u>X</u>_____ Abnormal _____ Describe. _____

   e. Heat: Normal _____ Abnormal <u>X</u>_____ Describe. <u>DIMINISHED RESPONSE LT FOOT</u>_____

   f. Cold: Normal _____ Abnormal <u>X</u>_____ Describe. <u>DIMINISHED RESPONSE LT FOOT</u>_____

   g. Any numbness? No _____ Yes <u>X</u>_____ Describe. <u>BILATERALLY IN FEET WHEN WALKING</u>_____

   h. Any tingling? No _____ Yes <u>X</u>_____ Describe. <u>"PINS AND NEEDLES IN FEET" WHEN WALKING</u>

6. Smell

   a. Right Nostril: Normal <u>X</u>_____ Abnormal _____ Describe. _____

   b. Left Nostril: Normal <u>X</u>_____ Abnormal _____ Describe. _____

7. Assess Cranial Nerves: Normal <u>X</u>_____ Abnormal _____
Describe deviations _____

8. Cerebellar Exam (Romberg, balance, gait, coordination, etc.): Normal _____ Abnormal <u>X</u>_____
Describe. <u>ROMBERG ABSENT, BALANCE GOOD, DOES NOT BEAR FULL WEIGHT ON LT FOOT</u>

9. Assess Reflexes: Normal <u>X</u>_____ Abnormal _____ Describe._____

10. Throat: Enlarged tonsils? No <u>X</u>_____ Yes _____ Location <u>NORMAL</u>_____
Tenderness? No <u>X</u>_____ Yes _____ Exudate on tonsils? No <u>X</u>_____ Yes _____ Color _____
Uvula midline? No _____ Yes <u>X</u>_____

11. Neck: Any enlarged lymph nodes? No <u>X</u>_____ Yes _____ Location and size _____

12. General Appearance

   a. Hair <u>BROWN, THINNING</u>_____

   b. Skin <u>PALE PINK, DRY, DECREASED TURGOR</u>_____
Eczema? No <u>X</u>_____ Yes _____

   c. Nails <u>TOENAILS AND FINGERNAILS DRY, THICK, AND BRITTLE</u>_____

   d. Body Odor <u>NONE</u>_____

13. History of multiple surgeries? No <u>X</u>_____ Yes _____; Reaction to latex? No <u>X</u>_____ Yes_____

14. Incisions healing well? No _____ Yes _____ N/A <u>X</u>_____

NUTRITIONAL–METABOLIC PATTERN

Subjective

1. Any weight gain in last 6 months? No _____ Yes <u>X</u>_____ Amount <u>20 LBS IN LAST 6 WEEKS</u>_____

2. Any weight loss in last 6 months? No <u>X</u>_____ Yes _____ Amount_____

3. Would you describe your appetite as: Good <u>X</u>_____ Fair _____ Poor _____

4. Do you have any food intolerances? No <u>X</u>_____ Yes _____ Describe._____

5. Do you have any dietary restrictions? (Check for those that are a part of a prescribed regimen as well as those that
patient restricts voluntarily; for example, to prevent flatus.)
No _____ Yes <u>X</u>_____ What <u>"SPECIAL DIET MY WIFE FIXES ME FOR DIABETES."</u>_____

6. Describe an average day's food intake for you (meals and snacks).

BREAKFAST: 3 PANCAKES WITH LOW SUGAR SYRUP, JUICE, BLACK COFFEE, SAUSAGE; LUNCH: SANDWICH, MILK OR SUGAR-FREE SOFT DRINK, POTATO CHIPS, FRUIT, "SOMETIMES A LITTLE CAKE OR PIE"; DINNER: CASSEROLE, ICED TEA, ROLLS WITH BUTTER, VEGETABLES AND DESSERT ("SURE DO LIKE MY ICE CREAM"). SNACKS: COOKIES AND JUICE

7. Describe an average day's fluid intake for you. "I DRINK ALL THE TIME," AT LEAST 4 LARGE GLASSES PER HOUR.

8. Describe food likes and dislikes LIKES: MEAT, DESSERTS, AND POTATOES; DISLIKES: VEGETABLES AND LOW SUGAR "STUFF"

9. Would you like to: Gain weight _____ Lose weight X _____ Neither _____

10. Any problems with:
    a. Nausea? No X _____ Yes _____ Describe. _____
    b. Vomiting? No X _____ Yes _____ Describe. _____
    c. Swallowing? No X _____ Yes _____ Describe. _____
    d. Chewing? No X _____ Yes _____ Describe. _____
    e. Indigestion? No X _____ Yes _____ Describe. _____

11. Would you describe your usual lifestyle as: Active _____ Sedate X _____

12. Any chronic health problems? No _____ Yes X _____ Describe. DIABETES MELLITUS

For breastfeeding mothers only:

13. Do you have any concerns about breastfeeding? No _____ Yes _____ Describe. _____

14. Are you having any problems with breastfeeding? No _____ Yes _____ Describe. _____

Objective

1. Skin Examination
   a. Warm _____ Cool X _____ Moist _____ Dry X _____
   b. Lesions? No _____ Yes X _____ Describe. 10 CM+ LT SHIN SEVERAL CM DEEP; RED 3 ROUND SCARS WITH ATROPHIED SKIN ON RT LEG; 1 ON LT LEG
   c. Rash? No X _____ Yes _____ Describe. _____
   d. Turgor: Firm _____ Supple _____ Dehydrated X _____ Fragile _____
   e. Color: Pale _____ ; Pink _____ ; Dusky _____ ; Cyanotic _____ ; Jaundiced _____ ; Mottled _____ ; Other PINK EXCEPT FOR LEGS. LEGS ARE CYANOTIC IN DEPENDENT POSITION; PALE WHEN ELEVATED.

2. Mucous Membranes
   a. Mouth
      (1) Moist _____ Dry X _____
      (2) Lesions? No X _____ Yes _____ Describe. _____
      (3) Color: Pale X _____ Pink _____
      (4) Teeth: Normal X _____ Abnormal _____ Describe. _____
      (5) Dentures? No _____ Yes _____ Upper _____ Lower _____ Partial X _____
      (6) Gums: Normal X _____ Abnormal _____ Describe. _____
      (7) Tongue: Normal X _____ Abnormal _____ Describe. _____
   b. Eyes
      (1) Moist _____ Dry X _____
      (2) Color of conjunctivae: Pale _____ Pink X _____ Jaundiced _____
      (3) Lesions? No X _____ Yes _____ Describe. _____

3. Edema
   a. General? No X _____ Yes _____ Describe. _____
      Abdominal Girth: _____ inches; Not measured X _____
   b. Periorbital? No X _____ Yes _____ Describe. _____
   c. Dependent? No _____ Yes X _____ Describe. BILATERAL ANKLES AND FEET WHEN DEPENDENT; LEGS SHINY; NO PITTING.
      Ankle Girth: Right _____ inches; Left _____ inches; Not measured X

4. Thyroid: Normal X _____ Abnormal _____ Describe. _____

5. Jugular vein distention? No X _____ Yes _____

6. Gag Reflex: Present X _____ Absent _____

7. Can the patient move self easily (turning, walking)? Yes _____ No X _____

Describe limitations <u>DOES NOT BEAR FULL WEIGHT ON LEG; TURNING OK</u>._____

8. Upon admission was the patient dressed appropriately for the weather? Yes <u>X</u>_____ No _____ Describe._____

For breastfeeding mothers only:

9. Breast Exam: Normal _____ Abnormal _____ Describe._____

10. Weigh the infant. Is the infant's weight within normal limits? Yes _____ No _____

ELIMINATION PATTERN

Subjective

1. What is your usual frequency of bowel movements? <u>ABOUT 3 TIMES PER WEEK</u>_____
   a. Have to strain to have BM? No <u>X</u>_____ Yes _____
   b. Same time each day? No <u>X</u>_____ Yes _____
2. Has the number of bowel movements changed in the past week? No <u>X</u>_____ Yes _____
   Increased _____ Decreased _____
3. Character of stool:
   a. Consistency: Hard _____ Soft <u>X</u>_____ Liquid _____
   b. Color: Brown <u>X</u>_____ Black _____ Yellow _____ Clay colored _____
   c. Bleeding with bowel movements? No <u>X</u>_____ Yes _____
4. History of constipation? No <u>X</u>_____ Yes _____ How often_____
   Use bowel movement aids (laxatives, suppositories, diet)? No <u>X</u>_____ Yes _____ Describe._____
5. History of diarrhea? No <u>X</u>_____ Yes _____ When_____
6. History of incontinence? No <u>X</u>_____ Yes _____
   Related to increased abdominal pressure (coughing, laughing, sneezing)? No _____Yes _____
7. History of recent travel? No <u>X</u>_____ Yes _____Where?_____
8. Usual voiding pattern:
   a. Frequency (times/day) <u>FOR PAST 3 DAYS, 3–4/HOUR</u>_____
      Decreased _____ Increased <u>X</u>_____
   b. Change in awareness of need to void? No _____ Yes <u>X</u>_____
      Increased _____ Decreased <u>X</u>_____
   c. Change in urge to void? No _____ Yes <u>X</u>_____ Increased <u>X</u>_____ Decreased _____
   d. Any change in amount? No _____ Yes <u>X</u>_____ Decreased _____ Increased <u>X</u>_____
   e. Color: Yellow <u>VERY PALE</u>_____ Smoky _____ Dark _____
   f. Incontinence? No _____ Yes <u>X</u>_____ When <u>"IF TOO FAR FROM BATHROOM."</u>_____
      Difficulty holding voiding when urge to void develops? No _____ Yes <u>X</u>_____
      Have time to get to bathroom? Yes _____ No <u>X</u>_____
      How often does problem reaching bathroom occur? <u>EVERY VOIDING</u>_____
   g. Retention? No <u>X</u>_____ Yes _____ Describe._____
   h. Pain or burning? No <u>X</u>_____ Yes _____ Describe._____
   i. Sensation of bladder spasms? No <u>X</u>_____ Yes _____ When?_____

Objective

1. Auscultate abdomen.
   a. Bowel Sounds: Normal <u>X</u>_____ Increased _____ Decreased _____ Absent _____
2. Palpate abdomen.
   a. Tender? No <u>X</u>_____ Yes _____ Where?_____
   b. Soft? Yes <u>X</u>_____ No _____; Firm? Yes _____ No <u>X</u>_____
   c. Masses? No <u>X</u>_____ Yes _____ Describe._____
   d. Distention (include distended bladder)? No <u>X</u>_____ Yes _____ Describe. _____
   e. Overflow urine when bladder palpated? Yes _____ No <u>X</u>_____
3. Rectal Exam
   a. Sphincter tone: Describe. <u>WITHIN NORMAL LIMITS</u>_____
   b. Hemorrhoids? No <u>X</u>_____ Yes _____ Describe._____
   c. Stool in rectum? No _____ Yes <u>X</u>_____ Describe. <u>HEME NEGATIVE</u>_____
   d. Impaction? No <u>X</u>_____ Yes _____ Describe._____
   e. Occult blood? No <u>X</u>_____ Yes _____
4. Ostomy present? No <u>X</u>_____ Yes _____ Location_____

ACTIVITY–EXERCISE PATTERN

Subjective

1. Using the following Functional Level Classification, have the patient rate each area of self-care. (Code adapted by NANDA from Jones, E, et al: Patient Classification for Long-Term Care: Users' Manual, HEW Publication No. HRA-74-3107. November, 1974.)

    0 = Completely independent
    1 = Requires use of equipment or device
    2 = Requires help from another person, for assistance, supervision, or teaching
    3 = Requires help from another person and equipment or device
    4 = Dependent, does not participate in activity

    Feeding <u>0</u> ; Bathing-hygiene <u>0</u> ; Dressing-grooming <u>0</u> ;
    Toileting <u>0</u> ; Ambulation <u>0</u> ; Care of home <u>WIFE</u> ; Shopping <u>WIFE</u> ;
    Meal preparation <u>WIFE</u> ; Laundry <u>WIFE</u> ; Transportation <u>0</u> .

2. Oxygen use at home? No <u>X</u> Yes _____ Describe._____
3. How many pillows do you use to sleep on? <u>1</u>
4. Do you frequently experience fatigue? No _____ Yes <u>X</u> Describe. <u>"I'M TIRED AFTER GOING TO THE</u> <u>BATHROOM SO MUCH."</u>
5. How many stairs can you climb without experiencing any difficulty (can be individual number or number of flights)? <u>1 FLIGHT</u>
6. How far can you walk without experiencing any difficulty? <u>1 BLOCK; "MY FOOT HURTS IF I TRY TO WALK</u> <u>TOO FAR."</u>
7. Any history of falls? No <u>X</u> Yes _____ How often?_____
8. Has assistance at home for care of self and maintenance of home? No _____ Yes <u>X</u>
    Who <u>WIFE</u>
    If no, would like to have or believes needs to have assistance? No _____ Yes _____
    With what activities?_____
9. Occupation (if retired, former occupation) <u>MAIL CARRIER</u>
10. Describe your usual leisure time activities-hobbies. <u>GARDENING, FISHING, READING</u>
11. Any complaints of weakness or lack of energy? No _____ Yes <u>X</u>
    Describe. <u>GOING TO THE BATHROOM SO MUCH "WEARS ME OUT."</u>
12. Any difficulties in maintaining activities of daily living? No _____ Yes <u>X</u>
    Describe. <u>"ALL I DO IS DRINK AND PEE."</u>
13. Any problems with concentration? No <u>X</u> Yes _____ Describe._____
14. If in wheelchair, do you have any problems manipulating the wheelchair? No ___Yes ___ N/A <u>X</u> Describe._____
15. Can you move yourself from site to site with no problems? No _____ Yes <u>X</u> Describe._____

Objective

1. Cardiovascular
    a. Cyanosis? No _____ Yes <u>X</u> Where? <u>LEGS WHEN DEPENDENT</u>
    b. Pulses: Easily palpable?
        Carotid: Yes <u>X</u> No _____; Jugular: Yes <u>X</u> No _____; Temporal: Yes <u>X</u> No _____;
        Radial: Yes <u>X</u> No _____; Femoral: Yes <u>X</u> No _____; Popliteal: Yes <u>X</u> No _____;
        Post tibial: Yes_____ No <u>X</u> ; Dorsalis pedis: Yes_____ No <u>X</u>
    c. Extremities:
        (1) Temperature: Cold _____ Cool <u>X</u> Warm _____ Hot _____
        (2) Capillary Refill: Normal _____ Delayed <u>X</u>
        (3) Color: Pink _____ Pale <u>X</u> Cyanotic <u>X</u> Other _____
            Describe. <u>PALE WHEN RAISED; CYANOTIC WHEN DEPENDENT</u>
        (4) Homans' sign? No <u>X</u> Yes _____
        (5) Nails: Normal ___ Abnormal <u>X</u> Describe. <u>TOENAILS AND FINGERNAILS DRY, THICK, BRITTLE</u>
        (6) Hair Distribution: Normal <u>X</u> Abnormal _____ Describe. _____
        (7) Claudication? No _____ Yes <u>X</u> Describe. <u>NUMBNESS AND TINGLING IN FEET</u>
    d. Heart: PMI Location <u>4TH ICS LCL</u>
        (1) Abnormal rhythm? No <u>X</u> Yes _____ Describe. _____
        (2) Abnormal sounds? No <u>X</u> Yes _____ Describe. _____

2. Respiratory
   a. Rate <u>20/MIN</u>_____ ; Depth: Shallow _____ Deep <u>X</u>_____ Abdominal _____ Diaphragmatic <u>X</u>_____
   b. Have the patient cough. Any sputum? No <u>X</u>_____ Yes _____ Describe. _____
   c. Fremitus? No <u>X</u>_____ Yes _____
   d. Any chest excursion? No <u>X</u>_____ Yes _____ Equal _____ Unequal _____
   e. Auscultate chest:
      Any abnormal sounds (rales, rhonchi)? No <u>X</u>_____ Yes ____ Describe. _____
   f. Have the patient walk in place for 3 minutes (if permissible):
      (1) Any shortness of breath after activity? No <u>X</u>_____ Yes _____
      (2) Any dyspnea? No X_____ Yes _____
      (3) BP after activity 108 / 74 in (right; <u>left</u>) arm
      (4) Respiratory rate after activity <u>25</u>____
      (5) Pulse rate after activity <u>110</u>_____
3. Musculoskeletal
   a. Range of motion: Normal _____ Limited <u>X</u>_____ Describe. <u>LIMITED IN LOWER EXTREMITIES</u>_____
   b. Gait: Normal ____ Abnormal <u>X</u>_____ Describe. <u>DOES NOT BEAR FULL WEIGHT ON LEFT ANKLE</u>_____
   c. Balance: Normal <u>X</u>_____ Abnormal _____ Describe._____
   d. Muscle Mass/Strength: Normal _____ Increased _____ Decreased <u>X</u>_____ Describe. <u>ATROPHY IN BOTH</u>
      <u>LEGS, ESPECIALLY IN AREA OF WOUNDS</u>_____
   e. Hand Grasp: Right: Normal <u>X</u>____ Decreased _____
                  Left: Normal <u>X</u>____ Decreased _____
   f. Toe Wiggle: Right: Normal <u>X</u>___ Decreased _____
                  Left: Normal <u>X</u>___ Decreased _____
   g. Posture: Normal <u>X</u>_____ Kyphosis _____ Lordosis _____
   h. Deformities? No <u>X</u>_____ Yes _____ Describe._____
   i. Missing limbs? No <u>X</u>_____ Yes _____ Where?_____
   j. Uses mobility assistive devices (walker, crutches, etc.)? No <u>X</u>_____ Yes _____ Describe._____
   k. Tremors? No <u>X</u>_____ Yes _____ Describe._____
   l. Traction or casts present? No <u>X</u>_____ Yes _____ Describe._____
   m. Easily turns in bed? No _____ Yes <u>X</u>_____
4. Spinal cord injury? No <u>X</u>_____ Yes _____ Level_____
5. Paralysis present? No <u>X</u>_____ Yes _____ Where?_____
6. Conduct developmental assessment. Normal _____ Abnormal _____ Describe. <u>NOT DONE</u>_____
7. Responds appropriately to stimuli? Yes <u>X</u>_____ No _____ Describe._____
8. Are there any abnormal movements? No <u>X</u>_____ Yes _____ Describe._____
9. Frequent locomotion? Yes _____ No <u>X</u>_____
10. Episodes of trespassing or getting lost? Yes _____ No <u>X</u>_____

SLEEP–REST PATTERN

Subjective

1. Usual sleep habits: Hours/night <u>6</u> ; Naps? No _____ Yes <u>X</u>_____ A.M. _____ P.M. <u>X</u>_____
   Feel rested? Yes <u>X</u>_____ No _____ Describe._____
2. Any problems:
   a. Difficulty going to sleep? No <u>X</u>_____ Yes_____
   b. Awakening during night? No _____ Yes <u>X (TO GO TO THE BATHROOM)</u>_____
   c. Early awakening? No <u>X</u>_____ Yes_____
   d. Insomnia? No <u>X</u>_____ Yes _____ Describe._____
3. Methods used to promote sleep: Medication? No <u>X</u>_____ Yes _____ Name_____
   Warm fluids? No <u>X</u>_____ Yes _____ What?_____
   Relaxation techniques? No <u>X</u>_____ Yes _____

Objective
None

COGNITIVE–PERCEPTUAL PATTERN

Subjective

1. Pain
   a. Location (have the patient point to area) <u>LEFT SHIN</u>
   b. Intensity (have the patient rank on scale of 0–10) <u>5</u>
   c. Radiation? No _____ Yes <u>X</u> _____ To where <u>UP LEG</u>
   d. Timing (how often; related to any specific events) <u>"ACHES ALL THE TIME"; INCREASED PAIN WITH WALK-</u>
      <u>ING OR IF TOUCH WOUND</u>
   e. Duration <u>AS ABOVE</u>
   f. What do you do to relieve pain at home? <u>ELEVATE, TAKE AN ADVIL</u>
   g. When did pain begin? <u>"TWO WEEKS AGO"</u>
2. Decision Making
   a. Find decision making: Easy <u>X</u> Moderately easy _____ Moderately difficult _____ Difficult _____
   b. Inclined to make decisions: Rapidly <u>X</u> Slowly _____ Delay _____
   c. Difficulty choosing between options? Yes _____ No <u>X</u> _____ Describe. _____
3. Knowledge level
   a. Can define what current problem is? Yes <u>X</u> _____ No _____
   b. Can restate current therapeutic regimen? Yes <u>X</u> _____ No _____

Objective

1. Review sensory and mental status completed in Health Perception–Health Management Pattern.
2. Any overt signs of pain? No ___ Yes <u>X</u> Describe. <u>WINCES WHEN TRIES TO BEAR WEIGHT ON LEFT LEG</u>
3. Any fluctuations in intercranial pressure? Yes _____ No <u>X</u>

SELF-PERCEPTION AND SELF-CONCEPT PATTERN

Subjective

1. What is your major concern at the current time? <u>"I'M TIRED OF DOING NOTHING BUT DRINKING AND</u>
   <u>PEEING"</u>
2. Do you think this admission will cause any lifestyle changes for you? No _____ Yes <u>X</u>
   What? <u>"HELP ME GET BETTER"</u>
3. Do you think this admission will result in any body changes for you? No _____ Yes <u>X</u>
   What? <u>"HEAL MY LEG"</u>
4. My usual view of myself is: Positive <u>X</u> Neutral _____ Somewhat negative _____
5. Do you believe you will have any problems dealing with your current health situation? No <u>X</u> Yes ___ Describe. _____
6. On a scale of 0–5, rank your perception of your level of control in this situation <u>4</u>
7. On a scale of 0–5, rank your usual assertiveness level <u>5</u>
8. Have you recently experienced a loss? No <u>X</u> Yes _____ Describe. _____

Objective

1. During assessment, the patient appears: Calm _____ Anxious _____ Irritable <u>X</u> Withdrawn ____ Restless _____
2. Did any physiologic parameters change: Face reddened? No <u>X</u> Yes _____
   Voice volume changed? No <u>X</u> Yes _____ Louder _____ Softer _____
   Voice quality changed? No <u>X</u> Yes _____ Quavering _____ Hesitation _____ Other _____
3. Body language observed <u>GUARDS LEFT SHIN</u>
4. Is current admission going to result in a body structure or function change for the patient? No _____ Yes _____
   Unsure at this time <u>X</u>
5. Is the patient expressing any fears about dying? Yes _____ No <u>X</u>
6. Is the patient expressing worries about the impact of his or her death on his or her family and/or friends?
   Yes _____ No <u>X</u>

ROLE-RELATIONSHIP PATTERN

Subjective

1. Does the patient live alone? Yes _____ No <u>X</u> _____ Lives with: <u>WIFE</u>
2. Is the patient married? Yes <u>X</u> _____ No _____; Children? No <u>X</u> Yes _____; # of children_____

Age(s) of children_____

Were any of the children premature? No _____ Yes _____ Describe. N/A _____

3. How would you rate your parenting skills: Not applicable X_____

No difficulty with _____ Average _____ Some difficulty with _____ Describe._____

4. Any losses (physical, psychological, social) in past year? No _____ Yes X _____

Describe. EARLY RETIREMENT _____

5. How is the patient handling this loss at this time? "DOING FINE, JUST NEED TO GET FEET IN SHAPE SO I CAN DO WHAT I WANT NOW THAT I HAVE THE TIME."_____

6. Do you believe this admission will result in any type of loss? No X_____ Yes _____ Describe. _____

7. Has the patient recently received a diagnosis related to a chronic physical or mental illness? No X_____ Yes_____

8. Is the patient verbally expressing sadness? No X_____ Yes _____

9. Ask both the patient and family: Do you think this admission will cause any significant changes in (the patient's) usual family role? No X_____ Yes _____ Describe._____

10. How would you rate your usual social activities? Very active _____ Active X_____ Limited _____ None _____

11. How would you rate your comfort in social situations? Comfortable X_____ Uncomfortable _____

12. What activities/jobs, etc., do you like to do? GARDENING, FISHING, PLAYING CARDS AND DOMINOES _____

13. What activities/jobs, etc., do you dislike doing? ANY HOUSEWORK OR COOKING AND HAVING TO PEE ALL THE TIME_____

14. Does the person use alcohol or drugs? No X_____ Yes _____ Kind_____

Amount_____

15. Is the patient in the role of primary caregiver for another person? No X_____ Yes _____

Objective

1. Speech Pattern

   a. Is English the patient's native language? Yes X_____ No _____

   Native language is_____; Interpreter needed? No X_____ Yes _____

   b. During interview have you noted any speech problems? No X_____ Yes _____ Describe._____

2. Family Interaction

   a. During interview have you observed any dysfunctional family interactions? No X_____ Yes _____ Describe._____

   b. If the patient is a child, is there any physical or emotional evidence of physical or psychosocial abuse?

   No _____ Yes _____ Describe._____

   c. If the patient is a child, is there evidence of attachment behaviors between the parents and child?

   Yes _____ No _____ Describe. N/A _____

   d. Any signs or symptoms of alcoholism? No X_____ Yes _____ Describe. _____

SEXUALITY–REPRODUCTIVE PATTERN

Subjective

Female

1. Date of LMP_____; Any pregnancies? Para_____ Gravida_____ Menopause? No _____ Yes _____ Year_____

2. Use birth control measures? No_____ N/A _____ Yes _____ Type_____

3. Any history of vaginal discharge, bleeding, lesions? No _____ Yes _____ Describe._____

4. Pap smear annually? Yes _____ No _____ Date of last pap smear_____

5. Date of last mammogram_____

6. History of STD (sexually transmitted disease)? No _____ Yes _____ Describe._____

If admission secondary to rape:

7. Is the patient describing numerous physical symptoms? No _____ Yes _____ Describe._____

8. Is the patient exhibiting numerous emotional reactions? No _____ Yes _____ Describe._____

9. What has been your primary coping mechanism to handle this rape episode?_____

10. Have you talked to persons from the rape crisis center? Yes _____ No _____

   If no, does the patient want you to contact them for her? No _____ Yes _____

   If yes, was this contact of assistance? No _____ Yes _____

Male

1. Any history of prostate problems? No X_____ Yes _____ Describe._____

2. Any history of penile discharge, bleeding, lesions? No X_____ Yes _____ Describe._____

3. Date of last prostate exam? <u>LAST ADMISSION</u>

4. History of STD (sexually transmitted disease)? No <u>X</u>_____ Yes _____ Describe._____

Both

1. Are you experiencing any problems in sexual functioning? No _____ Yes <u>X</u>_____
   Describe. <u>IMPOTENCY FOR PAST SEVERAL MONTHS</u>

2. Are you satisfied with your sexual relationship? Yes _____ No <u>X</u>_____
   Describe. <u>IMPOTENT</u>

3. Do you believe this admission will have any impact on sexual functioning? No _____ Yes <u>X</u>_____
   Describe. <u>"GET MY DIABETES UNDER CONTROL AND PROBLEM WILL BE HELPED."</u>

Objective

Review admission physical exam for results of pelvic and rectal exams. If results not documented, nurse should perform exams. Check history to see whether admission resulted from a rape.

COPING–STRESS TOLERANCE PATTERN

Subjective

1. Have you experienced any stressful or traumatic events in the past year in addition to this admission?
   No _____ Yes <u>X</u>_____ Describe. <u>NUMEROUS ADMISSIONS AND I MISS WORK SOME</u>

2. How would you rate your usual handling of stress: Good _____ Average <u>X</u>_____ Poor _____

3. What is the primary way you deal with stress or problems? <u>YELL OR AVOID SITUATION. "I DON'T LIKE TO TALK ABOUT IT."</u>

4. Have you or your family used any support or counseling groups in the past year?
   No <u>X</u>_____ Yes _____ Group Name_____
   Was support group helpful? Yes _____ No _____ Additional comments_____

5. What do you believe is the primary reason behind the need for this admission? <u>"TO GET MY DIABETES UNDER CONTROL AGAIN; I GUESS I'M A SLOW LEARNER."</u>

6. How soon, after first noting symptoms, did you seek health care assistance? <u>3 WEEKS</u>

7. Are you satisfied with the care you have been receiving at home? Yes <u>X</u>_____ No _____
   Comments <u>"MY WIFE HAS ALWAYS TAKEN GOOD CARE OF ME AND I DIDN'T WANT TO HAVE THOSE PEOPLE (V.N.A.) COMING TO MY HOUSE."</u>

8. Ask primary caregiver: What is your understanding of the care that will be needed when the patient goes home? <u>WIFE NOT PRESENT AT THIS TIME</u>

Objective

1. Observe behavior. Are there any overt signs of stress (e.g., crying, wringing of hands, clenched fists, etc.)? Describe. <u>CLENCHED FISTS</u>

2. Has the patient threatened to kill himself or herself? Yes _____ No <u>X</u>_____

3. Ask the family: Has the patient demonstrated any marked changes in behavior, attitude or school performance?
   Yes _____ No <u>X</u>_____

VALUE–BELIEF PATTERN

Subjective

1. Are you satisfied with the way your life has been developing? Yes _____ No <u>X</u>_____
   Comments <u>"WAS O.K. UNTIL THIS DIABETES DEVELOPED."</u>

2. Will this admission interfere with your plans for the future? No <u>X</u>_____ Yes _____
   How? _____

3. Religion: Protestant <u>X</u>_____ Catholic _____ Jewish _____ Islam _____ Buddhist _____

4. Will this admission interfere with your spiritual or religious practices? No <u>X</u>_____ Yes _____
   How? _____

5. Any religious restrictions to care (diet, blood transfusions)? <u>NO</u>

6. Would you like to have your (pastor, priest, rabbi, hospital chaplain) contacted to visit you?
   No <u>X</u>_____ Yes _____ Which?_____

7. Have your religious beliefs helped you to deal with problems in the past? No _____ Yes <u>X</u>_____
   Comments <u>NONE</u>

Objective

1. Observe behavior. Is the patient exhibiting any signs of alterations in mood (e.g., anger, crying, withdrawal, etc.)?
   No _____ Yes <u>X</u>_____ What <u>CLENCHED FISTS</u>_____

GENERAL

1. Is there any information we need to have that I have not covered in this interview?
   No <u>X</u>_____ Yes _____ Comments_____
2. Do you have any questions you need to ask me concerning your health, plan of care, or this agency?
   No <u>X</u>_____ Yes _____ Questions_____
3. What is the first problem you would like to have assistance with? <u>STOP ME FROM HAVING TO GO TO THE BATH-</u>
   <u>ROOM ALL THE TIME</u>_____

Index

Note: Page numbers followed by f indicate figures; page numbers followed by t indicate tables.